MW00838260

Sturdevant's Art and Science of Operative Dentistry

Sturdevant's Art and Science of Operative Dentistry

Seventh Edition

André V. Ritter, DDS, MS, MBA

Thomas P. Hinman Distinguished Professor
Department of Operative Dentistry
The University of North Carolina at Chapel Hill School of Dentistry
Chapel Hill, North Carolina

Lee W. Boushell, DMD, MS

Associate Professor
Department of Operative Dentistry
The University of North Carolina at Chapel Hill School of Dentistry
Chapel Hill, North Carolina

Ricardo Walter, DDS, MS

Clinical Associate Professor
Department of Operative Dentistry
The University of North Carolina at Chapel Hill School of Dentistry
Chapel Hill, North Carolina

ELSEVIER

ELSEVIER

3251 Riverport Lane
St. Louis, Missouri 63043

STURDEVANT'S ART AND SCIENCE OF OPERATIVE DENTISTRY,
SEVENTH EDITION   ISBN: 978-0-323-47833-5
Copyright © 2019 by Elsevier Inc. All rights reserved.

No part of this publication may be reproduced or transmitted in any form or by any means, electronic or
mechanical, including photocopying, recording, or any information storage and retrieval system, without
permission in writing from the publisher. Details on how to seek permission, further information about the
Publisher's permissions policies and our arrangements with organizations such as the Copyright Clearance Center
and the Copyright Licensing Agency, can be found at our website: www.elsevier.com/permissions.

This book and the individual contributions contained in it are protected under copyright by the Publisher (other
than as may be noted herein).

Notices

Practitioners and researchers must always rely on their own experience and knowledge in evaluating and using
any information, methods, compounds or experiments described herein. Because of rapid advances in the
medical sciences, in particular, independent verification of diagnoses and drug dosages should be made. To the
fullest extent of the law, no responsibility is assumed by Elsevier, authors, editors or contributors for any
injury and/or damage to persons or property as a matter of products liability, negligence or otherwise, or from
any use or operation of any methods, products, instructions, or ideas contained in the material herein.

Previous editions copyrighted 2013, 2006, 2002, 1995, 1985, and 1968.

International Standard Book Number: 978-0-323-47833-5

Senior Content Strategist: Jennifer Flynn-Briggs
Senior Content Development Manager: Ellen Wurm-Cutter
Associate Content Development Specialist: Laura Klein
Publishing Services Manager: Julie Eddy
Senior Project Manager: David Stein
Design Direction: Bridget Hoette

Printed in China

Last digit is the print number: 9   8   7   6   5   4   3   2   1

Working together
to grow libraries in
developing countries

www.elsevier.com • www.bookaid.org

This book is dedicated to the art and science of Operative Dentistry. Our focus with this edition is to provide students, teachers, and practicing colleagues with a comprehensive and evidence-based resource for Operative Dentistry and related disciplines.

We also dedicate the seventh edition to the editors and contributors of the previous editions. Much of their work can still be found in this edition.

Finally, we dedicate this book to Drs. Clifford Sturdevant, Roger Barton, and John Brauer, who were the editors for The Art and Science of Operative Dentistry, First Edition, 1968. We hope that they would be proud to see how far their legacy has extended.

Contributors

Sumitha N. Ahmed, BDS, MS
Clinical Assistant Professor
Department of Operative Dentistry
The University of North Carolina at Chapel Hill School of
    Dentistry
Chapel Hill, North Carolina

Lee W. Boushell, DMD, MS
Associate Professor
Department of Operative Dentistry
The University of North Carolina at Chapel Hill School of
    Dentistry
Chapel Hill, North Carolina

Terence E. Donovan, DDS
Professor
Department of Operative Dentistry
The University of North Carolina at Chapel Hill School of
    Dentistry
Chapel Hill, North Carolina

Dennis J. Fasbinder, DDS
Clinical Professor
Cariology, Restorative Sciences, and Endodontics
University of Michigan School of Dentistry
Ann Arbor, Michigan

Andréa G. Ferreira Zandoná, DDS, MSD, PhD
Associate Professor
Department of Operative Dentistry
The University of North Carolina at Chapel Hill School of
    Dentistry
Chapel Hill, North Carolina

Harald O. Heymann, DDS, MEd
Professor
Department of Operative Dentistry
The University of North Carolina at Chapel Hill School of
    Dentistry
Chapel Hill, North Carolina

Patricia A. Miguez, DDS, MS, PhD
Assistant Professor
Department of Operative Dentistry
The University of North Carolina at Chapel Hill School of
    Dentistry
Chapel Hill, North Carolina

Thiago Morelli, DDS, MS
Clinical Assistant Professor
Department of Periodontology
The University of North Carolina at Chapel Hill School of
    Dentistry
Chapel Hill, North Carolina

Gisele F. Neiva, DDS, MS, MS
Clinical Associate Professor
Cariology, Restorative Sciences, and Endodontics
The University of Michigan School of Dentistry
Ann Arbor, Michigan

Gustavo Mussi Stefan Oliveira, DDS, MS
Clinical Assistant Professor
Department of Operative Dentistry
The University of North Carolina at Chapel Hill School of
    Dentistry
Chapel Hill, North Carolina

Joe C. Ontiveros, DDS, MS
Professor and Head, Esthetic Dentistry
Restorative Dentistry and Prosthodontics
University of Texas School of Dentistry at Houston
Houston, Texas

Rade D. Paravina, DDS, MS, PhD
Professor
Department of Restorative Dentistry and Prosthodontics
Director, Houston Center for Biomaterials and Biomimetics
    (HCBB)
Ralph C. Cooley DDS Distinguished Professor in Biomaterials
University of Texas School of Dentistry at Houston
Houston, Texas

Jorge Perdigão, DMD, MS, PhD
Professor
Department of Restorative Sciences
Division of Operative Dentistry
University of Minnesota School of Dentistry
Minneapolis, Minnesota

Richard B. Price, BDS, DDS, MS, PhD, FRCD(C), FDS RCS (Edin)
Professor and Head Division of Fixed Prosthodontics
Dental Clinical Services
Dalhousie University
Halifax, Nova Scotia, Canada

André V. Ritter, DDS, MS, MBA
Thomas P. Hinman Distinguished Professor
Department of Operative Dentistry
The University of North Carolina at Chapel Hill School of Dentistry
Chapel Hill, North Carolina

Frederick A. Rueggeberg, DDS, MS
Professor and Section Director, Dental Materials
Restorative Sciences
Dental College of Georgia at Augusta University
Augusta, Georgia

Daniel A. Shugars, DDS, PhD, MPH
Professor Emeritus
Department of Operative Dentistry
The University of North Carolina at Chapel Hill School of Dentistry
Chapel Hill, North Carolina

Gregory E. Smith, DDS, MSD
Professor Emeritus
Department of Restorative Sciences
College of Dentistry
University of Florida
Gainesville, Florida

John R. Sturdevant, DDS
Associate Professor
Department of Operative Dentistry
The University of North Carolina at Chapel Hill School of Dentistry
Chapel Hill, North Carolina

Taiseer A. Sulaiman, BDS (Hons), PhD
Assistant Professor
Department of Operative Dentistry
The University of North Carolina at Chapel Hill School of Dentistry
Chapel Hill, North Carolina

Edward J. Swift, Jr., DMD, MS
Associate Dean for Education
Professor
Department of Operative Dentistry
The University of North Carolina at Chapel Hill School of Dentistry
Chapel Hill, North Carolina

Ricardo Walter, DDS, MS
Clinical Associate Professor
Department of Operative Dentistry
The University of North Carolina at Chapel Hill School of Dentistry
Chapel Hill, North Carolina

Aldridge D. Wilder, Jr., BS, DDS
Professor
Department of Operative Dentistry
The University of North Carolina at Chapel Hill School of Dentistry
Chapel Hill, North Carolina

Contributors to Past Editions

Stephen C. Bayne, MS, PhD
Professor and Chair
Department of Cariology, Restorative Sciences, and Endodontics
School of Dentistry
University of Michigan
Ann Arbor, Michigan

R. Scott Eidson, DDS
Clinical Associate Professor
Department of Operative Dentistry
The University of North Carolina at Chapel Hill School of Dentistry
Chapel Hill, North Carolina

Jeffrey Y. Thompson, PhD
Professor
Section of Prosthodontics
Director
Biosciences Research Center
College of Dental Medicine
Nova Southeastern University
Ft. Lauderdale, Florida

Foreword

Dr. Clifford Sturdevant had a brass plaque on his desk that read "If it's almost right it's wrong!" This commitment to excellence also was the mantra upon which his classic textbook, *The Art and Science of Operative Dentistry*, was first written and published in 1968. This textbook has been the basis for training dental students in the fine art and clinical science of Operative Dentistry for 50 years. In light of this significant landmark, which coincides with the publication of this new Seventh Edition, we believe it is important to present the evolution of the various editions of the textbook from a historical perspective.

The First Edition (Sturdevant, Barton, Brauer, 1968) was meant "to present the significant aspects of Operative Dentistry and the research findings in the basic and clinical sciences that have immediate application" in the field of Operative Dentistry. It is important to note that Dean Brauer pointed out in his preface that beyond having the knowledge and skills needed to perform a procedure, the practitioner must also have high moral and ethical standards, essential and priceless ingredients. Since the First Edition, this textbook series has always attempted to present artistic and scientific elements of Operative Dentistry in the context of ethical standards for patient care.

It is also worth noting that the First Edition was printed and bound in "landscape" format so that it could more easily be used as a manual in the preclinical laboratory and would always remain open to the desired page. The handmade 5X models used to illustrate the various steps in cavity preparation were created by two dental students enrolled at The University of North Carolina at Chapel Hill School of Dentistry during the writing of the First Edition. Illustrations of these models have continued to be used in later editions, and the models themselves have served as important teaching materials for decades.

Although the techniques, materials, armamentarium, and treatment options continue to evolve, many of the principles of Operative Dentistry described in the First Edition are still pertinent today. An understanding of these principles and the ability to meticulously apply them are critical to providing the outstanding dental treatment expected by our patients.

The Second Edition (Sturdevant, Barton, Sockwell, Strickland, 1985) expanded on many techniques (e.g., acid etching) using experience and published research that had occurred since publication of the First Edition. The basics of occlusion were emphasized and presented in a way that would be helpful to the dental student and practitioner. A chapter on treatment planning and sequencing of procedures, as well as a chapter providing a thorough treatise on the use of pins, was included. Information on silicate cement, self-curing acrylic resin, and the baked porcelain inlay was eliminated for obvious reasons. A chapter on endodontic therapy and the chapter on the "dental assistant" were no longer included. Chapters on (1) tooth-colored restorations and (2) additional conservative

and esthetic treatments explained the changes and improvements that occurred in the areas of esthetic options available to patients. In the chapter on gold inlay/onlay restorations, increased emphasis was given to the gold onlay restorations for Class II cavity preparations.

The Third Edition (Sturdevant, Roberson, Heymann, J. Sturdevant, 1995) placed a new emphasis on cariology and the "medical model of disease" with regard to risk assessment and managing the high-risk caries patient. This important concept laid the foundation for what is still taught today with regard to identifying risk factors and defining a treatment plan based on caries risk assessment. The Third Edition also included new expanded chapters on infection control, diagnosis and treatment planning, and dental materials. In light of the growing interest in the area of esthetic dentistry, a variety of conservative esthetic treatments were introduced including vital bleaching, microabrasion and macroabrasion, etched porcelain veneers, and the novel all-porcelain bonded pontic. Additionally, an entirely new section on tooth-colored inlays and onlays was included that chronicled both lab-processed resin and ceramic restorations of this type and those fabricated chairside with CAD/CAM systems.

With the Fourth Edition of this text (Roberson, Heymann, Swift, 2002), Dr. Clifford Sturdevant's name was added to the book title to honor his contributions to the textbook series and the discipline of Operative Dentistry. In this edition, a particular emphasis was placed on bonded esthetic restorations. Consequently, an entirely new chapter was included on fundamental concepts of enamel and dentin adhesion. This chapter was intended to provide foundational information critical to the long-term success of all types of bonded restorations.

The Fifth Edition (Roberson, Heymann, Swift, 2006) continued with the renewed emphasis on the importance of adhesively bonded restorations and focused on scientific considerations for attaining optimal success, particularly with posterior composites. Concepts such as the "C Factor" and keys to reducing polymerization effects were emphasized along with factors involved in reducing microleakage and recurrent decay.

The Sixth Edition (Heymann, Swift, Ritter, 2013) represented a transition from a large printed edition, as in the past, to a smaller, streamlined printed version that focused on concepts and techniques immediately essential for learning contemporary Operative Dentistry. The same amount of information was included, but many chapters such as those addressing biomaterials, infection control, pain control, bonded splints and bridges, direct gold restorations, and instruments and equipment were available for the first time in a supplemental online format.

With this new Seventh Edition of *Sturdevant's Art and Science of Operative Dentistry*, fundamental concepts and principles of contemporary Operative Dentistry are maintained and enhanced, but vital new areas of content also have been incorporated. Diagnosis, classification, and management of dental caries have been significantly updated in light of the latest clinical and epidemiological research. Similarly, content on adhesive dentistry and composite resins has been updated as a result of the evolving science in these fields.

An entirely *new* chapter on light curing and its important role in the clinical success of resin composite restorations has been added. Moreover, a *new* scientifically based chapter details the important elements of color and shade matching and systematically reviews how the dental clinician is better able to understand the many co-variables involved in color assessment. It also reviews how best to improve shade matching of esthetic restorations to tooth structure.

In an attempt to better optimize restorative treatment outcomes involving periodontal challenges, a *new* chapter has been included that addresses these principles. Periodontology Applied to Operative Dentistry chronicles the various clinical considerations involving conditions such as inadequate crown length, lack of root coverage, and other vexing problems requiring interdisciplinary treatment to optimize success.

Finally, the Seventh Edition of this text addresses the ever-evolving area of digital dentistry with a *new* chapter, Digital Dentistry in Operative Dentistry. This chapter reviews the various technologies involved in scanning and image capture for both treatment planning and restorative applications. Additionally, the authors review various types of digital restorative systems for both chairside and modem-linked laboratory-based fabrication of restorations. In recognition of the rapid movement to digital dentistry, this chapter is a vital addition to a textbook whose tradition has been always to reflect the latest technologies and research findings in contemporary Operative Dentistry.

Since its inception 50 years ago, the Sturdevant text has been a dynamic document, with content that has included innovative information on the latest materials and techniques. Over this time period, numerous internationally recognized experts have addressed many specific topics as authors and co-authors of various chapters. It also should be pointed out that with all editions of the textbook, the authors of the various chapters are themselves actively involved in teaching students preclinical and clinical Operative Dentistry. Moreover, they are "wet-fingered dentists" who also practice Operative Dentistry for their individual patients.

In summary, for 50 years *Sturdevant's Art and Science of Operative Dentistry* has been a major resource guiding educators in the teaching of contemporary Operative Dentistry. Each edition of this text has striven to incorporate the latest technologies and science based on the available literature and supporting research. The Seventh Edition is a superb addition to this tradition, which will most assuredly uphold the standard of publication excellence that has been the hallmark of the Sturdevant textbooks for half a century.

Harald O. Heymann, DDS, MEd
Kenneth N. May, Jr., DDS

Since the publication of the First Edition in 1968, The University of North Carolina's *The Art and Science of Operative Dentistry* has been considered a major Operative Dentistry textbook in many countries, and it has been translated in several languages. The widespread use of this textbook in dental education is a testimony to both its success and its value for dental students and dental educators alike.

With the Seventh Edition we attempted to elevate the level of excellence this textbook series is known for. All relevant content from the previous editions is still here (from cariology and treatment planning to biomaterials and clinical techniques for amalgam and composite restorations). However, most chapters were significantly revised to reflect current scientific and clinical evidence, and several chapters were virtually rewritten by new contributors who are more engaged in the specific content areas. The chapter on biomaterials, in addition to being significantly revised, appears again in print in the Seventh Edition, making it easier for the reader to access the information while reading the print version of the textbook. Additionally, many chapters were condensed into more streamlined and concise single chapters (for example, three of the "composite chapters" from the Sixth Edition are now concisely presented in a single "composite chapter" in this new edition; a similar approach was used for the "amalgam chapters").

In addition, four new and relevant chapters were added (Light Curing of Restorative Materials, Color and Shade Matching in Operative Dentistry, Periodontology Applied to Operative Dentistry, and Digital Dentistry in Operative Dentistry) to bring the textbook in line with disciplines that ever more interface with Operative Dentistry, emphasizing the increased role of an interdisciplinary approach to modern Operative Dentistry. Each of these new chapters is authored by recognized authorities in the respective topics, and considerably broaden the scope of the Seventh Edition.

The new edition also features an Expert Consult website that includes a full online version of the print text, as well as five additional online-only chapters and technique videos.

Expanding on a significant layout facelift that started with the Sixth Edition, the Seventh Edition offers an increased number of color images, line drawings that were further revised and improved

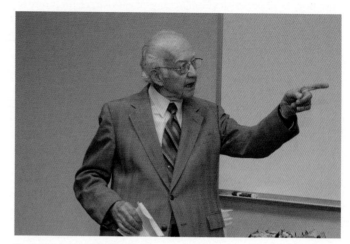

Dr. Clifford Sturdevant.

for increased text comprehension, and a reorganization of chapter sequence. Furthermore, redundant and outdated information has been deleted. All these updates enhance the user experience and make the Seventh Edition an even user-friendlier textbook for the wide range of readers—students, teachers, and practitioners/colleagues.

Many hours of diligent work have been invested so as to offer you the best possible Operative Dentistry textbook at this point in time. We have sought to honor the long-standing tradition of *The Art and Science of Operative Dentistry* textbook series and to bring you updated, clinically relevant and evidence-based information. To publish this edition on the year we commemorate the 50th anniversary of the publication of the First Edition is a milestone for Operative Dentistry in general and for The University of North Carolina at Chapel Hill's Department of Operative Dentistry in particular. We are honored to have had the opportunity to work on and present the Seventh Edition.

The Editors

Acknowledgments

The editors would like to thank:
- Our spouses and families for their love, understanding, and support during this revision.
- The University of North Carolina at Chapel Hill's Operative Dentistry staff, faculty, and graduate students, whose support was invaluable to make this effort possible.
- The many colleagues who contributed with illustrations—their names are referenced throughout the textbook.
- The team at Elsevier (Jennifer Flynn-Briggs, Laura Klein, David Stein, Ellen Wurm-Cutter, Julie Eddy, and Jodi Bernard) for the support, encouragement, and expertise during the revision process. Their professionalism and guidance are reflected in every page of this work.

Contents

1

Clinical Significance of Dental Anatomy, Histology, Physiology, and Occlusion

LEE W. BOUSHELL, JOHN R. STURDEVANT

A thorough understanding of the histology, physiology, and occlusal interactions of the dentition and supporting tissues is essential for the restorative dentist. Knowledge of the structures of teeth (enamel, dentin, cementum, and pulp) and their relationships to each other and to the supporting structures is necessary, especially when treating dental caries. The protective function of the tooth form is revealed by its impact on masticatory muscle activity, the supporting tissues (osseous and mucosal), and the pulp. Proper tooth form contributes to healthy supporting tissues. The contour and contact relationships of teeth with adjacent and opposing teeth are major determinants of muscle function in mastication, esthetics, speech, and protection. The relationships of form to function are especially noteworthy when considering the shape of the dental arch, proximal contacts, occlusal contacts, and mandibular movement.

Teeth and Supporting Tissues

Dentitions

Humans have primary and permanent dentitions. The primary dentition consists of 10 maxillary and 10 mandibular teeth. Primary teeth exfoliate and are replaced by the permanent dentition, which consists of 16 maxillary and 16 mandibular teeth.

Classes of Human Teeth: Form and Function

Human teeth are divided into classes on the basis of form and function. The primary and permanent dentitions include the incisor, canine, and molar classes. The fourth class, the premolar, is found only in the permanent dentition (Fig. 1.1). Tooth form predicts the function; class traits are the characteristics that place teeth into functional categories. Because the diet of humans consists of animal and plant foods, the human dentition is called *omnivorous*.

Incisors

Incisors are located near the entrance of the oral cavity and function as cutting or shearing instruments for food (see Fig. 1.1). From a proximal view, the crowns of these teeth have a relatively triangular shape, with a narrow incisal surface and a broad cervical base. During mastication, incisors are used to shear (cut through) food.

Incisors are essential for proper esthetics of the smile, facial soft tissue contours (e.g., lip support), and speech (phonetics).

Canines

Canines possess the longest roots of all teeth and are located at the corners of the dental arches. They function in the seizing, piercing, tearing, and cutting of food. From a proximal view, the crown also has a triangular shape, with a thick incisal ridge. The anatomic form of the crown and the length of the root make canine teeth strong, stable abutments for fixed or removable prostheses. Canines not only serve as important guides in occlusion, because of their anchorage and position in the dental arches, but also play a crucial role (along with the incisors) in the esthetics of the smile and lip support.

Premolars

Premolars serve a dual role: (1) They are similar to canines in the tearing of food, and (2) they are similar to molars in the grinding of food. Although first premolars are angular, with their facial cusps resembling canines, the lingual cusps of the maxillary premolars and molars have a more rounded anatomic form (see Fig. 1.1). The occlusal surfaces present a series of curves in the form of concavities and convexities that should be maintained throughout life for correct occlusal contacts and function. Although less visible than incisors and canines, premolars still play an important role in esthetics.

Molars

Molars are large, multicusped, strongly anchored teeth located nearest the temporomandibular joint (TMJ), which serves as the fulcrum during function. These teeth have a major role in the crushing, grinding, and chewing of food to dimensions suitable for swallowing. They are well suited for this task because they have broad occlusal surfaces and anchorage (Figs. 1.2 and 1.3). Premolars and molars are important in maintaining the vertical dimension of the face (see Fig. 1.1).

Structures of Teeth

Teeth are composed of enamel, the pulp–dentin complex, and cementum (see Fig. 1.3). Each of these structures is discussed individually.

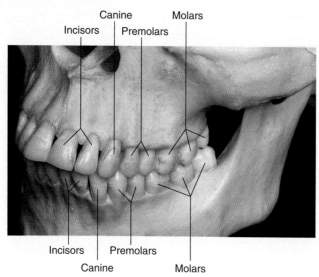

• **Fig. 1.1**   Maxillary and mandibular teeth in maximum intercuspal position. The classes of teeth are incisors, canines, premolars, and molars. Cusps of mandibular teeth are one half cusp anterior of corresponding cusps of teeth in the maxillary arch. (From Logan BM, Reynolds P, Hutchings RT: *McMinn's color atlas of head and neck anatomy*, ed 4, Edinburgh, 2010, Mosby.)

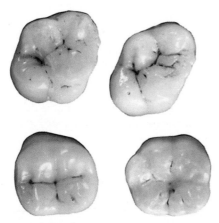

• **Fig. 1.2**   Occlusal surfaces of maxillary and mandibular first and second molars after several years of use, showing rounded curved surfaces and minimal wear.

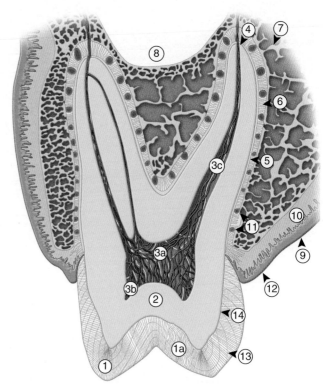

• **Fig. 1.3**   Cross section of the maxillary molar and its supporting structures. *1*, Enamel; *1a*, gnarled enamel; *2*, dentin; *3a*, pulp chamber; *3b*, pulp horn; *3c*, pulp canal; *4*, apical foramen; *5*, cementum; *6*, periodontal fibers in periodontal ligament; *7*, alveolar bone; *8*, maxillary sinus; *9*, mucosa; *10*, submucosa; *11*, blood vessels; *12*, gingiva; *13*, lines of Retzius; *14*, dentinoenamel junction (DEJ).

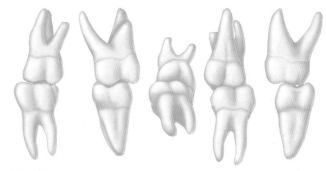

• **Fig. 1.4**   Maxillary and mandibular first molars in maximum intercuspal contact. Note the grooves for escape of food.

Enamel

Enamel formation, *amelogenesis*, is accomplished by cells called *ameloblasts*. These cells originate from the embryonic germ layer known as *ectoderm*. Enamel covers the anatomic crown of the tooth, varies in thickness in different areas, and is securely attached to the dentin by the dentinoenamel junction (DEJ) (see Fig. 1.3). It is thicker at the incisal and occlusal areas of the crown and becomes progressively thinner until it terminates at the cementoenamel junction (CEJ). The thickness also varies from one class of tooth to another, averaging 2 mm at the incisal ridges of incisors, 2.3 to 2.5 mm at the cusps of premolars, and 2.5 to 3 mm at the cusps of molars.

Cusps on the occlusal surfaces of posterior teeth begin as separate ossification centers, which form into developmental lobes. Adjacent developmental lobes increase in size until they begin to coalesce. Grooves and fossae result in the areas of coalescence (at the junction of the developmental lobes of enamel) as cusp formation nears completion. The strategic placement of the grooves and fossae complements the position of the opposing cusps so as to allow movement of food to the facial and lingual surfaces during mastication. A functional cusp that opposes a groove (or fossa) occludes on enamel inclines on each side of the groove and not in the depth of the groove. This arrangement leaves a V-shaped escape path between the cusp and its opposing groove for the movement of food during chewing (Fig. 1.4).

Enamel thickness varies in the area of these developmental features and may approach zero depending on the effectiveness of adjacent cusp coalescence. Failure or compromised coalescence of the enamel of the developmental lobes results in a deep invagination in the groove area of the enamel surface and is termed *fissure*. Noncoalesced enamel at the deepest point of a fossa is termed *pit*.

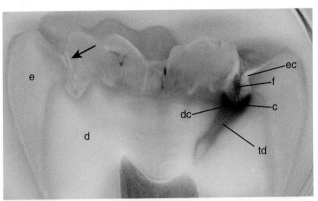

• **Fig. 1.5** Fissure *(f)* at junction of lobes allows accumulation of food and bacteria predisposing the tooth to dental caries *(c)*. Enamel *(e)*, dentin *(d)*, enamel caries lesion *(ec)*, dentin caries lesion *(dc)*, transparent dentin *(td)*; early enamel demineralization *(arrow)*.

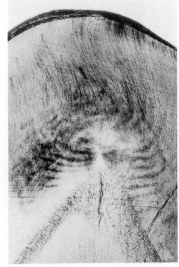

• **Fig. 1.6** Gnarled enamel. (From Berkovitz BKB, Holland GR, Moxham BJ: *Oral anatomy, histology and embryology*, ed 4, Edinburgh, 2009, Mosby.)

Fissures and/or pits represent non–self-cleansing areas where acidogenic biofilm accumulation may predispose the tooth to dental caries (Fig. 1.5).

Chemically, enamel is a highly mineralized crystalline structure. Hydroxyapatite, in the form of a crystalline lattice, is the largest mineral constituent (90%–92% by volume). Other minerals and trace elements are present in smaller amounts. The remaining constituents of tooth enamel include organic matrix proteins (1%–2%) and water (4%–12%) by volume.

Structurally, enamel is composed of millions of enamel rods (or "prisms"), rod sheaths, and a cementing interrod substance. Enamel rods, which are the largest structural components, are formed linearly by successive apposition of enamel in discrete increments. The resulting variations in structure and mineralization are called *incremental striae of Retzius* and may be considered growth rings that form during amelogenesis (see Fig. 1.3). The striae of Retzius appear as concentric circles in horizontal sections of a tooth. In vertical sections, the striae are positioned transversely at the cuspal and incisal areas in a symmetric arc pattern, descending obliquely to the cervical region and terminating at the DEJ. When these circles are incomplete at the enamel surface, a series of alternating grooves, called *imbrication lines of Pickerill*, are formed. Elevations between the grooves are called *perikymata*; they are continuous around a tooth and usually lie parallel to the CEJ and each other. Rods vary in number from approximately 5 million for a mandibular incisor to about 12 million for a maxillary molar. In general, the rods are aligned perpendicularly to the DEJ and the tooth surface in the primary and permanent dentitions except in the cervical region of permanent teeth, where they are oriented outward in a slightly apical direction. Microscopically, the enamel surface initially has circular depressions indicating where the enamel rods end. These concavities vary in depth and shape, and gradually wear smooth with age. Additionally, a structureless outer layer of enamel about 30 μm thick may be commonly identified toward the cervical area of the tooth crown and less commonly on cusp tips. There are no visible rod (prism) outlines in this area and all of the apatite crystals are parallel to one another and perpendicular to the striae of Retzius. This layer, referred to as *prismless enamel*, may be more heavily mineralized.

Each ameloblast forms an individual enamel rod with a specific length based on the specific type of tooth and the specific coronal location within that tooth. Enamel rods follow a wavy, spiraling course, producing an alternating clockwise and counterclockwise

arrangement for each group or layer of rods as they progress radially from the dentin toward the enamel surface. They initially follow a curving path through one third of the enamel next to the DEJ. After that, the rods usually follow a more direct path through the remaining two thirds of the enamel to the enamel surface. Groups of enamel rods may entwine with adjacent groups of rods and follow a curving irregular path toward the tooth surface. These constitute *gnarled enamel*, which occurs near the cervical regions and also in incisal and occlusal areas (Fig. 1.6). Gnarled enamel is not subject to fracture as much as is regular enamel. This type of enamel formation does not yield readily to the pressure of bladed, hand-cutting instruments in tooth preparation. The orientation of the enamel rod heads and tails and the gnarling of enamel rods provide strength by resisting, distributing, and dissipating impact forces.

Changes in the direction of enamel rods, which minimize the potential for fracture in the axial direction, produce an optical appearance called *Hunter-Schreger bands* (Fig. 1.7). These bands appear to be composed of alternate light and dark zones of varying widths that have slightly different permeability and organic content. These bands are found in different areas of each class of teeth. Because the enamel rod orientation varies in each tooth, Hunter-Schreger bands also have a variation in the number present in each tooth. In anterior teeth, they are located near the incisal surfaces. They increase in numbers and areas of teeth, from canines to premolars. In molars, the bands occur from near the cervical region to the cusp tips. In the primary dentition, the enamel rods in the cervical and central parts of the crown are nearly perpendicular to the long axis of the tooth and are similar in their direction to permanent teeth in the occlusal two thirds of the crown.

Enamel rod diameter near the dentinal borders is about 4 μm and about 8 μm near the surface. This diameter difference accommodates the larger outer surface of the enamel crown compared with the dentinal surface at the DEJ. Enamel rods, in transverse section, have a rounded head or body section and a tail section, forming a repetitive series of interlocking rods. Microscopic (~5000×) cross-sectional evaluation of enamel reveals that the rounded head portion of each rod lies between the narrow tail portions of two adjacent prisms (Fig. 1.8). Generally, the rounded

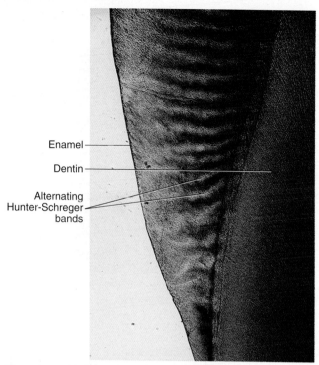

Enamel

Dentin

Alternating
Hunter-Schreger
bands

• **Fig. 1.7** Photomicrograph of enamel Hunter-Schreger bands. Photographed obtained by reflected light. (Modified from Chiego DJ Jr: *Essentials of oral histology and embryology: A clinical approach*, ed 4, St Louis, 2014, Mosby.)

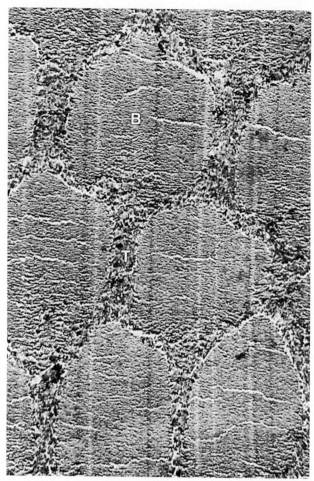

• **Fig. 1.8** Electron micrograph of cross section of rods in mature human enamel. Crystal orientation is different in "bodies" (B) than in "tails" (T). Approximate level of magnification ×5000. (From Meckel AH, Griebstein WJ, Neal RJ: Structure of mature human dental enamel as observed by electron microscopy, *Arch Oral Biol* 10(5):775–783, 1965.)

head portion is oriented in the incisal or occlusal direction; the tail section is oriented cervically. The final act of the ameloblasts, upon the completion of enamel rod formation, is the secretion of a membrane layer that covers the ends of the enamel rods. This layer is referred to as *Nasmyth membrane*, or *primary enamel cuticle*. Ameloblasts degenerate upon completion of Nasmyth membrane, which covers the newly erupted tooth and is worn away by mastication and cleaning. The membrane is replaced by an organic deposit called the *pellicle*, which is a precipitate of salivary proteins. Microorganisms may attach to the pellicle to form a biofilm (bacterial plaque), which, if acidogenic in nature, may become a precursor to dental disease.

Each enamel rod contains millions of small, elongated apatite crystallites that vary in size and shape. The crystallites are tightly packed in a distinct pattern of orientation that gives strength and structural identity to the enamel rod. The long axis of the apatite crystallites within the central region of the head (body) is aligned almost parallel to the rod long axis, and the crystallites incline with increasing angles (65 degrees) to the rod axis in the tail region.

The susceptibility of these crystallites to acidic conditions, from the caries process or as a result of an etching procedure, may be correlated with their orientation. Acid-induced mineral dissolution (demineralization) occurs more in the head region of each rod. The tail region and the periphery of the head region are relatively resistant to acidic demineralization. The crystallites are irregular in shape, with an average length of 160 nm and an average width of 20 to 40 nm. Each apatite crystallite is composed of thousands of unit cells that have a highly ordered arrangement of atoms. A crystallite may be 300 unit cells long, 40 cells wide, and 20 cells thick in a hexagonal configuration (Fig. 1.9). An organic matrix surrounds individual crystals.

Although enamel is a hard, dense structure, it is permeable to certain ions and molecules. The route of passage may be through structural units such as rod sheaths, enamel cracks, and other defects that are hypomineralized and rich in organic content. Water plays an important role as a transporting medium through the small intercrystalline spaces. Enamel tufts are hypomineralized structures of interrod substance between adjacent groups of enamel rods that project from the DEJ (Fig. 1.10). These projections arise in dentin, extend into enamel in the direction of the long axis of the crown, and may play a role in the spread of dental caries. Enamel lamellae are thin, leaflike faults between the enamel rod groups that extend from the enamel surface toward the DEJ, sometimes extending into dentin (see Fig. 1.10). They contain mostly organic material and may predispose the tooth to the entry of bacteria and subsequent development of dental caries. Enamel permeability decreases with age because of changes in the enamel matrix, a decrease referred to as *enamel maturation*.

Enamel is soluble when exposed to acidic conditions, but the dissolution is not uniform. Solubility of enamel increases from the enamel surface to the DEJ. When fluoride ions are present during enamel formation or are topically applied to the enamel surface, the solubility of surface enamel is decreased. Fluoride

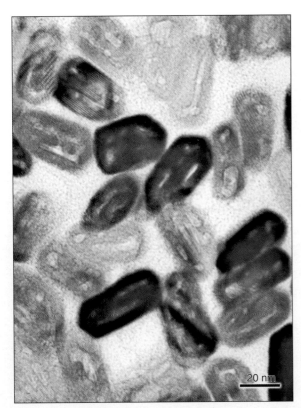

• **Fig. 1.9**   Electron micrograph of mature, hexagon-shaped enamel crystallites. (From Nanci A: *Ten Cate's oral histology: development, structure, and function*, ed 7, St Louis, 2008, Mosby.)

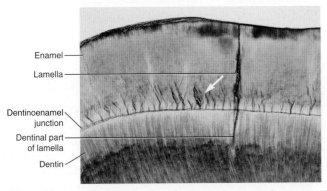

• **Fig. 1.10**   Microscopic view through lamella that goes from enamel surface into dentin. Note the enamel tufts *(arrow)*. (From Fehrenbach MJ, Popowics T: *Illustrated dental embryology, histology, and anatomy*, ed 4, St. Louis, 2016, Saunders. Courtesy James McIntosh, PhD, Assistant Professor Emeritus, Department of Biomedical Sciences, Baylor College of Dentistry, Dallas, TX.)

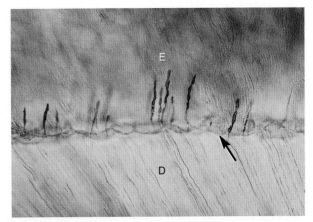

• **Fig. 1.11**   Microscopic view of scalloped dentoenamel junction (DEJ; *arrow*). *E*, Enamel; *D*, dentin. (From Fehrenbach MJ, Popowics T: *Illustrated dental embryology, histology, and anatomy*, ed 4, St. Louis, 2016, Saunders. Courtesy James McIntosh, PhD, Assistant Professor Emeritus, Department of Biomedical Sciences, Baylor College of Dentistry, Dallas, TX.)

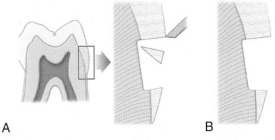

• **Fig. 1.12**   A, Enamel rods unsupported by dentin base are fractured away readily by pressure from hand instrument. B, Cervical preparation showing enamel rods supported by dentin base.

concentration decreases toward the DEJ. Fluoride is able to affect the chemical and physical properties of the apatite mineral and influence the hardness, chemical reactivity, and stability of enamel, while preserving the apatite structures. Trace amounts of fluoride stabilize enamel by lowering acid solubility, decreasing the rate of demineralization, and enhancing the rate of remineralization.

Enamel is the hardest substance of the human body. Hardness may vary over the external tooth surface according to the location; also, it decreases inward, with hardness lowest at the DEJ. The density of enamel also decreases from the surface to the DEJ. Enamel is a rigid structure that is both strong and brittle (high elastic modulus, high compressive strength, and low tensile strength). The ability of the enamel to withstand masticatory forces depends on a stable attachment to the dentin by means of the DEJ. Dentin is a more flexible substance that is strong and resilient (low elastic modulus, high compressive strength, and high tensile strength), which essentially increases the fracture toughness of the more superficial enamel. The junction of enamel and dentin (DEJ) is scalloped or wavy in outline, with the crest of the waves penetrating toward enamel (Fig. 1.11). The rounded projections of enamel fit into the shallow depressions of dentin. This interdigitation may contribute to the durable connection of enamel to dentin. The DEJ is approximately 2 μm wide and is comprised of a mineralized complex of interwoven dentin and enamel matrix proteins. In addition to the physical, scalloped relationship between the enamel and dentin, an interphase matrix layer (made primarily of a fibrillary collagen network) extends 100 to 400 μm from the DEJ into the enamel. This matrix-modified interphase layer is considered to provide fracture propagation limiting properties to the interface between the enamel and the DEJ and thus overall structural stability of the enamel attachment to dentin.[1] Enamel rods that lack a dentin base because of caries or improper preparation design are easily fractured away from neighboring rods. For optimal strength in tooth preparation, all enamel rods should be supported by dentin (Fig. 1.12).

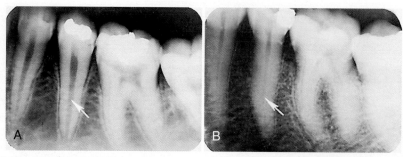

• **Fig. 1.13** Pulp cavity size. A, Premolar radiograph of young person. B, Premolar radiograph of older person. Note the difference in the size of the pulp cavity *(arrows)*.

Pulp–Dentin Complex

Pulp and dentin tissues are specialized connective tissues of mesodermal origin, formed from the dental papilla of the tooth bud. Many investigators consider these two tissues as a single tissue, which forms the pulp–dentin complex, with mineralized dentin constituting the mature end product of cell differentiation and maturation.

Dental pulp occupies the pulp cavity in the tooth and is a unique, specialized organ of the human body that serves four functions: (1) formative (developmental), (2) nutritive, (3) sensory (protective), and (4) defensive/reparative. The formative function is the production of primary and secondary dentin by odontoblasts. The nutritive function supplies mineral ions, proteins, and water to dentin through the blood supply to odontoblasts and their processes. The sensory function is provided by nerve fibers within the pulp that mediate the sensation of pain. Dentin nervous nociceptors are unique because various stimuli elicit only pain as a response. The pulp usually does not differentiate between heat, touch, pressure, or chemicals. Motor nerve fibers initiate reflexes in the muscles of the blood vessel walls for the control of circulation in the pulp. The defensive/reparative function is discussed in the subsequent section on *The Pulp-Dentin Complex: Response to Pathologic Challenge.*

The pulp is circumscribed by dentin and is lined peripherally by a cellular layer of odontoblasts adjacent to dentin. Anatomically, the pulp is divided into (1) coronal pulp located in the pulp chamber in the crown portion of the tooth, including the pulp horns that are located beneath the incisal ridges and cusp tips, and (2) radicular pulp located in the pulp canals in the root portion of the tooth. The radicular pulp is continuous with the periapical tissues through the apical foramen or foramina of the root. Accessory canals may extend from the pulp canals laterally through the root dentin to periodontal tissue. The shape of each pulp conforms generally to the shape of each tooth (see Fig. 1.3).

The pulp contains nerves, arterioles, venules, capillaries, lymph channels, connective tissue cells, intercellular substance, odontoblasts, fibroblasts, macrophages, collagen, and fine fibers.[2] The pulp is circumscribed peripherally by a specialized odontogenic area composed of the odontoblasts, the cell-free zone, and the cell-rich zone.

Knowledge of the contour and size of the pulp cavity is essential during tooth preparation. In general, the pulp cavity is a miniature contour of the external surface of the tooth. Pulp cavity size varies with tooth size in the same person and among individuals. With advancing age, the pulp cavity usually decreases in size. Radiographs are an invaluable aid in determining the size of the pulp cavity and any existing pathologic condition (Fig. 1.13). A primary

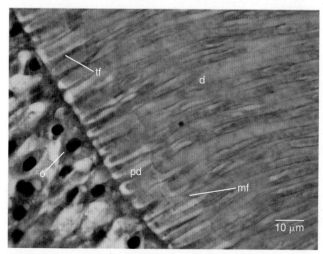

• **Fig. 1.14** Odontoblasts *(o)* have cell processes (Tomes fibers [tf]) that extend through the predentin *(pd)* into dentin *(d). mf*, Mineralization front.

objective during operative procedures must be the preservation of the health of the pulp.

Dentin formation, *dentinogenesis*, is accomplished by cells called *odontoblasts*. Odontoblasts are considered part of pulp and dentin tissues because their cell bodies are in the pulp cavity, but their long, slender cytoplasmic cell processes (Tomes fibers) extend well (100–200 µm) into the tubules in the mineralized dentin (Fig. 1.14).

Because of these odontoblastic cell processes, dentin is considered a living tissue, with the capability of reacting to physiologic and pathologic stimuli. Odontoblastic processes occasionally cross the DEJ into enamel; these are termed *enamel spindles* when their ends are thickened (Fig. 1.15). Enamel spindles may serve as pain receptors, explaining the sensitivity experienced by some patients during tooth preparation that is limited to enamel only.

Dentin forms the largest portion of the tooth structure, extending almost the full length of the tooth. Externally, dentin is covered by enamel on the anatomic crown and cementum on the anatomic root. Internally, dentin forms the walls of the pulp cavity (pulp chamber and pulp canals) (Fig. 1.16). Dentin formation begins immediately before enamel formation. Odontoblasts generate an extracellular collagen matrix as they begin to move away from adjacent ameloblasts. Mineralization of the collagen matrix, facilitated by modification of the collagen matrix by various noncollagenous proteins, gradually follows its secretion. The most recently formed layer of dentin is always on the pulpal surface.

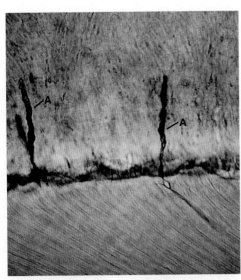

• **Fig. 1.15** Longitudinal section of enamel. Odontoblastic processes extend into enamel as enamel spindles *(A)*. (From Berkovitz BKB, Holland GR, Moxham BJ: *Oral anatomy, histology and embryology*, ed 4, Edinburgh, 2009, Mosby. Courtesy of Dr. R. Sprinz.)

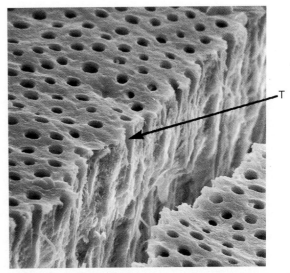

• **Fig. 1.17** Ground dentinal surface, acid-etched with 37% phosphoric acid. The artificial crack shows part of the dentinal tubules *(T)*. The tubule apertures are opened and widened by acid application. (From Brännström M: *Dentin and pulp in restorative dentistry*, London, 1982, Wolfe Medical.)

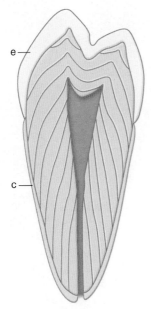

• **Fig. 1.16** Pattern of formation of primary dentin. This figure also shows enamel *(e)* covering the anatomic crown of the tooth and cementum *(c)* covering the anatomic root.

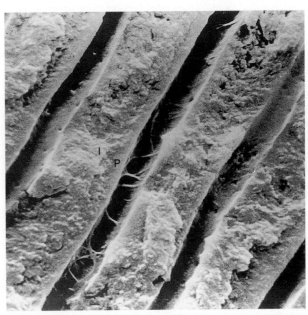

• **Fig. 1.18** Dentinal tubules in cross section, 1.2 mm from pulp. Peritubular dentin *(P)* is more mineralized than intertubular dentin *(I)*. (From Brännström M: *Dentin and pulp in restorative dentistry*, London, 1982, Wolfe Medical.)

This unmineralized zone of dentin is immediately next to the cell bodies of odontoblasts and is called *predentin* (see Fig. 1.14). Dentin formation begins at areas subjacent to the cusp tip or incisal ridge and gradually spreads, at the rate of ~4 μm/day, to the apex of the root (see Fig. 1.16). In contrast to enamel formation, dentin formation continues after tooth eruption and throughout the life of the pulp. The dentin forming the initial shape of the tooth is called *primary dentin* and is usually completed 3 years after tooth eruption (in the case of permanent teeth).

The dentinal tubules are small canals that remain from the process of dentinogenesis and extend through the entire width of dentin, from the pulp to the DEJ (Figs. 1.17 and 1.18). Each tubule contains the cytoplasmic cell process (Tomes fiber) of an odontoblast and is lined with a layer of peritubular dentin, which is much more mineralized than the surrounding intertubular dentin (see Fig. 1.18).

The surface area of dentin is much larger at the DEJ and dentinocemental junction than it is on the pulp cavity side. Because odontoblasts form dentin while progressing inward toward the pulp, the tubules are forced closer together. The number of tubules increases from 15,000 to 20,000/mm² at the DEJ to 45,000 to 65,000/mm² at the pulp.[3] The lumen of the tubules also varies from the DEJ to the pulp surface. In coronal dentin, the average diameter of tubules at the DEJ is 0.5 to 0.9 μm, but this increases to 2 to 3 μm near the pulp (Fig. 1.19).

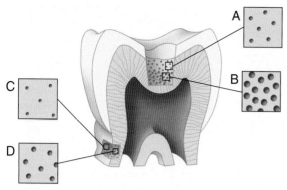

• **Fig. 1.19** Tubules in superficial dentin close to the dentoenamel junction (DEJ) *(A)* are smaller and more sparsely distributed compared with deep dentin *(B)*. The tubules in superficial root dentin *(C)* and deep root dentin *(D)* are smaller and less numerous than those in comparable depths of coronal dentin.

The course of the dentinal tubules is a slight S-curve in the tooth crown, but the tubules are straighter in the incisal ridges, cusps, and root areas (Fig. 1.20). Tubules are generally oriented perpendicular to the DEJ. Along the tubule walls are small lateral openings called *canaliculi* or lateral canals. The lateral canals are formed as a result of the presence of secondary (lateral) branches of adjacent odontoblastic processes during dentinogenesis. Near the DEJ, the tubules are divided into several branches, forming an intercommunicating and anastomosing network (Fig. 1.21).

After the primary dentin is formed, dentin deposition continues at a reduced rate (~0.4 μm/day) even without obvious external stimuli, although the rate and amount of this physiologic secondary dentin vary considerably among individuals. In secondary dentin, the tubules take a slightly different directional pattern in contrast to the primary dentin (Fig. 1.22). The secondary dentin forms on all internal aspects of the pulp cavity, but in the pulp chamber, in multirooted teeth, it tends to be thicker on the roof and floor than on the side walls.[4]

The walls of the dentinal tubules (peritubular dentin) in the primary dentin gradually thicken, through ongoing mineral deposition, with age. The dentin therefore becomes harder, denser, and, because tubular fluid flow becomes more restricted as the lumen spaces become smaller, less sensitive. The increased amount of mineral in the primary dentin is defined as *dentin sclerosis*. Dentin sclerosis resulting from aging is called *physiologic dentin sclerosis*.

Human dentin is composed of approximately 50% inorganic material and 30% organic material by volume. The organic material is approximately 90% type I collagen and 10% noncollagenous proteins. Dentin is less mineralized than enamel but more mineralized than cementum or bone. The mineral content of dentin increases with age. The mineral phase is composed primarily of hydroxyapatite crystallites, which are arranged in a less systematic manner than are enamel crystallites. Dentinal crystallites are smaller than enamel crystallites, having a length of 20 to 100 nm and a width of about 3 nm, which is similar to the size seen in bone and cementum.[4] Dentin is significantly softer than enamel but harder than bone or cementum. The hardness of dentin averages one fifth that of enamel, and its hardness near the DEJ is about three times greater than near the pulp. Although dentin is a hard, mineralized tissue, it is flexible, with a modulus of elasticity of approximately 18 gigapascals (GPa).[5] This flexibility helps support the more brittle, less resilient enamel. Dentin is not as prone to fracture as is the enamel rod structure. Often small "craze lines"

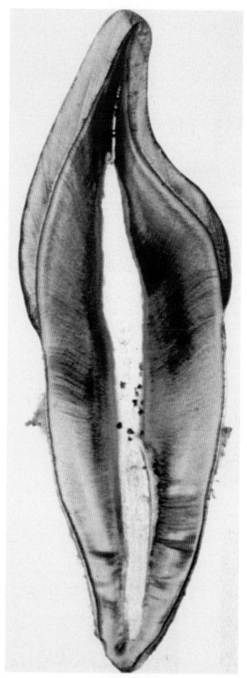

• **Fig. 1.20** Ground section of human incisor. Course of dentinal tubules is in a slight S-curve in the crown, but straight at the incisal tip and in the root. (From Young B, Lowe JS, Stevens A, Heath JW: *Wheater's functional histology: a text and colour atlas*, ed 5, Edinburgh, 2006, Churchill Livingstone.)

are seen in enamel, indicating minute fractures of that structure. The craze lines usually are not clinically significant unless associated with cracks in the underlying dentin. The ultimate tensile strength of dentin is approximately 98 megapascals (MPa), whereas the ultimate tensile strength of enamel is approximately 10 MPa. The compressive strength of dentin and enamel are approximately 297 and 384 MPa, respectively.[5]

During tooth preparation, dentin usually is distinguished from enamel by (1) color and opacity, (2) reflectance, (3) hardness, and (4) sound. Dentin is normally yellow-white and slightly darker

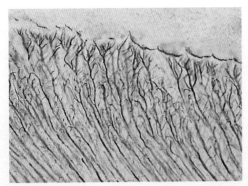

• **Fig. 1.21**   Ground section showing dentinal tubules and their lateral branching close to the dentoenamel junction (DEJ). (From Berkovitz BKB, Holland GR, Moxham BJ: *Oral anatomy, histology, and embryology*, ed 4, Edinburgh, 2010, Mosby.)

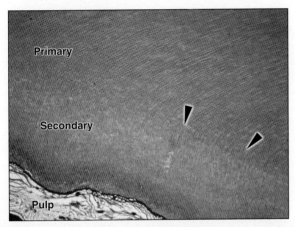

• **Fig. 1.22**   Ground section of dentin with pulpal surface at right. Dentinal tubules curve sharply as they move from primary to secondary dentin. Dentinal tubules are more irregular in shape in secondary dentin. (From Nanci A: *Ten Cate's oral histology: development, structure, and function*, ed 8, St. Louis, 2013, Mosby.)

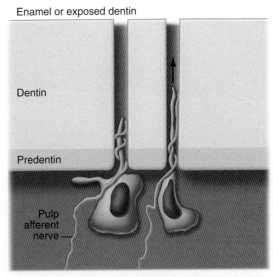

• **Fig. 1.23**   Stimuli that induce rapid fluid movements in dentinal tubules distort odontoblasts and afferent nerves *(arrow),* leading to a sensation of pain. Many operative procedures such as cutting or air-drying induce rapid fluid movement.

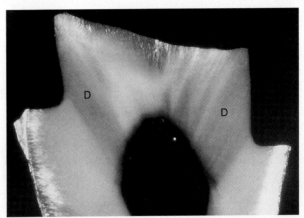

• **Fig. 1.24**   Ground section of MOD (mesio-occluso-distal) tooth preparation of a third molar. Dark blue dye was placed in the pulp chamber under pressure after tooth preparation. Dark areas of dye penetration *(D)* show that the dentinal tubules of axial walls are much more permeable than those of the pulpal floor of preparation.

than enamel. In older patients, dentin is darker, and it can become brown or black when it has been exposed to oral fluids, old restorative materials, or slowly advancing caries. Dentin surfaces are more opaque and dull, being less reflective to light than similar enamel surfaces, which appear shiny. Dentin is softer than enamel and provides greater yield to the pressure of a sharp explorer tine, which tends to catch and hold in dentin.

Dentin sensitivity is perceived whenever nociceptor afferent nerve endings, in close proximity to odontoblastic processes within the dental tubules, are depolarized. The nerve transduction is most often interpreted by the central nervous system as pain. Physical, thermal, chemical, bacterial, and traumatic stimuli are remote from the nerve fibers and are detected through the fluid-filled dentinal tubules, although the precise mechanism of detection has not been conclusively established. The most accepted theory of stimulus detection is the *hydrodynamic theory*, which suggests that stimulus-initiated rapid tubular fluid movement within the dentinal tubules accounts for nerve depolarization.[6] Operative procedures that involve cutting, drying, pressure changes, osmotic shifts, or changes in temperature result in rapid tubular fluid movement, which is perceived as pain (Fig. 1.23).

Dentinal tubules are filled with dentinal fluid, a transudate of plasma that contains all components necessary for mineralization

to occur. These components include water, matrix proteins, matrix-modifying proteins, and mineral ions. The vital dental pulp has a slight positive pressure that results in continual dentinal fluid flow toward the external surface of the tooth. Enamel and cementum, though semipermeable, provide an effective layer serving to protect the underlying dentin and limit tubular fluid flow. When enamel or cementum is removed during tooth preparation, the protective layer is lost, allowing increased tubular fluid movement toward the cut surface. Permeability studies of dentin indicate that tubules are functionally much smaller than would be indicated by their measured microscopic dimensions as a result of numerous constrictions along their paths (see Fig. 1.18).[7] Dentin permeability is not uniform throughout the tooth. Coronal dentin is much more permeable than root dentin. There also are differences within coronal dentin (Fig. 1.24).[8] Dentin permeability primarily depends on the remaining dentin thickness (i.e., length of the tubules) and the diameter of the tubules. Because the tubules are shorter, more

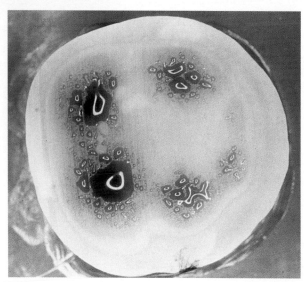

• **Fig. 1.25** Horizontal section in the occlusal third of a molar crown. Dark blue dye was placed in the pulp chamber under pressure. Deep dentin areas (over pulp horns) are much more permeable than superficial dentin. (From Pashley DH, Andringa HJ, Derkson GD, Derkson ME, Kalathoor SR: Regional variability in the permeability of human dentin, *Arch Oral Biol* 32:519–523, 1987, with permission from Pergamon, Oxford, UK.)

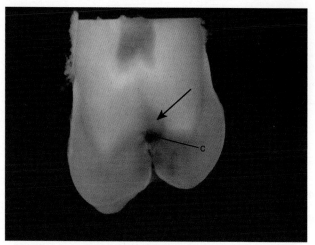

• **Fig. 1.26** Transparent dentin *(arrow)* beneath a caries lesion *(c)*.

numerous, and larger in diameter closer to the pulp, deep dentin is a less effective pulpal barrier compared with superficial dentin (Fig. 1.25).

The Pulp–Dentin Complex: Response to Pathologic Challenge

The pulp–dentin complex responds to tooth pathology through pulpal immune-inflammation defense systems and dentin repair/formation. The defensive and reparative functions of the pulp are mediated by an extremely complex host-defense response to bacterial, chemical, mechanical, and/or thermal irritation.[9] Primary odontoblasts are the first to respond to lesion formation and communicate with the deeper pulp tissue (via cytokines and chemokines) such that an adaptive and innate inflammatory reaction begins. Mild to moderate injury normally causes a reversible inflammatory response in the pulp, referred to as *reversible pulpitis,* which resolves when the pathology is removed. Moderate to severe injury (e.g., deep caries) may cause the degeneration of the affected odontoblastic processes and death of the corresponding primary odontoblasts. Toxic bacterial products, molecules released from the demineralized dentin matrix, and/or high concentrations of inflammatory response mediators may signal death of the primary odontoblasts. In cases of severe injury, an irreversible inflammatory response of the pulp *(irreversible pulpitis)* will ultimately result in capillary dilation, local edema, stagnation of blood flow, anoxia, and ultimately pulpal necrosis (see Chapter 2).

Very early host-defense processes in primary dentin seek to block the advancement of a caries lesion by means of the precipitation of mineral in the lumens of the dentinal tubules of the affected area. The physical occlusion of the tubular lumens increases the ability of light to pass through this localized region (i.e., increases its transparency). This dentin is referred to as *transparent dentin* (Fig. 1.26).[10] Dentin in this area is not as hard as normal primary dentin because of mineral loss in the intertubular dentin (see Chapter 2). Successful host-defense repair processes result in the

remineralization of the intertubular dentin, in addition to the mineral occlusion of the dentinal tubules, such that the final hardness of the dentin in this affected area is greater than normal primary dentin. The increased overall mineralization of this caries-affected primary dentin is referred to as *reactive dentin sclerosis.*

Deep dentin formation processes occur simultaneously with the pulpal inflammatory response and result in the generation of *tertiary dentin* at the pulp–dentin interface. The net effect of these processes is to increase the thickness/effectiveness of the dentin as a protective barrier for the pulp tissue. Two types of tertiary dentin form in response to lesion formation. In the case of mild injury (e.g., a shallow caries lesion), primary odontoblasts initiate increased formation of dentin along the internal aspect of the dentin beneath the affected area through secretion of *reactionary tertiary dentin* (or "reactionary dentin"). Reactionary dentin is tubular in nature and is continuous with primary and secondary dentin.

More severe injury (e.g., a deep caries lesion) causes the death of the primary odontoblasts. When therapeutic steps successfully resolve the injury, replacement cells (variously referred to as *secondary odontoblasts, odontoblast-like cells,* or *odontoblastoid cells*) differentiate from pulpal mesenchymal cells. The secondary odontoblasts subsequently generate *reparative tertiary dentin* (or "reparative dentin") as a part of the ongoing host defense. Reparative dentin usually appears as a localized dentin deposit on the wall of the pulp cavity immediately subjacent to the area on the tooth that had received the injury (Fig. 1.27). Reparative dentin is generally atubular and therefore structurally different from the primary and secondary dentin.

Cementum

Cementum is a thin layer of hard dental tissue covering the anatomic roots of teeth. It is formed by cells known as *cementoblasts,* which develop from undifferentiated mesenchymal cells in the connective tissue of the dental follicle. Cementum is slightly softer than dentin and consists of about 45% to 50% inorganic material (hydroxyapatite) by weight and 50% to 55% organic matter and water by weight. The organic portion is composed primarily of collagen and protein polysaccharides. *Sharpey fibers* are portions of the principal collagen fibers of the periodontal ligament embedded in cementum and alveolar bone to attach the tooth to the alveolus (Fig. 1.28). Cementum is avascular.

Cementum is yellow and slightly lighter in color than dentin. It is formed continuously throughout life because, as the superficial

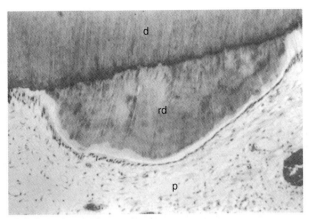

• **Fig. 1.27** Reparative dentin in response to a caries lesion. *d*, Dentin; *rd*, reparative dentin; *p*, pulp. (From Trowbridge HO: Pulp biology: Progress during the past 25 years, *Aust Endo J* 29(1):5–12, 2003.)

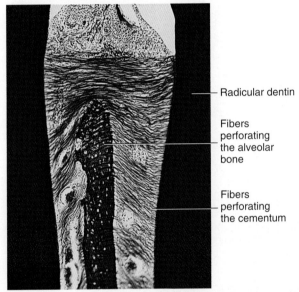

• **Fig. 1.28** Principal fibers of periodontal ligament continue into surface layer of cementum as Sharpey fibers. (Modified from Chiego DJ Jr: *Essentials of oral histology and embryology: A clinical approach*, ed 4, St Louis, 2014, Mosby.)

layer of cementum ages, a new layer of cementum is deposited to keep the attachment intact. *Acellular cementum* (i.e., there are no cementoblasts) is predominately associated with the coronal half of the root. *Cellular cementum* is more frequently associated with the apical half of the root. Cementum on the root end surrounds the apical foramen and may extend slightly onto the inner wall of the pulp canal. Cementum thickness may increase on the root end to compensate for attritional wear of the occlusal or incisal surface and passive eruption of the tooth.

The cementodentinal junction is relatively smooth in the permanent tooth. The attachment of cementum to dentin, although not completely understood, is very durable. Cementum joins enamel to form the CEJ. In about 10% of teeth, enamel and cementum do not meet, and this can result in a sensitive area as the openings of the dentinal tubules are not covered. Abrasion, erosion, caries, scaling, and restoration finishing/polishing procedures may denude dentin of its cementum covering. This may lead to sensitivity to various stimuli (e.g., heat, cold, sweet substances, sour substances).

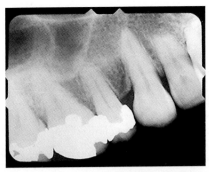

• **Fig. 1.29** Radiograph showing root resorption on lateral incisor after orthodontic tooth movement.

Cementum is capable of repairing itself to a limited degree and is not resorbed under normal conditions. Some resorption of the apical portion of the root cementum and dentin may occur, however, if orthodontic pressures are excessive and movement is too fast (Fig. 1.29).

Physiology of Tooth Form

Function

Teeth serve four main functions: (1) mastication, (2) esthetics, (3) speech, and (4) protection of supporting tissues. Normal tooth form and proper alignment ensure efficiency in the incising and reduction of food. The various tooth classes—incisors, canines, premolars, and molars—perform specific functions in the masticatory process and in the coordination of the various muscles of mastication. The form and alignment of anterior teeth contribute to the esthetics of personal physical appearance. The form and alignment of anterior and posterior teeth assist in the articulation of certain sounds so as to effect proper speech. Finally, the form and alignment of teeth assist in the development and protection of supporting gingival tissue and alveolar bone.

Contours

Facial and lingual surfaces possess a degree of convexity that affords protection and stimulation of supporting tissues during mastication. The convexity generally is located at the cervical third of the crown on the facial surfaces of all teeth and the lingual surfaces of incisors and canines. Lingual surfaces of posterior teeth usually have their height of contour in the middle third of the crown. Normal tooth contours act in deflecting food only to the extent that the passing food stimulates (by gentle massage) and does not irritate (abrade) supporting soft tissues. If these curvatures are too great, tissues usually receive inadequate stimulation by the passage of food. Too little contour may result in trauma to the attachment apparatus. Normal tooth contours must be recreated in the performance of operative dental procedures. Improper location and degree of facial or lingual convexities may result in iatrogenic injury, as illustrated in Fig. 1.30, in which the proper facial contour is disregarded in the design of the cervical area of a mandibular molar restoration. Overcontouring is the worst offender, usually resulting in increased plaque retention that leads to a chronic inflammatory state of the gingiva.

Proper form of the proximal surfaces of teeth is just as important to the maintenance of periodontal tissue health as is the proper form of facial and lingual surfaces. The proximal height of contour serves to provide (1) contacts with the proximal surfaces of adjacent teeth, thus preventing food impaction, and (2) adequate embrasure space (immediately apical to the contacts) for gingival tissue, supporting bone, blood vessels, and nerves that serve the supporting structures (Fig. 1.31).

Proximal Contact Area

When teeth initially erupt to make proximal contact with previously erupted teeth, a contact *point* is present. The contact point increases in size to become a proximal contact *area* as the two adjacent tooth surfaces abrade each other during physiologic tooth movement (Figs. 1.32 and 1.33).

The physiologic significance of properly formed and located proximal contacts cannot be overemphasized; they promote normal healthy interdental papillae filling the interproximal spaces. Improper contacts may result in food impaction between teeth, potentially increasing the risk of periodontal disease, caries, and tooth movement. In addition, retention of food is objectionable because of its physical presence and the halitosis that results from food decomposition. Proximal contacts and interdigitation of maxillary and mandibular teeth, through occlusal contact areas, stabilize and maintain the integrity of the dental arches.

The proximal contact area is located in the incisal third of the approximating surfaces of maxillary and mandibular central incisors (see Fig. 1.33). It is positioned slightly facial to the center of the proximal surface faciolingually (see Fig. 1.32). Proceeding posteriorly from the incisor region through all the remaining teeth, the contact area is located near the junction of the incisal (or occlusal) and middle thirds or in the middle third. Proximal contact areas typically are larger in the molar region, which helps prevent gingival food impaction during mastication. Adjacent surfaces near the proximal contacts (embrasures) usually have remarkable symmetry.

Embrasures

Embrasures are V-shaped spaces that originate at the proximal contact areas between adjacent teeth and are named for the direction toward which they radiate. These embrasures are (1) facial, (2) lingual, (3) incisal or occlusal, and (4) gingival (see Figs. 1.32 and 1.33).

Initially, the interdental papilla fills the gingival embrasure. When the form and function of teeth are ideal and optimal oral

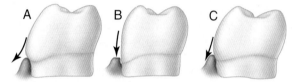

• **Fig. 1.30** Contours. Arrows show pathways of food passing over facial surface of mandibular molar during mastication. A, Overcontour deflects food from gingiva and results in understimulation of supporting tissues. B, Undercontour of tooth may result in irritation of soft tissue. C, Correct contour permits adequate stimulation and protection of supporting tissue.

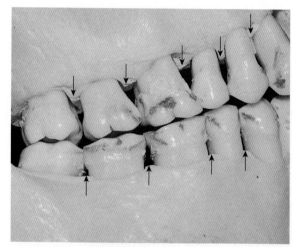

• **Fig. 1.31** Portion of the skull, showing triangular spaces beneath proximal contact areas. These spaces are occupied by soft tissue and bone for the support of teeth.

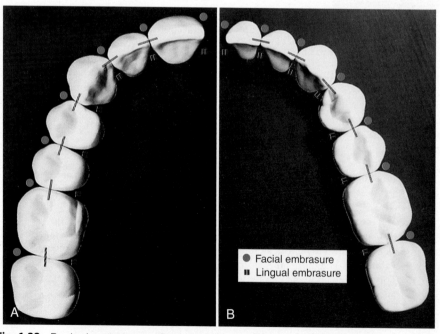

● Facial embrasure
‖ Lingual embrasure

• **Fig. 1.32** Proximal contact areas. Black lines show positions of contact faciolingually. A, Maxillary teeth. B, Mandibular teeth. Facial and lingual embrasures are indicated.

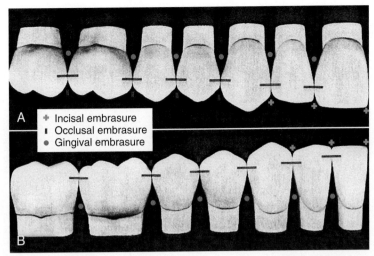

• **Fig. 1.33** Proximal contact areas. Black lines show positions of contact incisogingivally and occluso-gingivally. Incisal, occlusal, and gingival embrasures are indicated. A, Maxillary teeth. B, Mandibular teeth.

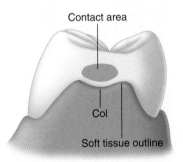

• **Fig. 1.34** Relationship of ideal interdental papilla to molar contact area.

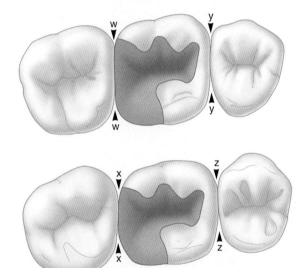

• **Fig. 1.35** Embrasure form. *w*, Improper embrasure form caused by overcontouring of restoration resulting in unhealthy gingiva from lack of stimulation. *x*, Good embrasure form. *y*, Frictional wear of contact area has resulted in decrease of embrasure dimension. *z*, When the embrasure form is good, supporting tissues receive adequate stimulation from foods during mastication.

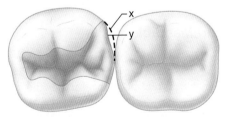

• **Fig. 1.36** Embrasure form. *x*, Portion of tooth that offers protection to underlying supporting tissue during mastication. *y*, Restoration fails to establish adequate contour for good embrasure form.

health is maintained, the interdental papilla may continue in this position throughout life. When the gingival embrasure is filled by the papilla, trapping of food in this region is prevented. In a facio-lingual vertical section, the papilla is seen to have a triangular shape between anterior teeth, whereas in posterior teeth, the papilla may be shaped like a mountain range, with facial and lingual peaks and the col ("valley") lying beneath the contact area (Fig. 1.34). This col, a central faciolingual concave area beneath the contact, is more vulnerable to periodontal disease from incorrect contact and embrasure form because it is covered by nonkeratinized epithelium.

The correct relationships of embrasures, cusps to sulci, marginal ridges, and grooves of adjacent and opposing teeth provide for the escape of food from the occlusal surfaces during mastication. When an embrasure is decreased in size or absent, additional stress is created on teeth and the supporting structures during mastication. Embrasures that are too large provide little protection to the supporting structures as food is forced into the interproximal space by an opposing cusp (Fig. 1.35). A prime example is the failure to restore the distal cusp of a mandibular first molar when placing a restoration (Fig. 1.36). Lingual embrasures are usually larger than facial embrasures; and this allows more food to be displaced lingually because the tongue can return the food to the occlusal surface more easily than if the food is displaced facially into the buccal vestibule (see Fig. 1.32). The marginal ridges of adjacent posterior teeth should be at the same height to have proper contact and embrasure forms. When this relationship is absent, it may

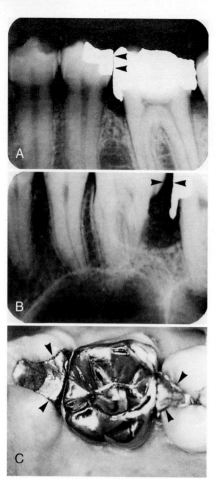

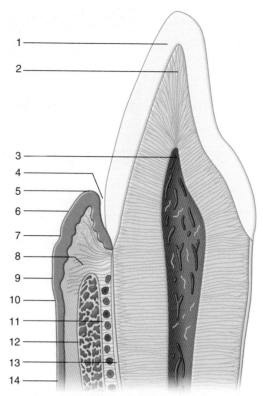

• **Fig. 1.37** Poor anatomic restorative form. A, Radiograph of flat contact/amalgam gingival excess and resultant vertical osseous loss. B, Radiograph of restoration with amalgam gingival excess and absence of contact resulting in osseous loss, adjacent root caries. C, Poor embrasure form and restoration margins.

• **Fig. 1.38** Vertical section of a maxillary incisor illustrating supporting structures: *1*, enamel; *2*, dentin; *3*, pulp; *4*, gingival sulcus; *5*, free gingival margin; *6*, free gingiva; *7*, free gingival groove; *8*, lamina propria of gingiva; *9*, attached gingiva; *10*, mucogingival junction; *11*, periodontal ligament; *12*, alveolar bone; *13*, cementum; *14*, alveolar mucosa.

cause an increase in the problems associated with inadequate proximal contacts and faulty embrasure forms.

Preservation of the curvatures of opposing cusps and surfaces in function maintains masticatory efficiency throughout life (see Fig. 1.2). Correct anatomic form renders teeth more self-cleansing because of the smoothly rounded contours that are more exposed to the cleansing action of foods and fluids and the frictional movement of the tongue, lips, and cheeks. Failure to understand and adhere to correct anatomic form may contribute to the breakdown of the restored system (Fig. 1.37).

Maxilla and Mandible

The human maxilla is formed by two bones, the maxilla proper and the premaxilla. These two bones form the bulk of the upper jaw and the major portion of the hard palate and help form the floor of the orbit and the sides and base of the nasal cavity. They contain 10 maxillary primary teeth initially and later contain 16 maxillary permanent teeth in the alveolar process (see Figs. 1.1 and 1.3, label 7).

The mandible, or the lower jaw, is horseshoe shaped and relates to the skull on either side via the TMJs. The mandible is composed of a body of two horizontal portions joined at the midline symphysis mandibulae and the rami, the vertical parts. The coronoid process

and the condyle make up the superior border of each ramus. The mandible initially contains 10 mandibular primary teeth and later 16 mandibular permanent teeth in the alveolar process. Maxillary and mandibular bones comprise approximately 38% to 43% inorganic material and 34% organic material by volume. The inorganic material is hydroxyapatite, and the organic material is primarily type I collagen, which is surrounded by a ground substance of glycoproteins and proteoglycans.

Oral Mucosa

The oral mucosa is the mucous membrane that covers all oral structures except the clinical crowns of teeth. It is composed of two layers: (1) the stratified squamous epithelium and (2) the supporting connective tissue, called *lamina propria*. (See the lamina propria of the gingiva in Fig. 1.38, *indicator 8*.) The epithelium may be keratinized, parakeratinized, or nonkeratinized, depending on its location. The lamina propria varies in thickness and supports the epithelium. It may be attached to the periosteum of alveolar bone, or it may be interposed over the submucosa, which may vary in different regions of the mouth (e.g., the floor of the mouth, the soft palate). The submucosa, consisting of connective tissues varying in density and thickness, attaches the mucous membrane to the underlying bony structures. The submucosa contains glands, blood vessels, nerves, and adipose tissue.

Oral mucosa is classified into three major functional types: (1) masticatory mucosa, (2) lining or reflective mucosa, and (3) specialized mucosa. The masticatory mucosa comprises the free and attached gingiva (see Fig. 1.38, *indicators 6 and 9*) and the mucosa of the hard palate. The epithelium of these tissues is keratinized, and the lamina propria is a dense, thick, firm connective tissue containing collagen fibers. The hard palate has a distinct submucosa except for a few narrow specific zones. The dense lamina propria of the attached gingiva is connected to the cementum and periosteum of the bony alveolar process (see Fig. 1.38, *indicator 8*).

The lining or reflective mucosa covers the inside of the lips, cheek, and vestibule, the lateral surfaces of the alveolar process (except the mucosa of the hard palate), the floor of the mouth, the soft palate, and the ventral surface of the tongue. The lining mucosa is a thin, movable tissue with a relatively thick, nonkeratinized epithelium and a thin lamina propria. The submucosa comprises mostly thin, loose connective tissue with muscle and collagenous and elastic fibers, with different areas varying from one another in their structures. The junction of the lining mucosa and the masticatory mucosa is the mucogingival junction, located at the apical border of the attached gingiva facially and lingually in the mandibular arch and facially in the maxillary arch (see Fig. 1.38, *indicator 10*). The specialized mucosa covers the dorsum of the tongue and the taste buds. The epithelium is nonkeratinized except for the covering of the dermal filiform papillae.

Periodontium

The periodontium consists of the oral hard and soft tissues that invest and support teeth. It may be divided into (1) the gingival unit, consisting of free and attached gingiva and the alveolar mucosa, and (2) the attachment apparatus, consisting of cementum, the periodontal ligament, and the alveolar process (see Fig. 1.38).

Gingival Unit

As mentioned, the free gingiva and the attached gingiva together form the masticatory mucosa. The free gingiva is the gingiva from the marginal crest to the level of the base of the gingival sulcus (see Fig. 1.38, *indicators 4 and 6*). The gingival sulcus is the space between the tooth and the free gingiva. The outer wall of the sulcus (inner wall of the free gingiva) is lined with a thin, nonkeratinized epithelium. The outer aspect of the free gingiva in each gingival embrasure is called *gingival* or *interdental papilla*. The free gingival groove is a shallow groove that runs parallel to the marginal crest of the free gingiva and usually indicates the level of the base of the gingival sulcus (see Fig. 1.38, *indicator 7*).

The attached gingiva, a dense connective tissue with keratinized, stratified, squamous epithelium, extends from the depth of the gingival sulcus to the mucogingival junction. A dense network of collagen fibers connects the attached gingiva firmly to cementum and the periosteum of the alveolar process (bone).

The alveolar mucosa is a thin, soft tissue that is loosely attached to the underlying alveolar bone (see Fig. 1.38, *indicators 12 and 14*). It is covered by a thin, nonkeratinized epithelial layer. The underlying submucosa contains loosely arranged collagen fibers, elastic tissue, fat, and muscle tissue. The alveolar mucosa is delineated from the attached gingiva by the mucogingival junction and continues apically to the vestibular fornix and the inside of the cheek.

Clinically, the level of the gingival attachment and gingival sulcus is an important factor in restorative dentistry. Soft tissue health must be maintained by teeth having the correct anatomic form and position to prevent recession of the gingiva and possible abrasion and erosion of the root surfaces. The margin of a tooth preparation should not be positioned subgingivally (at levels between the marginal crest of the free gingiva and the base of the sulcus) unless dictated by caries, previous restoration, esthetics, or other preparation requirements.

Attachment Apparatus

The tooth root is attached to the alveolus (bony socket) by the periodontal ligament (see Fig. 1.38, *indicator 11*), which is a complex connective tissue containing numerous cells, blood vessels, nerves, and an extracellular substance consisting of fibers and ground substance. Most of the fibers are collagen, and the ground substance is composed of a variety of proteins and polysaccharides. The periodontal ligament serves the following functions: (1) attachment and support, (2) sensory, (3) nutritive, and (4) homeostatic. Bundles of collagen fibers, known as *principal fibers of the ligament*, serve to connect between cementum and alveolar bone so as to suspend and support the tooth. Coordination of masticatory muscle function is achieved, through an efficient proprioceptive mechanism, by the sensory nerves located in the periodontal ligament. Blood vessels supply the attachment apparatus with nutritive substances. Specialized cells of the ligament function to resorb and replace cementum, the periodontal ligament, and alveolar bone.

The alveolar process—a part of the maxilla and the mandible—forms, supports, and lines the sockets into which the roots of teeth fit. Anatomically, no distinct boundary exists between the body of the maxilla or the mandible and the alveolar process. The alveolar process comprises thin, compact bone with many small openings through which blood vessels, lymphatics, and nerves pass. The inner wall of the bony socket consists of the thin lamella of bone that surrounds the root of the tooth and is termed *alveolar bone proper*. The second part of the bone is called *supporting alveolar bone*, which surrounds and supports the alveolar bone proper. Supporting bone is composed of two parts: (1) the cortical plate, consisting of compact bone and forming the inner (lingual) and outer (facial) plates of the alveolar process, and (2) the spongy base that fills the area between the plates and the alveolar bone proper.

Occlusion

Occlusion literally means "closing"; in dentistry, the term means the contact of teeth in opposing dental arches when the jaws are closed (static occlusal relationships) and during various jaw movements (dynamic occlusal relationships). The size of the jaw and the arrangement of teeth within the jaw are subject to a wide range of variation. The locations of contacts between opposing teeth (occlusal contacts) vary as a result of differences in the sizes and shapes of teeth and jaws and the relative position of the jaws. A wide variety of occlusal schemes are found in healthy individuals. Consequently, definition of an ideal occlusal scheme is fraught with difficulty.[11] Repeated attempts have been made to describe an ideal occlusal scheme, but these descriptions are so restrictive that few individuals can be found to fit the criteria. Failing to find a single adequate definition of an ideal occlusal scheme has resulted in the conclusion that "in the final analysis, optimal function and the absence of disease is the principal characteristic of a good occlusion."[11] The dental relationships described in this section conform to the concepts of normal, or usual, occlusal schemes and include common variations of tooth-and-jaw relationships. The masticatory system (muscles, TMJs, and teeth) is highly adaptable and usually able to successfully function over a wide range of differences in jaw size and tooth alignment. Despite this great adaptability, however, some patients are highly sensitive to changes in tooth contacts (which influence the masticatory muscles and TMJs), which may be brought about by orthodontic and restorative dental procedures.

Occlusal contact patterns vary with the position of the mandible. Static occlusion is defined further by the use of reference positions that include fully closed, terminal hinge (TH) closure, retruded, protruded, and right and left lateral extremes. The number and location of occlusal contacts between opposing teeth have important effects on the amount and direction of muscle force applied during mastication and other parafunctional activities such as mandibular clenching, tooth grinding, or a combination of both (bruxism). In extreme cases, these forces damage the teeth and/or their supporting tissues. Forceful tooth contact occurs routinely near the limits or borders of mandibular movement, showing the relevance of these reference positions.[12]

Tooth contact during mandibular movement is termed *dynamic occlusal relationship*. Gliding or sliding contacts occur during mastication and other mandibular movements. Gliding contacts may be advantageous or disadvantageous, depending on the teeth involved, the position of the contacts, and the resultant masticatory muscle response. The design of the restored tooth surface will have important effects on the number and location of occlusal contacts, and both static and dynamic relationships must be taken into consideration. The following sections discuss common arrangements and variations of teeth and the masticatory system. Mastication and the contacting relationships of anterior and posterior teeth are described with reference to the potential restorative needs of teeth.

General Description

Tooth Alignment and Dental Arches

In Fig. 1.39A, the cusps have been drawn as blunt, rounded, or pointed projections of the crowns of teeth. Posterior teeth have one, two, or three cusps near the facial and lingual surfaces of each tooth. Cusps are separated by distinct developmental grooves and sometimes have additional supplemental grooves on cusp inclines. Facial cusps are separated from the lingual cusps by a deep groove, termed *central groove*. If a tooth has multiple facial cusps or multiple lingual cusps, the cusps are separated by facial or lingual developmental grooves. The depressions between the cusps are termed *fossae* (singular, *fossa*). Cusps in both arches are aligned in a smooth curve. Usually, the maxillary arch is larger than the mandibular arch, which results in maxillary cusps overlapping mandibular cusps when the arches are in maximal occlusal contact (see Fig. 1.39B). In Fig. 1.39A, two curved lines have been drawn over the teeth to aid in the visualization of the arch form. These curved lines identify the alignment of similarly functioning cusps or fossae. On the left side of the arches, an imaginary arc connecting the row of facial cusps in the mandibular arch have been drawn and labeled *facial occlusal line*. Above that, an imaginary line connecting the maxillary central fossae is labeled *central fossa occlusal line*. The mandibular facial occlusal line and the maxillary central fossa occlusal line coincide exactly when the mandibular arch is fully closed into the maxillary arch. On the right side of the dental arches, the maxillary lingual occlusal line and mandibular central fossa occlusal line have been drawn and labeled. These lines also coincide when the mandible is fully closed.

In Fig. 1.39B, the dental arches are fully interdigitated, with maxillary teeth overlapping mandibular teeth. The overlap of the maxillary cusps may be observed directly when the jaws are closed. *Maximum intercuspation (MI)* refers to the position of the mandible when teeth are brought into full interdigitation with the maximal number of teeth contacting. Synonyms for MI include *intercuspal contact*, *maximum closure*, and *maximum habitual intercuspation (MHI)*.

In Fig. 1.39C (proximal view), the mandibular facial occlusal line and the maxillary central fossa occlusal line coincide exactly. The maxillary lingual occlusal line and the mandibular central fossa occlusal line identified in Fig. 1.39A also are coincidental. The cusps that contact opposing teeth along the central fossa occlusal line are termed *functional cusps* (synonyms include supporting, holding, or stamp cusps); the cusps that overlap opposing teeth are termed *nonfunctional cusps* (synonyms include nonsupporting or nonholding cusps). The mandibular facial occlusal line identifies the mandibular functional cusps, whereas the maxillary facial cusps are nonfunctional cusps. These terms are usually applied only to posterior teeth to distinguish the functions of the two rows of cusps. In some circumstances, the functional role of the cusps may be reversed, as illustrated in Fig. 1.40C.2. Posterior teeth are well suited to crushing food because of the mutual cusp–fossa contacts (Fig. 1.41D).

In Fig. 1.39D, anterior teeth are seen to have a different relationship in MI, but they also show the characteristic maxillary overlap. Incisors are best suited to shearing food because of their overlap and the sliding contact on the lingual surface of maxillary teeth. In MI, mandibular incisors and canines contact the respective lingual surfaces of their maxillary opponents. The amount of horizontal (overjet) and vertical (overbite) overlap (see Fig. 1.40A.2) can significantly influence mandibular movement and the cusp design of restorations of posterior teeth. Variations in the growth and development of the jaws and in the positions of anterior teeth may result in open bite, in which vertical or horizontal discrepancies prevent teeth from contacting (see Fig. 1.40A.3).

Anteroposterior Interarch Relationships

In Fig. 1.39E, the cusp interdigitation pattern of the first molar teeth is used to classify anteroposterior arch relationships using a system developed by Angle.[13] During the eruption of teeth, the tooth cusps and fossae guide the teeth into maximal contact. Three interdigitated relationships of the first molars are commonly observed. See Fig. 1.39F for an illustration of the occlusal contacts that result from different molar positions. The location of the mesiofacial cusp of the maxillary first molar in relation to the mandibular first molar is used as an indicator in Angle classification. The most common molar relationship finds the maxillary mesiofacial cusp located in the mesiofacial developmental groove of the mandibular first molar. This relationship is termed Angle Class I. Slight posterior positioning of the mandibular first molar results in the mesiofacial cusp of the maxillary molar settling into the facial embrasure between the mandibular first molar and the mandibular second premolar. This is termed Class II and occurs in approximately 15% of the U.S. population. Anterior positioning of the mandibular first molar relative to the maxillary first molar is termed Class III and is the least common. In Class III relationships, the mesiofacial cusp of the maxillary first molar fits into the distofacial groove of the mandibular first molar; this occurs in approximately 3% of the U.S. population. Significant differences in these percentages occur in people in other countries and in different ethnic groups.

Although Angle classification is based on the relationship of the cusps, Fig. 1.39G illustrates that the location of tooth roots in alveolar bone determines the relative positions of the crowns and cusps of teeth. When the mandible is proportionally similar in size to the maxilla, a Class I molar relationship is formed; when the mandible is proportionally smaller than the maxilla, a Class

A. Dental arch cusp and fossa alignment

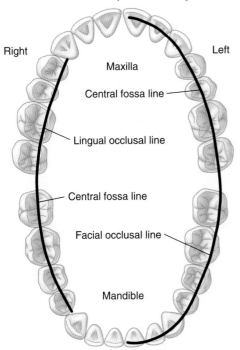

1. The maxillary lingual occlusal line and the mandibular central fossa line are coincident.
2. The mandibular facial occlusal line and the maxillary central fossa line are coincident.

B. Maximum intercuspation (MI): the teeth in opposing arches are in maximal contact

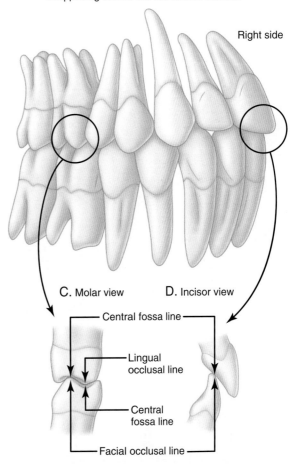

Right side

C. Molar view   D. Incisor view

Central fossa line

Lingual occlusal line

Central fossa line

Facial occlusal line

E. Facial view of anterior-posterior variations

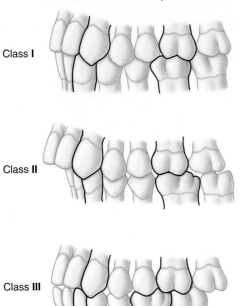

Class I

Class II

Class III

F. Molar Classes I, II, and III relationships

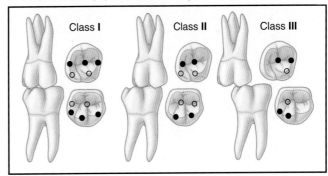

Class I   Class II   Class III

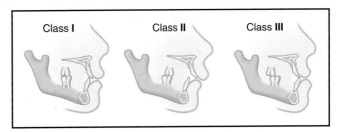

Class I   Class II   Class III

G. Skeletal Classes I, II, and III relationships

• **Fig. 1.39**   Dental arch relationships.

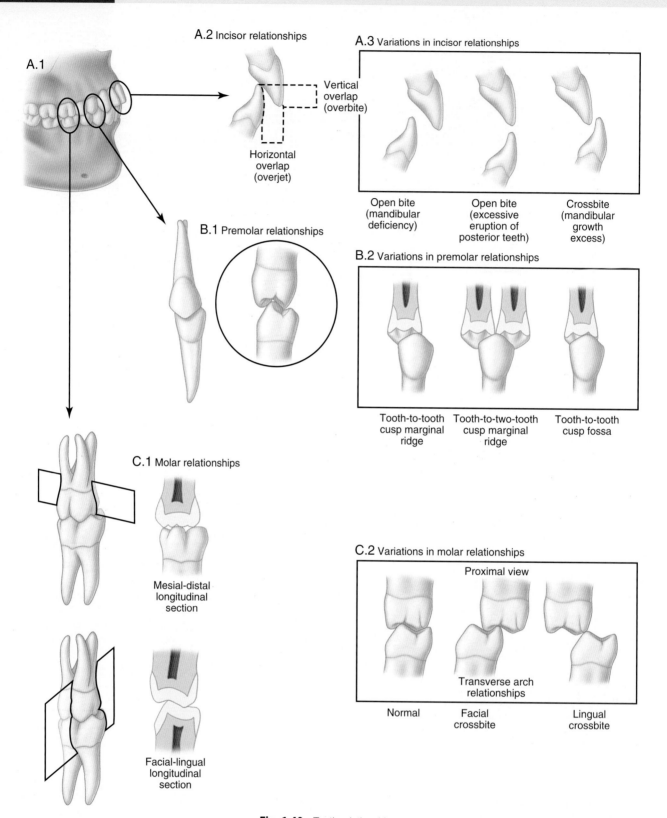

• **Fig. 1.40** Tooth relationships.

II relationship is formed; and when the mandible is relatively greater than the maxilla, a Class III relationship is formed.

Interarch Tooth Relationships

Fig. 1.40 illustrates the occlusal contact relationships of individual teeth in more detail. In Fig. 1.40A.2, incisor overlap is illustrated.

The overlap is characterized in two dimensions: (1) horizontal overlap (overjet) and (2) vertical overlap (overbite). Differences in the sizes of the mandible and the maxilla can result in clinically significant variations in incisor relationships, including open bite as a result of mandibular deficiency or excessive eruption of posterior teeth, and crossbite as a result of mandibular growth excess (see

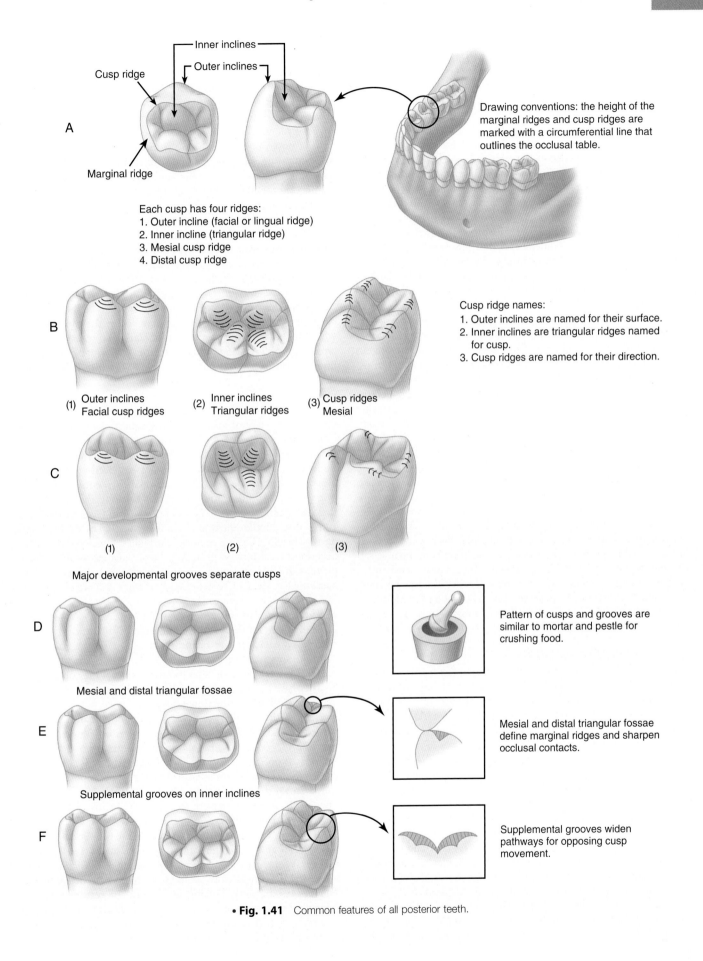

A

Inner inclines
Outer inclines
Cusp ridge
Marginal ridge

Drawing conventions: the height of the marginal ridges and cusp ridges are marked with a circumferential line that outlines the occlusal table.

Each cusp has four ridges:
1. Outer incline (facial or lingual ridge)
2. Inner incline (triangular ridge)
3. Mesial cusp ridge
4. Distal cusp ridge

B

(1) Outer inclines
Facial cusp ridges

(2) Inner inclines
Triangular ridges

(3) Cusp ridges
Mesial

Cusp ridge names:
1. Outer inclines are named for their surface.
2. Inner inclines are triangular ridges named for cusp.
3. Cusp ridges are named for their direction.

C

(1)　(2)　(3)

Major developmental grooves separate cusps

D

Pattern of cusps and grooves are similar to mortar and pestle for crushing food.

Mesial and distal triangular fossae

E

Mesial and distal triangular fossae define marginal ridges and sharpen occlusal contacts.

Supplemental grooves on inner inclines

F

Supplemental grooves widen pathways for opposing cusp movement.

• **Fig. 1.41** Common features of all posterior teeth.

Fig. 1.40A.3). These variations have significant clinical effects on the contacting relationships of posterior teeth and resultant masticatory activity during various jaw movements because the anterior teeth are not contributing to mandibular guidance.

Fig. 1.40B.1 illustrates a normal Class I occlusion, in which each mandibular premolar is located one half of a tooth width anterior to its maxillary antagonist. This relationship results in the mandibular facial cusp contacting the maxillary premolar mesial marginal ridge and the maxillary premolar lingual cusp contacting the mandibular distal marginal ridge. Because only one antagonist is contacted, this is termed *tooth-to-tooth relationship*. The most stable maxillary/mandibular tooth relationship results from the contact of the functional cusp tips against the two marginal ridges, termed *tooth-to-two-tooth contact*. Variations in the mesiodistal root position of teeth produce different relationships (see Fig. 1.40B.2). When the mandible is slightly distal to the maxilla (termed Class II tendency), each functional cusp tip occludes in a stable relationship with the opposing mesial or distal fossa; this relationship is a cusp–fossa contact.

Fig. 1.40C illustrates Class I molar relationships in more detail. Fig. 1.40C.1 shows the mandibular facial cusp tips contacting the maxillary marginal ridges and the central fossa triangular ridges. A faciolingual longitudinal section reveals how the functional cusps contact the opposing fossae and shows the effect of the developmental grooves on reducing the height of the nonfunctional cusps opposite the functional cusp tips. During lateral movements, the functional cusp is able to move through the facial and lingual developmental groove spaces without contact. Faciolingual position variations are possible in molar relationships because of differences in the growth of the width of the maxilla or the mandible.

Fig. 1.40C.2 illustrates the normal molar contact position, facial crossbite, and lingual crossbite relationships. Facial crossbite in posterior teeth is characterized by the contact of the maxillary facial cusps in the opposing mandibular central fossae and the mandibular lingual cusps in the opposing maxillary central fossae. Facial crossbite (also termed *buccal crossbite*) results in the reversal of roles of the cusps of the involved teeth. In this reversal example, the mandibular lingual cusps and maxillary facial cusps become functional cusps, and the maxillary lingual cusps and mandibular facial cusps become nonfunctional cusps. Lingual crossbite results in a poor molar relationship that provides little functional contact.

Posterior Cusp Characteristics

Four cusp ridges may be identified as common features of all cusps. The outer incline of a cusp faces the facial (or the lingual) surface of the tooth and is named for its respective surface. In the example using a mandibular second premolar (see Fig. 1.41A), the facial cusp ridge of the facial cusp is indicated by the line that points to the outer incline of the cusp. The inner inclines of the posterior cusps face the central fossa or the central groove of the tooth. The inner incline cusp ridges are widest at the base and become narrower as they approach the cusp tip. For this reason, they are termed *triangular ridges*. The triangular ridge of the facial cusp of the mandibular premolar is indicated by the arrow to the inner incline. Triangular ridges are usually set off from the other cusp ridges by one or more supplemental grooves. In Fig. 1.41B.1 and C.1, the outer inclines of the facial cusps of the mandibular and maxillary first molars are highlighted. In Fig. 1.41B.2 and C.2, the triangular ridges of the facial and lingual cusps are highlighted.

Mesial and distal cusp ridges extend from the cusp tip mesially and distally and are named for their directions. Mesial and distal cusp ridges extend downward from the cusp tips, forming the characteristic facial and lingual profiles of the cusps as viewed from the facial or lingual aspect. At the base of the cusp, the mesial or distal cusp ridge abuts to another cusp ridge, forming a developmental groove, or the cusp ridge turns toward the center line of the tooth and fuses with the marginal ridge. Marginal ridges are elevated, the rounded ridges being located on the mesial and distal edges of the tooth's occlusal surface (see Fig. 1.41A). The occlusal table of posterior teeth is the area contained within the mesial and distal cusp ridges and the marginal ridges of the tooth. The occlusal table limits are indicated in the drawings by a circumferential line connecting the highest points of the curvatures of the cusp ridges and marginal ridges.

The unique shape of cusps produces the characteristic form of individual posterior teeth. The mandibular first molars have longer triangular ridges on the distofacial cusps, causing a deviation of the central groove (see Fig. 1.41B.2). The mesiolingual cusp of a maxillary molar is much larger than the mesiofacial cusp. The distal cusp ridge of the maxillary first molar mesiolingual cusp curves facially to fuse with the triangular ridge of the distofacial cusp (see Fig. 1.41C.2). This junction forms the oblique ridge, which is characteristic of maxillary molars. The transverse groove crosses the oblique ridge where the distal cusp ridge of the mesiolingual cusp meets the triangular ridge of the distofacial cusp.

Functional Cusps

In Fig. 1.42, the lingual occlusal line of maxillary teeth and the facial occlusal line of mandibular teeth mark the locations of the functional cusps. These cusps contact opposing teeth in their corresponding faciolingual center on a marginal ridge or a fossa. Functional cusp–central fossa contact has been compared to a mortar and pestle because the functional cusp cuts, crushes, and grinds fibrous food against the ridges forming the concavity of the fossa (see Fig. 1.41D). Natural tooth form has multiple ridges and grooves ideally suited to aid in the reduction of the food bolus during chewing. During chewing, the highest forces and the longest duration of contact occur at MI. Functional cusps also serve to prevent drifting and passive eruption of teeth—hence the term *holding cusp*. The functional cusps (see Fig. 1.42) are identified by five characteristic features:[14]

1. They contact the opposing tooth in MI.
2. They maintain the vertical dimension of the face.
3. They are nearer the faciolingual center of the tooth than nonfunctional cusps.
4. Their outer (facial) incline has the potential for contact.
5. They have broader, more rounded cusp ridges with greater dentin support than nonfunctional cusps.

Because the maxillary arch is larger than the mandibular arch, the functional cusps are located on the maxillary lingual occlusal line (see Fig. 1.42D), whereas the mandibular functional cusps are located on the mandibular facial occlusal line (see Fig. 1.42A and B). Functional cusps of both arches are more robust and better suited to crushing food than are the nonfunctional cusps. The lingual tilt of posterior teeth increases the relative height of the functional cusps with respect to the nonfunctional cusps (see Fig. 1.42C), and the central fossa contacts of the functional cusps are obscured by the overlapping nonfunctional cusps (see Fig. 1.42E and F). A schematic showing removal of the nonfunctional cusps allows the functional cusp–central fossa contacts to be studied (see Fig. 1.42G and H). During fabrication of restorations, it is important that functional cusps are not contacting opposing teeth in a manner that results in lateral deflection. Rather, restorations should provide contacts on plateaus or smoothly concave fossae

Synonyms for
functional
cusps include:
1. Centric cusps
2. Holding cusps
3. Stamp cusps

A. Mandibular arch

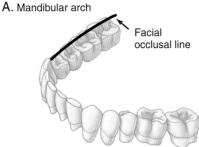

Facial
occlusal line

The mandibular arch is smaller than
the maxillary arch, so the functional
cusps are located on the facial occlusal
line. The mandibular lingual cusps that
overlap the maxillary teeth are
nonsupporting cusps.

B. Mandibular right quadrant

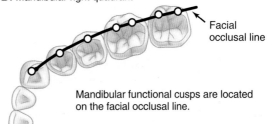

Facial
occlusal line

Mandibular functional cusps are located
on the facial occlusal line.

C. Proximal view of molar
teeth in occlusion

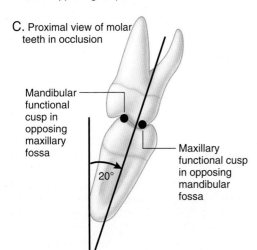

Mandibular
functional
cusp in
opposing
maxillary
fossa

20°

Maxillary
functional cusp
in opposing
mandibular
fossa

D. Maxillary right quadrant

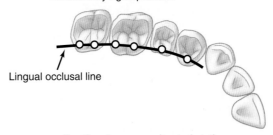

Lingual occlusal line

Functional cusps are located on the
lingual occlusal line in maxillary arch.

E. Lingual view of left dental arches in
occlusion

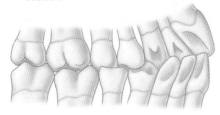

G. Mandibular nonfunctional cusps
removed

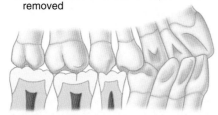

Maxillary functional cusps occluding in
opposing fossae and on marginal ridges

F. Facial view of left dental arches in
occlusion

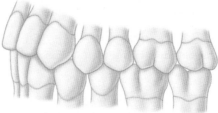

H. Maxillary nonfunctional cusps removed

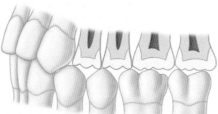

Mandibular functional cusps occluding in
opposing fossae and on marginal ridges

Functional cusp features:
1. Contact opposing tooth in MI
2. Support vertical dimension
3. Nearer faciolingual center of
   tooth than nonsupporting
   cusps
4. Outer incline has potential for
   contact
5. More rounded than
   nonsupporting cusps

• **Fig. 1.42** Functional cusps.

so that masticatory forces are directed approximately parallel to the long axes of teeth (i.e., approximately perpendicular to the occlusal plane).

Nonfunctional Cusps

Fig. 1.43 illustrates that the nonfunctional cusps form a lingual occlusal line in the mandibular arch (see Fig. 1.43D) and a facial occlusal line in the maxillary arch (see Fig. 1.43B). Nonfunctional cusps overlap the opposing tooth without contacting the tooth. Nonfunctional cusps are located, when viewed in the anteroposterior plane, in facial (lingual) embrasures or in the developmental groove of opposing teeth, creating an alternating arrangement when teeth are in MI (see Fig. 1.43E and F). The maxillary premolar nonfunctional cusps also play an essential role in esthetics. In the occlusal view, the nonfunctional cusps are farther from the faciolingual center of the tooth than are the functional cusps and have less dentinal support. Nonfunctional cusps have sharper cusp ridges that may serve to shear food as they pass close to the functional cusp ridges during chewing strokes. The overlap of the maxillary nonfunctional cusps helps keep the soft tissue of the cheek out and away from potential trauma from the occlusal table. Likewise, the overlap of the mandibular nonfunctional cusps helps keep the tongue out from the occlusal table. Therefore, the position of the maxillary and mandibular nonfunctional cusps help to prevent self-injury during chewing.

Mechanics of Mandibular Motion

Mandible and Temporomandibular Joints

The mandible articulates with a depression in each temporal bone called *glenoid fossa*. The joints are termed *temporomandibular joints (TMJs)* because they are named for the two bones (temporal and mandible) forming the articulation. The TMJs allow the mandible to move in all three planes (Fig. 1.44A).

A TMJ is similar to a ball-and-socket joint, but it differs from a true mechanical ball-and-socket joint in some very important aspects. The ball part (the mandibular condyle) is smaller than the socket (the glenoid fossa) (see Fig. 1.44B). The space resulting from the size difference is filled by a tough, pliable, and movable stabilizer termed the *articular disc*. The disc separates the TMJ into two articulating surfaces lubricated by synovial fluid in the superior and inferior joint spaces. Rotational opening of the mandible occurs as the condyles rotate under the discs (see Fig. 1.44C). Rotational movement occurs between the inferior surface of the discs and the condyle. During wide opening or protrusion of the mandible, the condyles move or slide anteriorly in addition to the rotational opening (see Fig. 1.44D and E). The TMJ is referred to as a *ginglymoarthrodial joint* because it has hinge (ginglymus) capability as well as sliding/gliding/translating (arthrodial) capability.

The discs move anteriorly with the condyles during opening and produce a sliding movement in the superior joint space between the superior surface of the discs and the articular eminences (see Fig. 1.44B). TMJs allow free movement of the condyles in the anteroposterior direction but resist lateral displacement. The discs are attached firmly to the medial and lateral poles of the condyles in normal, healthy TMJs (see Fig. 1.45B). The disc–condyle arrangement of the TMJ allows simultaneous sliding and rotational movement in the same joint.

Because the mandible is a semirigid, U-shaped bone with joints on both ends, movement of one joint produces a reciprocal movement in the other joint. The disc–condyle complex is free to move anteroposterior, providing sliding movement between the disc and the glenoid fossa. One condyle may move anteriorly, while the other remains in the fossa. Anterior movement of only one condyle produces reciprocal lateral rotation in the opposite TMJ.

The TMJ does not behave like a rigid joint as those on articulators (mechanical devices used by dentists to simulate jaw movement and reference positions [see the subsequent section on *Articulators and Mandibular Movement*s]). Because soft tissues cover the two articulating bones and an intervening disc composed of soft tissue is present, some resilience is to be expected in the TMJs. In addition to resilience, normal, healthy TMJs have flexibility, allowing small posterolateral movements of the condyles. In healthy TMJs, the movements are restricted to slightly less than 1 mm laterally and a few tenths of a millimeter posteriorly.

When morphologic changes occur in the hard and soft tissues of a TMJ because of disease, the disc–condyle relationship is possibly altered in many ways, including distortion, perforation, or tearing of the disc, and remodeling of the soft tissue articular surface coverings or their bony support. Diseased TMJs have unusual disc–condyle relationships, different geometry, and altered jaw movements and reference positions. Textbooks on TMJ disorders and occlusion should be consulted for information concerning the evaluation of diseased joints.[15] The remainder of this discussion of the movement and position of the mandible is based on normal, healthy TMJs and does not apply to diseased joints.

Review of Normal Masticatory Muscle Function and Mandibular Movement

Masticatory muscles work together to allow controlled, subtle movements of the mandible. The relative amount of muscle activity depends on the interarch relationships of maxillary and mandibular teeth as well as the amount of resistance to movement.[16-19] Primary muscles involved in mandibular movements include the anterior temporalis, middle temporalis, posterior temporalis, superficial masseter, deep masseter, superior lateral pterygoid, inferior lateral pterygoid, medial pterygoid, and digastric muscles.[17,18,20] The suprahyoid, infrahyoid, mylohyoid, and geniohyoid muscles also are involved in mandibular movements but not usually included in routine clinical examinations.[18,21] The relative amount of muscle activity of the various muscles has been identified through the use of electromyographic technology, in which electrodes were placed in the evaluated muscles,[17,18,22] as well as on the skin immediately adjacent to the muscles of interest.[12,17,18,20,21-30] The strategic three-dimensional arrangement of the muscles and the corresponding force vectors allow for the complete range of finely controlled mandibular movements. The reader should consult an appropriate human anatomy textbook to identify the location, size, shape, three-dimensional orientation, and bony insertion of the various muscles discussed in this section.

Simple jaw opening requires the activation of digastric and inferior lateral pterygoid muscles.[17,18,22] Fine control of opening is accomplished by simultaneous mild antagonistic activity of the medial pterygoid.[17,18] When resistance is applied to jaw opening, mild masseter activation allows further stabilization and fine control.[17,18]

Jaw closure requires the activation of the masseter and medial pterygoid.[18] Once teeth come into contact, the temporalis (anterior, middle, and posterior) muscles activate as well.[17,18] The masseter, medial pterygoid, and temporalis muscles act to elevate the mandible and are generally referred to as *elevator muscles*. Clenching involves maximum activation of the masseter and temporalis, moderate activation of the medial pterygoid and superior lateral pterygoid,

A. Maxillary arch

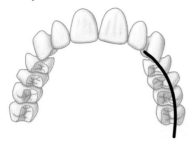

The maxillary arch is larger than the mandibular arch causing the maxillary facial line (nonfunctional cusps) to overlap the mandibular teeth.

B. Maxillary left quadrant

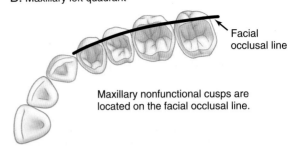

Facial occlusal line

Maxillary nonfunctional cusps are located on the facial occlusal line.

C. Molar teeth in occlusion

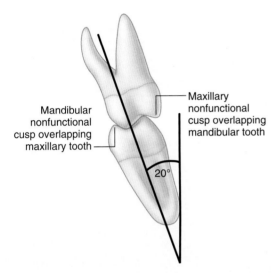

Mandibular nonfunctional cusp overlapping maxillary tooth

Maxillary nonfunctional cusp overlapping mandibular tooth

20°

D. Mandibular left quadrant

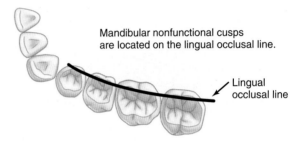

Mandibular nonfunctional cusps are located on the lingual occlusal line.

Lingual occlusal line

Nonfunctional cusp features:
1. Do not contact opposing tooth in MI
2. Keep soft tissue of tongue or cheek off occlusal table
3. Farther from faciolingual center of tooth than supporting cusps
4. Outer incline has no potential for contact
5. Have sharper cusp ridges than supporting cusps

E. Views of left dental arches in occlusion showing interdigitation of nonfunctional cusps

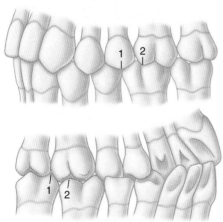

Nonfunctional cusp location:
1. Opposing embrasure
2. Opposing developmental groove

F. Views of left dental arches in occlusion showing facial and lingual occlusal lines

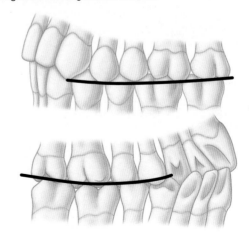

• **Fig. 1.43** Nonfunctional cusps.

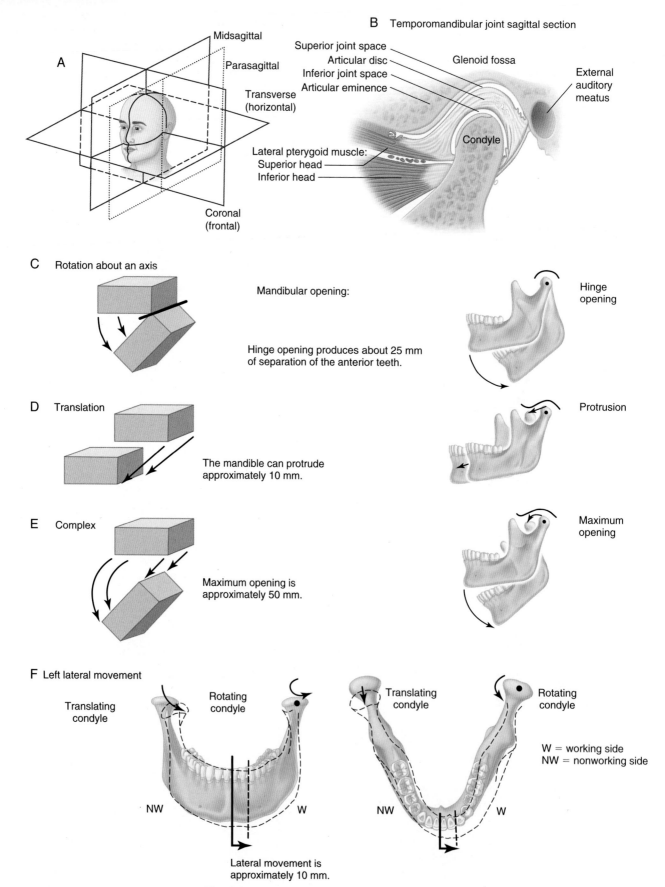

• **Fig. 1.44**   Types and directions of mandibular movements.

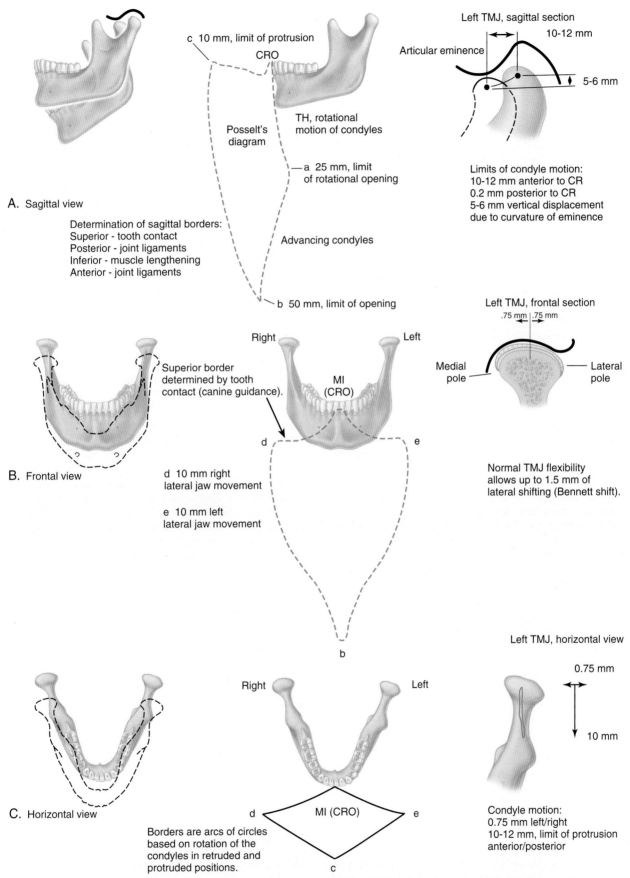

c 10 mm, limit of protrusion
CRO

Left TMJ, sagittal section
10-12 mm
Articular eminence
5-6 mm

TH, rotational
motion of condyles

Posselt's
diagram

a 25 mm, limit
of rotational opening

A. Sagittal view

Determination of sagittal borders:
Superior - tooth contact
Posterior - joint ligaments
Inferior - muscle lengthening
Anterior - joint ligaments

Advancing condyles

b 50 mm, limit of opening

Limits of condyle motion:
10-12 mm anterior to CR
0.2 mm posterior to CR
5-6 mm vertical displacement
due to curvature of eminence

Right   Left

Superior border
determined by tooth
contact (canine guidance).

MI
(CRO)

d   e

Left TMJ, frontal section
.75 mm   .75 mm
Medial
pole
Lateral
pole

B. Frontal view

d 10 mm right
lateral jaw movement

e 10 mm left
lateral jaw movement

Normal TMJ flexibility
allows up to 1.5 mm of
lateral shifting (Bennett shift).

b

Left TMJ, horizontal view

0.75 mm

10 mm

Right   Left

d   MI (CRO)   e

C. Horizontal view

Borders are arcs of circles
based on rotation of the
condyles in retruded and
protruded positions.

c

Condyle motion:
0.75 mm left/right
10-12 mm, limit of protrusion
anterior/posterior

• **Fig. 1.45**   Capacity of mandibular movement. (Mandible drawings are not to scale with border diagrams.) CO=MI (i.e., there is no functional shift and, therefore, is termed centric relation occlusion [CRO]).

and recruitment of the inferior lateral pterygoid, digastrics, and mylohyoid muscles.[17,18,22] In general, the superficial masseter has slightly higher activity than the deep masseter during clenching.[20] Coactivation of cooperating and antagonistic muscles allows for controlled force to be applied to teeth.[17]

Protrusion requires maximum bilateral activation of the inferior lateral pterygoid, with moderate activation of the medial pterygoid, masseter, and digastric muscles. During protrusion minimal activation of the temporalis and superior lateral pterygoid occurs. The superior lateral pterygoid has muscle fibers that insert into the temporomandibular disc as well as the neck of the mandibular condyle (see Fig. 1.44).[22] It is important to note that minimal activation of the superior lateral pterygoid is necessary if the temporomandibular disc is to rotate to the top of the condylar head as the condyle translates down the articular eminence during mandibular protrusive or excursive movements.[17]

Incisal biting with posterior disclusion requires maximum bilateral activity of the superficial masseter to force the incisors toward each other, as well as maximum activity of the inferior lateral pterygoid to maintain the protruded position of the condylar head down the slope of the articular eminence.[17] Incisal biting also requires moderate activity of the anterior temporalis, medial pterygoid, anterior digastric, and superior lateral pterygoid.[17] Note that the shift in the level of activity of the superior lateral pterygoid from protrusion to incisal biting indicates a dual role in condylar positioning and temporomandibular disc positioning or stabilization. The middle and posterior temporalis regions have minimal activity during incisal biting.[18]

Retrusion of the mandible requires bilateral maximum activation of the posterior and middle temporalis as well as moderate activity of the anterior temporalis and anterior digastric.[17,18] The superior lateral pterygoid is maximally active when the mandible is retruded and posterior teeth are clenched.[17] The masseter has minimal activity in retrusion.[17] The inferior lateral pterygoid and the medial pterygoid have minimal to no activity during retrusion.[17,18]

Excursive movement of the mandible to the right requires moderate to maximal activity of the left inferior lateral pterygoid and medial pterygoid muscles as well as the right posterior temporalis, middle temporalis, and anterior digastric.[17-19] In addition to these, the right superior lateral pterygoid, right anterior temporalis, and left anterior digastric are minimally to moderately active.[17-19] Activation of the right superior lateral pterygoid provides resistance to right condyle distalization as well as positional support of the right temporomandibular disc. The right superficial masseter, right inferior lateral pterygoid, right medial pterygoid, left superior lateral pterygoid, left anterior temporalis, left middle temporalis, left posterior temporalis, and left superficial masseter all have minimal activity.[17-19] Minimal activity of the left superior lateral pterygoid allows the disc to shift distally, as needed, so as to remain between the condylar head and the articular eminence while translation or rotation of the left condylar head occurs. Activation of the elevator muscles on the left side provides for the translating left condyle–disc complex to remain in contact with the articular eminence. Movement of the mandible to the left follows the same pattern of coordinated muscle activity except in reverse.

Wide opening requires bilateral moderate to maximal activity of the inferior lateral pterygoid and anterior digastric muscles.[17] In addition to these, the medial pterygoid muscles are minimally to moderately active.[17] The temporalis, masseter, and superior lateral pterygoid muscles have minimal to no activity during wide opening.[17,18]

During mastication, the typical mandibular movement involves opening with corresponding bilateral anterior, inferior, and rotating condylar motion.[12,31] As closure begins, the entire mandible moves laterally.[12] As closure continues, the working-side condyle shifts back to its terminal hinge position before the teeth occlude and remains nearly stationary.[12] As the closure continues, the working-side condyle shifts medially while the nonworking-side condyle shifts superiorly, distally, and laterally to its terminal hinge position.[12] The medial shift of the working-side condyle may be caused by the influence of the superior lateral pterygoid muscle contraction. The opening and closing paths of the incisors vary from individual to individual and also depend on the consistency of the food being masticated.[12] The realistic normal lower limit for the incisal opening in patients between 10 and 70 years of age is 40 mm.[32]

To describe mandibular motion, its direction and length must be specified in three mutually perpendicular planes. By convention, these planes are sagittal, coronal (frontal), and transverse (horizontal) (see Fig. 1.44A). The midsagittal plane is a vertical (longitudinal) plane that passes through the center of the head in an anteroposterior direction. A vertical plane off the center line, such as a section through the TMJ, is termed *parasagittal plane*. The coronal plane is a vertical plane perpendicular to the sagittal plane. The transverse plane is a horizontal plane that passes from anterior to posterior and is perpendicular to the sagittal and frontal planes. Mandibular motion is described in each of these planes.

Types of Motion

Centric relation (CR), in healthy TMJs, is the location of the mandible when the condyles are positioned superiorly and anteriorly in the glenoid fossae. In CR, the thinnest avascular portion of the TMJ discs are in an anterosuperior position on the condylar head, and are adjacent to the beginning of the slopes of the articular eminences (see Fig. 1.44B). This position is independent of tooth contacts.

Rotation is a simple motion of an object around an axis (see Fig. 1.44C). The mandible is capable of rotation about an axis through centers located in the condyles. The attachments of the discs to the poles of the condyles permit the condyles to rotate under the discs. Rotation with the condyles positioned in CR is termed *terminal hinge (TH) movement*. Maximum rotational opening in TH is limited to approximately 25 mm measured between the incisal edges of anterior teeth. Initial tooth contact during a TH closure provides a reference point termed *centric occlusion (CO)*. Many patients have a small slide from CO to MI, referred to as a *functional shift*, which may have forward and lateral components. CR is used in dentistry as a reproducible reference position for major restorative reconstruction of the maxillary and mandibular occlusal planes and also when fabricating full dentures. The reproducibility of the CR position allows the establishment of simultaneous contact of all functional cusps in maximum intercuspation while the mandible is in CR. This occlusion is termed *centric relation* occlusion (CRO). CRO allows maximum osseous support of the mandibular condyles and even distribution of occlusal loading forces, generated by the elevator muscles, across the whole dentition. The functional cusps in CRO are termed *centric cusps*. The nonfunctional cusps in CRO are termed *noncentric cusps*.

Translation is the bodily movement of an object from one place to another (see Fig. 1.44D). The mandible is capable of translation by the anterior movement of the disc–condyle complex from the TH position forward and down the articular eminence and back. Simultaneous, direct anterior movement of both condyles, or mandibular forward thrusting, is termed *protrusion*. The pathway followed by anterior teeth during protrusion may not be smooth or straight because of contact between anterior teeth and sometimes posterior teeth. (See the superior border of Posselt diagram in Fig. 1.45A.) Protrusion is limited to approximately 10 mm by the ligamentous attachments of masticatory muscles and the TMJs.

Fig. 1.44E illustrates complex motion, which combines rotation and translation in a single movement. Most mandibular movement during speech, chewing, and swallowing consists of rotation and translation. The combination of rotation and translation allows the mandible to open 50 mm or more.

Fig. 1.44F illustrates the left lateral movement of the mandible. It is the result of forward translation of the right condyle and rotation of the left condyle. Right lateral movement of the mandible is the result of forward translation of the left condyle and rotation of the right condyle.

Capacity of Motion of the Mandible

In 1952, Posselt recorded mandibular motion and developed a diagram (termed *Posselt diagram*) to illustrate it (see Fig. 1.45A).[33] By necessity, the original recordings of mandibular movement were done outside of the mouth, which magnified the vertical dimension but not the horizontal dimension. Modern systems using digital computer techniques can record mandibular motion in actual time and dimensions and then compute and draw the motion as it occurred at any point in the mandible and teeth.[12] This makes it possible to accurately reconstruct mandibular motion simultaneously at several points. Three of these points are particularly significant clinically: incisor point, molar point, and condyle point (Fig. 1.46A).[34] The incisor point is located on the midline of the mandible at the junction of the facial surface of mandibular central incisors and the incisal edge. The molar point is the tip of the mesiofacial cusp of the mandibular first molar on a specified side. The condyle point is the center of rotation of the mandibular condyle on the specified side.

Limits of Mandibular Motion: The Borders

In Fig. 1.45A, the limits for movement of the incisor point are illustrated in the sagittal plane. The mandible is not drawn to scale with the drawing of the sagittal borders. This particular diagram is drawn in CRO (i.e., CO coincides with MI). The starting point for this diagram is CRO, the contact of all teeth when the condyles are in CR. The posterior border of the diagram from CRO to *a* in Fig. 1.45A is formed by the rotation of the mandible around the condyle points. This border from CRO to *a* is the TH movement. *Hinge axis* is the term used to describe an imaginary line connecting the centers of rotation in the condyles (condyle points) and is useful for reference to articulators (see upcoming section, *Articulators and Mandibular Movements*). The hinge-axis position (also referred to as CR) is a reproducible reference position and rotational, mandibular closure movement on this axis is used when restorative procedures require recreation of the occlusal relationships of multiple teeth. The inferior limit to this hinge opening occurs at approximately 25 mm and is indicated by *a* in Fig. 1.45A. The superior limit of the posterior border occurs at tooth contact and is identified as CRO.

At point *a* in Fig. 1.45A, further rotation of the condyles is impossible because of the stretch limits of the joint capsule, ligamentous attachments to the condyles, and the mandible-opening muscles. Further opening can be achieved only by translation of the condyles anteriorly, producing the line *a-b*. Maximum opening (point *b*) in adults is approximately 50 mm. These measures are important diagnostically. Mandibular opening limited to 25 mm

suggests blockage of condylar translation, usually the result of a disc disorder(s). Limitation of opening in the 35- to 45-mm range suggests masticatory muscle hypertonicity. The line CRO-*a-b* represents the maximum retruded opening path. This is the posterior border, or the posterior limit of mandibular opening. The line *b-c* represents the maximum protruded closure. This is achieved by a forward thrust of the mandible that keeps the condyles in their maximum anterior positions while closing the mandible.

Retrusion, or posterior movement of the mandible, results in the irregular line *c*-CRO. The irregularities of the superior border are caused by tooth contacts; the superior border is a tooth-determined border. Protrusion is a reference mandibular movement starting from CRO and proceeding anteriorly to point *c*. Protrusive mandibular movements are used by dentists to evaluate occlusal relationships of teeth and restorations. The complete diagram, CRO-*a-b-c*-CRO, represents the maximum possible motion of the incisor point in all directions in the sagittal plane. The area of most interest to dentists is the superior border produced by tooth contact. (Mandibular movement in the sagittal plane is illustrated in more detail in Fig. 1.46.)

The motion of the condyle point during chewing is strikingly different from the motion of the incisor point. Motion of the condyle point is a curved line that follows the articular eminence. The maximum protrusion of the condyle point is 10 to 12 mm anteriorly when following the downward curve of the articular eminence. The condyle point does not drop away from the eminence, as a result of controlled/coordinated elevator muscle activity, during mandibular movements. Chewing movements in the sagittal plane are characterized by a nearly vertical up-and-down motion of the incisor point, whereas the condyle points move anteriorly and then return posteriorly over a curved surface (see Fig. 1.46B).

In the frontal view shown in Fig. 1.45B, the incisor point and chin are capable of moving about 10 mm to the left or right. This lateral movement—or excursion—is indicated by the lines MI-*d* to the right and MI-*e* to the left. Points *d* and *e* indicate the limit of the lateral motion of the incisor point. Lateral movement is often described with respect to only one side of the mandible for the purpose of defining the relative motion of mandibular teeth to maxillary teeth. In a left lateral movement, the left mandibular teeth move away from the midline, and the right mandibular teeth move toward the midline.

Mandibular pathways directed away from the midline are termed *working* (synonyms include *laterotrusion* and *functional*), and mandibular pathways directed toward the midline are termed *nonworking* (synonyms include *mediotrusion*, *nonfunctional*, and *balancing*). The terms *working* and *nonworking* are based on observations of chewing movements in which the mandible is seen to shift during closure toward the side of the mouth containing the food bolus. The side of the jaw where the bolus of food is placed is termed *the working side*. The working side is used to crush food, whereas the nonworking side is without a food bolus. Working side also is used in reference to jaws or teeth when the patient is not chewing (e.g., in guided test movements directed laterally). The term also may identify a specific side of the mandible (i.e., the side toward which the mandible is moving). During chewing, the working-side closures start from a lateral position and are directed medially to MI.

The left lateral mandibular motion indicated by the line MI-*e* (see Fig. 1.45B) is the result of rotation of the left condyle (working-side condyle) and translation of the right condyle (nonworking-side condyle) to its anterior limit (see Fig. 1.44F). The translation of

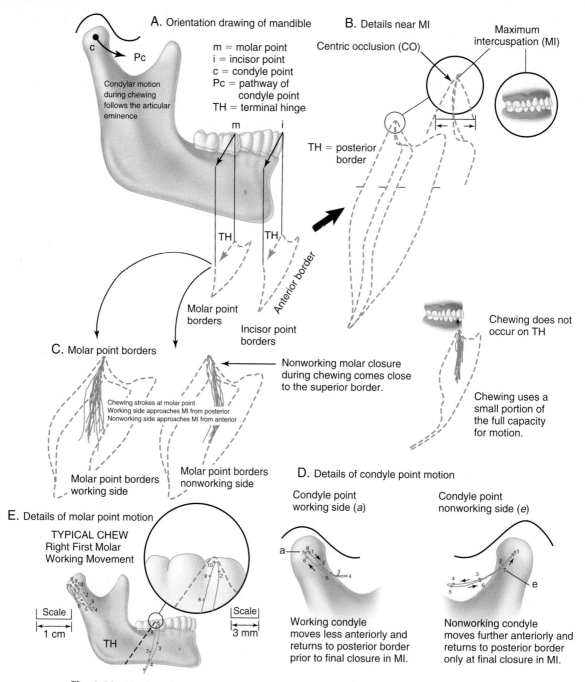

A. Orientation drawing of mandible

Condylar motion during chewing follows the articular eminence

m = molar point
i = incisor point
c = condyle point
Pc = pathway of condyle point
TH = terminal hinge

B. Details near MI

Maximum intercuspation (MI)

Centric occlusion (CO)

TH = posterior border

Chewing does not occur on TH

Chewing uses a small portion of the full capacity for motion.

C. Molar point borders

Nonworking molar closure during chewing comes close to the superior border.

Chewing strokes at molar point
Working side approaches MI from posterior
Nonworking side approaches MI from anterior

Molar point borders working side

Molar point borders nonworking side

Molar point borders

Incisor point borders

Anterior border

D. Details of condyle point motion

Condyle point working side (*a*)

Condyle point nonworking side (*e*)

Working condyle moves less anteriorly and returns to posterior border prior to final closure in MI.

Nonworking condyle moves further anteriorly and returns to posterior border only at final closure in MI.

E. Details of molar point motion

TYPICAL CHEW
Right First Molar
Working Movement

Scale
1 cm

Scale
3 mm

• **Fig. 1.46** Mandibular capacity for movement: sagittal view. CO≠MI (i.e., there is a functional shift).

the nonworking condyle in a right lateral motion of the mandible can be seen in the horizontal view in Fig. 1.47A and B. The line *e-b* in Fig. 1.45B is completed by mandibular opening that is the result of rotation of both condyles and translation of the working condyle to its maximum anterior position. The line *b-d*-MI represents similar motions on the right side.

The vertical displacement in the incisor point line from MI to *e* or *d*, shown in Fig. 1.45B, is the result of teeth, usually canines, gliding over each other. Vertical displacement of the mandible secondary to gliding contact of canine teeth is termed *canine guidance* and has significance for restorative procedures. The gliding tooth contact supplied by canine guidance provides some of the vertical separation of posterior teeth during lateral jaw movements and prevents potentially damaging collisions of their cusps secondary

to the increased elevator muscle activity that occurs when posterior teeth come into contact. When the canine guidance is shallow, the occlusal surface of posterior teeth must be altered to prevent potentially damaging contacts during lateral or protrusive movements.

Flexibility in the TMJs allows the condyles to move slightly to the working side during the closing stroke. This lateral shift of the condylar head, illustrated in the frontal view of a right TMJ in Fig. 1.45B, is termed *Bennett shift* or *lateral shift* and varies from patient to patient (see Fig. 1.47B–D). The magnitude of the shift in normal TMJs varies from 0 to 1.5 and normally has little effect on posterior teeth. Excessive lateral shift may be associated with morphologic changes of the TMJs. Excessive lateral condylar shifting coupled with shallow canine guidance poses a significant problem,

Lateral movement is produced by anterior translation of one condyle, producing rotation about the center in the opposite condyle.

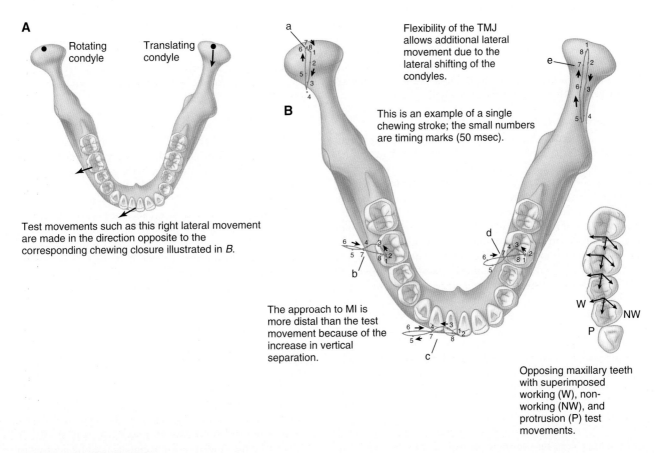

A

Rotating condyle

Translating condyle

Test movements such as this right lateral movement are made in the direction opposite to the corresponding chewing closure illustrated in *B*.

B

Flexibility of the TMJ allows additional lateral movement due to the lateral shifting of the condyles.

This is an example of a single chewing stroke; the small numbers are timing marks (50 msec).

The approach to MI is more distal than the test movement because of the increase in vertical separation.

Opposing maxillary teeth with superimposed working (W), non-working (NW), and protrusion (P) test movements.

Nonworking condyle movement:
1. Condylar translation with rotation about the center of the opposite condyle
2. Solid line indicates the change in the condylar path due to progressive shifting of the center of rotation in the opposite condyle
3. Solid line indicates the condylar path resulting from immediate shifting of the center of rotation of the opposite condyle
4. Observed motion of the condyle during chewing: note shifting as closing is initiated and the return to normal position at the end of closure

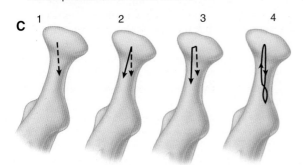

C 1 2 3 4

Effect of shifting at first molar:
1. Little change on working side
2. Wide lateral motion on nonworking side

Left lateral movement with shifting

D

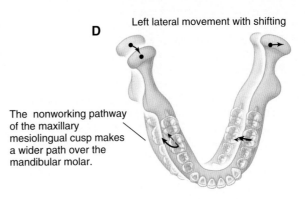

The nonworking pathway of the maxillary mesiolingual cusp makes a wider path over the mandibular molar.

• **Fig. 1.47** Mandibular capacity for movement: horizontal view.

however, for restorative procedures because the resulting lateral mandibular movements are flat; consequently, little separation of posterior teeth occurs, resulting in increased contact of posterior teeth as well as associated increased elevator muscle activity.

In Fig. 1.45C, the horizontal view illustrates the capability of the mandible to translate anteriorly. Extreme left lateral motion is indicated by MI-*e* produced by rotation of the left condyle (working condyle) and translation of the right condyle (nonworking condyle) to its anterior limit. From point *e*, protrusion of the left condyle moves the incisor point to *c*, the maximum protruded position where both condyles have translated.

Sagittal View

In Fig. 1.46, the drawing of the mandible is used to orient the sagittal border diagrams in a patient who has a functional shift between CO and MI. Recall CO is the tooth contact that occurs when the TMJs are in CR and that, in many patients, a small anterior or anterolateral slide may occur from CO to MI. Projected below the mandible are diagrams of the incisor point (*i*) and molar point (*m*) borders (see Fig. 1.46A). The molar point borders are similar to the incisor point diagram but are shorter in the vertical dimension because the molar point is closer to the TMJ. Closure of the jaw on the posterior border is termed *TH closure*. TH closure is a simple arc of a circle with a radius equal to the length from the incisor point to the center of the hinge axis (condyle point *c*). The area near MI is enlarged to illustrate the details of the TH closure (see Fig. 1.46B). CO and MI are located fairly close to each other in this case. In the magnified view, teeth may be seen to guide the mandible from CO to MI. The gliding (sliding) functional shift typically is 1 to 2 mm long and may occur on any of the posterior teeth. The horizontal component of this slide varies and may only be a few tenths of a millimeter. The primary concern is that the functional shift may position the condyle(s) on the slope of the articular eminence, a position that requires constant protrusive muscle activity to maintain.[17,22]

The clinical significance of the shift between CO and MI has been a source of debate in dentistry, resulting in extensive literature on the topic.[35,36] Clinical ramifications may include an increased risk of the development of pathologic changes in the TMJs and/or pain associated with the muscles of mastication. It has been observed that asymmetrical shifts between CO and MI were related to symptoms and signs of temporomandibular disorders, whereas symmetrical shifts were not.[32] It has been noted that increasing symptoms and signs of temporomandibular disorders were associated with increasing functional shift distance from CO to MI.[37] However, a shift of greater than 2 mm, mediotrusive posterior tooth interferences, and a large overjet were only weakly associated with masticatory muscle pain, suggesting other factors in addition to occlusal relationships may be involved.[38,39] Failure to recognize that some patients have damaged TMJs may further complicate the determination of the clinical significance of a CO–MI slide. Damage to the TMJs as a consequence of arthritic processes or internal derangements may change the relationship of CO to MI.

Chewing movements at the incisor point involve an almost vertical opening and a loop slightly to the posterior on closing, using only a small percentage of the total area of the sagittal border diagram. During chewing, the only border contact occurs at MI. The closing strokes never approach TH, indicating that at least one condyle (on the nonworking side) remains advanced during the closing stroke. The condyle point moves along the pathway *Pc* during all movements other than TH (see Fig. 1.46). In contrast

to the nearly vertical closing strokes at incisor point, the sagittal closing strokes at the molar point involve an anterior component on the working side and a posterior component on the nonworking side. This difference in molar point movement is caused by the deviation of the jaw to the working side during closure, illustrated by the difference in motion of the working-side and nonworking-side condyles. The nonworking-side closing strokes closely approach the superior border, indicating the potential for undesirable posterior tooth contact and increased elevator muscle activity (as well as increased activity of the superior lateral pterygoid muscle) on the nonworking side (see Fig. 1.46C).

Horizontal View

Fig. 1.47A shows a horizontal view (or occlusal view when referring to teeth) of the mandible with superimposed incisor, molar, and condyle point test movements. Chewing movements are characterized by wide lateral movement of the mandible to the working side during closure (see Fig. 1.47B). When viewed from above, the pathways of the molar and incisor points are typically in a figure-8 pattern, with an S-shaped lateral opening motion and a straight medial closing stroke. Important differences exist in the directions of closure for the molar point on the working and nonworking sides. During closure on the working side (labeled *b* in Fig. 1.47B), mandibular teeth medially approach maxillary teeth from a slightly posterior position and move slightly anteriorly into MI. During closure on the nonworking side (the contralateral side, labeled *d* in Fig. 1.47B), mandibular molar teeth approach the maxillary teeth in a medial-to-lateral direction from a slightly anterior position and move slightly posteriorly into MI. The closing strokes are the same pathways generated by guided (test) lateral mandibular movements used to check the occlusion except the directions traveled are opposite (see Fig. 1.47B, *inset*). On the inset drawing of the maxillary left teeth in Fig. 1.47B, the working, nonworking, and protrusive pathways are marked *W*, *NW*, and *P*. These are the guided test movements used by dentists to assess the occlusal contact of teeth during function.

The horizontal, enlarged view of the mandible showing condyle point movement (working side labeled *a*; nonworking side labeled *e*) during chewing is important because it illustrates the lateral shift of the condyles during the closing stroke (see Fig. 1.47B). Opening, in the typical chewing motion illustrated here, involves movement of both condyle points on the midsagittal path, producing the vertical drop in the incisor point seen in the sagittal view. Lateral opening may be seen in normal children and adults with worn and flattened teeth. As closing is initiated, the mandible shifts laterally, moving both condyle points to the working side. The nonworking condyle movement closely approaches its medial border during the closing stroke (see Fig. 1.47C). During final closure, when teeth are brought into MI, the condyle points return to their starting positions. Contact and gliding on the inclines of teeth are responsible for bringing the mandible into its final, fully closed position (MI).

Allowance for lateral displacement of the condyles during lateral jaw movements is built into semiadjustable articulators in the form of a Bennett angle or progressive lateral shift adjustment. The progressive lateral shift allows the condyles to shift gradually during lateral mandibular movement. As a result of mandibular movement studies, more recent articulator models have replaced the progressive lateral shift with immediate shift. Shifting of the mandible, as depicted by the shift in the condyle points, results in a similar shift at the teeth that cannot be simulated by progressive shift (see Fig. 1.47C).

The superior border of the incisor point tracing is determined by the canine teeth, but the molar point superior border is influenced by the pathway of the condyle point. Canine guidance and articular eminence slope are mechanically coupled to produce the superior border of the molar point tracing but they do not contribute equally. The canine is primarily responsible for the superior border of molar point on the working pathway (away from the midline). The nonworking side articular eminence has the dominant influence on the nonworking pathway (toward the midline) on the molar point superior border.

If the molar cusps are higher than the border, then they will collide during chewing. This is more likely to occur on the nonworking side.

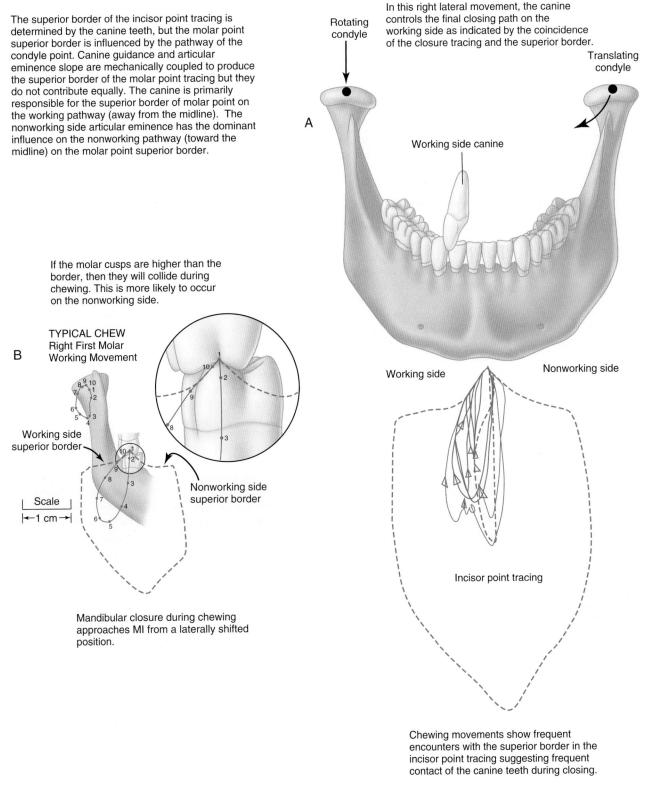

In this right lateral movement, the canine controls the final closing path on the working side as indicated by the coincidence of the closure tracing and the superior border.

Rotating condyle

Translating condyle

Working side canine

A

Working side   Nonworking side

Incisor point tracing

TYPICAL CHEW
Right First Molar
Working Movement

B

Working side
superior border

Nonworking side
superior border

Scale
|← 1 cm →|

Mandibular closure during chewing approaches MI from a laterally shifted position.

Chewing movements show frequent encounters with the superior border in the incisor point tracing suggesting frequent contact of the canine teeth during closing.

• **Fig. 1.48** Mandibular capacity for movement: frontal view.

Frontal View

In Fig. 1.48A, lateral movement of the mandible on the superior border is controlled by three elements—the rotating condyle, the translating condyle, and the working-side canine. During chewing closures, mandibular teeth approach maxillary teeth from a lateral position. Frequent contact with the border occurs in the incisor and molar point tracings, indicating that lateral tooth gliding is common during chewing. This gliding contact occurs on the teeth having the highest projecting cusps that form the superior border (usually canines).

The incisor point tracing is projected below the drawing of the mandible in Fig. 1.48A. The chewing strokes show the gliding contact on the border. The incisor-point superior border is shaped by the lingual surfaces of the guiding teeth, which most frequently are maxillary canines. In Fig. 1.48B, the lateral side of the molar-point superior border is shaped by the working-side tooth guidance, which is usually the maxillary canine. The medial side of the molar-point superior border is predominately formed by the nonworking condyle moving down the articular eminence. The shape of the superior border at the molar point is the critical factor for determining the location and height of the molar cusps during restorative procedures. It is easy to visualize the effect of changes in the cusp height when viewing the close-up of molar teeth in the magnified inset.

Articulators and Mandibular Movements

Figs. 1.49, 1.50, 1.51, and 1.52 illustrate the scientific basis for the use of articulators to aid in diagnostic evaluation of occlusion and fabrication of dental restorations.[37,40-42] In these figures, the characteristics of chewing movements and dentist-guided test movements are compared with the characteristics of movements produced by simple articulators. This may be done by comparing the cusp movement near MI produced by the articulator with the cusp movement observed in chewing studies or guided movements of patients. Additionally, the changes in cusp movement near MI that occur because of variations in the adjustment of articulators are discussed with respect to their effects on dental restorations.

Fig. 1.49 illustrates the relationship between condylar movement and articulator settings. Together, the horizontal condylar guidance setting and the medial-wall setting of an articulator supply sufficient information to approximate the condyle movement near MI. The horizontal condylar guidance setting approximates the slope of the articular eminence; the medial-wall setting approximates the lateral shift. Collectively, these two settings are referred to as *posterior guidance.*

Posterior guidance alone is not sufficient to simulate mandibular movements near MI because tooth guidance also is involved in forming the superior border. Full-arch casts mounted in the articulator, with the use of techniques that correctly position the maxillary cast relative to the artificial TMJs, supply the information concerning anterior guidance from canines and incisors. The mechanical coupling of the anterior guidance and posterior guidance settings provides sufficient information to simulate the movement of posterior teeth on the superior border.

Research has identified that the slope of the articular eminence ranges approximately 25 to 70 degrees from the axis-orbital plane (see Fig. 1.50A and B).[43] Adjustable articulators have been designed based on these observations and allow establishment of patient-specific setting of horizontal condylar inclination. Furthermore, left/right individual settings allow for differences that may exist in the relative movements of the two condyles (see Fig. 1.50C and D). The condyles move anteriorly and inferiorly while in contact with the curved surface of the simulated articular eminence within the condylar housing of the articulator. More recent designs of semiadjustable articulators have adopted curved surfaces to simulate the curvature of the articular eminence. Only the first few millimeters of movement have significant effects on the posterior teeth. Horizontal condylar guidance (supplied by the articulator) and anterior guidance (supplied by the mounted casts) are mechanically coupled to produce the separation of posterior teeth. The combined guidance determines the amount of (or lack of) vertical separation of posterior teeth

as the mandible leaves or enters MI during protrusion and lateral movements.

Lateral mandibular movements also produce separation of posterior teeth. Horizontal guidance of the nonworking condyle coupled with working-side canine guidance determines the amount of vertical separation of posterior teeth on both sides as the mandible leaves or enters MI during lateral movements (see Fig. 1.48). This information may be used to design restorations with the proper cusp location and height to avoid collisions during chewing and other mandibular movements.

The slope of the articular eminence varies considerably among individuals. The effect of different slopes may be evaluated by altering the horizontal condylar guidance on articulators. Increasing the horizontal condylar guidance increases the steepness of the mandibular molar movement in protrusion. The movement of the maxillary mesiolingual cusp relative to the mandibular molar is plotted in Fig. 1.50E–G for 20-, 30-, and 50-degree slopes.[44] The effect of removing the anterior guidance (*a*) is drawn on the same grid. The loss of anterior guidance has the greatest effect when the horizontal condylar guidance is shallow (20 degrees) and has the least effect when the horizontal condylar guidance is steep (50 degrees). Anterior guidance has an additive effect on the molar pathway at all degrees of horizontal guidance. This is an important observation because alteration of the anterior guidance may occur during dental treatment that involves the guiding surfaces of the anterior teeth. There may be a therapeutic advantage to increasing anterior guidance, by restorative or orthodontic means, to facilitate the separation of posterior teeth in patients who have shallow horizontal guidance. The articulator may be used to diagnose the need to alter the anterior guidance and to design restorations that avoid cusp collisions in mandibular movements.

TMJ lateral shift may be measured clinically and transferred to an adjustable articulator. A series of tracings of guided movements from different patients is shown in Fig. 1.51A.[45,46] All the tracings are parallel after the first few millimeters of movement. The difference from one patient to the next is the result of the amount of lateral shift. Fig. 1.51B illustrates simulations of arcs at different degrees of lateral shift; the similarity of lines *a*, *b*, and *c* to the lines similarly marked in Fig. 1.51A should be noted. None of the tracings of lateral condylar movement exhibits the "progressive" lateral shift indicated by the dashed line in Fig. 1.51B. Fig. 1.51C illustrates the underside of a condylar housing of an articulator. Shifting the medial wall simulates TMJ lateral shift and allows movements similar to those illustrated in Fig. 1.51A. Fig. 1.51D illustrates how movements *a*, *b*, and *c* were made for Fig. 1.51B by shifting the medial wall of the condylar housing on the articulator. Increasing lateral shift of the TMJ results in significant changes in movement of the molar point near MI (see Fig. 1.51E). The working-side movement is least affected because it is already a directly lateral movement. The nonworking molar-point movement is changed in the lateral and horizontal components. The lateral pathway is extended progressively more laterally in patients with excessive lateral shift of the TMJs. The horizontal effect is a "flattening" of the pathway by reduction of the vertical separation. These effects are illustrated by tracings of molar-point movement on an articulator as the amount of lateral shift is increased from "*a*" to "*b*" to "*c*." The effect of increasing lateral shift is to increase the likelihood of collisions of the mesiolingual cusps of the maxillary molars with the mandibular distofacial cusps of the molars on the nonworking side (see Fig. 1.51E and F). These types of undesirable contact between the opposing functional cusps are termed *nonworking interferences.*

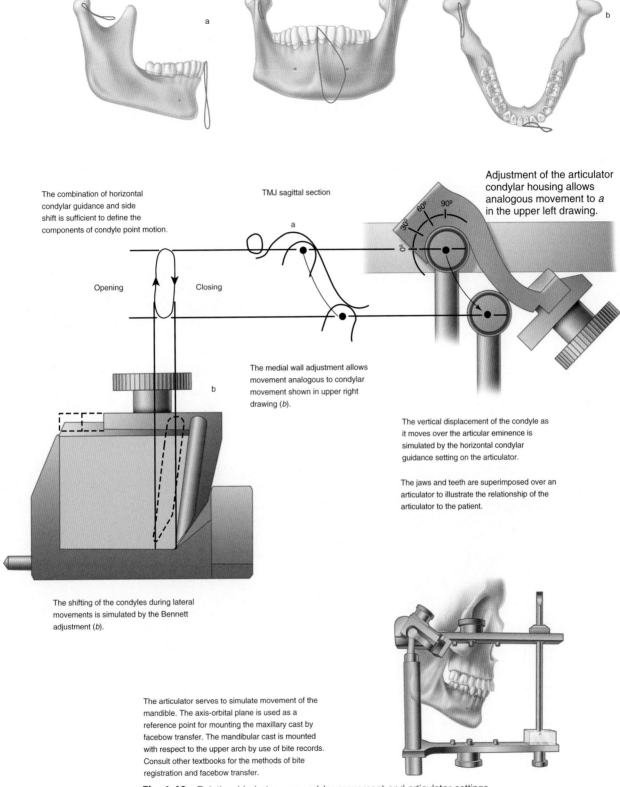

a

b

The combination of horizontal condylar guidance and side shift is sufficient to define the components of condyle point motion.

TMJ sagittal section

Adjustment of the articulator condylar housing allows analogous movement to *a* in the upper left drawing.

a

90°

60°

30°

0°

Opening

Closing

b

The medial wall adjustment allows movement analogous to condylar movement shown in upper right drawing (*b*).

The vertical displacement of the condyle as it moves over the articular eminence is simulated by the horizontal condylar guidance setting on the articulator.

The jaws and teeth are superimposed over an articulator to illustrate the relationship of the articulator to the patient.

The shifting of the condyles during lateral movements is simulated by the Bennett adjustment (*b*).

The articulator serves to simulate movement of the mandible. The axis-orbital plane is used as a reference point for mounting the maxillary cast by facebow transfer. The mandibular cast is mounted with respect to the upper arch by use of bite records. Consult other textbooks for the methods of bite registration and facebow transfer.

• **Fig. 1.49** Relationship between condylar movement and articulator settings.

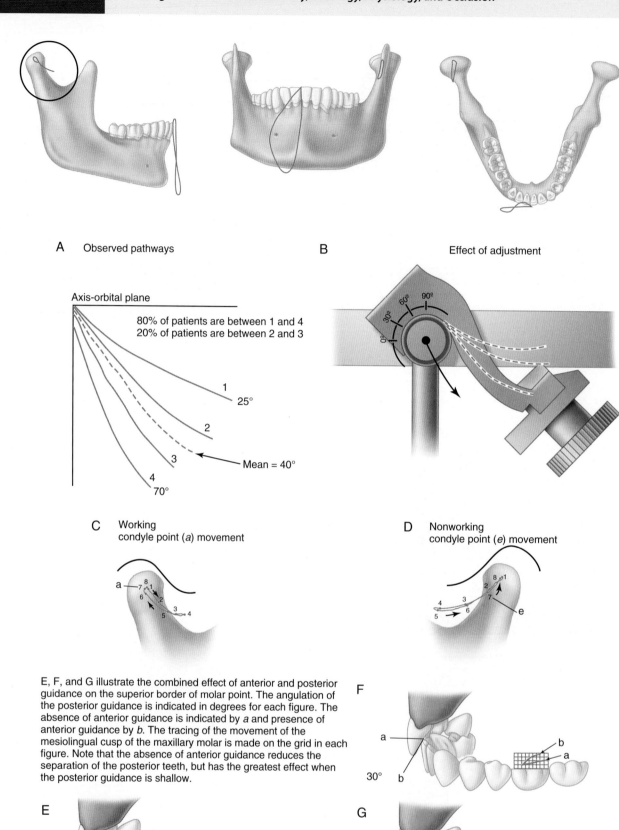

A Observed pathways

Axis-orbital plane

80% of patients are between 1 and 4
20% of patients are between 2 and 3

1
25°

2

3
Mean = 40°

4
70°

B Effect of adjustment

30° 60° 90°
0°

C Working condyle point (*a*) movement

D Nonworking condyle point (*e*) movement

E, F, and G illustrate the combined effect of anterior and posterior guidance on the superior border of molar point. The angulation of the posterior guidance is indicated in degrees for each figure. The absence of anterior guidance is indicated by *a* and presence of anterior guidance by *b*. The tracing of the movement of the mesiolingual cusp of the maxillary molar is made on the grid in each figure. Note that the absence of anterior guidance reduces the separation of the posterior teeth, but has the greatest effect when the posterior guidance is shallow.

F

30°

E

20°

G

50°

• **Fig. 1.50** Horizontal condylar guidance.

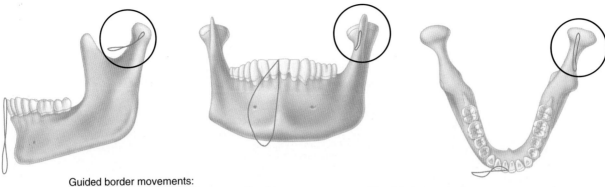

Guided border movements:
1. Follow chewing pathway in reverse direction
2. Differences are due to amount of side shift
3. Progressive side shift was not observed

Simulated movements:
1. Are arcs of circles
2. Differ by side shift
3. Are comparable to guided movements

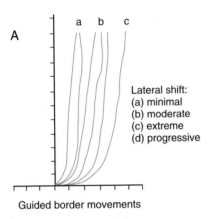

A

Lateral shift:
(a) minimal
(b) moderate
(c) extreme
(d) progressive

Guided border movements

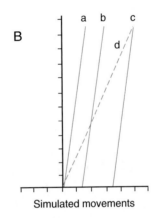

B

Simulated movements

Underside of condylar housing condylar ball movement at extreme side shift

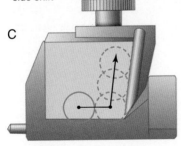

C

Maxillary molar; showing change in nonworking movement of mandibular distofacial cusp with increasing lateral shift

Adjustment of the lateral shift to produce simulated movements above

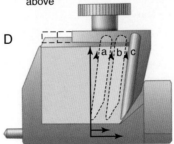

D

Mandibular molar; showing change in nonworking movement of maxillary mesiolingual cusp with increasing lateral shift

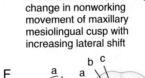

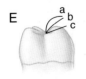

E

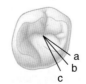

F

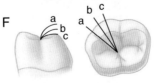

• **Fig. 1.51** Lateral condylar guidance: the medial wall.

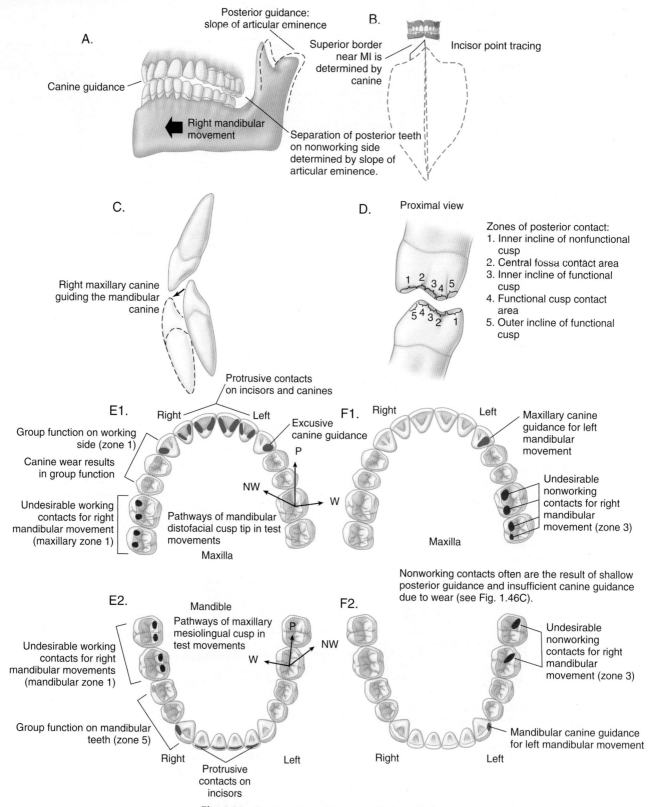

• **Fig. 1.52** Tooth contacts during mandibular movement.

Tooth Contacts During Mandibular Movements

Dentists must design restorations capable of withstanding the forces of mastication. Evaluation of the location, direction, and area of tooth contacts during various mandibular movements is an essential part of the preoperative evaluation of teeth to be restored. Anterior teeth support gliding contacts, whereas posterior teeth support the heavy forces applied during chewing and clenching. Fig. 1.52 shows a variety of tooth contact relationships. In Fig. 1.52A, a right mandibular movement is illustrated, showing the separation of the posterior teeth on the left, or nonworking, side. This separation of posterior teeth results from the combined effects of the canine guidance and the slope of the articular eminence on the nonworking side. The effect of the canine guidance is illustrated in the incisor point tracing in Fig. 1.52B. The superior border on either side of MI is determined by the shape of the lingual surfaces of maxillary canine teeth. Guiding contact between the right canines is illustrated in Fig. 1.52C. A variety of areas on posterior teeth may contact opposing teeth during mandibular movements. In Fig. 1.52D, the opposing surfaces of molar teeth are divided into five areas:

1. *Inner incline of the nonfunctional cusp.* This area has the potential for undesirable contact in working-side movements by contacting the outer aspect of the functional cusp (area 5).
2. *Fossa or marginal ridge contact area.* This is the main contact area for the opposing functional cusp.
3. *Inner incline of the functional cusp.* This area has the potential for undesirable contact during nonworking movements.
4. *Contact area of the functional cusp.* This is the main cusp contact area.
5. *Outer aspect of the functional cusp.* This area sometimes participates in working-side movements by contacting the inner incline of the nonfunctional cusp (area 1).

Anterior Tooth Contacts

During anterior movement of the mandible (i.e., protrusion), the lower anterior teeth glide along the lingual surfaces of maxillary anterior teeth (see Fig. 1.52E and F). The combination of the anterior guidance (slope and vertical overlap of anterior teeth) and the slope of the articular eminence (horizontal condylar guidance on the articulator) determines the amount of vertical separation of posterior teeth as the mandible moves anteriorly. Some texts refer to this separation as *disocclusion* (or *disclusion*) of posterior teeth. Multiple contacts between the opposing dental arches on anterior teeth are desirable in protrusion movements. With protrusion, multiple contacts serve to prevent excessive force on any individual pair of gliding teeth. Posterior tooth contact during protrusion is not desirable because it may overload the involved teeth secondary to the increased elevator muscle activity that occurs when posterior teeth come into contact. It has been shown that when anterior teeth are in contact and posterior teeth are discluded, elevator muscles are less active.[16-19,23,27,30,47]

Articulator-mounted casts may be used to assess the superior border near MI, which is the critical zone for tooth contact. This information is useful during the fabrication of indirect restorations because the position and height of the restored cusps can be evaluated and adjusted in the laboratory, which minimizes the chairside time and effort required to adjust the completed restorations.

Posterior Tooth Contacts

In idealized occlusal schemes designed for restorative dentistry, posterior teeth should contact only in MI such that the force that results from maximum activation of the elevator muscles is distributed evenly over multiple teeth.[16-19,23,27,28,30,47] Any movement of the mandible should result in the separation of posterior teeth by the combined effects of anterior guidance and the slope of the articular eminence (horizontal condylar guidance on the articulator). The immediate separation of posterior teeth during protrusion or excursion results in a decrease in the level of activity and force being generated by the elevator muscles.[16,18,19,21,23,27,30,47]

Forceful contact of individual posterior tooth cusps during chewing and clenching may lead to muscle discomfort, damage

to teeth and supporting structures, or both in some patients. In patients with shallow anterior guidance or open bite, restoration without the introduction of undesirable tooth contacts is more difficult. Articulator-mounted casts may be used to assess and solve restorative problems that are difficult to manage by direct intraoral techniques.

The preferred occlusal relationship for restorative purposes is one that limits the working-side contact to canines only. This is directly related to the observation that, compared with canine guidance alone, guidance from canines *and* posterior teeth will result in greater activation of the anterior temporalis muscle and longer activation of the masseter and temporalis muscles during excursive movements.[27,30,47]

Tooth contact posterior to the canine on the working side may occur naturally in worn dentitions. As canines are shortened by wear, separation of posterior teeth diminishes. Lateral mandibular movements in worn dentitions successively bring into contact more posterior teeth as the heights of canines decrease. Multiple tooth contacts during lateral jaw movements are termed *group function*. Right-sided group function is illustrated in Fig. 1.52E, compared with left canine guidance contact in Fig. 1.52F. Because the amount of torque and wear imposed on teeth increases closer to the muscle attachments on the mandible, molar contact in group function is undesirable (see Fig. 1.52E and F). It has been observed that facial cusps of the maxillary premolars and molars (Maxillary Zone 1, nonfunctional cusps) and lingual cusps of mandibular molars (Mandibular Zone 1, nonfunctional cusps) have increased incidence of fracture.[48] This finding is consistent with the increased elevator muscle activity that occurs as posterior teeth come into contact and that the bulk of dentin supporting the nonfunctional cusps is considerably less than that of the functional maxillary and mandibular cusps. Group function limited to premolars may be a therapeutic goal when the bony support of canines is compromised by periodontal disease or Class II occlusions in which canine guidance is impossible.

The nonworking side is opposite the working side and normally does not contain a food bolus during chewing. During chewing closures, mandibular teeth on the nonworking side close from an anteromedial position and approach MI by moving posterolaterally. Contact of the molar cusps on the nonworking side may overload these teeth, compromise the ipsilateral TMJ, or both because of a resultant increase in the activity of the masseter, anterior temporalis, and posterior temporalis muscles and the ipsilateral superior lateral pterygoid.[16-18,20] Each of these muscles counteracts the action of the nonworking-side inferior lateral pterygoid, which is responsible (along with the contralateral posterior temporalis and digastric muscles) for effecting the down and forward translation of the nonworking-side condyle. Additional activity of the ipsilateral superior lateral pterygoid muscle should not occur during condylar translation when the TMJ disc needs to rotate posteriorly toward the top of the condylar head to maintain its position between the condyle and the articular eminence. Great variation exists among patients in the level of masticatory system tolerance to nonworking-side contacts. Questions remain as to whether the presence of a nonworking-side posterior contact always represents an interference to mandibular function. The predictable, normal physiologic muscle response to nonworking-side tooth contact (along with the potential negative sequelae of tooth wear, tooth fracture, masticatory muscle pain and/or TMJ internal disc derangement) leads to the conclusion that avoidance of these contacts is an important goal for restorative procedures in the posterior dentition. Undesirable nonworking-side contacts are illustrated in Fig. 1.52F.

Neurologic Correlates and Control of Mastication

This summary of neurologic control is based on an excellent review by Lund.[49] The control of mastication depends on sensory feedback. Sensory feedback serves to control the coordination of the lips, tongue, and mandibular movement during manipulation of the food bolus through all stages of mastication and preparation for swallowing. Physiologists divide an individual chewing cycle into three components: *opening, fast closing,* and *slow closing.* The slow-closing segment of chewing is associated with the increased forces required for crushing food. The central nervous system receives several types of feedback from muscle spindles, periodontal receptors, and touch receptors in the skin and mucosa. This feedback controls the mandibular closing muscles during the slow-closing phase. Sensory feedback often results in inhibition of movement (e.g., because of pain). During mastication, some sensory feedback from teeth is excitatory, causing an increase in the closing force as the food bolus is crushed. An upper limit must, however, be present where inhibition occurs; this prevents the buildup of excessive forces on teeth during the occlusal stage.

A group of neurons in the brainstem produces bursts of discharges at regular intervals when excited by oral sensory stimuli. These bursts drive motor neurons to produce contractions of the masticatory muscles at regular intervals, resulting in rhythmic mandibular movement. The cluster of neurons in the brainstem that drives the rhythmic chewing is termed *central pattern generator.* The chewing cycles illustrated in Figs. 1.46, 1.47, and 1.48 are caused by central pattern generator rhythms. Oral sensory feedback can modify the basic central pattern generator pattern and is essential for the coordination of the lips, tongue, and mandible. Sensory input from the periodontal and mucosal receptors maintains the rhythmic chewing. Coactivation of the opening and closing muscles serves to protect the dentition from excessively forceful contact, makes the mandible more rigid, and probably serves to brace the condyles while the food is crushed.

References

1. Dusevich V, Xu C, Wang Y, et al: Identification of a protein-containing enamel matrix layer which bridges with the dentin-enamel junction of adult human teeth. *Arch Oral Biol* 57(12):1585–1594, 2012.
2. Digka A, Lyroudia K, Jirasek T, et al: Visualisation of human dental pulp vasculature by immunohistochemical and immunofluorescent detection of CD34: a comparative study. *Aust Endod J* 32:101–106, 2006.
3. Garberoglio R, Brännström M: Scanning electron microscopic investigation of human dentinal tubules. *Arch Oral Biol* 21:355–362, 1976.
4. Scott JH, Symons NBB: *Introduction to dental anatomy,* ed 9, Philadelphia, 1982, Churchill Livingstone.
5. Craig RG, Powers JM: *Restorative dental materials,* ed 12, St Louis, 2006, Mosby.
6. Brännström M: *Dentin and pulp in restorative dentistry,* London, 1982, Wolfe Medical.
7. Michelich V, Pashley DH, Whitford GM: Dentin permeability: comparison of function versus anatomic tubular radii. *J Dent Res* 57:1019–1024, 1978.
8. Sturdevant JR, Pashley DH: Regional dentin permeability of class I and II cavity preparations (abstract no. 173). *J Dent Res* 68:203, 1989.
9. Farges J-C, Alliot-Licht B, Renard E, et al: Dental pulp defence and repair mechanisms in dental caries. *Mediat Inflam* 2015. http://dx.doi.org/10.1155/2015/230251. Article ID 230251.
10. Boushell LW, Nagaoka H, Nagaoka H, et al: Increased matrix metalloproteinase-2 and bone sialoprotein response to human coronal caries. *Caries Res* 45:453–459, 2011, doi:10.1159/000330601.
11. Mohl ND, Zarb GA, Carlsson GE, et al: The dentition. In Mohl ND, Zarb GA, Carisson GE, et al, editors: *A textbook of occlusion,* Chicago, 1988, Quintessence.
12. Gibbs CH, Messerman T, Reswick JB, et al: Functional movements of the mandible. *J Prosthet Dent* 26(5):604–620, 1971.
13. Angle EH: Classification of malocclusion. *Dent Cosmos* 41:248–264, 350–357, 1899.
14. Kraus BS, Jorden E, Abrams L: *Dental anatomy and occlusion,* ed 1, Baltimore, 1969, Williams & Wilkins.
15. Dawson PE: *Functional occlusion: from TMJ to smile design,* St Louis, 2007, Mosby.
16. Belser UC, Hannam AG: The influence of altered working-side occlusal guidance on masticatory muscles and related jaw movement. *J Prosthet Dent* 53(3):406–413, 1985.
17. Gibbs CH, Mahan PE, Wilkinson TM, et al: EMG activity of the superior belly of the lateral pterygoid muscle in relation to other jaw muscles. *J Prosthet Dent* 51(5):691–702, 1984.
18. Vitti M, Basmajian JV: Integrated actions of masticatory muscles: simultaneous EMG from eight intramuscular electrodes. *Anat Rec* 187:173–190, 1976.
19. Williamson EH, Lundquist DO: Anterior guidance: its effect on electromyographic activity of the temporal and masseter muscles. *J Prosthet Dent* 49(6):816–823, 1983.
20. Santana U, Mora MJ: Electromyographic analysis of the masticatory muscles of patients after complete rehabilitation of occlusion with protection by non-working side contacts. *J Oral Rehabil* 22:57–66, 1995.
21. Valenzuela S, Baeza M, Miralles R, et al: Laterotrusive occlusal schemes and their effect on supra- and infrahyoid electromyographic activity. *Angle Orthod* 76(4):585–590, 2006.
22. Mahan PE, Wilkinson TM, Gibbs CH, et al: Superior and inferior bellies of the lateral pterygoid muscle and EMG activity at basic jaw positions. *J Prosthet Dent* 50(5):710–718, 1983.
23. Borromeo GL, Suvinen TI, Reade PC: A comparison of the effects of group function and canine guidance interocclusal device on masseter muscle electromyographic activity in normal subjects. *J Prosthet Dent* 74(2):174–180, 1995.
24. Graham GS, Rugh JD: Maxillary splint occlusal guidance patterns and electrographic activity of the jaw-closing muscles. *J Prosthet Dent* 59(1):73–77, 1988.
25. Hannam AG, De Cou RE, Scott JD, et al: The relationship between dental occlusion, muscle activity and associated jaw movement in man. *Arch Oral Biol* 22:25–32, 1977.
26. Leiva M, Miralles R, Palazzi C, et al: Effects of laterotrusive occlusal scheme and body position on bilateral sternocleidomastoid EMG activity. *J Craniomandibular Practice* 21(2):99–109, 2003.
27. Manns A, Chan C, Miralles R: Influence of group function and canine guidance on electromyographic activity of elevator muscles. *J Prosthet Dent* 57(4):494–501, 1987.
28. Manns A, Miralles R, Valdivia J, et al: Influence of variation in anteroposterior occlusal contacts on electromyographic activity. *J Prosthet Dent* 61:617–623, 1989.
29. Rugh JD, Drago CJ: Vertical dimension: a study of clinical rest position and jaw muscle activity. *J Prosthet Dent* 45(6):670–675, 1981.
30. Shupe RJ, Mohamed SE, Christensen LV, et al: Effects of occlusal guidance on jaw muscle activity. *J Prosthet Dent* 51(6):811–818, 1984.
31. Huang BY, Whittle T, Peck CC, et al: Ipsilateral interferences and working-side condylar movements. *Arch Oral Biol* 51:206–214, 2006.
32. Solberg WK, Woo MW, Houston JB: Prevalence of mandibular dysfunction in young adults. *J Am Dent Assoc* 98:25–34, 1979.
33. Posselt U: Studies in the mobility of the mandible. *Acta Odont Scand* 10(Suppl 10):1952.

34. Gibbs CH, Lundeen HC: Jaw movements and forces during chewing and swallowing and their clinical significance. In Lundeen HC, Gibbs CH, editors: *Advances in occlusion*, Bristol, 1982, John Wright PSG.

35. Celenza FV, Nasedkin JN: *Occlusion: the state of the art*, Chicago, 1978, Quintessence.

36. Keshvad A, Winstanley RB: An appraisal of the literature on centric relation. *J Oral Rehabil* 28:55–63, 2001.

37. Crawford SD: Condylar axis position, as determined by the occlusion and measured by the CPI instrument, and signs and symptoms of temporomandibular dysfunction. *Angle Orthod* 69(2):103–116, 1999.

38. Landi N, Manfredini D, Tognini F, et al: Quantification of the relative risk of multiple occlusal variables for muscle disorders of the stomatognathic system. *J Prosthet Dent* 92:190–195, 2004.

39. Pahkala R, Qvarnstrom M: Can temporomandibular dysfunction signs be predicted by early morphological or functional variables? *Eur J Orthod* 26(4):367–373, 2004.

40. Griffiths RH: Report of the president's conference on the examination, diagnosis, and management of temporomandibular disorders. *J Am Dent Assoc* 106:75–77, 1983.

41. Kim SK, Kim KN, Chang IT, et al: A study of the effects of chewing patterns on occlusal wear. *J Oral Rehabil* 28:1048–1055, 2001.

42. Mongelli de Fantini S, Batista de Paiva J, Neto JR, et al: Increase of condylar displacement between centric relation and maximal habitual intercuspation after occlusal splint therapy. *Braz Oral Res* 19(3): 176–182, 2005.

43. Lundeen HC, Wirth CG: Condylar movement patterns engraved in plastic blocks. *J Prosthet Dent* 30:866–875, 1973.

44. Lundeen HC, Shryock EF, Gibbs CH: An evaluation of mandibular border movements: their character and significance. *J Prosthet Dent* 40:442–452, 1978.

45. Lundeen TF, Mendosa MA: Comparison of Bennett shift measured at the hinge axis and an arbitrary hinge axis position. *J Prosthet Dent* 51:407–410, 1984.

46. Lundeen TF, Mendosa MA: Comparison of two methods for measurement of immediate Bennett shift. *J Prosthet Dent* 51:243–245, 1984.

47. Akoren AC, Karaagaclioglu L: Comparison of the electromyographic activity of individuals with canine guidance and group function occlusion. *J Oral Rehabil* 22:73–77, 1995.

48. Bader JD, Martin JA, Shugars DA: Incidence rates for complete cusp fracture. *Comm Dent Oral Epidemiol* 29:346–353, 2001.

49. Lund JP: Mastication and its control by the brain stem. *Crit Rev Oral Biol Med* 2:33–64, 1991.

2

Dental Caries: Etiology, Clinical Characteristics, Risk Assessment, and Management

ANDRÉA G. FERREIRA ZANDONÁ, ANDRÉ V. RITTER, R. SCOTT EIDSON[a]

This chapter presents basic definitions and information on dental caries, clinical characteristics of the caries lesion, caries risk assessment, and caries management, in the context of clinical operative dentistry.

What Is Dental Caries?

Dental caries is a preventable, chronic, and biofilm-mediated disease modulated by diet. This multifactorial, oral disease is caused primarily by an imbalance of the oral flora (biofilm) due to the presence of fermentable dietary carbohydrates on the tooth surface over time. Traditionally, this tooth-biofilm-carbohydrate interaction has been illustrated by the classical Keyes-Jordan diagram (Fig. 2.1).[1] However, dental caries onset and activity are in fact much more complex than this three-way interaction, as not all persons with teeth, biofilm, and consuming carbohydrates will have caries lesions over time. Several modifying risk and protective factors influence the dental caries process, as will be discussed later in this chapter.

At the tooth level, dental caries activity is characterized by localized demineralization and loss of tooth structure, the *caries lesion* (Figs. 2.2 and 2.3). In health, the microbiome is in symbiosis, the oral commensals striving in a neutral pH. Some bacteria in the biofilm metabolize refined carbohydrates for energy and produce organic acid by-products. These organic acids, if present in the biofilm ecosystem for extended periods, can lower the pH in the biofilm to below a critical level (5.5 for enamel, 6.2 for dentin). This low pH has effects both on the biofilm composition and at the tooth surface level (Fig. 2.4).[132] With extended periods of low pH there is a shift in the microbiome to bacteria that are acidogenic and acidophilic, causing a dysbiosis in the microbiome. This change in turn will lead to further acidification of the environment. The low pH drives calcium and phosphate from the tooth to the biofilm in an attempt to reach equilibrium, hence resulting in a net loss of minerals by the tooth, or *demineralization*. When the pH in the biofilm returns to neutral and the concentration of soluble calcium and phosphate is supersaturated relative to that in the tooth, mineral can then be added back to partially demineralized enamel in a process called *remineralization*. Thus at the tooth surface and subsurface level, dental caries lesions result from a dynamic process of damage (demineralization) and restitution (remineralization) of the tooth matter. These events take place several times a day over the life of the tooth and are modulated by many factors including number and type of microbial flora in the biofilm, diet, oral hygiene, genetics, dental anatomy, dentin and enamel composition, use of fluorides and other chemotherapeutic agents, saliva composition, salivary flow, and buffering capacity. These factors are highly individual and tooth specific, and will differ from person to person, tooth to tooth in the same individual, and site to site on a same tooth. The balance between demineralization and remineralization has been illustrated in terms of pathologic factors (i.e., those favoring demineralization) and protective factors (i.e., those favoring remineralization) (Fig. 2.5).[2] Individuals in whom the balance tilts predominantly toward protective factors (remineralization) are much less likely to develop dental caries lesions than those in which the balance is tilted toward pathologic factors (demineralization). *Understanding the balance between demineralization and remineralization is key to caries management.*

Repeated demineralization events may result from a predominantly pathologic environment causing the localized dissolution and destruction of the calcified dental tissues, evidenced as a caries lesion. The ongoing demineralization at the enamel subsurface level leads to a collapse of the surface and hence the formation of a cavitation in the enamel surface. Severe demineralization of dentin results in the exposure of the protein matrix, which is denatured initially by host matrix metalloproteinases (MMPs) and subsequently degraded by MMPs and other bacterial proteases. Demineralization of the inorganic phase (dentin mineral), and denaturation and degradation of the organic phase (primarily dentin collagen) result in dentin cavitation.[3]

It is essential to understand that caries lesions, or cavitations in teeth, are signs of an underlying condition, an imbalance between protective and pathologic factors favoring the latter. In clinical practice it is very easy to lose sight of this fact and focus entirely on the restorative treatment of caries lesions, failing to treat the underlying cause of the disease (Table 2.1). Although symptomatic treatment is important for many reasons, failure to identify and

---

[a]Dr. Eidson was an inactive author in this edition.

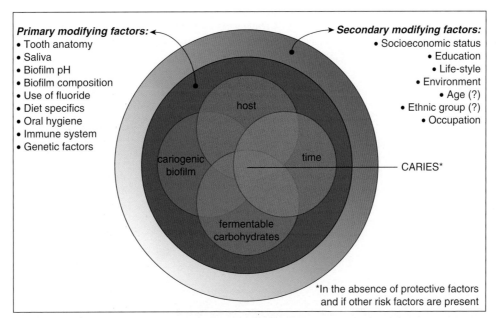

Primary modifying factors:
- Tooth anatomy
- Saliva
- Biofilm pH
- Biofilm composition
- Use of fluoride
- Diet specifics
- Oral hygiene
- Immune system
- Genetic factors

Secondary modifying factors:
- Socioeconomic status
- Education
- Life-style
- Environment
- Age (?)
- Ethnic group (?)
- Occupation

host

cariogenic biofilm

time

CARIES*

fermentable carbohydrates

*In the absence of protective factors and if other risk factors are present

• **Fig. 2.1**   Modified Keyes-Jordan diagram. As a simplified description, dental caries is a result of the interaction of cariogenic oral flora (biofilm) with fermentable dietary carbohydrates on the tooth surface (host) over time. However, dental caries onset and activity are, in fact, much more complex, as not all persons with teeth, biofilm, and who are consuming carbohydrates will have caries over time. Several modifying risk factors and protective factors influence the dental caries process. (Modified from Keyes PH, Jordan HV: Factors influencing initiation, transmission and inhibition of dental caries. In Harris RJ, editor: *Mechanisms of hard tissue destruction*, New York, 1963, Academic Press.)

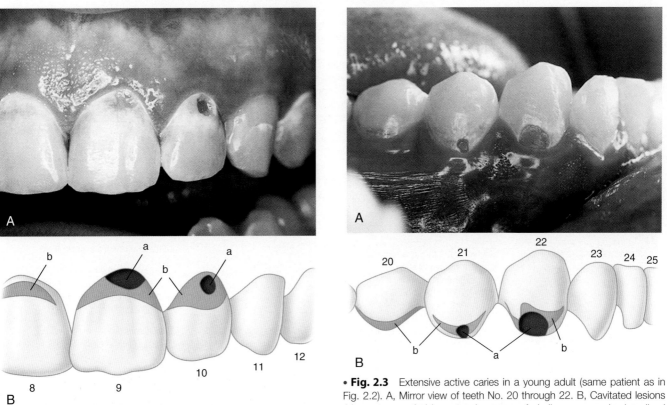

• **Fig. 2.2**   A, Young adult with multiple active initial and cavitated caries lesions involving teeth No. 8 through 10. B, Cavitated areas *(a)* are surrounded by areas of extensive demineralization that are chalky and opaque *(b)*. Some areas of initial (noncavitated) caries have superficial stain.

• **Fig. 2.3**   Extensive active caries in a young adult (same patient as in Fig. 2.2). A, Mirror view of teeth No. 20 through 22. B, Cavitated lesions *(a)* are surrounded by extensive areas of chalky, opaque demineralized areas *(b)*. The presence of smooth-surface lesions such as these is associated with rampant caries. Occlusal and interproximal smooth-surface caries usually occur in advance of facial smooth-surface lesions. The presence of these types of lesions should alert the dentist to the possibility of a high caries risk patient and possibly extensive caries activity elsewhere in the mouth. The interproximal gingiva is swollen red and would bleed easily on probing. These gingival changes are the consequence of long-standing irritation from the biofilm adherent to the teeth.

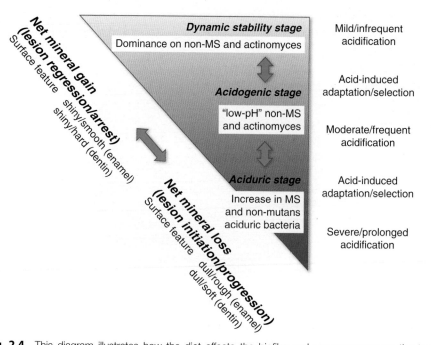

• **Fig. 2.4** This diagram illustrates how the diet affects the biofilm and consequences on the tooth surface. In health, the biofilm is in symbiosis. A person who has only occasional consumption of fermentable carbohydrates will have a resident microbiome dominated by nonmutans streptococci and actinomyces in a dynamic stability stage that is adapting to the relatively minor changes in pH. As the diet changes to more frequent exposures to fermentable carbohydrates, the microbiome adapts to the more acidic environment in an acidogenic stage, where bacteria that favor low pH flourish. In diets with frequent exposures to fermentable carbohydrates this constant acid-induced adaptation and selection of the microbiome continues and leads to an aciduric stage where there is an increase in MS and nonmutans aciduric bacteria, thus leading to a dysbiosis of the microbiome. At one end of the spectrum, in an environment with severe and prolonged acidification and aciduric bacteria, there is a net mineral loss at the tooth surface, enamel, or dentin, causing lesion initiation or lesion progression, while at the other end of the spectrum with only mild acidification there is a net mineral gain at the tooth surface and consequently lesion regression or arrest. Certainly this is a simplified explanation of the changes in the biofilm as the microbiome adapts to the acidic environment due to cariogenic diets, which does not consider the many other factors that are at play to either halt the process or boost the process. (From Takahashi N1, Nyvad B. The role of bacteria in the caries process: ecological perspectives, *J Dent Res* 90(3):294–303, 2011. doi:10.1177/0022034510379602)

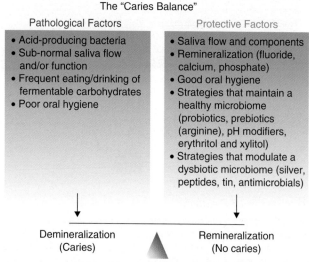

• **Fig. 2.5** The caries balance. The balance between demineralization and remineralization is illustrated in terms of pathologic factors (i.e., those favoring demineralization) and protective factors (i.e., those favoring remineralization). (Modified from Featherstone JDB: Prevention and reversal of dental caries: role of low level fluoride, *Community Dent Oral Epidemiol* 27:31–40, 1999.)

TABLE 2.1	Caries Management Based on the Medical Model	
Primary Etiology	**Cariogenic Biofilm Resultant From a Cariogenic Diet**
Symptoms	Demineralization lesions in teeth
Treatment, therapeutic	Improvement of host resistance by (1) biofilm modification, (2) elevating biofilm pH, and (3) enhancing remineralization
Treatment, symptomatic	Remineralization/arrest of lesions, restoration of cavitated lesions
Posttreatment assessment, therapeutic	Reevaluation of etiologic conditions and primary and secondary risk factors; and continuous management based on findings
Posttreatment assessment, symptomatic	Examination of teeth for new lesions, assessment of lesion activity, assessment of lesion progression

manage the underlying causative factors of dental caries allows the disease to continue and increases the chance of treatment failure. Caries management efforts must be directed not only at the tooth level (traditional or surgical treatment) but also at the total-patient level (caries management by risk assessment). *Restorative treatment does not cure the caries process.* Instead, identifying and managing the risk factors for caries must be the primary focus, in addition to the restorative repair of damage caused by caries.

This chapter emphasizes the components of a caries management program that is based first on risk assessment and then on modifying the biofilm ecology to enhance protective factors and minimize pathologic factors.[4] This chapter also presents information on clinical characteristics of the caries lesion as they relate to clinical operative dentistry. Use of correct and consistent terms when referring to caries and caries lesions is important. Box 2.1 summarizes the most common terms used in this textbook to define caries lesions based on their location, cavitation status, and activity status. More

in-depth information on the dental caries process can be found elsewhere.[133]

Ecologic Basis of Dental Caries: The Role of the Biofilm

Dental plaque is a term historically used to describe the soft, tenacious film accumulating on the surface of teeth. Dental plaque has been more recently referred to as the *dental biofilm* or simply the *biofilm*, which is a more complete and accurate description of its composition (bio) and structure (film).[5] The biofilm is composed mostly of bacteria, their by-products, extracellular matrix, and water (Figs. 2.6, 2.7, 2.8, 2.9, and 2.10). Biofilm is not adherent food debris, as was widely and erroneously thought, nor does it result from the haphazard collection of opportunistic microorganisms. The accumulation of the biofilm on teeth is a highly organized

---

• BOX 2.1 Caries Lesion Definitions

- **Caries lesion.** Tooth demineralization as a result of the caries process. Other texts may use the term *carious lesion*. Laypeople may use the term *cavity*.
- **Smooth-surface caries.** A caries lesion on a smooth tooth surface.
- **Pit-and-fissure caries.** A caries lesion on a pit-and-fissure area.
- **Occlusal caries.** A caries lesion on an occlusal surface.
- **Proximal caries.** A caries lesion on a proximal surface.
- **Enamel caries.** A caries lesion in enamel, typically indicating that the lesion has not penetrated into dentin. (Note that many lesions detected clinically as enamel caries may very well have extended into dentin histologically.)
- **Dentin caries.** A caries lesion into dentin.
- **Coronal caries.** A caries lesion in any surface of the anatomic tooth crown.
- **Root caries.** A caries lesion in the root surface.
- **Primary caries.** A caries lesion not adjacent to an existing restoration or crown.
- **Secondary caries.** A caries lesion adjacent to an existing restoration, crown, or sealant. Other term used is *caries adjacent to restorations and sealants* (CARS). Also referred to as recurrent caries, implying that a primary caries lesion was restored but that the lesion reoccurred.
- **Residual caries.** Refers to carious tissue that was not completely excavated prior to placing a restoration. Sometimes residual caries can be difficult to differentiate from secondary caries.
- **Cavitated caries lesion.** A caries lesion that results in the breaking of the integrity of the tooth, or a cavitation.
- **Initial caries lesion.** A caries lesion that has not been cavitated. In enamel caries, initial caries lesions are also referred to as noncavitated or "white spot" lesions. (Clinically, the distinction between a cavitated and a noncavitated caries lesion is not as simple as it may seem. Although historically any roughness detectable with a sharp explorer has been considered a cavitated lesion, more recent caries detection guidelines establish that only lesions in which a blunt probe penetrates without pressure are to be considered cavitated. This distinction has important implications on lesion management, because most initial caries lesions can be arrested or remineralized, while most cavitated lesions require restorative intervention.)
- **Moderate caries lesion.** A caries lesion that may or may not have cavitated but that has not reached the inner one-third of dentin. This can be observed clinically by microcavitations in the enamel or a gray shadow.
- **Advanced (deep) caries lesion.** A definitely cavitated lesion exposing dentin. For the purposes of this protocol any lesion that has reached the inner one-third of the dentin will be considered an advanced lesion.

- **Active caries lesion.** A caries lesion that is considered to be biologically active—that is, a lesion in which tooth demineralization is in frank activity at the time of examination.
- **Inactive caries lesion.** A caries lesion that is considered to be biologically inactive at the time of examination—that is, in which tooth demineralization caused by caries may have happened in the past but has stopped and is currently stalled. Also referred to as *arrested caries*, meaning that the caries process has been arrested but that the clinical signs of the lesion itself are still present.
- **Rampant caries.** Term used to describe the presence of extensive and multiple cavitated and active caries lesions in the same person. Typically used in association with "baby bottle caries," "radiation therapy caries," or "meth-mouth caries." These terms refer to the etiology of the condition.
- **Primary dentin.** Sound, normal dentin that forms during tooth development; it is usually completed 3 years after tooth eruption. Histologically, primary dentin has tubules with smooth odontoblastic processes, with no intratubular crystals. The intertubular dentin has normal cross-banded collagen and normal dense apatite crystals. Clinically, primary dentin is hard, cannot be easily penetrated with a blunt explorer, and can only be cut by a bur or a sharp cutting instrument.
- **Secondary dentin.** Sound, normal dentin that forms physiologically on all internal aspects of the pulp cavity throughout the life of the tooth. Histologically, secondary dentin resembles primary dentin. Clinically, secondary dentin is similar to primary dentin.
- **Tertiary dentin.** Dentin that forms in response to stimuli such as caries, attrition, and operative procedures. Also known as reparative or reactive dentin. Usually appears as a localized dentin deposit on the wall of the pulp space immediately subjacent to the area of the tooth that has received the injury. Tertiary dentin is less mineralized than primary and secondary dentin, and contains irregular dentinal tubules. Clinically, tertiary dentin is not as hard as primary dentin.
- **Sclerotic dentin.** Dentin that forms in response to stimuli such as aging or mild irritation (slow advancing caries). When responding to initial caries demineralization events, crystalline material precipitates in intratubular and intertubular dentin. Sclerotic dentin walls off a lesion by blocking (sealing) the dentinal tubules. This zone can be seen even before the demineralization reaches the dentin and it may not be present in rapidly advancing lesions. Clinically, sclerotic dentin is dark and harder than normal dentin.
- **Leathery dentin.** Term used to describe the clinical presentation of the transition zone between soft and firm dentin (see next section). Technically leathery dentin is part of the firm dentin zone.

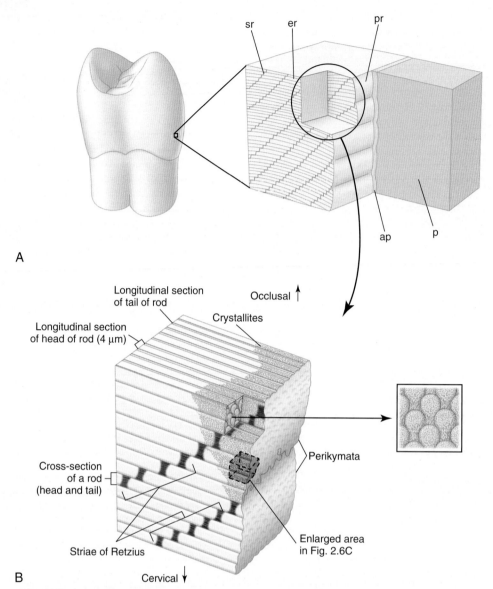

• **Fig. 2.6** A, Composite diagram illustrating the relationship of biofilm *(p)* to the enamel in a smooth-surface initial (noncavitated) lesion. A relatively cell-free layer of precipitated salivary protein material, the acquired pellicle *(ap)* covers the perikymata ridges *(pr)*. The biofilm bacteria attach to the pellicle. Overlapping perikymata ridges can be seen on the surface of enamel (see Fig. 2.7). (Figs. 2.9 and 2.10 are photomicrographs of cross sections of biofilm.) The enamel is composed of rodlike structures *(er)* that course from the inner dentinoenamel junction (DEJ) to the surface of the crown. Striae of Retzius *(sr)* can be seen in cross sections of enamel. B, Higher power view of the cutout portion of enamel in *A*. Enamel rods interlock with each other in a head-to-tail orientation. The rod heads are visible on the surface as slight depressions on the perikymata ridges. The enamel rods comprise tightly packed crystallites. The orientation of the crystallites changes from being parallel to the rod in the head region to being perpendicular to the rod axis in the tail end. Striae of Retzius form a descending diagonal line, descending cervically.

and ordered sequence of events. Bacteria seem to occupy the same spatial niche on most individuals. A "hedgehog" formation has been recently characterized[209] because of the spine of radially oriented filaments. The filaments are a mass of *Corynebacterium* filaments with *Streptococcus* at the periphery. Actinomyces are usually found at the base of the biofilm suggesting that *Corynebacterium* attaches to a preexisting biofilm containing *Actinomyces*. In any case it is notable that each taxon is localized in a precise and well-defined spatial zone indicating that the microbes in the oral biofilm have a precise and well-tuned interaction[209] (see Fig. 2.6D).

Many of the organisms found in the mouth are not found elsewhere in nature. Survival of microorganisms in the oral environment depends on their ability to adhere to a surface. Free-floating organisms are cleared rapidly from the mouth by salivary flow and frequent swallowing. Although a few specialized organisms, primarily streptococci, are particularly able to adhere to oral surfaces such

Text continued on p. 48

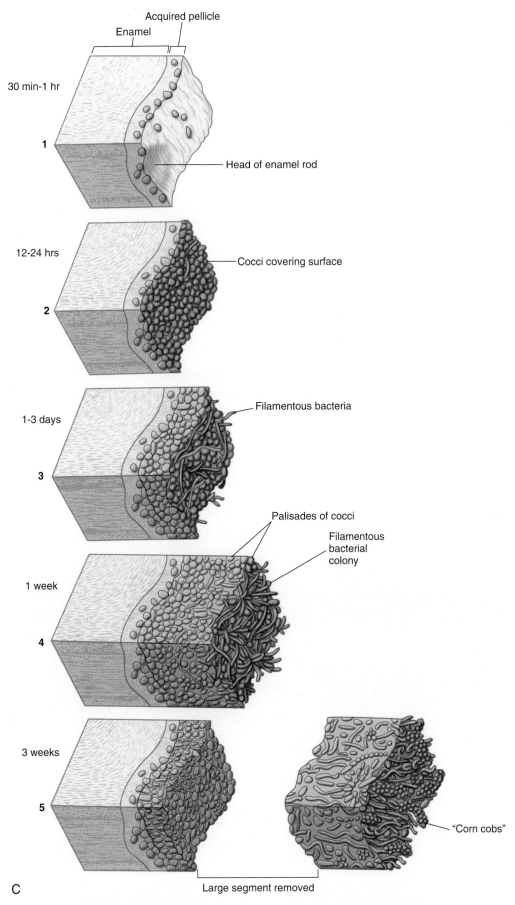

C

Large segment removed

• **Fig. 2.6, cont'd**   C, Drawings 1 through 5 illustrate the various stages in colonization during plaque formation on the shaded enamel block shown in *B*. The accumulated mass of bacteria on the tooth surface may become so thick that it is visible to the unaided eye. Such plaques are gelatinous and tenaciously adherent; they readily take up disclosing dyes, aiding in their visualization for oral hygiene instruction. Thick plaque biofilms (*4* and *5*) are capable of great metabolic activity when sufficient nutrients are available. The gelatinous nature of the plaque limits outward diffusion of metabolic products and serves to prolong the retention of organic acid metabolic by-products.   *Continued*

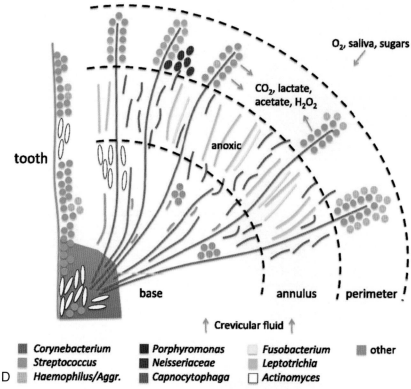

O_2, saliva, sugars

CO_2, lactate, acetate, H_2O_2

anoxic

tooth

base · annulus · perimeter

↑ Crevicular fluid ↑

▨ *Corynebacterium*	■ *Porphyromonas*	▨ *Fusobacterium*	■ other
▨ *Streptococcus*	▨ *Neisseriaceae*	▨ *Leptotrichia*	
D ▨ *Haemophilus/Aggr.*	▨ *Capnocytophaga*	□ *Actinomyces*	

• Fig. 2.6, cont'd D, This illustrates how different taxons inhabit specific niches on the biofilm creating microenvironments. There is a fine-tuned synergy among the cells in the oral microbial communities. The environment and the biochemical gradients drive the selection process. This can be exemplified by the the role of *Streptococcus*. Where *Streptococcus* predominate they create an environment rich in CO_2, lactate, and acetate, containing peroxide and having low oxygen. This environment is advantageous for the growth of bacteria such as *Fusobacterium* and *Leptotrichia*. (From Welch JL, Rossetti BJ, Riekem CW, et al: Biogeography of a human oral microbiome at the micron scale, *Proc Natl Acad Sci USA* 9;113(6):E791–E800, 2016. doi:10.1073/pnas.1522149113)

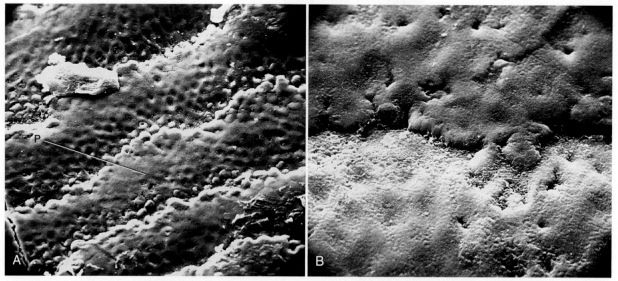

• Fig. 2.7 A, Scanning electron microscope view (600×) of overlapping perikymata *(P)* in sound enamel from unerupted molar. B, Higher power view (2300×) of overlapped site rotated 180 degrees. Surface of noncavitated enamel lesions has "punched-out" appearance. (From Hoffman S: Histopathology of caries lesions. In Menaker L, editor: *The biologic basis of dental caries*, New York, 1980, Harper & Row.)

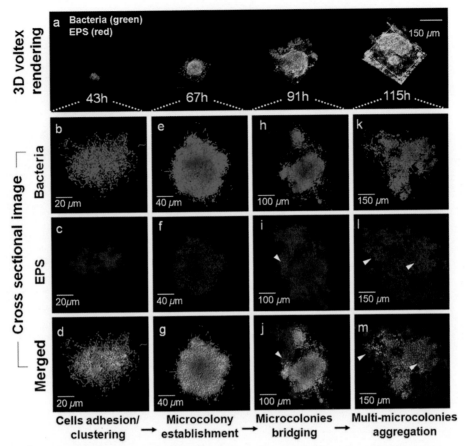

• **Fig. 2.8**   Representative 3-D rendering images of mixed-species biofilms in an environment with 1% (W/V) sucrose. The images show the evolution of the microcolonies over time and the arrangement with the EPS matrix. (From Xiao J, Klein MI, Falsetta ML, et al: The exopolysaccharide matrix modulates the interaction between 3D architecture and virulence of a mixed-species oral biofilm, *PLoS Pathog* 8(4):e1002623, 2012. https://doi.org/10.1371/journal.ppat.1002623)

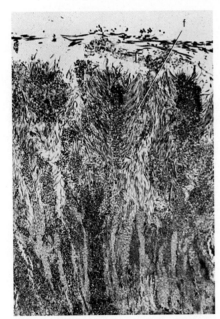

• **Fig. 2.9**   Plaque biofilm formation at 1 week. Filamentous bacteria *(f)* appear to be invading cocci microcolonies. Plaque near gingival sulcus has fewer coccal forms and more filamentous bacteria (860×). (From Listgarten MA, Mayo HE, Tremblay R: Development of dental plaque on epoxy resin crowns in man. A light and electron microscopic study, *J Periodontol* 46(1):10–26, 1975.)

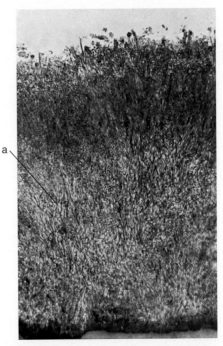

• **Fig. 2.10**   At 3 weeks old, plaque biofilm is almost entirely composed of filamentous bacteria. Heavy plaque formers have spiral bacteria *(a)* associated with subgingival plaque (660×). (From Listgarten MA, Mayo HE, Tremblay R: Development of dental plaque on epoxy resin crowns in man. A light and electron microscopic study, *J Periodontol* 46(1):10–26, 1975.)

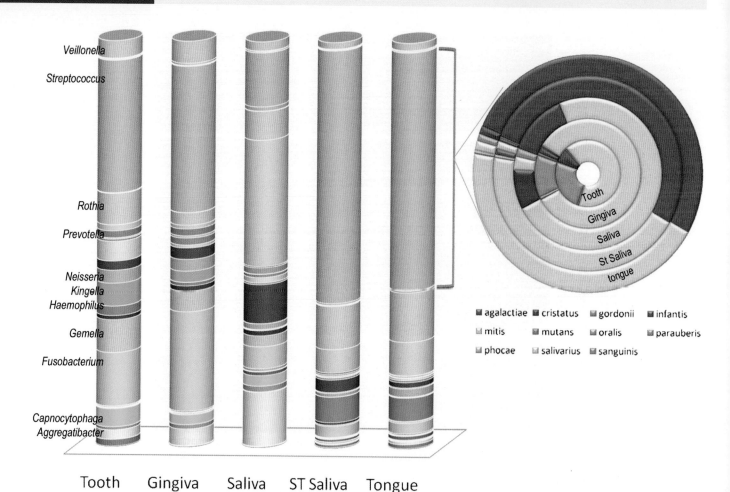

Veillonella
Streptococcus
Rothia
Prevotella
Neisseria
Kingella
Haemophilus
Gemella
Fusobacterium
Capnocytophaga
Aggregatibacter

Tooth

Gingiva
Saliva
St Saliva
tongue

■ agalactiae ■ cristatus ■ gordonii ■ infantis
◩ mitis ◩ mutans ◩ oralis ■ parauberis
◩ phocae ◩ salivarius ◩ sanguinis

Tooth   Gingiva   Saliva   ST Saliva   Tongue

• **Fig. 2.11** Approximate proportional distribution of predominant cultivable flora of five oral habitats. (From Simón-Soro Á, Tomás I, Cabrera-Rubio R, et al: Microbial geography of the oral cavity, *J Dent Res* 92:616, 2013. DOI:10.1177/0022034513488119.)

as the mucosa and tooth structure, over 700 different species of bacteria have been identified in the oral biofilm. Oral biofilm from healthy teeth have a higher diversity than from carious teeth.[134]

Significant differences exist in the biofilm communities found in various habitats (ecologic environments) within the oral cavity (Fig. 2.11A and B). The organisms also have unique contributions to the ecosystem (see Fig. 2.11B). Mature biofilm communities have tremendous metabolic potential and are capable of rapid anaerobic metabolism of any available carbohydrate (Fig. 2.12). However, because of the highly structured bacterial microcolonies embedded in an exopolysaccharide (EPS)-rich matrix, there are acidic regions in the biofilm that are not neutralized by saliva buffers.[210]

Many distinct habitats may be identified on individual teeth, with each habitat containing a unique biofilm community (Table 2.2; see Fig. 2.11A). Although the pits and fissures on the crown may harbor a relatively simple population of streptococci, the root surface in the gingival sulcus may harbor a complex community dominated by filamentous and spiral bacteria. Even within the same anatomic location there can be a considerable difference in bacterial diversity.[134] For example the mesial surface of a molar may be carious and have a biofilm dominated by large populations of mutans streptococci (MS) and lactobacilli, whereas the distal surface may lack these organisms and be caries free. Generalization about biofilm communities is difficult.

Recent evidence indicates that there are no specific pathogens that correlate with dental caries, but rather microbial communities.[135] Nevertheless, the general activity of biofilm growth and maturation is predictable and sufficiently well known to be of therapeutic importance in the prevention of dental caries.

Professional tooth cleanings are intended to control the biofilm (plaque) and prevent caries (and periodontal) disease. However, after professional removal of all organic material and bacteria from the tooth surface, a new coating of organic material begins to accumulate immediately. Within 2 hours, a cell-free, organic film, the acquired enamel pellicle (AEP) (see Fig. 2.6A and C), can cover the previously denuded area completely. The pellicle is formed primarily from the selective precipitation of various components of saliva, particularly selective enzymes. The functions of the pellicle are believed to be (1) to protect the enamel, (2) to reduce friction between teeth, and (3) to provide a matrix for remineralization.[6] Although the pellicle exhibits antibacterial activity due to the presence of several enzymes, it can also function as a facilitator of bacterial cononization.[136]

Tooth Habitats for Cariogenic Biofilm

The tooth surface is unique because it is not protected by the surface-shedding mechanisms (continual replacement of epithelial cells) used throughout the remainder of the digestive tract. The

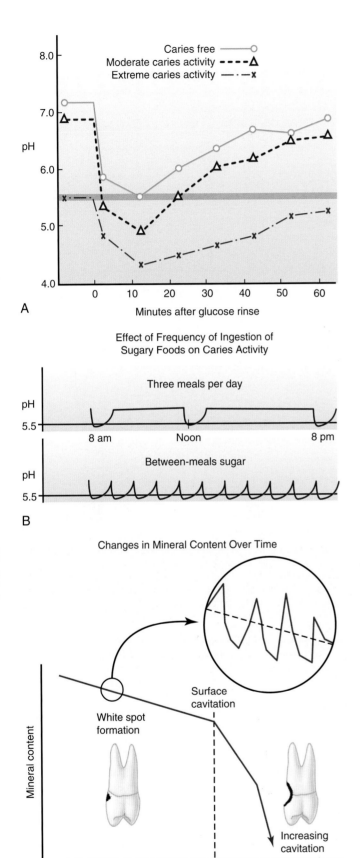

A

Effect of Frequency of Ingestion of Sugary Foods on Caries Activity

B

Changes in Mineral Content Over Time

C

• **Fig. 2.12** A, Mature biofilm communities have tremendous metabolic potential and are capable of rapid anaerobic metabolism of any available carbohydrates. Classic studies by Stephan show this metabolic potential by severe pH drops at the plaque-enamel interface after glucose rinse. It is generally agreed that a pH of 5.5 is the threshold for enamel demineralization. Exposure to a glucose rinse for an extreme caries activity plaque results in a sustained period of demineralization (pH 5.5). Recording from a slight caries activity biofilm shows a much shorter period of demineralization. B, The frequency of sucrose exposure for cariogenic biofilm greatly influences the progress of tooth demineralization. The top line illustrates pH depression, patterned after Stephan's curves in A. Three meals per day results in three exposures of biofilm acids, each lasting approximately 1 hour. The biofilm pH depression is relatively independent of the quantity of sucrose ingested. Between-meal snacks or the use of sweetened breath mints results in many more acid attacks, as illustrated at the bottom. The effect of frequent ingestion of small quantities of sucrose results in a nearly continuous acid attack on the tooth surface. (The clinical consequences of this behavior can be seen in Fig. 2.37.) C, In active caries, a progressive loss of mineral content subjacent to the cariogenic biofilm occurs. Inset illustrates that the loss is not a continuous process. Instead, alternating periods of mineral loss (demineralization) occur, with intervening periods of remineralization. The critical event for the tooth is cavitation of the surface, marked by the vertical dashed line. This event marks an acceleration in caries destruction of the tooth and irreversible loss of tooth structure. An intervention is usually required to arrest the lesion, often of the restorative nature. (A, Adapted and redrawn from Stephan RM: Intra-oral hydrogen-ion concentration associated with dental caries activity, *J Dent Res* 23:257, 1944.)

tooth surface is stable and covered with the pellicle of precipitated salivary glycoproteins, enzymes, and immunoglobulins. It is the ideal surface for the attachment of many oral streptococci. If left undisturbed, biofilm rapidly builds up to sufficient depth to produce an anaerobic environment adjacent to the tooth surface. Given the right conditions (that is, a conducive diet and poor oral hygiene) these tooth habitats will become favorable for harboring pathogenic biofilm and include (1) pits and fissures (Fig. 2.13); (2) the smooth enamel surfaces immediately gingival to the proximal contacts and in the gingival third of the facial and lingual surfaces of the clinical crown (Fig. 2.14); (3) root surfaces, particularly near the cervical line; and (4) subgingival areas (Fig. 2.15). These sites correspond to the locations where caries lesions are most frequently found.

Pits and Fissures

Pits and fissures are particularly susceptible surfaces for caries lesion initiation (Figs. 2.16, 2.17, 2.18, 2.19, 2.20; see also Figs. 2.13 to 2.15). The pits and fissures provide excellent mechanical shelter for organisms and harbor a community dominated by *S. sanguis* and other streptococci.[7] The relative proportion of MS most probably determines the cariogenic potential of the pit-and-fissure community. In susceptible patients, sealing the pits and fissures just after tooth eruption may be the most important strategy in their resistance to dental caries on those surfaces.

Smooth Enamel Surfaces

The proximal enamel surfaces immediately gingival to the contact area are the second most susceptible areas to dental caries lesions (Figs. 2.21 and 2.22; see also Figs. 2.14 and 2.19). These areas are protected physically and are relatively free from the effects of mastication, tongue movement, and salivary flow. The types and

TABLE 2.2	Oral Habitats[a]		
Habitat	**Predominant Species**	**Environmental Conditions Within Biofilm**	
Mucosa	S. mitis S. sanguis S. salivarius	Aerobic pH approximately 7 Oxidation-reduction potential positive	
Tongue	S. salivarius S. mutans S. sanguis	Aerobic pH approximately 7 Oxidation-reduction potential positive	
Teeth (noncarious)	S. sanguis	Aerobic pH 5.5 Oxidation-reduction negative	
Gingival crevice	Fusobacterium Spirochaeta Actinomyces Veillonella	Anaerobic pH variable Oxidation-reduction very negative	
Enamel caries	S. mutans	Anaerobic pH <5.5 Oxidation-reduction negative	
Dentin caries	S. mutans Lactobacillus	Anaerobic pH <5.5 Oxidation-reduction negative	
Root caries	Actinomyces	Anaerobic pH <5.5 Oxidation-reduction negative	

[a]The microenvironmental conditions in the habitats associated with host health are generally aerobic, near neutrality in pH, and positive in oxidation-reduction potential. Significant microenvironmental changes are associated with caries and periodontal disease. The changes are the result of the biofilm community metabolism.

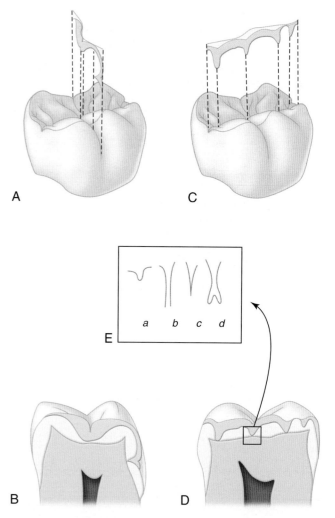

• **Fig. 2.13** Developmental pits, grooves, and fissures on the crowns of the teeth can have complex and varied anatomy. A and B, The facial developmental groove of the lower first molar often terminates in a pit. The depth of the groove and the pit varies. C and D, The central groove extends from the mesial pit to the distal pit. Sometimes grooves extend over the marginal ridges. E, The termination of pits and fissures may vary from a shallow groove (a) to complete penetration of the enamel (b). The end of the fissure may end blindly (c) or open into an irregular chamber (d). The physical nature of the pit and fissures allows for biofilm to remain stagnated. Additionally, the decreased thickness of enamel (and sometimes absence of enamel) at the bottom of the pit and fissure make these surfaces especially susceptible to dental caries.

numbers of organisms composing the proximal surface biofilm community vary. Important ecologic determinants for the biofilm community on the proximal surfaces are the topography of the tooth surface, the size and shape of the gingival papillae, and the oral hygiene and diet of the patient. A rough surface (caused by caries lesions, a poor-quality restoration, or a structural defect) restricts adequate biofilm removal. This situation favors the occurrence and progression of caries lesions and/or periodontal disease at the site.

Root Surfaces

The proximal root surface, particularly near the cementoenamel junction (CEJ), often is unaffected by the action of hygiene procedures such as flossing because it may have concave anatomic surface contours (fluting) and occasional roughness at the termination of the enamel. These conditions, when coupled with exposure to the oral environment (as a result of gingival recession), favor the formation of mature, cariogenic biofilm and proximal root-surface caries lesions. Likewise, the facial or lingual root surfaces

(particularly near the CEJ), when exposed to the oral environment (because of gingival recession), are often both neglected in hygiene procedures and usually not rubbed by the bolus of food. Consequently, these root surfaces also frequently harbor cariogenic biofilm. Root-surface caries lesions are more common in older patients because of niche availability and other factors sometimes associated with senescence, such as decreased salivary flow due to multiple medications and poor oral hygiene as a result of lowered manual dexterity and decreased motivation. Caries lesions originating on the root are alarming because they (1) have a comparatively rapid progression, (2) are often asymptomatic, (3) are closer to the pulp, and (4) are more difficult to restore.

Text continued on p. 58

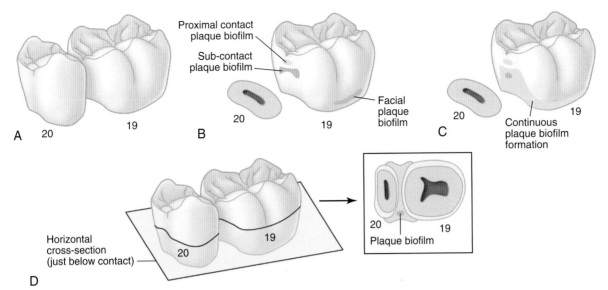

• **Fig. 2.14**   Biofilm formation on posterior teeth and associated caries lesions. A, Teeth No. 19 and 20 in contacting relationship. B, The crown of tooth No. 20 has been removed at the cervix. The proximal contact and subcontact biofilm can be seen on the mesial surface of tooth No. 19. The biofilm on the facial surfaces is illustrated. C, During periods of unrestricted growth, the biofilms on the mesial and facial surfaces become part of a continuous ring of biofilm around teeth. D, A horizontal cross section through teeth No. 19 and 20 with heavy biofilm. Inset shows the interproximal space below the contact area filled with gelatinous biofilm. This mass of interproximal biofilm concentrates the effects of biofilm metabolism on the adjacent tooth smooth surfaces. All interproximal surfaces are subject to biofilm accumulation and acid demineralization. In patients exposed to fluoridated water, most interproximal lesions become arrested at a stage before cavitation.

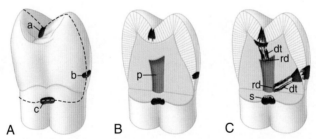

• **Fig. 2.15**   A, Caries lesions may originate at many distinct sites: pits and fissures *(a)*, smooth surface of crown *(b)*, and root surface *(c)*. Proximal surface lesion of crown is not illustrated here because it is a special case of smooth-surface lesion. Histopathology and progress of facial (or lingual) and proximal lesions are identical. Dotted line indicates cut used to reveal cross sections illustrated in *B* and *C*. Lesions illustrated here are intended to be representative of each type. No particular association between these lesions is implied. B, In cross section, the three types of lesions show different rates of progression and different morphology. Caries lesion progression and morphology follows the inclination of the enamel rods and/or dentinal tubules. Pit-and-fissure lesions have small sites of origin visible on the occlusal surface but have a wide base. Overall shape of a pit-and-fissure lesion is an inverted V. In contrast, a smooth-surface lesion is V shaped with a wide area of origin and apex of the V directed toward pulp *(p)*. Root caries begins directly on dentin. Root-surface lesions can progress rapidly because dentin is less resistant to caries attack. C, Although advanced caries lesions produce considerable histologic change in enamel, dentin and pulp changes in dentin can be seen even before the lesion reached the dentin. Bacterial invasion of lesion results in extensive demineralization and proteolysis of the dentin. Clinically, this necrotic dentin appears soft, wet, and mushy. Deeper pulpally, dentin is demineralized and is structurally intact. This tissue appears to be dry and leathery in texture. Two types of pulp–dentin response are illustrated. Under pit-and-fissure lesions and smooth-surface lesions, odontoblasts have died, leaving empty tubules called dead tracts *(dt)*. New odontoblasts have been differentiated from pulp mesenchymal cells. These new odontoblasts have produced reparative dentin *(rd)*, which seals off dead tracts. Another type of pulp–dentin reaction is sclerosis *(s)*—occlusion of the tubules by peritubular dentin. This is illustrated under root-caries lesion.

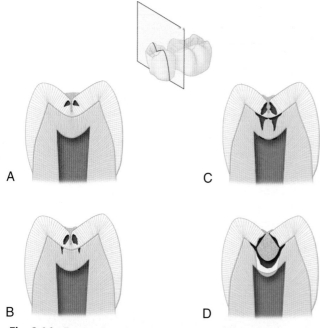

• **Fig. 2.16** Progression of caries in pits and fissures. A, Initial lesions develop on the lateral walls of the fissure. Demineralization follows the direction of the enamel rods, spreading laterally as it approaches the dentinoenamel junction (DEJ). B, Soon after the initial enamel lesion occurs, a reaction can be seen in the dentin and pulp. Forceful probing of the lesion at this stage can result in damage to the weakened porous enamel and accelerate the progression of the lesion. Clinical detection at this stage should be based on observation of discoloration and opacification of the enamel adjacent to the fissure. These changes can be observed by careful cleaning and drying of the fissure. C, Initial cavitation of the opposing walls of the fissure cannot be seen on the occlusal surface. Opacification can be seen that is similar to the previous stage. Remineralization of the enamel because of trace amounts of fluoride in the saliva may make progression of pit-and-fissure lesions more difficult to detect. D, Extensive cavitation of the dentin and undermining of the covering enamel darken the occlusal surface (see Fig. 2.17).

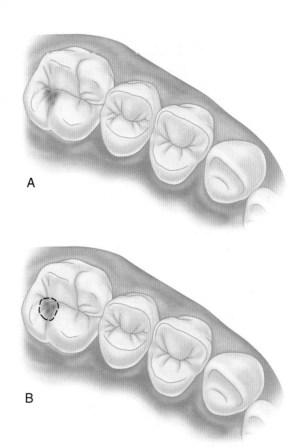

• **Fig. 2.17** A, Maxillar first molar has undermined discolored enamel owing to extensive pit-and-fissure caries. Note the dark shadow due to the dentin demineralization underneath the enamel. The lesion began as illustrated in Fig. 2.16 and has progressed to the stage illustrated in Fig. 2.16D. B, Discolored enamel is outlined by the broken line in the central fossa region.

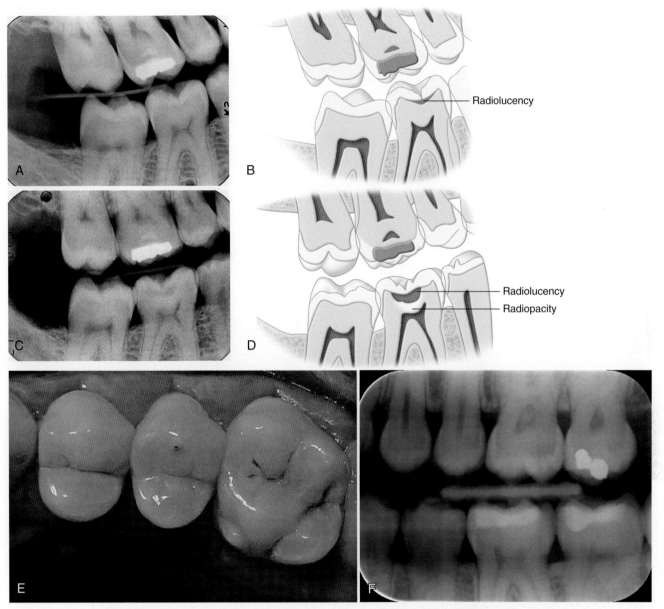

• **Fig. 2.18** Progression of pit-and-fissure caries. A, The mandibular right first molar (tooth No. 30) was sealed. Note radiolucent areas under the occlusal enamel in A and B. The sealant failed, and caries progressed slowly during the next 5 years; the only symptom was occasional biting-force pain. This underscores the need to monitor the sealant for failures. C and D, Note the extensive radiolucency under the enamel and an area of increased radiopacity below the lesion, suggesting sclerosis. Conversely, a well-sealed surface can prevent lesion progression. E and F, This maxillar first molar (tooth No. 14) with a shadow and a radiolucency indicative of dental caries was sealed as part of a clinical study.

Continued

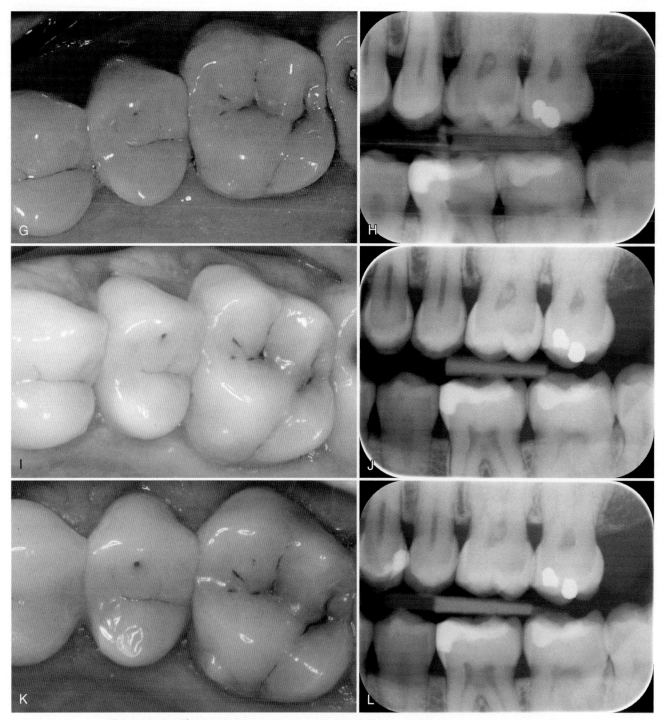

• **Fig. 2.18, cont'd**   G–J, The tooth was followed clinically and by bitewing radiographs over the next 8 years. K and L, No progression of the lesion was observed. (E–L, Courtesy Dr. Azam Bakhshandeh, Department of Odontology, Faculty of Health and Medical Sciences, University of Copenhagen, Department of Cariology, Endodontics, and Pediatric Dentistry, Copenhagen, Denmark.)

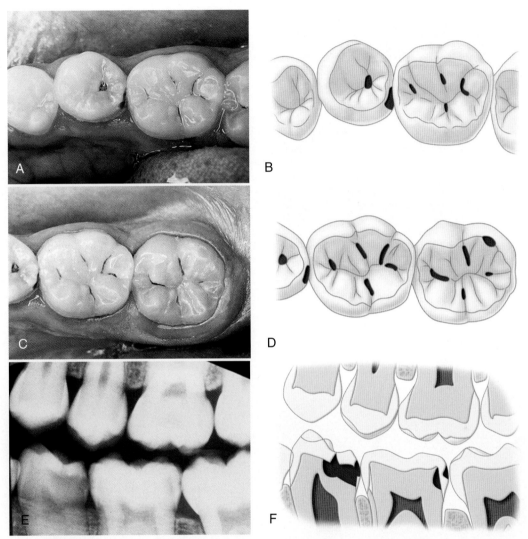

• **Fig. 2.19**   A young patient with extensive caries. A and B, The occlusal pits of the first molar and second premolar are carious. An interproximal caries lesion is seen on the second premolar. The second premolar is rotated almost 90 degrees, bringing the lingual surface into contact with the mesial surface of the first molar. Normally, the lingual surfaces of mandibular teeth are rarely affected by caries, but here tooth rotation makes the lingual surface a proximal contact and consequently produces an interproximal habitat, which increases the susceptibility of the surface to caries. C and D, The first and second molars have extensive caries lesions in the pits and fissures. E and F, On the bitewing radiograph, not only can the extensive nature of the caries lesion in the second premolar be seen but also seen is a lesion on the distal aspect of the first molar, which is not visible clinically. (Dark areas in B, D, and F indicate caries.)

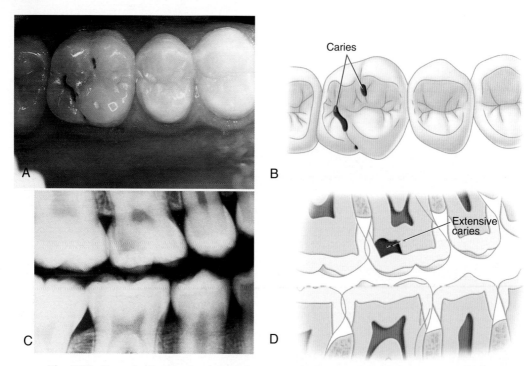

• **Fig. 2.20** Example of occlusal caries that has undermined enamel. Note the dark shadow from the dentin next to the stained fissure. A and B, Clinical example. C and D, A bitewing radiograph further confirms the extensive area of demineralization undermining the distofacial cusp.

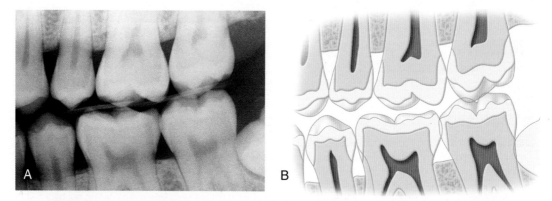

• **Fig. 2.21** Bitewing radiograph of normal teeth, free from caries. Note the uniform density of the enamel on the interproximal surfaces. A third molar is impacted on the distal aspect of the lower second molar. The interproximal bone levels are uniform and located slightly below the cementoenamel junctions, suggesting a healthy periodontium.

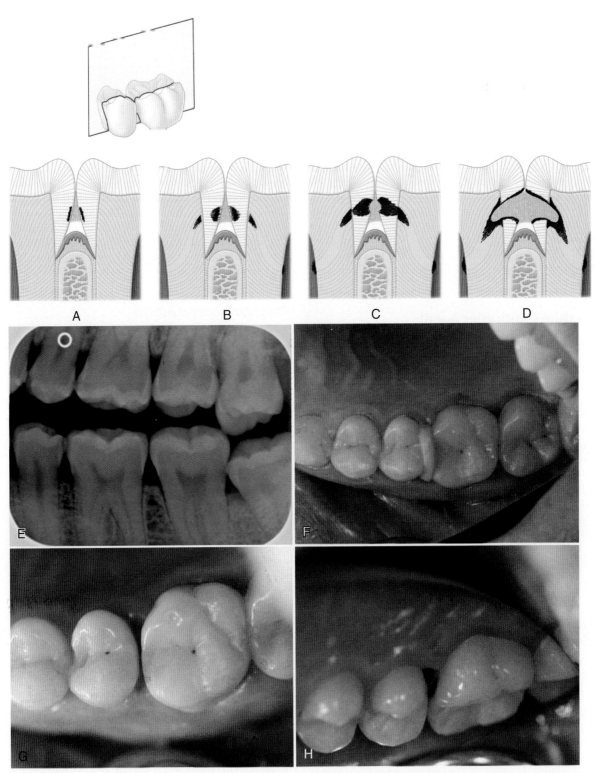

• **Fig. 2.22** Longitudinal sections (see inset for A) showing initiation and progression of caries on interproximal surfaces. A, Initial demineralization (indicated by the shading in the enamel) on the proximal surfaces is difficult to detect clinically or radiographically. The lesions develop right below the contact surface. Flossing of the interproximal area and thorough drying will allow for the best conditions to detect these lesions clinically. B, When proximal caries lesions first become detectable radiographically, the enamel surface is likely still to be intact. An intact surface is essential for successful remineralization and arrest of the lesion. Demineralization of the dentin (indicated by the shading in the dentin) occurs before cavitation of the surface of the enamel. Treatment designed to promote remineralization can be effective up to this stage. C, Cavitation of the enamel surface is a critical event in the caries process in proximal surfaces. After cavitation, lesion arrest becomes more difficult and virtually impossible in an interproximal surface contact. Restorative treatment to repair the damaged tooth surface is required. Cavitation can be diagnosed only by clinical observation. The use of a sharp explorer to detect cavitation is problematic because excessive force in application of the explorer tip during inspection of the proximal surfaces can damage weakened enamel and accelerate the caries process by iatrogenic cavitation. Separation of the teeth using orthodontic separators can be used to provide more direct visual inspection of suspect surfaces. Fiberoptic illumination although not specific for cavitation can facilitate detection; an orange shadow can be seen when lesions reach the dentin. D, Advanced cavitated lesions require prompt restorative intervention to prevent pulpal disease, limit tooth structure loss, and remove the nidus of infection of odontopathic organisms. E, Radiographic image showing radiolucency on distal of tooth No. 13 and mesial of tooth No. 14. F, An orthodontic separator was placed and left in place for 3 days. G, Clinical image of the teeth after separation. H, There was no evidence of cavitation on either surface.

Oral Hygiene and Its Role in the Dental Caries Process

Oral hygiene, accomplished primarily by proper tooth brushing and flossing, is another ecologic determinant of dental caries onset and activity. Careful mechanical cleaning of teeth disrupts the biofilm and leaves a clean enamel surface. The cleaning process does not destroy most of the oral bacteria but merely removes them from the surfaces of teeth. Large numbers of these bacteria subsequently are removed from the oral cavity during rinsing and/ or swallowing after flossing and brushing, but sufficient numbers remain to recolonize teeth. Some fastidious organisms and obligate anaerobes may be killed by exposure to oxygen during tooth cleaning; however, no single species is likely to be entirely eliminated. Although all the species that compose mature biofilm continue to be present, most of these are unable to initiate colonization on the clean tooth surface.

Saliva: Nature's Anticaries Agent

Saliva is an extremely important substance for the proper digestion of foods, and it also plays a key role as a natural anticaries agent (Table 2.3). The importance of saliva for oral health is dramatically noted after therapeutic radiation to the head and neck. After radiation, salivary glands become fibrotic and produce little or no saliva, leaving the patient experiencing an extremely dry mouth (xerostomia) (*xero*, dry; *stoma*, mouth), a condition termed *hyposalivation*. Such patients may experience near-total destruction of the teeth in just a few months after radiation treatment.[8,9] Patients that have autoimmune disease (e.g., Sjögren syndrome) also suffer from hyposalivation and experience severe xerostomia, and can experience the same devastating effects of hyposalivation on their dentition. In addition, many common medications are capable of reducing salivary flow and increasing caries risk (Table 2.4). Salivary protective mechanisms that maintain the normal oral flora and tooth surface integrity include bacterial clearance, direct antibacterial activity, buffers, and remineralization.[10]

Bacterial Clearance

Secretions from various salivary glands pool in the mouth to form whole or mixed saliva. The amount of saliva secreted varies greatly over time. When secreted, saliva remains in the mouth for a short time before being swallowed. While in the mouth, saliva lubricates oral tissues and bathes teeth and the biofilm. The secretion rate of saliva may have a bearing on dental caries susceptibility and calculus formation. Adults produce 1 to 1.5 L of saliva a day, very little of which occurs during sleep. The flushing effect of this salivary flow is, by itself, adequate to remove virtually all microorganisms not adherent to an oral surface. The flushing is most effective during mastication or oral stimulation, both of which produce large volumes of saliva. Large volumes of saliva also can dilute and buffer biofilm acids.

Direct Antibacterial Activity

Salivary glands produce an impressive array of antimicrobial products (see Table 2.3). Lysozyme, lactoperoxidase, lactoferrin, and agglutinins possess antibacterial activity. These salivary proteins are not part of the immune system but are part of an overall protection scheme for mucous membranes that occurs in addition to immunologic control. These protective proteins are present continuously at relatively uniform levels, have a broad spectrum of activity, and do not possess the "memory" of immunologic mechanisms. However, it is important to note that the normal resident oral flora apparently has developed resistance to most of these antibacterial mechanisms.

Although the antibacterial proteins in saliva play an important role in the protection of soft tissue in the oral cavity from infection by pathogens, they have little effect on dental caries because similar levels of antibacterial proteins can be found in caries-active and caries-free individuals.[11,12] It is suggested that dental caries susceptibility in healthy individuals is not related to saliva composition.

TABLE 2.3 Elements of Saliva That Control Biofilm Communities

Names	Action	Effects on Biofilm Community
Salivary Enzymes		
Amylase	Cleaves—1,4 glucoside bonds	Increases availability of oligosaccharides
Lactoperoxidase	Catalyzes hydrogen peroxide–mediated oxidation; adsorbs to hydroxyapatite in active form	Lethal to many organisms; suppresses biofilm formation on tooth surfaces
Lysozyme	Lyses cells by degradation of cell walls, releasing peptidoglycans; binds to hydroxyapatite in active conformation	Lethal to many organisms; peptidoglycans activate complement; suppresses biofilm formation on tooth surfaces
Lipases	Hydrolysis of triglycerides to free fatty acids and partial glycerides	Free fatty acids inhibit attachment and growth of some organisms
Nonenzyme Proteins		
Lactoferrin	Ties up free iron	Inhibits growth of some iron-dependent microbes
Secretory immunoglobulin A(IgA) (smaller amounts of IgM, IgG)	Agglutination of bacteria inhibits bacterial enzymes	Reduces numbers in saliva by precipitation; slows bacterial growth
Glycoproteins (mucins)	Agglutination of bacteria	Reduces numbers in saliva by precipitation

TABLE 2.4 Medications With Potential to Cause Hyposalivation or Dry Mouth (Xerostomia)

Action/Medication Group	Medicaments	Action/Medication Group	Medicaments
Sympathomimetic		**Anticholinergic, Dehydration**	
Antidepressants	Venlafaxine	Diuretics	Furosemide
	Duloxetine		Bumetanide
	Reboxetine		Torsemide
	Bupropion		Ethacrynic acid
Anticholinergic		**Sympathomimetic**	
Tricyclic antidepressants	Amitriptyline	Antihypertensive agents	Metoprolol
	Clomipramine		Moxonidine
	Amoxapine		Rilmenidine
	Protriptyline		
	Doxepin	Appetite suppressants	Fenfluramine
	Imipramine		Sibutramine
	Trimipramine		Phentermine
	Nortriptyline		
	Desipramine	Decongestants	Pseudoephedrine
Muscarinic receptor antagonists	Oxybutynin	Bronchodilators	Tiotropium
Alpha-receptor antagonists	Tamsulosin	Skeletal muscle relaxants	Tizanidine
	Terazosin	Antimigraine agents	Rizatriptan
		Synergistic Mechanism	
Antipsychotics	Promazine	Opioids, hypnotics	Opium
	Triflupromazine		Cannabis
	Mesoridazine		Tramadol
	Thioridazine		Diazepam
	Clozapine		
	Olanzapine	**Unknown**	
Antihistamines	Aziridine	H2 antagonists, proton pump inhibitors	Cimetidine
	Brompheniramine		Ranitidine
	Chlorpheniramine		Famotidine
	Cyproheptadine		Nizatidine
	Dexchlorpheniramine		Omeprazole
	Hydroxyzine		
	Phenindamine	Cytotoxic drugs	Fluorouracil
	Cetirizine	Anti-HIV drugs, protease inhibitors	Didanosine
	Loratadine		

Adapted from the Kois Center, Support Materials, Always Pages, http://koiscenter.com/store/supmatlist.aspx, accessed January 13, 2012.

Individuals with decreased salivary production (owing to illness, medication, or irradiation) may have significantly higher caries susceptibility (see Table 2.4).

Buffer Capacity

The volume and buffering capacity of saliva available to tooth surfaces have major roles in dental caries protection.[13] The buffering capacity of saliva is determined primarily by the concentration of bicarbonate ion. Buffering capacity can be estimated by titration techniques and may be a useful method for assessment of saliva in caries-active patients. Simple commercial kits are available for chairside tests. The benefit of the buffering is to reduce the potential for acid formation; however, in pathogenic biofilms there are highly compartmentalized clusters of acidic pH and neutral pH that make neutralization by saliva difficult.[210, 211]

In addition to buffers, saliva contains molecules that contribute to increasing biofilm pH. These include urea and sialin, the latter of which is a tetrapeptide that contains lysine and arginine. Hydrolysis of either of these basic compounds results in production of ammonia, causing the pH to increase.

Because saliva is crucial in controlling the oral flora and the mineral content of teeth, salivary testing should be done on patients with signs and symptoms of hyposalivation. Signs include lack of saliva pool on the floor of the mouth, gingivitis and mucositis (including burning mouth syndrome), cheilitis (inflammation and fissuring of the lips and/or the tongue), fissure in the soft mucosa, fungal infections in the mouth such as thrush, glossodynia (painful tongue), sialadenitis (salivary gland infection), saliva that seems thick and stringy, and several caries lesions especially in uncommon areas such as the lower central incisors. Symptoms include complaints of "cotton mouth" (xerostomia); bad breath; difficulty chewing, speaking, and swallowing; a changed sense of taste; and problems wearing dentures.

Remineralization

Saliva and biofilm fluid are supersaturated with calcium and phosphate ions. Without a means to control precipitation of these ions, the teeth literally would become encrusted with mineral deposits. Saliva contains statherin, a proline-rich peptide that stabilizes calcium and phosphate ions and prevents excessive deposition of these ions on teeth.[14] This supersaturated state of the saliva provides a constant opportunity for remineralizing enamel and can help protect teeth in times of cariogenic challenges.

Diet and Dental Caries

High-frequency exposure to fermentable carbohydrates such as sucrose may be the most important factor in producing cariogenic biofilm and ultimately caries lesions. Frequent ingestion of fermentable carbohydrates begins a series of changes in the local tooth environment, essentially changing the composition of the biofilm, thus favoring the growth of highly acidogenic bacteria that eventually leads to caries lesion formation (see Fig. 2.4). In contrast, when ingestion of fermentable carbohydrates is severely restricted or absent, biofilm growth typically does not lead to caries lesions. Dietary sucrose plays a leading role in the development of pathogenic biofilms and may be the most important factor in disruption of the normal healthy ecology of dental biofilm communities. Sucrose in particular allows the formation of extracellular polysaccharides, which render the biofilm viscous and sticky. Because the eventual metabolic product of cariogenic diet is acid, in addition to caries lesions the exposure to acidity from other sources (e.g., dried fruits, fruit drinks, or other acidic foods and drinks) also may result in dental erosion. The dietary emphasis must include all intakes that result in acidity, not just sucrose.

Clinical Characteristics of the Caries Lesion

As discussed, the caries lesion results from disequilibrium between the demineralization and remineralization processes. However, caries lesions appear in a variety of different clinical presentations depending on lesion location, severity, and progression rate or activity of the demineralization process, among other factors. Clinically, caries lesions can be present on various tooth surfaces, can be cavitated or noncavitated, active or inactive, and vary depending on their severity (initial, moderate, or severe). For a complete description of current caries classification criteria based on lesion severity and activity, see Chapter 3. The following sections will summarize these characteristics.

Clinical Sites for Caries Initiation

The characteristics of a caries lesion vary with the nature of the surface on which the lesion develops. There are three distinctly different clinical sites for caries lesion initiation: (1) developmental pits and fissures of enamel, which are the most susceptible sites; (2) smooth enamel surfaces that shelter cariogenic biofilm; and (3) root surfaces (see Fig. 2.15). Each of these areas has distinct surface morphology and environmental conditions. Consequently each area has a distinct biofilm population. The diagnosis, treatment, and prevention of these different lesion types should take into account the different etiologic factors operating at each site.

Pits and Fissures

Bacteria rapidly colonize the pits and fissures of newly erupted teeth. The type and nature of the organisms prevalent in the oral cavity determine the type of organisms colonizing pits and fissures and are instrumental in determining the outcome of the colonization. Large variations exist in the microflora found in pits and fissures, suggesting that each site can be considered a separate ecologic system. Numerous gram-positive cocci, especially *S. sanguis*, are found in the pits and fissures of newly erupted teeth, whereas

large numbers of MS usually are found in carious pits and fissures.

The shape of the pits and fissures contributes to their high susceptibility to caries lesion. The long, narrow fissure prevents adequate biofilm removal (see Fig. 2.13). Considerable morphologic variation exists in these structures. Some pits and fissures end blindly, others open near the dentin, and others penetrate entirely through the enamel.

Pit-and-fissure caries lesions typically "expand" as they penetrate into the enamel. The entry site may appear much smaller than the actual lesion, making clinical detection difficult. Caries lesions of pits and fissures develop from demineralization on their walls, known as *wall lesions* (see Fig. 2.16A–C). Progression of the dissolution of the walls of a pit-and-fissure lesion is similar in principle to that of the smooth-surface lesion because a wide susceptible surface area extends inward, paralleling the enamel rods. A lesion originating in a pit or fissure affects a greater area of the dentinoenamel junction (DEJ) than does a comparable smooth-surface lesion. In cross section, the gross appearance of a pit-and-fissure lesion is an inverted V with a narrow entrance and a progressively wider area of involvement closer to the DEJ (see Fig. 2.16D).

Smooth Enamel Surfaces

The smooth enamel surfaces of teeth present a less favorable site for cariogenic biofilm attachment. Cariogenic biofilm usually develops only on the smooth surfaces that are near the gingiva or are under proximal contacts. The proximal surfaces are particularly susceptible to caries lesion formation because of the extra shelter provided to resident cariogenic biofilm owing to the proximal contact area immediately occlusal to it (Fig. 2.22 and 2.23). Lesions starting on smooth enamel surfaces have a broad area of origin and a conical, or pointed, extension toward the DEJ. The path of ingress of the lesion is roughly parallel to the long axis of the enamel rods in the region. A cross section of the enamel portion of a smooth-surface lesion shows a V shape, with a wide area of origin and the apex of the V directed toward the DEJ. After the demineralization reaches the DEJ, when there is enamel cavitation and bacterial contamination, the bacterial metabolic activity within the lesion causes rapid dentin demineralization both laterally and pulpally (see Fig. 2.22).[142,143]

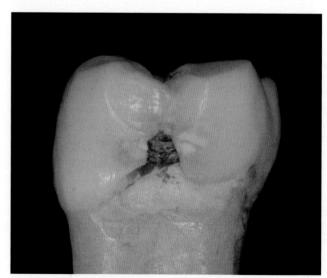

• **Fig. 2.23**   Extracted tooth showing extensive caries lesion just gingival to the proximal contact area. (Note the slightly "flat" contact area adjacent to marginal ridge.)

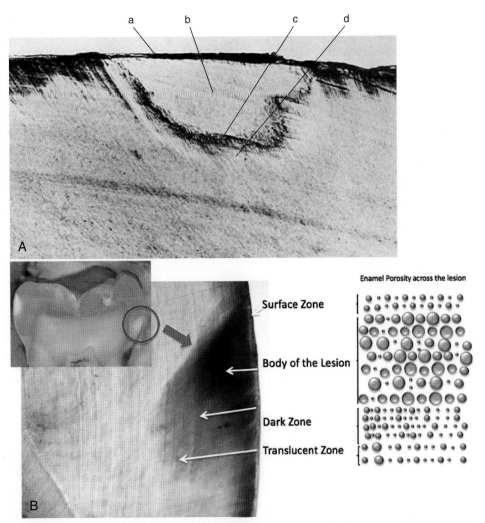

• **Fig. 2.24** A, Cross section of small caries lesion in enamel examined by transmitted light (100×). Surface *(a)* appears to be intact. Body of lesion *(b)* shows enhancement of striae of Retzius. Dark zone *(c)* surrounds body of lesion, whereas translucent zone *(d)* is evident over entire advancing front of lesion. B, The porosity of the lesion changes across the different zones. Thus a sharp explorer can easily penetrate the outer enamel and cause a small cavitation on an active lesion. (A, From Silverstone LM, et al. editors: *Dental caries,* London and Basingstoke, 1981, Macmillan, Ltd. Reproduced with permission of Palgrave Macmillan. B, Courtesy Dr. Masatoshi Ando.)

Root Surfaces

The root surface is rougher than enamel and readily allows cariogenic biofilm formation in the absence of good oral hygiene. The cementum covering the root surface is extremely thin and provides little resistance to caries lesion activity. In addition, the critical pH for dentin is higher than for enamel, so demineralization is likely to start even before the pH reaches the critical level for enamel (pH = 5.5). Root caries lesions have less well-defined margins than coronal caries lesions, tend to be U shaped in cross section, and progress more rapidly than coronal caries lesions because of the lack of protection from an enamel covering. In recent years, the prevalence of root caries has increased significantly because of the increasing number of older persons who retain more teeth, experience gingival recession, and usually have cariogenic biofilm on the exposed root surfaces.[15-18]

Caries Lesion Progression

The progression and morphology of the caries lesion vary depending on the site of origin and the conditions in the mouth (see Figs. 2.15, 2.16, and 2.22). The time for progression from a noncavitated caries lesion to a cavitated caries lesion on smooth surfaces is estimated to be 18 months (± 6 months).[19] Peak rates for the incidence of new lesions occur 3 years after the eruption of the tooth. Occlusal pit-and-fissure lesions develop in less time than smooth-surface caries lesions. Poor oral hygiene and frequent exposures to sucrose-containing or acidic food can produce noncavitated initial ("white spot") lesions (first clinical evidence of demineralization) in 3 weeks. Radiation-induced *hyposalivation* (dry mouth) can lead to development of caries lesions in 3 months from the onset of the radiation. Caries lesion progression in healthy individuals is usually slow compared with the progression in compromised persons.

Enamel Caries Lesions

An understanding of the enamel composition and histology is helpful to understand enamel caries histopathology (see Chapter 1; Figs. 2.24, 2.25, and 2.26). On clean, dry teeth the earliest evidence of caries lesion on the smooth enamel surface of a crown

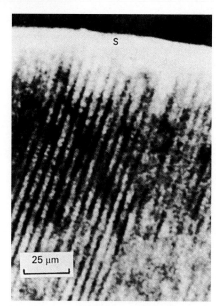

• **Fig. 2.25** Microradiograph (150×) of cross section of small caries lesion in enamel. Well-mineralized surface (s) is evident. Alternating radiolucent and radiopaque lines indicate demineralization between enamel rods. (From Silverstone LM, et al, editors: *Dental caries*, London and Basingstoke, 1981, Macmillan, Ltd. Reproduced with permission of Palgrave Macmillan.)

is the initial lesion or a "white spot" (Fig. 2.27; see also Figs. 2.2 and 2.3). These lesions usually are observed on the facial and lingual surfaces of teeth. Initial lesions are chalky white, opaque areas that are revealed only when the tooth surface is desiccated and are termed *noncavitated enamel caries lesions* or *initial lesions*. These areas of enamel lose their translucency because of the extensive subsurface porosity caused by demineralization. Care must be exercised in distinguishing white spots of initial caries lesions from developmental white spot hypocalcifications or other developmental defects of enamel. Initial (white spot) caries lesions partially or totally disappear visually when the enamel is hydrated (wet), whereas hypocalcified enamel is affected less by drying and wetting (Table 2.5). Hypocalcified enamel does not represent a clinical problem except for its potential esthetically objectionable appearance. The surface texture of an initial lesion is unaltered and is undetectable by tactile examination with an explorer. A more advanced lesion develops an irregular surface that is rougher than the unaffected, normal enamel. Softened chalky enamel that can be chipped away with an explorer is a sign of active caries. However, injudicious use of an explorer tip can cause actual cavitation in a previously noncavitated area, requiring, in most cases, restorative intervention. Similar initial lesions occur on the proximal smooth surfaces, although their detection by visual examination is more challenging. Tooth separation with orthodontic separators can facilitate visual

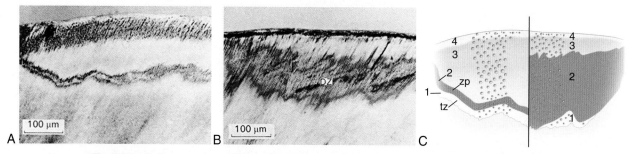

• **Fig. 2.26** A, Cross section of initial caries lesion in enamel examined in quinoline with polarized light (100×). Advancing front of lesion appears as a dark band below body of lesion. B, Same section after exposure to artificial calcifying solution examined in quinoline and polarized light. Dark zone (DZ) covers a much greater area after remineralization has occurred (100×). C, Schematic diagram of A and B. Left side indicates small extent of zones 1 and 2 before remineralization. Small circles indicate relative sizes of pores in each zone. Right side indicates increase in zone 2, the dark zone, after remineralization. This micropore system must have been created where previously the pores were much larger. (From Silverstone LM, et al, editors: *Dental caries*, London and Basingstoke, 1981, Macmillan, Ltd. Reproduced with permission of Palgrave Macmillan. *C* was redrawn.)

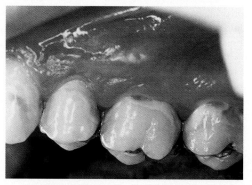
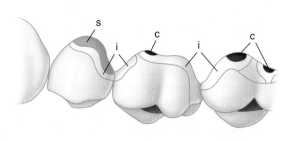

• **Fig. 2.27** Facial and lingual smooth-surface caries. This patient has high caries activity with rapidly advancing caries lesions. Cariogenic biofilm extends entirely around the cervical areas of the posterior teeth. Several levels of caries involvement can be seen, including cavitation (c); initial (noncavitated) white spot lesions (i); and stained, roughened, partially remineralized initial (noncavitated) lesions (s).

TABLE 2.5	Clinical Characteristics of Normal and Altered Enamel			
	Hydrated	**Desiccated**	**Surface Texture**	**Surface Hardness**
Normal Enamel	Translucent	Translucent	Smooth	Hard
Hypocalcified Enamel	Opaque	Opaque	Smooth	Hard
Active Initial Caries	Translucent (early lesions) Opaque (more established initial lesions)	Opaque Opaque	Rough Rough	Softened Softened
Arrested Initial Caries	Shiny and/or dark	Shiny and/or dark	Smooth	Hard
Active Moderate Caries	Opaque	Opaque	Rough	Softened
Arrested Moderate Caries	Shiny and/or dark	Shiny and/or dark	Smooth	Hard
Active Advanced Caries	Opaque	Opaque	Rough	Softened
Arrested Advanced Caries	Shiny and/or dark	Shiny and/or dark	Smooth	Leathery or hard

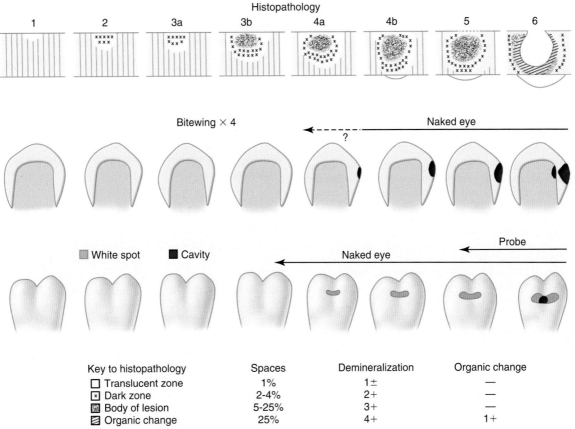

• **Fig. 2.28** Schematic representation of developmental stages of enamel caries lesion correlated with radiographic and clinical examination. Cavitation occurs late in development of the lesion. Before cavitation remineralization is possible, lesion arrest is possible at *any* stage given the right conditions. (Redrawn from Darling AI: The pathology and prevention of caries, *Br Dent J* 107:287–302, 1959. Reproduced by kind permission of the editor.)

examination of proximal tooth surfaces. Initial enamel lesions sometimes may be seen on radiographs as a faint radiolucency that is limited to the superficial enamel. When a proximal lesion is clearly visible radiographically, the lesion may have advanced significantly, and histologic alteration of the underlying dentin probably already has occurred, whether the lesion is cavitated or not (Fig. 2.28).

It has been shown experimentally and clinically that initial enamel caries lesions can remineralize[20,21] whether the dentin is involved or not. Table 2.5 and Table 2.6 list the characteristics of enamel at various stages of demineralization. Initial, noncavitated enamel lesions retain most of the original crystalline framework of the enamel rods, and the etched crystallites serve as nucleating agents for remineralization. Calcium and phosphate ions from

	Biofilm	Enamel Structure	Nonrestorative, Therapeutic Treatment (e.g., Remineralization, Antimicrobial, pH control)	Restorative Treatment
Normal Enamel	Normal	Normal	Not indicated	Not indicated
Hypocalcified Enamel	Normal	Abnormal, but not weakened	Not indicated	Only for esthetics
Noncavitated Caries	Cariogenic	Porous, weakened	Yes	Not indicated
Active Caries	Cariogenic	Cavitated, very weak	Yes	Yes
Inactive Caries	Normal	Remineralized, strong	Not indicated	Only for esthetics

TABLE 2.6 Clinical Significance of Enamel Lesions

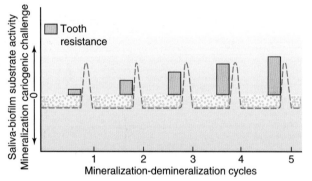

Local mechanism of enamel adaptation to the cariogenic challenge

• **Fig. 2.29** Diagrammatic representation of enamel adaptation reaction. Enamel interacts with its fluid environment in periods of undersaturation and supersaturation, presented here as periodic cycles. Undersaturation periods dissolve most soluble mineral at the site of cariogenic attack, whereas periods of supersaturation deposit most insoluble minerals if their ionic components are present in immediate fluid environment. As a result, under favorable conditions of remineralization, each cycle could lead toward higher enamel resistance to a subsequent challenge. (Redrawn from Koulouirides T: In Menaker L, editor: *The biologic basis of dental caries*, New York, 1980, Harper & Row.)

saliva can penetrate the enamel surface and precipitate on the highly reactive crystalline surfaces in the enamel lesion. The supersaturation of saliva with calcium and phosphate ions serves as the driving force for the remineralization process. Artificial and natural caries lesions of human enamel have been shown to regress to earlier histologic stages after exposure to conditions that promote remineralization. The presence of trace amounts of fluoride ions during this remineralization process greatly enhances the precipitation of calcium and phosphate, resulting in the remineralized enamel becoming more resistant to subsequent caries activity because of the incorporation of more acid-resistant fluorapatite (Fig. 2.29). Remineralized (arrested) lesions may be observed clinically as either intact, smooth white lesions or discolored, usually brown or black, spots (Fig. 2.30). The change in color is presumably caused by trapped organic debris and metallic ions within the enamel. These discolored, remineralized, arrested caries lesion areas are more resistant to subsequent caries activity than the adjacent unaffected enamel. They should not be restored unless they are esthetically objectionable.

Cavitated enamel lesions can be initially detected as subtle breakdown of the enamel surface. These lesions are very sensitive to probing and can be easily enlarged by using sharp explorers and excessive probing force. More advanced cavitated enamel lesions are more obviously detected as enamel breakdown. Although theoretically any caries lesion given the right conditions can be arrested and have their progression to larger lesions forestalled, once cavitation occurs removal of the biofilm is more difficult and many will require a sealant or restorative intervention. When the tooth surface cavitates, a more retentive site becomes available to the biofilm community. The cavitation of the tooth surface produces a synergistic acceleration of the growth of the cariogenic biofilm community and the expansion of the demineralization with ensuing expanded cavitation. This sheltered, highly acidic, and anaerobic environment provides an ideal niche for cariogenic bacteria. This situation results in a rapid and progressive destruction of the tooth structure.

Dentin Caries Lesions

An understanding of the dentin composition and histology is helpful to understand the histopathology of dentin caries lesions (see Chapter 1; Fig. 2.31). Progression of dental caries in dentin is different from progression in enamel because of the structural differences of dentin (Figs. 2.32, 2.33, and 2.34; see also Fig. 2.31). Dentin contains much less mineral and possesses microscopic tubules that provide a pathway for the ingress of bacteria and egress of minerals.

When enamel demineralization advances to the DEJ, rapid lateral expansion of the caries lesion along the DEJ may occur if there is bacterial contamination. This process is still poorly understood, but it likely occurs only when there is enamel cavitation. For many years this "lateral spread" has been attributed to the DEJ's lower mineral content compared to primary dentin.[137] More recently, it has been shown that a high concentration of MMPs is found at the DEJ. MMPs are implied in dentin caries lesion progression, although this may be a host defense mechanism and not necessarily linked to an increase in caries susceptibility.[138] What is known is that the increased susceptibility to demineralization observed at the DEJ on lesions that have reached dentin is a result of bacterial metabolic activity within the dentinal lesion.[139-141]

Increasing demineralization of the body of the enamel lesion results in the weakening and eventual collapse of the surface enamel. The resulting cavitation provides an even more protective and retentive habitat for the cariogenic biofilm, accelerating the progression of the lesion. The DEJ provides less resistance to the carious process than either enamel or dentin. The dentin contamination by bacterial metabolites leads to the lateral spread of the lesion at

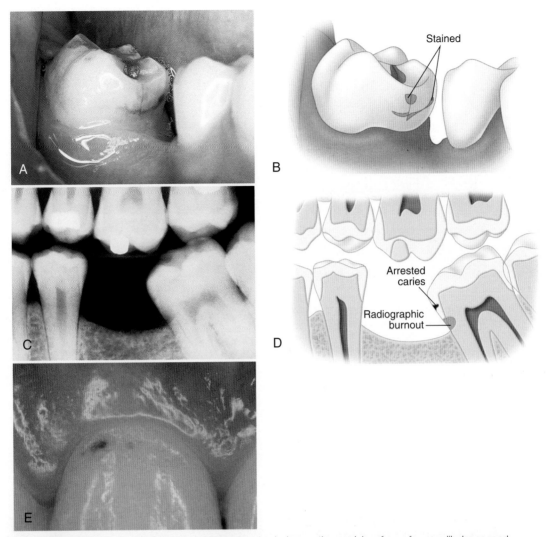

• **Fig. 2.30** A and B, Example of arrested caries lesion on the mesial surface of a mandibular second molar. The area below the proximal contact (A and B, mirror view of tooth No. 18) is partly opaque and stained. Clinically the surface is hard and intact, yet the area is more radiolucent than the enamel above or below the stain. C and D, In a different clinical case, caries diagnosis based only on the radiograph would lead to a false-positive diagnosis (i.e., caries lesion present when it is not). The radiolucency is caused by the broad area of subsurface demineralization that extends from the facial to the lingual line angles. The x-ray beam was directed parallel to the long axis of demineralization and consequently produced a sharply demarcated zone of radiolucency in the enamel. This example illustrates the shortcomings of radiographic diagnosis. Were there not visual access to the mesial surface of the second molar, it would be easy to diagnose active caries incorrectly and consequently restore the tooth. E, Cavitated inactive (arrested) enamel caries lesion on the cervical one third of a central incisor of a 27-year-old patient with low caries risk. This lesion, if not esthetically offensive, does not require a restoration and should be monitored.

the DEJ, producing the characteristic second cone of caries activity in dentin (see Figs. 2.16 and 2.22).[143] Figs. 2.31, 2.35, 2.36, 2.37, and 2.38 illustrate advanced lesions with soft, infected dentin. Because of these characteristics, dentin caries is **V** shaped in cross section with a wide base at the DEJ and the apex directed pulpally. Caries lesions advance more rapidly in dentin than in enamel because dentin provides much less resistance to acid demineralization owing to less mineralized content and the presence and orientation of the dentinal tubules.

The dental caries process produces a variety of responses in dentin including pain, sensitivity, demineralization, and remineralization. Often pain is not reported even when caries lesions invade dentin except when deep lesions bring the bacterial infection close to the pulp. Episodes of short-duration pain may be felt occasionally during earlier stages of dentin caries lesion progression. The pain is caused by stimulation of pulp tissue by the rapid movement of fluid through the dentinal tubules that have been opened to the oral environment by cavitation. When bacterial invasion of the dentin is close to the pulp, toxins and possibly a few bacteria enter the pulp, resulting in inflammation of the pulpal tissues, increased pulpal pressure, and thus pulpal pain.

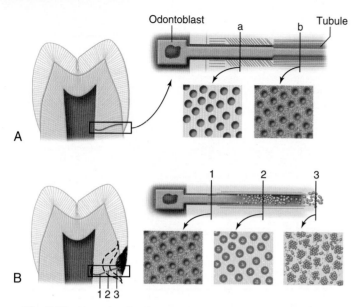

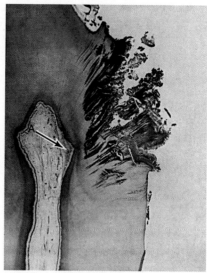

• **Fig. 2.31** Normal and carious dentin. A, Normal dentin has characteristic tubules that follow a wavy path from the external surface of dentin, below enamel or cementum, to the inner surface of dentin in the pulp tissue of the pulp chamber or pulp canal. Dentin is formed from the external surface and grows inward. As dentin grows, odontoblasts become increasingly compressed in the shrinking pulp chamber, and the number of associated tubules becomes more concentrated per unit area. The more recently formed dentin near the pulp (a) has large tubules with little or no peritubular dentin and calcified intertubular dentin filled with collagen fibers. Older dentin, closer to the external surface (b), is characterized by smaller, more widely separated tubules and a greater mineral content in intertubular dentin. The older dentin tubules are lined by a uniform layer of mineral termed *peritubular dentin*. These changes occur gradually from the inner surface to the external surface of the dentin. Horizontal lines indicate predentin; diagonal lines indicate increasing density of minerals; darker horizontal lines indicate densely mineralized dentin and increased thickness of peritubular dentin. The transition in mineral content is gradual, as indicated in Fig. 2.25. B, Carious dentin undergoes several changes. The most superficial infected zone of carious dentin (3) is characterized by bacteria filling the tubules and granular material in the intertubular space. The granular material contains very little mineral and lacks characteristic cross-banding of collagen. As bacteria invade dentinal tubules, if carbohydrates are available, they can produce enough lactic acid to remove peritubular dentin. This doubles or triples the outer diameter of the tubules in infected dentin zone. Pulpal to (below) the infected dentin is a zone where the dentin appears transparent in mounted whole specimens. This zone (2) is the advancing demineralization front, affected carious dentin, and is characterized by loss of mineral in the intertubular and peritubular dentin. Many crystals can be detected in the lumen of the tubules in this zone. The crystals in the tubule lumen render the refractive index of the lumen similar to that of the intertubular dentin, making the zone transparent. Normal dentin (1) is found pulpal to (below) transparent dentin.

• **Fig. 2.32** Cross section of demineralized specimen of advanced caries in dentin. Reparative dentin (A) can be seen adjacent to the most advanced portion of lesion. (From Boyle P: *Kornfeld's histopathology of the teeth and their surrounding structures*, Philadelphia, 1955, Lea & Febiger.)

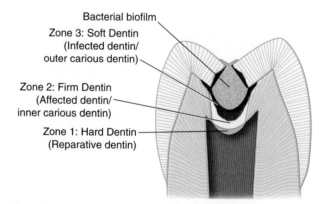

• **Fig. 2.33** Cross section of occlusal caries. The occlusal enamel appears intact, with a small opening in the occlusal fissure. Enamel is darkened where it is undermined by demineralization. The surface of enamel may not be clinically cavitated, but usually some discoloration is observed at the entrance of the fissure. The lesion is filled with a bacterial plug containing high numbers of MS and lactobacilli. When there is a break in the enamel, the dentin underneath the enamel will be highly contaminated below the plug. Deeper dentin is not as heavily contaminated but is extensively demineralized. Reparative dentin is being formed below the lesion.

The pulp–dentin complex reacts to caries activity by attempting to initiate remineralization and blocking of the open tubules. These reactions result from odontoblastic activity and the physical process of demineralization and remineralization. The pulp–dentin complex reaction occurs even before the lesion has reached the dentin. Dentin can react defensively (by repair) to low-intensity and moderate-intensity caries lesion progression as long as the pulp remains vital and has adequate blood circulation. Dentin reaction can happen through remineralization of intertubular dentin and apposition of peritubular dentin or by reparative dentin, as described in the next paragraphs.

In slowly advancing caries lesions, a vital pulp can repair demineralized dentin by remineralization of the intertubular dentin and by apposition of peritubular dentin. Initial stages of caries lesions or mild caries activity produce long-term, low-level acid demineralization of dentin. Direct exposure of the pulp tissue to microorganisms is not a prerequisite for an inflammatory response. Toxins and other metabolic by-products, especially hydrogen ion,

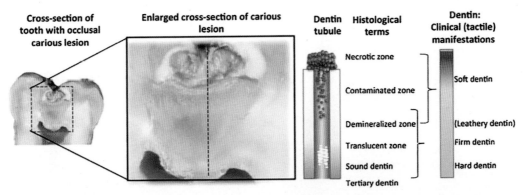

• **Fig. 2.34** A cross section of a caries lesion in dentin and the histologic and clinical manifestations (adapted from Ogawa et al, 1983). The most superficial outer layer of dentin is heavily contaminated, necrotic, with irreversible demineralization and denatured collagen fibers. Clinically this is very soft, wet dentin. This soft, contaminated layer gets progressively harder as the dentin approaches the pulp. The still demineralized dentin (formerly affected dentin) can feel leathery to the touch or firm, but not as hard as sound dentin or tertiary dentin (closest to the pulp, dentin formed in reaction to the caries process). During caries excavation, the goal is to remove only the soft, outer carious dentin (infected dentin), while the inner carious dentin (affected dentin) is remineralizable and can be maintained. (For orientation of layers on tooth, see Fig 2.35.) (Modified from Ogawa K, Yamashita Y, Ichijo T, et al: The ultrastructure and hardness of the transparent layer of human carious dentin. *J Dent Res* 62(1):7–10, 1983.)

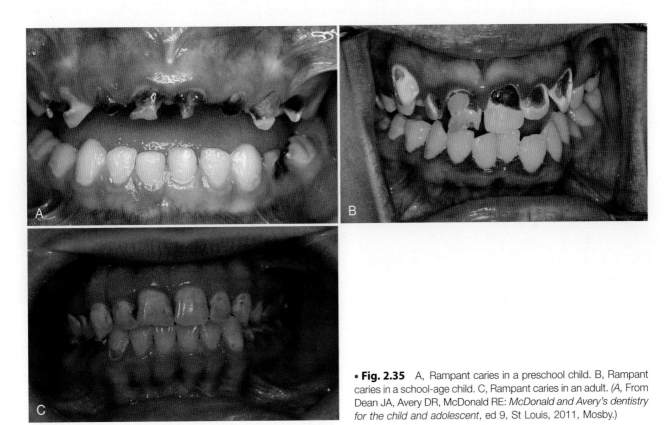

• **Fig. 2.35** A, Rampant caries in a preschool child. B, Rampant caries in a school-age child. C, Rampant caries in an adult. (*A,* From Dean JA, Avery DR, McDonald RE: *McDonald and Avery's dentistry for the child and adolescent,* ed 9, St Louis, 2011, Mosby.)

can penetrate via the dentinal tubules to the pulp. Even when the lesion is limited to enamel, the pulp can be shown to respond with inflammatory cells.[22,23] Dentin responds to the stimulus of its first caries demineralization episode by deposition of crystalline material from the intertubular dentin in the lumen of the tubules in the advanced demineralization front (formally called affected dentin) (see Figs. 2.31 and 2.34). The refractive index of the dentin changes and the intertubular dentin with more mineral content

than normal dentin is termed *sclerotic dentin.* The apparent function of the sclerotic dentin is to wall off a lesion by blocking (sealing) the tubules. The permeability of sclerotic dentin is greatly reduced compared with that of normal dentin because of the decrease in the tubule lumen diameter.[24] Hypermineralized areas may be seen on radiographs as zones of increased radiopacity (often S shaped, following the course of the tubules) ahead of the advancing, infected portion of the lesion. Sclerotic dentin formation may also be seen

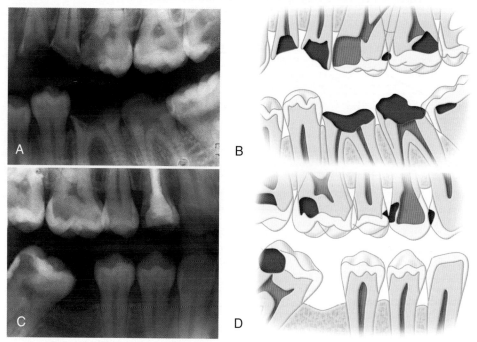

Dark areas indicate caries

• **Fig. 2.36** Rampant caries in a 21-year-old man. Although occlusal and interproximal lesions exist in the patient, the progress of the occlusal lesions produced the most tooth destruction. The potential for developing occlusal lesions could have been reduced by earlier application of sealants. This extensive amount of caries was the result of the patient's excessive fear of bad breath. In an attempt to keep his breath smelling fresh, he kept sugar-containing breath mints in his mouth most of the day. (Dark areas in B and D indicate caries.)

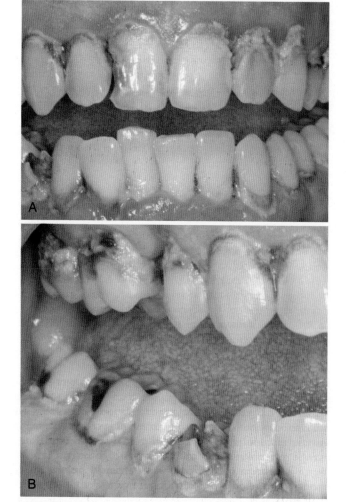

• **Fig. 2.37** Acute, rampant caries in both anterior (A) and posterior (B) teeth.

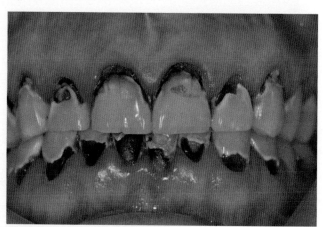

• **Fig. 2.38** Advance cavitated active caries lesions on a 35-year-old patient with high caries risk. (Courtesy Dr. Ayesha Swarn, DDS, Operative Dentistry Graduate Program at UNC School of Dentistry.)

under an old restoration. Sclerotic dentin is usually shiny and darker in color but feels hard to the explorer tip. By contrast, normal, freshly cut dentin lacks a shiny, reflective surface and allows some penetration from a sharp explorer tip. This repair by sclerotic dentin occurs only if the tooth pulp is vital.

When these affected tubules become completely occluded by the mineral precipitate, they appear clear when a histologic section of the tooth is evaluated. This portion of dentin has been termed *translucent dentin* (see Zones of Dentinal Caries Lesions) and is the result of mineral loss in the intertubular dentin and precipitation of this mineral in the tubule lumen. Consequently, translucent dentin is softer than normal dentin (see Fig. 2.34)[25] and is called "firm" (affected) dentin, in contrast to sound dentin that is "hard" dentin.

More intense caries activity results in bacterial invasion of dentin. The most superficial (closer to the tooth surface) zone of the carious dentin is the necrotic zone. This very soft (infected) dentin contains a wide variety of pathogenic materials or irritants, including high acid levels, hydrolytic enzymes, bacteria, and bacterial cellular debris. These materials can cause the degeneration and death of odontoblasts and their tubular extensions below the lesion and a mild inflammation of the pulp. The pulp may be irritated sufficiently from high acid levels or bacterial enzyme production to cause the formation (from undifferentiated mesenchymal cells) of replacement odontoblasts (secondary odontoblasts). These cells produce reparative dentin (reactionary or tertiary dentin) on the affected portion of the pulp chamber wall (see Figs. 2.31B and 2.33). This dentin is different from the normal dentinal apposition that occurs throughout the life of the tooth by primary (original) odontoblasts. The structure of reparative dentin varies from well-organized tubular dentin (less often) to very irregular atubular dentin (more often), depending on the severity of the stimulus. Reparative dentin is an effective barrier allowing limited diffusion of material through the tubules and is an important step in the repair of dentin. Severe stimuli also can result in the formation within the pulp chamber of unattached dentin, termed *pulp stones*, in addition to reparative dentin.

The success of dentinal reparative responses, either by remineralization of intertubular dentin and apposition of peritubular dentin or by reparative dentin, depends on the severity of the caries challenge and the ability of the pulp to respond. The pulpal blood supply may be the most important limiting factor to the pulpal responses. Acute, rapidly advancing caries lesions with high levels of acid production overpower host defenses of the pulp and result in infection, abscess, and death of the pulp. Compared with other oral tissues, the pulp is poorly tolerant of inflammation. Small, localized infections in the pulp produce an inflammatory response involving capillary dilation, local edema, and stagnation of blood flow. Because the pulp is contained in a sealed chamber, and its blood is supplied through narrow root canals, any stagnation of blood flow can result in local anoxia and necrosis. The local necrosis leads to more inflammation, edema, and stagnation of blood flow in the immediately adjacent pulp tissue, which becomes necrotic in a cascading process that rapidly spreads to involve the entire pulp.

Maintenance of pulp vitality depends on the adequacy of pulpal blood supply. Recently erupted teeth with large pulp chambers and short, wide canals with large apical foramina have a much more favorable prognosis for surviving pulpal inflammation than fully formed teeth with small pulp chambers and small apical foramina.

Zones of Dentin Caries Lesions

Although enamel and dentin have distinct characteristics, the reaction observed in dentin is a direct response of the pulp to external insults to the enamel.[133] Since enamel is a microporous solid, stimuli in the tooth surface are transmitted to the pulp. The first defense of the pulp is tubular sclerosis, which consists of mineral deposition in the peritubular dentin and in the dentinal tubule's lumen. Wear and age can also cause tubular sclerosis. This process only occurs in vital pulps. Caries progression in dentin proceeds through three changes: (1) Weak organic acids demineralize dentin and expose its organic matrix; (2) the organic matrix of dentin, particularly collagen, is denatured and degraded; and (3) the loss of matrix structural integrity is followed by invasion of bacteria. Three different zones of dentin have been described in moderate and advanced caries lesions (see Figs. 2.33 and 2.35):

- **Soft Dentin (formerly infected dentin).** Also called *outer carious dentin*, soft (infected) dentin is primarily characterized by bacterial contamination. This is the carious dentin closer to the tooth surface, characterized by the presence of bacteria, low mineral content, and irreversibly denatured collagen. Histologically this zone may be referred to as *necrotic* and *contaminated*. While soft dentin typically does not self-repair, the advance front of the soft dentin zone (near firm dentin) is characterized by superficial bacterial invasion and the caries process can still be stalled when a good restorative seal is obtained. Clinically, soft dentin lacks structure and can be easily excavated with hand and rotary instrumentation.

- **Firm Dentin (formerly affected dentin).** Also called *inner carious dentin*, firm (affected) dentin is primarily characterized by demineralization of intertubular dentin and of initial formation of intratubular fine crystals at the advancing front of the caries lesion. As the tubule lumen becomes filled with minerals it will give a "transparent" appearance in a section observed in a light microscope. Histologically this zone may be referred to as *demineralized*. Because of the caries demineralization process, firm dentin is softer than hard, normal dentin. Although organic acids attack the mineral and organic contents of dentin, the collagen cross-linking remains intact in this zone and can serve as a template for remineralization of intertubular dentin. Therefore, provided that the pulp remains vital, firm (affected) dentin is remineralizable. Clinically, firm dentin is resistant to hand excavation and can only be removed by exerting pressure. The transition between soft and firm dentin can have a leathery texture, particularly in slowly advancing lesions, and has been called *leathery dentin*. Clinically, leathery dentin does not deform upon pressure from an instrument but can be excavated with hand instruments such as spoons and curette without much pressure.

- **Hard Dentin.** Hard dentin represents the deepest zone of a caries lesion—assuming the lesion has not yet reached the pulp—and may include *tertiary dentin, sclerotic dentin, and normal (or sound) dentin*. Clinically this dentin is hard, cannot be easily penetrated with a blunt explorer, and can only be removed by a bur or a sharp cutting instrument. (See definitions in Box 2.1 for histologic characteristics of hard, tertiary, and sclerotic dentin.)

These dentin caries zones are most clearly distinguished in slowly advancing lesions. In rapidly progressing caries lesions (see Figs. 2.36, 2.37, and 2.38), the difference between the zones becomes less distinct.

Caries Risk Assessment and Management

Although it is very important to detect caries lesions, caries detection and caries diagnosis are not exclusively a tooth-centered process.

It is critical to remember that clinicians treat the entire patient and not just individual teeth and caries lesions. As noted earlier in this chapter, dental caries is a multifactorial medical disease process, and the caries lesions are the expression of a disease process that involves the patient as a whole. Equally important in the management of the caries disease is the ability to individualize caries diagnosis and treatment or interventions for each patient. To do this, the clinician must formulate a caries risk assessment profile that is based on the individual patient's current risk factors and risk indicators. A *risk factor* is defined as an environmental, behavioral, or biologic factor that directly increases the probability that a disease will occur and the absence or removal of which reduces the possibility of disease.[37,38] Risk factors are part of the causal chain of the disease process, or they expose the host to the causal chain; but once the disease occurs, removal of a risk factor may not always result in the disease process being halted. Any definition of risk factor must clearly establish that the exposure has occurred before the outcome or before the conditions are established that make the outcome likely. This means that longitudinal studies are necessary to demonstrate risk factors. Terms such as *risk indicators* and *risk markers* are also used in the caries literature to refer to risk factors, putative risk factors, or something else entirely. *Risk indicators* may refer to existing signs of the disease process, or signs that the disease process has occurred, but are not part of the disease causal chain. For example, existing caries lesions would be risk indicators, as they indicate a risk status, but are not per se part of the causal chain so they are not risk factors. Multiple risk factors (and indicators) have been studied, reviewed, and validated in the assessment of risk for development of future caries disease, but caries risk assessment is not an exact science. Because caries is a complex multifactorial disease, no single risk factor (or indicator, or marker) is highly predictive of future caries. However, caries risk assessment is necessary to identify what (if any) interventions are needed to lower the patient's caries risk and activity—which is the ultimate goal of caries management when using the medical model.[39,40] A discussion of different risk factors will be included in this section of the chapter.

Caries risk assessments are specific for adults and adolescents older than 6 years and for children under 6 years of age. It is very important to spend time with the patient to uncover all relevant risk factors and indicators currently present. Some risk and protective factors can be adjusted and modified by either the patient or the clinician, such as sucrose intake and fluoride exposure; other risk factors are not easily modifiable, such as hyposalivation as the result of a needed medication or an existing condition such as Sjögren syndrome. Understanding and controlling risk factors and protective factors can be very important in the prevention of new caries lesion formation and to slow or arrest the progression of existing caries lesions.

No consensus exists on exactly how to define the risk categories for caries risk assessments. Examples of terms used to describe risk assessment are "at risk," "low risk," "medium risk," "high risk," and "extreme risk." Assignment of these terms is typically based on the subjective judgment of the clinician with general rules applied, based on the clinician's previous clinical experiences and training. If a clinician finds no detectable or active caries lesions and minimum or no identifiable risk factors, that patient would be assigned a *low caries risk*. In this situation, in the current state of the patient's health, the protective factors for not developing caries lesions outweigh the risk factors that could lead to new caries lesions. The strongest predictor for caries risk for patients in the *at-risk* and *high-risk* categories are the number of caries lesions being detected for the patient over the last 2 to 3 years along with past history of caries lesions in the patient's lifetime.[39]

Historically, dentistry has used a surgical model for dental caries management, which mainly contemplated the biomechanical excision (removal, excavation) of caries lesions and the restoration of the resultant *tooth preparation* to form and function with a restorative material. Management of caries disease by a surgical model consisted of detecting cavitations and "treating" them with excavation and restorations. Eventually it became apparent that dealing only with the end result of the disease and not addressing its etiology for each individual patient was not successful in controlling the caries disease process. Since surgical management alone was not successful, a system has been developed using caries management strategies. This system looks at individualized caries risk assessments and uses this information to design treatment plans according to the risk assessment findings. These assessments look at each patient's unique set of pathologic and protective factors. *Caries management by risk assessment* (CAMBRA) represents a management philosophy that manages the caries disease process using a medical model. This process provides an individualized evaluation of a patient's pathologic factors and protective factors and assesses the patient's risk for developing future disease. The risk assessment is then used to develop an *individualized* evidence-based caries management plan that involves aspects of nonsurgical therapeutics and dental surgical interventions. Both risk assessment and patient-centered interventions are based on the concept of caries balance as discussed earlier in this chapter (see Fig. 2.1). The caries balance model is based on minimizing pathologic factors while maximizing protective factors to attain a balance that favors no disease occurring, or health. With the use of CAMBRA for patient management, mounting evidence suggests that early damage to teeth may be reversed and that the incidence of disease manifestations can be significantly reduced or prevented. CAMBRA is a concept that has gained interest in the United States, and is evolving into the standard of care in caries management.[4,41,144,145] Additionally, the International Caries Classification and Management System (ICCMS)[146-148] has endeavored to merge caries detection and assessment with an individualized management plan. Another caries risk assessment method that has been validated for children is the Cariogram.[149,150]

Caries Risk Assessment

The clinical examination process for diagnosis and detection of caries lesions is discussed in detail in Chapter 3. The caries risk assessment is an important part of this overall process of patient care. The clinician must gather all appropriate data from both the interview with the patient and the clinical examination for caries detection to formulate an individualized caries risk assessment. Part of the caries risk assessment identifies the risk (causative) factors, but does not predict the caries outcome. Risk factors can exist for a patient without the disease being expressed at the time of the examination. The predictive model part of the risk assessment looks at the assessment of caries progression in the future. Risk factors are associated with the variables that have value for prediction purposes, which means that the risk factor is present *before* the disease occurs. As discussed, risk indicators are existing signs of the disease process. They are examples of what is happening with the patient's current state of oral health, not how disease occurred. Risk indicators are clinical observations and detection modalities used to identify risk-level status. Examples include visible cavitations in pits and fissures or in proximal surfaces of teeth, brown spots, active initial lesions, or cavitated lesions on free smooth surfaces, as well as any restorations in the past 3 years. The ideal caries risk assessment method should be inexpensive and easy to use but at the same time have high predictive value. It should be valuable in decision making for caries management in the use of nonsurgical therapeutics and surgical interventions that serve the patient in a cost-effective and health-promoting manner.

One of the roles of caries risk assessment in caries management is to assist in determining the current caries lesion activity. Caries lesions may be detected significantly before frank cavitation occurs. The diagnosis of caries lesions should include whether they are actively progressing. An inactive lesion may be visible clinically or radiographically; however, it may not be active or progressing over time. With a positive shift in protective factors, change in oral hygiene, or reduction of pathologic factors, it is possible for caries lesions to change in density, size, hardness, and clinical appearance. These inactive lesions are arrested and may not require operative intervention. Assessment by the clinician of all the pathologic and protective factors in the patient's current history will greatly aid in the decision regarding current activity. A thorough risk assessment allows for a more predictive analysis of current and future disease activity and assists in deciding on nonsurgical or surgical interventions. Caries risk assessment helps the clinician to identify the etiologic causes of the disease for a specific patient at a specific point in time, and to determine the frequency and treatment protocols for patient follow-up visits. Restorative decisions in terms of material used and cavity preparation design are also influenced by the information gathered in the risk assessment process. The data gathered establish an important baseline for use in future reassessments to help the clinician and the patient measure the effectiveness of the caries management treatment protocol used for the patient. The systematic use of risk assessment profiles is essential in uncovering risk factors that are present before disease manifestation. This information may be useful in the prevention of caries lesions in patients who have risk factors present but no disease expression and then experience a lifestyle change that adds additional risk factors. The new risk factors then become a tipping point for the caries balance equation toward disease expression. For instance, a patient who frequently consumes high-sugar soft drinks during the day (risk factor) suddenly is prescribed a hyposalivation-inducing medication (additional risk factor) that increases caries risk. The informed patient would have the option of making the decision to eliminate a modifiable risk factor (soft drinks) before expression of the disease and before the introduction of the hyposalivation-inducing medication considering this risk assessment.

The incorporation of risk assessments in routine patient care and in each patient's caries management program is necessary because of the multifactorial nature of the caries disease. No one factor is able to predict the probability of a patient developing caries lesions. When developing a preventive and restorative caries management plan, consideration of the whole patient is essential to successful outcomes. In addition, recorded specific risk assessment profiles provide patients with an educational tool that empowers them to be an important part of managing their disease. Finally, risk assessments provide a means for both the clinician and the patient to monitor and measure the proposed caries management protocols over time and evaluate and adjust the protocols as needed. Risk assessments lead to better treatment outcomes for patients.

Knowing certain factors pertaining to the patient's history is key in establishing a caries risk assessment. Factors that have been identified as contributing to caries risk include age, gender, fluoride exposure, home care, smoking habits, alcohol intake, medications, dietary habits, economic and educational status, and general health. Increased smoking, alcohol consumption, use of medications, and sucrose intake result in increased risk for caries development.[42] Children and older adults have increased risks. Decreased fluoride exposure, lower economic status, and lower educational attainment also increase risk. Poor general health also increases the risk. A strong body of evidence suggests that past caries experience is the best predictor of future caries activity.[43] Information that is important and obtained in the patient history interview would be biologic and environmental factors that include, but are not limited to, medical history including current and past diseases, current medications, and history of hyposalivation from medications or conditions; dental history including past history of dental caries, dental phobias, and history of dental conditions; current home care practices and how well this is done; current diet and exposure to sucrose and other fermentable carbohydrates; and current exposure to topical fluoride products in toothpaste, mouth rinses, and fluoridated water supply. Some of these factors are explored in more detail in the following sections.

Fig. 2.39A and B present two examples of caries risk assessment forms that can be used as part of the initial caries diagnosis process; Fig. 2.39C is an example of a caries assessment form that can be used to facilitate communication of the findings with patients. This latter caries assessment form is a useful tool to measure changes and determine the effectiveness of caries management procedures. All of these forms can be incorporated into an electronic patient management system for increased efficiency.

Social, Economic, and Education Status

Social status and economic status are not directly involved in the disease process but are important because they affect the expression and management of the caries disease. The socioeconomic status and educational status of the patient have implications on the necessary compliance and behavioral changes that can decrease risk for caries development. Socioeconomic status and educational status are predictive at the population level but are generally inaccurate at the individual level.

Diet Analysis

Increased frequency of sugar intake in the form of fermentable carbohydrates increases risk for caries by modifying the biofilm to support a lower pH environment. The frequent use of candies and lozenges during the day or night increases the risk. Sugar-containing acidic beverages, including sport drinks, fruit juices, and soft drinks, all contribute to increased risk. Frequent ingestion of fermentable carbohydrates can change the microbiome profile of the biofilm favoring acidogenic and aciduric bacteria and by influencing the pH of the biofilm to support cariogenic bacteria (see Fig. 2.4).

Salivary Analysis

Salivary flow rate, buffering capacity, and pH all can be measured by various methods (tests). The caries risk predictive value for these tests is not fully demonstrated by strong evidence in all circumstances. Patients with normal salivary flow and adequate buffering capacity may still develop and/or have caries. However, when patients have dry mouth symptoms and a salivary flow analysis leads to a diagnosis of hyposalivation, the decreased salivary flow is a predictive risk factor for root caries in older patients with recession and for increased caries in general in other populations. As discussed, saliva has numerous effects in protection against

ADA American Dental Association®

America's leading advocate for oral health

Caries Risk Assessment Form (Age >6)

Patient Name:

Birth Date: | **Date:**

Age: | **Initials:**

		Low Risk	Moderate Risk	High Risk
	Contributing Conditions	Check or Circle the conditions that apply		
I.	**Fluoride Exposure** (through drinking water, supplements, professional applications, toothpaste)	☐Yes	☐No	
II.	**Sugary Foods or Drinks** (including juice, carbonated or non-carbonated soft drinks, energy drinks, medicinal syrups)	Primarily at mealtimes ☐		Frequent or prolonged between meal exposures/day ☐
III.	**Caries Experience of Mother, Caregiver and/or other Siblings** (for patients ages 6-14)	No carious lesions in last 24 months ☐	Carious lesions in last 7-23 months ☐	Carious lesions in last 6 months ☐
IV.	**Dental Home:** established patient of record, receiving regular dental care in a dental office	☐Yes	☐No	
	General Health Conditions	Check or Circle the conditions that apply		
I.	**Special Health Care Needs** (developmental, physical, medical or mental disabilities that prevent or limit performance of adequate oral health care by themselves or caregivers)	☐No	Yes (over age 14) ☐	Yes (ages 6-14) ☐
II.	**Chemo/Radiation Therapy**	☐No		☐Yes
III.	**Eating Disorders**	☐No	☐Yes	
IV.	**Medications that Reduce Salivary Flow**	☐No	☐Yes	
V.	**Drug/Alcohol Abuse**	☐No	☐Yes	
	Clinical Conditions	Check or Circle the conditions that apply		
I.	**Cavitated or Non-Cavitated** (incipient) **Carious Lesions or Restorations** (visually or radiographically evident)	No new carious lesions or restorations in last 36 months ☐	1 or 2 new carious lesions or restorations in last 36 months ☐	3 or more carious lesions or restorations in last 36 months ☐
II.	**Teeth Missing Due to Caries in past 36 months**	☐No		☐Yes
III.	**Visible Plaque**	☐No	☐Yes	
IV.	**Unusual Tooth Morphology** that compromises oral hygiene	☐No	☐Yes	
V.	**Interproximal Restorations - 1 or more**	☐No	☐Yes	
VI.	**Exposed Root Surfaces** Present	☐No	☐Yes	
VII.	**Restorations with Overhangs** and/or **Open Margins; Open Contacts** with Food Impaction	☐No	☐Yes	
VIII.	**Dental/Orthodontic Appliances** (fixed or removable)	☐No	☐Yes	
IX.	**Severe Dry Mouth (Xerostomia)**	☐No		☐Yes

Overall assessment of dental caries risk: ☐ Low   ☐ Moderate   ☐ High

Patient Instructions:

© American Dental Association, 2009, 2011. All rights reserved.

A

• **Fig. 2.39** A, Example of a caries risk assessment form recommended by the American Dental Association. B, Example of a caries risk assessment form used by the University of North Carolina, Department of Operative Dentistry. C, Another caries assessment form used by the University of North Carolina, Department of Operative Dentistry. This form is very useful for patient communication and compliance. (*A, Copyright 2009, 2011 the American Dental Association.*)

Caries Risk Initial Assessment

Name _____

Date _____

Risk	Low Risk	At Risk	High Risk
Risk Rating Score	≤ 3	≥4 and ≤8	≥9

Patient Interview Assessment

Dental History

			Risk Rating
1. Had non emergency dental care in last year	yes	no	-1
2. Brushes teeth at least twice daily	yes	no	-3
3. Uses fluoridated toothpaste or product daily	yes	no	-3
4. New caries lesions within the last 3 years	yes	no	8
5. Patient has teeth sensitive to hot, cold, sweets	yes	no	3
6. Patient avoids brushing any part of mouth	yes	no	3

Supplemental notes for dental history

Dietary Assessment

1. Water supply currently fluoridated	yes	no	-2
2. Frequent snacking with sugary foods, acidic foods, fermentable carb foods	yes	no	8
3. Sugary drinks including soft drinks, juice, sports drinks, medicinal syrups	yes	no	8
4. Tobacco use of any kind	yes	no	3
5. Excessive alcohol or recreational drug use	yes	no	8
6. Eating disorders	yes	no	5

Supplemental notes for dietary assessment

Xerostomia Assessment

1. Patient is aware of dry mouth or reduced saliva	yes	no	10
2. Medications taken that reduce salivary flow	yes	no	8
3. Medical conditions affecting salivary flow/content	yes	no	8
4. Saliva flow or content visibly abnormal	yes	no	10

Xerostomia Assessments with scores of 8-10 indicate baseline salivary testing is required

Patient Clinical Assessment

Clinical Oral Findings

1. Readily visible biofilm/plaque	yes	no	5
2. Visible cavitated lesions	yes	no	10
3. Interproximal enamel lesions or radiolucencies	yes	no	10
4. Visible white spots	yes	no	5
5. Visible brown spots or non cavitated caries lesions	yes	no	3
6. Deep pits or grooves	yes	no	5
7. Radiographic cavitated lesions	yes	no	10
8. Restorations with overhangs and/or margin concerns or open contacts	yes	no	3
9. Prosthesis ortho, fixed, or removable	yes	no	3

Clinical Assessments with scores of 10 indicate that baseline bacterial testing is required

Risk Rating Total = _____

10. Clinician's impression of patient's risk	low	at risk	high

This is clinician's impression of patient's risk if different than would be indicated by risk factors marked. Describe in box below.

Patient Compliance Assessment

Patient's attitude and general assessment of patient's ability to comply for each of the following categories:

Oral hygiene compliance patient limitations	yes	no
Dietary recommendation patient limitations	yes	no
Therapeutic homecare products limitations	yes	no
Special needs health care (physical or mental compliance issues)	yes	no

This is clinician's assessment of any perceived limitations for the patient to comply with oral hygiene, dietary, or using home care products. Could be lifestyle, physical, or economic reasons. Describe in box below.

Patient Clinical In Office Tests Indicated From Risk Score

Cariscreen Meter	completed	at risk	low risk	reading _____
GC America Saliva Check	completed	at risk	low risk	
GC America Strep Mutans	completed	at risk	low risk	
GC America Plaque Indicator	completed	at risk	low risk	
UNC Biologic Testing Lab	completed	at risk	low risk	

Notes from oral findings, patient's attitude, office tests, special circumstances that would influence caries risk or management

B

• **Fig. 2.39, cont'd**

Continued

Caries Assessment Testing Results

PREPARED FOR

Name_____

Date_____

PREPARED BY

_____.

Your Risk Scores: Risk predicts your likelihood of developing future disease. Green is low risk and means you are unlikely to develop a cavity whereas red means you are very likely to develop a cavity unless your risk factors are managed. We will use these results to work with you to develop an individualized plan to control your disease.

Existing Dental Conditions

Your dental condition score is based on current areas of decay, number of cavities in the last three years, exposed root surfaces, crowns and fillings that are defective. Your score will also be higher if you wear partial dentures or other appliances.

Saliva Assessment Testing

Saliva pH Testing

>6.8   6.0-6.6   <5.8

Saliva Flow and Buffering

Normal   Abnormal

Your saliva is the main protective factor in the caries risk disease state equation. Yellow and Red results can produce an increased incidence of cavities. If the pH of the saliva is low, it sets the stage for the bacteria to grow that cause cavities to form in your mouth. If the quantity of the saliva is below normal, the healing ability of the saliva to remineralize your teeth after acidic food and beverages is greatly reduced. This can, in most incidences, result in a dry mouth that is uncomfortable when eating and lead to an increase in cavities on the roots and other surfaces of your teeth. Any change in saliva content, amount, or pH can increase your risk for cavities to form even if you have not had cavities in the past. New medications and medical conditions can cause your saliva to change rapidly.

Plaque Assessment Testing

Plaque pH Testing

>6.8   6.0-6.6   <5.8

Biofilm Activity

<1500   1500-2000   >2000

Visible Plaque

Low   High

Plaque or biofilm is the mass of bacteria that is always changing and clings to the surfaces of your teeth. Plaque is one of the main risk factors that result in cavities. For plaque to produce the acid that dissolves your teeth and form cavities, it has to be in an acidic state, or in other words, have a low pH. The more acidic, the more damage that can result. The type of bacteria in the plaque also influences how easy it is for the damage to occur. The biofilm activity measures the amount of the "bad" bacteria present in the plaque. The higher the number, the more bacteria are present that cause the cavities to form. The amount of plaque on your teeth means more bacteria are present in your mouth. More bacteria produce higher amounts of acid to demineralize your teeth and cause them to decay.

Dietary Habits

Frequency of Snacking

< 1   2-3   >3

Frequency of sweetened beverages and sport drinks

< 1   2-3   >3

A key factor in how you control your disease and prevent cavities is how you eat and what beverages you consume. Snacking with sweet foods or high carbohydrate foods that can form sugars causes the plaque to become acidic. This results in more bacteria forming that produce even more acid. All of this acid dissolves your teeth and forms the cavities. Sweetened drinks or drinks high in acid content also produce low pH plaque and more bacteria. Soft drinks and sports drinks like Gatorade are very low in pH. The more you drink, the more acid the plaque and bacteria produce to cause the cavities in your teeth.

C

• **Fig. 2.39, cont'd**

caries, including inhibition of bacteria, eliminating (clearing of) bacteria from the tooth surface, dilution of bacterial products, buffering of bacterial acids, and offering a reparative environment with necessary calcium and phosphate minerals after bacteria-induced demineralization. Since all of these benefits are missing when patients have salivary hypofunction, patients with "dry mouth" are at higher risk for caries. These patients are more susceptible to dietary changes that are associated with lower pH foods and beverages or foods and beverages containing fermentable carbohydrates, since the protective factors of saliva are diminished in patients with hyposalivation.

Dental Clinical Analysis (Dental Exam)

The dental examination identifies risk indicators more than risk factors. This is important as many of the indicators are directly related to the current caries activity. Risk indicators and current caries activity drive the decision-making process toward the type of intervention that the clinician would prescribe. Visible cavitated caries lesions and active initial lesions on teeth are both indicators of caries risk. Visible biofilm may also be considered a risk factor for caries development. Other examination findings that would influence increased risk for caries are exposed root surfaces; deep pits or grooves; fixed, removable prosthesis or orthodontic appliances used; and existing restorations with open contacts, open margins, rough surfaces, or overhangs.

Bacterial Biofilm Analysis

Use of supplemental tests to analyze the bacterial component of the biofilm has little value to determine the patient's risk level. For example, the presence of *MS* or lactobacilli in saliva or plaque as a sole predictor for caries in primary teeth has been shown to have low sensitivity but high specificity. The measurement of adenosine triphosphate (ATP) activity of the biofilm bacteria as a surrogate measure of caries activity has also not been identified to be a strong predictor of risk. Although these bacterial tests may be useful for patient communication by providing insight into the specifics of the biofilm (bacterial types and resultant environment), the predictive value (for caries risk) of the evidence of the tests requires further validation by controlled research studies.

Risk Assessment Considerations for Children Under 6 Years Old

In addition to all the above mentioned risk factors for adults and adolescents, there are age-specific risk factors and indicators that should be considered for children under 6 years. These include presence of active caries in the primary caregiver in the past year, feeding on demand past 1 year of age, bedtime bottle or sippy cup with anything other than water, no supervised brushing, and severe enamel hypoplasia.

Caries Management and Protocols or Strategies for Prevention

Caries risk assessment is only meaningful if used in conjunction with a corresponding caries management program. The caries prevention or management program should comprise a menu of prevention therapies and interventions that should be recommended on the basis of the level of caries risk (Table 2.7 and Box 2.2) and address the patient's risk factors. However, as discussed in the previous section, no caries risk assessment system is perfect. Therefore, in addition to the outcome of the caries risk assessment tool, the clinician needs to use his or her best clinical judgment, coupled with the best available research evidence, to design a preventive or therapeutic program that works for the patient. Needless to say, this is a dynamic process, so monitoring and

TABLE 2.7	Suggested Risk-Based Interventions for Adults[a]	
Caries Risk Category	**Office-Based Interventions**	**Home-Based Interventions**
High	3-month recare examination and oral prophylaxis Fluoride varnish at each recare visit Individualized oral hygiene instructions and use of specialized cleaning aids (e.g., powered toothbrush, Waterpik) Dietary counseling Bitewing radiographs every 6–12 months[b]	Brush with prescription fluoride dentifrice (e.g., 1/1%/5000 ppm NaF) Use sugar substitutes (e.g., xylitol, erythritol) Apply calcium-phosphate compounds (e.g., MI Paste) On selected cases use agents to modulate a dysbiotic microbiome (e.g., xylitol gum or lozenge, chlorhexidine rinse). Use agents to encourage a healthy microbiome (probiotics, prebiotics, like arginine) If xerostomic, increase salivary function (e.g., xylitol gum, rinses, oral moisturizers)
Moderate	4–6 month recare examination and oral prophylaxis Fluoride varnish at each recall Reinforce proper oral hygiene Dietary counseling	Brush with fluoride dentifrice (e.g., 1450 ppm fluoride) OTC fluoride rinse (e.g., 0.05% NaF)
Low	9–12 month recare examination and oral prophylaxis Reinforce good oral hygiene	Brush with fluoride dentifrice

NaF, Sodium fluoride; *OTC,* over the counter; *ppm,* parts per million.

[a]These are general guidelines and should be customized based on the specific patient's needs and on weight of individual risk factors uncovered with a caries risk assessment instrument.

[b]Data from US Department of Health and Human Services, Public Health Service, Food and Drug Administration; and American Dental Association, Council on Dental Benefit Programs, Council on Scientific Affairs. The selection of patients for dental radiographic examinations. Rev. ed. 2004.

Available at www.ada.org/prof/resources/topics/radiography.asp. Accessed January 20, 2012.

Modified from Shugars DA, Bader JD: *MetLife quality resource guide: risk-based management of dental caries in adults,* ed 3, Bridgewater, NJ, 2009–2012, Metropolitan Life Insurance Co., p. 6.

• BOX 2.2 Sample Preventive Protocol for a High-Risk Patient With Cavitated Caries Lesions

1. A comprehensive oral and radiographic evaluation is conducted charting caries lesions, periodontal pocket probing, existing restorations, and oral cancer exam; the medical and dental histories are reviewed. In this hypothetical patient, multiple caries lesions, poor oral hygiene, and generalized marginal gingivitis are noted.
2. A caries risk assessment is completed with emphasis on discovering the risk factors that are contributing to the causative aspect of the caries problem and discovering the risk factors for the patient that are predictors of future caries risk. A discussion of these risk factors with the patient is essential for understanding of the caries disease process and the patient's role and the provider's role in controlling the disease.
3. Diagnosis and treatment planning procedures are completed and discussed with the patient.
4. Nonoperative and operative treatments will be completed in three phases: (i) a control phase, (ii) a definitive treatment phase, and (iii) a maintenance reassessment phase.
5. CONTROL PHASE (2–4 weeks):
   a. Oral hygiene procedures are explained and reviewed at each patient visit. The frequency of the visits in this initial phase is determined by severity of the disease. This could be weekly or more frequent, depending on the provider's evaluation. When attempting behavior modification, repetition is essential. Review of patient's current home care techniques and frequency of home care are reviewed along with lifestyle issues that might impede compliance. Use of a powered toothbrush and an oral irrigator for possibly improving patient compliance and technique are discussed. Evaluation of the patient's motivation along with the person's mental and physical capacity to comply with recommendations for home care must be noted and considered by the provider. Specific recommendations are listed for the patient to use at home, and the patient agrees that this is practical for his or her life situation.
   b. Prescription fluoride toothpaste is prescribed (5000 parts per million [ppm]) and the patient is instructed to brush with it three times per day and to use according to given instructions (do not rinse after use, only expectorate excess). Any products used for home care should be carefully reviewed for the pH of the product. Products with pH lower than 6 should be carefully considered whether their use would contribute to the pH shift of the biofilm to pathologic for caries lesion formation.
   c. A diet analysis is completed, analyzed, and reviewed with the patient. Cariogenic foods and beverages are identified and alternatives suggested. Also acidic foods and beverages that are contributing to the pH shift to a lower oral pH environment are identified and discussed. Options for foods that have impact to raise the oral pH are suggested, such as foods rich in arginine. Again the patient's motivation and abilities to fit the necessary diet modifications into his or her lifestyle must be evaluated and discussed.
   d. A microbiologic survey may be completed for patient motivation. This can be accomplished using either the adenosine triphosphate (ATP) chairside device or formal saliva samples to identify specific mutans streptococci (MS) and lactobacilli counts.
   e. A saliva analysis is conducted to determine stimulated flow rate, salivary pH and buffering capacity, and viscosity. Treatment protocols for hyposalivation are recommended for patients with an analysis that indicates deficiencies in the above areas. Patients with low salivary pH would need to use baking soda rinses during the day and use xylitol gum or other recommended products to raise pH levels, increase flow, and increase buffering capacity.
   f. Caries control (described elsewhere in this chapter) is completed. This may involve use of silver diamine fluoride (SDF) for cavitated lesions or partial caries removal and interim restoration of all cavitated caries lesions (usually during one appointment and restoring with glass ionomer) or a combination of both. This is critical to reduce the bacterial load and prevent further progression on the lesion.

   g. A prophylaxis is performed and 5% sodium fluoride (NaF) varnish is applied to all teeth.
   h. If SDF is used, the lesion should be reassessed 1 to 2 weeks after first application to determine if it has arrested. If the lesion has not arrested a new application of SDF is advised. Lesions that will not be restored need to have a new SDF application every 6 months.
   i. The microbiologic testing, if done, may be repeated 2 to 4 weeks after initiation of treatment. A reduction in counts can be a great motivational tool for patients to continue with their modifications in behavior (diet or oral hygiene). Diet analysis is followed up and reviewed again. Successes in diet modifications are positively reinforced. Shortcomings in diet modifications are discussed and options explored with the patient to rectify diet issues, where needed. Home care regimens are reviewed again with patients and refined. It is important to listen to the patient and work to incorporate diet and home care into the patient's lifestyle and abilities to mentally and physically comply with the recommendations.
6. DEFINITIVE TREATMENT PHASE:
   a. The glass ionomer provisional restorations are replaced (usually by quadrants) with definitive restorations.
   b. Oral hygiene procedures are reinforced at each visit. Flossing and brushing three times per day with prescription toothpaste is recommended.
   c. Patients with root caries may benefit from chewing xylitol chewing gum with at least 1 gram of xylitol per piece three to six times per day, preferably after meals and snacks.
   d. Some patients with low salivary flow or low salivary buffering capacity may benefit from applying casein phosphopeptide–amorphous calcium phosphates (CPP-ACP) to teeth after brushing and flossing prior to retiring to bed.
   e. If reduced salivary flow rates are considered to be a major etiologic factor, the patient should be instructed to chew sugar-free mints several times a day or use other recommended products for xerostomia treatment. Prescribing pilocarpine or other salivary stimulant should be considered.
   f. When all definitive restorations are completed, the patient then enters the maintenance reassessment phase.
7. MAINTENANCE REASSESSMENT PHASE:
   a. The patient should be recalled every 3 months. Oral hygiene and home care procedures are reviewed and evaluated. Recommendations for improvement and modifications to home care are evaluated and discussed.
   b. Prophylaxis followed by fluoride varnish application is accomplished.
   c. Caries risk assessment is completed again; changes are noted in risk factors that have been controlled and those risk factors still listed as causative and predictive factors.
   d. Diet analysis and recommendations from previous visits are reviewed and evaluated.
   e. Patient continues use of prescription 5000-ppm toothpaste, CPP-ACP paste, and xylitol chewing gum as advised. Any other recommendations to changes or additions to the product protocols are reviewed, discussed, and implemented.
   f. Every 6 months, salivary evaluations are repeated. Microbiologic evaluations may also be repeated to keep patient motivation.
   g. Bitewing radiographs are taken on an annual basis or more frequently if new lesions continue to be detected.
   h. It is critical for the patient to understand that caries is a disease that is only controlled and not "cured." The protocol that is determined to be currently successful may have to be periodically reviewed, updated, and changed. More importantly, the patient will be much like a patient with diabetes, requiring lifetime medication and therapy, diet control, and lifestyle management for disease stability, and will need to be dedicated to a lifetime of careful management of caries risk factors to keep the disease controlled.

TABLE 2.8	Health History Factors Associated With Increased Caries Risk
History Factor	Risk-Increasing Observations
Age	Childhood, adolescence, senescence
Fluoride exposure	No fluoride in public water supply No fluoride toothpaste
Smoking	Risk increases with amount smoked
Alcohol	Risk increases with amount consumed
General health	Chronic illness and debilitation decreases ability to give self-care
Medication	Medications that reduce salivary flow

TABLE 2.9	Clinical Examination Findings Associated With Increased Caries Risk
Clinical Examination	Risk-Increasing Findings
General appearance	Appearance: sick, obese, or malnourished
Mental or physical disability	Inability or unwillingness to comply with dietary and oral hygiene instruction
Mucosal membranes	Dry, red, glossy mucosa, suggesting decreased salivary flow
Active caries lesions	Cavitation and softening of enamel and dentin; circumferential chalky opacity at gingival margins
Plaque biofilm	High plaque scores
Gingiva	Puffy, swollen, and inflamed gingiva; bleeds easily
Existing restorations	Large numbers, indicating past high caries rate; poor quality, indicating increased habitat for cariogenic organisms

periodic reassessment and reevaluation of the disease activity and prevention or management program are critical.

Management of dental caries and its consequences remains the predominant activity of dentists; however, preventive and diagnostic services are increasing.[44,45] Although these activities relate to a variety of dental problems, diagnosis and prevention of caries are major parts of these increases. In a modern practice model, the restoration of a caries lesion can no longer be considered a cure for dental caries. Rather, the practitioner must identify patients who have active caries lesions and patients at high risk for caries and institute appropriate preventive and treatment measures. This section presents some measures that may reduce the likelihood of a patient developing caries lesions. Depending on the risk status of the patient and the risk factors at play for the specific patient, the dentist must decide which of these to institute. With this paradigm shift, dentistry is focusing increasingly on limiting the need for restorative treatment.

Preventive treatment methods are designed to limit tooth demineralization caused by cariogenic bacteria, preventing initial lesions and progression of initial lesions into cavitated lesions. These methods include (1) limiting pathogen growth and altering metabolism of the biofilm, (2) increasing the resistance of the tooth surface to demineralization, and (3) increasing biofilm pH. A caries prevention and management program is a complex process involving multiple interrelated factors (Tables 2.8, 2.9, 2.10, and 2.11; see also Table 2.7 and Box 2.2). The primary goals of a caries prevention program are (1) to modulate the biofilm into a non-pathogenic biofilm and (2) to create an environment conducive to remineralization. Prevention should start with a consideration to maintain the patient with a noncariogenic biofilm. Although the general health of the patient, fluoride exposure history, and function of the immune system and salivary glands have a significant impact on the patient's caries risk, the patient may have little control over these factors. The patient usually is capable of controlling other factors such as diet, oral hygiene, use of agents to modulate the biofilm, and dental care (which may include use of sealants and restorations). This section presents a variety of factors that may have an impact on caries prevention.

General Health

The patient's general health has a significant impact on overall caries risk. Declining health signals the need for increased preventive measures, including more frequent recalls. Every patient has an effective surveillance and destruction system for "foreign" bacteria.

The effectiveness of a patient's immune system depends on overall health status. Patients undergoing radiation or chemotherapy treatment have significantly decreased immunocompetence and are at risk for increased caries.

Medically compromised patients should be examined for changes in the following: plaque index, salivary analysis, oral mucosa, gingiva, and teeth. Early signs of increased risk include increased biofilm; puffy, bleeding gingiva; dry mouth with red, glossy mucosa; and initial caries lesions on teeth. Decreased saliva flow is common during acute and chronic systemic illnesses and is responsible for the dramatic increase in biofilm. Ambulatory patients with chronic illnesses often take multiple medications, which individually or in combination may reduce salivary flow significantly (see Table 2.4). Saliva should be tested for flow and buffering capacities when signs or symptoms are detected from an oral examination.

Diet

Dietary sucrose has two important detrimental effects on how biofilm affects caries. First, frequent ingestion of foods containing sucrose provides a change in the biofilm profile from a noncariogenic biofilm to a cariogenic biofilm.[151] Second, mature biofilm exposed frequently to sucrose rapidly metabolizes it into organic acids, resulting in a profound and prolonged decline in pH. Caries activity is most strongly stimulated by the frequency, rather than the quantity, of sucrose ingested. The message that excessive and frequent sucrose intake can cause caries has been widely disseminated and is well known by laypeople. Despite this knowledge, dietary modification for the purpose of caries control has failed as a public health measure. For an individual patient, dietary modification may be effective if the patient is properly motivated and supervised. Evidence of new caries activity in adolescent and adult patients indicates the need for dietary counseling. The goals of dietary counseling should be to identify the sources of sucrose and acidic foods in the diet and to reduce the frequency of ingestion of both. Minor dietary changes such as substitution of sugar-free foods for snacks are more likely to be accepted than more dramatic changes. Rampant (or acute) caries (a rapidly developing process usually involving several teeth) is a sign of gross dietary inadequacy, a

TABLE 2.10   Methods of Caries Treatment by the Medical Model

Method and Indications	Rationale	Techniques or Material
A. Limit Cariogenic Substrate **Indications**: Frequent sucrose exposure Poor-quality diet	Reduce number, duration, and intensity of acid attacks Reduce selection pressure for mutans streptococci (MS)	Diet diary Eliminate sucrose from between-meal snacks Substantially reduce or eliminate sucrose from meals
B. Modify Microflora **Indications**: High MS counts High lactobacilli counts	Modify a dysbiotic biofilm and encourage a healthy biofilm Reduce overall biofilm burden to improve gingival health	Bactericidal mouthrinse (chlorhexidine) Topical fluoride treatments; probiotics and prebiotics
C. Disorganize Plaque Biofilm **Indications**: High plaque biofilm scores Puffy red gingiva High bleeding point score	Prevents plaque biofilm succession Decreases plaque biofilm mass Promotes buffering	Brushing Flossing Other oral hygiene aids as necessary (e.g., electric toothbrush)
D. Modify Tooth Surface **Indications**: Noncavitated lesions Surface roughening	Increase resistance to demineralization Decrease plaque biofilm retention	Systemic fluorides Topical fluorides Smooth surface
E. Stimulate Saliva Flow **Indications**: Dry mouth with little saliva Red mucosa Medication that reduces salivary flow	Increases clearance of substrate and acids Promotes buffering	Eat noncariogenic foods that require lots of chewing Sugarless chewing gum Medications to stimulate salivary flow Use dry mouth topical agents, oral lubricants, etc.
F. Seal Susceptible Surfaces **Indications**: Moderate and high caries risk individuals Teeth with susceptible anatomy (deep grooves) Initial noncavitated enamel lesions in high-risk patients (smooth-surface sealants)	Prevents colonization (infection) of pit-and-fissure system with cariogenic plaque biofilm Inhibits progression of smooth-surface lesion	Use pit-and-fissure and smooth-surface resin sealants
G. Restore Active Cavitated Surfaces **Indications**: Cavitated lesions Defective restorations	Eliminate nidus of cariogenic biofilm Deny habitat for cariogenic biofilm reinfection	Apply SDF to caries lesions as indicated Restore all cavitated lesions Correct all defects (e.g., marginal crevices, proximal overhangs)

TABLE 2.11   Treatment Strategies

Examination Findings	Nonrestorative, Therapeutic Treatment	Restorative Treatment	Follow-up[a]
Normal (no lesions)	None	None	1-year clinical examination
Hypocalcified enamel (developmental white spot)	None for nonhereditary lesions; hereditary lesions (dentinogenesis imperfecta) may require special management	Treatment is elective; esthetics (restore defects)	1-year clinical examination
Noncavitated enamel lesions only; bitewing radiographs indicated (demineralized white spot)	Techniques A–E in Table 2.9, as indicated	Seal defective pits and fissures as indicated	3 months; evaluate: oral flora, mutans streptococci (MS) counts, progression of white spots, presence of cavitations
Possible cavitated lesions (active caries) and other noncavitated lesions present; bitewing radiographs indicated	Techniques A–E in Table 2.9, as indicated	Techniques F and G (restorations, sealants) in Table 2.9 as indicated	3 months; evaluate: oral flora, MS counts, progression of white spots, presence of new cavitations, pulpal response
Inactive caries; no active (new cavitations) or noncavitated lesions	None	Treatment is elective; esthetics (restore defects)	1-year clinical examination

[a]These are only generalized follow-up times. Particular circumstances may dictate shorter or longer follow-up intervals, depending on presence of primary and secondary modifying risk factors (see Fig. 2.1).

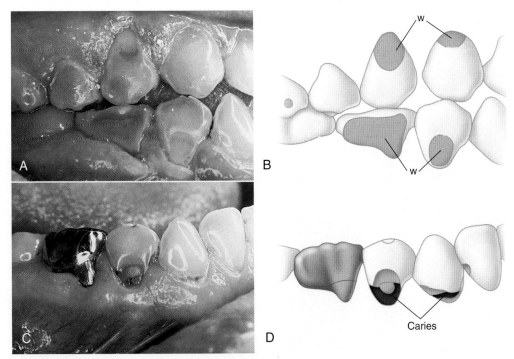

• **Fig. 2.40**   Erosion wear and poor home care leading to caries. A young female patient with severe wear on the facial surfaces of posterior teeth. This patient subsequently was found to have a hiatal hernia with frequent regurgitation of stomach acids. Too vigorous brushing and acid demineralization of teeth accelerated the loss of tooth structure (*A* and *B*). Areas of severe wear *(w)* exhibit dentin hypersensitivity. Dentin pain was the symptom that caused the patient to seek dental care. Advising the patient to reduce vigorous tooth brushing resulted in cessation of all brushing. Caries activity rapidly occurred (*C* and *D*).

complete absence of oral hygiene practice, systemic illness, or a combination of these pathologic factors. Rampant caries that is present primarily on proximal surfaces may point more to diet as the main driving factor, whereas rampant caries in the cervical and interproximal areas may point to diet and hygiene as the driving factors. The presence of rampant caries indicates the need for comprehensive patient evaluation. Textbooks on dental caries, nutrition, and medicine should be consulted as needed.

For high-risk patients, a formal diet analysis should routinely be undertaken to identify cariogenic foods and beverages that are frequently ingested. This analysis may take place by asking the patient to recall everything that was ingested in the past 24 hours (the "24-hour diet interview"). Alternatively, a more detailed diet analysis may be facilitated by requesting the patient to record a diet diary, which consists usually of a 5- to 7-consecutive-day period with 2 days surveyed being weekend days as patients' diets frequently change considerably on weekends. A form should be provided to the patient that divides each day into six segments (breakfast, morning, lunch, afternoon, dinner, and evening), and the patient should be instructed to write down everything ingested, including medications, the amount, and the time of consumption. The diary is then analyzed by the dentist, and a discussion is held with the patient to suggest appropriate alternatives.[46] The dentist should focus on type of cariogenic foods and time intervals between their consumption as well as length of exposure of each cariogenic episode. For example, if a patient were to record "10:00 AM 1 soda," the dentist should clarify the type of soda consumed, the quantity of soda, and the duration of time to finish the soda. An 8-oz glass of sugar-containing soda consumed over a 5-minute period will have a different impact than a 20-oz glass sipped over a 2-hour period.

Oral Hygiene

Biofilm-free tooth surfaces do not decay. Daily removal of biofilm by dental flossing and tooth brushing with a fluoridated toothpaste is the best patient-based measure for preventing caries and periodontal disease (Figs. 2.40 and 2.41). Löe established supragingival plaque as the etiologic agent of gingivitis.[47] Longstanding gingivitis may lead to damage of the epithelial attachment and progression to more serious periodontal disease. Although plaque scores are not reliable indicators of caries risk, the presence of biofilm over a lesion may help assess lesion activity.[152,153] Effective biofilm control by oral hygiene measures using a fluoridated toothpaste results in resolution of the gingival inflammation and remineralization of any initially demineralized enamel surface.

Mechanical biofilm disorganization by brushing and flossing has the advantage of not eliminating the normal oral flora. Topical antibiotics may control oral biofilm, but long-term use predisposes the host to infection by antibiotic-resistant pathogens such as *Candida albicans*. Frequent mechanical biofilm removal does not engender the risk of infection by opportunistic organisms; rather it changes the species composition of biofilm in the selection for pioneering organisms and the denial of habitat to potential pathogens. The oral flora on the teeth of patients with good biofilm control has a high percentage of *S. sanguis* or *S. mitis* and is much less cariogenic than older, mature biofilm communities, which have a significantly higher percentage of MS.

Krasse showed that a combination of oral hygiene and diet counseling is effective in children.[48] In this classic study, children in two schools were monitored for *Lactobacillus* levels. The children in one school were given feedback about their *Lactobacillus* levels and proper preventive oral hygiene and dietary instruction. After

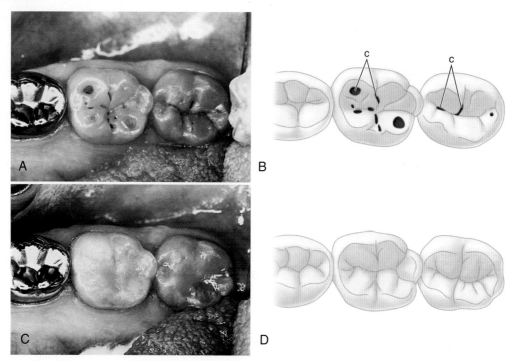

• **Fig. 2.41** A and B, Photograph of the occlusal surfaces of the teeth illustrated in Fig. 2.40. C and D, After cessation of oral hygiene procedures, caries (c) rapidly developed in the exposed dentin and fissures on the occlusal surfaces. Caries was treated conservatively by excavation of softened dentin and restoration of the excavations and fissures with composite.

18 months, the children in the school receiving preventive counseling had an average of 3.3 new restorations, whereas the control schoolchildren, who received no counseling, averaged 8.2 new restorations. This study is an excellent demonstration that good oral hygiene and dietary improvements may be effective when using microbiologic testing as a motivational tool.

Rigid oral hygiene programs should be prescribed only to high-risk persons with evidence of active disease. Overzealous, universal application of oral hygiene training programs is frustrating to dentists and their patients. High-risk patients should receive intensive oral hygiene training usually with a prescription-strength fluoridated toothpaste (5000 parts per million [ppm] F), dietary instruction, and preventive dental treatment, as necessary, to control the progress of disease. Adults with a low caries experience probably require less frequency of daily flossing and brushing.

Biofilm control requires a little dexterity and a lot of motivation. Some knowledge of tooth contours, embrasure form, proximal contacts, and tooth alignment is helpful in optimal biofilm control. Instruction should include the selection and use of mechanical aids based on patient needs. Professional tooth cleanings can have an important effect on caries reduction. One study divided grade school students into three treatment groups: control, monthly professional cleaning, and twice-a-month professional cleaning.[49] In students with low MS levels, the once-a-month cleaning group showed ~50% fewer new carious surfaces (0.8 surfaces/student) than the control group (1.8 surfaces/student). In the high MS group, the control group had the most new caries (2.5 surfaces/student), whereas the once-a-month cleaning group had similar levels (0.96 surfaces/student) to the low MS group, and the twice-a-month cleaning group had almost one tenth the number of new lesions (0.34 surfaces/student) as the control group. This study showed that professional biofilm removal on grade school students,

even only once every 2 weeks, dramatically reduces the development of new caries lesions. There is little evidence that professional prophylaxis at the usual 6-month intervals reduces dental caries levels; therefore it is important to customize recall intervals to the patient risk. Equal or greater reductions may be expected in patients who practice proper oral hygiene methods for biofilm removal.

Another adjunct to regular brushing and flossing is the regular use of electric toothbrushes and oral irrigation devices. A recent study has demonstrated these devices are effective in the removal of biofilm and, more importantly, change the composition of the biofilm in a favorable direction when used regularly.[50] Since most patients are not very efficacious on judicious removal of biofilm, brushing may be viewed more as a delivery mechanism for fluoride. Recommendations of brushing for at least 2 minutes and not rinsing may increase compliance and improve outcomes. Additionally, simple suggestions, like feeling tooth surfaces with the tongue to assess if the biofilm was removed, may improve awareness and assist in efficacy.

Fluoride Exposure

The highest level of evidence for caries prevention and reduction supports the exposure of teeth to fluoride. Fluoride in trace amounts increases the resistance of tooth structure to demineralization and is particularly important for caries prevention (Fig. 2.42). When fluoride is available during cycles of tooth demineralization, it is a major factor in reduced caries activity.[51] Fluoride seems to be an essential nutrient for humans and is required only in very small quantities. Laboratory animals fed a completely fluoride-free diet develop anemia and reduced reproduction after four generations. When available to humans, fluoride produces spectacular decreases in caries incidence. The availability of fluoride for caries risk reduction has primarily been achieved through the fluoridation of

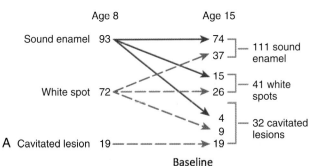

	Baseline			Cavitation at Follow-up		
	Backer Dirks, 1966	Ferreira Zandona et al, 2012		Backer Dirks, 1966	Ferreira Zandona et al, 2012	
	Class V lesions	Class V lesions	All surfaces	Class V lesions	Class V lesions	All surfaces
Sound	93	7905	59335	4%	1%	2%
Initial	72	737	3207	13%	10%	24%
B Enamel Cavities		10	275		20%	67%

• **Fig. 2.42**   A, Initial (white spot) lesions of enamel (stage 3 in Fig. 2.28) may remineralize, remain unchanged, or progress to cavitated lesions. In this study, done in a community with a fluoridated public water supply, only 9 of 72 noncavitated lesions became cavitated. More than half of noncavitated lesions (37 of 72) regressed to become indistinguishable from normal enamel. B, White spot lesions of enamel (stage 3 in Fig. 2.28) may remineralize, remain unchanged, or progress to cavitated lesions. A comparison of a study done in a community with a fluoridated public water supply published in 1966 (Backer Dirks, 1966) versus a study completed in a nonfluoridated community published in 2012 (Ferreira Zandona et al, 2012). The 1966 study followed 184 smooth surfaces (buccal) over a 7-year period. The 2012 followed 62,812 surfaces over a 4-year period, of those 8652 were buccal surfaces. In both studies only a very small portion of sound surfaces cavitate (4% versus 1%–2%). Most initial lesions in enamel on smooth surfaces will not progress to cavitation (only 13% progressed to cavitation in 1966 and only 10% in 2012). When other surfaces are included the number of lesions that progress to cavitation more than double (24%) but it still represents only one fourth of all initial lesions. On smooth surfaces even when enamel cavities are considered, only 20% progress to cavitation exposing the dentin; and, when all surfaces are included, 30% of enamel cavities do not progress to cavitations exposing the dentin. (A, Redrawn from Backer Dirks O: Posteruptive changes in dental enamel. *J Dent Res* 45:503–511, 1966.)

community water systems. Fluoride exposure may occur by means of diet, toothpastes, mouth rinses, and professional topical applications. The optimal fluoride level for public water systems is 0.7 mg per liter of water.[52] The percentage of the U.S. population with public fluoridated community water systems has increased from 62% (140 million) in 1999 to 66% (162 million) in 2000, to 69% (184 million) in 2006,[23,54] to 74% (284 million) in 2014. Public water fluoridation has been one of the most successful public health measures instituted in the United States. For communities that have fluoridated water systems, the annual cost averages about $0.70 per person.[53] For every $1 spent on water fluoridation, $6 of health savings are realized. The U.S. Public Health Service recommends 0.7 ppm of fluoride in public water programs to reap the benefits of water fluoridation and reduce the risk of fluorosis. Excessive fluoride exposure (≥10 ppm) results in fluorosis, which initially causes enamel to become white but may eventually cause a brownish discoloration, a condition termed *mottled enamel.*

Fluoride exerts its anticaries effect by three different mechanisms. First, the presence of fluoride ion greatly enhances the precipitation into tooth structure of fluorapatite from calcium and phosphate ions present in saliva. This insoluble precipitate replaces the soluble salts containing manganese and carbonate that were lost because of bacteria-mediated demineralization. This exchange process results

in the enamel becoming more acid resistant (see Fig. 2.29). Second, initial caries lesions are remineralized by the same process. Third, fluoride has antimicrobial activity. In low concentrations, fluoride ion inhibits the enzymatic production of glucosyltransferase. Glucosyltransferase promotes glucose to form extracellular polysaccharides, which increases bacterial adhesion. Intracellular polysaccharide formation also is inhibited, preventing storage of carbohydrates by limiting microbial metabolism between the host's meals. In high concentrations (12,000 ppm) used in topical fluoride treatments, fluoride ion is directly toxic to some oral microorganisms, including MS. Suppression of growth of MS after a single topical fluoride treatment may last several weeks.[55] It is possible to lengthen this suppression greatly by a change in dietary habits (especially eliminating sucrose) and by the patient's conscientious application of a good oral hygiene program.

All fluoride exposure methods (Table 2.12) are effective to some degree. The clinician's goal is to choose the most effective combination for each patient. This choice must be based on the patient's age, caries experience, general health, and oral hygiene. Children with developing permanent teeth benefit most from systemic fluoride treatments via the public water supply. In regions without adequate fluoride in the water supply, dietary supplementation of fluoride is indicated for children and sometimes for adults. The amount of fluoride supplement must be determined individually. This is

TABLE 2.12 **Fluoride Treatment Modalities**[a]

Route	Method of Delivery	Concentration (ppm)	Caries Reduction (%)
Systemic Topical	Public water supply	0.7	50–60
	Self-application		
	Low-dose/high-frequency rinses (0.05% sodium fluoride daily)	225	30–40
	High-potency–low-frequency rinses (0.2% sodium fluoride weekly)	900	30–40 after 2 years
	Fluoridated dentifrices (daily)	1000–1450	20
	Prescription-strength fluoridated dentifrices (daily)	4950	32
	Professional application		
	Acidulated phosphate fluoride gel (1.23%) annually or semiannually	12,300	40–50
	Sodium fluoride solution (2%)	20,000	40–50
	Sodium fluoride varnish (5%)	22,500	30
	Stannous fluoride solution (8%)	80,000	40–50
	Silver diamine fluoride (SDF) (38%)	44,800	~96.1 for caries arrest ~70.3 for caries prevention

ppm, Parts per million.

[a]Caries reduction estimates for topically administered fluorides indicate their effectiveness when used individually. When they are combined with systemic fluoride treatment, they can provide some additional caries protection.

of particular importance in rural areas with individual wells because the fluoride content of well water can vary greatly within short distances.

Topical application of fluoride should be done periodically for children and adults who are at high risk for caries development. The periodicity varies with the case. Teeth can be cleaned free of biofilm before the application of topical fluorides. Flossing followed by tooth brushing is recommended for this purpose. Pumicing of teeth (professional prophylaxis) is able to remove a considerable amount of the fluoride-rich surface layer of enamel and may be counterproductive. Acidulated phosphate fluoride gel is effective, but a potential risk of swallowing excessive amounts of fluoride exists, particularly in young children. Acidulated phosphate fluoride is available in thixotropic gels and has a long shelf life. Stannous fluoride (8% F), another option, has a bitter, metallic taste; may burn the mucosa; and has a short shelf life. Although the tin ion in stannous fluoride may be responsible for staining the teeth, it may also be beneficial in arresting root caries. Topical fluoride agents should be applied according to the manufacturer's recommendations and always under supervision so as to limit ingestion.

Various fluoride varnishes are available and are successful in preventing caries. Varnishes provide a high uptake of the fluoride ion into enamel and are widely accepted as the vehicle of choice for fluoride delivery to young adults and older adults alike. Fluoride varnishes are professionally applied and may provide the most cost-effective means of delivery of fluoride to teeth. These varnishes are effective bactericidal and caries-preventive agents. Fluoride varnishes were developed several decades ago in an attempt to improve fluoride application techniques and benefits. European countries have used fluoride varnishes for many years. Numerous randomized clinical trials conducted outside the United States point to the efficacy and safety of fluoride varnishes as caries-preventive agents.[56-64] Fluoride varnish enables the deposition of large amounts of fluoride on an enamel surface, especially on a demineralized enamel surface. Calcium fluoride precipitates on the surface, and often fluorapatite is formed. The high concentration of surface fluoride also may provide a reservoir for fluoride, which promotes remineralization. Although additional research on fluoride varnishes is needed, the use of a fluoride varnish as a caries-preventive

agent should be expanded because it has advantages over other topical fluoride vehicles in terms of safety, ease of application, and fluoride concentration at the enamel surface.[6] The American Dental Association (ADA) Council on Scientific Affairs recently endorsed the use of fluoride-containing varnishes as caries prevention agents.[65]

Current evidence indicates that fluoride varnishes with the concentration of 5% sodium fluoride are the most efficacious of all topically applied fluoride products.[58,66] For patients with a high risk of caries, fluoride varnish should be applied every 3 months. For moderate-risk patients, application every 6 months is indicated. Fluoride varnish is not indicated for low-risk patients.

When applying fluoride varnish, the clinician dries off saliva from teeth and applies a thin layer of fluoride varnish directly onto teeth. Because the fluoride varnish sets when contacting moisture, thorough isolation of the area is not required. Only tooth brushing, rather than prophylaxis, is necessary before application. The main disadvantage of fluoride varnish is that a temporary change in tooth color may occur. Patients should avoid eating for several hours and avoid brushing until the next morning after the varnish has been applied.

Self-administered fluoride rinses have an additive effect (about 20% reduction) when used in conjunction with topical or systemic fluoride treatment. Fluoride rinses are indicated in high-risk patients and patients exhibiting a recent increase in caries activity. Two varieties of fluoride rinses have similar effectiveness: (1) high dose–low frequency and (2) low dose–high frequency. High-dose (0.2% F)–low-frequency rinses are best used in supervised weekly rinsing programs based in public schools. Low-dose (0.05% F)–high-frequency rinses are best used by individual patients at home. A high-risk or caries-active patient should be advised to use the rinse daily. The optimal application time is in the evening. The rinse should be forced between teeth many times and then expectorated, not swallowed. Eating and drinking should be avoided after the rinse.

Routine use of over-the-counter fluoride containing dentifrice three times per day is recommended for all patients. These toothpastes generally contain 0.32% sodium fluoride (1450 ppm). For moderate-risk and high-risk patients 6 years or older, prescription dentifrices containing higher concentrations of fluoride are recommended. These products typically contain 1.1% sodium fluoride

(5000 ppm) and can be safely used up to three times per day in this age group.[67] For most benefit, patients should be instructed to not rinse after brushing and avoid eating or drinking for 30 minutes after use.

Silver Diamine Fluoride

Silver diamine fluoride (SDF) is a topical solution used as a caries-arresting and antihypersensitivity agent.[154,155]

SDF was recently cleared by the US Food and Drug Administration (FDA) as an antihypersensitivity agent and is used off-label to arrest caries lesions. Both silver and fluoride play active roles in their mechanisms of arresting caries development and treatment of tooth hypersensitivity.[156-158] Silver has an antibacterial action that slows demineralization and enhances remineralization.[159] SDF, due to its ease of use, has been recommended to arrest large cavitated lesions, allowing not only conservation of tooth structure, but delivery of treatment to groups of patients that either do not have access to traditional restorative care or to whom delivery of the standard treatment is challenging. The main drawback of SDF is that with the precipitation of silver, the carious dentin becomes stained black. Some researchers have studied the use of SDF on root caries and have found it to be effective at preventing root caries lesions.[160]

Application of SDF usually only requires removal of the biofilm and application of the product with a microbrush for 3 minutes, then either rinsing the area with water or covering the lesion with fluoride varnish. Gingival tissues and lips should be covered with petroleum jelly to avoid staining. This approach may give patients who would otherwise be unable to receive treatment a low-cost alternative to arrest caries lesions and preserve their dentition (Fig. 2.43). However, the anticaries effect of SDF may be reduced over time. It has been reported that up to 50% of arrested lesions were "reactivated" by 24 months after one application of SDF.[161] The authors reported that this was likely due to the biofilm-retaining nature of these cavitated lesions. Thus there is a rationale for restoring these arrested lesions from both the caries management approach and for function and esthetics.

Immunization

For many years, investigators have been trying to develop an effective anticaries vaccine. Several prototypes have been tested in animals, but at this time neither the safety nor the efficacy of such a vaccine has been demonstrated in humans.[68,69]

Even if an anticaries vaccine was developed, some concerns remain, which may affect its widespread use. First, the potential adverse effects of a vaccine must be identified. The safety of such

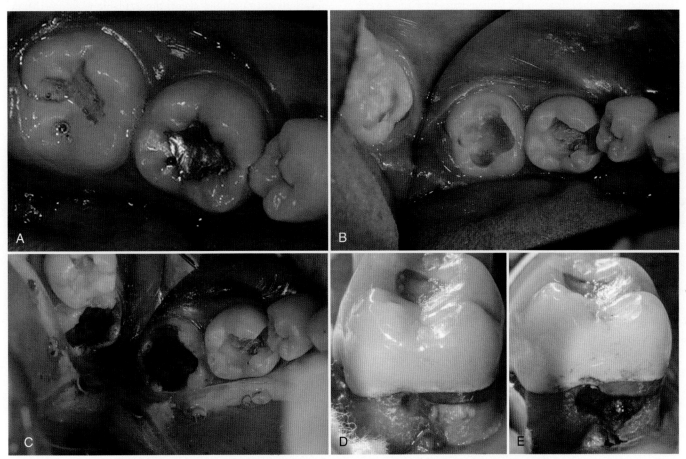

• **Fig. 2.43**   A, Young high caries risk patient. Tooth No. 17 with extensive caries lesion. Tooth was asymptomatic and roots were still developing. B, Unsupported enamel was removed, soft caries was left on the pulpal floor to avoid exposing the pulp. C, SDF was applied and left for 3 minutes. Darkened dentin can be observed. Tooth was restored with amalgam and remained asymptomatic. D, Tooth with PFM crown and secondary root caries on distal surface with difficult access for restoration. E, SDF applied and darkened dentin can be observed. (A–C, Courtesy Dr. Nguyen Ngoc, resident Graduate Operative Program at UNC; D and E, Courtesy Dr. Epure, resident Graduate Operative Dentistry Program at UNC.)

a vaccine has not yet been shown; concerns about a possible cross-reaction with human heart tissue remain. Second, its cost must be compared with that of public water fluoridation, which is inexpensive and already effective at reducing caries. Vaccination may be no more effective than fluoride therapy, which has a proven safety record. It may however be practical to use a caries vaccine when public water fluoridation is impractical in developed countries, and it may be useful in developing countries. Third, limitations imposed by governmental regulatory agencies may affect the widespread use of an anticaries vaccine.

Saliva

Saliva, as noted earlier in this chapter, provides an effective first line of defense against dental caries. Saliva works by diluting acid produced in biofilm, washing the acid away (swallowing), buffering the produced acid (bicarbonate + phosphate), and assisting in remineralization (calcium + phosphate). Saliva also works by forming a pellicle. When normal salivary flow rates are compromised, patients are usually at high risk for developing caries.

Normal aging does not result in reduced salivary flow rates; however, many older patients have compromised salivary flow rates as a result of medications taken for systemic conditions. Many commonly prescribed medications have hyposalivation as a potential side effect. A recent study has indicated that 63% of the 200 most commonly prescribed drugs in the United States have the adverse effect of reduced salivary flow rates.[70]

One important strategy for the prevention of caries in such patients is to increase the salivary flow rate and, by this, the concomitant buffering capacity. For these patients, gathering initial baseline data on salivary flow rates is critical. Commercial kits are available for the assessment of salivary flow. These kits provide data on simulated flow rates, the pH of saliva, and the level of buffering capacity. If saliva samples are sent for microbiologic testing, specific MS and lactobacilli counts may be determined. Specific strategies for improving flow rates and reducing bacterial counts may then be initiated. Subsequent retesting is necessary to identify the relative efficacy of the strategies.

When attempting to improve salivary flow rates, a consultation with the patient's physician may be in order. It may be possible that a less xerogenic drug be prescribed or the dose of a current drug reduced. Changing the time of taking the medication(s) may be useful. Prescribing salivary stimulants such as pilocarpine or cevimeline may be very beneficial in patients with functioning salivary glands but who have medication-induced hyposalivation.

Other strategies to improve salivary flow rates include increased water intake, use of sugar-free candies/mints several times a day, and/or use of xylitol chewing gum. Xylitol will be discussed in the next section.

Chemical Agents

Chemical agents to help modulate the biofilm have been proposed. These agents have been shown to reduce MS levels but this alone has not been shown to modify caries outcomes.[71] Prior to initiating procedures to reduce the numbers of cariogenic bacteria in the oral cavity, bacterial testing should be conducted to determine baseline microbiologic variables. Saliva samples may be tested for specific MS and lactobacilli levels; commercial devices may help evaluate the level of ATP in the biofilm. Bacterial counts or ATP levels are not reliable risk indicators but can be useful as motivational tools for patients.

Various antimicrobial agents are available (Table 2.13). As discussed, fluoride has antimicrobial effects. Two differing strategies have been suggested for reducing bacterial counts. The traditional approach is the use of chlorhexidine (CHX) mouthwash, varnish, or both, along with prescription fluoride toothpaste. When using this approach, it may be prudent to use toothpaste free from sodium laurel sulfate (SLS), which causes the foaming action in dentifrices. Although data are equivocal, evidence demonstrates that SLS reduces the ability of CHX to reduce biofilm formation.[72] Although CHX decreases MS, there is no evidence that it decreases caries incidence in the absence of fluoride.

CHX was first available in the United States as a rinse and was first used for periodontal therapy. It was prescribed as a 0.12%

TABLE 2.13	Antimicrobial Agents			
	Mechanism of Action	Spectrum of Antibacterial Activity	Persistence in Mouth	Adverse Effects
Antibiotics				
Vancomycin	Blocks cell wall synthesis	Narrow	Short	Increases gram-negative flora
Kanamycin	Blocks protein synthesis	Broad	Short	Can increase caries activity
Actinobolin	Blocks protein synthesis	Streptococci	Long	Unknown
Bis Biguanides				
Alexidine	Antiseptic; prevents bacterial adherence	Broad	Long	Bitter taste; stains teeth and tongue brown; mucosal irritation
Chlorhexidine	Antiseptic; prevents bacterial adherence	Broad	Long	Bitter taste; stains teeth and tongue brown; mucosal irritation
Halogens				
Iodine	Bactericidal	Broad	Short	Metallic taste
Fluoride	1–10 parts per million (ppm) reduces acid production; 250 ppm bacteriostatic; 1000 ppm bactericidal	Broad	Long	Increases enamel resistance to caries attack; fluorosis in developing teeth with chronic high doses

rinse to high-risk patients for short-term use. It is also available as a varnish, and the most effective mode of varnish use is as a professionally applied material.[73] Chlorhexidine gluconate (0.12%) solution is effective in its ability to chelate cations and, as a result, disrupts cell adhesion, cell membrane function, and the ability of MS to uptake glucose and produce glucans and its metabolism resulting in a decrease in MS counts. Emilson concluded that CHX varnishes provide effective reduction in MS, although recent evidence is not as conclusive in favor of a CHX rinse.[74,75] Despite some favorable evidence, because there is only a weak correlation with a reduction in caries, CHX currently has very limited application as a regularly used caries management antimicrobial agent.

Xylitol is a natural five-carbon sugar obtained from birch trees. MS cannot ferment (metabolize) xylitol, so no acid is produced. Over time xylitol reduces the number of MS in the biofilm. It is usually recommended that patients chew two pieces of xylitol gum containing a total of 1 g xylitol 3 to 6 minutes after eating or snacking. Chewing any sugar-free gum after meals reduces the acidogenicity of the biofilm because chewing stimulates salivary flow, which improves the buffering of the pH drop that occurs after eating.[80] Reductions in caries rates are greater however when xylitol is used as the sugar substitute.[81] Although there is some suggestion that xylitol may reduce caries rate,[82] enhance remineralization, and help arrest dentinal caries,[78,79,162] studies in adults have not been able to confirm its role on caries control[163] except for root caries.[164] The evidence supporting the use of xylitol products for the purpose of caries reduction in both adults and children is very weak.[165]

A myriad of other chemical agents have been suggested to selectively kill gram-positive cariogenic coaggregates of bacteria. Among these are propolis, nutraceutical phenols from licorice root, arginine, and bactericidal products such as sodium hypochlorite 0.2% in the form of an oral rinse.[166-168] However, despite the effect of these strategies on decreasing cariogenic bacteria counts, they have not been shown to actually decrease caries incidence in the absence of fluoride. Caries is a biofilm disease modulated by diet; therefore changes to bacterial counts will have a short-term impact on the caries process. In the absence of other changes, for example a significant reduction in fermentable carbohydrate intake, the biofilm microbiome will continue to adapt to the acidogenic and aciduric environment caused by a highly cariogenic diet; and these antimicrobial strategies will have little impact on caries outcomes.

Calcium and Phosphate Compounds

Amorphous calcium-phosphate (ACP) products have become commercially available and reportedly have the potential to remineralize tooth structure.[83] ACP is a reactive and soluble calcium phosphate compound that releases calcium and phosphate ions to convert to apatite and remineralize the enamel when it comes in contact with saliva. Forming on the tooth enamel and within the dentinal tubules, ACP provides a reservoir of calcium and phosphate ions in the saliva.[84] Casein phosphopeptide (CPP) is a milk-derived protein that binds to the tooth's biofilm and is used to stabilize ACP. Remineralization products that use CPP as a vehicle to deliver and maintain a supersaturation state of ACP at or near the tooth surface have recently been introduced. Some of these products contain other caries-preventive agents such as fluoride and xylitol (e.g., MI Paste Plus, GC America, Alsip, IL). Gum, lozenges, and topically applied solutions containing CPP-ACP have also been reported to remineralize white spots.[85,86] Mounting evidence indicates that CPP-ACP complexes, when used regularly, are effective

in enamel remineralization[87-90]; however, most of these studies have not looked at its effect independent of fluoride. The CPP-ACP products must not be prescribed to patients with allergies to dairy (milk) proteins.

Probiotics

One novel approach for reducing dental caries that has emerged in recent years is that of probiotics. The fundamental concept is to inoculate the oral cavity with bacteria that will compete with cariogenic bacteria and eventually replace them. Obviously the probiotic bacteria must not produce significant adverse effects.

A number of commercial products have been introduced and have been demonstrated to be safe in short-term studies. However, their relative level of efficacy remains unknown. It has been speculated that for the probiotic microorganisms to gain dominance, existing pathogens must first be eliminated. The concept of probiotics holds significant promise but considerably more research is required.

Sealants

Although fluoride treatments are most effective in preventing smooth-surface caries, they are less effective in preventing pit-and-fissure caries. The use of sealants is an effective preventive treatment for caries in pit-and-fissure areas.[91] Sealants have three important preventive effects. First, sealants mechanically fill pits and fissures with a resin-based polymer. Second, because the pits and fissures are physically closed off from the oral environment with the sealant resin, MS and other cariogenic organisms no longer have access to their preferred habitat. Third, sealants render the surface of the tooth, where the pits and fissures are located, easier to clean by toothbrushing and mastication (Figs. 2.44 and 2.45).

Based on the available scientific literature, pit-and-fissure sealants are appropriate for prevention of caries in susceptible teeth and, within limits, for arresting initial caries lesions.[92-96] There is mounting evidence that sealing initial lesions is an effective means to arrest dental caries.[169]

Another strategy recently introduced is the use of extremely low-viscosity resin sealants for the infiltration of white-spot caries lesions on smooth surfaces[97] (Fig. 2.46). In situ studies demonstrate the ability of resin sealants, also called *infiltrants*, to prevent further demineralization under cariogenic conditions.[98] Resin infiltrants have reportedly been used in free (i.e., facial and lingual) as well as in interproximal enamel surfaces. However, similar to the sealant technique used in pit-and-fissure areas, the technique requires careful attention to detail. A practice-based randomized clinical research trial has indicated that infiltration was more effective at preventing lesion progression than instructions on oral hygiene, flossing, and fluoride use.[170]

Restorations

The status of a patient's existing restorations may have an important bearing on the outcome of preventive measures and caries treatment. Old restorations that are rough and plaque retentive should be smoothed and polished. If the marginal integrity is inadequate, then the restoration should be repaired or replaced. Restoration defects such as overhangs, open proximal contacts, and defective contours contribute to plaque formation and retention. These defects should be corrected, usually by replacement of the defective restoration. Detection of caries around restorations and sealants (CARS) ("secondary caries") may be difficult around old restorations. Discoloration of the enamel adjacent to a restoration suggests the potential for CARS, but is not a definitive diagnosis. This condition

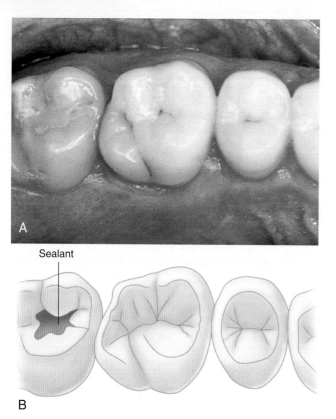

• **Fig. 2.44** A and B, Sealant applied to the central fossa of a maxillary second molar. This tooth was treated because of the appearance of chalky enamel and softening in the central fossa. A highly filled sealant was used (see Fig. 2.43).

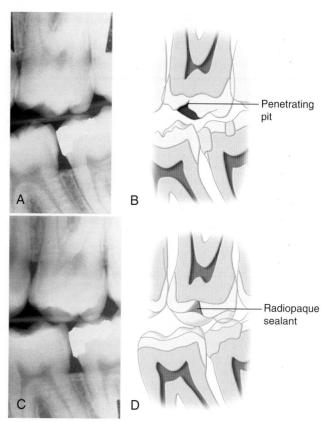

• **Fig. 2.45** A and B, Radiograph of a maxillary first molar with a deep central fossa pit that appears to penetrate to the dentin. C and D, The central pit was sealed with a highly filled, radiopaque sealant. The sealant is readily visible on the radiograph.

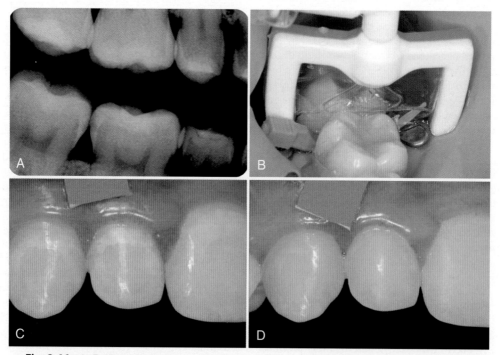

• **Fig. 2.46** A, Radiographic image of first mandibular molar with a proximal lesion on distal surface. B, Tooth was infiltrated according to manufacturer's instructions (Icon, DMG America). C and D, Clinical images of smooth-surface lesions on anterior teeth before and after infiltration, with Icon. (A, Courtesy Dr. Andrea Cortes, Operative Dentistry Specialization Program, El Bosque University. B, Courtesy Dr. Olga Lucia Zarta (chair) and Dr. Ainimsay Benitez (resident), Operative Dentistry Specialization Program, Dental School, El Bosque University, Bogotá, Colombia. C and D, Reprinted with permission from Meyer-Lueckel H, Paris, *Zahnmedizin up2date* 267–290, 2017.)

appears as a localized opalescent area next to the restoration margins. (*Exception:* A bluish color of facial or lingual enamel that directly overlies an old, otherwise acceptable amalgam restoration does not indicate replacement unless there is a need for improvement of esthetics. Such a discoloration may be caused by the amalgam itself.) Because metallic restorations are radiopaque, the radiolucency of CARS may be masked. The restoration of cavitated active caries lesions is preventive only because it removes large numbers of cariogenic organisms and some of the sites in which they may be protected, and it restores adequate tooth contours and surface smoothness that may facilitate oral hygiene. As emphasized earlier, the placement of a restoration into a cavitated carious tooth does not cure the caries process.

Although caries diagnostic and preventive measures have been improved and are more widely used, the repair of destruction caused by the caries process still is necessary for many patients. The treatment regimen is dictated by the patient's caries status. If the patient is at high risk for caries development, treatment should consist of restorative procedures concomitant with many of the preventive measures described previously. The damage done by caries may be repaired while at the same time seeking to lower the patient's risk status for further caries development. Sometimes, patients present with active caries lesions in numerous teeth. Because these teeth may be in jeopardy and because of the large numbers and sites of cariogenic bacteria, arresting medication for caries control (e.g., SDF) or restorative treatment for caries control may be indicated, as described later in this section. This procedure rapidly eliminates the caries lesions, providing better assessment of the pulpal responses of some teeth and greater success of the preventive measures instituted. Later, teeth may be restored with more definitive restorations.

Once caries has produced cavitation of the tooth surface, unless the cariogenic biofilm can be removed from a cavitated caries lesion or the lesion has been treated with SDF, preventive measures will be inadequate to prevent further progression of the lesion. Excision of the lesion (tooth preparation) and proper tooth restoration will not only stop the progression of active, cavitated lesions but also restore tooth function and esthetics.

Clinical Considerations for Caries Removal

Under normal operative clinical circumstances, in a vital permanent tooth with no symptoms or signs of pulpal pathology, the extent of the dentin caries removal (excavation) is dictated primarily by lesion severity and depth:

- Moderate lesions (lesions not reaching the inner one third of dentin and with no anticipated risk of pulp exposure) should be excavated to a caries-free DEJ and firm dentin.
- Advanced (deep) lesions (lesions reaching the inner one third of dentin and with anticipated risk of pulp exposure) should be excavated to a caries-free DEJ and soft dentin, following a selective caries removal (SCR) protocol.[171,172]

For a complete description of current caries classification criteria based on lesion severity and activity, please see Chapter 3. The SCR protocol is a professionally recognized and accepted tooth-level caries control treatment,[173-176] and it can be used on any tooth with an advanced (deep) caries lesion that is deemed restorable, and for which the pulpal and periapical areas are deemed healthy. Selective caries removal consists of complete caries removal peripherally to a sound, caries-free DEJ; axially and pulpally, caries is removed to within approximately 1 mm of the pulp within soft dentin; a glass ionomer (e.g., Fuji IX, GC America, Alsip, IL) temporary restoration or a definitive restoration is then placed.

Growing evidence suggests that temporization followed by reentry does not contribute to improved clinical outcomes[27, 28]; therefore current research supports the placement of a definitive restoration.[30,177-181] Selective caries removal allows a restoration to be placed while avoiding pulpal exposure.[26] Avoiding a pulpal exposure has a great impact on the lifetime prognosis of the tooth and long-term treatment costs.[182] Although the residual dentin thickness cannot be accurately assessed clinically, its preservation is a significant factor in avoiding pulpal distress.[183,184]

In slowly advancing lesions, it is expedient to remove the soft (infected) dentin until the readily identifiable hard (sclerotic) dentin is reached. In rapidly advancing lesions (see Figs. 2.36, 2.37, and 2.43A), little clinical evidence (as determined by texture or color change) exists to indicate the extent of the soft (infected) dentin. For deep lesions, this lack of clinical evidence may result in an excavation that risks pulp exposure. In a tooth with a deep advanced caries lesion, no history of spontaneous pain, normal responses to thermal stimuli, and a vital pulp, a deliberate, selective caries lesion removal (as noted) may be indicated. This procedure is supported by a large body of evidence.[26-34,99-123,185-192]

Removal of the bacterial infection has been seen as an essential part of all operative procedures; however, even removal of dentin up to hard dentin in deep, advanced caries lesions does not ensure a "sterile" dentin as bacteria have been found to be present in all dentinal layers in deep caries lesions. Nevertheless, even when bacteria are present, compounding evidence indicates that when a good seal is present the lesion will arrest[193-196] (see Fig. 2.18E–L). Therefore it is not necessary to remove all of the dentin that has been compromised by the caries process. Although caries detection solutions such as 1% acid red 52 (acid rhodamine B or food red 106) in propylene glycol[35] have been developed to help stain the infected layer, these dyes bind and stain the demineralized dentin matrix and do not stain bacteria exclusively. Complete removal of all stained tooth structure in the preparation therefore ultimately leads to significantly larger preparations than the traditional visual-tactile method of evaluating for caries removal, so their use is no longer recommended.[197-199]

The following are additional clinical considerations for caries lesion removal:

a. Regardless of which protocol is used for caries removal (caries removal to firm dentin or selective caries removal to soft dentin), the tooth may be restored with a final restoration (Figs. 2.47 and 2.48). However, the patient should be clearly informed that in the treatment of advanced (deep) dentin caries some leathery and soft dentin may remain under the restoration. This remaining caries-affected dentin has many implications, including higher risk for endodontic complications[205] (not because "caries was left under the restoration" but because deep caries was present to begin with) and a radiographic presentation that may suggest secondary or residual caries.

b. Although there is overwhelming scientific evidence in support of the SCR protocol, this is still a controversial clinical procedure in certain countries[32] with potential liability implications as well as implications for clinical board examinations, most of which still require complete caries removal (excavation) to hard dentin as a criteria for a successful clinical board examination.

c. The patient should be clearly informed of the risks and benefits of the selective caries removal to soft dentin protocol, and provide informed consent. If the patient is not willing to accept the risks, then the alternative, either complete caries removal with a higher risk of complications (endodontic therapy, postoperative sensitivity) or tooth extraction, should be presented.

d. A sealed tooth-restoration interface is critical for the success of the restorative procedure (see Fig. 2.18E–L). When a proper seal is NOT obtained, or when/if the seal is compromised, marginal leakage and ingress of bacteria/fluids/nutrients will allow lesion progression. This is particularly critical when soft dentin remains under the restoration.

e. When excavating advanced (deep) dentin caries, if a caries-free DEJ cannot be obtained, a protective restoration (sedative filling, temporary restoration) should be used and tooth restorability should be reassessed. A permanent restoration should not be used unless a sound DEJ (or peripheral dentin margin) is reached (see Figs. 2.47 and 2.48).

f. In slowly advancing lesions, it is practical to remove the soft (infected) dentin until firm (demineralized, affected) dentin is reached. Despite being demineralized, with adequate marginal seal, the lesion may arrest and the affected dentin may

remineralize. This allows for the most conservative tooth preparation without jeopardizing the restoration.

g. The pulpal diagnoses outlined here rely on signs and symptoms of pulp pathology using the best diagnostic tools available. However, actual pulpal status is difficult to determine

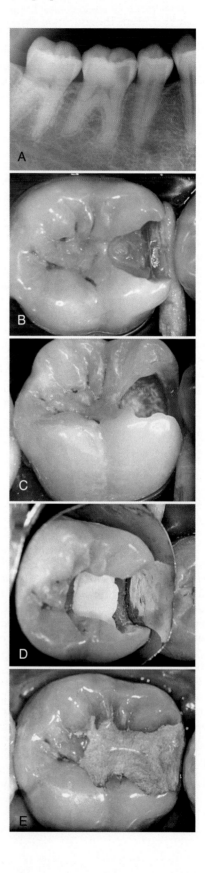

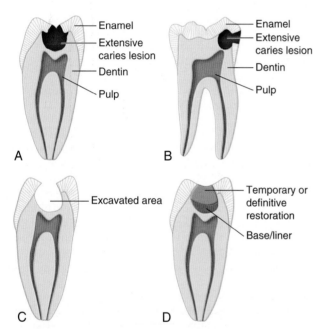

• **Fig. 2.47** Schematic representation of caries-control procedure. A and B, Faciolingual (A) and mesiodistal (B) cross sections of mandibular first molar show extensive preoperative occlusal and proximal caries lesions. C, Tooth after excavation of extensive caries. Note remaining unsupported enamel. D, Temporary amalgam restoration inserted after appropriate liner or base.

• **Fig. 2.48** A, Preoperative clinical radiograph illustrating extensive caries lesion in the proximal and occlusal regions of the mandibular right first molar. Initial caries excavation of tooth. B, Remaining caries requires further excavation. Also, note the wedge in place, protecting rubber dam and soft tissue; it has been lightly shaved by a bur. C, Remaining unsupported enamel under mesiolingual cusp. D, Tooth ready for placement of temporary restoration. Carious involvement required further extension than that seen in B and C. Liner or base material has been applied to deepest excavated areas, and matrix, appropriately wedged, has been placed. E, Temporary restoration completed for caries-control procedure. Caries has been eliminated, the pulp adequately protected, and interarch and intraarch positions of tooth maintained by caries-control procedure.

clinically—bacteria and toxins progressing ahead of caries may cause areas of undetectable and asymptomatic pulpal necrosis or irreversible pulpitis.

h. Use of calcium hydroxide (or other liner/base materials) after caries removal and before use of a protective or final restoration does not appear to improve outcomes.[200]

i. Teeth that are restorable only by use of full cuspal coverage restoration generally are not appropriate for the SCR technique because of the difficulty of evaluating the tooth for possible failures such as continuing caries activity under the full coverage restoration. Another concern is the cost of rectifying failures.

j. This protocol recognizes that exposures will occur despite admonitions to leave soft and leathery (infected) dentin rather than expose the pulp. Whenever there is a pulp exposure, the treatment should be consistent with existing endodontic guidelines for vital pulp exposures.

k. Advances in vital pulp therapy may allow successful endodontic therapy of pulp exposures without the need for root canal treatment. With the advent of tricalcium silicates, the prognosis of pulp capping (partial and full pulpotomy of permanent mature teeth) has tremendously improved. Recent observational and randomized trials, as well as systematic reviews and meta-analyses, have shown that these procedures have success for pulp vitality that exceeds 90%.[201-203] Complete caries removal with the option of vital pulp therapy should be one of the options offered to the patient during the informed consent process.

l. The SCR protocol can be applied either on a single tooth being treated or to several teeth in a caries control phase treatment. High caries risk patients with multiple cavitated caries lesions can benefit from a treatment plan designed specifically to gain control over the rapid progression of their disease. The term *caries control* refers to a procedure in which multiple teeth with acute threatening caries are treated quickly by (1) applying a medication (e.g., SDF) to arrest the caries lesions or (2) removing the infected tooth structure, medicating the pulp if necessary, and restoring the defect(s) with a temporary or definite material. The intent of caries-control procedures is immediate, corrective intervention of advanced caries lesions so as to prevent pulpal disease and avoid possible sequelae such as toothache, root canal therapy, or more complex ultimate restorations.

This allows the caries process in these cavitated lesions to be essentially arrested and the overall bacterial load to be reduced. Caries-control procedures must be accompanied by other preventive measures (Table 2.14). Teeth rapidly treated by caries-control procedures subsequently may be treated by using routine restorative techniques if appropriate pulpal responses are obtained.

Root Caries Management

It is clear that the baby boom generation of North America is aging. In the year 1900, 3% of the US population was over 60 years of age, whereas in the year 2000, 13% of the population was over 60 years.[124] In the year 2030, it is estimated that at least 20% of the population will be 60 years or older. Root caries is a pervasive problem in a high percentage of older patients.[125,126] Many of these patients have had extensive restorative dentistry done in their lifetimes. Approximately 38% of patients between the ages of 55 and 64 years have root caries, and 47% of those between 65 and 74 years have experienced root caries.[127] The incidence of root caries in old-older adults (over 75 years) is even higher.[128]

TABLE 2.14	Caries-Control Restoration
Initial treatment	Caries risk assessment
	Education and motivation
	Thorough evaluation and documentation of lesions
	Temporization of all large cavitated lesions by caries-control restorations
	Specific nonrestorative, therapeutic treatment (see Table 2.10)
	Plaque control (see Table 2.10, technique C)
	Dietary control (see Table 2.10, technique A)
Preliminary assessment	Gingival response as a marker of plaque biofilm control effectiveness
	Arrest of cavitated lesions with SDF as indicated
	Pulpal response of teeth with selective caries-excavation and restoration
	Assessment of patient compliance with medications, oral hygiene, and dietary control measures
Follow-up care	Careful clinical evaluation of teeth
	Replacement of caries-control restorations with permanent restorations
	Monitoring of plaque biofilm and mutans streptococci (MS) levels
	Further antimicrobial treatment and dietary reassessment as indicated by new cavitations, noncavitated lesions, or high MS levels

One of the primary etiologic factors for these patients is their use of prescription drugs for a wide variety of systemic medical problems. It has been estimated that 63% of the 200 most commonly prescribed medications have dry mouth as an adverse effect. It is the subsequent reduction in salivary flow rates and concomitant diminished buffering capacity resulting from use of these medications that is primarily responsible for the increase in root caries in older patients.

The critical pH of dentin (pH at which dentin begins to demineralize) is between 6.2 and 6.7, whereas that of enamel is about 5.5.[129] As a result, root dentin will demineralize in very weak acids, and root caries progresses at about twice the rate of coronal caries. Thus it is critical that all older patients receive thorough clinical and radiographic examinations on a regular basis.

As described previously in this chapter, a caries risk assessment should be carried out for all older patients. Factors that increase the risk for root caries include the following:

1. Gingival recession
2. Poor oral hygiene
3. Cariogenic diet
4. Presence of multiple restorations or multiple missing teeth
5. Existing caries
6. Xerogenic medications
7. Compromised salivary flow rates

Once it has been determined that a patient is at high risk for root caries, an aggressive preventive protocol should be considered. This protocol is based upon four primary strategies for the prevention of root caries. The *first* strategy is to improve salivary flow rates and increase the buffering capacity. The *second* strategy is to modulate a cariogenic biofilm in the oral cavity. The *third* strategy is to reduce the quantity and numbers of exposures of ingested refined carbohydrates, and the *fourth* is to attempt to remineralize initial lesions and prevent new lesions from developing. In addition to following the aforementioned protocol, three additional considerations are important:

1. Use of powered toothbrushes and irrigation devices. It is critical that patients susceptible to root caries practice meticulous oral hygiene. However, many of these patients have physical and visual deficiencies, which makes it difficult for them to adequately cleanse the mouth. For these patients, a powered toothbrush may be advantageous.[207] Additionally, daily use of a water irrigation device (Waterpik, Water Pik Inc., Fort Collins, CO) may be beneficial. Although the device will not remove biofilm, studies have shown that daily use will change the composition of the biofilm in a beneficial way. However, since the toothbrush essentially provides the means of fluoride delivery, use of a water irrigation device alone is not indicated unless used with a fluoridated rinse (e.g., ACT).

2. Restoration of all root caries lesions with a fluoride-releasing material. Resin-modified glass ionomer materials are preferred for definitive restorations of active root caries lesions primarily because they bond effectively to both enamel and dentin and they act as reservoirs for fluoride, which may be re-released into the oral cavity.[130,131] These materials may be effective as anticaries materials only if patients reload the material a minimum of three times a day by brushing with fluoride-containing toothpaste or by using other fluoride-containing products.[208] Alternatively these same root caries lesions can be arrested by application of SDF (see Fig. 2.43D and E).

3. Educating patients of the necessity for three exposures to fluoride per day and for reloading the fluoride-releasing materials can assist in motivating them to improved levels of compliance.[208]

In summary, many older patients are experiencing an epidemic of root caries, primarily as a result of the hyposalivatory effects of medications prescribed for systemic illnesses. Many root caries lesions occur in locations that make them difficult if not impossible to restore. The dental profession has a strong track record of prevention, and it is clear that with root caries, prevention is much better than restoration.

Summary

Caries management efforts must be directed not at the tooth level (traditional or surgical treatment) but at the total-patient level (medical model of treatment). Restorative treatment does not cure the caries process. Instead, identifying and eliminating the causative factors for caries must be the primary focus, in addition to the restorative repair of damage caused by caries.

Much of the remainder of this textbook presents information on when and how to restore tooth defects. Many tooth defects are the result of caries activity. Only implementation of appropriate caries-preventive measures will lower the probability that caries lesions will recur. Tooth restorations are preventive in the sense that they remove numerous cariogenic organisms in the affected site and eliminate a protected habitat for other cariogenic bacteria; however, they primarily repair the tooth damage caused by caries and have only a limited impact on the patient's overall caries risk.

Acknowledgments

The authors would like to thank Professor JM ("Bob") ten Cate PhD, University of Amsterdam, for his review of the Ecologic Basis of Dental Caries: The Role of the Biofilm section of this chapter.

References

1. Keyes PH: Research in dental caries. *J Am Dent Assoc* 76(6):1357–1373, 1968.
2. Featherstone JD: The caries balance: The basis for caries management by risk assessment. *Oral Health Prev Dent* 2(Suppl 1):259–264, 2004.
3. Chaussain-Miller C, Fioretti F, Goldberg M, et al: The role of matrix metalloproteinases (MMPs) in human caries. *J Dent Res* 85(1):22–32, 2006.
4. Young DA, Kutsch VK, Whitehouse J: A clinician's guide to CAMBRA: A simple approach. *Compend Contin Educ Dent* 30(2):92–94, 96, 98, passim, 2009.
5. Marsh PD: Dental plaque as a biofilm and a microbial community—implications for health and disease. *BMC Oral Health* 6(Suppl 1):S14, 2006.
6. Hannig C, Hannig M: The oral cavity—a key system to understand substratum-dependent bioadhesion on solid surfaces in man. *Clin Oral Invest* 13(2):123–139, 2009.
7. Juhl M: Three-dimensional replicas of pit and fissure morphology in human teeth. *Scand J Dent Res* 91(2):90–95, 1983.
8. Brown LR: Effects of selected caries preventive regimes on microbial changes following radiation-induced xerostomia in cancer patients. *Microbiol Abstr Spec Suppl* 1:275, 1976.
9. Dreizen SBL: Xerostomia and dental caries. *Microbiol Abstr Spec Suppl* 1263, 1976.
10. Mandel ID: Salivary factors in caries prediction, *Sp. Suppl. Microbiology Abstracts.* In Bibby BG, Shern RJ, editors: *Proceedings "Methods of Caries Prediction"*, ed 4, Arlington, Va, 1978, Information Retrieval, Inc, pp 147–162.
11. Arnold RR, Russell JE, Devine SM, et al: Antimicrobial activity of the secretory innate defense factors lactoferrin, lactoperoxidase, and lysozyme. In Guggenheim B, editor: *Cariology today*, Basel, 1984, Karger, pp 75–88.
12. Mandel I, Ellison SA: Naturally occurring defense mechanism in saliva. In Tanzer JM, editor: *Animal models in cariology (supplement to Microbiology Abstracts)*, Washington, DC, 1981, Information Retrieval.
13. van Houte J: Microbiological predictors of caries risk. *Adv Dent Res* 7(2):87–96, 1993.
14. Hay DI: Specific functional salivary proteins. In Guggenheim B, editor: *Cariology today*, Basel, 1984, Karger.
15. Ritter AV, Shugars DA, Bader JD: Root caries risk indicators: A systematic review of risk models. *Community Dent Oral Epidemiol* 38(5):383–397, 2010.
16. Du M, Jiang H, Tai B, et al: Root caries patterns and risk factors of middle-aged and elderly people in China. *Community Dent Oral Epidemiol* 37(3):260–266, 2009.
17. Saunders RH, Jr, Meyerowitz C: Dental caries in older adults. *Dent Clin North Am* 49(2):293–308, 2005.
18. Berry TG, Summitt JB, Swift EJ, Jr: Root caries. *Oper Dent* 29(6):601–607, 2004.
19. Parfitt GJ: The speed of development of the carious cavity. *Br Dent J* 100:204–207, 1956.
20. Backer DO: Posteruptive changes in dental enamel. *J Dent Res* 45:503, 1966.

21. Silverstone LM: In vitro studies with special reference to the enamel surface and the enamel-resin interface. In Silverstone LM, Dogon IC, editors: *Proceedings of an international symposium on the acid etch tecnique*, St Paul, MN, 1975, North Central.

22. Baum LJ: Dentinal pulp conditions in relation to caries lesions, *Int Dent J* 20:309–337, 1970.

23. Brannstrom M, Lind PO: Pulpal response to early dental caries. *J Dent Res* 44(5):1045–1050, 1965.

24. Pashley DH: Clinical correlations of dentin structure and function. *J Prosthet Dent* 66(6):777–781, 1991.

25. Ogawa K, Yamashita Y, Ichijo T, et al: The ultrastructure and hardness of the transparent layer of human carious dentin. *J Dent Res* 62(1):7–10, 1983.

26. Hayashi M, Fujitani M, Yamaki C, et al: Ways of enhancing pulp preservation by stepwise excavation—a systematic review. *J Dent* 39(2):95–107, 2011.

27. Bjorndal L, Reit C, Bruun G, et al: Treatment of deep caries lesions in adults: Randomized clinical trials comparing stepwise vs. direct complete excavation, and direct pulp capping vs. partial pulpotomy. *Eur J Oral Sci* 118(3):290–297, 2010.

28. Ricketts DN, Pitts NB: Novel operative treatment options. *Monogr Oral Sci* 21:174–187, 2009.

29. Hilton TJ: Keys to clinical success with pulp capping: a review of the literature. *Oper Dent* 34(5):615–625, 2009.

30. Thompson V, Craig RG, Curro FA, et al: Treatment of deep carious lesions by complete excavation or partial removal: A critical review. *J Am Dent Assoc* 139(6):705–712, 2008.

31. Bjorndal L: Indirect pulp therapy and stepwise excavation. *J Endod* 34(7 Suppl):S29–S33, 2008.

32. Oen KT, Thompson VP, Vena D, et al: Attitudes and expectations of treating deep caries: A PEARL Network survey. *Gen Dent* 55(3):197–203, 2007.

33. Miyashita H, Worthington HV, Qualtrough A, et al: Pulp management for caries in adults: Maintaining pulp vitality. *Cochrane Database Syst Rev* (2):CD004484, 2007.

34. Maltz M, Oliveira EF, Fontanella V, et al: Deep caries lesions after incomplete dentine caries removal: 40-month follow-up study. *Caries Res* 41(6):493–496, 2007.

35. Fusayama T: Two layers of carious dentin: Diagnosis and treatment. *Oper Dent* 4(2):63–70, 1979.

36. Kuboki Y, Liu CF, Fusayama T: Mechanism of differential staining in carious dentin. *J Dent Res* 62(6):713–714, v, 1983.

37. Beck JD, Kohout F, Hunt RJ: Identification of high caries risk adults: Attitudes, social factors and diseases. *Int Dent J* 38(4):231–238, 1988.

38. Beck JD: Risk revisited. *Community Dent Oral Epidemiol* 26(4):220–225, 1998.

39. Fontana M, Zero DT: Assessing patients' caries risk. *J Am Dent Assoc* 137(9):1231–1239, 2006.

40. Steinberg S: Understanding and managing dental caries: A medical approach. *Alpha Omegan* 100(3):127–134, 2007.

41. Steinberg S: Adding caries diagnosis to caries risk assessment: The next step in caries management by risk assessment (CAMBRA). *Compend Contin Educ Dent* 30(8):522, 24–26, 28 passim, 2009.

42. Domejean-Orliaguet S, Gansky SA, Featherstone JD: Caries risk assessment in an educational environment. *J Dent Educ* 70(12):1346–1354, 2006.

43. Hausen H: Caries prediction—state of the art. *Community Dent Oral Epidemiol* 25(1):87–96, 1997.

44. Riley JL, 3rd, Gordan VV, Rindal DB, et al: General practitioners' use of caries-preventive agents in adult patients versus pediatric patients: Findings from the dental practice-based research network. *J Am Dent Assoc* 141(6):679–687, 2010.

45. Riley JL, 3rd, Gordan VV, Rindal DB, et al: Preferences for caries prevention agents in adult patients: Findings from the dental practice-based research network. *Community Dent Oral Epidemiol* 38(4):360–370, 2010.

46. Kidd EA: The use of diet analysis and advice in the management of dental caries in adult patients. *Oper Dent* 20(3):86–93, 1995.

47. Löe H: Human research model for the production and prevention of gingivitis. *J Dent Res* 50:256, 1971.

48. Krasc B: *Caries risk*, Chicago, 1985, Quintessence.

49. Klock B, Krasse B: Effect of caries-preventive measures in children with high numbers of S. mutans and lactobacilli. *Scand J Dent Res* 86(4):221–230, 1978.

50. Gorur A, Lyle DM, Schaudinn C, et al: Biofilm removal with a dental water jet. *Compend Contin Educ Dent* 30(Spec1):1 6, 2009.

51. Brown LJ, Lazar V: The economic state of dentistry. Demand-side trends. *J Am Dent Assoc* 129(12):1685–1691, 1998.

52. HHS US Department of Health & Human Services: New Assessments and Actions on Fluoride: Accessed 06/07/2011: http://www.hhs.gov/news/press/2011pres/01/20110107a.html.

53. American Dental Association Sc: *Key dental facts*, Chicago, 2004, American Dental Association.

54. Populations receiving optimally fluoridated public drinking water—United States, 1992-2006. *MMWR Morb Mortal Wkly Rep* 57(27):737–741, 2008.

55. Svanberg M, Westergren G: Effect of SnF2, administered as mouthrinses or topically applied, on *Streptococcus mutans, Streptococcus sanguis* and lactobacilli in dental plaque and saliva. *Scand J Dent Res* 91(2):123–129, 1983.

56. Beltran-Aguilar ED, Goldstein JW, Lockwood SA: Fluoride varnishes. A review of their clinical use, cariostatic mechanism, efficacy and safety. *J Am Dent Assoc* 131(5):589–596, 2000.

57. Centers for Disease Control and Prevention: Recommendations for using fluoride to prevent and control dental caries in the United States. *MMWR Morb Mortal Wkly Rep* 50(RR–14):1–30, 2001.

58. Newbrun E: Topical fluorides in caries prevention and management: A North American perspective. *J Dent Educ* 65(10):1078–1083, 2001.

59. Weintraub JA: Fluoride varnish for caries prevention: Comparisons with other preventive agents and recommendations for a community-based protocol. *Spec Care Dentist* 23(5):180–186, 2003.

60. Borutta A, Kunzel W, Rubsam F: The caries-protective efficacy of 2 fluoride varnishes in a 2-year controlled clinical trial [translation]. *Dtsch Zahn Mund Kieferheilkd Zentralbl* 79(7):543–549, 1991.

61. Borutta A, Reuscher G, Hufnagl S, et al: Caries prevention with fluoride varnishes among preschool children [translation]. *Gesundheitswesen* 68(11):731–734, 2006.

62. Castellano JB, Donly KJ: Potential remineralization of demineralized enamel after application of fluoride varnish. *Am J Dent* 17(6):462–464, 2004.

63. Haugejorden O, Nord A: Caries incidence after topical application of varnishes containing different concentrations of sodium fluoride: 3-year results. *Scand J Dent Res* 99(4):295–300, 1991.

64. Seppa L: Effects of a sodium fluoride solution and a varnish with different fluoride concentrations on enamel remineralization in vitro. *Scand J Dent Res* 96(4):304–309, 1988.

65. Hutter JW, Chan JT, Featherstone JD, et al: Professionally applied topical fluoride. Executive summary of evidence-based clinical recommendations. *J Am Dent Assoc* 137(8):1151–1159, 2006.

66. Alaluusua S, Kleemola-Kujala E, Gronroos L, et al: Salivary caries-related tests as predictors of future caries increment in teenagers. A three-year longitudinal study. *Oral Microbiol Immunol* 5(2):77–81, 1990.

67. Professionally applied topical fluoride: Evidence-based clinical recommendations. *J Am Dent Assoc* 137(8):1151–1159, 2006.

68. Lehner T, Challacombe SJ, Caldwell J: An immunological investigation into the prevention of caries in deciduous teeth of rhesus monkeys. *Arch Oral Biol* 20(5–6):305–310, 1975.

69. Taubman MA, Smith DJ: Effects of local immunization with glucosyltransferase fractions from *Streptococcus mutans* on dental caries in rats and hamsters. *J Immunol* 118(2):710–720, 1977.

70. Sreebny LM, Schwartz SS: A reference guide to drugs and dry mouth—2nd edition. *Gerodontology* 14(1):33-47, 1997.

71. Swarn A, Ritter AV, Donovan T, et al: Caries risk evaluation: Correlation between chair-side, laboratory and clinical tests. *J Dent Res* 89(SpecialB, USB of abstracts #4272):2010.

72. Barkvoll P, Rolla G, Svendsen K: Interaction between chlorhexidine digluconate and sodium lauryl sulfate in vivo. *J Clin Periodontol* 16(9):593-595, 1989.

73. Emilson CG: Potential efficacy of chlorhexidine against mutans streptococci and human dental caries. *J Dent Res* 73(3):682-691, 1994.

74. Slot DE, Vaandrager NC, Van Loveren C, et al: The effect of chlorhexidine varnish on root caries: A systematic review. *Caries Res* 45(2):162-173, 2011.

75. Ashley P: Effectiveness of chlorhexidine varnish for preventing caries uncertain. *Evid Based Dent* 11(4):108, 2010.

76. Reference deleted in pages.

77. Reference deleted in pages.

78. Tanzer JM: Xylitol chewing gum and dental caries. *Int Dent J* 45(1 Suppl 1):65-76, 1995.

79. Trahan L: Xylitol: A review of its action on mutans streptococci and dental plaque–its clinical significance. *Int Dent J* 45(1 Suppl 1):77-92, 1995.

80. Edgar WM: Saliva and dental health. Clinical implications of saliva: Report of a consensus meeting. *Br Dent J* 169(3-4):96-98, 1990.

81. Hayes C: The effect of non-cariogenic sweeteners on the prevention of dental caries: A review of the evidence. *J Dent Educ* 65(10):1106-1109, 2001.

82. Deshpande A, Jadad AR: The impact of polyol-containing chewing gums on dental caries: A systematic review of original randomized controlled trials and observational studies. *J Am Dent Assoc* 139(12):1602-1614, 2008.

83. Tung MS, Eichmiller FC: Amorphous calcium phosphates for tooth mineralization. *Compend Contin Educ Dent* 25(9 Suppl 1):9-13, 2004.

84. Chow LC, Takagi S, Vogel GL: Amorphous calcium phosphate: The contention of bone. *J Dent Res* 77(1):6, author reply 7, 1998.

85. Cai F, Shen P, Morgan MV, et al: Remineralization of enamel subsurface lesions in situ by sugar-free lozenges containing casein phosphopeptide-amorphous calcium phosphate. *Aust Dent J* 48(4):240-243, 2003.

86. Morgan MV, Adams GG, Bailey DL, et al: The anticariogenic effect of sugar-free gum containing CPP-ACP nanocomplexes on approximal caries determined using digital bitewing radiography. *Caries Res* 42(3):171-184, 2008.

87. Reynolds EC: Remineralization of enamel subsurface lesions by casein phosphopeptide-stabilized calcium phosphate solutions. *J Dent Res* 76(9):1587-1595, 1997.

88. Reynolds EC, Cai F, Shen P, et al: Retention in plaque and remineralization of enamel lesions by various forms of calcium in a mouthrinse or sugar-free chewing gum. *J Dent Res* 82(3):206-211, 2003.

89. Yengopal V, Mickenautsch S: Caries preventive effect of casein phosphopeptide-amorphous calcium phosphate (CPP-ACP): A meta-analysis. *Acta Odontol Scand* 67(6):1-12, 2009.

90. Llena C, Forner L, Baca P: Anticariogenicity of casein phosphopeptide-amorphous calcium phosphate: A review of the literature. *J Contemp Dent Pract* 10(3):1-9, 2009.

91. Simonsen RJ: Cost effectiveness of pit and fissure sealant at 10 years. *Quintessence Int* 20(2):75-82, 1989.

92. Tinanoff N, Douglass JM: Clinical decision making for caries management in children. *Pediatr Dent* 24(5):386-392, 2002.

93. Ahovuo-Saloranta A, Hiiri A, Nordblad A, et al: Pit and fissure sealants for preventing dental decay in the permanent teeth of children and adolescents. *Cochrane Database Syst Rev* (3):CD001830, 2004.

94. Beauchamp J, Caufield PW, Crall JJ, et al: Evidence-based clinical recommendations for the use of pit-and-fissure sealants: A report of the American Dental Association Council on Scientific Affairs. *J Am Dent Assoc* 139(3):257-268, 2008.

95. Bader JD, Shugars DA, Bonito AJ: Systematic reviews of selected dental caries diagnostic and management methods. *J Dent Educ* 65(10):960-968, 2001.

96. Simonsen RJ: Pit and fissure sealant: Review of the literature. *Pediatr Dent* 24(5):393-414, 2002.

97. Paris S, Meyer-Lueckel H: Masking of labial enamel white spot lesions by resin infiltration—a clinical report. *Quintessence Int* 40(9):713-718, 2009.

98. Paris S, Meyer-Lueckel H: Inhibition of caries progression by resin infiltration in situ. *Caries Res* 44(1):47-54, 2010.

99. Swift EJ: Treatment options for the exposed vital pulp. *Pract Periodontics Aesthet Dent* 11:735-739, 1999.

100. Banerjee A, Watson TF, Kidd EA: Dentine caries: Take it or leave it? *Dent Update* 27(6):272-276, 2000.

101. Bjorndal L: Buonocore Memorial Lecture. Dentin caries: Progression and clinical management. *Oper Dent* 27(3):211-217, 2002.

102. Bjorndal L: Indirect pulp therapy and stepwise excavation. *Pediatr Dent* 30(3):225-229, 2008.

103. Bjorndal L, Kidd EA: The treatment of deep dentine caries lesions. *Dent Update* 32(7):402-404, 407-410, 413, 2005.

104. Bjorndal L, Larsen T: Changes in the cultivable flora in deep carious lesions following a stepwise excavation procedure. *Caries Res* 34(6):502-508, 2000.

105. Bjorndal L, Larsen T, Thylstrup A: A clinical and microbiological study of deep carious lesions during stepwise excavation using long treatment intervals. *Caries Res* 31(6):411-417, 1997.

106. Bjorndal L, Thylstrup A: A practice-based study on stepwise excavation of deep carious lesions in permanent teeth: A 1-year follow-up study. *Community Dent Oral Epidemiol* 26(2):122-128, 1998.

107. Foley J, Evans D, Blackwell A: Partial caries removal and cariostatic materials in carious primary molar teeth: A randomised controlled clinical trial. *Br Dent J* 197(11):697-701, discussion 689, 2004.

108. Innes NP, Evans DJ, Stirrups DR: The Hall Technique; a randomized controlled clinical trial of a novel method of managing carious primary molars in general dental practice: Acceptability of the technique and outcomes at 23 months. *BMC Oral Health* 7:18, 2007.

109. Kidd EA: How "clean" must a cavity be before restoration? *Caries Res* 38(3):305-313, 2004.

110. Kidd EA, Fejerskov O: What constitutes dental caries? Histopathology of carious enamel and dentin related to the action of cariogenic biofilms. *J Dent Res* 83(SpecC):C35-C38, 2004.

111. Leksell E, Ridell K, Cvek M, et al: Pulp exposure after stepwise versus direct complete excavation of deep carious lesions in young posterior permanent teeth. *Endod Dent Traumatol* 12(4):192-196, 1996.

112. Maltz M, de Oliveira EF, Fontanella V, et al: A clinical, microbiologic, and radiographic study of deep caries lesions after incomplete caries removal. *Quintessence Int* 33(2):151-159, 2002.

113. Mertz-Fairhurst EJ, Adair SM, Sams DR, et al: Cariostatic and ultraconservative sealed restorations: Nine-year results among children and adults. *ASDC J Dent Child* 62(2):97-107, 1995.

114. Mertz-Fairhurst EJ, Curtis JW, Jr, Ergle JW, et al: Ultraconservative and cariostatic sealed restorations: Results at year 10. *J Am Dent Assoc* 129(1):55-66, 1998.

115. Mertz-Fairhurst EJ, Schuster GS, Fairhurst CW: Arresting caries by sealants: Results of a clinical study. *J Am Dent Assoc* 112(2):194-197, 1986.

116. Mertz-Fairhurst EJ, Schuster GS, Williams JE, et al: Clinical progress of sealed and unsealed caries. Part II: Standardized radiographs and clinical observations. *J Prosthet Dent* 42(6):633-637, 1979.

117. Mertz-Fairhurst EJ, Schuster GS, Williams JE, et al: Clinical progress of sealed and unsealed caries. Part I: Depth changes and bacterial counts. *J Prosthet Dent* 42(5):521-526, 1979.

118. Mjor IA: Pulp-dentin biology in restorative dentistry. Part 7: The exposed pulp. *Quintessence Int* 33(2):113–135, 2002.
119. Pinheiro SL, Simionato MR, Imparato JC, et al: Antibacterial activity of glass-ionomer cement containing antibiotics on caries lesion microorganisms. *Am J Dent* 18(4):261–266, 2005.
120. Ricketts D: Management of the deep carious lesion and the vital pulp dentine complex. *Br Dent J* 191(11):606–610, 2001.
121. Ricketts DN, Kidd EA, Innes N, et al: Complete or ultraconservative removal of decayed tissue in unfilled teeth. *Cochrane Database Syst Rev* (3):CD003808, 2006.
122. Uribe S: Partial caries removal in symptomless teeth reduces the risk of pulp exposure. *Evid Based Dent* 7(4):94, 2006.
123. van Amerongen WE: Dental caries under glass ionomer restorations. *J Public Health Dent* 56(3 Spec No):150 154, discussion 161–163, 1996.
124. Shay K: The evolving impact of aging America on dental practice. *J Contemp Dent Pract* 5(4):101–110, 2004.
125. Leake JL: Clinical decision-making for caries management in root surfaces. *J Dent Educ* 65(10):1147–1153, 2001.
126. Thomson WM: Dental caries experience in older people over time: What can the large cohort studies tell us? *Br Dent J* 196(2):89–92, discussion 87, 2004.
127. Winston AE, Bhaskar SN: Caries prevention in the 21st century. *J Am Dent Assoc* 129(11):1579–1587, 1998.
128. Berkey DB, Berg RG, Ettinger RL, et al: The old-old dental patient: The challenge of clinical decision-making. *J Am Dent Assoc* 127(3):321–332, 1996.
129. Surmont PA, Martens LC: Root surface caries: An update. *Clin Prev Dent* 11(3):14–20, 1989.
130. Burgess JO, Gallo JR: Treating root-surface caries. *Dent Clin North Am* 46(2):385–404, vii–viii, 2002.
131. Haveman CW, Redding SW: Dental management and treatment of xerostomic patients. *Tex Dent J* 115(5):43–56, 1998.
132. Takahashi N, Nyvad B: The role of bacteria in the caries process: ecological perspectives. *J Dent Res* 90(3):294–303, 2011.
133. Ferjeskov O, Nyvad B, Kidd E, editors: *Dental Caries: The disease and its clinical management*, 3rd ed, Oxford, 2015, Wiley-Blackwell.
134. Simón-Soro A, Tomás I, Cabrera-Rubio R, et al: Mira AMicrobial geography of the oral cavity. *J Dent Res* 92(7):616–621, 2013.
135. Ling Z, Kong J, Jia P, et al: Analysis of oral microbiota in children with dental caries by PCR-DGGE and barcoded pyrosequencing. *Microb Ecol* 60(3):677–690, 2010.
136. Hannig C, Hannig M, Attin T: Enzymes in the acquired enamel pellicle. *Eur J Oral Sci* 113(1):2–13, 2005.
137. Silverstone LM, Hicks MJ: The structure and ultrastructure of the carious lesion in human dentin. *Gerodontics* 1(4):185–193, 1985.
138. Boushell LW, Nagaola H, Yamauchi M: Increased Matrix Metalloproteinase-2 and Bone Sialoprotein Response to Human Coronal Caries. *Caries Res* 45:453–459, 2011.
139. Bjørndal L, Kidd EA: The treatment of deep dentine caries lesions. *Dent Update* 32(7):402–413, 2005.
140. Bjørndal L, Thylstrup A: A structural analysis of approximal enamel caries lesions and subjacent dentin reactions. *Eur J Oral Sci* 103(1):25–31, 1995.
141. Ekstrand KR, Ricketts DN, Kidd EA: Do occlusal carious lesions spread laterally at the enamel-dentin junction? A histopathological study. *Clin Oral Investig* 2(1):15–20, 1998.
142. Bjørndal L, Kidd EA: The treatment of deep dentine caries lesions. *Dent Update* 32(7):402–413, 2005.
143. Ekstrand KR, Ricketts DN, Kidd EA: Do occlusal carious lesions spread laterally at the enamel-dentin junction? A histopathological study. *Clin Oral Investig* 2(1):15–20, 1998.
144. Doméjean S, Featherstone JDB, White J: Validation of the CDA CAMBRA caries risk assessment: a six-year retrospective study. *J Calif Dent Assoc* 39:709–715, 2011.
145. Cheng J, Chaffee BW, Cheng NF, et al: Understanding treatment effect mechanisms of the CAMBRA randomized trial in reducing caries increment. *J Dent Res* 94(1):44–51, 2015.
146. Ismail AI, Pitts NB, Tellez M, et al: The International Caries Classification and Management System (ICCMS™) An Example of a Caries Management Pathway. *BMC Oral Health* 15(Suppl 1):S9, 2015.
147. Pitts NB, Ekstrand KR, Foundation ICDAS: International Caries Detection and Assessment System (ICDAS) and its International Caries Classification and Management System (ICCMS) - methods for staging of the caries process and enabling dentists to manage caries. *Community Dent Oral Epidemiol* 41(1):e41–e52, 2013.
148. Ismail AI, Tellez M, Pitts NB, et al: Caries management pathways preserve dental tissues and promote oral health. *Community Dent Oral Epidemiol* 41(1):e12–e40, 2013.
149. Campus G, Cagetti MG, Sale S, et al: Cariogram validity in schoolchildren: a two-year follow-up study. *Caries Res* 46:16–22, 2012.
150. Petersson GH, Isberg PE, Twetman S: Caries risk profiles in schoolchildren over 2 years assessed by Cariogram. *Int J Paediatr Dent* 20:341–346, 2010.
151. Takahashi N, Nyvad B: Ecological hypothesis of dentin and root caries. *Caries Res* 50:422–431, 2016.
152. Ekstrand KR, Martignon S, Ricketts DJN, et al: Detection and activity assessment of primary coronal caries lesions: a methodologic study. *Oper Dent* 32(3):225–235, 2007.
153. Nyvad B, Machiulskiene V, Baelum V: Reliability of a new caries diagnostic system differentiating between active and inactive caries lesions. *Caries Res* 33(4):252–260, 1999.
154. Yamaga R, Nishino M, Yoshida S, et al: Diammine silver fluoride and its clinical application. *J Osaka Univ Dent Sch* 12:1–20, 1972.
155. Horst JA, Ellenikiotis H, Milgrom PL: UCSF Protocol for Caries Arrest Using Silver Diamine Fluoride: Rationale, Indications and Consent. *J Calif Dent Assoc* 44(1):16–28, 2016.
156. Mei ML, Ito L, Cao Y, et al: Inhibitory effect of silver diamine fluoride on dentine demineralisation and collagen degradation. *J Dent* 41(9):809–817, 2013.
157. Mei ML, Li QL, Chu CH, et al: Antibacterial effects of silver diamine fluoride on multi-species cariogenic biofilm on caries. *Ann Clin Microbiol Antimicrob* 12:4, 2013.
158. Markowitz K, Pashley DH: Discovering new treatments for sensitive teeth: the long path from biology to therapy. *J Oral Rehabil* 35(4):300–315, 2008.
159. Rosenblatt A, Stamford TC, Niederman R: Silver diamine fluoride: a caries "silver-fluoride bullet." *J Dent Res* 88(2):116–125, 2009.
160. Tan HP, Lo ECM, Dyson JE, et al: Randomized clinical trial on arresting dental root caries through silver diamine fluoride applications in community-dwelling elders. *Br Dent J* 221(7):409, 2016.
161. Yee R, Holmgren C, Mulder J, et al: Efficacy of silver diamine fluoride for Arresting Caries Treatment. *J Dent Res* 88(7):644–647, 2009.
162. Campus G, Cagetti MG, Sale S: Six months of high-dose xylitol in high-risk caries subjects–a 2-year randomised, clinical trial. *Clin Oral Invest* 17:785–791, 2013.
163. Bader JD, Vollmer WM, Shugars DA, et al: Results from the Xylitol for Adult Caries Trial (X-ACT). *J Am Dent Assoc* 144(1):21–30, 2013.
164. Ritter AV, Bader JD, Leo MC, et al: Tooth-surface-specific effects of xylitol: randomized trial results. *J Dent Res* 92(6):512–517, 2013.
165. Riley P, Moore D, Ahmed F, et al: Xylitol-containing products for preventing dental caries in children and adults. *Cochrane Database Syst Rev* 26(3):2015.
166. Bueno-Silva B, Koo H, Falsetta ML, et al: Effect of neovestitol–vestitol containing Brazilian red propolis on accumulation of biofilm in vitro and development of dental caries in vivo. *J Bioadhesion Biofilm Res* 29:1233–1242, 2013.
167. Ástvaldsdóttir Á, Naimi-Akbar A, Davidson T, et al: Arginine and Caries Prevention: A Systematic Review. *Caries Res* 50(4):383–393, 2016.
168. Bader JD, Shugars DA, Bonito AJ: A systematic review of selected caries prevention and management methods. *Community Dent Oral Epidemiol* 29:399–411, 2001.

169. Wright JT, Tampi MP, Graham L, et al: Sealants for preventing and arresting pit-and-fissure occlusal caries in primary and permanent molars. A systematic review of randomized controlled trials—a report of the American Dental Association and the American Academy of Pediatric Dentistry. *J Am Dent Assoc* 147(8):631–645, e18, 2016.

170. Meyer-Lueckel H, Balbach A, Schikowsky C, et al: Pragmatic RCT on the Efficacy of Proximal Caries Infiltration. *J Dent Res* 95(5):2016.

171. Innes NP, Frencken JE, Bjorndal L, et al: Managing Carious Lesions: Consensus Recommendations on Terminology. *Adv Dent Res* 28(2):49–57, 2016.

172. Schwendicke F, Frencken JE, Bjorndal L, et al: Managing Carious Lesions: Consensus Recommendations on Carious Tissue Removal. *Adv Dent Res* 28(2):58–67, 2016.

173. Schwendicke F, Frencken JE, Bjorndal L, et al: Managing Carious Lesions: Consensus Recommendations on Carious Tissue Removal. *Adv Dent Res* 28(2):58–67, 2016.

174. Banerjee A, Watson TF, Kidd EA: Dentine caries: take it or leave it? *Dent Update* 27(6):272–276, 2000.

175. Bjorndal L: Buonocore Memorial Lecture. Dentin caries: progression and clinical management. *Oper Dent* 27(3):211–217, 2002.

176. Bjorndal L: Indirect pulp therapy and stepwise excavation. *Pediatr Dent* 30(3):225–229, 2008.

177. Oen KT, Thompson VP, Vena D, et al: Attitudes and expectations of treating deep caries: a PEARL Network survey. *Gen Dent* 55(3):197–203, 2007.

178. Pinheiro SL, Simionato MR, Imparato JC, et al: Antibacterial activity of glass-ionomer cement containing antibiotics on caries lesion microorganisms. *Am J Dent* 18(4):261–266, 2005.

179. Ricketts D: Management of the deep carious lesion and the vital pulp dentine complex. *Br Dent J* 191(11):606–610, 2001.

180. Ricketts DN, Kidd EA, Innes N, et al: Complete or ultraconservative removal of decayed tissue in unfilled teeth. *Cochrane Database Syst Rev* (3):2006.

181. van Amerongen WE: Dental caries under glass ionomer restorations. *J Public Health Dent* 56(3 Spec No):150–154, discussion 61-63, 1996.

182. Banerjee A, Watson TF, Kidd EA: Dentine caries: take it or leave it? *Dent Update* 27(6):272–276, 2000.

183. Bjorndal L: Indirect pulp therapy and stepwise excavation. *J Endod* 34(7 Suppl):S29–S33, 2008.

184. Bjorndal L, Kidd EA: The treatment of deep dentine caries lesions. *Dent Update* 32(7):402–413, 2005.

185. Oen KT, Thompson VP, Vena D, et al: Attitudes and expectations of treating deep caries: a PEARL Network survey. *Gen Dent* 55(3):197–203, 2007.

186. Pinheiro SL, Simionato MR, Imparato JC, et al: Antibacterial activity of glass-ionomer cement containing antibiotics on caries lesion microorganisms. *Am J Dent* 18(4):261–266, 2005.

187. Ricketts D: Management of the deep carious lesion and the vital pulp dentine complex. *Br Dent J* 191(11):606–610, 2001.

188. Ricketts DN, Kidd EA, Innes N, et al: Complete or ultraconservative removal of decayed tissue in unfilled teeth. *Cochrane Database Syst Rev* (3):2006.

189. Ricketts DN, Pitts NB: Novel operative treatment options. *Monogr Oral Sci* 21:174–187, 2009.

190. Thompson V, Craig RG, Curro FA, et al: Treatment of deep carious lesions by complete excavation or partial removal: a critical review. *J Am Dent Assoc* 139(6):705–712, 2008.

191. Uribe S: Partial caries removal in symptomless teeth reduces the risk of pulp exposure. *Evid Based Dent* 7(4):94, 2006.

192. van Amerongen WE: Dental caries under glass ionomer restorations. *J Public Health Dent* 56(3 Spec No):150–154, discussion 61-63, 1996.

193. Bjorndal L, Larsen T: Changes in the cultivable flora in deep carious lesions following a stepwise excavation procedure. *Caries Res* 34(6):502–508, 2000.

194. Maltz M, Garcia R, Jardim JJ, et al: Randomized trial of partial vs. stepwise caries removal: 3-year follow-up. *J Dent Res* 91(11):1026–1031, 2012.

195. Alves LS, Fontanella V, Damo AC, et al: Qualitative and quantitative radiographic assessment of sealed carious dentin: a 10-year prospective study. *Oral Surg Oral Med Oral Pathol Oral Radiol Endod* 109(1):135–141, 2010.

196. Lima KC, Coelho LT, Pinheiro IVA, et al: Microbiota of dentinal caries as assessed by reverse-capture checkerboard analysis. *Caries Res* 45:21–30, 2011.

197. Banerjee A, Kidd EA, Watson TF: In vitro validation of carious dentin removed using different excavation criteria. *Am J Dent* 16(4):228–230, 2003.

198. Hamama HH, Yiu CK, Burrow MF, et al: Chemical, morphological and microhardness changes of dentine after chemomechanical caries removal. *Aust Dent J* 58(3):283–292, 2013.

199. Hamama HH, Yiu CK, Burrow MF, et al: Systematic Review and Meta-Analysis of Randomized Clinical Trials on Chemomechanical Caries Removal. *Oper Dent* 40(4):E167–E178, 2015.

200. Corralo DJ, Maltz M: Clinical and ultrastructural effects of different liners/restorative materials on deep carious dentin: a randomized clinical trial. *Caries Res* 47(3):243–250, 2013.

201. Alqaderi H, Lee CT, Borzangy S, et al: Coronal pulpotomy for cariously exposed permanent posterior teeth with closed apices: A systematic review and meta-analysis. *J Dent* 44:1–7, 2016.

202. Hoefler V, Nagaoka H, Miller CS: Long-term survival and vitality outcomes of permanent teeth following deep caries treatment with step-wise and partial-caries-removal: A Systematic Review. *J Dent* 54(11):25–32, 2016.

203. Reference deleted in pages.

204. Reference deleted in pages.

205. Schwendicke F, Meyer-Lückel H, Dorfer C, et al: Failure of incompletely excavated teeth: a systematic review. *J Dent* 41(7):569–580, 2013.

206. Zanini M, Hennequin M, Cousson PY: A Review of Criteria for the Evaluation of Pulpotomy Outcomes in Mature Permanent Teeth. *J Endod* 42(8):1167–1174, 2016.

207. Yaacob M, Worthington HV, Deacon SA, et al: Powered versus manual toothbrushing for oral health. *Cochrane Database Syst Rev* (6):2014.

208. Haveman CW, Summitt JB, Burgess JO, et al: Three restorative materials and topical fluoride gel used in xerostomic patients: A clinical comparison. *J Amer Dent Assoc* 134:177–184, 2003.

209. Welch JL, Rossetti BJ, Riekem CW, et al: Biogeography of a human oral microbiome at the micron scale. *Proc Natl Acad Sci USA* 113(6):E791–E800, 2016.

210. Xiao J, Klein MI, Falsetta ML, et al: The exopolysaccharide matrix modulates the interaction between 3D architecture and virulence of a mixed-species oral biofilm. *PLoS Pathog* 8(4):e1002623, 2012.

211. Koo H, Falsetta ML, Klein MI: The exopolysaccharide matri: A virulence determinant of cariogenic biofilm. *J Dent Res* 92(12):1065–1073, 2013.

3

Patient Assessment, Examination, Diagnosis, and Treatment Planning

LEE W. BOUSHELL, DANIEL A. SHUGARS, R. SCOTT EIDSON[a]

This chapter provides an overview of the process through which a clinician completes patient assessment, clinical examination, diagnosis, and treatment planning for operative dentistry procedures. The chapter assumes that the reader has a background in oral medicine and an understanding of how to perform complete (comprehensive) extraoral and intraoral hard and soft tissue examinations, as well as an understanding of the etiology, characteristics, risk assessment, and management of dental caries as presented in Chapter 2. It is not in the scope of this chapter to incorporate the details of other aspects of a complete dental examination, such as periodontal, occlusal, and esthetic examinations. Appropriate textbooks that cover the specifics of these areas, in health and disease, should be consulted.

Any discussion of diagnosis and treatment must begin with an appreciation of the role of the dentist in helping patients maintain their oral health. This role is summarized by the Latin phrase "primum non nocere," which means "do no harm." This phrase represents a fundamental principle continually embraced by those in the healing arts over many centuries.

The implication of this concept for operative dentistry is that, before we recommend treatment, we must be reasonably confident that the patient will be better off as a result of our intervention. However, how can we be reasonably confident when we realize that few, if any, of the tests we perform or the assessments of risk that we make are completely accurate? To make matters even more challenging, none of the treatments we provide is without adverse outcomes and none will likely last for the life of the patient. The answer is that we must acknowledge that the information or evidence we have is not perfect and that we must be clear about the possible consequences of our decisions. If we are informed and clear about options and their consequences, then we reduce the chances of doing any harm.

The success of operative treatment depends heavily on an appropriate plan of care, which, in turn, is based on a comprehensive analysis of the patient's reasons for seeking care and on a systematic assessment of the patient's current conditions and risk for future problems. This information is then combined with the best available evidence on approaches to management of the patient's needs so that an appropriate plan of care may be offered.

The collection of this information and the determinations based on examination findings should be comprehensive and accomplished in a stepwise manner. Simply put, skipping steps may lead to overlooking potentially important parts of the patient's individual needs. These steps include reasons for seeking care, medical and dental histories, clinical examination for the detection of abnormalities, establishing diagnoses (which includes assessing risk), and determining prognosis. All of these steps must occur before a sound and appropriate plan of care may be developed and recommended.

Growing attention to using only the most effective and appropriate treatment has spawned interest in numerous research efforts. Research that provides information on treatments that work best in certain situations is expanding the knowledge base of dentistry and has led to an interest in translating the results of that research into practice activities that enhance care for patients. This movement has been termed *evidence-based dentistry* and is defined as the "conscientious, explicit, and judicious use of current best evidence in making decisions about the care of individual patients."[1] Systematic reviews emerging from the focus on evidence-based dentistry will provide practitioners with a distillation of the available knowledge about various conditions and treatments. It is incumbent on the authors of the systematic review to openly discuss the strengths and weaknesses of the reviewed studies as well as the relative value of their conclusions for application in dental care. Currently, the American Dental Association (ADA) has developed a website (http://ebd.ada.org/) that may be used by dental professionals for evidence-based dentistry decision making. This website helps clinicians identify systematic reviews, describes the preferred method for assembling the best available scientific evidence, and provides an appraisal of the evidence through critical summaries. As evidence-based dentistry continues to expand, professional associations will become more active in the development of guidelines to assist dentists and their patients in making informed and appropriate decisions.

General Considerations

It is difficult to overstate the importance of gaining comprehensive insight into each patient. Dentistry has, by its very origins, been heavily focused on reconstruction of damaged areas. However, nothing that we design and create has the ability to withstand the wet, warm, salty, thermally cycled, and cyclically loaded environment of the oral cavity for the whole life of the patient. Therefore the emphasis in dentistry has shifted toward understanding and maintaining conditions consistent with a healthy stomatognathic

---

[a]Dr. Eidson was an inactive author in this edition.

system so that steps may be taken to prevent dental disease. The specific circumstances of each individual must be considered in light of the known requirements of optimal oral health. Gaining insight into individual circumstances begins with proper patient assessment. Medical and dental health survey questions are excellent basic tools designed to facilitate this process. Responses to the broad overview questions (generally referred to as the "medical history" and "dental history") then enable specific exploration of previous or current conditions unique to the individual patient, that may represent risk factors or indicators for dental disease, as well as the primary reason (i.e., the chief concern) that prompted the patient to seek the assistance of the dentist. This interview process is then followed by the clinical gathering of additional information by means of strategic examination. The examination is the "hands-on" process of observing the patient's extraoral and intraoral structures and detecting of symptoms and signs of abnormal conditions or disease. During the clinical examination, the dentist must be keenly sensitive to subtle symptoms (that the patient reports), signs (that the dentist detects), and variations from normal to detect pathologic conditions and determine etiologic factors. The discovery of additional risk factors/indicators may occur during the examination. The combined patient assessment and examination information is then used to formulate diagnoses (and risk profiles), which are a determination or judgment of health versus disease, variations from normal, and likelihood for the development of additional disease. The dentist must be committed to comprehensive and meticulous attention to detail.

Patient Assessment

Medical History

The patient or legal guardian completes a standard, comprehensive medical history form. This form is an integral part of the preexamination patient interview, which helps identify conditions that could alter, complicate, or contraindicate proposed dental procedures. The practitioner should identify (1) communicable diseases that require special precautions, procedures, or referral; (2) allergies or medications, which may contraindicate the use of certain drugs; (3) systemic diseases, cardiac abnormalities, or joint replacements, which may require prophylactic antibiotic coverage or other treatment modifications; and (4) physiologic changes associated with aging, which may alter clinical presentation and influence treatment. The practitioner also might identify a need for medical consultation or referral before initiating dental care. All of this information is carefully detailed in the patient's permanent record and is used, as needed, to shape subsequent treatment recommendations.

Dental History

The dental history is a review of previous dental experiences and current dental problems. Review of the dental history often reveals information about past dental problems, previous dental treatment, and the patient's responses to treatments. Frequency of dental care and perceptions of previous care may be indications of the patient's future behavior. If a patient has difficulty tolerating certain types of procedures or has encountered problems with previous dental care, an alteration of the treatment or environment might help avoid future complications. It is crucial to understand past experiences in order to provide optimal care in the future. Also, this discussion might lead to identification of specific problems such as areas of food impaction, inability to floss, areas of pain, and

broken restorations or tooth structure. Finally, the date, type, and diagnostic quality of available radiographs should be recorded so as to ascertain the need for additional radiographs and to minimize the patient's exposure to ionizing radiation.

Chief Concern

Before initiating any treatment, the patient's chief concerns, or the problems that initiated the patient's visit, should be identified and clearly understood. Concerns are recorded essentially verbatim in the dental record. The patient should be encouraged to discuss all aspects (symptoms) of the current problem(s), including onset, duration, and related factors they are experiencing. This information is vital to establishing which specific diagnostic tests are required, determining the cause, selecting appropriate treatment options for the concerns, and building a sound relationship with the patient.

Examination

It is somewhat artificial to discuss *examination* as a separate entity from patient assessment for aspects of the patient "examination" begin during initial conversations with the patient. Careful observation of extraoral symmetry of the patient's physical appearance of the head and neck areas, mandibular movement during speech, ability to articulate sounds, and tendencies to smile provides vital information relative to overall presence or absence of abnormalities or disease. These observations occur while reviewing/clarifying information reported in the medical and dental history and while listening to the patient's chief concern(s). By definition, these early observations are all extraoral in nature.

Many examination data recording systems utilize organizational logic that begins with "extraoral examination" followed by "intraoral examination" so as to facilitate the recording of observational information (what the dentist observes while interacting with the patient). Utilization of clinical photography to capture full face and profile images is particularly useful in this process. Any observations will ultimately be followed by the physical examination necessary to assess extraoral aspects of the muscles of mastication, temporomandibular joints (TMJs), lymphnodes, and other vital structures, which will then be followed by intraoral examination.

Examination of Esthetic Appearance

Examination of esthetic appearance may be described as the evaluation of tooth color, form, display, and position in relation to the face. Evaluation must include discussion of realistic esthetic expectations when considering treatment options with the patient. Attaining the desired esthetic outcomes may be complicated by maximum tooth display and excessive or uneven tissue display. Risk of patient dissatisfaction with treatment outcomes may be lowered by careful attention to the establishment of intrafacial, intraarch, and interarch tooth positions that have been identified as consistent with maximum esthetics. This is accomplished in light of the reality that when individual teeth are correct in their anatomic shape, and positioned in the face and arches for optimum function, then the overall esthetic result will be optimal ("form follows function"). Tooth color evaluation becomes a factor if teeth are more visible when smiling or at the resting position of lips. Darker colored teeth, teeth with enamel intrinsic staining, and conditions such as tetracycline staining all increase the risk for not satisfying the esthetic expectations of patients with tooth color concerns. Symmetry of gingival margins becomes very important in patients who display a large amount of gingival tissue when smiling. Lack of symmetry increases the risk of not meeting the patient's esthetic expectations. Presence of multiple risk factors requires in-depth, careful consideration of the various components/relationships of the stomatognathic system, the ability to develop an interdisciplinary treatment plan, and excellent listening skills so as to identify realistic options consistent with the patient's overall esthetic expectations. All of this must be accomplished without compromising the short- and long-term dental health of the patient ("*do no harm*"). In many of these situations, conservative direct or indirect enamel-supported restorations are more appropriate for long-term risk management than are more aggressive preparations that remove relatively more tooth structure.

Examination of Occlusion

A careful examination of the patient's current occlusal scheme, along with potential impact on the muscles of mastication and TMJs, must occur before planning and implementing restorative care (see Chapter 1). This examination includes identification of signs of occlusal trauma, such as heavy wear facets, enamel cracks, or tooth mobility, and notation of occlusal abnormalities that may be contributing to pathologic conditions such as bone loss. Identification of the current relative health of the stomatognathic system then allows consideration of the potential ability of the proposed restorative treatment to achieve harmonious function of each component of the system. Careful analysis may identify need for modification of the current occlusal scheme prior to the initiation of any definitive restorative care.

The static and dynamic occlusion must be examined carefully (see Chapter 1) in light of the observation that there is no "ideal" occlusion and that most patients may have the ability to adapt to their occlusion without clinical symptoms. However, the clinician must understand the normal physiologic response of the muscles of mastication to various occlusal interrelationships and be able to identify where, for a specific patient, pathology (of the dentition, muscles of mastication, and/or TMJs) is present and what modifications may be indicated. A description of the patient's static anatomic occlusion in maximum intercuspation, including the relationship between molars and canines (Angle Class I, II, or III), and the amount of vertical overlap (overbite) and horizontal overlap (overjet) of anterior teeth should be recorded. This should include assessment of the presence and specifics of any functional shift from centric relation occlusion to maximum intercuspation. The presence of missing teeth and the relationship of the maxillary and mandibular midlines should be determined. The appropriateness of the occlusal plane and the positions of malposed teeth should be identified. Supererupted teeth, spacing, fractured teeth, and marginal ridge discrepancies should be noted. The dynamic functional occlusion in all movements of the mandible (right, left, forward, and all excursions in between) should be evaluated. The evaluation also includes assessing the relationship of teeth in centric relation, which is the orthopedic position of the joint where the condyle head is in its most anterior and superior position against the articular eminence within the glenoid fossa. Functional movements of the mandible are evaluated to determine if canine guidance or group function exists. The presence and amount of anterior guidance is evaluated to note the degree of potential posterior disclusion. Teeth are examined for abnormal wear patterns that are excessive and not age appropriate. If signs of abnormal or premature wear are present, the patient is queried as to awareness of any contributing parafunction habits such as grinding or clenching. Nonworking-side excursive contacts are recorded and related to any findings of masticatory muscle myositis and/or ipsilateral TMJ disc issues. Working-side excursive contacts are recorded and related to areas of cusp fracture development. Protrusive contacts on all posterior teeth molars are noted. Heavy wear facets on posterior cuspal inclines, mobility of teeth, or fremitus during function is identified and classified as primary or secondary occlusal traumatism. Full analysis of the occlusion may require articulated diagnostic models. Movement of the mandible from maximum intercuspation to maximum opening is observed and maximum unassisted opening is measured; any "clicking or popping" of the joint disc(s) during mandibular movements is noted and related to any history of trauma, nonworking occlusal interferences, or other possible pathologic changes. Bimanual loading of the joints and palpation of the condyle lateral poles and retrocondylar areas (during wide mandibular opening) are completed to further test for tenderness/pain as signs of inflammation. The occlusal relationships of the teeth are assessed for the presence of an unusually tall and narrow cusp (a "plunger cusp") that "plunges" deep into the occlusal plane of the opposing arch. A plunger cusp might contact the lower of two adjacent marginal ridges of different levels, contacting directly between two adjacent marginal ridges in maximum intercuspation, or be positioned in a deep fossa. It may increase the likelihood of food impaction and tooth or restoration fracture.

The results of the occlusal examination should be included in the dental record and considered in the restorative treatment plan. Acceptable aspects of the occlusion must be preserved and not altered during treatment. When possible, improvement of the occlusion (elimination of interferences), based on knowledge of the physiologic masticatory muscle response to various relationships, is desirable; occlusal interferences must not be perpetuated in the restorative treatment.

Examination of Teeth and Restorations

Preparation for Clinical Examination

A trained assistant familiar with the terminology, notation system, and charting procedure may survey the patient's teeth and existing restorations and record the information to save chair time for the dentist. The dentist subsequently performs the examination and confirms the charting. Proper instruments, including a mirror, an explorer, and a periodontal probe, and the ability to air-dry the surfaces of the teeth are required. Every accessible surface of each tooth must be inspected for localized changes in color, texture, and translucency. A routine for charting should be established, such as starting in the upper right quadrant with the most posterior tooth and progressing around the maxillary and mandibular arches. Dental floss is useful in identifying overhanging restorations, improper proximal contours, and open contacts. The clinical examination is performed systematically in a clean, dry, well-illuminated mouth. A cotton roll in the vestibular space and another under the tongue maintain dryness and improve visualization of the teeth and adjacent gingiva (Fig. 3.1). Heavy biofilm accumulation may require flossing and a toothbrush prophylaxis to aid in the examination process. Occasionally a gross debridement must be schedule before final clinical examination of the teeth may be accomplished.

Clinical Examination for Caries

Contemporary caries management, which encompasses expanded nonoperative approaches and conservative operative interventions,

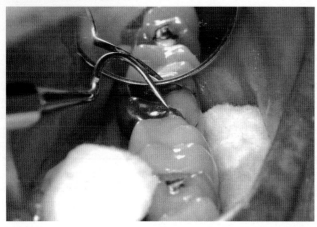

• **Fig. 3.1** Accurate clinical examination requires a clean, dry, well-illuminated mouth. Cotton rolls are placed in the vestibular space and under the tongue to maintain dryness and enhance visibility.

relies on enhanced risk assessment and improved lesion detection and classification. Clinical caries lesion detection has been found lacking; thus improvement is needed.[2] One means of addressing these concerns has been the development of a visual system for caries lesion detection and classification. The International Caries Detection and Assessment System (ICDAS) was developed to serve as a guide for standardized visual caries assessment that could be used for clinical practice, clinical research, education, and epidemiology (Fig. 3.2). In the United States, the Caries Management by Risk Assessment (CAMBRA) movement, as discussed in Chapter 2, embraces the principles of the ICDAS for visual examination and assessment of caries lesions. The ICDAS has been further condensed by the American Dental Association into the Caries Classification System (ADA CCS)[3] (see Fig. 3.2). Assessment of dental caries also requires identification of caries lesion activity so as to make decisions relative to treatment recommendations (Table 3.1). The objective of improved detection and classification systems is to accurately identify those early enamel lesions that are most likely to be reversed by remineralization. Therefore appropriate nonoperative care may be attempted, and lesions that require operative treatment may be identified as early as possible in the disease process. With this approach, restoration

ADA CCS		Initial		Moderate		Extensive	
Occlusal Protocol * **							
ICDAS code	0	1	2	3	4	5	6
	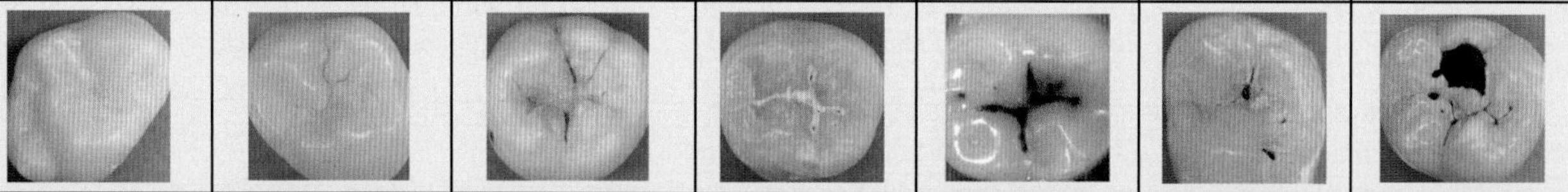						
Definitions	Sound tooth surface; no caries change after air drying (5 sec); or hypoplasia, wear, erosion, and other noncaries phenomena	First visual change in enamel; seen only after air drying or colored, change "thin" limited to the confines of the pit and fissure area	Distinct visual change in enamel; seen when wet, white or colored, "wider" than the fissure/fossa	Localized enamel breakdown with no visible dentin or underlying shadow; discontinuity of surface enamel, widening of fissure	Underlying dark shadow from dentin, with or without localized enamel breakdown	Distinct cavity with visible dentin; frank cavitation involving less than half of a tooth surface	Extensive distinct cavity with dentin; cavity is deep and wide involving more than half of the tooth
Histologic depth		Lesion depth in P/F was 90% in the outer enamel with only 10% into dentin	Lesion depth in P/F was 50% inner enamel and 50% into the outer 1/3 dentin	Lesion depth in P/F with 77% in dentin	Lesion depth in P/F with 88% into dentin	Lesion depth in P/F with 100% in dentin	Lesion depth in P/F 100% reaching inner 1/3 dentin
Sealant/restoration Recommendation for low risk	Sealant optional DIAGNOdent may be helpful	Sealant optional DIAGNOdent may be helpful	Sealant optional or caries biopsy if DIAGNOdent is 20-30	Sealant or minimally invasive restoration needed	Minimally invasive restoration	Minimally invasive restoration	Minimally invasive restoration
Sealant/restoration Recommendation for moderate risk	Sealant optional DIAGNOdent may be helpful	Sealant recommended DIAGNOdent may be helpful	Sealant optional or caries biopsy if DIAGNOdent is 20-30	Sealant or minimally invasive restoration needed	Minimally invasive restoration	Minimally invasive restoration	Minimally invasive restoration
Sealant/restoration Recommendation for high risk * and extreme risk **	Sealant recommended DIAGNOdent may be helpful	Sealant recommended DIAGNOdent may be helpful	Sealant optional or caries biopsy if DIAGNOdent is 20-30	Sealant or minimally invasive restoration needed	Minimally invasive restoration	Minimally invasive restoration	Minimally invasive restoration

* Patients with one (or more) cavitated lesion(s) are high-risk patients. ** Patients with one (or more) cavitated lesion(s) and xerostomia are extreme-risk patients.

*** All sealants and restorations to be done with a minimally invasive philosophy in mind. Sealants are defined as confined to enamel. Restoration is defined as in dentin. A two-surface restoration is defined as a preparation that has one part of the preparation in dentin and the preparation extends to a second surface (note: the second surface does not have to be in dentin). A sealant can be either resin-based or glass ionomer. Resin-based sealants should have the most conservatively prepared fissures for proper bonding. Glass ionomer should be considered where the enamel is immature, or where fissure preparation is not desired, or where rubber dam isolation is not possible. Patients should be given a choice in material selection.

• **Fig. 3.2** American Dental Association Caries Classification System (ADA CCS) and International Caries Detection and Assessment System (ICDAS) chart showing visual caries detection. (Modified from Young DA, Nový BB, Zeller GG, et al.: The American Dental Association Caries Classification System for Clinical Practice, A report of the American Dental Association Council on Scientific Affairs, *J Am Dent Assoc* 146(2):79–86, 2015; and Jenson L, Budenz AW, Featherstone JD, et al.: Clinical protocols for caries management by risk assessment, *J Calif Dent Assoc* 35:714, 2007.)

TABLE 3.1	Characteristics of Active and Inactive Caries Lesions	
	CARIES LESION ACTIVITY ASSESSMENT DESCRIPTORS	
Activity Assessment Factor	Likely to Be Inactive/Arrested	Likely to Be Active
Location of the Lesion	Lesion is not in a plaque stagnation area	Lesion is in a plaque stagnation area (pit/fissure, approximal, gingival)
Plaque Over the Lesion	Not thick or sticky	Thick and/or sticky
Surface Appearance	Shiny; color: brown-black	Matte/opaque/loss of luster; color: white-yellow
Tactile Feeling	Smooth, hard enamel/ hard dentin	Rough enamel/soft dentin
Gingival Status (If the Lesion is Located Near the Gingiva)	No inflammation, no bleeding on probing	Inflammation, bleeding on probing

From Young DA, Nový BB, Zeller GG, et al.: The American Dental Association Caries Classification System for Clinical Practice, A report of the American Dental Association Council on Scientific Affairs, *J Am Dent Assoc* 146(2):79–86, 2015.

will result in the removal of the minimum amount of tooth structure.

Caries lesions may be detected by visual changes in tooth surface texture or color or in tactile sensation when an explorer is used judiciously to detect surface roughness by gently stroking across the tooth surface. Current thinking finds that the use of an explorer in this manner might have some relevance for assessing caries activity. However, it cannot be overemphasized that the *explorer must not be used to determine a "stick"* (i.e., a resistance to withdrawal from a fissure or pit). This improper use of a sharp explorer has been shown to irreversibly damage the tooth by turning a sound, remineralizable subsurface lesion into a possible cavitation that is prone to progression. Forcing an explorer into pits and fissures also theoretically risks cross-contamination from one probing site to another. In contrast, for assessment of root caries, an explorer is valuable for detecting root surface softness. Additional methods used in caries lesion identification include radiographs, which show changes in tooth density from normal, and adjunctive tests that use various technologies to aid in caries lesion detection and caries activity (discussed in later sections).

Occlusal Surfaces

Caries lesions are most prevalent in the faulty pits and fissures of the occlusal surfaces where the developmental enamel lobes of posterior teeth partially or completely failed to coalesce (Fig. 3.3A). It is important to remember the distinction between primary occlusal grooves and fossae and occlusal fissures and pits. Primary occlusal grooves and fossae are smooth "valley or saucer" landmarks that result from complete coalescence of developmental enamel lobes (see Chapter 1). Normally, such grooves and fossae are not susceptible to caries because they are not niches for biofilm and

frequently are cleansed by the rubbing action of food during mastication. Conversely, occlusal fissures and pits are deep, tight crevices or holes in enamel, where the lobes failed to coalesce partially or completely. Fissures and pits are detected visually and may frequently be stained but not diseased.

As noted earlier, sharp explorers previously have been used to evaluate fissures and pits in an attempt to diagnose fissure/pit caries. However, numerous studies have found that the use of a sharp explorer for this purpose did not increase diagnostic validity compared with visual inspection alone.[4-7] The use of the dental explorer for this purpose was found to fracture enamel and serve as a source for transferring pathogenic bacteria among various teeth.[8,9] Therefore the use of a sharp explorer in diagnosing pit-and-fissure caries is contraindicated as part of the detection process.

An occlusal surface is examined visually and radiographically.[10,11] The visual examination is conducted in a dry, well-illuminated field. Direct vision is used to observe how light passes into the surface of the tooth structure. The occlusal surface is diagnosed as diseased if external chalkiness (enamel caries) or subsurface opacity (dentin caries) or cavitation of tooth structure, forming the fissure or pit, is seen. At times a brown-gray discoloration, radiating peripherally from the fissure or pit, is present (see Fig. 3.3A, enamel area adjacent to the central pit/lingual fissure) indicating caries progression in dentin below the translucent enamel. In contrast, it is common to observe nondiseased occlusal surfaces with narrow grooves or fossae that exhibit superficial staining, but no visual changes in light reflection through the enamel immediately adjacent (see Fig. 3.3A, distal aspect of central groove and distal fossa area) and with no radiographic evidence of caries. The superficial staining is extrinsic and occurs over several years of oral exposure in a person with low caries risk. Caries lesions occasionally develop on cusp tips (see Fig. 3.3B). Typically, these are the result of developmental enamel defects or following loss of enamel (exposure of dentin) due to erosion, abrasion, or parafunction. The presence of caries in these self-cleansing areas usually indicates that the patient is at high risk of developing additional caries (see Risk Assessments and Profiles in the Diagnosis section to come). Carious pits and fissures also occur on the occlusal two thirds of the facial or lingual surface of posterior teeth and on the lingual surface of maxillary incisors.

The clinical interpretation of subtle changes in the appearance of tooth structure is aided by simultaneous consideration of the patient's overall caries risk, along with the patient's previous patterns of susceptibility. The patient's medical history, dental history, oral hygiene, diet, and age, among other caries risk factors and indicators, may suggest a prediction of current and future caries activity. In addition, occlusal caries lesions tend to occur bilaterally.

The ICDAS uses a two-stage process to record the status of the caries lesion. The first is a code for the severity of the caries lesion and the second is for the restorative status of the tooth. The status of the caries severity is determined visually on a scale of 0 to 6:

0 = sound tooth structure
1 = first visual change in enamel
2 = distinct visual change in enamel
3 = enamel breakdown, no dentin visible
4 = dentinal shadow (not cavitated into dentin)
5 = distinct cavity with visible dentin
6 = extensive distinct cavity with visible dentin

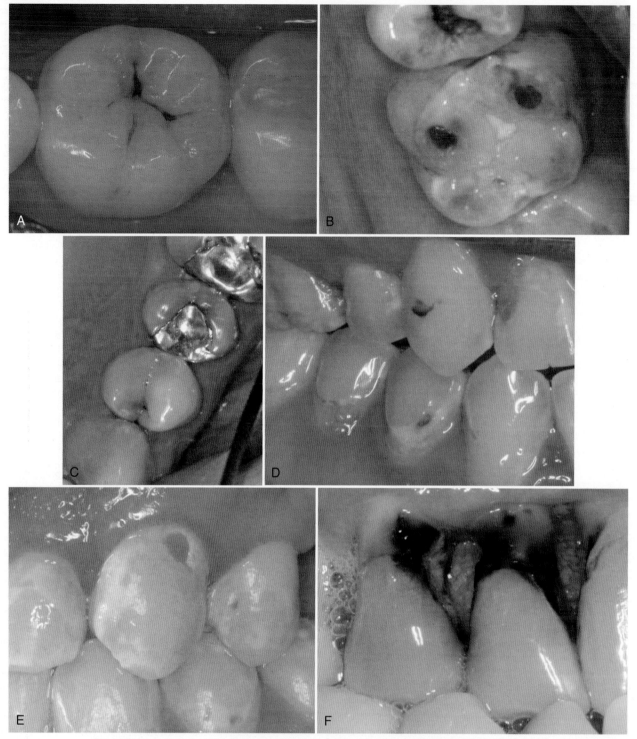

• **Fig. 3.3** Caries may be diagnosed clinically by careful inspection. A, Loss of translucency and change in color of occlusal enamel resulting from a carious fissure. B, Caries lesions on cusp tips. C, White chalky appearance or shadow under marginal ridge (distal #4 and mesial #5). D, Incipient smooth-surface caries lesion, or a white spot, has intact surface. E, Smooth-surface caries may appear white or dark, depending on the degree of extrinsic staining. F, Root-surface caries.

This severity code is paired with a restorative/sealant code 0 to 8:

0 = not sealed or restored
2 = sealant, partial
3 = sealant, full; tooth-colored restoration

4 = amalgam restoration
5 = stainless steel restoration
6 = ceramic, gold, PFM (porcelain-fused-to-metal) crown or veneer
7 = lost or broken restoration
8 = temporary restoration

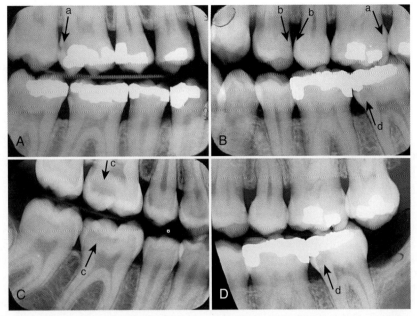

• **Fig. 3.4** Caries may be diagnosed radiographically as translucencies in the enamel or dentin. A and B, Proximal caries tends to occur bilaterally (*a*) and on adjacent surfaces (*b*). C, Occlusal caries (*c*). D, Recurrent caries gingival to an existing restoration (*d*). This same recurrent caries (*d*) also is shown in B. Note that there are additional radiolucencies (consistent with caries lesion development) that are not identified with arrows.

See Fig. 3.2 for examples of ADA CCS and ICDAS coding for caries lesion severity. The details of the ICDAS system for detection, and training to use the system with an online tutorial, are available at www.icdas.org.

Proximal Surfaces

Early proximal surface caries, one form of smooth-surface caries, is usually diagnosed radiographically (Fig. 3.4A and B). It also may be detected by careful visual examination after tooth separation or through fiberoptic transillumination.[12] When the caries lesion has progressed through the proximal surface enamel and has demineralized dentin, a white opaque appearance or a shadow under the marginal ridge may become evident (see Fig. 3.3C). Careful probing with an explorer on the proximal surface may detect cavitation, which is defined as a break in the surface contour of enamel. The combined use of all examination methods may be helpful in arriving at an accurate final diagnosis.

Brown spots on intact, hard proximal surface enamel adjacent to and usually gingival to the contact area are often seen in older patients, in whom caries activity is low. These discolored areas are a result of extrinsic staining during earlier caries demineralizing episodes, each followed by a remineralization episode. These areas are no longer carious and are usually more resistant to caries as a result of fluorohydroxyapatite formation. Restorative treatment of these areas is not indicated. Inactive proximal caries lesions sometimes are difficult to correctly diagnose because of faint radiographic evidence revealing previous mineral loss.

Proximal surface caries in anterior teeth may be identified by radiographic examination, visual inspection (with optional transillumination), or probing with an explorer. Transillumination is accomplished by placing the mirror or light source on the lingual aspect of teeth and directing the light through teeth. Small early enamel proximal lesions may be detectable only on the radiograph (see Fig. 3.4B). More advanced proximal lesions appear as a dark area along the marginal ridge when the light is directed through the tooth. In addition to transillumination, tactile exploration of anterior teeth is appropriate to detect cavitation because the proximal surfaces generally are more visible and accessible than in the posterior regions.

Another form of smooth-surface caries may occur on the facial and lingual surfaces of the teeth of patients with high caries activity, particularly in the cervical areas that are less accessible for cleaning. The earliest clinical evidence of early enamel lesions on these surfaces is a white spot that is visually different from the adjacent translucent enamel that appears when the surface is dried. Rewetting results in partial or total disappearance. This appearing–disappearing phenomenon distinguishes the smooth-surface early enamel lesion from the enamel white spot that results from *nonhereditary enamel hypocalcification* (see section on clinical examination for additional defects). Both types of white spots are undetectable tactilely because the surface is intact, smooth, and hard. For white spot lesions, nonsurgical remineralization therapies (discussed in Chapter 2) should be instituted to promote remineralization.

The presence of several facial (or lingual) smooth-surface caries lesions within a patient's dentition suggests a high caries rate, which means that if the existing risk factors are not addressed, the patient is at high risk for developing more lesions in the future. In a caries-susceptible patient, the gingival third of the facial surfaces of maxillary posterior teeth and the gingival third of the facial and lingual surfaces of mandibular posterior teeth should be evaluated carefully because these surfaces are often at a greater risk for caries. Advanced smooth-surface caries exhibits discoloration and demineralization and feels soft as the explorer is translated across the suspicious area. The discoloration may range from white to dark brown, with rapidly progressing caries usually being light in color. Slowly progressing caries, in a patient with low caries activity, darkens over time because of extrinsic staining and physical changes in the structure of the dentin collagen matrix. Remineralization of the decalcified tooth structure will return the tactile hardness of the lesion and is an evidence that the caries has been arrested. The dentin in an arrested remineralized lesion has become sclerotic (see Chapter 1). Such an arrested lesion at times may be rough, although cleanable, and restoration is not indicated except to address the esthetic concerns of the patient or to assist with patient control of biofilm accumulation. These lesions are inactive but remain susceptible to new caries activity in the future.

Cervical Areas

In patients with attachment loss, extra care must be taken to inspect for root-surface caries. A combination of root exposure, dietary changes, systemic diseases, and medications that affect the amount and character of saliva may predispose a patient, especially an older individual, to root-surface caries. Lesions are often found at the cementoenamel junction (CEJ) or more apically on cementum or exposed dentin in older patients or in patients who have undergone periodontal surgery (see Fig. 3.3F). Early in its development, root caries appears as a well-defined, discolored area adjacent to the gingival margin, typically near the CEJ. Root caries is softer than the adjacent tooth structure, and lesions typically spread laterally around the CEJ. Although no clinical criteria are universally accepted for the diagnosis of root caries, it is generally agreed that softened cemental or dentinal tooth structure compared with the surrounding surface is characteristic.[13] Active root caries is detected by the presence of softening and cavitation.[14,15] Although root-surface caries may be detected on radiographic examination, a careful, thorough clinical examination is crucial. A difficult diagnostic challenge is the patient who has attachment loss with no gingival recession, limiting accessibility for clinical inspection of the proximal root surfaces. Proximal root-surface lesions often progress rapidly and are best diagnosed using quality bitewing radiographs. Differentiation of a caries lesion from a radiolucent artifact created by radiographic cervical burnout is, however, essential.[12,13]

Clinical Examination of Amalgam Restorations

Evaluation of existing restorations should be accomplished systematically in a clean, dry, well-lit field. Clinical evaluation of amalgam restorations requires visual observation, application of tactile sense with the explorer, use of dental floss, interpretation of radiographs, and knowledge of the probabilities that a given condition is sound or at risk for further breakdown. At least 11 distinct conditions might be encountered when amalgam restorations are evaluated: (1) amalgam "blues," (2) proximal overhangs, (3) marginal ditching, (4) voids, (5) fracture lines, (6) lines indicating the interface between abutted amalgam restorations placed at separate times, (7) improper anatomic contours, (8) marginal ridge incompatibility, (9) improper proximal contacts, (10) improper occlusal contacts, and (11) recurrent caries lesions.

Discolored areas or "amalgam blues" are often seen through the enamel in teeth that have amalgam restorations. This bluish hue results either from the leaching of amalgam corrosion products into the dentinal tubules or from the color of underlying amalgam seen through translucent enamel. The latter occurs when the enamel has little or no dentin support, such as in undermined cusps, marginal ridges, and regions adjacent to proximal margins. When other aspects of the restoration are sound, amalgam blues do not indicate caries, do not warrant classifying the restoration as defective, and require no further treatment. Replacement of the restoration may be considered, however, for elective improvement of esthetics or for areas under heavy functional stress that may require a cusp coverage restoration designed to prevent possible tooth fracture.

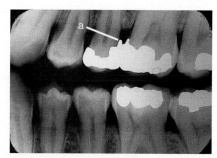

• **Fig. 3.5** Proximal restoration overhang (*a*) may be diagnosed radiographically.

Proximal overhangs are diagnosed visually, tactilely, and radiographically (Fig. 3.5). The amalgam–tooth junction is evaluated by moving the explorer back and forth across it. If the explorer stops at the junction and then moves outwardly onto the amalgam, an overhang is present. Overhangs also may be confirmed by the catching or tearing of unwaxed dental floss. Such an overhang likely represents an area of biofilm accumulation, provides an obstacle to good oral hygiene, and may contribute to chronic inflammation of adjacent soft tissue. This type of overhang should be corrected, and often indicates the need for restoration replacement.

Marginal gap formation (or "ditching") is the deterioration of the amalgam–tooth interface as a result of enamel wear and/or restoration edge fracture (Fig. 3.6A). Improper tooth preparation may predispose an amalgam restoration to ditching. It can be diagnosed visually or by the explorer dropping into an opening as it crosses the margin. Shallow ditching less than 0.5 mm deep usually is not a reason for restoration replacement because the area is self-cleaning and not prone to caries development.[16] Such a restoration usually looks worse than it really is. The ongoing self-sealing property of amalgam allows the restoration to continue serving adequately if it can be satisfactorily cleaned and maintained. If the ditch is too deep to be cleaned or jeopardizes the integrity of the remaining restoration or tooth structure, the restoration should be replaced.[16] However, marginal gaps near the gingival wall frequently become areas of secondary caries development and correction of these areas is indicated.[17]

Localized voids, which result from poor condensation of the amalgam, may also occur at the margins of amalgam restorations. If the void is at least 0.3 mm deep and is located in the gingival third of the tooth crown, the restoration is judged as defective and should be repaired or replaced. Accessible small voids in other marginal areas where the enamel is thicker may be corrected by enamel recontouring or repairing with a small restoration.

A careful clinical examination is able to detect the presence of a fracture line across the occlusal portion of an amalgam restoration. A line that occurs in the isthmus region generally indicates a fractured amalgam, and the defective restoration must be replaced (Fig. 3.7A). Procedures involved with replacement must ensure adequate thickness of the amalgam restoration and rounding of the internal line angles (e.g., the axiopulpal line angle) so as to limit the likelihood of recurrence of a fracture on the occlusal surface (see Fig. 3.7B). Care must be taken to correctly evaluate any such line, however, especially if it is in the midocclusal area because this may be an interface line, a manifestation of two abutted restorations accomplished at separate appointments (see Fig. 3.7A). If other aspects of the abutted restorations are satisfactory, replacement is unnecessary.

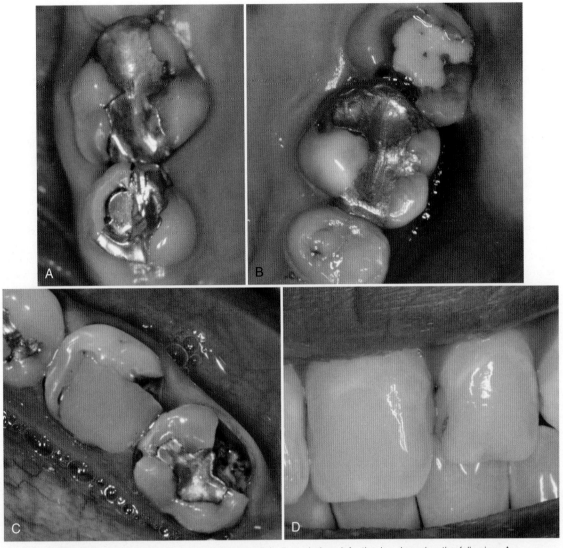

• **Fig. 3.6** Restorations may be diagnosed clinically as being defective by observing the following. A, Deep marginal ditching. B, Improper contour. C, Recurrent caries. D, Esthetically unappealing dark staining.

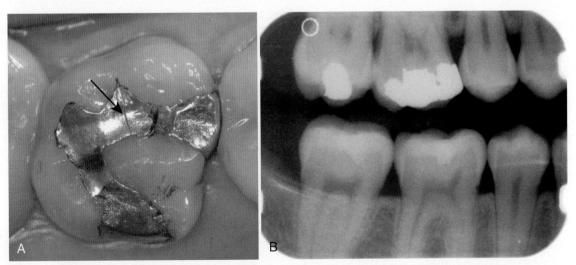

• **Fig. 3.7** Lines across the occlusal surface of an amalgam restoration. A, Fracture line indicates replacement. An interface line (arrow) indicates two restorations placed at separate appointments, which, by itself, is insufficient indication for replacement. B, Radiograph revealing thin amalgam area, which allowed material flexure and subsequent fracture.

Amalgam restorations should duplicate the normal anatomic contours of teeth. Restorations that impinge on soft tissue, have inadequate embrasure form or proximal contact, or prevent the use of dental floss should be classified as defective, indicating recontouring or replacement (see Fig. 3.6B).

The marginal ridge portion of the amalgam restoration should be compatible with the adjacent marginal ridge. Both ridges should be at approximately the same level and display correct occlusal embrasure form for passage of food to the facial and lingual surfaces and for proper proximal contact area (see Chapter 1). If the marginal ridges are incompatible and are associated with poor tissue health, food impaction, or the inability of the patient to floss, the restoration is defective and should be recontoured or replaced.

The proximal surface of an amalgam restoration should recreate the normal height of contour such that it comes into contact with the adjacent tooth at the proper occlusogingival and faciolingual area with correct adjacent embrasure form (a "closed" contact). The use of floss is helpful in assessing the intensity of a closed contact. If the proximal contact of any restoration is suspected to be inadequate, it should be evaluated visually by trial angulations of a mouth mirror (held lingually when viewing from the facial aspect, etc.) to reflect light and see if a space where the contact should occur ("open" contact) is present. For this viewing, the contact must be free of saliva. If the contact is open and is associated with poor interproximal tissue health, food impaction, or both, the restoration should be classified as defective and should be replaced or repaired. An open contact typically is annoying to the patient, so correcting the problem usually is an appreciated service.

Recurrent caries adjacent to the marginal area of the restoration is detected visually, tactilely, or radiographically and is an indication for repair or replacement (see Figs. 3.4D and 3.6C). The same criteria for initial proximal and occlusal caries lesions apply for the diagnosis of and intervention for recurrent caries lesions around restorations.

Improper occlusal contacts on an amalgam restoration may cause deleterious occlusal loading (and predisposition to fracture or pain on biting from hyperocclusion), undesirable tooth movement, or both. Premature occlusal contacts may be seen as a "shiny" spot on the surface of the restoration or detected by occlusal marking paper. Such a condition warrants correction by selective occlusal adjustment.

Clinical Examination of Indirect Metal Restorations

Indirect metal restorations should be evaluated clinically in the same manner as amalgam restorations. Any aspect of the restoration that is not satisfactory, that is causing harm to tissue or occlusal function, should be noted and considered for recontouring, repair, or replacement.

Clinical Examination of Composite and Other Tooth-Colored Restorations

Tooth-colored restorations (direct and indirect) should be evaluated clinically in the same manner as amalgam and cast-metal restorations. The presence of improper contour or inadequate proximal contact, overhanging margin, recurrent caries, or occlusal interference should be noted and considered for correction. Corrective procedures include recontouring, polishing, repairing, or replacement of the restoration.

One of the main concerns with anterior teeth is esthetics. If a tooth-colored restoration has dark marginal staining or is discolored to the extent that it is esthetically unappealing to the patient, the restoration should be judged as defective (see Fig. 3.6D). Marginal staining that is judged to be noncarious may be corrected by a small repair restoration along the margin. Occasionally, the staining is superficial and may be removed by resurfacing or removal of restoration excess extending beyond the preparation margins.

Clinical Examination of Dental Implants and Implant-Supported Restorations

Baseline radiographs that reveal the initial levels of implant bone support should be obtained when the implant is restored. Percussion of the restoration should reveal a clinical sound consistent with integration. Probing depths associated with the implant fixture should be consistent with the thickness of the local gingival tissue. The gingival tissue should be assessed for signs of inflammation (redness, edema, tenderness, bleeding on probing). The marginal adaptation between implant restorations and their abutments should allow for optimal biofilm removal. Any deviation from normal should be noted. Many edentulous areas receive implants that are generally smaller than the roots of the teeth they are replacing. Therefore the restorations of the implants require modified cervical contours. Implant restorations should be evaluated for proper cervical (especially proximal) contours that limit food impaction or biofilm accumulation.

Chronic inflammation (periimplantitis), secondary to the presence of residual dental cement or biofilm accumulation, of the tissue immediately adjacent to the implant fixture/restoration may lead to localized bone loss around an implant and impact its long-term survival. Periimplantitis has a multifactorial etiology. See Chapter 11, and a textbook dedicated to dental implantology, for additional information.

Clinical Examination for Additional Defects

A thorough clinical examination occasionally identifies localized noncavitated, hard white areas on the facial (Fig. 3.8) or lingual surfaces or on the cusp tips of teeth. Generally, these are hypocalcified areas of enamel resulting from childhood fever, trauma, or fluorosis that occurred during the developmental stages of tooth formation. These areas are diagnosed as *nonhereditary developmental enamel hypoplasia*. Another cause of hypocalcification is arrested and remineralized incipient caries, which leaves an opaque, discolored, and hard surface. When smooth and cleanable, such areas do not warrant restorative intervention unless they are esthetically offensive to the patient. These areas remain visible whether the tooth is wet or dry, and should not be confused with the opaque white smooth-surface incipient caries lesions that appear when

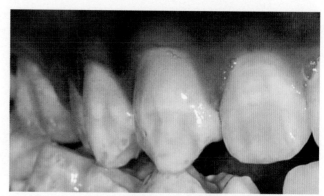

• **Fig. 3.8** Nonhereditary hypocalcified areas on facial surfaces. These areas may result from numerous factors but do not warrant restorative intervention unless they are esthetically offensive or cavitation is present.

teeth are air-dried. Care must be exercised in distinguishing nonhereditary developmental enamel hypoplasia from an early enamel caries lesion.

Rare genetic disorders affecting enamel and dentin may be discovered during clinical examination. Defective enamel organization and calcification, which results in teeth that are compromised in appearance and strength, is referred to as *amelogenesis imperfecta*. Defective dentin formation and a compromised dentinoenamel junction (DEJ) resulting in early loss of clinically normal enamel is referred to as *dentinogenesis imperfecta*. Additional information on these genetic disorders may be found in textbooks on oral pathology.

The loss of surface tooth structure by chemical action in the continued presence of demineralizing agents with low pH (Fig. 3.9) is defined as *erosion*. The resulting defective surface is usually smooth. Although erosive agents are the predominant causative factors, it is thought that toothbrushing and/or other abrasive agents in the diet may accelerate the loss of tooth structure, which

is generally referred to as *erosive tooth wear*. It is necessary to document the severity of the tooth structure loss and the specific areas that have been affected. If the defects are only on the lingual of upper teeth, the diagnosis would be different from finding defects on the occlusal surfaces of lower molars. Exogenous acidic agents such as lemon juice (through sucking on lemons) may cause crescent-shaped or dished defects (rounded as opposed to angular) on the surfaces of teeth exposed to the agent (see Fig. 3.9A), whereas endogenous acidic agents, such as gastric fluids, cause generalized erosion on the lingual, incisal, and occlusal surfaces (see Fig. 3.9B). Erosion processes may also be involved in the loss of the tooth structure with a clinical presentation of "cupped-out" areas on occlusal surfaces. These defective areas are associated with the binge–purge syndrome in bulimia, or with gastroesophageal reflux disease (GERD). Many patients with GERD are often not aware of their gastric symptoms or do not associate them with the problems with their teeth. Consultation with a physician to obtain a proper diagnosis of GERD may assist in the diagnosis and

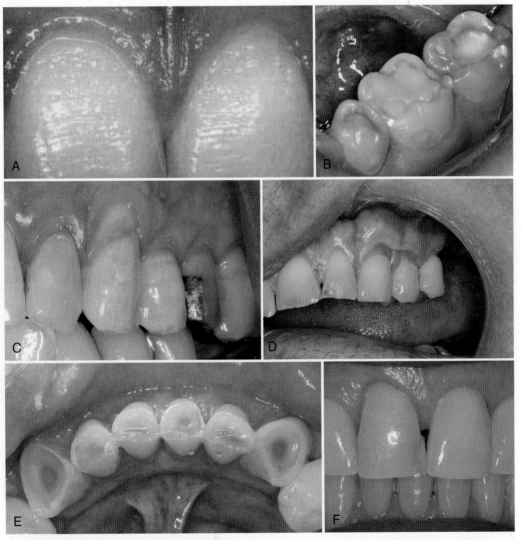

• **Fig. 3.9**   Erosion. A, Crescent-shaped defects on enamel facial surfaces caused by exogenous demineralizing agent (from sucking on lemons several years previous to the time of the photograph). B, Generalized erosion caused by endogenous fluids. C, Rounded cervical lesions associated with toothbrush abrasion. D, Idiopathic erosion lesions in cervical areas are hypothesized to be associated with abnormal occlusal forces. E, Generalized attrition caused by excessive functional or parafunctional mandibular movements. F, Enamel craze lines.

management of erosion. Other sources of erosion may be use of sports drinks, herbal teas, and vomiting associated with chemotherapy, and, in the case of alcoholism, the presence of stomach contents in the mouth during periods of excessive alcohol consumption. It is necessary to document the erosion process as it progresses over time through the use accurate study models, photography, and/or digital scanning technology. Risk assessments for erosion should be included in the assessment of the patient, as indicated. The flow and buffering capacity of the individual patient's saliva impact the rate of progression of erosive tooth wear. Understanding, identifying, and diagnosing tooth damage secondary to erosion (erosive tooth wear) is essential if management of the disease process is to be successful.[18]

Abnormal tooth surface loss resulting from direct frictional forces between teeth and external objects or from frictional forces between contacting teeth in the presence of an abrasive medium is termed *abrasion*. Habitual chewing on hard objects (e.g., paper clips, pens, pencils) or chronic use of agents with high abrasivity (e.g., smokeless tobacco, inadequately washed vegetables) may result in loss of occlusal-surface tooth structure.

The loss of tooth structure in the cervical areas (*abrasion*) is commonly seen as a rounded notch in the gingival portion of the facial aspects of teeth (see Fig. 3.9C). In contrast to cervical lesions that develop from abrasion processes, *idiopathic erosion lesions* ("*abfractions*") are cervical, wedge-shaped defects (angular as opposed to rounded) similar to the defects customarily associated with abrasion but in which one of the possible causative factors may include excessive flexure of the tooth as a result of heavy, eccentric occlusal forces (see Fig. 3.9D). The heavy occlusal loading may also lead to the development of a pronounced occlusal wear facet. It is hypothesized that the flexural force produces tension stress in the affected wedge-shaped region on the tooth side away from the tooth-bending direction, resulting in loss of the surface tooth structure by microfractures, which is termed *abfracture*.[19] Proponents of this hypothesis add that microfractures may increase the rate of tooth structure loss during abrasion from tooth brushing and/or from acids in the diet or biofilm. Opponents of this hypothesis note that these cervical lesions have been detected in individuals who do not have any apparent evidence of heavy occlusal forces (such as wear facets and/or fremitus). The general consensus among experts is that the etiology of these lesions is multifactorial and that well-designed clinical research studies are required to gain better understanding relative to the etiology of cervical abrasion and abfraction defects, which are generally referred to as noncarious cervical lesions (NCCLs).[20] The presence of such defects does not automatically warrant intervention.

The mechanical wear of the incisal or occlusal tooth structure that results from functional or parafunctional movements of the mandible is termed *attrition*. Although a certain degree of attrition is expected with age, it is important to note abnormally advanced attrition (see Fig. 3.9E). If abnormal attrition is present, the patient's functional movements should be evaluated and inquiry made with regard to potential parafunctional habits such as tooth grinding or clenching/grinding *(bruxism)*. Heavy occlusal loading from clenching may result in the presence of "craze lines" that are limited to enamel (i.e., do not progress through the DEJ into dentin; see Fig. 3.9F). Craze lines are not sensitive and do not require treatment but may be evidence of excessive masticatory muscle activity (see Chapter 1). The etiology of the parafunction may include stress, airway issues, and/or sleep apnea. In some older patients, the enamel of the cusp tips (or incisal edges) is worn off, resulting in cupped-out areas because the exposed, softer dentin wears faster than the surrounding enamel, though there may also be an erosive component to the process. Sometimes, these areas are an annoyance because of food retention or the presence of peripheral, ragged, sharp enamel edges. The sharp edges may result in tongue or cheek biting; rounding these edges does not completely resolve the problem but may improve comfort. Slowing such wear by appropriate restorative treatment may be indicated.

The examination process may reveal areas of horizontal or vertical fracture development. Awareness of extreme variations in dental anatomy aids in the identification of fracture-prone areas. For example, deep developmental fissures that cross between marginal or cusp ridges may predispose posterior teeth to fracture. Early fractures may be invisible upon initial assessment. Appropriate dye materials or transillumination may aid in detecting the line of fracture within the tooth structure. Cusp isolation/loading devices and techniques must be utilized so as to identify fractures that involve the dentin and are symptomatic (i.e., fractures that are actively propagating). Teeth with active, symptomatic fractures should be considered for full coverage of the occlusal surface. Fractures that have been present for a period of time become stained and thereby visible during examination; they should be considered at risk for further propagation into dentin. Any tooth that has extensive caries, or restoration, and remaining cusps with little dentin support should be identified as being susceptible to future fracture and considered for a cusp-protecting restoration (Fig. 3.10). Complete cusp fracture is a common occurrence in posterior teeth. In general, the most frequently fractured cusps are the nonfunctional cusps (see Chapter 1). Specifically, the most frequently fractured teeth are mandibular molars and second premolars, with the lingual (nonfunctional) cusps fracturing more often than the facial (functional) cusps. Maxillary premolars also frequently fracture, and similar to mandibular teeth, the facial (nonfunctional) cusps fracture more often than the lingual (functional) cusps. The mesiofacial (nonfunctional) and distolingual (small functional) cusps are the most commonly fractured cusps in maxillary molars.[21] A study of fracture severity found that 95% of the fractures

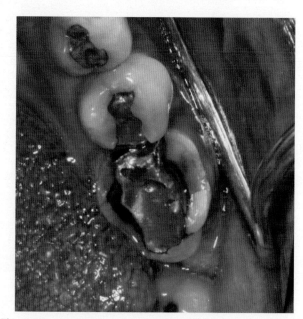

• **Fig. 3.10** Extensively restored teeth with weakened and fractured cusps. Note the distal developmental fissure in the second molar, which further predisposes the distal cusps to fracture.

exposed dentin, 25% were below the CEJ, and 3% resulted in pulp exposure. The consequences of posterior tooth fracture were found to vary, with maxillary premolar and mandibular molar fractures being generally more severe. Most fractures were treated with direct or indirect restorations or recontouring and polishing; 3% of the fractured teeth were extracted, and 4% received endodontic treatment.[22] Risk factors for nontraumatic fracture of posterior teeth were found to be the presence of a stained fracture in enamel and an increase in the proportion of the volume of the natural tooth crown occupied by a restoration.[23,24] The examination process should notate the presence and activity of all fracture areas.

The dental examination also may reveal dental anomalies that include variations in size, shape, structure, or number of teeth—such as dens in dente, macrodontia, microdontia, gemination, concrescence, dilaceration, amelogenesis imperfecta, and dentinogenesis imperfecta. An in-depth discussion of these anomalies is beyond the scope of this text. The reader should consult an oral pathology textbook for additional information.

Radiographic Examination of Teeth and Restorations

Radiographs are an indispensable part of the contemporary dentist's diagnostic armamentarium. The use of diagnostic ionizing radiation is, however, not without risks. Cumulative exposure to ionizing radiation potentially may result in adverse effects. The diagnostic yield or potential benefit that might be gained from a radiograph must be weighed against the financial costs and the potential adverse effects of exposure to radiation. Several technologies, particularly digital radiography, are now available and are designed to enhance diagnostic yield and reduce radiation exposure.

The ADA, in collaboration with the Food and Drug Administration (FDA), developed guidelines for the prescription of dental radiographic examinations to serve as an adjunct to the dentist's professional judgment with regard to the best use of diagnostic imaging. Radiographs help the dental practitioner evaluate and definitively diagnose many oral diseases and conditions. However, the dentist must weigh the benefits of taking dental radiographs against the risk of exposing a patient to ionizing radiation, the effects of which accumulate from multiple sources over time. The dentist, being aware of the patient's health history and vulnerability to oral disease, is in the best position to make this judgment. For this reason, guidelines are intended to serve as a resource for the practitioner and are not intended to be standards of care, requirements, or regulations. The ADA/FDA guidelines help direct the type and frequency of radiographs needed according to patient condition and risk factors (Table 3.2).

Generally, patients at higher risk for caries or periodontal disease should receive more frequent and more extensive radiographic surveys. A systematic review of methods of diagnosing dental caries lesions found that although radiographs were useful in detecting lesions, they do have limitations.[25] For the examination of occlusal surfaces, radiographs had moderate sensitivity and good specificity for diagnosing dentinal lesions; however, for enamel lesions, the sensitivity was poor and the specificity was reduced (see the section on Diagnosis for description of these terms). Studies of the radiographic examination of proximal surfaces found that there was moderate sensitivity and good specificity for the detection of cavitated lesions and low to moderate sensitivity and moderate to high specificity for enamel or dentinal lesions. Before rendering a diagnosis and deciding on treatment, information obtained from radiographs should be confirmed or augmented through clinical examination findings if at all possible.

For diagnosis of proximal surface caries, restoration overhangs, or poorly contoured restorations, posterior bitewing and anterior periapical radiographs are most helpful. When interpreting the radiographic presentation of proximal tooth surfaces, it is necessary to know the normal anatomic picture presented in a radiograph before any abnormalities may be diagnosed. In a radiograph, a proximal caries lesion usually appears as a dark area or a radiolucency in the enamel slightly apical to the contact (see Fig. 3.4A). This radiolucency is typically triangular and has its apex toward the DEJ.

Moderate-to-deep occlusal caries lesions may be seen as a radiolucency extending into dentin (see Fig. 3.4C). Because the specificity of radiographs for detecting dentinal lesions on occlusal surfaces is relatively good at 80% (very few false positives), when a radiolucency is apparent beneath the occlusal enamel surface emanating from the DEJ a diagnosis of caries is appropriate. However, because the sensitivity of radiographs for dentinal lesions on the occlusal surface is rather low (50%), the absence of a radiolucency does not mean that a lesion is not present. In these situations, the clinician should rely more on the results of the visual examination and the findings of any adjunctive tests (discussed later).

Some defective aspects of restorations, including improper contour, overhangs (see Fig. 3.5), and recurrent caries lesions gingival to restorations (see Fig. 3.4D), may also be identified radiographically. The height and integrity of the marginal periodontium may be evaluated using bitewing radiographs. Pulpal abnormalities such as pulp stones and internal resorption may be identified in various radiographs. Periapical radiographs are helpful in identifying changes in the periapical periodontium that are consistent with periapical abscesses, dental granulomas, or cysts. Impacted third molars, supernumerary teeth, and other congenital or acquired abnormalities also may be discovered on periapical radiographic examination. The sensitivity and specificity of dental radiographs vary, however, according to the diagnostic task (e.g., surface of the tooth being examined, proximal versus occlusal; and depth, enamel versus dentin).

Radiographs aid in determining the relationship between the margins of existing or proposed restorations and bone. A biologic width of at least 2 mm is required for the junctional epithelium and the connective tissue attachments located between the base of the sulcus and the alveolar bone crest (Fig. 3.11A). In addition to this physiologic dimension, the restoration margin should be placed occlusally as far away as possible from the base of the sulcus. Restoration margins that encroach on the biologic width, by being placed deep in the sulcus, are inaccessible for biofilm removal and result in chronic inflammation. The inflammatory state may be clinically detected as clinical redness, swelling, and bleeding on probing or flossing in the area. Localized loss of osseous support will occur and the biologic width will reorganize further apically. The osseous loss and reorganization will result in deeper periodontal probing depths, which in turn will further limit effective biofilm removal. For these reasons, the final position of a proposed gingival margin, which is dictated by the existing restoration, caries, or retention features, must be estimated before restoration to determine if crown-lengthening procedures are indicated (see Fig. 3.11B). Surgical crown lengthening procedures involve the surgical removal of the gingiva, bone, or both to create a longer clinical crown and provide more tooth structure for placing the restoration margin and for increasing retention form. Another possible treatment option may be to orthodontically extrude the tooth so that the restoration margins do not violate the biologic width. Restorative procedures must be accomplished such that the periodontal health may be maintained.

Dental radiographs should always be interpreted cautiously. The dental radiograph is a two-dimensional image of a three-dimensional mass; thus a facial or lingual lesion (or radiolucent tooth-colored restoration) may be radiographically superimposed over the proximal area, mimicking a proximal caries lesion (false positive). The general finding that approximately 25% mineral loss has to occur before a radiolucency begins to appear on a radiograph means that a caries lesion may be present and not detected (false negative). Misdiagnosis may occur when cervical burnout (the radiographic picture of the normal structure and contour of the cervical third of the crown) mimics a caries lesion. Finally, although a caries lesion may be more extensive clinically

than it appears radiographically, it is estimated that over half of radiographically detected proximal lesions (in the outer half of dentin) are likely to be noncavitated and treatable with remineralization measures.[26] Radiographic findings must always be clinically verified (if possible) prior to the finalization of a diagnosis and treatment plan.

Adjunctive Aids for Examining Teeth and Restorations

Magnification in Operative Dentistry

Clinical dentistry often requires the viewing and evaluation of small details in teeth, intraoral and perioral tissues, restorations, and study casts. Unaided vision is often inadequate to view details

---

TABLE 3.2	Guidelines for Prescribing Dental Radiographs

The recommendations in this chart are subject to clinical judgment and may not apply to every patient. They are to be used by dentists only after reviewing the patient's health history and completing a clinical examination. Because every precaution should be taken to minimize radiation exposure, protective thyroid collars and aprons should be used, whenever possible. This practice is strongly recommended for children, women of childbearing age, and pregnant women.

Type of Encounter	Patient Age and Dental Developmental Stage				
	Child With Primary Dentition (Prior to Eruption of First Permanent Tooth)	Child With Transitional Dentition (After Eruption of First Permanent Tooth)	Adolescent With Permanent Dentition (Prior to Eruption of Third Molars)	Adult, Dentate or Partially Edentulous	Adult, Edentulous
New patient* being evaluated for dental diseases and dental development	Individualized radiographic exam consisting of selected periapical/occlusal views and/or posterior bitewings if proximal surfaces cannot be visualized or probed. Patients without evidence of disease and with open proximal contacts may not require a radiographic exam at this time.	Individualized radiographic exam consisting of posterior bitewings with panoramic exam or posterior bitewings and selected periapical images.	Individualized radiographic exam consisting of posterior bitewings with panoramic exam or posterior bitewings and selected periapical images. A full mouth intraoral radiographic exam is preferred when the patient has clinical evidence of generalized dental disease or a history of extensive dental treatment.		Individualized radiographic exam, based on clinical signs and symptoms.
Recall patient* with clinical caries or at increased risk for caries^^	Posterior bitewing exam at 6- to 12-month intervals if proximal surfaces cannot be examined visually or with a probe.			Posterior bitewing exam at 6- to 18-month intervals.	Not applicable
Recall patient* with no clinical caries and not at increased risk for caries**	Posterior bitewing exam at 12- to 24-month intervals if proximal surfaces cannot be examined visually or with a probe.		Posterior bitewing exam at 18- to 36-month intervals.	Posterior bitewing exam at 24- to 36-month intervals.	Not applicable
Recall patient* with periodontal disease	Clinical judgment as to the need for and type of radiographic images for the evaluation of periodontal disease. Imaging may consist of, but is not limited to, selected bitewing and/or periapical images of areas where periodontal disease (other than nonspecific gingivitis) can be identified clinically.				Not applicable
Patient for monitoring of growth and development	Clinical judgment as to need for and type of radiographic images for evaluation and/or monitoring of dentofacial growth and development.		Clinical judgment as to need for and type of radiographic images for evaluation and/or monitoring of dentofacial growth and development. Panoramic or periapical exam to assess developing third molars.	Usually not indicated	

TABLE 3.2	Guidelines for Prescribing Dental Radiographs—cont'd
Patient with other circumstances including, but not limited to, proposed or existing implants, pathology, restorative/endodontic needs, treated periodontal disease, and caries remineralization	Clinical judgment as to need for and type of radiographic images for evaluation and/or monitoring in these circumstances.

*Clinical situations for which radiographs may be indicated include but are not limited to:

A. Positive Historical Findings
  1. Previous periodontal or endodontic treatment
  2. History of pain or trauma
  3. Familial history of dental anomalies
  4. Postoperative evaluation of healing
  5. Remineralization monitoring
  6. Presence of implants or evaluation for implant placement
B. Positive Clinical Symptoms/Signs
  1. Clinical evidence of periodontal disease
  2. Large or deep restorations
  3. Deep caries lesions
  4. Malposed or clinically impacted teeth
  5. Swelling
  6. Evidence of dental/facial trauma
  7. Mobility of teeth
  8. Sinus tract ("fistula")
  9. Clinically suspected sinus pathology
  10. Growth abnormalities
  11. Oral involvement in known or suspected systemic disease
  12. Positive neurologic findings in the head and neck
  13. Evidence of foreign objects
  14. Pain and/or dysfunction of the temporomandibular joint and/or muscles of mastication
  15. Facial asymmetry
  16. Abutment teeth for fixed or removable partial prosthesis
  17. Unexplained bleeding

  18. Unexplained sensitivity of teeth
  19. Unusual eruption, spacing, or migration of teeth
  20. Unusual tooth morphology, calcification, or color
  21. Unexplained absence of teeth
  22. Clinical erosion

**Factors increasing risk for caries may include but are not limited to:
  1. High level of caries experience or demineralization
  2. History of recurrent caries
  3. High titers of cariogenic bacteria
  4. Existing restoration(s) of poor quality
  5. Poor oral hygiene
  6. Inadequate fluoride exposure
  7. Prolonged nursing (bottle or breast)
  8. Frequent high sucrose content in diet
  9. Poor family dental health
  10. Developmental or acquired enamel defects
  11. Developmental or acquired disability
  12. Xerostomia
  13. Genetic abnormality of teeth
  14. Many multisurface restorations
  15. Chemotherapy/radiation therapy
  16. Eating disorders
  17. Drug/alcohol abuse
  18. Irregular dental care

From American Dental Association, US Food and Drug Administration: The selection of patients for dental radiograph examinations. Available on www.ada.org. Document created November 2004.

needed to make treatment decisions. Magnification aids such as loupes provide a larger image size for improved visual acuity, while allowing proper upright posture to be maintained with less eye fatigue.

When choosing loupes, several parameters should be considered.[27-29] Magnification (power) describes the increase in image size. Most dentists use magnifications of 2× to 4×. The lower power systems of 2× to 2.5× allow multiple quadrants to be viewed, whereas the higher power systems of 3× to 4× enable viewing of several teeth or a single tooth. In general, higher magnification systems are heavier, have a narrower field of view, are more expensive, and require more light than lower power systems. The use of small, lightweight light-emitting diode (LED) headlamps attached to the eyeglass frame or headband offer the considerable visual advantage of added illumination when used with loupes.

Working distance (focal length) is the distance from the eye to the object when the object is in focus. This parameter should be considered carefully before selecting loupes because the desired working distance depends on the dentist's height, arm length, and seating preferences. Dentists of average height typically choose a working distance of 13 to 14 inches (33–35 cm), whereas tall dentists and those who prefer to work farther away from the patient use working distances of 14 to 16 inches (35–40 cm).

Depth of focus, or the difference between the far and near focus limits of the working distance, depends on the magnification. Typically, the lower the magnification, the greater is the depth of focus.

Many choices of magnification loupes are currently available for dentistry. The simplest magnifiers are the diopter single-lens loupes, which are single-piece plastic pairs of lenses that clip onto eyeglass frames. These loupes are inexpensive and lightweight and may provide magnification of up to 2.5×. However, images may be distorted, and working lengths less than ideal. The more commonly used dental loupe is binocular with lenses mounted on an eyeglass frame. Binocular loupes typically have Galilean and prismatic optics that provide 2×, 3.5×, 4×, and greater magnification. Prescription lenses may be placed in the eyeglass frames for all loupe types. Most models also have side shields or a wraparound design for eye protection and infection control. Two mounting systems are currently available for binocular loupes: (1) flip-up and (2) fixed or through-the-lens types.

Dental microscopes, though limited primarily to endodontic practices in the past, are now being used in some restorative dentistry practices. Compared with high powered loupes, dental microscopes allow the clinician to view intraoral structures at a higher level of magnification while maintaining a broader field of view. Because very small areas may be seen, microscopes are used in detail-oriented procedures such as the finishing of porcelain restoration margins, identifying minute caries lesions, and minimizing the removal of sound tooth structure. Generally, microscopes include five or six levels of magnification that typically range from 2.5× to 20×. Manufacturers of dental microscopes include Carl Zeiss, Inc. (Dublin, CA); Global Surgical Corporation (St. Louis, MO); and Seiler Precision Microscope Instrument Company (St. Louis, MO).

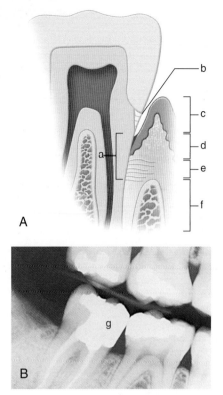

• **Fig. 3.11** A, Biologic width (*a*) is the physiologic dimension needed for the junctional epithelium (*d*) and the connective tissue attachment (*e*), which is measured from the base of the sulcus (*c*) to the level of the bone crest (*f*). The margin of the restoration (*b*) must not violate this dimension. B, Tooth with an existing restoration (*g*) that encroaches on the biologic width requires crown-lengthening procedures before placement of a new restoration.

Cost, size of the equipment, and perceived lack of value to the clinician are factors that have limited the use of microscopes in operative dentistry practice.

Photography in Operative Dentistry

Photography in dentistry has many uses and, with newer digital technologies, is becoming mainstream in dental practice. Photography is an excellent tool for documentation and evaluation. Intraoral cameras and single-lens reflex (SLR) digital cameras provide opportunities to document existing esthetic conditions such as color, shape, and position of teeth. Close-up images of existing pits and fissures provide the opportunity to image current conditions for the purpose of future reevaluation and detection of changes that may be developing. Photographs of preparations of deep caries lesions provide documentation to aid in future diagnosis of tooth conditions. Digital documentation with photographs, and ability to process and store images in an electronic patient record, is easy and cost effective.

Diagnostic Study Models

Study models are helpful in evaluating a patient's clinical status in many situations. Study models are able to provide an understanding of occlusal relationships, help in developing the treatment plan, and serve as a tool for educating the patient. Accurately mounted study models provide an opportunity for a thorough evaluation of the tooth interdigitation, the functional occlusion, and any occlusal abnormalities. Study models allow further

evaluation of the plane of occlusion; tilted, rotated, or extruded teeth; crossbites; plunger cusps; wear facets and defective restorations; coronal contours; proximal contacts; and embrasure spaces between teeth. The ability to obtain virtual study models via digital impression technology has increased the ease and level of diagnostic evaluation, especially in situations where the use of conventional impression techniques/materials may not be an option (such as in patients with a hyperactive gag reflex). Combined with clinical and radiographic findings, study casts allow the practitioner to carefully reflect on findings and develop a treatment plan without the patient present, thus saving valuable chair time. When a proposed treatment plan is discussed with the patient, study models are a valuable educational medium in helping the patient understand and visualize existing conditions and the need for the proposed treatment.

Caries Detection Technologies

In addition to the traditional methods of caries detection, several new technologies have emerged and show promising results for the clinical detection and diagnosis of caries lesions. These devices may have the potential to replace the tactile portion of caries detection, where explorers are used to try to estimate the depth of the caries lesions into the pits and fissures. However, these devices have two limitations. The first is that they are only indicated for use on unrestored pits and fissures. The second is that their diagnostic accuracy has not been firmly established. The technologies currently approved by the FDA include laser-induced fluorescence, light-induced fluorescence, and alternating current (AC) impedance spectroscopy (ACIST).[10,30]

The DIAGNOdent device (KaVo Dental Corporation, Charlotte, NC) uses laser fluorescence technology, with the intention of detecting and measuring bacterial products and changes in tooth structure in a caries lesion. This compact and portable device, which requires a clean, dry occlusal surface, yields a numerical score from 0 to 99. The manufacturer has recommended threshold scores that represent the presence and extent of a lesion. A systematic review found that the "device is clearly more sensitive than traditional diagnostic methods, but the increased likelihood of false-positive diagnoses limits its usefulness as a principal diagnostic method."[31]

Another system currently available for caries lesion detection is the CamX Spectra Caries Detection Aid (Air Techniques, Melville, NY). This system claims to detect caries lesions by measuring increased light-induced fluorescence. Special LEDs project high-energy violet or blue light onto the tooth surface. Light of this wavelength supposedly stimulates porphyrins—metabolites unique to cariogenic bacteria—to appear distinctly red, while healthy enamel fluoresces to appear green. Using this fluorescent technology, the data captured by the Spectra system are analyzed by imaging software, which highlights the lesions in different color ranges and defines the potential caries activity on a scale of 0 to 5.

The CarieScan PRO (CarieScan, LLC, Charlotte, NC) is a device for the detection and monitoring of caries by the application and analysis of ACIST (AC Impedance Spectroscopy Technology). The CarieScan PRO claims to enable clinicians to evaluate demineralized tooth structure using ACIST by providing information about tissue being healthy, in the early stages of demineralization, or already significantly decayed. The device provides a color scale and a numerical scale to determine the severity of the caries lesion and is accompanied by management recommendations that range from therapeutic prevention to operative intervention appropriate for the extent of the demineralization.

Although these technologies appear promising, the standard of care remains visual inspection of well-illuminated, clean and dry teeth, with use of radiographs as indicated.[32] An ideal diagnostic test accurately detects when a tooth surface is healthy (specificity); when a lesion or demineralization is present (sensitivity); and if demineralization is present, whether or not it is active and whether or not it has cavitated the surface (see section on Diagnosis). Except for the presence of frank cavitation in more advanced lesions, none of the available approaches to detecting caries or determining lesion activity is completely accurate. Thus the clinician must take all of the available diagnostic information together—visual, tactile, radiographic, and so on—along with the respective reported levels of accuracy and combine that with an assessment of the patient's overall caries status to make a final diagnosis of the presence and extent of a caries lesion.

Diagnosis

Dental Disease; Interpretation and Use of Diagnostic Findings

As discussed in Chapter 2, dental caries is a multifactorial, transmissible, infectious oral disease caused primarily by the complex interaction of cariogenic oral flora (biofilm) with fermentable dietary carbohydrates on the tooth surface over time. *Caries lesions are the result of the caries disease process, not the cause.*

The diagnostic effort of health care professionals has been enhanced by the use of principles adopted from clinical epidemiology. This analytic approach relies on "2 × 2" contingency tables (Fig. 3.12) derived from clinical trials data. Such studies compare the results of a diagnostic test with the results obtained from a "gold standard" (knowledge of the actual condition) to determine how well a test identifies the "true," or actual, condition. The results of the diagnostic test, positive or negative, are shown across the rows of the table, and the results of a "gold standard" or the "truth" are displayed in the columns. Cell A of the table contains the cases that the test identifies as being positive (or diseased) that actually are positive (i.e., confirmed by the "gold standard"). These cases are termed *true positives.* Cell B contains all cases for which a positive finding from the diagnostic test is present, but where the actual condition is negative. Therefore this cell denotes *false positives.* Cell C includes the cases identified by the diagnostic test as not being diseased, but actually are diseased, as determined by

the "gold standard." Findings in this cell are termed *false negatives.* The final cell, cell D, includes *true negatives,* where the diagnostic test accurately identifies nondiseased cases that are truly negative as confirmed by the "gold standard." A perfect diagnostic test would result in all cases being assigned to cells A or D with no false positives (cell B) or false negatives (cell C).

When the basics of this table are understood, the information it yields may be put to good use by the diagnostician. The first concept is test *sensitivity,* which is calculated as the number of true positives (A) divided by the number of total positive cases (A + C, i.e., the number of times where disease was actually present regardless of the diagnostic test results). Sensitivity indicates the proportion of individuals with disease in any group or population that is identified positively by the test. In contrast, *specificity* refers to the proportion of individuals without disease properly classified by the diagnostic test and is the ratio of true negatives (D) to all negatives (B + D). Sensitivity and specificity will not vary on the basis of the prevalence of disease, that is, the proportion of cases in a population. Rather, these statistics indicate what proportions of existing disease and absence of disease will be correctly identified in any group of individuals.

A test with low sensitivity indicates that a high probability exists that many of the individuals with negative results have the disease and go undiagnosed. Conversely, a test with high sensitivity means that most of those who actually have disease will be identified as such. Tests with high specificity suggest that patients without the disease are highly likely to test negative. Tests with low specificity will misclassify a sizable proportion as diseased when many are actually free of disease.

Very few tests have *both* high sensitivity and high specificity, so trade-offs are inevitable. The clinician must weigh the seriousness of the disease that is left untreated (in cases of low sensitivity) against the invasiveness of the treatment (in cases of low specificity). In the former, low sensitivity may be acceptable for tests diagnosing slowly progressing, nonfatal conditions but unacceptable for conditions that progress rapidly or are life threatening. In the latter, low specificity may not be acceptable if the treatment is invasive and irreversible, but more acceptable if the treatment is noninvasive and temporary. In the case of dental caries, all things being equal, this means that the clinician may accept a less sensitive test (i.e., miss some initial lesions [cell C]) because caries usually progresses slowly over years. But given that operative treatment is invasive and irreversible, a highly specific test (i.e., few false positives [cell B]) means that fewer healthy teeth will be incorrectly treated.

The dentist should be mindful of the fact that except in cases of relatively large caries lesions, *the accuracy of the methods used to detect lesions (visual inspection, radiographs, caries detection devices, etc.) are all prone to inaccuracies* (Box 3.1). These inaccuracies result in false-positive and false-negative findings. This situation raises the question, "What are the implications of these inaccuracies for clinical decision making?" False-positive findings may result in the surgical treatment of a sound tooth, and false-negative findings will result in a diseased surface receiving remineralization treatment instead of operative treatment. The former situation is irreversible and should be avoided, whenever possible. In the latter situation, false negatives will receive remineralization therapy, regular monitoring, and, if a lesion develops, may be treated operatively at a later time, if needed. This reasonable approach takes into consideration that caries lesions generally do not progress rapidly.[33-35] Thus the clinician should strive to reduce the number of false positives by making sure that strong diagnostic evidence supports the presence

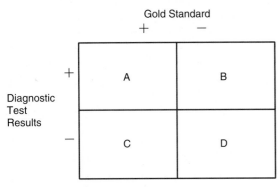

Gold Standard

Cell A = true positives
Cell B = false positives
Cell C = false negatives
Cell D = true negatives

• **Fig. 3.12** Contingency table for interpretation of diagnostic tests.

• BOX 3.1   Assessing the Accuracy of a Diagnostic Test for Caries

Contingency Table for Diagnostic Test Evaluation
Histologic Gold Standard
    Caries
    No caries
Diagnostic Test
    Caries
        True positive (TP)
        False positive (FP)
    No caries
        False negative (FN)
        True negative (TN)

Desirable and Undesirable Outcomes Resulting from Diagnostic Tests with Low Sensitivity or Specificity

Example 1
Diagnosing 100 teeth (90 healthy and 10 carious) with a diagnostic test having a high sensitivity (0.80) and low specificity (0.50) would result in the following:
Desirable outcomes:
    Correctly detect 8 of 10 carious teeth (TP)
    Correctly diagnose 45 of 90 healthy teeth (TN)
Undesirable outcomes:
    Fail to detect 2 of 10 carious teeth (FN)
    Fail to diagnose 45 healthy teeth as carious (FP)

Example 2
Diagnosing 100 teeth (90 healthy and 10 carious) with a diagnostic test having low sensitivity (0.50) and high specificity (0.80) would result in the following:
Desirable outcomes:
    Correctly detect 5 of 10 carious teeth (TP)
    Correctly diagnose 72 of 90 healthy teeth (TN)
Undesirable outcomes:
    Fail to detect 5 of 10 carious teeth (FN)
    Fail to diagnose 18 healthy teeth as carious (FP)

---

of cavitation or dentin penetration before recommending irreversible operative treatment.

These concepts are widely used in medical practice. Although many of the necessary research studies have not been conducted to develop probabilities for dental conditions, interest in the use of clinical epidemiology in the dental profession has been growing. In the future, more research studies will be conducted so as to provide this information to clinicians, and one should be prepared to take advantage of their use.

Risk Assessments and Profiles

The patient assessment and examination process allows opportunity to identify factors and indicators that increase likelihood (risk) of future problems, given the patient's current behaviors, clinical conditions, and so on (see Chapter 2).[36,37] *Risk assessments* help organize the data relative to multiple causative factors. Few diseases or dental conditions are caused by a single factor. Rather, most diseases and dental conditions have been shown to be associated with numerous behavioral or sociodemographic, physical or environmental, microbiologic, or host factors. In addition, every patient has a different set of risk factors. This presents a challenge to determining the likelihood that a disease or condition would occur in the future or that some form of dental treatment or therapeutics would decrease the chances of disease occurrence. Many risk assessments use terms such as *low risk, medium risk,*

and *high risk* to associate a level of risk with a category. This is sometimes expressed by using color-coded categories: red for high risk, yellow for medium risk, and green for low risk. Categories simplify the concept for the patient, as they are easily understood while discussing assessments and their implications for treatment recommendations.

Patients who possess risk factors and risk indicators should be considered to be at risk for dental caries even if the examination does not reveal any caries lesions.[33] A patient at high risk for dental caries should receive aggressive intervention to remove or alter as many risk factors as possible. Alternatively, regular monitoring and reassessment might be appropriate for a patient at low risk for dental caries. Risk assessment is a relatively young science in the dental profession, but as more research is completed, evidence is quickly validating this approach to patient care. Approaches to patient care using risk assessments and disease management such as CAMBRA are becoming the recognized standard of care. The CAMBRA guidelines were developed over several years as an evidence-based approach to preventing, reversing, and, when necessary, repairing early damage to teeth caused by caries. Refer to Chapter 2 for more information on how CAMBRA is used to determine caries risk and how this determination helps the clinician in the decision-making process for surgical or nonsurgical therapeutic interventions.

In relation to operative dentistry, risk assessments are made for caries, erosive tooth wear, and structural problems of teeth such as fractures. However, risk assessments should be established for other areas of the stomatognathic system such as periodontal disease, functional occlusal and TMJ issues, and for the "risk" involved in satisfying the patient's esthetic expectations. All treatment for patients should be designed to lower their risk for problems in each of these areas. Dental treatment in any one of the abovementioned areas may improve risk status in that area but at a cost of increased risk in another area. For example, preparation of teeth for full-coverage crowns might reduce occlusal or esthetic risk but at a cost of increasing risk for future caries or pulpal pathology. Taken together, risk assessments provide a *risk profile* that helps guide preventive and operative recommendations that are made to the patient with the goal of mitigating as many risk factors as possible.

Prognosis

Prognosis is the term used to describe the prediction of the probable course and outcome of a disease or condition as well as the outcome expected from an intervention, be it preventive or operative. Prognosis may also be used to estimate the likelihood of recovery from a disease or condition. In operative dentistry, prognosis may be used to describe the likelihood of success of a particular treatment procedure in terms of time of service, functional value, comfort, and esthetic value for the patient. A prognosis may be described as *excellent, good, fair, poor,* or even *hopeless.* Prognosis for a disease or condition is largely dependent on the risk factors and indicators that are present in the patient. However, other variables, such as the skill of the dentist and the current status of the disease before beginning treatment, also have an effect on the prognosis. For example, a patient with severe caries may be willing to eliminate all of the modifiable risk factors, but if the disease is too advanced, the long-term prognosis for the affected teeth may still be poor. It is important for the clinician to take into account the entire risk profile of the patient in all areas of the person's medical and dental health when trying to establish a prognosis. Once the dentist and the patient have a good understanding of the current condition(s), the patient's risk profile, and all associated prognoses, they will be able to work together as a team to identify treatment options and establish a treatment plan.

Treatment Planning

General Considerations

Patient assessment, examination, and diagnosis result in a listing of dental problems, an inventory of existing risk factors (or indicators), and an accurate prognosis for each tooth and for the patient's overall oral health. The dentist then begins to consider various options in light of the paramount principle in dentistry: to *do no harm*. Clinicians must have a sound knowledge of the current evidence relative to the risks and benefits of their treatment recommendations. One option that must always be included is recommend that there not be any intervention. Another consideration, based on the patient–dentist interaction, particular needs/desires of the patient, and/or the skill/comfort level of the dentist, is to recommend referral to another practitioner. With regard to operative dentistry procedures, the decision to recommend surgical or nonsurgical intervention depends on the determination that a tooth is diseased, a restoration is defective, or the tooth or restoration is at some increased risk of further deterioration if the intervention does not occur. If any of these conditions exists, intervention is recommended to the patient. There may be multiple possible means by which to resolve the diagnosed disease or defect. Identification of treatment alternatives involves establishing a list of one or more reasonable interventions from the set of possible alternatives. Treatment alternatives for a specific condition may include, for example, periodic reevaluation to monitor the condition, chemotherapeutics (e.g., applications of fluoride to promote remineralization or antimicrobials to reduce bacteria), recontouring defective restorations or irregular tooth surfaces, repair of an existing restoration, and restoration of caries lesions or other defects. The list of reasonable treatment alternatives is based on current evidence of the effectiveness of treatments, prevailing standards of care, and clinical and nonclinical patient factors. If the decision is made to recommend intervention then identification and selection among treatment alternatives, with the patient's involvement, enables creation of the *treatment plan.*

The treatment plan is a carefully sequenced series of services designed to eliminate or control etiologic factors, repair existing damage, and create a functional, maintainable environment. An appropriate treatment plan depends on thorough evaluation of the patient, the expertise of the dentist, and a prediction of the patient's response to treatment. The treatment plan will also include strategies designed to reduce the patient's risk for future caries or other oral disease. Selection of specific components of the treatment plan is accomplished in consultation with the patient. The patient is advised of the reasonable treatment alternatives and related risks and benefits. After the patient is fully informed, the dentist and patient select a course of action that is most appropriate.

Treatment plans are influenced by many factors, including patient preferences, motivation, systemic health, emotional status, and financial resources. The treatment plan is also influenced by the dentist's knowledge, experience, and training; laboratory support; dentist–patient compatibility; availability of specialists; and the patient's functional, esthetic, and technical demands. Finally, a treatment plan is not a static list of services. Rather, it is often a multiphase and dynamic series of activities. Success of the treatment plan is determined by its ability to meet the patient's initial and long-term needs. A treatment plan should allow for reevaluation and be adaptable to meet the changing needs, preferences, and health conditions of the patient.

In the context of planning dental treatment, the clinician should recommend invasive operative treatment only when the benefits outweigh the risks of adverse outcomes. Restorations that require permanent removal of tooth structure have a limited lifespan. Studies have shown that the average lifespan of a restoration ranges from 5 to more than 15 years.[38] When the restoration is subsequently replaced additional tooth structure is removed, regardless of how carefully the operator removes the existing restoration. This situation results in what has been termed *the cycle of re-restoration*, which leads to larger and more invasive restorations over the course of a patient's life.[39]

As a general rule, remineralization therapies, as well as sealants in the case of pits and fissures, are the preferred methods of managing coronal lesions that are neither cavitated nor involve dentin. Remineralization is also recommended for root-surface lesions in which a break in the surface contour of the exposed root surface has not occurred. However, it is very important to note that *remineralization requires a high level of patient compliance with the therapeutic regimen and frequent recall visits to assess the success of the treatment*. If lesion progression is detected at recall, then operative intervention is warranted.

There are exceptions to the general rule of managing noncavitated enamel lesions with remineralization. Remineralization requires a shift in the delicate balance of the oral biofilm and therefore depends heavily on changes in patient behavior (e.g., improved home care, diet) and the timely application of antimicrobial agents, fluoride, and other remineralizing agents. Thus, when it is clear that the patient is unwilling or unable to follow the prescribed remineralization regimen of home care and professional care, it is often appropriate to remove the lesion(s) surgically and restore the defect or to seek to arrest the lesion (see Chapter 2).

If confirmed cavitation of the enamel or demineralization penetrating into the dentin on coronal surfaces is present or a break exists in the contour of exposed root and softening of the surface, then operative treatment is usually recommended. One exception to this general guideline is the lesion that is deemed arrested.

Treatment Plan Sequencing/Phasing

Proper sequencing is a crucial component of a successful treatment plan. Certain treatments must follow others in a logical order, whereas other treatments may or must occur concurrently and require coordination. Complex treatment plans often are sequenced in phases, including an urgent phase, a control phase, a reevaluation phase, a definitive phase, and a maintenance phase (that includes reassessment and recare). For most patients, the first three phases are accomplished simultaneously. Generally, the principle of "greatest need" guides the order in which treatment is sequenced. This principle suggests that what the patient needs most is performed first—with pain, bleeding, and swelling at the beginning of the treatment plan and elective esthetic procedures at the end. The process of treatment planning requires that the dentist develop an ever-increasing, comprehensive knowledge of dental disease management in the context of individualized patient care. Study of textbooks devoted to this discipline is indicated.[40]

Urgent Phase

The urgent phase of care begins with a thorough review of the patient's medical history and current condition. A patient presenting with swelling, pain, bleeding, or infection should have these problems managed as soon as possible, before initiation of subsequent phases.

Control Phase

A control phase is appropriate when the patient presents with multiple pressing problems and extensive active disease or when the prognosis is unclear. The goals of this phase are to remove etiologic factors, eliminate the ecologic niches of pathogens, and stabilize the patient's dental health. These goals are accomplished by (1) removal of active disease such that inflammation may resolve, (2) correction of conditions that prevent or limit hygiene efforts, (3) elimination of potential causes of disease, and (4) initiation of preventive activities. Examples of control phase treatment include extractions, endodontics, periodontal debridement and scaling, occlusal adjustment, caries arrest and/or removal, replacement or repair of defective restorations such as those with gingival overhangs, and use of caries control measures, as discussed in Chapter 2.

The dentist should develop a plan for the management and prevention of dental caries as part of the control phase. After the patient's caries status and caries risk have been determined, chemical, surgical, behavioral, mechanical, and dietary techniques may be used to improve host resistance and alter the oral flora.[40] Chapter 2 presents a detailed discussion of caries diagnosis, prevention, treatment, and control.

Reevaluation Phase

The reevaluation phase allows time between the control and definitive phases for resolution of inflammation and healing. Initial treatment and pulpal responses are reevaluated during this phase as the relative effectiveness of control phase treatment may influence and modify the definitive phase treatment plan. This phase is used to reinforce home care habits and assess motivation for further treatment.

Patients with an overall low risk profile, who only require minor alterations in diet, behaviors, and exposure to remineralization agents, may not require a formal control phase/reevaluation phase process. The treatment plan for these patients may start with a plan to definitively address immediate concerns while simultaneously implementing minor changes and reinforcing habits consistent with dental health.

Definitive Phase

The patient enters the definitive phase of treatment only after the dentist reassesses initial efforts to control disease and, with the patient, determines the need for further care. This phase may include endodontic, periodontal, orthodontic, and surgical procedures. The patient's active disease must be under control, and preventive efforts habitually established, before fixed or removable prosthodontic treatment. This phase is discussed in more detail in the section on interdisciplinary considerations in operative treatment planning.

Maintenance (Reassessment and Recare) Phase

The maintenance phase includes regular reassessment (synonyms include reevaluation, periodic) examinations that may reveal the need for adjustments to prevent future breakdown, provide an opportunity to reinforce home care, and plan recare treatment steps where disease has returned. Examinations for reassessment most frequently occur as part of strategically planned (recall) appointments for biofilm removal (dental prophylaxis). The frequency of reevaluation examinations depends, in large part, on the patient's risk for dental disease. A patient with a low risk profile may have longer intervals (e.g., 9–12 months) between recall visits. In contrast, patients at high risk profile should be recalled and examined much more frequently (e.g., 3–4 months).

Interdisciplinary Considerations in Operative Treatment Planning

When an operative procedure is performed during the control or definitive phases, general guidelines help determine when the operative treatment should occur relative to other forms of care. Following is a discussion on sequencing operative care with endodontic, periodontal, orthodontic, surgical, and prosthodontic treatments.

Endodontics

All teeth to be restored with large restorations should have a pulpal and periapical evaluation. If indicated, teeth should have endodontic treatment before restoration is completed. Also, a tooth previously endodontically treated, that shows no evidence of healing or has an inadequate filling or a filling exposed to oral fluids, should be evaluated for retreatment before restorative therapy is initiated.[41]

Periodontics

Generally, periodontal treatment should precede operative care, especially when improved oral hygiene and initial scaling/root planing procedures create (through reduction of gingival inflammation) a more desirable environment for performing operative treatment. A tooth with a questionable periodontal prognosis should not receive an extensive restoration until periodontal treatment provides a more favorable prognosis. If a tooth has a good periodontal prognosis, then operative treatment may occur before or after periodontal therapy, as long as the operative treatment is not compromised by the existing tissue condition. Treatment of deep caries lesions often requires caries control (see Chapter 2). Caries control may utilize temporization, creation of a foundation, or root canal therapy/foundation before periodontal therapy. The correction of gross restorative defects in restoration contours (e.g., open contact resulting from restoration undercontour, gingival overhang, poor embrasure form, occlusal interference resulting in increased mobility) is considered a part of initial periodontal therapy, and such corrections enable a more favorable tissue response. If periodontal surgical procedures are required, indirect restorations such as inlays or onlays, crowns, and prostheses should be delayed until the surgical phase is completed. Teeth planned for cast restorations may, however, be prepared and temporized before periodontal surgery. This approach permits confirmation of the restored tooth prognosis before surgery and allows improved access for the surgical procedure.

Patients with gingivitis and early periodontitis generally respond favorably to improved oral hygiene and scaling/root planing procedures. Patients with more advanced periodontitis might require removal (or at least minimization) of associated risk factors/indicators through surgical steps that eliminate/reduce sulcular depths or various regenerative procedures to resolve their periodontal disease. Steps to increase the zones of attached gingiva and eliminate abnormal frenal tension should be achieved by corrective periodontal surgical procedures around teeth receiving restorations with subgingival margins. In addition, any teeth requiring restorations that may encroach on the biologic width of the periodontium should have appropriate crown-lengthening surgical procedures performed before the final restoration is placed. Usually, a minimum of 6 weeks is required after the surgery before final restorative procedures are undertaken.

Orthodontics

Orthodontic therapy, such as realignment or extrusion, may be required to provide improved interdental spacing, stress distribution, function, and esthetics. All caries lesions should be corrected with amalgam or composite restorations before orthodontic treatment begins. Few indications exist for cast restorations before orthodontic treatment is completed. In addition, patients undergoing orthodontic treatment should receive more intense focus (especially by the orthodontist) on the minimization/elimination of risk factors for caries and gingival/periodontal disease. The orthodontic treatment plan should include shorter recall intervals for biofilm removal, examination, and oral hygiene reinforcement.

Oral Surgery

In most instances, impacted, unerupted, and/or hopelessly diseased teeth should be removed before operative treatment. Oral surgery procedural steps required for third molar removal may jeopardize new restorations placed on second molars. In addition, soft tissue lesions, complicating exostoses, and improperly contoured ridge areas should be eliminated or corrected before final restorative care.

Fixed, Removable, and Implant Prosthodontics

Direct restorations should be completed, if possible, before placing indirect restorations. Large amalgam or composite foundation restorations must have secondary retention features (grooves, slots, pins) placed further from the external surface of the tooth so that the retention of the foundation material is not compromised during preparation for the indirect restoration. In removable prosthodontics, tooth preparations and restorations should allow for the design of the removable partial denture. This includes allowance for rests, guide planes, and clasps. The design of the direct restoration and the selection of appropriate restorative materials must be compatible with the design of the contemplated removable prosthesis. In cases where dental implants have been or will be placed, direct restorations should be planned and executed to allow necessary mesial, distal, and vertical (occlusal) space for implant-supported indirect restorations. Implant restorations may sometimes have unusual proximal contours, and adjacent amalgam or composite restorations should be designed to allow the best possible proximal contact relationships.

Treatment of Abrasion, Erosion, Abfraction, and Attrition

Abraded or eroded areas should be considered for restoration only if one or more of the following is true: (1) The area is affected by caries, (2) the defect is sufficiently deep to compromise the structural integrity of the tooth, (3) intolerable sensitivity exists and is unresponsive to conservative desensitizing measures, (4) the defect contributes to a gingival or periodontal problem (chronic biofilm accumulation), (5) the area is to be involved in the design of a removable partial denture, (6) the depth of the defect is such that there is increased risk of pulpal involvement, (7) the defect is actively progressing, or (8) the patient desires esthetic improvement. Areas of significant occlusal attrition that have exposed dentin, are sensitive, or annoying should be considered for restoration or at least protection from additional loss of tooth structure. The

creation of an occlusal guard, for nocturnal use, may be indicated with a diagnosis of sleep-related bruxism. A treatment plan for definitive indirect restorations must include an occlusal analysis (which requires articulated diagnostic models) as part of the comprehensive examination. Careful consideration of related information from the patient assessment and examination process is essential if all aspects of the etiology are to be identified and risk factors reduced. Also, occlusal guard therapy should be considered for nocturnal protection of indirect restorations completed as part of the definitive phase.

Treatment of Root-Surface Caries

Root caries is common in older adults and in patients who have had periodontal therapy. Increases in the number of older patients in the patient population and tooth retention have contributed to this growing problem. Areas with root-surface caries usually should be restored when clinical and/or radiographic evidence of cavitation exists. Care must be exercised, however, to distinguish the active from the arrested (inactive) root-surface lesion. The arrested root-surface lesion may have sclerotic dentin that has darkened from extrinsic staining, is firm to the touch of an explorer, may be rough but is cleanable. Successful caries arrest usually occurs in patients whose oral hygiene or diet has improved such that the balance between demineralization and remineralization has become favorable. Generally, these lesions should not be restored except when the patient expresses esthetic concerns. If it is determined that the lesion needs restoration, it may be restored with tooth-colored materials or amalgam, depending on demands of the restorative material, preferences of the patient, and caries risk.

Prevention is preferred over restoration. It is recommended that appropriate preventive steps, such as improvement in diet/oral hygiene and fluoride treatment (with or without cementoplasty/dentinoplasty to eliminate surface roughness), be taken so as to limit carious breakdown and the need for restoration.

Treatment of Root-Surface Sensitivity

It is not unusual for patients to complain of root-surface sensitivity, which is an annoying sharp pain usually associated with gingival recession and exposed root surfaces. The most widely accepted explanation of this phenomenon is the *hydrodynamic theory*. This theory postulates that rapid dentinal tubule fluid movement toward the external surface of the tooth elongates odontoblastic processes (which extend from the pulp through the predentin and into dentin) and associated afferent nerve fibers. The elongation of the nerve fibers results in depolarization and the perception of pain (see Chapter 1). Causes of such fluid shifts include temperature changes, air-drying, and extreme osmotic gradients. Treatment methods that reduce rapid fluid shifts, by partially or totally occluding the ends of the exposed dentinal tubules, may help reduce the perceived sensitivity.

Dentinal hypersensitivity may become a problem when periodontal surgery causes clinical exposure of root surfaces (such that dentinal tubules are exposed and open). Numerous forms of nonsurgical treatment, such as fluoride varnishes, oxalate solutions, glutaraldehyde/HEMA-based desensitizers, resin-based adhesives, sealants, and desensitizing toothpastes that contain potassium nitrate, have been used to occlude the open tubules and, thereby, provide relief. When nonsurgical methods fail to provide relief, direct restorative treatment that physically covers the exposed dentin is indicated.

Treatment by Repair and Recontour of Existing Restorations

Amalgam, composite, or indirect restorations often may be repaired or recontoured as opposed to completely removed and replaced. Growing evidence suggests that the removal and replacement of restorations result in the cycle of re-restoration, which leads to increasingly larger tooth preparations and the resultant trauma to the tooth and supporting structures.[39] In addition, resurfacing or repair of composites and repair of cast restorations has been shown to be effective.[42-44] Also, amalgam restorations with localized defects may be repaired with amalgam or with sealant resins.[17,42] If a restoration has an isolated carious defect, and complete removal of the caries lesion has been confirmed, then it is acceptable and often preferable to restore the isolated area without replacement of the whole restoration. In many instances, recontouring or resurfacing the existing restoration may delay replacement and is an acceptable form of treatment.

Treatment by Replacement of Existing Restorations

Indications for replacing restorations include the following: (1) marginal void(s), especially in the gingival one third, that cannot be repaired and predispose to caries formation; (2) poor proximal contour or a gingival overhang that contributes to periodontal breakdown; (3) a marginal ridge discrepancy that contributes to food impaction; (4) overcontouring of a facial or lingual surface resulting in biofilm accumulation gingival to the height of contour and resultant inflammation of gingiva overprotected from the cleansing action of food bolus or toothbrush; (5) poor proximal contact that is either open or improper in location or size, resulting in interproximal food impaction and inflammation of impacted gingival papilla; (6) recurrent caries that cannot be treated adequately by a repair restoration; and (7) superficial marginal gap formation (ditching) deeper than 0.5 mm that predisposes to caries.[44]

Indications for replacing tooth-colored restorations include (1) improper contours that cannot be repaired, (2) large voids, (3) deep marginal staining, (4) recurrent caries, and (5) unacceptable esthetics.[44] Bonded restorations that have superficial marginal staining may be corrected by shallow, narrow, marginal repair.

Treatment With Amalgam Restorations

Dental amalgam still is recognized as one of the most successful direct restorative materials and is especially indicated for patients deemed to be moderate or high caries risk.[45] Inaccurate information with regard to the safety of amalgam has resulted in controversy among health care providers, environmentalists, legislators, and the general population. Although the use of amalgam is considered safe by multiple independent agencies, the release of elemental mercury does contribute to environmental levels. Therefore responsible handling is important. Chapter 10 presents the current indications for amalgam restorations and Chapter 13 presents a more complete discussion of legitimate mercury concerns and the safe use of dental amalgam.

Treatment With Direct Composite and Other Tooth-Colored Restorations

Direct composite restorations are indicated for the treatment of many lesions in anterior and posterior teeth. Successful treatment outcomes require meticulous attention to detail with regard to the enamel/dentin substrate and the properties of the specific adhesive system/composite resin being used. Correct application will result in the rewarding creation of form, function, and lifelike appearance of missing tooth structure. Determination of patient caries risk is important when considering the use of composite resin-based restorations. A systematic review has identified that the likelihood of development of recurrent caries adjacent to composite resin restorations is at least twice that of amalgam restorations in high caries risk patients.[45] Detailed indications for composite and other tooth-colored restorations are presented in Chapter 8.

Treatment With Indirect Cast-Metal Restorations

Partial- or full-coverage indirect cast-metal (primarily gold alloy) onlay restorations still remain among the most predictable and dependable restorations available to dentistry. These are the conservative restoration of choice for compromised teeth in high stress areas. The benefit of these restorations is that they cover and reinforce cusps without removal of healthy tooth structure in the middle and cervical areas of the facial and lingual surfaces (see Online Chapter 18). Indirect cast-metal restoration of the total clinical crown of teeth allows complete control of all contours and, thereby, the creation of anatomic shape consistent with optimal occlusal function and gingival health.

Treatment With Indirect Tooth-Colored Restorations

Properly designed porcelain-fused-to-metal (PFM) indirect restorations have clinically proven, long-term success in the restoration of individual teeth and edentulous areas. The use of ceramic materials without metal substrates has steadily increased in recent years. Partial-coverage bonded indirect tooth-colored restorations may be indicated for the restoration of large defects in low stress areas when esthetics and optimal control of contours is necessary. Full-coverage bonded indirect tooth-colored restorations also may be selected for the conservative restoration of weakened posterior teeth in low stress, esthetically critical areas.

The use of tooth-colored, zirconia-based, indirect restorations has steadily increased over the last two decades. *In vitro* and short-term *in vivo* research studies suggest that the clinical durability of these crowns may allow use as an alternative to indirect cast-metal or PFM restorations. However, there are currently no published long-term randomized, controlled clinical trials verifying this to actually be the case. These restorations may be generated through the use of traditional impression/dental laboratory techniques or through the use of computer-assisted digital impression, design and manufacturing processes. Indirect tooth-colored restorations are covered in more detail in Chapter 12.

Treatment of Esthetic Concerns

Interest in smile esthetics is growing among many segments of the population. As a result, a range of treatments has been developed to manage a wide array of esthetic concerns. Chapter 9 describes conservative esthetic treatments, which include selective recontouring of anterior teeth, vital bleaching, and microabrasion. These conservative approaches have well-documented outcomes. In addition to these conservative techniques, advances in direct composite restorations have permitted the closure of diastemas, recontouring of teeth, and other tooth additions by means other than extensive full-coverage indirect restorations.

Treatment Considerations for Older Patients

In the past, older adults constituted a relatively minor proportion of the population. Older individuals used dental services infrequently because most were edentulous, had limited financial resources, and delayed unmet dental needs until they became symptomatic. Today, individuals 65 years and older represent a rapidly growing segment of the population. Older individuals now are better educated consumers, have greater financial resources, are more prevention minded, and have retained more teeth as compared with their predecessors. However, older individuals are living with increasingly more complex medical, mental, emotional, and social conditions that affect their ability to care for their dentition and periodontium. These conditions must be considered when planning dental treatment. Financial and social barriers prevent some older individuals from seeking oral health care. Although, as a group, older adults enjoy greater financial resources, many remain on restricted budgets and are faced with tough decisions regarding the spending of limited resources. Transportation to and from the dental office becomes complicated for those who no longer drive. A comprehensive review of geriatric dentistry is beyond the scope of this chapter; rather, some issues that are important for treatment planning for older patients are highlighted.[46-48]

Clear and effective communication is crucial. Many older adults have hearing loss and dentists must speak more distinctly and at a higher volume. Patients with memory loss appreciate written summaries and instructions that assist them in remembering details of the visit and planned treatment when they leave the dental office. The use of large simple fonts in written communications is particularly helpful to patients with diminished visual acuity.

An accurate medical history, risk assessment, and integration of dental and medical care are particularly important considerations for older patients. Many chronic diseases of the cardiovascular, respiratory, endocrine, renal, gastrointestinal, musculoskeletal, immune, and neurologic systems are associated with aging, influence dental disease, and complicate dental treatment decision making. Cardiovascular disease, Alzheimer disease, depression, osteoarthritis, rheumatoid arthritis, osteoporosis, cancer, and diabetes are a few of the diseases that commonly affect older adults, and their medical management increases in complexity with advancing years. It is estimated that older individuals living in community settings take an average of four medications each day; six of the top 10 drugs prescribed in 2001 were used to treat age-related chronic conditions.[46,47] Many of these medications have the potential for adverse drug reactions and drug interactions. Oral adverse effects include dry mouth (xerostomia), increased bleeding of tissues, lichenoid reactions, tissue overgrowth, and hypersensitivity reactions. The dentist must be aware of the impact these medications may have on dental treatment planning and management. Consultation with the patient's physician is highly recommended so as to gain understanding of these medical, mental, and emotional conditions and their potential impact on dental treatment. The dentist should recognize the impact of polypharmacy on salivary flow, especially the use of xerostomic medications, and discuss with the physician the potential substitution of medications with fewer xerostomic effects.

Oral changes associated with undernourishment, immunosuppression, dehydration, smoking, alcohol use, disease, medications, and dental problems lead to a depressed sense of taste and smell in older patients.[49] Perceptions of salty and bitter tastes and olfactory function decline with age, whereas perceptions of sweet and sour tastes do not. As a result, food may become tasteless and unappetizing, and more sugars, fats, and salts are added in an attempt to increase flavor. Undernourished individuals are encouraged to consume calorie-rich, complete-nutrition beverages, which also are rich in refined carbohydrates. Smoking reduces the taste of foods by causing physical coating of the tongue and regression of the taste buds on the tongue and olfactory receptors in the roof of the nasal cavity over time. Inadequate fluid intake may lead to chronic dehydration and altered taste perception. These practices increase the risk of dental disease in this population. Dietary assessment and counseling are crucial in older patients to identify inadequate diets and suggest modifications that enhance taste and smell while lowering the risks of dental disease. Herb seasonings may enhance the flavor of foods in lieu of sugar and salt. Salivary stimulants, citrus-flavored candies containing xylitol or other sugar replacements, tongue brushing or scraping, and smoking cessation are some additional measures that may promote taste and olfactory perception in older adults.

Dental and periodontal diseases may progress more rapidly in older adults.[47] Dental caries, particularly root caries, is the most significant reason for tooth loss in older adults. Ineffective plaque removal, xerostomia, soft sugar-rich diets, fixed and removable prostheses, abrasions at the CEJ, gingival recession, and chronic periodontal inflammation (with increased activity of collagenolytic enzymes) make root surfaces more prone to caries compared with other surfaces. Root-surface restorations are challenging to successfully perform and are at risk of recurrent decay in the future. Careful selection of restoration design, materials, and finishing is essential if the patient is to be able to perform successful biofilm removal and thereby maximize the longevity of restorations. Also, many dental practitioners prefer to intervene more aggressively with dental treatment rather than take a "watchful waiting" approach. As more teeth are being retained and have large restorations at risk of fracture or recurrent decay, attention must be placed on developing cost-effective and innovative means of restoring teeth, particularly for older individuals on a limited budget. The cost-effective use of silver diamine fluoride (SDF) to arrest caries, even though the treated area becomes darkly stained, may be an optimal treatment option in this population (see Chapter 2).

Prevention of dental disease increases in importance but becomes more challenging in older adults. Physical limitations such as arthritis, Parkinson disease, vision impairment, and other chronic illnesses reduce the patients' ability to clean their teeth and periodontal tissues effectively. Powered rotation–oscillation toothbrushes and manual toothbrushes with larger handles, for easier gripping, are recommended for patients with decreased manual dexterity. Consistent use of fluoride-containing dentifrices and other remineralization products, antimicrobial mouthrinses, oral pH management, flossing, oral irrigation, and chewing of xylitol gum may reduce the risk of developing dental caries and periodontal infection.[50] Written reminders are useful to serve as aids for older patients who forget to brush their teeth because of memory loss associated with Alzheimer disease. Because many older individuals may have never been taught how to effectively clean their teeth, the dentist must observe their technique and instruct them in proper oral hygiene procedures to be performed after each meal. Dentists must carefully inform patients in the proper application method of 5000-ppm fluoride toothpastes. Incorrect application (e.g., rinsing/eating/drinking immediately after brushing) severely limits any potential benefit.

A unique aspect of aging is an increasing reliance on the assistance of caregivers with activities of daily living. As a result, the dentist must work with caregivers who provide dental care for patients in the home, assisted living facility, nursing home, and hospital settings. The dental professional may need to spend more time educating and training the caregiver, rather than the patient, in the importance of oral hygiene and effective plaque removal techniques.

Treatment Plan Approval

Informing patients well about their conditions and treatment options and then obtaining their consent has become an integral part of contemporary dental practice.[51] One aspect of informed consent is to provide patients with the necessary information about the alternative therapies available to manage their oral conditions. For nearly all conditions, usually more than one treatment alternative is available. These alternatives, with their advantages and disadvantages, should be presented to the patient. In addition, the patient should be informed of the risks associated with each alternative therapy. Dentists must remember that a reasonable alternative often is *not* to intervene directly with restorative care. Rather, based on the nature of dental disease progression, elimination or reduction of risk factors/indicators may need to be the initial focus while monitoring the condition. Even these intentional efforts are part of a treatment plan and must be included in the informed consent process. Proactive conservative steps, in the case of caries, may be to attempt to remineralize or arrest the lesion(s). Finally, the cost of treatment alternatives should be discussed with the patient. Treatment may proceed when the dentist is sure that the patient has a full and complete understanding of the alternative treatments, their associated risks and benefits, and the results of possible nontreatment.[51-53]

Summary

Proper assessment, examination, diagnosis, and treatment planning play a crucial role in the delivery of quality dental care. Each patient must be evaluated (examined) individually in a thorough and systematic fashion. After the patient's preferences, risks, and condition(s) are understood and recorded, a treatment plan may be developed and implemented. A successful treatment plan carefully sequences and integrates all necessary procedures indicated for the patient. Few absolutes exist in treatment planning; the available information must be considered carefully and incorporated into a sequenced approach that fits the desires/needs of the individual. Patients must have an active role in the process; they must be informed of the findings, advised of the risks and benefits of proposed treatment, and given the opportunity to decide the course of treatment. The process of patient assessment, examination, diagnosis, and treatment planning represents one of the greatest challenges in dentistry and is rewarding for both the patient and the dentist if done properly (i.e., thoroughly and with the patient's best interests in mind).

References

1. Sackett DL, Rosenberg WM, Gray JA, et al: Evidence-based medicine: What it is and what it isn't. *Br Med J* 312:71–72, 1996.
2. Bader JD, Shugars DA: Systematic review of selected dental caries diagnostic and management methods. *J Dent Educ* 65:960–968, 2001.
3. Young DA, Nový BB, Zeller GG, et al: The American Dental Association Caries Classification System for Clinical Practice, A report of the American Dental Association Council on Scientific Affairs. *J Am Dent Assoc* 146(2):79–86, 2015.
4. Kidd EAM, Ricketts DN, Pitts NB: Occlusal caries diagnosis: A changing challenge for clinicians and epidemiologists. *J Dent* 21:323–331, 1993.
5. Lussi A: Validity of diagnostic and treatment decisions of fissure caries. *Caries Res* 25:296–303, 1991.
6. Penning C, van Amerongen JP, Seef RE, et al: Validity of probing for fissure caries diagnosis. *Caries Res* 26:445–449, 1992.
7. Pretty I, Maupome G: A closer look at diagnosis in clinical dental practice: Part 1. Reliablity, validity, specificity, and sensitivity of diagnostic procedures. *J Can Dent Assoc* 70:251–255, 2004.
8. Ekstrand K, Qvist V, Thylstrup A: Light microscope study of the effect of probing occlusal surfaces. *Caries Res* 21:368–374, 1987.
9. Yassin OM: In vitro studies of the effect of a dental explorer on the formation of an artificial carious lesion. *J Dent Child* 62:111–117, 1995.
10. Ashley PF, Blinkhorn AS, Davies RM: Occlusal caries diagnosis: An in vitro histological validation of the Electronic Caries Monitor (ECM) and other methods. *J Dent* 26:83–88, 1998.
11. Kidd EA, Joyston-Bechal S, Beighton D: Diagnosis of secondary caries: a laboratory study. *Br Dent J* 176:135–139, 1994.
12. Hintze H, Wenzel A, Danielsen B, et al: Reliability of visual examination, fiber-optic transillumination, and bite-wing radiography, and reproducibility of direct visual examination following tooth separation for the identification of cavitated carious lesions in contacting approximal surfaces. *Caries Res* 32:204–209, 1998.
13. Katz RV: The clinical identification of root caries. *Gerodontology* 5:21–24, 1986.
14. Newwitter DS, Katz RV, Clive JM: Detection of root caries: Sensitivity and specificity of a modified explorer. *Gerodontics* 1:65–67, 1985.
15. Newbrun E: Problems in caries diagnosis. *Int Dent J* 43:133–142, 1993.
16. Kidd EAM, Joyston-Bechal S, Beighton D: Marginal ditching and staining as a predictor of secondary caries around amalgam restorations: A clinical and microbiological study. *J Dent Res* 74:1206–1211, 1995.
17. Mjor IA: Frequency of secondary caries at various anatomical locations. *Oper Dent* 10:88–92, 1985.
18. Lussi A, Ganss C. Erosive tooth wear: from diagnosis to therapy, 2nd edition, revised and extended, Monographs in oral science, ISSN 0077-0892; vol. 25.
19. Grippo JO, Simring M, Coleman TA: Abfraction, abrasion, biocorrosion, and the enigma of noncarious cervical lesions: A 20-year perspective. *J Esthet Restor Dent* 24:10–25, 2012, doi:10.1111/j.1708-8240.2011.00487.x.
20. Senna P, Del Bel Cury A, Rösing C: Non-carious cervical lesions and occlusion: a systematic review of clinical studies. *J Oral Rehab* 39(6):450–462, 2012, doi:10.1111/j.1365-2842.2012.02290.x.
21. Bader JD, Martin JA, Shugars DA: Incidence rates for complete cusp fracture. *Community Dent Oral Epidemiol* 29:346–353, 2001.
22. Bader JD, Shugars DA, Sturdevant JR: Consequences of posterior cusp fracture. *Gen Dent* 52:128–131, 2004.
23. Bader JD, Shugars DA, Martin JA: Risk indicators for posterior tooth fracture. *J Am Dent Assoc* 135:883–892, 2004.
24. Sturdevant JR, Bader JD, Shugars DA, et al: A simple method to estimate restoration volume as a possible predictor for tooth fracture. *J Prosthet Dent* 90:162–167, 2003.

25. Matteson SR, Joseph LP, Bottomley W, et al: The report of the panel to develop radiographic selection criteria for dental patients. *Gen Dent* 39:264–270, 1991.

26. Dove SB: Radiographic diagnosis of caries. *J Dent Educ* 65:985–990, 2001.

27. Christensen GJ: Magnification in dentistry: Useful tool or another gimmick? *J Am Dent Assoc* 134:1647–1650, 2003.

28. Forgie A: Magnification: What is available, and will it aid your clinical practice? *Dent Update* 28:125–130, 2001.

29. Strassler HE, Syme SE, Serio F, et al: Enhanced visualization during dental practice using magnification systems. *Compend Cont Educ Dent* 19:595–612, 1998.

30. Ferreira-Zandona AG, Analoui M, Beiswanger BB, et al: An in vitro comparison between laser fluorescence and visual examination for detection of demineralization in occlusal pits and fissures. *Caries Res* 32:210–218, 1998.

31. Bader J, Shugars D: Systematic review of the performance of the DIAGNOdent device for caries detection. *J Am Dent Assoc* 135:1413–1426, 2004.

32. Pretty IA, Ekstrand KR: Detection and monitoring of early caries lesions: a review. *Eur Arch Paediatr Dent* 17(1):13–25, 2016.

33. Axelsson P: *Diagnosis and risk prediction of dental caries*, Chicago, 2000, Quintessence Publishing.

34. American Dental Association Council: Access, Prevention and Interprofessional Relations: Caries diagnosis and risk assessment: a review of preventive strategies and management. *J Am Dent Assoc* 126(Special Suppl):1995.

35. Hamilton JC, Dennison JB, Stoffers KW, et al: Early treatment of incipient carious lesions: a two-year clinical evaluation. *J Am Dent Assoc* 133:1643–1651, 2002.

36. Burt BA: Definition of Risk. *J Dent Edu* 65(10):1007–1008, 2001.

37. Hunter PB: Risk factors in dental caries. *Int Dent J* 38(4):211–217, 1988.

38. Downer MC, Azli NA, Bedi R, et al: How long do routine dental restorations last? A systematic review. *Br Dent J* 187:432–439, 1999.

39. Brantley CF, Bader JD, Shugars DA, et al: Does the cycle of rerestoration lead to larger restorations? *J Am Dent Assoc* 126:1407–1413, 1995.

40. Stefanac SJ, Nesbit SP: *Diagnosis and treatment planning in Dentistry*, ed 3, St Louis, 2017, Elsevier Publishing.

41. Madison M, Wilcox LR: An evaluation of coronal microleakage in endodontically-treated teeth: Part III. In vivo study. *J Endod* 14:455–458, 1998.

42. Mertz-Fairhurst EJ, Call-Smith KM, Shuster GS, et al: Clinical performance of sealed composite restorations placed over caries compared with sealed and unsealed amalgam restorations. *J Am Dent Assoc* 115:689–694, 1987.

43. Fitch DR, Boyd WJ, McCoy RB, et al: Amalgam repair of cast gold crown margins: A microleakage assessment. *Gen Dent* 30:328–333, 1982.

44. Anusavice K: Criteria for placement and replacement of dental restorations: An international consensus report. *Int Dent J* 38:193–194, 1988.

45. Rasines Alcaraz MG, Veitz-Keenan A, Sahrmann P, et al: Direct composite resin fillings versus amalgam fillings for permanent or adult posterior teeth (Review). *Cochran Database of Systematic Reviews* (3):Art. No.:CD005620, 2014.

46. DeBiase CB, Austin SL: Oral health and older adults. *J Dent Hyg* 77:125–145, 2003.

47. Ettinger RL: The unique oral health needs of an aging population. *Dent Clin North Am* 41:633–649, 1997.

48. American Dental Association Council: Access, prevention and interprofessional relations: Providing dental care in long-term dental care facilities: A resource manual, 1997. Chicago, American Dental Association.

49. Winkler S, Garg AK, Mekayarajjananonth T, et al: Depressed taste and smell in geriatric patients. *J Am Dent Assoc* 130:1759–1765, 1999.

50. Simons D, Brailsford SR, Kidd EA, et al: The effect of medicated chewing gums and oral health in frail elderly people: a one-year clinical trial. *J Am Geriatr Soc* 50:1348–1353, 2002.

51. Sfikas PM: Informed consent and the law. *J Am Dent Assoc* 129:1471–1473, 1998.

52. Christensen GJ: Educating patients: a new necessity. *J Am Dent Assoc* 124:86–87, 1993.

53. Christensen GJ: Educating patients about dental procedures. *J Am Dent Assoc* 126:371–372, 1995.

4

Fundamentals of Tooth Preparation

LEE W. BOUSHELL, RICARDO WALTER

Teeth require intervention (i.e., need some type of preparation) for various reasons: (1) caries lesion progression to the point that loss of tooth structure requires restoration; (2) tooth fracture compromising form and function with or without associated pain or sensitivity; (3) congenital malformation or improper position in need of reestablishment of form or function; (4) previous restoration with inadequate occlusal or proximal contact, defective (open) margins, or poor esthetics; or (5) as part of fulfilling other restorative needs (see Chapter 3). Every effort must be made to limit the risk of iatrogenic damage to adjacent tooth surfaces while seeking to prepare and restore caries lesions or defects. Teeth requiring intervention are prepared such that various restorative materials have the most predictable outcome.

This chapter defines tooth preparation and the historical classification of anatomic locations affected by caries lesions. Consideration is given to factors that directly impact preparation design, followed by description of the logic and procedural organization of preparation steps. Additional factors that must be considered in overall care of the patient may indirectly impact preparation design (Box 4.1; see Online Chapter 15). Chapters that are devoted to the preparation and restoration of specific lesions/defects elaborate on these additional factors. The ability to utilize the information presented here requires working knowledge of dental anatomy and a solid understanding of concepts presented in Chapters 1, 2, and 3.

In the past, most restorative treatment was for cavitated caries lesions, and the term *cavity* was used to describe a caries lesion that had progressed to the point that there was a breach in the surface integrity of the tooth. Likewise, when the affected tooth was treated, the cutting or preparation of the remaining tooth structure (to receive a restorative material) was referred to as *cavity preparation*. Currently, many indications for treatment are not related to carious destruction, and the preparation of the tooth no longer is referred to as *cavity preparation*, but as *tooth preparation*.

Tooth Preparation: Definition and Foundational Concepts

Tooth preparation is the mechanical alteration of a defective, injured, or diseased tooth such that placement of restorative material reestablishes normal form (and therefore function) including esthetic corrections, where indicated. Generally, the objectives of tooth preparation are to (1) conserve as much healthy tooth structure as possible, (2) remove all defects while simultaneously providing protection of the pulp–dentin complex, (3) form the tooth

preparation so that, under the forces of mastication, the tooth or the restoration (or both) will not fracture and the restoration will not be displaced, and (4) allow for the esthetic placement of a restorative material where indicated.

G.V. Black presented a classification of tooth preparations according to diseased anatomic areas involved and by the associated type of treatment.[1] Black's classification originally was based on the observed frequency of caries lesions in various surface areas of teeth. These classifications were designated as Class I, Class II, Class III, Class IV, and Class V. Since Black's original classification, an additional class has been added, Class VI. Although the relative frequency of caries lesion locations may have changed over the years, the original classification is still used in the diagnosis of caries lesions (e.g., Class I Caries). In addition, the various classes are used to identify lesion-associated preparations and restorations (e.g., a Class I amalgam preparation or a Class I amalgam restoration).

All preparations required to treat pit-and-fissure caries are termed *Class I preparations*. These include preparations on (1) occlusal surfaces of premolars and molars, (2) occlusal two thirds of the facial and lingual surfaces of molars, and (3) the lingual surfaces of maxillary incisors. Preparations required to correct caries lesions that develop in the proximal surfaces of posterior teeth are termed *Class II preparations*. Preparations required to correct caries lesions that develop in the proximal surfaces of anterior teeth that do not include the incisal edge are termed *Class III preparations*. Preparations required to correct caries lesions or other defects that develop in the proximal surfaces of anterior teeth that include the incisal edge are termed *Class IV preparations*. Preparations required to correct caries lesions or other defects that develop in the gingival third of the facial or lingual surfaces of all teeth are termed *Class V preparations*. Preparations required to correct caries lesions or other defects that develop in the incisal edges of anterior teeth or the occlusal cusp tips of posterior teeth are termed *Class VI preparations*.

Much of the rationale supporting the development of tooth preparation techniques was introduced by Black.[1] Modifications of Black's principles of tooth preparation have resulted from the influence of Bronner, Markley, J. Sturdevant, Sockwell, and C. Sturdevant; from improvements in restorative materials, instruments, and techniques; and from the increased knowledge and application of preventive measures for caries.[2-6] Tooth preparation design takes into consideration the nature of the tooth (the structure of enamel, the structure of dentin, the position of the pulp in the pulp–dentin complex, the enamel connection to the dentin) *and* the nature of material to be used for restoration of the defect. For example, a diamond abrasive cutting instrument may be chosen to increase the roughness, and thereby surface area, of prepared walls and

---

• BOX 4.1   **Factors to Consider Before and During Tooth Preparation**

Patient Factors

- Desires
- Home care
- Risk status
- Age
- Cooperation
- Anesthesia

Anatomical Factors

- Enamel rod orientation
- Dentin thickness
- Pulp location
- Coronal contours
- Extent of previous restoration

Procedural Factors

- Operator skill
- Instrument design
- Type of rotary cutting instrument
- Ability to isolate

Lesion/Defect Factors

- Bone support
- Occlusion
- Severity
- Gingival status
- Pulpal status
- Fracture development

Restorative Material Factors

- Physical properties
- Color characteristics
- Cost effectiveness

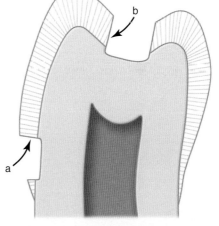

• **Fig. 4.1**   All enamel walls must consist of either full-length enamel rods on sound dentin (a) or full-length enamel rods on sound dentin supported on preparation side by shortened rods also on sound dentin (b).

margins when planning for an adhesively retained composite resin restoration (see Online Fig. 14.24).

Highly mineralized enamel depends on the resiliency of its dentin support. Every preparation is designed to conserve as much dentin as possible for the strength of the enamel and the protection of the pulp. The durable attachment between enamel and dentin (the dentinoenamel junction [DEJ]) enables enamel to withstand the rigors of mastication. When caries (or any defect) has compromised the DEJ, then associated superficial enamel becomes prone to fracture under cyclic occlusal loading. Most preparation designs remove enamel that has lost its attachment to the underlying dentin (see Chapter 8 for exceptions). The nature of enamel formation (see Chapter 1) requires that the preparation walls be, at minimum, oriented 90 degrees to the external surface of the enamel so as to maintain a continuous connection with the essential supporting dentin beneath (Fig. 4.1, *a*). An enamel wall with this configuration is able to withstand the forces associated with occlusal loading. An even more durable wall configuration results when the preparation has full-length enamel rods buttressed by shorter enamel rods on the preparation side of the wall (Fig. 4.1, *b*). Tooth preparations must also include design features that take into account the physical limitations of the planned restorative material.

Dental restorative materials are best considered in terms of their ability to survive the stresses of the oral environment in comparison with natural tooth structure. Natural tooth structure is able to withstand the cyclic loading of mastication because of its ability to undergo small amounts of flexure without fracture or separation of the enamel from the dentin. Ideal restorative materials would be able to mimic the durability of natural tooth structure. All current restorative materials fall short of the ideal. Tooth preparation design takes into consideration that dental restorative materials are structurally either polycrystalline or polymeric.

Restorative materials that are *polycrystalline* in nature (e.g., dental amalgam, glass-ceramic) have very limited ability to flex without fracturing. Therefore they are prone to fracture when occlusal loading causes material flexure. Preparations for polycrystalline materials require removal of diseased tooth structure followed by

a design that allows enough material thickness such that flexure under occlusal load will not occur. This process usually results in a preparation with fairly uniform (at least uniformly minimal) depths. Polycrystalline materials generally require a minimum thickness of 1.5 to 2.0 mm so as to withstand occlusal loading without flexure. The periphery of preparations for polycrystalline materials are designed to allow thickness (i.e., bulk) of the margins (edges) of the planned restoration. The design of the cavosurface margins for these materials is therefore as close to 90 degrees as possible as this marginal configuration allows maximum thickness of the polycrystalline material that will subsequently be placed in the preparation (Fig. 4.2; also see Fig. 1.12). Preparations for polycrystalline restorative materials often require strategic, additional removal of healthy tooth structure to allow for material limitations.

Restorative materials that are *polymeric* in nature (e.g., composite resin) have greater ability to flex without fracture. Therefore they are not prone to fracture when occlusal loading causes material flexure. Preparations for polymeric restoratives generally only require removal of the diseased tooth structure as these materials have no minimum material thickness requirement. The thin restoration will flex as needed. The periphery of preparations for polymeric materials do not require any particular design to allow for bulk of material at the margins of the planned restoration. Polymeric restorative materials may be as thin as is required to replace lost tooth structure and reestablish normal anatomy. For this reason, preparations for polymeric restorative materials generally allow maximum conservation of natural tooth structure and therefore are considered to be "minimally invasive" by design. The attachment between polymeric materials and enamel remains stable over time. However, the attachment between polymeric materials and dentin deteriorates over time.

Tooth preparations are usually limited to the clinical crowns of teeth. The *clinical crown* is the portion of the tooth (usually predominantly covered by enamel) that is exposed in the oral cavity. Frequently tooth preparation leaves much of the clinical crown surface uninvolved and is referred to as an *intracoronal tooth preparation*. The appearance of the completed preparation has been conceptually described as "boxlike" (Fig. 4.3). The goal of the operative dentist is always maximum conservation of any remaining

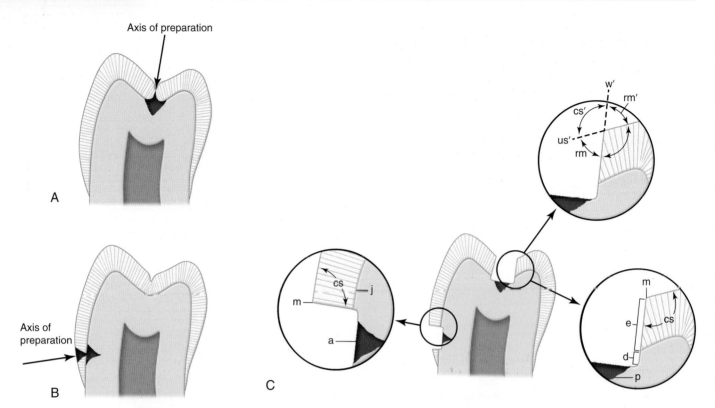

• **Fig. 4.2** Diagram of caries lesion development in the occlusal pit/fissure area (ICDAS 4) of a tooth (A) and in the smooth surface area on the facial (B). Sectional view (C) of initial stage of tooth preparations for lesions in A and B when planning for a polycrystalline restorative material such as amalgam. C, The preparation cavosurface angle (*cs*), axial wall (*a*), pulpal wall (floor) (*p*), enamel wall (*e*), dentinal wall (*d*), preparation margin (*m*), and DEJ (*j*). Note, in the upper exploded view, that the cavosurface angle (*cs*) may be visualized by imaginary projections of the preparation wall (*w'*) and of the unprepared surface (*us'*) contiguous with the margin, forming angle *cs'*. Angles *cs* and *cs'* are equal because opposite angles formed at the intersection of two straight lines are equal. Likewise, minimal restorative material angle *rm* is equal to angle *rm'*. Polycrystalline restorative materials require *rm* to approach 90 degrees. Note the axis of preparation aligned with the long axis of the mandibular posterior tooth crown.

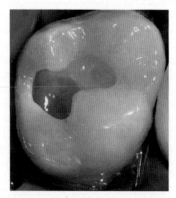

• **Fig. 4.3** Intracoronal preparation with "boxlike" appearance.

clinical crown knowing that the tooth has already been weakened from the carious loss of tooth structure. Controlled, conservative removal of any remaining tooth structure, based on the needs of the restorative material, is always accomplished with the awareness that the intracoronal restoration will *not* add strength to the tooth over the long term, regardless of the nature of the restorative material being used.

When carious destruction of the clinical crown is severe (i.e., the remaining enamel has lost a large amount of the dentinal support), additional efforts to encircle and reinforce the remaining tooth structure are required. These additional preparation efforts most frequently require removal of most or all of the remaining enamel and therefore include the whole *anatomic crown*. All external enamel surfaces are involved and the preparation effort is therefore referred to as an *extracoronal preparation*. In concept, all the enamel (at least the correct physical dimensions and frequently the physical appearance) is to be replaced. In addition, missing dentin may need to be replaced with an appropriate restorative material to act as a dentin substitute. The dentin substitute, along with remaining healthy dentin, acts to support the new restorative material that is replacing the enamel. The goal of the extracoronal preparation is to create enough physical space for the planned restorative material to restore the natural anatomy of the affected tooth. In general, the appearance of a completed extracoronal preparation is reminiscent of a tree stump and is referred to as "stumplike" (Fig. 4.4). The actual amount of space required depends directly on the physical properties of the restorative material to be used. The extracoronal restoration generally reestablishes the anatomy of the crown of the tooth (clinical or anatomic crown, depending on whether any enamel is remaining) and is therefore termed a "crown." The crown must extend well

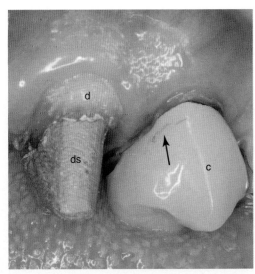

• **Fig. 4.4** Extracoronal "stumplike" tooth preparation with dentin (*d*) and dentin substitute (core component of a cast post and core, *ds*). The adjacent tooth has been restored with a full porcelain-fused-to-metal crown (*c*). Note staining that has subsequently developed in areas of iatrogenic damage *(arrow).*

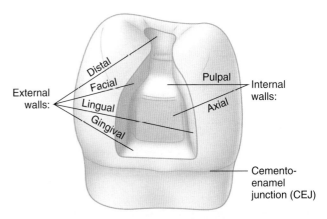

• **Fig. 4.5** The external and internal walls (floors) for Class II tooth preparation required to treat occlusal and mesioproximal caries lesions.

beyond any dentin substitute (i.e., include remaining adjacent healthy tooth structure) if the restorative process is to successfully reestablish the strength required for durable function of the restored tooth. The more extensive the preparation, the greater the risk of iatrogenic damage of adjacent structures or restorations during procedures. Further information relative to extracoronal tooth preparations and restorations may be identified in textbooks devoted to this subject.

Dentistry has developed terminology useful in the communication of all aspects of preparation design and associated procedures. Tooth preparation terminology effectively describes preparation aspects with regard to complexity, anatomic location, three-dimensional orientation, and geometry.

Tooth Preparation: Terminology

A tooth preparation is termed *simple* if only one tooth surface is involved, *compound* if two or three surfaces are involved, and *complex* if a preparation involves four or more surfaces. A preparation takes the name of the involved tooth surface(s)—for example, a defect on the occlusal surface is treated with an occlusal preparation. When discussing or writing a term denoting a combination of two or more surfaces, the *-al* ending of the prefix word is changed to an *-o*. For example, the angle formed by the lingual and incisal surfaces of an anterior tooth would be termed *linguoincisal line angle* and the tooth preparation involving the mesial and occlusal surfaces is termed *mesioocclusal preparation.* The preparation involving the mesial, occlusal, and distal surfaces is a *mesioocclusodistal preparation.* For brevity in records and communication, the description of a tooth preparation is abbreviated by using the first letter, capitalized, of each tooth surface involved. Examples are as follows: (1) A simple tooth preparation involving an occlusal surface is an "O"; (2) a compound preparation involving the mesial and occlusal surfaces is an "MO"; and (3) a complex preparation involving the mesial, occlusal, distal, and lingual surfaces is an "MODL."

The process of creating a preparation in a tooth results in the formation of preparation walls or floors (Fig. 4.5). An *internal wall* is a prepared surface that does not extend to the external

tooth surface. There are two types of internal walls. The *axial wall* is an internal wall that is oriented parallel to the long axis of the tooth. The *pulpal wall* is an internal wall that is oriented perpendicular to the long axis of the tooth and is located occlusal to the pulp. This internal wall may also be referred to as the *pulpal floor.* An *external wall* is a prepared surface that extends to the external tooth surface. Such a wall takes the name of the tooth surface (or aspect) that the wall is adjacent to (Fig. 4.5). The external wall that is approximately horizontal (i.e., perpendicular to the occlusal forces that are directed occlusogingivally and generally parallel to the long axis of the tooth crown) may also be referred to as a preparation *floor* (e.g., a gingival floor; see Fig. 4.5). The *enamel wall* is that portion of a prepared external wall consisting of enamel (see Fig. 4.2C). The *dentinal wall* is that portion of a prepared external wall consisting of dentin, in which mechanical retention features may be located (see Fig. 4.2C). Tooth preparation features or sections that are parallel (or nearly so) to the long axis of the tooth crown are commonly described as *vertical,* such as vertical height of cusps, or vertical walls. The term *longitudinal* may be used in lieu of *vertical.* Tooth preparation features that are perpendicular (or nearly so) to the long axis of the tooth are termed *horizontal* or *transverse.*

The junction of two or more prepared surfaces is referred to as the *angle.* This transition area from one surface to another is designed to be smooth and rounded, rather than abrupt or sharp, to limit stress concentration. A *line angle* is the junction of two planar surfaces of different orientation along a line (Figs. 4.6 and 4.7). An *internal* line angle is the line angle whose apex points into the tooth. The *external* line angle is the line angle whose apex points away from the tooth. The *point angle* is the junction of three planar surfaces of different orientation (see Figs. 4.6 and 4.7).

The *cavosurface angle* is the angle of tooth structure formed by the junction of a prepared wall and the external surface of the tooth. The actual junction is referred to as *cavosurface margin.* The cavosurface angle may differ with the location on the tooth, the direction of the enamel rods on the prepared wall, or the type of restorative material to be used. In Fig. 4.2C, the cavosurface angle *(cs)* is determined by projecting the prepared wall in an imaginary line *(w')* and the unprepared enamel surface in an imaginary line *(us')* and noting the angle *(cs')* opposite to the cavosurface angle *(cs).* For better visualization, these imaginary projections may be formed by using two periodontal probes, one lying on the unprepared surface and the other on the prepared external tooth wall (Fig. 4.8).

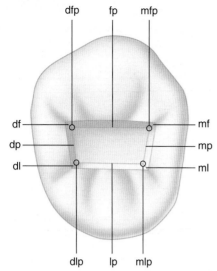

• **Fig. 4.6** Schematic representation (for descriptive purpose) of a Class I tooth preparation illustrating line angles and point angles. Line angles are faciopulpal (*fp*), distofacial (*df*), distopulpal (*dp*), distolingual (*dl*), linguopulpal (*lp*), mesiolingual (*ml*), mesiopulpal (*mp*), and mesiofacial (*mf*). Point angles are distofaciopulpal (*dfp*), distolinguopulpal (*dlp*), mesiolinguopulpal (*mlp*), and mesiofaciopulpal (*mfp*).

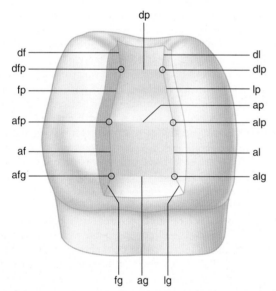

• **Fig. 4.7** Schematic representation (for descriptive purpose) of a Class II tooth preparation illustrating line angles and point angles. Line angles are distofacial (*df*), faciopulpal (*fp*), axiofacial (*af*), faciogingival (*fg*), axiogingival (*ag*), linguogingival (*lg*), axiolingual (*al*), axiopulpal (*ap*), linguopulpal (*lp*), distolingual (*dl*), and distopulpal (*dp*). Point angles are distofaciopulpal (*dfp*), axiofaciopulpal (*afp*), axiofaciogingival (*afg*), axiolinguogingival (*alg*), axiolinguopulpal (*alp*), and distolinguopulpal (*dlp*).

Tooth Preparation: Stages and Procedural Steps

Overview

It is imperative that the end result (i.e., the overall shape/goals of the preparation procedure) be envisioned/considered *before* the initiation of any step. The process of tooth preparation is

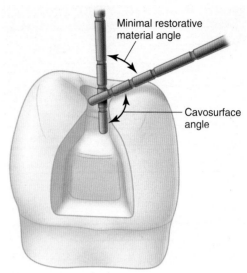

• **Fig. 4.8** Visualization of the cavosurface angle and the associated minimal restorative material angle for a typical amalgam tooth preparation.

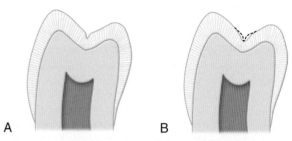

• **Fig. 4.9** A, Enameloplasty on area of imperfect coalescence of enamel. B, No more than one third of the enamel thickness should be removed.

conceptually divided into initial and final stages, each with several steps, so as to facilitate this mental discipline.

The initial stage of the preparation involves what is essentially a superficial surgical incision (with rotary instrumentation) into and through the enamel caries lesion to the depth of the DEJ followed by lateral extension of the preparation walls, at this limited depth, so as to fully expose the carious dentin lesion or defect. The lateral extension is controlled so as to only remove enamel with a compromised (demineralized) DEJ. The placement and orientation of the preparation walls are designed to resist fracture of the tooth or restorative material from masticatory forces principally directed parallel to the long axis of the tooth and to retain the restorative material in the tooth (except for a Class V preparation and Class III preparations with no component involving the occlusion).

Occasionally, very narrow grooves or fossae (that do not penetrate to any great depth into enamel) at the periphery of the preparation prevent the creation of preparation margins that are clearly defined and easily restored. Extension of the preparation to include these nondiseased irregularities would result in unnecessary removal of healthy tooth structure. A reasonable compromise may be to make a minor modification of the external enamel contours, in this peripheral area only, by selective removal of the surface enamel associated with the shallow, narrow developmental groove or fossa. The objective of this process, referred to as *enameloplasty*, is to create a smooth, saucer-shaped external surface that is self-cleansing or easily cleaned (Fig. 4.9 and Box 4.2).

• BOX 4.2 Enameloplasty and Prophylactic Odontotomy

Historically, enameloplasty was utilized as an ultraconservative procedure on the occlusal surfaces, which were deemed to be at risk of the development of a pit or fissure caries lesion. Extreme prudence was exercised in the selection of these areas and in the depth of enamel removed. This procedure was never used unless the area could be transformed into a cleansable groove (or fossa) by a minimal reduction of enamel, and unless occlusal contacts could be maintained. This procedure technically included a preparation stage but no restoration stage. Currently, clinical situations such as these (ICDAS 1 or 2) are managed by treatment with fluoride or placement of sealants. Research studies support the filling of fissures/pits and narrow grooves/fossae (i.e., "sealing") with low viscosity composite resin materials, without any mechanical alteration (enameloplasty) of the at-risk tooth anatomy.[9] Additionally, "prophylactic odontotomy" procedures were used in the past. These more aggressive procedures involved preparing developmental or structural imperfections of the enamel that were thought to be at increased risk of caries and filling the preparation with amalgam to prevent caries from developing in these sites. Prophylactic odontotomy is no longer advocated as a preventive measure.[42]

• BOX 4.3 Steps of Tooth Preparation

Initial Tooth Preparation Stage
Step 1: Initial depth and outline form
Step 2: Primary resistance form
Step 3: Primary retention form
Step 4: Convenience form

Final Tooth Preparation Stage
Step 5: Removal of defective restorative material and/or soft dentin
Step 6: Pulp protection
Step 7: Secondary resistance and retention forms
Step 8: External wall finishing
Step 9: Final procedures: debridement and inspection

Enameloplasty is accomplished as part of the initial preparation stage but does not involve extension of the preparation outline form and may be useful when creating a preparation to be restored with amalgam or glass-ceramic. Restorative material will not be placed into the recontoured area. The only difference in the restoration is that the thickness of the restorative material, at the enameloplastied margin, is slightly decreased because the pulpal depth of the preparation external wall is slightly decreased. This approach differs from including adjacent faulty (decalcified, discolored, poorly contoured) enamel areas, during preparation steps for composite restorations, as these defective areas are physically covered with adhesively bonded composite material as part of the restoration. Care is taken when choosing the area that will benefit from enameloplasty. Usually, a narrow groove should be included in the initial preparation extension if it penetrates to more than one third the thickness of the enamel in the area. If one third or less of the enamel depth is involved, the narrow groove may be removed by enameloplasty, thus limiting further extension of the tooth preparation. This procedure is also applicable to supplemental narrow grooves extending up cusp inclines. If the ends of these grooves were to be included in the tooth preparation, the cusp may be weakened to the extent that it would need to be reduced and covered with restorative material. Another instance in which enameloplasty may be indicated is the presence of a narrow groove that approaches or crosses a lingual or facial ridge. Inclusion of this narrow groove in the preparation would result in the involvement of two surfaces of the tooth, and use of the enameloplasty procedure may often limit the tooth preparation to one surface. Once the initial stage is completed, the final stage of preparation design may be accomplished.

The final stage is focused on (1) accurate management of the lesion/defect that has been isolated, (2) optimal protection of remaining tooth structure, and (3) preparation enhancements consistent with best long-term prognosis (durability) of the restoration. The goals of each step in the preparation stages must be thoroughly understood, and each step must be accomplished as

precisely as possible if optimal treatment outcomes are to be obtained. The stages and steps in tooth preparation are listed in Box 4.3. The sequence of these steps may need to be altered when extensive caries has increased the risk of pulpal involvement (see Chapter 2).

The concepts of initial and final stages of tooth preparation are utilized for caries lesions that have progressed into dentin, have compromised the dentinal support of enamel, and therefore require surgical intervention. The information presented is comprehensive and specific primarily for tooth preparations designed to receive direct restorative materials that are not adhesively attached to the tooth structure and are polycrystalline in nature (i.e., amalgam). Major differences that exist for other types of minimally invasive tooth preparations for polymeric restorative materials (composite resin) are noted.

Occlusal Contact Identification and Rotary Instrument Axis Alignment

Class I, II, III, IV, and VI preparations may involve surfaces that are brought into direct occlusal contact with opposing tooth structure during function. Identification of the precise area of occlusal contact is essential so as to prevent the placement of a preparation margin (and subsequent preparation/restoration interface) where the occlusal contact occurs. Occlusal contact on the preparation/restoration interface will increase the risk of early failure of the restoration. Identification of the occlusal contact areas may be accomplished by use of articulating paper (Fig. 4.10).

The anatomic orientation of caries lesion formation in the pit and fissure areas of posterior teeth requires alignment of the rotary instrument shank axis (through proper positioning of the handpiece) so that it is parallel with the long axis of the tooth crown *prior to* initiation of the preparation (see Online Chapter 14 for information on handpieces and rotary instruments, specifically Fig. 14.18). Correct alignment of the long axis of the shank limits the likelihood of iatrogenic removal, and thereby weakening, of adjacent healthy (occasionally referred to as "sound") coronal tooth structure. Most proximal caries lesions associated with posterior teeth also require that the shank axis be aligned parallel with the long axis of the tooth crown (Figs. 4.11 and 4.12; also see Fig. 4.2). Caries lesion formation associated with the facial or lingual surfaces of the dentition require that the shank axis be aligned perpendicular to the external surface of the tooth where the lesion is located (see Fig. 4.12B).

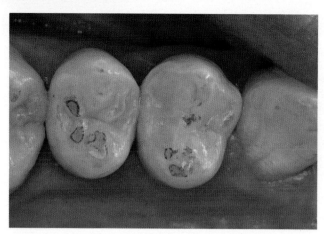

• **Fig. 4.10**   Occlusal contact areas identified through the use of articulating paper.

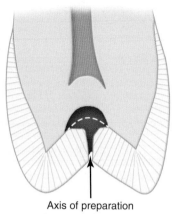

• **Fig. 4.11**   Diagram of a carious fissure. Note that the fissure is parallel to the long axis of the posterior tooth crown. The axis of the initial preparation into the carious fissure is aligned with the long axis of the tooth crown so as to prevent iatrogenic removal of adjacent healthy tooth structure.

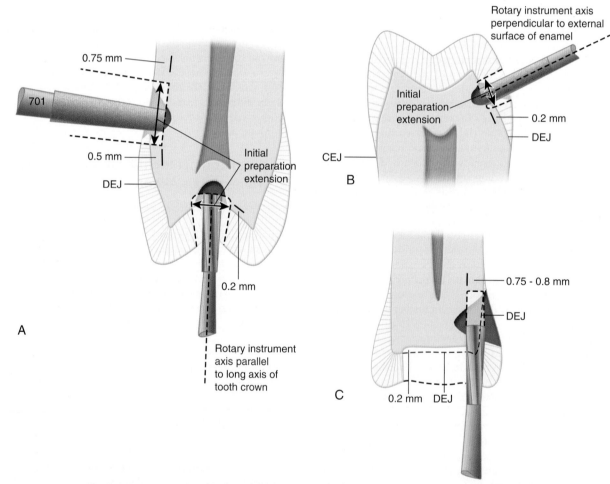

• **Fig. 4.12**   Initial tooth preparation stage for conventional preparations. A–C, Extensions in all directions are to healthy, mineralized ("sound") tooth structure, while maintaining a specific limited pulpal or axial depth regardless of whether end (or side) of rotary instrument is in a caries lesion or old restorative material. The dentinoenamel junction (DEJ) and the cementoenamel junction (CEJ) are indicated in B. In A, initial depth is approximately two thirds of 3-mm rotary instrument head length, or 2 mm, as related to prepared facial and lingual walls, but is half the rotary instrument (specifically the No. 245 carbide bur) head length, or 1.5 mm, as related to central fissure location.

Initial Tooth Preparation Stage: Steps 1-4

Step 1: Initial Depth and Outline Form

The first step in tooth preparation is to establish the *initial depth* and then, at that depth, extend the walls of the preparation until the junction between the enamel and supporting dentin is uncompromised (i.e., a "sound DEJ" has been reached; see Fig. 4.12). The peripheral walls determine the overall outline of the preparation, which is referred to as the *outline form*. It is essential that the outline form be visualized (i.e., mentally anticipated) as much as possible before any mechanical alteration of the tooth has begun. The initial depth of the preparation is 0.2 mm internal to the DEJ or 0.8 mm internal to the normal root surface (see Fig. 4.12). Establishment of the initial depth is always accomplished even when there is a large caries lesion (i.e., no healthy tooth structure immediately adjacent to the point of entry) or when previous restorative material is present. An exception to this initial depth of 0.2 mm internal to the DEJ is when the enamel is thin and greater depth is necessary for the strength of the restorative material that will be used. The initial preparation depth is 0.5 mm internal to the DEJ in any area where secondary retention features are being planned (see Step 7). Root-surface preparations may be shallower than 0.8 mm if the restorative material to be used does not require secondary retention features. Generally, the goals behind the establishment of initial depth and outline form on occlusal surfaces are the preservation of cuspal and marginal ridge strength (where possible). These goals are accomplished by limitation of the depth of the preparation into dentin and the minimization of faciolingual and mesiodistal extensions. Careless, iatrogenic removal of healthy dentin further compromises the diseased tooth and must be avoided. The outline form is designed, regardless of the type of tooth preparation, such that (1) all unsupported or weakened (friable) enamel is usually removed, (2) all faults are included, and (3) all preparation margins are usually placed in a position that allows inspection and finishing of the subsequent restoration margins. See Chapters 8 and 10 for exceptions to these general principles.

Black theorized that, in tooth preparations for smooth-surface caries, the initial preparation should be further extended to areas that are normally self-cleansing so as to prevent recurrence of caries around the periphery of the restoration.[1] This principle was known as *extension for prevention* and was broadened to include the extension necessary to remove remaining enamel imperfections, such as deep, noncarious fossae and grooves, on occlusal surfaces. The practice of extension for the prevention has virtually been eliminated, however, because of the relative caries immunity provided by preventive measures such as fluoride application and improved education relative to oral hygiene and diet. This change has fostered a more conservative tooth preparation philosophy. Current factors that dictate extension on smooth surfaces include (1) the extent of caries or injury and (2) the restorative material to be used. Likewise, extension for prevention to include the caries-prone areas on occlusal surfaces has been reduced by treatments that conserve tooth structure. Such treatments may include enameloplasty, application of pit-and-fissure sealant, and preventive resin or conservative composite restoration.[7]

Esthetic considerations not only affect the choice of restorative material but also the design of the tooth preparation in an effort to maximize the esthetic result of the restoration. Correcting or improving occlusal relationships also may necessitate altering the tooth preparation to accommodate such changes, even when the involved tooth structure is not faulty (i.e., a cuspal form may need

to be altered so as to improve occlusal relationships). Likewise, the adjacent tooth contour may dictate specific preparation extensions that enable the creation of appropriate proximal restoration form. Occasionally the tooth preparation outline for a new restoration contacts or extends slightly into a sound, existing restoration (e.g., a new MO abutting a sound DO). This approach is an acceptable practice (i.e., to have a margin of a new restoration placed into an existing, clinically acceptable restoration). Lastly, the desired cavosurface marginal configuration of the proposed restoration affects the outline form. Restorative materials that need beveled margins require tooth preparation outline form extensions that must anticipate the final cavosurface position and form that will result *after* the bevels have been placed.

Step 2: Primary Resistance Form

Primary resistance form may be defined as the shape and placement of the preparation walls (floors) that best enable the remaining tooth structure, as well as the anticipated restoration, to withstand masticatory forces primarily oriented parallel to the long axis of the tooth. Such floors may be purposefully prepared to provide a level supporting surface for the restoration, allowing a broader area for stress distribution. Primary resistance form is obtained through use of a preparation design that conserves as much healthy tooth structure as possible. Carefully controlled extension of the preparation walls allows conservation of the dentin support of adjacent cusps (and marginal ridges when possible), which helps to maintain maximum strength and therefore resistance to fracture during the cyclic loading of mastication. Transitions between the walls of the preparation (i.e., the internal line angles) are slightly rounded so as to limit stress concentration in these areas, which increases tooth resistance to fracture.[8,9] Rounding of external angles within the tooth preparation (e.g., axiopulpal line angles) limits the likelihood of stress concentration in the corresponding intaglio surface of restorative materials, which increases resistance to fracture of the restorative material. The relatively horizontal pulpal and gingival walls, prepared perpendicular to the tooth's long axis, help the restoration resist occlusal forces and limit the likelihood of tooth fracture from wedging effects caused by opposing cusps. It may be necessary to reduce cusps that no longer have sufficient dentin support and cover (or envelope) them with an adequate thickness of restorative material in order to provide resistance to fracture of the tooth and/or the restorative material. Preparation design must allow for adequate thickness of polycrystalline restorative materials to ensure adequate primary resistance to restoration fracture. The minimal occlusal thickness, for appropriate resistance to fracture, of amalgam is 1.5 to 2 mm and glass-ceramic is 2 mm. Polymeric restorative materials (e.g., composite resins) have no minimal thickness.

When developing the outline form in Class I and II preparations, the end of the cutting instrument prepares a relatively horizontal pulpal wall of uniform depth into the tooth (i.e., the pulpal wall follows the original occlusal surface contours and the DEJ, which are approximately parallel; see Fig. 4.12A and C). Similarly, in the proximal portion of Class II preparations, the end of the cutting instrument prepares a gingival wall (floor) that is approximately parallel to the occlusal surface and, thereby, relatively perpendicular to occlusal forces.

When an extensive caries lesion is present, facial or lingual extension of pulpal or gingival walls may require (1) reduction of weak cusps for coverage by the restorative material (Fig. 4.13) and/or (2) extension of the gingival floors around axial tooth line angles onto facial or lingual surfaces. These preparation modifications provide resistance to parallel and also obliquely (laterally) directed

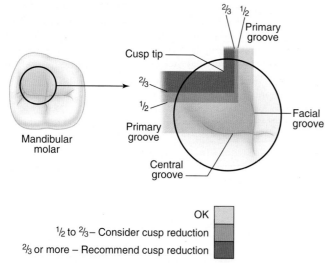

• Fig. 4.13 Rule for cusp reduction and coverage: If extension from a primary groove toward the cusp tip is no more than half the distance, no cusp reduction and coverage should be done; if the extension is one half to two thirds of the distance, consider cusp reduction and coverage; if the extension is more than two thirds of the distance, usually reduce the cusp and cover it with restorative material. Cusp reduction and coverage has also been referred to as "cusp capping."

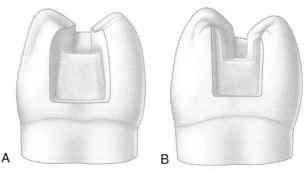

• Fig. 4.14 Basic primary retention form in Class II tooth preparations for amalgam (A) with vertical external walls of proximal and occlusal portions converging occlusally and for inlay (B) with similar walls slightly diverging occlusally.

occlusal forces. The decision to reduce a cusp should be approached judiciously. The most important aspect in the evaluation of a suspicious cusp is the judgment of the amount of remaining dentin support. Cusp reduction should be *considered* when the outline form has extended half the distance from a primary groove to a cusp tip. Cusp reduction is *strongly recommended* when the outline form has extended two thirds the distance from an adjacent primary groove to the cusp tip. The exception to reducing a cusp, where extension has been two thirds from a primary groove toward the cusp tip, is when the operator judges that adequate cuspal strength (adequate dentin support) remains. Reduction of cusps occurs as early as possible in the preparation process so as to improve access and visibility for the operator.

Special consideration is given to teeth that have lost an excessive amount of dentin support in the central area of the tooth secondary to endodontic procedures. Adjacent cusps may be considerably compromised and, as such, may need to be reduced, enveloped, and covered with restorative material to prevent subsequent catastrophic fracture when under occlusal load.[10,11] In general, the greater the occlusal load, the greater is the potential for future fracture of the tooth and/or restoration. The further posterior the tooth is, the greater is the effective occlusal load because of its closer location to the hinge axis (i.e., the temporomandibular joint [TMJ]).

Weakened, friable tooth structure always should be removed at this step in the preparation. Unsupported but not friable enamel may be left for esthetic reasons in anterior teeth where stresses are minimal and a bonded composite restoration is anticipated.

Step 3: Primary Retention Form

Primary retention form is the shape or form of the preparation that prevents displacement or removal of the restoration by tipping or lifting forces. In many respects, retention form and resistance form are accomplished at the same time (Fig. 4.14). The retention form

developed during initial tooth preparation may be adequate to retain the restorative material in the tooth.

The design of preparation primary retention form is directly related to the retention needs of the anticipated restorative material. Amalgam restoration of a Class I or II preparation is retained by developing external tooth walls that converge occlusally (see Fig. 4.14A). In this way, when the amalgam is placed in the preparation and hardens, it cannot be dislodged. However, excessive occlusal convergence of the external walls will result in unsupported enamel rods at the cavosurface margin and must be avoided. The external walls of Class III and V preparations diverge so as to provide strong enamel margins (see Figs. 1.12B and 4.12A and B). Retention of amalgam in these areas requires the creation of secondary features (coves or grooves) in the dentinal walls that serve to retain the restoration (see Step 7).

Composite restorations are primarily retained in the tooth by micromechanical and, depending on the adhesive, chemical bonding that is established between the restoration and the tooth structure. In such restorations, the preparation surface of the enamel and dentin are etched (demineralized) by creation of acidic conditions and then infiltrated with resin-based adhesive materials before placement of the composite.

Cast-metal intracoronal restorations, referred to as inlay restorations, rely on diverging vertical walls that are almost parallel and a luting cement to provide retention of the casting in the tooth (see Online Chapter 18). During the initial tooth preparation, the preparation walls are designed not only to provide for draw (for the casting to be placed into the tooth) but also to provide for an appropriate small angle of divergence (2–5 degrees per wall) from the line of draw (to enable retention of the luted restoration). The amount of divergence required depends on the length of the prepared walls: The greater the vertical height of the walls, the more divergence is permitted and recommended, but within the range described. The path of draw is usually designed to be perpendicular to the horizontal features of the preparation (see Fig. 4.14B).

Step 4: Convenience Form

Convenience form is the shape or form that provides adequate observation, accessibility, and ease in the preparation and restoration of the tooth. Severe caries destruction may necessitate the extension of distal, mesial, facial, or lingual walls so as to gain adequate access to deeper areas of the preparation. Extension of the proximal walls, so as to obtain clearance with an adjacent proximal surface, may afford better access for the finishing of preparation walls, the placement of the matrix, and the finishing of the restoration margins.

The arbitrary extension of facial margins on anterior teeth is usually contraindicated, however, for esthetic reasons. Clearance with the adjacent proximal surface is mandatory for glass-ceramic and cast gold restorations because of the need to finish the preparation walls, make an accurate impression of the prepared tooth, and accomplish insertion/finishing. Preparation extensions to increase the convenience of various procedures are always accomplished in light of the goal of conserving as much healthy tooth structure as possible.

Final Stage of Tooth Preparation: Steps 5-9

When the design of external wall orientation and position has fulfilled the objectives of initial tooth preparation, the preparation is carefully inspected for other needs. The preparation may be complete after the initial tooth preparation stage when the caries lesion (or other defect) is minimal. In this case the preparation will then only require (1) desensitization of the prepared dentin walls for amalgam or (2) modification of the surface of the enamel and dentin so as to create an adhesive interface for composite.

Step 5: Removal of Defective Restorative Material and/or Soft Dentin

Once the caries lesion has been fully exposed (via the initial preparation), careful pulpal and/or axial extension is accomplished so as to *remove defective restorative material and/or soft dentin* as indicated (see Chapter 2). Old restorative material may remain on the pulpal or axial walls after initial tooth preparation. This material should be removed if any of the following conditions are present: (1) the old material may negatively affect the esthetic result of the new restoration (i.e., old amalgam material left under a new composite restoration), (2) radiographic evidence indicates caries lesion development under the old material and clinical evaluation confirms the radiographic interpretation, (3) the tooth pulp was symptomatic preoperatively, (4) the dentin along the periphery of the remaining old restorative material is soft, or (5) retention of the existing material is compromised and the material is easily dislodged. If none of these conditions is present, it is acceptable to leave the remaining old restorative material to serve as a base, rather than risk unnecessary excavation in close proximity to the pulp, which may result in pulpal irritation or exposure. Removal of remaining old restorative material, when indicated, may be accomplished using sharp rotary instruments and light intermittent pressure with or without water irrigation/cooling. Water spray (along with high-volume evacuation) is used when removing old amalgam material to reduce exposure to mercury vapor.

In preparations that remain primarily in enamel, isolated faulty areas (remnants of diseased enamel fissure or pit) on the pulpal wall may require additional minimal extensions. When a pulpal or axial wall has been established at the proper initial tooth preparation position, and a small amount of carious tissue remains, only this tissue should be removed, leaving a rounded, concave area in the wall. The level or position of the wall peripheral to the excavation should not be altered.

Clinical decisions that guide carious tissue removal are based on the relative tactile hardness (firmness) of the dentin associated with the caries lesion. Carious dentin that has had some mineral loss, but not to the point of collagen exposure, is not as clinically hard as normal dentin and is referred to as *firm dentin*. Firm dentin, if isolated from the oral environment by some type of restoration, will remineralize and therefore should not be removed.[12]

If further demineralization causes exposure of the collagen matrix, subsequent enzymatic degradation of the matrix begins as a result of the activity of host matrix metalloproteinases (MMPs) and cysteine cathepsins. Denaturation of the collagen, by host proteolytic enzymes, allows subsequent collagen degradation (of the denatured collagen) by bacterial proteases. Bacterial proteases are not able to degrade intact, native collagen. The process of denaturation and degradation changes the three-dimensional structure of the collagen such that remineralization is no longer possible. Carious tissue that has been demineralized and structurally damaged to this level feels tactilely soft and is therefore referred to as *soft dentin*. Soft dentin (previously referred to as *infected dentin* because of high numbers of bacteria) no longer retains the physical properties necessary to survive in the rigors of the oral environment and must be removed except in the deepest areas of the preparation where removal would result in exposure of an asymptomatic, vital pulp (see Chapter 2, selective caries removal [SCR] protocol).

The use of color alone to determine how much dentin to remove is unreliable. For example, an area of dentin that has experienced episodes of demineralization and remineralization often clinically appears discolored, compared with normal dentin, yet may be firm to tactile exploration and should not be removed. Alternatively, acute (rapid) caries often manifests itself entirely within the normal range of color for dentin and is tactilely soft. The soft dentin requires removal except as indicated (see Chapter 2). Additionally, when the conditions in the lesion have allowed remineralization to occur, the dentin may be distinctly discolored or "stained." In this case host defenses not only have enabled remineralization of the dentin, which is often clinically comparable in firmness (hardness) with surrounding normal dentin, but also have, for the most part, successfully filled in the dentinal tubules with mineral. This resultant hypermineralized state of the dentin (mineralization above that which is found in normal dentin as the lumens of the dentinal tubules are filled with mineral in addition to the normal mineralization of the intertubular dentin) is referred to as *sclerotic dentin*. Sclerotic dentin should not be removed.

Removal of carious dentin is accomplished with awareness of the ability of the vital pulp to effect remineralization of dentin when the matrix (collagen) has not been denatured. Therefore every effort should be made to limit further pulpal irritation and limit the likelihood of pulpal involvement during the caries removal process. The use of sharp spoon excavators and sharp rotary instruments, with intermittent light pressure, may help limit pulpal irritation. Removal of carious tissue in a *moderate lesion* (i.e., a lesion that has not reached the inner one third of dentin) has a low risk of pulpal involvement. The pulpal and axial caries removal of a moderate lesion should therefore extend to where the dentin is firm to tactile sense (i.e., extend to *firm dentin*). Removal of a carious tissue in an *advanced lesion* (i.e., a lesion that has reached the inner one third of dentin) has a higher risk of pulpal involvement. The pulpal and axial caries removal of an advanced lesion should therefore extend to approximately 1 mm from the pulp with the recognition that dentin in this deep region may still be soft (*soft dentin*) to tactile sense. Carious dentin in more peripheral areas is removed until the dentin is firm.

In dentin, as the caries lesion progresses, a zone of demineralization precedes the invasion of, or infection by, bacteria. It is currently impossible to clinically identify the specific depth of the bacterial invasion. Previous notions of dentin excavation for the purpose of complete removal of all bacteria have resulted in exposure of pulp tissue that was not irreversibly inflamed, leading to overtreatment and increased frequency of adverse outcomes. It is not necessary that all dentin invaded by bacteria be removed. In moderate caries lesions, removal of the masses of bacteria and subsequent sealing of the preparation by a restoration at best destroy those comparatively few remaining microorganisms and at worst reduce them to inactivity or dormancy.[13] Even in advanced caries lesions, in which actual invasion of the pulp may have occurred, the recovery of the pulp requires only that a favorable balance be established between the virulence of the bacteria and the resistance of the host. This balance is best accomplished by utilization of the selective caries removal protocol (see Chapter 2). Caries removal in advanced lesions usually is immediately followed by efforts to afford protection to the pulp tissue adjacent to the deepest area of the preparation.

Step 6: Pulp Protection

Deep dentin is very porous and susceptible to desiccation. The thin remaining wall of dentin provides little protection from (1) heat generated by rotary instruments during subsequent steps, (2) noxious ingredients of various restorative materials, (3) thermal changes conducted through restorative materials, (4) forces transmitted through materials to the dentin, (5) galvanic shock, and (6) the ingress of bacteria and/or noxious bacterial toxins through microleakage.[14,15] Deep dentin also is a very poor substrate for subsequent bonding procedures. Therefore efforts to cover deep dentin, to limit dentinal tubular fluid flow, and to create a protective thermal/physical barrier are warranted. Various materials that have been utilized to establish this protective barrier include suspensions or dispersions of zinc oxide, calcium hydroxide, or resin-modified glass ionomer (RMGI) that are applied to the tooth surface.[15] These materials are referred to as *liners* when used in a relatively thin film.[15] The term *base* is used to describe the placement of materials, used in thicker dimensions, beneath permanent restorations to provide for mechanical, chemical, and thermal protection of the pulp. Examples of bases include zinc phosphate, zinc oxide–eugenol, polycarboxylate, and most commonly, some type of glass ionomer material (usually a RMGI). Generally, it is desirable to have approximately a 2-mm dimension of bulk between the pulp and a metallic restorative material. This bulk may include remaining dentin, liner, or base. Composite resin materials, which are thermal insulators, do not require the same bulk of material (dentin + liner/base) between the restoration and the pulp. Although the placement of liners and bases is not a step in tooth preparation, in the strict sense of the term, these serve to create an effective barrier over the deep pulpal/axial dentin prior to receiving the final restorative material.

If the removal of soft dentin does not extend deeper than 1 to 2 mm from the initially prepared pulpal or axial wall, usually no liner is indicated. If the excavation extends to within 0.5 mm of the pulp, a liner usually is selected to cover the deepest area of the dentin. The stimulation of reparative dentin (indirect pulp cap procedure) in this deep area with a calcium hydroxide ($CaOH_2$) liner may be effective.[16] Current evidence suggests that the actual type of material used for the liner is not as important as the overall effective sealing of the dentin with the liner (or base) and subsequent restoration.[17]

Zinc oxide–eugenol and calcium hydroxide liners (chemosetting types that harden) in thicknesses of approximately 0.5 mm or greater have adequate strength to resist condensation forces of amalgam and provide insulation against thermal extremes.[18] $CaOH_2$ liners must always be covered with a RMGI when used under amalgam restorations to prevent dissolution of the liner over time. In addition, $CaOH_2$ liners should be covered by a RMGI to protect the liner from dissolution from the phosphoric acid etchant used prior to composite placement.[14,19] Protection of the $CaOH_2$ liner with an RMGI base also prevents inadvertent displacement of the liner during subsequent procedural steps.

Very deep excavations may contain microscopic pulpal exposures that are not visible to the naked eye. Hemorrhage is the usual evidence of a vital pulp exposure, but with microscopic exposures, such evidence may be lacking. Nevertheless, these exposures may be large enough to allow direct pulpal access for bacteria or other restorative materials. The ability of a hard-setting $CaOH_2$ material to stimulate the formation of reparative dentin when in contact with pulpal tissue makes it the usual material of choice for application to very deep excavations and known pulpal exposures (direct pulp cap procedures).[16] Alternatively, mineral trioxide aggregate (MTA) liners have been found to be effective for direct pulp capping.[17,20] Liners and bases in exposure areas should be applied without pressure.

Usually, a RMGI is used for "base" needs. These materials effectively bond to tooth structure, release fluoride, and have sufficient strength. Placement and contouring of RMGI materials is readily accomplished. Mechanical retentive preparation features are not typically required for RMGI because of their chemical bond to the mineral phase of tooth structure. These materials are excellent for use under amalgam, gold, ceramic, and composite restorations. A base should never overfill the preparation and, thereby, compromise the minimum required thickness of the final restoration.

A liner may be utilized to seal off the dentin immediately adjacent to the pulp when traumatic fracture has occurred. The desired pulpal effects may include sedation and stimulation, the latter resulting in reparative dentin formation. The specific pulpal response desired dictates the choice of liner material. An appropriate text focused on the emergency management of dental trauma should be consulted for current treatment strategies.

Step 7: Secondary Retention and Resistance Forms

Placement of secondary retention and resistance forms, as part of a preparation, follows management of the caries lesion and any indicated pulpal protection. Each anatomically distinct area requiring restoration must be independently retentive. When the external walls of the preparation converge toward each other, as they approach the external surface of the tooth, then no additional or "secondary" retention is required. However, correctly oriented external walls (i.e., walls that have proper dentinal support of the enamel) may diverge as they approach the external surface of the tooth. For example, preparation of a proximal caries lesion on a posterior tooth will frequently result in facial, lingual, and gingival walls that diverge proximally. Preparation walls that diverge will not physically retain a restoration that is not bonded in place. Diverging walls will not resist forces that have the potential to result in the dislodgement of a restoration. Therefore it may become necessary to strategically modify internal aspects of the preparation so as to mechanically retain the restoration.

Because many preparation features that improve retention form also improve resistance form, and the reverse is true, they are presented together. The *secondary retention and resistance forms* are of two types: (1) mechanical preparation features and (2) treatments of the preparation walls with etching, priming, and adhesive materials. The second type is not really considered a part of tooth preparation but, rather, the first step for the insertion of the restorative material. Regardless, some general comments are presented about such treatments.

Mechanical Features

A variety of mechanical alterations to the preparation enhance retention form. These alterations require additional selective removal of healthy tooth structure.

Retention Grooves and Coves. Vertically oriented grooves associated with the facial and lingual aspects of a proximal preparation are used to provide additional retention for the proximal portions of some Class II amalgam restorations. Horizontally oriented retention grooves are prepared in most Class III and V preparations for amalgam and in some root-surface tooth preparations for amalgam and composite resin. Small retentive indentions, referred to as "coves," are utilized for retention in the incisal areas of Class III amalgams.

Historically, retention grooves in Class II preparations for amalgam restorations were recommended to increase retention of the proximal portion against movement secondary to creep. Also, it was thought that retention grooves may increase the resistance form of the restoration against fracture at the junction of the proximal and occlusal portions. *In vivo* studies do not substantiate the necessity of these grooves in proximocclusal preparations with occlusal dovetail outline forms or in MOD preparations.[4] They are recommended, however, for extensive tooth preparations for amalgam involving wide faciolingual proximal boxes resulting in notable proximal wall divergence, cusp reduction procedures, or both. Therefore mastery of the techniques of optimal groove design and placement is indicated.

Preparation Extensions. Additional retention of the restorative material may be obtained by arbitrarily extending the preparation for molars onto the facial or lingual surface to include a facial or lingual groove. Such an extension, when performed for cast-metal restorations, results in additional vertical (almost parallel) walls for retention. This preparation design may also enhance the resistance form of the remaining tooth by enveloping and contributing reinforcement.

Skirts. Skirts are preparation features used in cast gold restorations that extend the preparation around some, if not all, of the line angles of the tooth. When properly prepared, skirts provide additional, opposing vertical walls that increase retention of the restoration. The placement of skirts also enables increased resistance to fracture by allowing the envelopment of the remaining compromised tooth structure with the restorative material.

Beveled Enamel Margins

Some cast-metal and composite preparations include beveled marginal configurations. The bevels for cast-metal restorations are used primarily to afford a better junctional relationship between the metal and the tooth. Additionally, retention form may be slightly improved when opposing bevels are present. Enamel margins of some composite restorations may utilize a beveled or flared (>90 degrees) configuration so as to increase the retention form of the preparation by increasing the area of enamel available for bonding.

Steps, Amalgam Pins, Slots, and Pins

When the need for increased retention form for amalgam is unusually great (i.e., there is limited remaining tooth structure available to help retain the restoration), additional secondary features may be incorporated into the preparation. Careful orientation of remaining horizontal and vertical walls during tooth preparation results in "steps" that increase retention and resistance form of the restoration. Independently retentive holes with parallel walls (for "amalgam pins") and/or horizontal slots (with internal converging walls) may be effectively used when there is moderate vertical loss

of tooth structure. Severe vertical loss of structure associated with the line angles of the tooth may require the placement of metal pins. These pins are anchored in remaining sound dentin, protrude vertically above the remaining tooth structure, are subsequently encased during placement of the restorative material, and thereby enable retention and resistance form. Features that enhance the retention form of a preparation also enhance the resistance form (e.g., slots or pins placed in a manner such that, upon completion of the restoration, the structural integrity of the restoration enhances the structural integrity of the remaining tooth structure).

Use of Adhesives to Increase Retention and Resistance

Superficial demineralization of preparation walls and subsequent infiltration of the altered surface with resin-based adhesives allows for increased retention and resistance of restorations. The structural makeup of enamel allows the creation of a microscopically roughened mineral surface when superficially demineralized by acidic conditions. All adhesive systems have some means by which to effect the necessary demineralization. This essential, initial step is then followed by infiltration of the roughened surface with resin-based adhesive materials. Demineralization of the exposed dentin surface results in exposure of the dentin matrix (collagen), which may then be infiltrated with adhesive resin materials. Restorative materials (composite, glass-ceramic) may then be attached to this adhesive layer through material-specific mechanisms resulting in increased retention of the "bonded" restoration. The use of bonding systems with intracoronal restorations, while enhancing retention, does not increase the resistance form of the remaining tooth structure over the long term.

Retention of indirect restorations may be enhanced by the material used for cementation. Although not considered part of the tooth preparation, the cementation procedure does affect the retention of these restorations, and some cementing materials require pretreatment of the dentin, resulting in varying degrees of micro-mechanical bonding. Adhesive bonding of etchable glass-ceramic materials to enamel and dentin increase their resistance to fracture development when under occlusal load.

Step 8: External Wall Finishing

Finishing the external preparation walls is the further development, when indicated, of a specific design (e.g., degree of smoothness or roughness, the placement of a bevel) immediately adjacent to or including the cavosurface margin such that the anticipated restorative material has the greatest likelihood of clinical success. Proper finishing of the external walls allows the creation of an optimal marginal junction between the restorative material and the tooth structure. When this occurs there is a smooth transition across the marginal junction and both tooth and restorative material have maximal strength. Awareness of the point of contact of the opposing functional cusp is essential as occlusal contact directly on the marginal interface will result in early fatigue and failure of the margin. When the defect results in a preparation outline form that places the marginal interface at the point of contact, then the final position of the preparation outline is modified slightly so that the marginal junction is away from the occlusal contact (review section Occlusal Contact Identification and Rotary Instrument Axis Alignment).

It is appropriate, for clinical practicality, to consider that enamel rods are oriented perpendicular to the external tooth surface. Enamel walls that form a 90-degree angle with the cavosurface may be considered to have dentinal support and to be strong (see Figs. 4.1 and 4.2C). Enamel rods that do not run uninterrupted from the preparation margin to dentin tend to split off, leaving a V-shaped ditch along the cavosurface margin area of the restoration. Enamel rods incline slightly apically in the gingival third of the tooth crown and preparation design in this area should be modified so as to ensure strong enamel margins (Fig. 4.15).

When a preparation has extended onto the root surface (i.e., no enamel present), the root-surface cavosurface angle should be either 90 degrees (for amalgam, composite, or ceramic restorations) or beveled (for intracoronal cast-metal restorations). The 90-degree root-surface margin provides a butt joint relationship between the restorative material and the dentin (with overlying cementum) preparation wall, a configuration that provides appropriate strength to both.

An acute, abrupt change in a preparation wall outline form increases the difficulty of optimal adaptation of the restorative material. The outline form of all preparation walls should have smooth curves or straight lines. The line angle that forms where two walls meet, regardless of whether it is acute or obtuse, should be slightly curved ("softened") (Fig. 4.16).

The design of the cavosurface angle depends on the restorative material being used. Because of the low edge strength of amalgam and glass-ceramic, a 90-degree cavosurface angle produces maximal strength for these materials. Beveling a cavosurface margin would result in a thin, fracture-prone amalgam or ceramic margin and is contraindicated. On occlusal surfaces for Class I and II amalgam restorations, the incline planes of the cusp and the converging walls (for retentive purposes) of the preparation approximate the desirable 90-degree butt joint junction, even though the actual occlusal enamel margin may be greater than 90 degrees (see Figs. 4.1, 4.2, 4.8, and 4.12).

Beveling the external walls is a preparation technique used for some materials, such as intracoronal cast gold and composite restorations. As previously noted, beveling will result in the strongest type of enamel margin. When a bevel is used for indirect cast gold restorations, it may allow a better marginal seal in slightly undersized castings and may assist in the adaptation of castings that fail to seat by a small amount. In addition, a thin gold margin is more readily burnished and adapted to the preparation margin.

Beveling enamel margins in composite preparations is indicated primarily for large restorations that have increased retention needs and insufficient amount of prepared enamel for proper retention. The use of a beveled marginal form increases the surface area available for bonding, which increases the retention form of the preparation. Diamond instruments are utilized to create the bevel so as to maximize the surface area for bonding. The use of a beveled marginal form is useful for inclusion of minor surface defects just adjacent to the cavosurface margin as well as affords enhanced marginal sealing. The esthetic quality of composite restorations of anterior teeth may be improved by use of a bevel to create an area of gradual increase in composite thickness from the margin to the bulk of the restoration. Hand instruments such as enamel hatchets and margin trimmers may be used in planing enamel walls, cleaving off unsupported enamel, and establishing enamel bevels.

Step 9: Final Procedures: Debridement and Inspection

Debridement (cleaning) of the tooth preparation involves use of the air/water syringe to remove visible debris with water and then excess moisture with a few light bursts of air. In some instances, debris clings to walls and angles despite the aforementioned efforts, and it may be necessary to loosen this material with an explorer or small cotton pellet. It is important not to dehydrate the tooth by overuse of air as this may damage the odontoblasts associated with the desiccated tubules (Fig. 4.17). Complete debridement allows careful *inspection* of the preparation so as to ensure adherence to all principles of preparation design. Any final changes may then be accomplished, as indicated, followed by steps to disinfect the preparation.

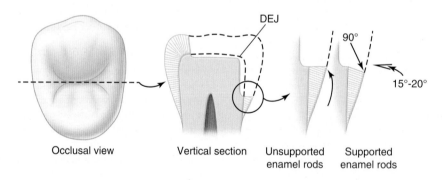

• **Fig. 4.15** Vertical section of Class II tooth preparation. Gingival floor enamel (and margin) is unsupported by dentin and friable unless removed.

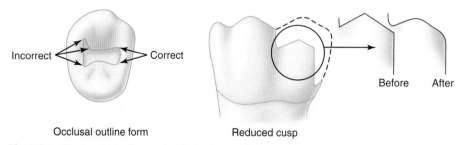

• **Fig. 4.16** The junctions of enamel walls (and respective margins) should be slightly rounded, whether obtuse or acute.

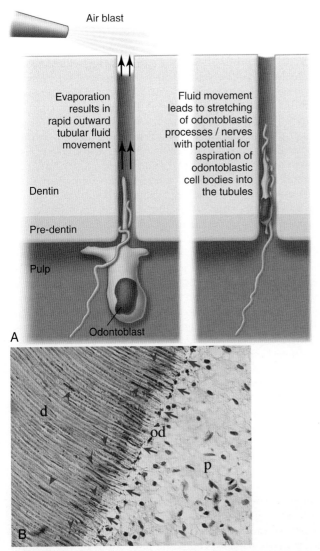

• Fig. 4.17 A, Excessive drying (desiccation) of tooth preparations may cause odontoblasts to be aspirated into dentinal tubules. B, Nuclei are seen as dark rods in dentinal tubules. Red arrowheads indicate the nuclei of the aspirated odontoblasts. Green arrows indicate location of the odontoblasts prior to them being drawn into the tubules from outward dentinal tubular fluid flow. *d*, dentin; *od*, odontoblasts; *p*, pulp. (B, From Mitsiadis TA, De Bari C, About I: Apoptosis in development and repair-related human tooth remodeling: A view from the inside, *Exp Cell Res* 314(4):869–877, 2008.)

Additional Concepts in Tooth Preparation

New techniques advocated for the restoration of teeth should be assessed on the basis of the fundamentals of tooth preparation presented in this chapter. All preparations in stress-bearing areas, once completed, should ensure healthy dentinal support of remaining enamel.

Tunnel Tooth Preparations for Amalgam, Composite Resin, and Glass Ionomers

In an effort to be conservative in the removal of tooth structure, some investigators advocate a "tunnel" tooth preparation. This preparation joins an occlusal lesion with a proximal lesion by means of a prepared tunnel under the involved marginal ridge. The objective of this approach is to remove the caries lesion and leave the marginal ridge essentially intact. However, the development of appropriately formed preparation walls and the excavation of the caries lesion may be compromised by lack of access and visibility. Preservation of the marginal ridge in a strong state is questionable, especially since the dentinal support (essential for enamel durability under occlusal loading) of the marginal ridge is no longer present or is compromised. Generally teeth that have been treated with tunnel preparations do not perform as well as those treated with preparations that remove the marginal ridge over the proximal lesion so as to gain access to the proximal caries lesion. Most currently published clinical trials focus on the use of glass ionomer materials to restore tunnel preparations and have found these materials to be inadequate for use as definitive, long-term restorations. It is currently unknown whether use of adhesively retained composite resin materials will result in better long-term clinical performance. This technique remains controversial and is not supported in this textbook.[12,21]

Adhesive Amalgam Restorations

In vitro research studies suggest that the use of adhesive systems may enhance resistance and retention forms of teeth with compound and complex amalgam preparations/restorations.[22,23] These techniques mechanically bond the amalgam material to tooth structure in the hope that this will increase the overall strength of the remaining tooth structure and improve the overall performance of the restoration. Although proposed bonding techniques vary, the essential procedure is to prepare the tooth in a fashion similar to that typical for amalgam and then utilize an adhesive to bond the amalgam restoration into the preparation. In addition, weakened remaining tooth structure is retained and bonded to the amalgam instead of reduced and covered with amalgam. The preparation walls, including the walls of compromised areas (where there is inadequate dentin support), are treated with specific adhesive lining materials that mechanically bond to the tooth and the amalgam. The amalgam is condensed into this adhesive material before polymerization, and a mechanical bond develops between the amalgam and adhesive. It has been suggested that this technique may limit the likelihood of the development of postoperative sensitivity, staining of the dental structure, secondary caries, fracture of the tooth, or partial/total loss of the restoration. However, no clinical improvement over normal, routine steps utilized in amalgam restoration has been demonstrated.[24-28] Therefore this book does not promote the use of bonded amalgams.

Preparation Treatments to Enhance Restoration

Disinfection, Desensitization, Stabilization

Disinfection of the preparation prior to insertion of the restorative material may be considered. Chlorhexidine (2 weight percent [wt%]) solutions have been successfully used in preparations for disinfection purposes. Disinfection procedures should not be considered absolutely essential. Investigators have verified the presence of bacteria in the dentinal tubules within the preparation walls. While it is true that the dentinal tubule lumens, which vary from 1 to

4 μm in diameter depending on the depth of the preparation, present a pathway for the entrance of bacteria, this fact in no way indicates that caries progression or restoration failure will result. The number of bacteria in the dentinal tubules is relatively small compared with the numerous microorganisms found in the superficial caries lesion. The caries lesion will not progress if the defect is correctly restored.[12]

Even when surface disinfection of the preparation has been attempted, it is doubtful that potential benefits will continue for any appreciable length of time because of the difference between the thermal coefficients of expansion of the tooth and restorative materials. Although differing in amounts, marginal leakage has been shown for current restorative materials.[18,29,30] Caries is unlikely to develop in association with marginal gaps that are less than 250 μm.[29] Limited protection from further carious activity may be afforded by some restorative materials.[31] The germicidal or protective effect may be from the fluoride content of some tooth-colored restorative materials or from the deposition of corrosion products at the interface between the preparation wall and an amalgam restoration.

The natural defense mechanisms of the tooth, which result in the mineralization of the dentinal tubules under a caries lesion, help limit the potential for invasion of any remaining bacteria. However, this natural occlusion of the dentinal tubules only will occur beneath a slowly progressing caries lesion. The precipitation of mineral in the dentinal tubules beneath a caries lesion (giving it a transparent appearance) creates a physical barrier to bacterial ingress. In addition to this host-defense mechanism, the presence of reparative dentin deposited as a result of pulpal insult constitutes a significant deterrent to bacterial invasion. Bacteria may transition into dormancy as the result of the more sealed environment of a restored tooth. When mineral occlusion of the dentinal tubules has not occurred, there is increased risk of pulpal sensitivity after the restoration has been placed. Therefore routine use of medicaments to occlude the dentinal tubules (i.e. "desensitizers") is recommended in the finalized preparation.

Desensitization may be accomplished by taking steps to limit rapid fluid movement in the dentinal tubules. Occlusion of the dentinal tubules limits the potential for rapid tubular fluid movement. Some desensitizers not only are effective disinfectants but also are able to occlude ("plug") the dentinal tubules by cross-linking and precipitating the proteins in the dentinal tubule fluid.[32-35] Preparations designed for amalgam restoration should be desensitized with a solution that contains 5% glutaraldehyde and 35% 2-hydroxyethyl methacrylate (HEMA) before amalgam placement.[36] The use of this type of desensitizer allows prevention of rapid fluid movement associated with osmotic gradients and temperature gradients. Osmotic gradients cause a rapid, transitory increase in the amount of marginal microleakage associated with recently placed amalgam restorations, which may result in sensitivity. Temperature gradients (amalgam is an excellent thermal conductor) also may result in rapid fluid movement in the dentinal tubules secondary to exposure to temperature extremes. Alternatively, there are some who advocate the use of an adhesive on the prepared tooth structure so as to limit rapid fluid movement by "sealing" the dentin before amalgam placement and in this way limit the potential for postoperative sensitivity.[37]

Composite restorations require some treatment of the preparation before insertion of the restorative material, which may primarily be considered as part of the restoration procedure (see Chapter 8); however, some discussion is appropriate at this point. Preparation wall treatment for composites includes the etching (surface demineralization) of enamel and dentin followed by placement of a resin-based adhesive. The smear layer that forms on wall surfaces during preparation is either altered or removed from the enamel and dentin during the etching process. Placement of the adhesive will allow subsequent formation of strong, durable mechanical bond between the etched enamel and the composite. In dentin, a hybrid layer is formed, which is characterized by an intermingling of the resin adhesive with exposed collagen fibrils of the intertubular dentin. This initially creates a strong mechanical bond between the composite and dentin. However, it has been identified that the bond to dentin deteriorates over time as a result of hydrolysis of the adhesive resin component of the hybrid layer and proteolytic degradation of the collagen component of the hybrid layer.[38] Therefore *stabilization* of the exposed collagen may be appropriate as an initial step in the restorative sequence.

Ongoing dental research has sought to optimize the long-term stability of the hybrid layer. For example, *in vivo* studies have shown that chlorhexidine (2 wt% solution) application to etched dentin is able to limit the activity of local collagenolytic enzymes (matrix metalloproteinases, or MMPs), which are able to degrade the exposed collagen matrix. Limiting the activity of the MMPs may help stabilize the hybrid layer, at least in Class I preparations for the short term.[39] Chlorhexidine is able to inactive MMPs that are exposed as a result of the etching process. However, additional new MMPs, being generated by ongoing odontoblastic activity, will remain active and able to degrade collagen that was demineralized but not adequately infiltrated with adhesive resin. Long-term hybrid layer stability, as a result of chlorhexidine use, has not been demonstrated. These findings, as well as the decision to incorporate chlorhexidine or other dentin protease inhibitors as an initial restorative step for hybrid layer stabilization, are to be considered in light of clinical studies that reveal the clinical performance of composite systems that did not use chlorhexidine is comparable with that of amalgam in patients who are low caries risk.[40] However, it has been found that, in high caries risk patients, composite restorations do not perform as well as amalgam restorations.[40,41] Therefore there may be advantages to the use of agents that stabilize and increase hybrid layer resistance to proteolytic activity as a first step of the restoration sequence.

The use of a 5% glutaraldehyde/35% HEMA solution theoretically may be used immediately after etching and before priming of the dentin for the following reasons: (1) to occlude dentinal tubules and, thereby, limit tubular fluid contamination during hybrid layer formation, (2) to cross-link the acid-exposed intertubular collagen so as to render it resistant to proteolytic degradation, and (3) to cross-link and inactivate noncollagenous proteins that are able to degrade collagen (MMPs and cathepsins). Recent *in vitro* evidence is in support of this theory.[35] However, potential cytotoxic effects of free glutaraldehyde and HEMA (i.e., not involved in the protein cross-linking and tubular occlusion) raise legitimate patient safety concerns. Removal of excess glutaraldehyde and HEMA by rinsing with water may significantly reduce any risk. The outward flow of dentinal tubular fluid may also tend to limit the potential for free glutaraldehyde and/or HEMA to diffuse toward and negatively impact pulpal tissue. Furthermore, it is necessary to recall that pulpal and axial dentin in an advanced lesion (see Step 5 above) has been damaged by the caries process and any bond to this deep dentin is compromised. Therefore deep dentin areas of the advanced lesion should be covered (i.e., sealed off) with a RMGI *prior* to any attempt at demineralization (either by total-etch or self-etch systems) of more peripheral dentin that might be followed by efforts (such as use of a 5% glutaraldehyde/35% HEMA solution) to stabilize and increase hybrid layer resistance to proteolytic activity as a part of the restorative sequence. Placement of the RMGI may theoretically limit the ability of any free glutaraldehyde or HEMA to gain access to tubules in closest proximity to the pulp. Additional testing to validate the safety and efficacy of this stabilization technique is indicated.

Summary

This chapter has addressed the principles of tooth preparation. Every effort should be made to conserve and protect remaining healthy natural tooth structure during the various steps of preparation. Tooth preparation is guided through careful consideration of the implications of many factors. Preparation design is strategically implemented so as to provide the subsequent restoration with an optimal chance of clinical success.

References

1. Black GV: *Operative dentistry*, ed 8, Woodstock, Ill, 1947–1948, Medico-Dental.
2. Bronner FJ: Mechanical, physiological, and pathological aspects of operative procedures. *Dent Cosmos* 73:577, 1931.
3. Markley MR: Restorations of silver amalgam. *J Am Dent Assoc* 43:133, 1951.
4. Sturdevant JR, Wilder AD, Roberson TM, et al: Clinical study of conservative designs for Class II amalgams (abstract 1549). *J Dent Res* 67:306, 1988.
5. Sockwell CL: Dental handpieces and rotary cutting instruments. *Dent Clin North Am* 15:219, 1971.
6. Sturdevant CM: *The art and science of operative dentistry*, ed 1, New York, 1968, McGraw-Hill.
7. Simonsen RJ: Preventive resin restoration. *Quintessence Int* 9:69–76, 1978.
8. Charbeneau GT, Peyton FA: Some effects of cavity instrumentation on the adaptation of gold castings and amalgam. *J Prosthet Dent* 8:514, 1958.
9. Marzouk MA: *Operative dentistry*, St Louis, 1985, Ishiyaku EuroAmerica.
10. Linn J, Messer HH: Effect of restorative procedures on the strength of endodontically treated molars. *J Endo* 20(10):479–485, 1994.
11. Hansen EK, Asmussen E, Christiansen NC: In vivo fractures of endodontically treated posterior teeth restored with amalgam. *Endod Dent Traumatol* 6(2):49–55, 1990.
12. Fejerskov O, Nyvad B, Kidd E, editors: *Dental caries: The disease and its clinical management*, 3rd ed, Oxford, 2015, Wiley Blackwell.
13. Reeves R, Stanley HR: The relationship of bacterial penetration and pulpal pathosis in carious teeth. *Oral Surg* 22:59, 1966.
14. Ritter AV, Swift EJ: Current restorative concepts of pulp protection. *Endod Topics* 5:41–48, 2003.
15. Murray PE, Hafez AA, Smith AJ, et al: Bacterial microleakage and pulp inflammation associated with various restorative materials. *Dent Mater* 18:470–478, 2002.
16. Swift EJ, Trope M, Ritter AV: Vital pulp therapy for the mature tooth—can it work? *Endod Topics* 5:49–56, 2003.
17. Hilton TJ: Keys to clinical success with pulp capping: A review of the literature. *Oper Dent* 34(5):615–625, 2009, doi:10.2341/09-132-0.
18. Craig RG, Powers JM, editors: *Restorative dental materials*, 11th ed, St. Louis, 2002, Mosby.
19. Goracci G, Giovani M: Scanning electron microscopic evaluation of resin-dentin and calcium hydroxide-dentin interface with resin composite restorations. *Quintessence Int* 27:129–135, 1996.
20. Resaratnam L: Review suggests direct pulp capping with MTA more effective than calcium hydroxide. *Evid Based Dent* 17(3):94–95, 2016, doi:10.1038/sj.ebd.6401194.
21. Wiegand A, Attin T: Treatment of proximal caries lesions by tunnel restorations. *Dent Mat* 23(12):1461–1467, 2007.
22. Boyer DB, Roth L: Fracture resistance of teeth with bonded amalgams. *Am J Dent* 7:91–94, 1994.
23. Zidan O, Abdel-Keriem U: The effect of amalgam bonding on the stiffness of teeth weakened by cavity preparation. *Dent Mater* 19:680–685, 2003.
24. Mach Z, Regent J, Staninec M, et al: The integrity of bonded amalgam restorations: A clinical evaluation after five years. *J Am Dent Assoc* 133:460–467, 2002.
25. Smales RJ, Wetherell JD: Review of bonded amalgam restorations, and assessment in a general practice over five years. *Oper Dent* 25:374–381, 2000.
26. Baratieri LN, Machado A, Van Noort R, et al: Effect of pulp protection technique on the clinical performance of amalgam restorations: Three-year results. *Oper Dent* 29:319–324, 2002.
27. Summitt JB, Burgess JO, Berry TG, et al: Six-year clinical evaluation of bonded and pin- retained complex amalgam restorations. *Oper Dent* 29:261–268, 2004.
28. Agnihotry A, Fedorowicz Z, Nasser M: Adhesively bonded versus non-bonded amalgam restorations for dental caries. *Cochrane Database Syst Rev* (3):CD007517, 2016, doi:10.1002/14651858.CD007517. pub3.
29. Dennison JB, Sarrett DC: Prediction and diagnosis of clinical outcomes affecting restoration margins. *J Oral Rehab* 39:301–318, 2012.
30. Mjör IA: Clinical diagnosis of recurrent caries. *J Amer Dent Assoc* 136:1426–1433, 2005.
31. Shay DE, Allen TJ, Mantz RF: Antibacterial effects of some dental restorative materials. *J Dent Res* 35:25, 1956.
32. Schüpbach P, Lutz F, Finger WJ: Closing of dentinal tubules by Gluma Desensitizer. *Eur J Oral Sci* 105:414–421, 1997.
33. Qin C, Xu J, Zhang Y: Spectroscopic investigation of the function of aqueous 2- hydroxyethylmethacrylate/glutaraldehyde solution as a dentin desensitizer. *Eur J Oral Sci* 114:354–359, 2006.
34. Munksgaard EC: Amine-induced polymerization of aqueous HEMA/ aldehyde during action as a dentin bonding agent. *J Dent Res* 69:1236–1239, 1990.
35. Lee J, Sabatini C: Glutaraldehyde collagen cross-linking stabilizes resin-dentin interfaces and reduces bond degradation. *Eur J Oral Sci* 125:63–71, 2017.
36. Boksman L, Swift EJ, Jr: Current usage of glutaraldehyde/HEMA. *J Esthet Rest Dent* 23(6):410–416, 2011, doi:10.1111/j.1708-8240. 2011.00490.x.
37. Ben-Amar A: Reduction of microleakage around new amalgam restorations. *J Am Dent Assoc* 119:725, 1989.
38. Pashley DH, Tay FR, Breschi L, et al: State of the art etch-and-rinse adhesives. *Dent Mater* 27:1–16, 2011.
39. Carrilho MRO, Geraldeli S, Tay F, et al: In vivo preservation of the hybrid layer by chlorhexidine. *J Dent Res* 86:529–533, 2007.
40. Opdam NJM, Bronkhorst EM, Loomans BAC, et al: 12-year Survival of Composite vs. Amalgam Restorations. *J Dent Res* 89:1063–1068, 2010, doi:10.1177/0022034510376071.
41. Rasiines Alcaraz MG, Veiz-Keenan A, Sahrmann P, et al: Direct composite fillings versus amalgam fillings for permanent or adult posterior teeth. *Cochran Database of Systematic Reviews* (3):Art. No.:CD005620, 2014, doi:10.1002/14651858.CD005620.pub2.
42. Hyatt TP: Prophylactic odontotomy: The ideal procedure in dentistry for children. *Dent Cosmos* 78:353, 1936.

5

Fundamental Concepts of Enamel and Dentin Adhesion

JORGE PERDIGÃO, RICARDO WALTER, PATRICIA A. MIGUEZ, EDWARD J. SWIFT, JR.

The classic concepts of operative dentistry were challenged in the 1980s and 1990s by the introduction of new adhesive techniques, first for enamel and then for dentin. This chapter discusses the differences in enamel and dentin adhesion and developments in adhesive systems over time. Current adhesive systems applied using several adhesion strategies with their indications and limitations, based on in vitro and clinical evidence, are discussed.

Basic Concepts of Adhesion

The American Society for Testing and Materials (specification D907) defines adhesion as "the state in which two surfaces are held together by interfacial forces which may consist of valence forces or interlocking forces or both."[1] The word *adhesion* comes from the Latin *adhaerere* ("to stick to"). An adhesive is a material, frequently a viscous fluid, that joins two substrates together by solidifying and transferring a load from one surface to the other. Adhesion or adhesive strength is the measure of the load-bearing capacity of an adhesive joint.[2] Four different mechanisms of adhesion have been described, as follows[3]:

1. *Mechanical adhesion*—interlocking of the adhesive with irregularities in the surface of the substrate, or adherend
2. *Adsorption adhesion*—chemical bonding between the adhesive and the adherend; the forces involved may be primary (ionic and covalent) or secondary (hydrogen bonds, dipole interaction, or van der Waals) valence forces
3. *Diffusion adhesion*—interlocking between mobile molecules, such as the adhesion of two polymers through diffusion of polymer chain ends across an interface
4. *Electrostatic adhesion*—an electrical double layer at the interface of a metal with a polymer that is part of the total bonding mechanism

In dentistry, bonding of resin-based materials to tooth structure is a result of four possible mechanisms, as follows[4]:

1. *Mechanical*—penetration of resin and formation of resin tags within the tooth surface
2. *Adsorption*—chemical bonding to the inorganic component (hydroxyapatite) or organic components (mainly type I collagen) of tooth structure
3. *Diffusion*—precipitation of substances on the tooth surfaces to which resin monomers can bond mechanically or chemically
4. A *combination* of the previous three mechanisms

For good adhesion, close contact must exist between the adhesive and the substrate (enamel or dentin). The surface tension of the adhesive must be lower than the surface energy of the substrate. Failures of adhesive joints occur in three locations, which are generally combined when an actual failure occurs: (1) cohesive failure in the substrate; (2) cohesive failure within the adhesive; and (3) adhesive failure, or failure at the interface of substrate and adhesive.

A major problem in bonding resins to tooth structure is that all methacrylate-based dental resins shrink during free-radical addition polymerization.[5] Dental adhesives must provide a strong initial bond to resist the stresses of resin shrinkage.

Trends in Restorative Dentistry

The introduction of enamel bonding, the increasing demand for restorative and nonrestorative esthetic treatments, and the ubiquity of fluoride have combined to transform the practice of operative dentistry.[6,7] The classic concepts of tooth preparation were advocated in the early 1900s,[8] but these have changed drastically. This transformation in philosophy has resulted in a more conservative approach to tooth preparation, with regard to not only the basic concepts of retention form but also the resistance form of the remaining tooth structure. Bonding techniques allow more conservative tooth preparations, less reliance on macromechanical retention, and less removal of unsupported enamel.

The availability of new scientific information on the etiology, diagnosis, and treatment of carious lesions and the introduction of reliable adhesive restorative materials have substantially reduced the need for extensive tooth preparations. With improvements in materials, indications for resin-based materials have progressively shifted from the anterior segment only to posterior teeth as well. Adhesive restorative techniques currently are used to accomplish the following:

1. Restore Class I, II, III, IV, V, and VI carious lesions or traumatic defects.
2. Change the shape and the color of anterior teeth (e.g., with full or partial resin veneers).[9,10]
3. Improve retention for porcelain-fused-to-metal (ceramometal) or metallic crowns.[11,12]
4. Bond all-ceramic restorations (Fig. 5.1).[13,14]
5. Seal pits and fissures.[15]
6. Bond orthodontic brackets.[16]

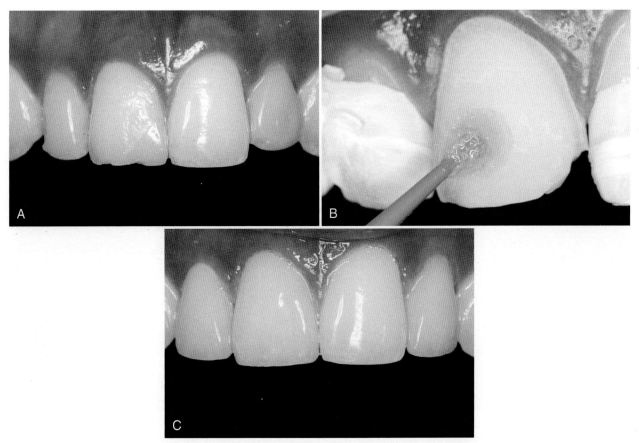

• **Fig. 5.1** A, Preoperative view of anterior teeth in a 24-year-old patient with defective composite restorations. The treatment plan included bonded porcelain veneers on teeth #7, #8, and #10 to match the natural aspect of tooth #9. B, Porcelain veneers were bonded with a two-step etch-and-rinse adhesive and a light-activated resin cement. C, Final aspect 1 week after the bonding procedure.

7. Bond splints for tooth luxations and periodontally involved anterior teeth and conservative tooth-replacement prostheses.[17-20]
8. Repair existing restorations (composite, amalgam, ceramic, or ceramometal).[21-24]
9. Provide foundations for crowns.[25,26]
10. Desensitize noncarious cervical lesions (NCCLs) and exposed root surfaces.[27-30]
11. Impregnate enamel and dentin making them less susceptible to caries.[31,32]
12. Bond fractured fragments of anterior teeth (Fig. 5.2).[33]
13. Bond prefabricated fiber, metal, and cast posts.[34]
14. Reinforce fragile endodontically treated roots internally.[35,36]
15. Seal root canals during endodontic therapy.[37,38]
16. Seal surgically resected root apices.[39,40]

Enamel Adhesion

Inspired by the industrial use of 85% phosphoric acid to facilitate adhesion of paints and resins to metallic surfaces, Buonocore envisioned the use of acids to etch enamel for sealing pits and fissures.[6,41] Since Buonocore's introduction of the acid-etch technique, many dental researchers have attempted to achieve methods for reliable and durable adhesion between resins and tooth structures.

Various concentrations of phosphoric acid have been used to etch enamel. Most current phosphoric acid gels have concentrations of 30% to 40%, with 37% being the most common, although some studies using lower concentrations have reported similar adhesion values.[42-45] An etching time of 60 seconds originally was recommended for permanent enamel using 30% to 40% phosphoric acid. Although one study concluded that shorter etch times resulted in lower bond strengths, other studies using scanning electron microscopy (SEM) showed that a 15-second etch resulted in a surface roughness similar to that provided by a 60-second etch.[46-49] Other in vitro studies have shown similar bond strengths and leakage for etching times of 15 and 60 seconds.[50-54]

As measured in the laboratory, shear bond strengths of composite to phosphoric acid-etched enamel usually exceed 20 megapascals (MPa) and can range up to 53 MPa, depending on the test method used.[55-58] Such bond strengths provide adequate retention for a broad variety of procedures and prevent leakage around enamel margins of restorations.[53]

Acid etching transforms the smooth enamel into an irregular surface (Fig. 5.3) and increases its surface-free energy. When a fluid resin-based material is applied to the irregular etched surface, the resin penetrates into the surface, aided by capillary action. Monomers in the material polymerize, and the material becomes interlocked with the enamel surface (Fig. 5.4).[41] The formation of resin microtags within the enamel surface is the fundamental mechanism of resin-enamel adhesion.[41,46,59] Fig. 5.5 shows a replica of an etched enamel surface visualized through the extensions of resin that penetrated the irregular enamel surface. The acid-etch technique has revolutionized the practice of restorative dentistry.

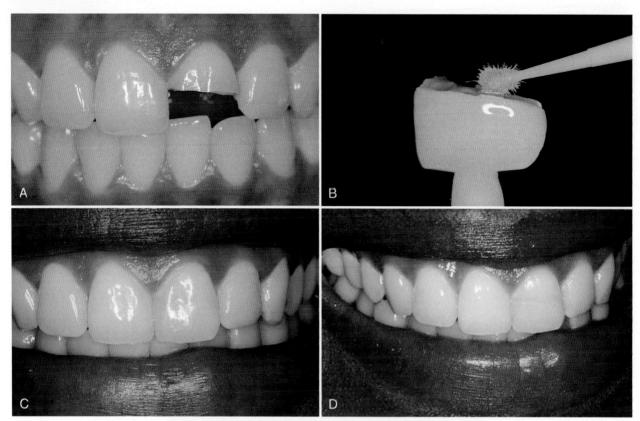

• **Fig. 5.2** A, Intraoral frontal view of a 20-year-old female presenting with complicated crown fracture on tooth #9 after endodontic treatment. The fracture extends subgingivally on the mesial aspect of the lingual surface. B, A two-step etch-and-rinse ethanol-based adhesive applied to the crown fragment and tooth. C, Extraoral view 6 months after rebonding. D, Extraoral view 3 years after rebonding. (From Macedo GV, Ritter AV: Essentials of rebonding tooth fragments for the best functional and esthetic outcomes, *Pediatr Dent* 31(2):110–116, 2009.)

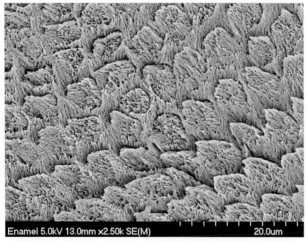

Enamel 5.0kV 13.0mm x2.50k SE(M) 20.0um

• **Fig. 5.3** Scanning electron micrograph of enamel etched with 35% phosphoric acid (3M Oral Care) for 15 seconds.

Dentin Adhesion

The classic concepts of operative dentistry were challenged in the 1980s and 1990s by the introduction of new adhesive techniques, first for enamel and then for dentin. Nevertheless, adhesion to dentin remains difficult. Adhesive materials can interact with dentin in different ways—mechanically, chemically, or both.[7,60-66] The importance of micromechanical bonding, similar to what occurs in enamel bonding, has become accepted.[60,67] Dentin adhesion relies primarily on the penetration of adhesive monomers into the network of collagen fibrils left exposed by acid etching (Fig. 5.6).[67,68] However, for adhesive materials that do not require etching, such as glass ionomer cements and some phosphate-based self-etch adhesives, chemical bonding between polycarboxylic or phosphate monomers and hydroxyapatite has been shown to be an important part of the bonding mechanism.[62-66] Contemporary strategies for bonding to dentin are summarized in Table 5.1.

Challenges in Dentin Bonding

Substrate

Bonding to enamel is a relatively simple process, without major technical requirements or difficulties. Bonding to dentin presents a much greater challenge. Several factors account for this difference between enamel and dentin bonding. Enamel is a highly mineralized tissue composed of more than 90% (by volume) hydroxyapatite, whereas dentin contains a substantial proportion of water and organic material, primarily type I collagen (Fig. 5.7).[69] Dentin also contains a dense network of tubules that connect the pulp with the dentinoenamel junction (DEJ) (Fig. 5.8). A cuff of hypermineralized dentin called *peritubular dentin* lines the tubules. The less mineralized intertubular dentin contains collagen fibrils with the characteristic collagen banding (Fig. 5.9). Intertubular dentin is penetrated by submicron channels, which allow the passage of

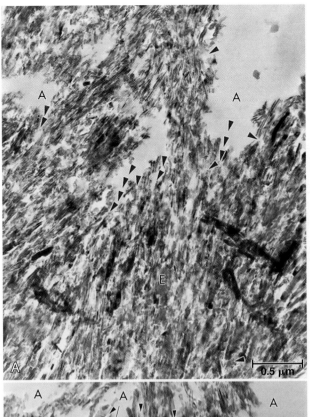

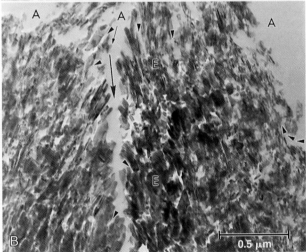

• **Fig. 5.4**   A and B, Transmission electron micrographs of the enamel-adhesive interface after application of Adper Single Bond (3M Oral Care) as per manufacturer's instructions. Acid etching with 35% phosphoric acid opened spaces between enamel prisms *(arrows),* allowing the permeation of resin monomers between the crystallites *(arrowheads). A,* Adhesive; *E,* enamel.

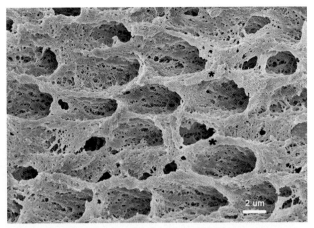

• **Fig. 5.5**   Replica of enamel etched with 35% phosphoric acid. Enamel was dissolved completely in 6N hydrochloric acid for 24 hours. The resin extensions correspond to the interprismatic spaces *(asterisks).*

tubular liquid and fibrils between neighboring tubules, forming intertubular anastomoses.

Dentin is an intrinsically hydrated tissue, penetrated by a maze of fluid-filled tubules. Movement of fluid from the pulp to the DEJ is a result of a slight but constant pulpal pressure.[70] Pulpal pressure has a magnitude of 25 to 30 mm Hg or 34 to 40 cm H_2O.[71,72] Dentinal tubules enclose cellular extensions from the odontoblasts and are in direct communication with the pulp (Fig. 5.10). Inside the tubule lumen, other fibrous organic structures such as the lamina limitans are present, which substantially decreases the functional radius of the tubule. The relative area occupied by

dentin tubules decreases with increasing distance from the pulp. The number of tubules decreases from about 45,000/mm² close to the pulp to about 20,000/mm² near the DEJ.[73] The tubules occupy an area of only 1% of the total surface near the DEJ, whereas they occupy 22% of the surface close to the pulp.[74] The average tubule diameter ranges from 0.63 μm at the periphery to 2.37 μm near the pulp.[75]

Adhesion can be affected by the remaining dentin thickness after tooth preparation. Bond strengths are generally less in deep dentin than in superficial dentin.[76-78] Some dentin adhesives, including one-step self-etch adhesives, do not seem to be affected by dentin depth.[79] When the concentration of cross-linked carboxyterminal telopeptide of type I collagen was evaluated using an immunoassay to detect the degree of collagen degradation, significantly increased degradation was measured for a two-step etch-and-rinse adhesive compared to a one-step self-etch adhesive.[80] In the same study, collagen in deep dentin underwent significantly more degradation than collagen in superficial dentin after thermal fatigue.[80] Degradation of collagen by dentin proteinases is known to negatively affect the bonded interface.

Whenever tooth structure is prepared with a bur or other instrument, residual organic and inorganic components form a "smear layer" of debris on the surface.[81,82] The smear layer fills the orifices of dentin tubules, forming "smear plugs" (Fig. 5.11), and decreases dentin permeability by nearly 90% in vitro.[83] The composition of the smear layer is basically hydroxyapatite and altered denatured collagen. This altered collagen can acquire a gelatinized consistency because of the friction and heat created by the preparation procedure.[84] Submicron porosity of the smear layer still allows for diffusion of dentinal fluid.[85] Removal of the smear layer and smear plugs with acidic solutions results in an increase of the fluid flow onto the exposed dentin surface. This fluid can interfere with adhesion because hydrophobic resins do not adhere to hydrophilic substrates, even if resin tags are formed in the dentin tubules.[7,86]

Several additional factors affect dentin permeability. Besides the use of vasoconstrictors in local anesthetics, which decrease pulpal pressure and fluid flow in the tubules, factors such as the radius and length of the tubules, the viscosity of dentin fluid, the pressure gradient, the molecular size of the substances dissolved in the tubular fluid, and the rate of removal of substances by the blood vessels in the pulp affect permeability. All of these variables

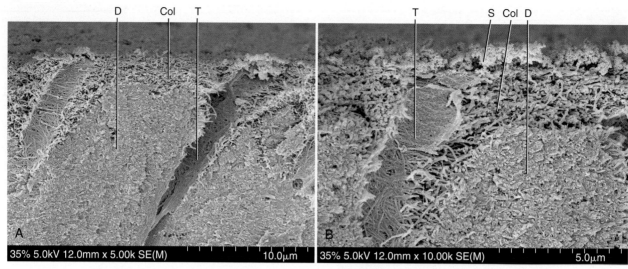

• **Fig. 5.6** A, Dentin etched with 35% phosphoric acid. B, Higher magnification view of etched dentin. *Col,* Collagen exposed by the acid; *D,* normal dentin; *T,* dentinal tubule; *S,* residual silica particles used as acid gel thickener.

TABLE 5.1	Current Strategies for Adhesion of Resins to Dentin		
	Etchant (E)	**Primer (P)**	**Bonding Agent (B)**
Three-step etch-and-rinse[a] E + P + B	Removes the smear layer Exposes intertubular and peritubular collagen Opens tubules in a funnel configuration Decreases surface-free energy	Includes bifunctional molecules (simultaneously hydrophilic and hydrophobic) Envelops the external surface of collagen fibrils Reestablishes surface-free energy to levels compatible with a more hydrophobic restorative material	Includes monomers that are mostly hydrophobic such as Bis-GMA; however, can contain a small percentage of hydrophilic monomers such as HEMA Copolymerizes with the primer molecules Penetrates and polymerizes into the interfibrillar spaces to serve as a structural backbone to the hybrid layer
Two-step etch-and-rinse E + [PB]	Removes the smear layer Exposes intertubular and peritubular collagen Opens tubules in a funnel configuration Decreases surface-free energy	Penetrates into the dentin tubules to form resin tags The first coat applied on etched dentin works as a primer—it increases the surface-free energy of dentin The second coat (and third, fourth, and so on) acts as the bonding agent used in three-step systems—it fills the spaces between the dense network of collagen fibrils	
Two-step self-etch [EP] + B	Enamel etch is typically shallow The self-etching primer (SEP) does not remove the smear layer, but fixes it and exposes about 0.5–1 μm of intertubular collagen because of its acidity (pH = 1.2–2) The smear plug is impregnated with acidic monomers, but it is not removed; some SEP monomers bond chemically to dentin When it impregnates the smear plug, the SEP prepares the pathway for the penetration of the subsequently placed fluid resin into the microchannels that permeate the smear plug	Uses the same type of bonding agent included in the three-step etch-and-rinse systems The resin tags form on resin penetration into the microchannels of the primer-impregnated smear plug	
One-step self-etch [EPB]	Etches enamel, but etch pattern is typically shallow Incorporates the smear layer into interface Being an aqueous solution of a phosphonated monomer, it demineralizes and penetrates dentin simultaneously, leaving a precipitate on the hybrid layer Forms a thin layer of adhesive, leading to low bond strengths; a multicoat approach is recommended; an extra layer of a hydrophobic bonding resin improves bond strengths and clinical performance Incompatible with self-cure composite resins unless coated with an hydrophobic bonding resin		

[a]Although the meaning of the two terms is the same, the term "etch-and-rinse" is preferred over "total-etch."

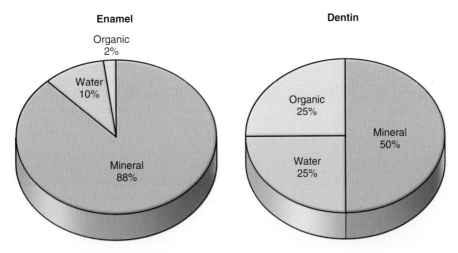

• **Fig. 5.7** Composition of enamel and dentin by volume percent.

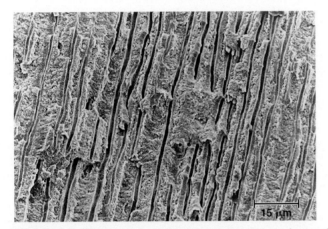

• **Fig. 5.8** Scanning electron micrograph of dentin that was fractured longitudinally to show dentinal tubules.

make dentin a dynamic substrate and consequently a difficult substrate for bonding.[74,87]

Stresses at the Resin–Dentin Interface

Composites shrink as they polymerize, creating considerable stresses within the composite mass, depending on the configuration of the preparation.[88-91] When the composite is bonded to one surface only (e.g., for a direct facial veneer), stresses within the composite are relieved by flow from the unbonded surface. Stress relief within a three-dimensional bonded restoration is limited however by its configuration factor (C-factor).[92] In an occlusal preparation, composite is bonded to five tooth surfaces—mesial, distal, buccal, lingual, and pulpal. The occlusal surface of the composite is the only "free" or unrestrained surface. In such a situation, the ratio between the number of bonded surfaces and the number of unbonded surfaces is 5:1, giving the restoration a configuration factor equal to 5. Stress relief is limited because flow can occur only from the single free surface.[92,93] Unrelieved stresses in the composite contribute to internal bond disruption and marginal gaps around restorations that may increase microleakage and potential postoperative sensitivity.[94] The C-factor might be partially responsible for the decrease in bond strengths observed when deep dentin is bonded as part of a three-dimensional preparation.[95]

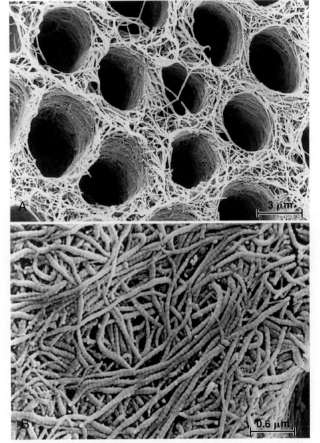

• **Fig. 5.9** A, Scanning electron micrograph of etched dentin showing exposed collagen fibrils. B, Higher magnification shows the characteristic collagen banding in intertubular collagen. Superficial collagen was dissolved by collagenase to remove the most superficial collagen fibrils that were damaged by tooth preparation.

In addition to the C-factor, the magnitude of the polymerization shrinkage stress depends on several other variables, including the rate of the polymerization reaction, the degree of conversion, the composite stiffness and its rate of acquisition of stiffness during polymerization, the nature and relative volume of the inorganic filler, the type of monomers in the composite, the composite

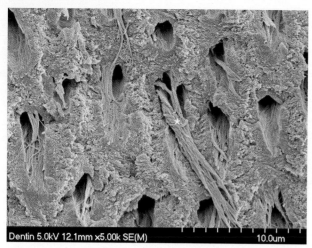

• **Fig. 5.10** Scanning electron micrograph of deep dentin displaying an odontoblastic process in a dentinal tubule *(asterisk)*.

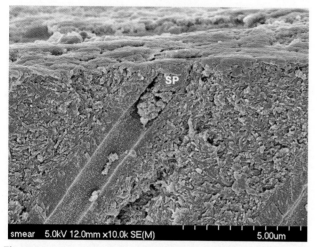

• **Fig. 5.11** Scanning electron micrograph of a smear plug blocking the entrance of a dentinal tubule. *SP,* Smear plug.

insertion technique, and the opacity of the composite.[96-100] It has been reported that immediate bond strengths of approximately 17 MPa are necessary to resist the contraction stresses that develop in the composite during polymerization, to prevent marginal debonding.[90,101] However, this magnitude of bond strengths may not be enough to counteract the polymerization contraction stresses in some composite restorations, as stiffer composite materials, in general, result in increased stresses than those generated by more elastic composite materials.[102]

The water absorption in composites results in partial relief of the contraction residual stresses from polymerization.[103] However, the magnitude of hygroscopic expansion from water absorption depends on the volume of the restoration and the specific monomers used in the composition of composites,[104,105] as more hydrophilic materials may actually result in a net expansion.[103] Composite materials that contain bisphenol A ethoxylated dimethacrylate (Bis-EMA) undergo less water sorption than composites with traditional monomers such as bisphenol A-glycidyl methacrylate (Bis-GMA) and urethane dimethacrylate (UDMA).[104] Silorane-based composites have the lowest hygroscopic expansion.[105]

Several clinical strategies have been suggested to reduce the effects of polymerization shrinkage stress, including control of curing light irradiance,[106,107] incremental insertion techniques,[102,108] and application of intermediate low-modulus liners.[109] None of these methods has been effective in completely eliminating the deleterious effects of polymerization shrinkage stress, which include cuspal deflection, tooth cracking, marginal leakage and gap formation, reduction of adhesive bond strengths, and decreased physical properties of the resin restorative material.[110] Nevertheless, polymerization shrinkage stresses of composites remain a concern, and stress relief in a restoration is important. Polymerization is initiated on the surface of the restoration, close to the light source, eliminating this surface as a potential stress relief pathway.[111] Several methods have been advocated to improve the flow capacity of composites used in Class II tooth preparations. One of those methods is the use of a flowable composite between the composite and the tooth wall. Conceptually, this flowable low-modulus composite would serve as a shock absorber and simultaneously protect the interface against fatigue stresses.[112,113] The use of flowable composites as an intermediate layer in NCCLs or as the gingival increment of Class II preparations however has not been proved effective clinically.[114-118] Likewise, the application of a glass ionomer cement base underneath posterior composite restorations does not improve the restoration survival rate at 18 years.[119] Also, modifications of the current resin-based composites have been proposed as a means to reduce stress without compromising mechanical properties.[120] Studies have shown that some commercial composites specifically designed to have reduced polymerization contraction and/or stress produce less deleterious outcomes on marginal adaptation and cuspal deflection.[121-123] However, further studies demonstrated that, in spite of the lower total shrinkage obtained with the recent low-shrinkage composite, shrinkage stress is not necessarily reduced.

Each time a restoration is exposed to wide temperature variations in the oral environment (e.g., drinking coffee and eating ice cream), the restoration undergoes volumetric changes of different magnitude compared with those of the tooth structure. This occurs because the linear coefficient of thermal expansion (CTE) of hybrid and microfilled composites is about two to three times and four times greater than that of dentin, respectively.[124-126] Microleakage around dentin margins is potentiated by this discrepancy in linear coefficient of thermal expansion between the restoration and the substrate.[127,128] Enamel bond strengths usually are sufficient to prevent the formation of marginal gaps by polymerization contraction stresses. These stresses might however be powerful enough to cause enamel defects at the margins.[107] Although the extension of the enamel cavosurface bevel helps improve the enamel peripheral seal in vitro and reduce the stresses,[88,129,130] recent systematic reviews have questioned the need for enamel beveling prior to acid etching.[131,132]

Loading and unloading of restored teeth can result in transitional or permanent interfacial gaps.[133] Additionally, the tooth substrate itself might be weakened by cyclic loading.[134] A study found that 71% of Class V composite restorations in third molars with antagonists had significantly more leakage than restorations placed in teeth without opposing contact.[135] Another study found that cyclic loading and preparation configuration significantly reduced the bond strengths of self-etch and etch-and-rinse adhesives.[136,137]

Development

Beginning

During the 1950s, it was reported that a resin containing glycerophosphoric acid dimethacrylate (GPDM) could bond to a hydrochloric acid–etched dentin surface.[138] (*Note:* A complete listing of the chemical names mentioned in this chapter is provided in

TABLE 5.2	Abbreviations Commonly Used in Dentin/Enamel Adhesion Literature and in This Chapter
Abbreviation	**Chemical Name**
Bis-EMA	Bisphenol A ethoxylated dimethacrylate
Bis-GMA	Bisphenol A-glycidyl methacrylate
EDTA	Ethylenediamine tetra-acetic acid
GPDM	Glycerophosphoric acid dimethacrylate
HEMA	Hydroxyethyl methacrylate
10-MDP	10-Methacryloyloxy decyl dihydrogen phosphate
4-META	4-Methacryloxyethyl trimellitate anhydride
NPG-GMA	N-phenylglycine glycidyl methacrylate
PENTA	Dipentaerythritol penta-acrylate monophosphate
Phenyl-P	2-(Methacryloxy) ethyl phenyl hydrogen phosphate
UDMA	Urethane dimethacrylate

Table 5.2.) The bond strengths of this primitive adhesion technique were severely reduced by immersion in water. A few years before that report, another researcher had used the same monomer chemically activated with sulfinic acid, and that combination would later be known commercially as Sevriton Cavity Seal (Amalgamated Dental Company, London, England).[139,140]

First Generation

The development of the surface-active comonomer NPG-GMA was the basis for Cervident (S.S. White Burs, Inc., Lakewood, NJ), which is considered the first-generation dentin bonding system.[141,142] Theoretically, this comonomer could chelate with calcium on the tooth surface to generate water-resistant chemical bonds of resin to dentinal calcium.[143,144] The in vitro dentin bond strengths of this material were, however, in the range of only 2 to 3 MPa.[145] Likewise, the in vivo results were discouraging as Cervident had poor clinical results when used to restore NCCLs without mechanical retention.[146]

Second Generation

In 1978, the Clearfil Bond System F[c] was introduced in Japan (Kuraray Co., Ltd., Osaka, Japan). Generally recognized as the first product of the second generation of dentin adhesives, it was a phosphate-ester material (phenyl-P and hydroxyethyl methacrylate [HEMA] in ethanol). Its mechanism of action was based on the polar interaction between negatively charged phosphate groups in the resin and positively charged calcium ions in the smear layer.[145] The smear layer was the weakest link in the system because of its relatively loose attachment to the dentin surface. Examination of both sides of failed bonds revealed the presence of smear layer debris.[147]

Several other phosphate-ester dentin bonding systems were introduced in the early 1980s, including Scotchbond (3M Dental Products, St. Paul, MN), Bondlite (Kerr Corporation, Orange, CA), and Prisma Universal Bond (DENTSPLY Caulk, Milford, DE). These second-generation dentin bonding systems typically had in vitro bond strengths of only 1 to 5 MPa, which was considerably below the 10-MPa value estimated as the threshold value for acceptable in vivo retention.[84,148] In addition to the problems caused

by the loosely attached smear layer, these resins were relatively devoid of hydrophilic groups and had large contact angles on intrinsically moist surfaces.[149] They did not wet dentin well, did not penetrate the entire depth of the smear layer, and therefore could not reach the superficial dentin to establish ionic bonding.[84] Whatever bonding did occur was due to interaction with calcium ions in the smear layer.[150]

The in vitro performance of second-generation adhesives after 6 months was unacceptable.[151] The bonding material tended to peel from the dentin surface after water storage, indicating that the interface between dentin and some types of chlorophosphate ester–based materials (e.g., second-generation dentin bonding systems) was unstable.[151,152] The in vivo performance of these materials was found to be clinically unacceptable 2 years after placement in cervical tooth preparations without additional retention, such as beveling and acid etching.[153,154]

Third Generation

The concept of phosphoric acid etching of dentin before application of a phosphate ester–type bonding agent was introduced by Fusayama et al. in 1979.[155] Because of the hydrophobic nature of the bonding resin however, acid etching did not produce a significant improvement in dentin bond strengths despite the flow of the resin into the open dentinal tubules.[86,156] Pulpal inflammatory responses were thought to be triggered by the application of acid on dentin surfaces, providing another reason to avoid etching.[157,158] Nevertheless, continuing the etched dentin philosophy, Kuraray introduced Clearfil New Bond in 1984. This phosphate-based material contained HEMA and a 10-carbon molecule known as *10-MDP* (10-methacryloyloxydecyl dihydrogen phosphate), which includes a long hydrophobic component and a short hydrophilic component.[143] Treatment of the smear layer with acidic primers was proposed using an aqueous solution of 2.5% maleic acid, 55% HEMA, and a trace of methacrylic acid (Scotchbond 2, 3M Dental Products).[95] Scotchbond 2 was the first dentin bonding system to receive "provisional" and "full acceptance" from the American Dental Association (ADA).[159] With this type of smear layer treatment, manufacturers effectively combined the dentin etching philosophy advocated in Japan with the more cautious approach advocated in Europe and the United States. The result was preservation of a modified smear layer with slight demineralization of the underlying intertubular dentin surface. Clinical results were mixed, with some reports of good performance and some reports of poor performance.[153,154]

The removal of the smear layer using chelating agents such as EDTA was recommended in the original Gluma system (Bayer Dental, Leverkusen, Germany) before the application of a primer solution of 5% glutaraldehyde and 35% HEMA in water. The effectiveness of this system might have been impaired however by the manufacturer's questionable recommendation of placing the composite over uncured unfilled resin.[154]

Most other third-generation materials were designed not to remove the entire smear layer, but to modify it and allow penetration of acidic monomers such as phenyl-P or PENTA (see Table 5.2). Despite promising laboratory results, some of the bonding mechanisms never resulted in satisfactory clinical results.[154]

Current Options for Resin–Dentin Bonding

Three-Step Etch-and-Rinse Adhesives

Although the smear layer acts as a "diffusion barrier" that reduces the permeability of dentin, it may be considered an obstacle that

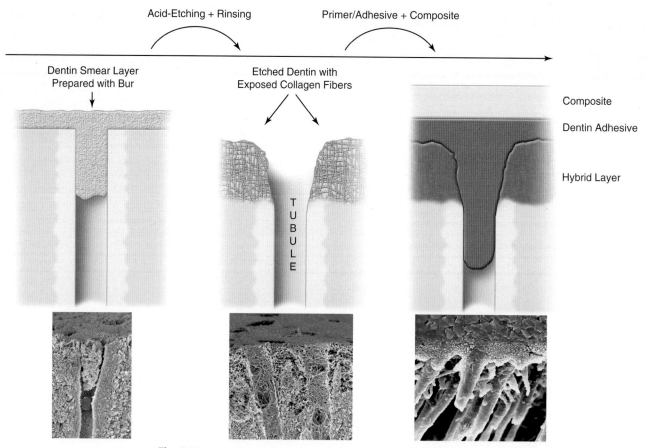

• **Fig. 5.12** Bonding of resin to dentin using an etch-and-rinse technique.

must be removed or chemically modified to permit resin bonding to the underlying dentin substrate.[65,83,160,161] Based on that consideration, a new generation of dentin adhesives was introduced for use on acid-etched dentin.[162] Removal of the smear layer via acid etching led to improvements in the in vitro bond strengths of resins to dentin.[163-166] Because the clinical technique involves simultaneous application of an acid to enamel and dentin, this method was originally known as the "total-etch" technique. Now more commonly called *etch-and-rinse technique*, it was the most popular strategy for dentin bonding during the 1990s and remains somewhat popular today (Fig. 5.12).

Application of acid to dentin results in partial or total removal of the smear layer and demineralization of the underlying dentin.[167] Acids demineralize intertubular and peritubular dentin, open the dentin tubules, and expose a dense filigree of collagen fibrils (see Fig. 5.6), increasing the microporosity of the intertubular dentin (Fig. 5.13).[67,167] Dentin is demineralized by up to approximately 7.5 μm depending on the type of acid, application time, and concentration.[67,167]

Despite the obvious penetration of early adhesives into the dentinal tubules, etching did not result in a significant improvement in bond strengths, possibly as a result of the hydrophobic nature of the phosphonated resin.[156] On the basis of concerns about the potential for inflammatory pulpal responses, acids were believed to be contraindicated for direct application on dentin, and the total-etch technique was not readily accepted in Europe or the United States. Adhesive systems based on the total-etch philosophy have proved successful however in vitro and in vivo.[154,168-170]

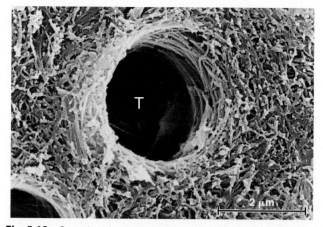

• **Fig. 5.13** Scanning electron micrograph of dentin that was kept moist after rinsing off the etchant. The abundant intertubular porosity serves as a pathway for the penetration of the dentin adhesive. *T*, Dentinal tubule.

Adhesive systems such as All-Bond 2 and All-Bond 3 (Bisco, Inc., Schaumburg, IL), OptiBond FL (Kerr Corporation), and Scotchbond Multi-Purpose (3M Oral Care, St. Paul, MN) (Table 5.3) are described by some authors as fourth-generation adhesives. However, because they include three essential components that are applied sequentially, they are more accurately described as three-step etch-and-rinse systems. The three essential components are (1) a phosphoric acid–etching gel that is rinsed off; (2) a primer

TABLE 5.3 Adhesive Systems Categorized by Adhesion Strategy

Type	Brand Names (Manufacturer)	COMPONENTS		
		1	2	3
Three-step etch-and-rinse	Adper Scotchbond Multi-Purpose (3M Oral Care) All-Bond 2 (Bisco, Inc.) All-Bond 3 (Bisco, Inc.) OptiBond FL (Kerr Corporation) Solobond Plus (Voco) Syntac (Ivoclar Vivadent)	Phosphoric acid	Hydrophilic primer	Bonding resin
Two-step etch-and-rinse	Admira Bond (Voco) Adper Single Bond Plus (3M Oral Care) ExciTE F (Ivoclar Vivadent) One-Step Plus (Bisco, Inc.) OptiBond SOLO Plus (Kerr Corporation) Prime & Bond NT (DENTSPLY Sirona) Prime & Bond XP (DENTSPLY Sirona)	Phosphoric acid	Combined (hydrophilic primer + bonding resin)	
Two-step self-etch	AdheSE (Ivoclar Vivadent) All-Bond SE (Bisco) Clearfil SE Bond (Kuraray Noritake Dental Inc) Clearfil SE Protect (Kuraray Noritake Dental Inc) OptiBond XTR (Kerr Corporation)		Self-etching primer	Bonding resin
One-step self-etch	Clearfil S³ Bond Plus (Kuraray Noritake Dental Inc) Futurabond M (Voco) iBond (Heraeus Kulzer) OptiBond All-in-One (Kerr Corporation) Xeno IV (DENTSPLY Sirona) Xeno V⁺ (DENTSPLY Sirona)	All-in-one Self-etch hydrophilic primer/bonding resin		
Two-step etch-and-rinse or One-step self-etch	Adhese Universal (Ivoclar Vivadent) All-Bond Universal (Bisco, Inc.) Clearfil Universal Bond (Kuraray Noritake Dental Inc) Futurabond U (Voco) One Coat 7 Universal (Coltene) Prime & Bond Elect (DENTSPLY Sirona) Scotchbond Universal Adhesive (3M Oral Care) Prime & Bond Active (DENTSPLY Sirona)	Phosphoric acid Self-etch hydrophilic primer/bonding resin	Hydrophilic bonding resin	

containing reactive hydrophilic monomers in ethanol, acetone, or water; and (3) a nonsolvated unfilled or filled resin bonding agent. Some authors refer to this third step as *adhesive*. It contains hydrophobic monomers such as Bis-GMA, frequently combined with hydrophilic molecules such as HEMA.

The acid-etching step not only alters the mineral content of the dentin substrate but also changes its surface-free energy.[77,162] The latter is an undesirable effect because for good interfacial contact, any adhesive must have a low surface tension, and the substrate must have a high surface-free energy.[84,152,171] Phosphoric acid etching of dentin removes hydroxyapatite, which has high surface energy, exposing the low surface energy collagen. A correlation exists between the ability of an adhesive to spread on the dentin surface and the concentration of calcium on that same surface.[172] The primer in a three-step system is designed to increase the critical surface tension of dentin, and a direct correlation between surface energy of dentin and shear bond strengths has been shown.[77]

When primer and bonding resin are applied to etched dentin, they penetrate the intertubular dentin, forming a resin–dentin interdiffusion zone or hybrid layer. They also penetrate and polymerize in the open dentinal tubules, forming resin tags. For most etch-and-rinse adhesives, the ultramorphologic characterization of the transition between the hybrid layer and the unaffected dentin

suggests that an abrupt shift from hybrid tissue to mineralized tissue occurs, without any empty space or pathway that could result in leakage (Figs. 5.14 and 5.15). The demarcation line seems to consist of hydroxyapatite crystals embedded in the resin from the hybrid layer (see Fig. 5.15B). For self-etch adhesive systems, the transition is more gradual, with a superficial zone of resin-impregnated smear residues and a deeper zone, close to the unaffected dentin, rich in hydroxyapatite crystals (Fig. 5.16).

Two-Step Etch-and-Rinse Adhesives

Much of the research and development (R&D) has focused on the simplification of the bonding procedure. A number of dental materials manufacturers market a simplified, two-step etch-and-rinse adhesive system. Some authors refer to these as fifth-generation adhesives. A separate etching step still is required. In vitro dentin bond strengths obtained with two-step etch-and-rinse adhesives have improved so much that they approach the level of enamel bonding.[56] However, three-step etch-and-rinse adhesives result in better laboratory and clinical performance than two-step etch-and-rinse adhesives.[170,173-175]

Numerous two-step etch-and-rinse adhesive systems are available (see Table 5.3), including One-Step Plus (Bisco, Inc.), Prime & Bond NT (DENTSPLY Sirona, York, PA, USA), Adper Single

Bond Plus (3M Oral Care), OptiBond SOLO Plus (Kerr Corporation), PQ1 (Ultradent Products, South Jordan, UT), ExciTE F (Ivoclar Vivadent, Schaan, Liechtenstein), One Coat Bond (Coltene, Altstätten, Switzerland), and Prime & Bond XP (DENTSPLY Sirona).

Different from three-step etch-and-rinse adhesives, these simplified etch-and-rinse materials do not contain a hydrophobic bonding agent as the last bonding step. The primer/adhesive single solution in two-step etch-and-rinse adhesives contains solvents and hydrophilic components from the primer that are mixed with the hydrophobic monomers from the bonding agent. For this reason, hydrolytic degradation, which directly relates to the hydrophilicity of the adhesive,[176] is more evident in two-step etch-and-rinse adhesives when compared to their nonsimplified predecessors.[174,176] Active rubbing application and the use of multiple coats of the adhesive have been shown to somewhat compensate for the lack of a hydrophobic resin bonding agent layer as the last step in two-step etch-and-rinse adhesives.[177,178]

Two-Step Self-Etch Adhesives

An alternative bonding strategy is the self-etch approach (Fig. 5.17; see Fig. 5.16).

Introduced in Japan, two-step self-etch adhesives (SEAs) contain an acidic monomer that functions as a self-etching primer and a hydrophobic nonsolvated bonding resin. The acidic primers include a phosphonated and/or carboxylated resin molecule that performs two functions simultaneously—etching and priming of dentin and enamel. In contrast to conventional etchants, the acidic primers are not rinsed off. The bonding mechanism of SEAs is based on the simultaneous etching and priming of enamel and dentin, forming a continuum in the substrate and incorporating smear plugs into the resin tags (Fig. 5.18).[179,180] In addition to simplifying the bonding technique, the elimination of rinsing and drying steps reduces the possibility of overwetting or overdrying dentin, either of which can affect adhesion adversely.[164,165] Also, water is always a component of the acidic primer because it is needed for the monomers to ionize and trigger demineralization of hard dental tissues; this makes SEAs less susceptible to variations in the degree of substrate moisture but more susceptible to chemical instability due to hydrolytic degradation.[176,181,182]

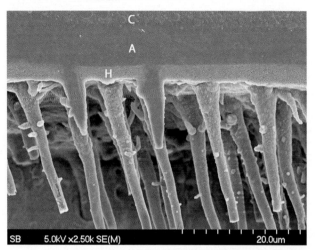

• **Fig. 5.14** Scanning electron micrograph of the transition between composite resin *(C)*–adhesive *(A)*, adhesive–hybrid layer *(H)*, and hybrid layer–dentin.

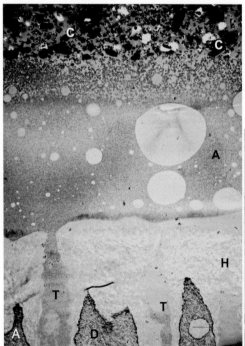
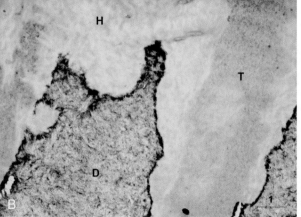

• **Fig. 5.15** Transmission electron micrograph of a resin–dentin interface formed by the etch-and-rinse adhesive Adper Single Bond Plus (3M Oral Care). This specimen was not decalcified or stained; the unaltered dentin appears darker and the hybrid layer appears lighter. A, General view showing the composite *(C)*, the adhesive *(A)*, the hybrid layer *(H)*, a filled resin tag *(T)*, and the unaffected dentin *(D)*. B, Higher magnification of the transition between the hybrid layer and unaffected dentin. Note the filler in the resin tag as small dark dots (nanofiller).

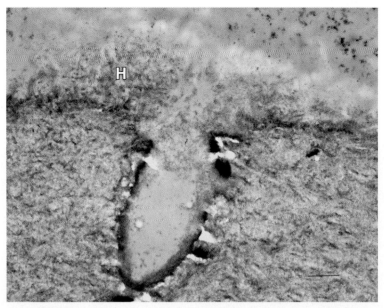

• **Fig. 5.16** Transmission electron micrograph of a resin–dentin interface formed with the two-step self-etch adhesive Clearfil SE Bond (Kuraray Noritake Dental Inc.). Residual hydroxyapatite crystals and residual components of the smear layer are embedded in the resin within the hybrid layer *(H)*.

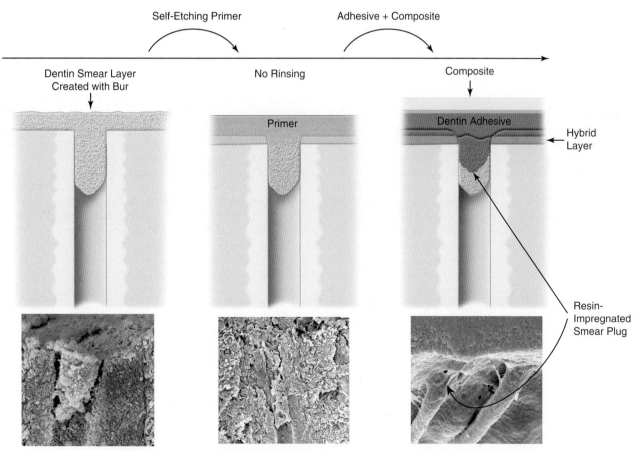

• **Fig. 5.17** Bonding to dentin using a self-etch primer.

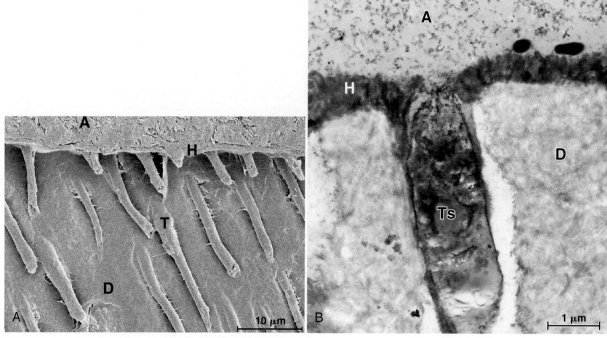

• **Fig. 5.18** *A,* Scanning electron micrograph of a resin–dentin interface formed with Clearfil SE Bond (Kuraray Noritake Dental Inc.) on chemical dissolution of the superficial dentin. *B,* Transmission electron micrograph of a resin–dentin interface formed with Clearfil SE Bond on EDTA decalcification and staining with uranyl acetate and lead citrate. *A,* Adhesive; *D,* residual dentin (appears gray in *B* because it was decalcified with EDTA); *H,* hybrid layer (appears dark in *B* because of decalcification followed by staining); *T,* resin tag; *Ts,* resin tag that incorporates the smear plug.

Because they are user friendly and do not require the etching and rinsing step, SEAs have become very popular.[183] One disadvantage is that some SEAs do not etch enamel as well as phosphoric acid, particularly if the enamel has not been instrumented.[184,185] However, some of the in vitro enamel bond strengths obtained with SEAs may not reflect their actual bonding effectiveness as the use of silicon carbide (Si-C) paper in in vitro experiments creates smear layers that are not clinically relevant.[160] If enamel is not etched adequately, the seal of enamel margins in vivo might be compromised.[186,187] When enamel bonds are stressed in the laboratory by thermal cycling, some of the first SEAs were more likely than etch-and-rinse systems to undergo deterioration.[188] This decrease in bond strengths with thermal fatigue might be a sign that a potential exists for enamel microleakage when SEAs are employed to bond to enamel. In a 10-year recall of an older generation SEA, 39 of 44 restorations had marginal discoloration.[189] The enamel bond strengths of some newer SEAs approach the enamel bond strengths of phosphoric acid–based adhesives however, suggesting that SEAs are gradually being developed to replace etch-and-rinse adhesive systems.

Several two-step SEAs are available, including AdheSE (Ivoclar Vivadent), All-Bond SE (Bisco, Inc.), Clearfil SE Bond or Clearfil SE Bond 2 (Kuraray Noritake Dental Inc., Tokyo, Japan), Clearfil SE Protect (Kuraray Noritake Dental Inc.), and OptiBond XTR (Kerr Corporation) (see Table 5.3). Clearfil SE Bond contains an aqueous mixture of a phosphoric acid ester monomer (10-MDP), with a much higher pH than that of phosphoric acid etchants.[190] Although the pH of a 34% to 37% phosphoric acid gel is much lower than 1.0, the pH of Clearfil SE Primer (Kuraray Noritake Dental Inc.) is 1.9 to 2.0.[167,191] SEAs have been classified according to their pH in three categories: *mild, moderate,* and *aggressive,* with Clearfil SE Bond being a mild SEA.[191] Mild SEAs tend to provide excellent dentin bond strengths and poorer enamel bonds, whereas more aggressive self-etch systems provide the reverse. Clearfil SE Bond resulted in 93% retention rate in Class V composite restorations at 13 years with selective enamel etching of the margins versus 86% without enamel etching, but the difference was not statistically significant.[192] Selective enamel etching improved marginal adaptation and marginal discoloration compared to the self-etch strategy.[192] In posterior restorations, Clearfil SE Bond resulted in 100% retention rate at 2 years with a tendency for deterioration of the composite margins compared with the etch-and-rinse control Adper Single Bond.[168] The clinical success of Clearfil SE Bond might be a result of its chemical composition, specifically the monomer 10-MDP, which has been shown to bond chemically to calcium in hydroxyapatite through a mechanism known as nanolayering.[65,193]

SEAs are less technique sensitive than are etch-and-rinse adhesives. Additionally, SEAs are less likely to result in a discrepancy between the depth of demineralization and the depth of resin infiltration because SEAs demineralize and infiltrate dentin simultaneously.[190] Recently, however, that concept has been challenged by showing that Clearfil SE Bond may also present partially demineralized dentin beneath the hybrid layer.[194] SEAs do not remove the smear layer from dentin completely (see Figs. 5.16 and 5.17), and in some cases smear layer remnants may interfere with in vitro bond strengths.[161] For some self-etch adhesives, collagen fibrils in the hybrid layer are not totally enveloped by the adhesive, leaving a partially demineralized dentin layer.[195] Strong one-step SEAs continue the demineralization of the adjacent dentin structure in the tubules, which may also result in exposed collagen fibers.[196] The presence of a hybrid layer that is not completely infiltrated by the adhesive may increase the stresses in resin–dentin interfaces.[194]

Research has been conducted on the potential for remineralization of the partially infiltrated demineralized collagen inside the hybrid layer. One of the methods used to remineralize exposed dentin collagen fibrils is the application of casein phosphopeptide-amorphous calcium phosphate (CPP-ACP), which has been shown to have the potential to induce biomimetic mineralization of dentin collagen fibrils.[197] Another method with promising results is to obtain intrafibrillar and interfibrillar remineralization of a 5-μm-thick layer of demineralized dentin with the inclusion of carboxylic acid–containing and phosphonic acid–containing polyelectrolytes as biomimetic analogues in a phosphate-containing fluid.[198] More recently it has been demonstrated that intermediate precursors of calcium phosphate biomineralization may be prefabricated for loading and release with the goal of achieving collagen intrafibrillar mineralization with released fluidic intermediate precursors.[199] These authors reported that collagen fibrils can be mineralized using polyacid-stabilized amorphous calcium phosphate loaded with amine-functionalized mesoporous silica nanoparticles. These nanoparticles may be included in the composition of dentin adhesives as controlled release devices for the delivery of the amorphous calcium phosphate prenucleation clusters to remineralize deficiently infiltrated hybrid layers.[200]

Despite the prevailing opinion that SEAs cause less postoperative sensitivity compared with etch-and-rinse systems, recent clinical studies have shown no relationship between the type of adhesive and the occurrence of postoperative sensitivity.[201-206]

One-Step Self-Etch Adhesives

Continuing the trend toward simplification, no-rinse self-etch materials that incorporate the fundamental steps of etching, priming, and bonding into one solution have become increasingly popular. In contrast to conventional adhesive systems that contain an intermediate light-cured, low-viscosity bonding resin to join the composite restorative material to the primed dentin–enamel substrate, these one-step SEAs contain uncured ionic monomers that contact the composite restorative material directly.[207,208] Their acidic unreacted monomers are responsible in part for the incompatibility between these simplified adhesives and self-cured composites (discussed later).[209] Additionally, one-step SEAs tend to behave as semipermeable membranes, facilitating hydrolytic degradation of the resin–dentin interface.[181] Because these adhesives must be acidic enough to be able to demineralize enamel and penetrate dentin smear layers, the hydrophilicity of their resin monomers, usually organophosphates and carboxylates, also is high. Some of these resin monomers are too hydrophilic, which makes them liable to water degradation.[176,210]

One-step SEAs, which have etching, priming, and bonding functions delivered in a single solution, include AdheSE One F (Ivoclar Vivadent), All-Bond SE (Bisco Inc.), Bond Force (Tokuyama Dental Corporation Inc., Tokyo, Japan), Clearfil S³ Bond Plus (Kuraray Noritake Dental Inc.), iBOND Self-Etch (Heraeus Kulzer GmbH, Hanau, Germany), OptiBond All-in-One (Kerr Corporation), and Xeno IV (DENTSPLY Sirona) (see Table 5.3). The pH of one-step SEAs affects their clinical properties. Also, application of multiple coats significantly increases dentin bond strengths and decreases leakage, suggesting that some of the one-step SEAs might not coat the dentin surface uniformly.[211]

The in vitro and clinical behavior of one-step SEAs improves with the addition of an extra coat of a hydrophobic bonding layer.[212-214] In a clinical study in Class V lesions, the one-step SEA iBond resulted in 40% retention rate at 18 months.[212] For the group to which an extra layer of a thick bonding resin was added (Scotchbond Multi-Purpose Adhesive), the retention rate increased to 83.3% at 18 months. This behavior of one-bottle SEAs may be related to their behavior as semipermeable membranes in vitro and in vivo.[181,215] Simplified SEAs do not provide a hermetic seal for vital deep dentin as demonstrated by transudation of dentinal fluid across the polymerized adhesives to form fluid droplets on the surface of the adhesive.[176]

Universal Adhesives

Dentists have used dentin adhesives following the adhesion strategy recommended by the respective manufacturer. With the advent of universal adhesives dentists are now using the same dentin adhesive for different adhesion strategies (i.e., self-etch, etch-and-rinse, or selective enamel etch adhesive), according to each specific clinical situation. Because of their multistrategy approach, this new generation of one-bottle dental adhesives has become very popular in dentistry.

These adhesives are basically one-step self-etch adhesives that can be used under different adhesion strategies (see Table 5.3).[216-218] As one-step SEAs, universal adhesives also benefit from the application of an extra hydrophobic bonding resin.[219] The major difference between traditional one-step SEAs and universal adhesives is that most universal adhesives contain 10-MDP (and/or other monomers), which is capable of bonding ionically to hydroxyapatite through nanolayering.[65,220] The 10-MDP molecule forms stable calcium-phosphate salts without causing strong decalcification. The chemical bonding formed by 10-MDP is more stable in water than that of other monomers used in the composition of SEAs, such as 4-META and phenyl-P.[221] Because the nature of the chemical bonding provided by 10-MDP depends on the concentration of this molecule, the extent of chemical bonding in universal adhesives is very weak compared to that observed for the two-step SEA Clearfil SE Bond.[220] Additionally, the presence of HEMA may hamper the chemical bonding ability of 10-MDP–containing universal adhesives,[222] because it reduces the formation of MDP-Ca salts.

The active application (rubbing) of 10-MDP–containing adhesives results in more intense nanolayering than passive application.[65] It has also been shown that active application results in higher bond strengths to intact enamel for most universal adhesives compared to passive application.[223] These improvements from rubbing the adhesive on the bonding substrate may be caused by higher concentration of 10-MPD molecules in intimate contact with the hydroxyapatite crystals in addition to higher rate of solvent evaporation from the enamel and dentin surfaces.[65]

Differences in the hydroxyapatite structure in dentin and enamel dictate the interaction pattern of 10-MDP with these substrates. The lesser amount and smaller hydroxyapatite crystals in dentin and their criss-cross orientation compared to a more parallel orientation in enamel makes dentin more receptive to the chemical interaction between 10-MDP and hydroxyapatite. This interaction discloses the formation of a nanolayered structure, which is reduced in enamel compared to dentin.[65]

Universal adhesives show signs of interfacial bonding degradation after 12-month water storage when applied either as self-etch or etch-and-rinse adhesives, although the self-etch strategy caused less nanoleakage.[224] In spite of the simplification of the bonding protocol, universal adhesives will likely undergo the same degradation pattern observed with older one-step SEAs.[218]

Moist Versus Dry Dentin Surfaces With Etch-and-Rinse Adhesives

Because vital dentin is inherently wet, complete drying of dentin is difficult to achieve clinically.[165,225] Water has been considered an obstacle for attaining an effective adhesion of resins to dentin, so research has shifted toward the development of dentin adhesives that are compatible with humid environments. The "moist bonding" technique used with etch-and-rinse adhesives prevents the spatial alterations (i.e., collagen collapse) that occur on drying demineralized dentin (Fig. 5.19; compare with Fig. 5.13).[165] Such alterations might prevent the monomers from penetrating the labyrinth of nanochannels formed by dissolution of hydroxyapatite crystals between collagen fibrils.[226,227]

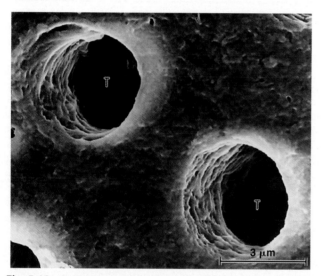

• **Fig. 5.19**   Scanning electron micrograph of dentin collagen after acid etching with 35% phosphoric acid. Dentin was air-dried. The intertubular porosity disappeared as a consequence of the collapse of the collagen secondary to the evaporation of water that served as a backbone to keep collagen fibrils raised.

The use of etch-and-rinse adhesive systems on moist dentin is made possible by incorporation of the organic solvents acetone or ethanol in the primers or adhesives. Because the solvent can displace water from the dentin surface and the moist collagen network, it promotes the infiltration of resin monomers throughout the nanospaces of the dense collagen web. The moist bonding technique has been shown repeatedly to enhance bond strengths of etch-and-rinse adhesives in vitro because water preserves the porosity of the collagen network available for monomer interdiffusion.[165,225,228] Studies showed that the excess water after rinsing the etching gel can be removed with a damp cotton pellet, high-volume suction, disposable brush, or laboratory tissue paper without adversely affecting bond strengths.[229,230] If the dentin surface is dried with air in vitro, the collagen mesh may undergo immediate collapse and prevent resin monomers from penetrating (Fig. 5.20).[231,232]

When etched dentin is dried using an air syringe, in vitro bond strengths decrease substantially, especially for acetone-based and (to a lesser extent) ethanol-based dentin adhesive systems.[164,232,233] When water is removed, the elastic characteristics of collagen may be lost. While in a wet state, wide gaps separate the collagen molecules from each other.[234] In a dry state, the molecules are arranged more compactly. This is because extrafibrillar spaces in hydrated type I collagen are filled with water, whereas dried collagen has fewer extrafibrillar spaces open for the penetration of the monomers included in the adhesive systems.[235] During air-drying, water that occupies the interfibrillar spaces previously filled with hydroxyapatite crystals is lost by evaporation, resulting in a decrease of the volume of the collagen network to about one third of its original volume.[231] Under the scanning electron microscope, the adhesive does not seem to penetrate etched intertubular dentin that has been dried.[232] Under the transmission electron microscope (TEM), collagen fibrils coalesce into a structure without individualized interfibrillar spaces.[232] When air-dried demineralized dentin is rewetted with water, the collagen matrix may reexpand and recover its primary dimensions to the levels of the original hydrated state.[227,231,236] This spatial reexpansion is a result of the spaces between fibrils being refilled with water, but also reexpansion occurs because type I collagen itself is capable of undergoing expansion on rehydration.[237] The stiffness of decalcified dentin increases when the tissue is dehydrated chemically in water-miscible solvents or physically in air.[227] The increase in stiffness is reversed when specimens are

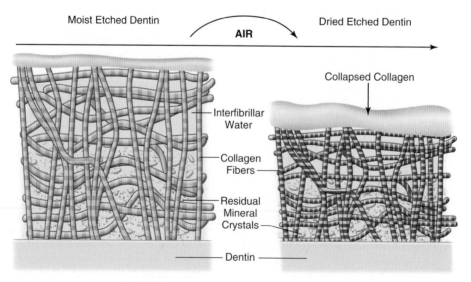

Moist Etched Dentin   AIR →   Dried Etched Dentin

Collapsed Collagen

Interfibrillar Water

Collagen Fibers

Residual Mineral Crystals

Dentin

• **Fig. 5.20**   Collapse of etched dentin by air-drying.

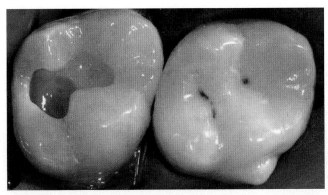

• **Fig. 5.21** Clinical aspect of moist dentin—a glistening appearance without accumulation of water. (From Rubinstein S, Nidetz A: The art and science of the direct posterior restoration: Recreating form, color, and translucency, *Alpha Omegan* 100(1):30–35, 2007.)

rehydrated in water. Rewetting dentin after air-drying to check for the enamel frosty aspect is an acceptable clinical procedure.[68,238] In addition, pooled moisture should not remain on the tooth because excess water can dilute the primer and render it less effective.[233,239] A glistening hydrated surface is preferred (Fig. 5.21).[240]

Although having adequate dentin surface moisture is important, agitation of the hydrophilic primer/adhesive during application of two-step etch-and-rinse adhesives may be critical for optimal adhesive infiltration into the demineralized collagen network. That procedure also may aid in the evaporation of residual water in the adhesive and hybrid layers preventing nanoleakage.[177,178,215] It is speculated that active rubbing of the adhesive compresses the demineralized collagen network, which is filled with the adhesive upon pressure release and expansion of the collagen. A recent clinical trial compared the performance of Prime & Bond NT using no rubbing action, slight rubbing action, and vigorous rubbing action in the restoration of NCCLs. While retention rates of 82.5% were found for the no rubbing action and slight rubbing action groups, 92.5% of the restorations in the vigorous rubbing action group were retained after 24 months of clinical service.[177]

In case universal adhesives are applied using an etch-and-rinse strategy, it may not be necessary to leave dentin moist for two reasons:

(1) Universal adhesives contain 10% to 20% water, which may be able to rewet dried dentin. Their bond strengths to dentin that has been air-dried for 10 seconds is similar to their bond strengths to moist dentin.[217]

(2) Manufacturers recommend the evaporation of the solvent with air for 5 seconds after the application of the universal adhesive (10 seconds for All-Bond Universal); however, 5 seconds is not enough to evaporate the water added to the composition of the adhesive.[241] If dentists leave dentin moist prior to applying universal adhesives, the amount of residual water left into the dentin substrate after air-drying will reduce bond strengths and substantially increase hydrolytic degradation of the bonded interface.[242]

Recently, some in vitro research has evaluated the possibility of replacing water with ethanol in the etched dentin collagen network, a technique known as "ethanol wet-bonding."[243,244] When acid-etched dentin is saturated with 100% ethanol instead of water, the bond strengths of both hydrophilic and hydrophobic resins increase significantly.[243,244] Although ethanol wet-bonding appears promising, it involves an extra step of replacing rinse water with 100% ethanol, and no clinical studies are available. Additionally,

the time needed to replace water with ethanol in the dentin collagen network would make the technique difficult to implement in a clinical setting.

Role of Water in Self-Etch Adhesives

Water plays different roles in the bonding mechanisms of self-etch adhesives and etch-and-rinse adhesives. Unlike etch-and-rinse adhesives, self-etch systems do not include separate acid-etching and rinsing steps. The functions of etching and priming are simultaneously performed by the acidic monomers. Water (10–30 weight percent [wt%]) is added to the hydrophilic formulations to ionize the acidic methacrylate monomers (usually phosphate or carboxylic) and to solubilize calcium and phosphate ions that form from the interaction of the monomers with dentin and enamel.[245,246] When SEAs are formulated, a compromise must be made to provide sufficient water for adequate ionization of the acidic monomers without lowering the monomer concentration to levels that would jeopardize the bonding efficacy. Increasing the water concentration from 0 to 60 volume percent (vol%) in the acidic primer resulted in improved acidic monomer ionization and increased depth of dentin demineralization created by the acidic monomers.[246] However, increasing the water concentration dilutes the concentration of the acidic monomer, thereby lowering the bonding efficacy of the respective adhesive system.

The mechanical properties of one-step SEAs might be significantly compromised in the presence of water, which is less likely to occur with two-step SEAs.[247] One-step SEAs have higher water absorption or solubility than two-step self-etch adhesives.[175,248]

Role of Proteins in Dentin Bonding

Despite efforts to generate new dental materials that can enhance dentin bonding, the stability of the hybrid layer and thus long-term acceptable bond strength are still a challenge. Stability of the hybrid layer due to hydrolytic degradation of dentin collagen fibrils that have been exposed by acid etching of dentin and not completely embedded by adhesive during the bonding procedure continues to be extensively studied. The degradation is enzyme driven and compromises the hybrid layer, which becomes the restoration's weakest link.[249,250] This observation is important because acid etching demineralizes dentin and may leave a layer of exposed collagen at the bottom of the hybrid layer.[251,252] However, it has been reported that when demineralized dentin is restored with an adhesive system, the demineralized layer might undergo remineralization within 4 months.[253]

Some evidence also suggests that phosphoric acid causes denaturation of collagen fibrils in dentin.[254,255] Concerns about potential effects of phosphoric acid on dentin collagen arose from its known susceptibility to other acids such as bacterial lactic acid in caries processes.[256] However, it has been demonstrated that treatment of collagen with phosphoric acid does not significantly alter the biochemistry of dentin collagen as per analyses of collagen intramolecular and intermolecular cross-links.[257] Although evidence suggests that longer etching times might denature the collagen fibril, the normal 15-second etch does not change the spatial configuration of the collagen molecule. Etching for 15 seconds does not compromise the bonding substrate.[258]

Collagen type I is the main organic component of dentin.[69] The mineralized dentin structure carries a well-compressive load, as mineral crystals minimize movement and deformation of the collagen. In physiologic conditions (dentin formation), particles are deposited within (intrafibrillar) and on the surface (interfibrillar) of collagen fibrils.[259,260] Structures such as bone and dentin have different mechanical properties from nonmineralized tissues. Mineralized structures are much stiffer, and although they tolerate compression well, they cannot extend much in tension.[261] When phosphoric acid treatment removes the mineral around and within collagen fibrils, the tension and compressive strength of the collagen change. Then, the cross-linking of collagen fibrils is extremely important in providing the mechanical and adaptive response.[262,263] In this regard, hydration also plays a major role. In hydrated and nonmineralized collagen, hydrogen bonds form between collagen and water, which allows for slipping and movement. However, as the collagen is dried, bonds form directly between collagen molecules and within fibrils, preventing sliding and stiffening the structure. With dehydration, the stress point lowers and collagen fibrils break more easily.[264] In dentin bonding, ideally collagen should be demineralized as minimally as possible, keeping the demineralized collagen hydrated and infiltrated with a hydrophilic adhesive to ensure proper penetration within the exposed collagen fibrils.

Ninety percent of the protein content of dentin is type I collagen and the remaining are noncollagenous proteins. The noncollagenous proteins fall into several categories: proteoglycans (PGs), SIBLINGs, growth factors, matrix metalloproteinases (MMPs), serum proteins, among others. A few of these noncollagenous proteins act as nucleators for mineral growth and dentin mineralization. The most characterized dentin mineral nucleator is dentin phosphoprotein (DPP). This protein is able to bind calcium and present it to collagen at the mineralization front during the formation of dentin.[265] It contains a large number of aspartic acid residues and thus is acidic. Biomimetic analogs of such proteins that are as acidic as DPP are able to create amorphous calcium phosphate precursors and to bind to dentin collagen.[266-269] Polyacrylic, polycarboxylic, and polyvinylphosphonic acids have been used as analogs of dentin noncollagenous phosphoproteins and have been able to induce intrafibrillar mineralization within hybrid layers when exposed to a remineralization media containing a calcium hydroxide–releasing material.[270-272]

Another noncollagenous protein category of importance in dentin bonding is the MMP family. Matrix metalloproteinases are zinc-dependent and calcium-dependent endopeptidases capable of degrading all extracellular matrix components.[273-275] In 1999, one study suggested that the direct inhibition of the MMP activity by chlorhexidine might explain the beneficial effects of chlorhexidine in the treatment of periodontitis.[276] Chlorhexidine was first used in dentin bonding as a dentin disinfectant prior to the application of the dentin adhesive. SEM revealed that chlorhexidine debris remained on the dentin surface and within the tubules of etched dentin after rinsing, but chlorhexidine had no significant effect on the dentin shear bond strengths.[277]

More recently, research has shifted toward the preservation of the hybrid layer through the inhibition of specific dentin proteases capable of degrading collagen, using chlorhexidine as a protease inhibitor.[278] Collagen fibrils that are not encapsulated by resin might be vulnerable to degradation by endogenous MMPs after acid etching.[273] Collagenolytic and gelatinolytic activities found in partially demineralized dentin imply the existence of MMP in human dentin.[273] Dentin contains gelatinases (MMP-2 and MMP-9), collagenase (MMP-8), and enamelysin (MMP-20).[273-275] These enzymes are trapped within the mineralized dentin matrix during odontogenesis.[273,275]

Dentin collagenolytic and gelatinolytic activities can be overcome by protease inhibitors, indicating that MMP inhibition might

preserve the integrity of the hybrid layer and reduce the rate of resin–dentin bond degradation within the first few months after restoration.[278,279] When chlorhexidine is used, the integrity of the hybrid layer and the magnitude of bond strengths are preserved in aged resin–dentin interfaces.[280-282] When phosphoric acid is applied without the subsequent application of chlorhexidine, it does not inhibit the collagenolytic activity of mineralized dentin. In contrast, the use of chlorhexidine after acid etching—even in very low concentrations—strongly inhibits that activity.

However, the role of MMPs in dentin bonding is not completely clear for several reasons: (1) The immunoreactivity of MMP-2 is localized preferably in predentin and around the DEJ in teeth from subjects age 12 to 30 years; (2) MMP-2 and MMP-9 are both gelatinases and are unable to degrade the collagen fibrils directly, so the initial degradation step has to be performed by another mechanism; (3) MMPs do not inhibit the degradation of bonded interfaces created by self-etch adhesives; and (4) preservation of the hybrid layer can occur even in the absence of MMP inhibitors.[283-285]

Microleakage and Nanoleakage

"Microleakage" is defined as the passage of bacteria and their toxins between restoration margins and tooth preparation walls. Clinically, microleakage becomes important when one considers that pulpal irritation is more likely caused by bacteria than by chemical toxicity of restorative materials.[286-288] An adhesive restoration might not bond sufficiently to etched dentin to prevent gap formation at margins.[289] Several studies have shown that the pulpal response to restorative materials is related to the degree of marginal leakage.[291-294] Bacteria are able to survive and proliferate within the fluid-filled marginal gaps under composite restorations. If the restoration is hermetically sealed, bacteria may not be able to survive.[286,293]

Despite the common presence of marginal gaps, their occurrence at the resin–dentin interface does not necessarily cause debonding of the restoration. Despite having shown excellent marginal seal in vitro, OptiBond (Kerr Corporation) does not completely seal the interface in vivo.[94] Other reports showed excellent clinical retention of OptiBond and OptiBond FL in Class V lesions at 12 and 13 years, respectively.[94,169,170] If a dentin adhesive system does not adhere intimately to the dentin substrate, an interfacial gap eventually develops; bacteria may penetrate through this gap and cause demineralization of the substrate around the restoration margins.[295] Despite the probability of an incomplete dentin margin seal, Class V clinical studies using etch-and-rinse dentin adhesive systems reported no findings of pulpal inflammation or necrosis.[76,154]

Important to point out is that in vitro microleakage measurements for a specific adhesive material often do not correlate with clinical behavior of the same material.[296] Additionally, silver nitrate penetration may be a particularly demanding test of marginal seal because silver ions are smaller than the bacteria that colonize the oral cavity.[297]

When all margins of the restoration are in enamel, the quality and integrity of the bonds remain unchanged with time, at least in vitro.[298] Degradation of the bonds might result from hydrolysis, which occurs either in the adhesive resin or in the collagen fibril that are not fully enveloped by the adhesive in the hybrid layer, especially when margins are in dentin.[298-300] The degree of degradation of the bonded interface is more pronounced with simplified adhesives (i.e., one-step self-etch and two-step etch-and-rinse

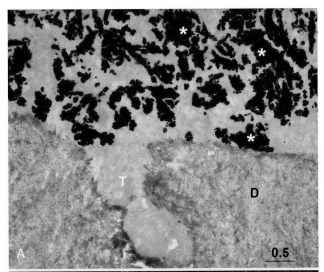

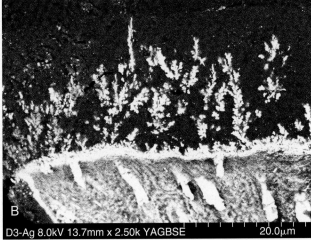

• **Fig. 5.22** Nanoleakage under the electron microscope. A, Spotted pattern in the hybrid layer formed by a one-step self-etch adhesive under the transmission electron microscope. B, Reticular pattern and "water trees" in the adhesive layer formed by a one-step self-etch adhesive under the scanning electron microscope in backscattered mode.

Biocompatibility

Besides demineralizing the dentin surface, phosphoric acid removes the smear layer and opens the orifices of the tubules (see Fig. 5.12).[67,305] Despite past apprehension about potential acid penetration into the dentin tubules and pulp space, the interaction of etchants with dentin is limited to the superficial 1 to 7 μm.[67,167] It is unlikely that the acid is directly responsible for any injury to the pulp.[306,307] Acid penetration occurs primarily along the tubules, with penetration of intertubular dentin occurring at a lower rate.[307,308] The effects of etchants on dentin are limited by the buffering effect of hydroxyapatite and other dentin components, including collagen, which may act as a barrier that reduces the rate of demineralization.[309,310] Marshall et al. elucidated the importance of pH with regard to the effects of acids on dentin surfaces.[307] Etching rates increase dramatically with lower pH. Small differences in pH between acidic gels of similar phosphoric acid concentration may be responsible for distinct depths of dentin demineralization. Manufacturers add thickeners to facilitate handling and other modifiers (e.g., buffers, surfactants, and colorants) to their etching gels, which may contribute to that phenomenon.

Several early studies suggested that acidic components included in restorative materials such as silicate cements would trigger adverse pulp reactions.[157,311] For several decades, the development of adhesive systems was limited by the belief that acids applied to dentin during restorative procedures caused pulpal inflammation. The use of bases and liners was considered essential to protect the pulp from the toxicity of restorative materials. This concept has, however, changed over the years.[286,287,312,313]

Dentin adhesive systems are well tolerated by the pulp-dentin complex in the absence of bacterial infection.[313] To prevent bacterial infection, restorations must be hermetically sealed. The pulp response to dentin adhesives, when teeth are restored in an ideal clinical environment, has been studied using histologic assessment of animal pulps or in human premolars extracted for orthodontic reasons and in third molars extracted for surgical reasons.[288,289,312-319] Some clinical studies also have reported normal pulp responses after the application of adhesive on the dentin-pulp complex when the pulp is macroscopically exposed, although reports involved only one tooth.[320,321] Another study showed that the newest dentin adhesive systems are not harmful when applied to exposed pulps.[322] Several reports have shown however that etching the pulp and applying a dentin adhesive directly on the exposed pulp tissue results in severe inflammation and eventual formation of pulpal abscesses.[323-326] The solution for this disparity would be long-term follow-up of patients in whom the pulp was treated with acid and adhesive. Ethical concerns do not allow the routine use of pulpal etching in patients. It is known however that the thicker the remaining dentin left between the pulpal aspect of the preparation and the pulp, the better the prognosis for that specific pulp.[324] The concept of pulp capping remains a controversial topic.

Adverse pulpal reactions after a restorative procedure are not caused by the material used in that procedure but by bacteria remaining in, or penetrating, the preparation. In some cases, adverse reactions are caused by a combination of factors, as follows:

1. Bacterial invasion of the pulp, either from the tooth preparation or from an existing carious lesion[286,327]
2. Bacterial penetration into the pulp caused by a faulty restoration[286]
3. Pressure gradient caused by excessive desiccation or by excessive pressure during cementation[328,329]
4. Traumatic injuries[330,331]

adhesives). A nearly 50% reduction in bond strengths of the 24-hour control has been reported at 1 year with a one-step SEA.[299]

The term "nanoleakage" has been used to describe small porosities in the hybrid layer or at the transition between the hybrid layer and the mineralized dentin that allow the penetration of minuscule particles of a silver nitrate dye.[301] When ammoniacal silver nitrate is used, silver deposits penetrate the hybrid layer formed by either etch-and-rinse or self-etch adhesive materials.[302] Penetration of ammoniacal silver nitrate results in two distinct patterns of nanoleakage: (1) a spotted pattern in the hybrid layer of self-etch adhesives, which might be caused by incomplete resin infiltration (Fig. 5.22A), and (2) a reticular pattern that occurs in the adhesive layer, most likely caused by areas where water was not totally removed from the bonding area (see Fig. 5.22B).[303] The term "water trees" is associated with porosities in the polymerized adhesive layer.[303] Silver uptake in hybrid layers formed by one-step SEAs is associated with areas of increased permeability within the polymerized resin from which water was incompletely removed. The residual water prevents complete polymerization.[303] There has been, however, some discussion regarding the clinical relevance of nanoleakage and the methods used to assess it.[304]

5. Iatrogenic tooth preparation—excessive pressure, heat, or friction[328,332]
6. Pulpal temperature rise induced during the polymerization of composites, especially flowable composites[333,334]
7. Stress derived from polymerization contraction of composites and adhesives[335]
8. Unpolymerized resin monomers[336]

With regard to the biocompatibility issue, tooth preparations with enamel peripheries are important. When all margins are in enamel, polymerization shrinkage stresses at the interface are counteracted by strong enamel adhesion. Marginal gaps are less likely to form, and the restoration is sealed against bacteria.

Relevance of In Vitro Studies

One of the major concerns with laboratory bond strength testing is the wide range of results obtained for the same material in different testing sites. It is not an uncommon occurrence for the same dentin adhesive system to have average shear bond strengths of 20 MPa in one laboratory and bond strengths less than 10 MPa in another.[84,142] Also, dentin bond strengths for a specific dentin adhesive vary depending on the specific test used—microtensile, shear, or microshear.[337] Some perplexity exists that no correlation can be established between bond strength and degree of resin penetration into the hybrid layer.[338,339] To illustrate this discrepancy, some reports have suggested that dentin adhesives do not penetrate the whole depth of the demineralized dentin layer but still result in bond strengths greater than 20 MPa.[340,341] Intuitively, one would expect an inverse relationship between bond strength and microleakage, but that relationship has not been confirmed.[342]

The microtensile bond strength testing methodology has become popular in recent decades.[343] This method allows for the assessment of bond strengths using bonded surfaces with a cross-sectional area in the range of 1 to 1.5 mm^2 or even less (Fig. 5.23). Microtensile testing has several advantages over conventional shear and tensile bond strength methods for the following reasons:

1. It permits the use of only one tooth to fabricate several bonded dentin-resin rods.
2. It allows for testing substrates of clinical significance, such as carious dentin, cervical sclerotic dentin, and enamel.[344]
3. It results in fewer defects occurring in the small-area specimens, as reflected in higher bond strengths.[345]
4. It allows for the testing of regional differences in bond strengths within the same tooth.[346]

However, the results of the microtensile bond strength methodology vary in function of several testing parameters, including storage time, the cross-sectional shape of the microspecimen, remaining dentin thickness, and jig design.[347,348]

Although in vitro bond strength studies are only rough categorizing tools for evaluating the relative efficacy of bonding materials, they are excellent tools for screening new materials and for comparing the same parameter among different adhesive systems.[349] The

results of in vitro bond strength tests have been validated with clinical results because improvements seen in the laboratory environment from the earlier generations to contemporary adhesive systems have been confirmed in clinical trials.[154]

A systematic analysis of the correlation between in vitro marginal adaptation and the outcome of clinical trials of Class V restorations revealed that the correlation is weak and only present for studies that used the same composite for the in vitro and in vivo evaluation.[350] Another systematic review found a correlation between bond strength data and clinical retention rates of Class V restorations, specifically when the bond strength specimens were aged prior to testing.[349] The clinical parameter in Class V restorations that is more directly related to bond strength data is marginal adaptation.[338] Clinical studies with dentin adhesive systems are expensive for manufacturers and take at least 18 months to 3 years. Cost is a major concern, in part because of the constant developments in the area of adhesion, making new materials quickly obsolete. No financial incentive exists for the manufacturer to invest in a clinical study of a material that may not be on the market by the time the study is concluded. Consequently, in vitro studies are still used predominantly by manufacturers to anticipate the clinical behavior of their materials.

Several factors contribute to the questionable use of in vitro tests to predict clinical behavior. Among others, variables including age and storage conditions of the teeth used, dentin depth, degree of sclerosis, tooth surface to be bonded, dentin roughness, and type of test used frequently are not controllable.[4,5,351,352] According to some authors, one of the major drawbacks of laboratory bond strength testing is the usual lack of simulated pulpal pressure to replicate the pulpal pressure that occurs in vivo. Other authors have reported, however, that the pulpal pressure does not interfere significantly with bond strength results.[353]

Clinical Performance

Several clinical factors may influence the success of an adhesive restoration. The mineral content of dentin increases in different situations, including aged dentin, dentin beneath a carious lesion, and dentin exposed to the oral cavity in NCCLs in which the tubules become obliterated with tricalcium phosphate crystals.[343,354,355] The dentin that undergoes these compositional changes is called sclerotic dentin and is much more resistant to acid etching than "normal" dentin.[163,356] Consequently, the penetration of a dentin adhesive is limited.[356-358] Irrespective of the use of a etch-and-rinse or a self-etch technique, bonding to sclerotic dentin in NCCLs has resulted in low bond strengths.[355,359] Additionally, the clinical effectiveness of dentin adhesives is less in sclerotic cervical lesions than in normal dentin.[360,361] Nevertheless, some specific dentin adhesives may perform better in sclerotic dentin than in normal dentin.[362]

Some evidence suggests that masticatory forces not only might cause NCCLs but also might contribute to the failure of Class V restorations.[359,363,364] Bruxism or any other eccentric movement may generate lateral forces that cause concentration of stresses around the cervical area of the teeth. Although this stress may be of very low magnitude, the fatigue caused by cyclic stresses may cause failure of bonds between resin and dentin. Considering the challenges to successfully bond to NCCLs, these have been used often as ultimate clinical test to assess adhesives.

The type of composite used might play an important role in clinical longevity of Class V, as well as Class II, restorations.[350,365] Composites shrink as they polymerize, but the amount of shrinkage

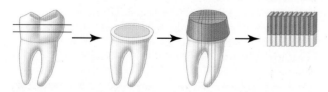

• **Fig. 5.23** Preparation of specimens for microtensile bond strength testing.

depends on the inorganic load of each specific composite. Microfilled composites have a low elastic (or Young) modulus, which means that they are better able to relieve stresses caused by polymerization or by tooth flexure.[366,367] Materials that have a higher Young modulus do not relieve stresses by flow; they are unable to compensate for the stresses accumulated during polymerization. These stresses subsequently might be transferred to the adhesive interface and cause debonding. As adhesives have improved however, restorative material stiffness might be less important. A 2-year clinical study of a three-step etch-and-rinse adhesive showed no difference in retention rates of Class V composite restorations based on stiffness of the restorative material.[368] Another clinical study reported that composite stiffness did not affect the clinical longevity of cervical composite restorations.[369]

A systematic review published in 2005[370] analyzed the literature published from January 1998 to May 2004 on the clinical effectiveness of adhesives to restore NCCLs to determine if simplified adhesives were as clinically effective as conventional three-step adhesives in terms of retention rate. Although GIC-based materials are usually outperformed by adhesively bonded restorations in in vitro studies, their clinical retention to tooth structure is more effective and durable than any other type of adhesive material. Three-step etch-and-rinse adhesives and two-step SEAs showed a clinically reliable clinical performance. The clinical effectiveness of two-step etch-and-rinse adhesives was less favorable, while the worst clinical performance was found for one-step SEAs.

A meta-analysis published in 2010, for which 50 clinical studies and 40 adhesive systems matched the inclusion criteria, reported that the clinical performance of dentin adhesives in NCCLs up to 3 years is significantly influenced by the type of adhesive system used and whether or not the dentin/enamel is roughened.[371] GIC-based materials, two-step SEAs, and three-step etch-and-rinse adhesives performed better than adhesives of the other categories. The use of rubber dam isolation did not increase the chance of survival of restorations in this meta-analysis.

Peumans et al.[174] conducted a systematic review in which they analyzed annual failure rates in NCCLs in publications, including AADR/IADR abstracts, up to 2013.[174] Dentin adhesive materials were divided into six main categories: three-step etch-and-rinse adhesives, two-step etch-and-rinse adhesives, two-step SEAs, one-step SEAs, GIC-based materials, and self-adhesive composites. Both classes of SEAs were further subdivided as "mild" and "intermediately strong" (pH ≥1.5) and "strong" (pH <1.5).[174] GIC-based materials had a 2% annual failure rate (AFR), which was the lowest for all adhesive classes analyzed. The AFR for two-step mild SEAs was 2.5% and for three-step etch-and-rinse adhesives was 3.1%. Higher AFRs were measured for one-step strong SEAs (5.4%), two-step etch-and rinse adhesives (5.8%), and two-step strong SEAs (7.9%). Selective enamel etching did not significantly influence the retention rate of SEAs.

Another recent meta-analysis analyzed prospective clinical trials on restorations of NCCLs with an observation period of at least 18 months.[132] Eighty-one studies involving 185 experiments for 47 adhesives matched the inclusion criteria. The respective authors concluded that 12.3% of the cervical restorations were lost, 27.9% exhibited marginal discoloration, and 34.6% exhibited marginal deterioration after 5 years of service. The clinical index[a] was 17.4% of failures after 5 years and 32.3% after 8 years; however, a great variability was measured for retention loss and marginal

discoloration. This meta-analysis concluded that roughened dentin and rubber-dam use resulted in a statistically significantly higher retention rate than unprepared dentin or no rubber dam. Enamel beveling however had no influence on any of the examined variables. Overall, one-step SEAs had a significantly worse clinical index than two-step SEAs and three-step etch-and-rinse adhesives.

Because universal adhesives are fairly recent materials, systematic reviews of clinical studies are not yet available. Two clinical trials have reported acceptable clinical effectiveness for the first universal adhesive introduced to the market, Scotchbond Universal Adhesive (Single Bond Universal in some regions) (3M Oral Care).[372,373] A 3-year clinical study compared this adhesive applied in different adhesion strategies (self-etch, selective enamel etch, etch-and-rinse applied on moist dentin, etch-and-rinse applied on air-dried dentin) and concluded that while there was no statistical difference among bonding strategies, there were signs of marginal degradation when the universal adhesive was applied in full self-etch mode.[372]

In summary, results from recent clinical studies and systematic reviews suggest that chemical bonding to dentin calcium may play a crucial role in stable adhesion to NCCLs, as GIC-based materials and mild two-step SEAs result in excellent retention rate. Roughening dentin in NCCLs may increase retention rate, whereas enamel beveling does not seem to be a significant factor. Although there is conflicting data on the influence of rubber-dam isolation, its use may decrease the failure rate of restorations in NCCLs. GIC-based materials are still the standard to restore NCCLs in terms of retention rate.

Incompatibility Issues With Self-Cure and Dual-Cure Composites

Chemically activated and dual-activated composites still have significant use in restorative dentistry, especially in areas of preparations with limited access to light. Examples include crown foundations, bonded posts, and ceramic and composite inlays, onlays, and crowns.

Several studies have reported incompatibility between specific light-cured adhesives and chemically activated composites.[209,374,375] In one study, Prime & Bond NT, which contains PENTA, a monomer with an acidic phosphate group, did not bond to a self-cured composite unless the adhesive was mixed with a sulfinic acid activator.[375] In another study, the reductions in mean bond strength of adhesives decreased by 45% to 91% when self-cured composite was used instead of light-cured composite.[374] The most drastic reduction was associated with Prime & Bond NT. The inhibition of polymerization of the self-cured composites by adhesives with specific compositions seems to be related directly to the pH of the adhesive.[374] One-Step, which caused the least reduction in bond strengths between self-cured and light-cured composite in that specific study, was the adhesive with the highest pH. Prime & Bond NT had the lowest (more acidic) pH.

Similarly, an adverse chemical interaction occurs between catalytic components of chemically cured composites and acidic one-step self-etch adhesives.[208,209] In contrast, despite the acidity of their primers, some two-step self-etch adhesives might be compatible with self-cure and dual-cure composites, owing to the presence of a thick resin layer that is less permeable and more hydrophobic than the layer formed with all-in-one systems.[208,209]

The issue related to the acidity of one-step adhesives also applies to recently introduced universal adhesives. This issue is particularly relevant because the indication for universal adhesives has been expanded to indirect restorations, including those made of

---

[a]Clinical index = (4xR + 2xMD + 1xMI) / 7 (R = Retention; MD = marginal discoloration; MI = detectable margins).

glass-matrix ceramics and oxide-based ceramics, without the need for additional primers.[376-378] While some current universal adhesives contain different functional monomers, the compatibility of universal adhesives with chemically activated and dual-cured resin-based composite materials has not been thoroughly investigated, especially taking into consideration that the pH of universal adhesives varies from to 1.6 to 3.2.[379,380] Among others, Clearfil Universal Bond (pH = 2.3, Kuraray Noritake Dental Inc.), One Coat 7 Universal (pH = 2.8, Coltene), Prime & Bond Elect (pH = 2.5, DENTSPLY Sirona), and Scotchbond Universal Adhesive (pH = 2.7, 3M Oral Care) are examples of universal adhesives for which the respective manufacturer recommends mixing the universal adhesive with a chemical activator when used with composite materials that contain a chemical activator, such as dual-cured buildup composite materials and dual-cured resin cements. AdheSE Universal (pH = 2.5–3, Ivoclar Vivadent) and All-Bond Universal (pH = 3.1–3.2, Bisco Inc.) are examples of universal adhesives for which the respective manufacturer does not recommend adding a chemical activator due the relatively high pH of the adhesive solution. The manufacturer of the universal adhesive Xeno Select (DENTSPLY Sirona, also known as Prime & Bond One Select in some countries) does not recommend this adhesive for any indirect restorations due to its low pH (1.6).[380]

All current universal adhesives that are recommended for indirect restorations resulted in high bond strengths to sandblasted zirconia if used in light-cured mode (without adding a dual-cured activator) with a dual-cured amine-free resin cement (NX3, Kerr Corporation).[380] This may explain why the manufacturer of Scotchbond Universal Adhesive recommends combining the adhesive with its proprietary amine-free dual-cured resin cement without the need to mix the adhesive with the respective chemical activator. The same adhesive must be mixed with the chemical activator if it is used with a conventional dual-cured resin cement based on the peroxide-amine redox system.

Expanded Clinical Indications for Dentin Adhesives

Desensitization

Dentin hypersensitivity is a common clinical condition that is difficult to treat because the treatment outcome is not consistently successful. Most authorities agree that the hydrodynamic theory best explains dentin hypersensitivity.[357] The equivalency of various hydrodynamic stimuli has been evaluated from measurements of the fluid movement induced in vitro and relating this to the hydraulic conductance of the same dentin specimen.[381] There are other mechanisms responsible for tooth sensitivity including those triggered by dental whitening agents.[382]

Patients may complain of discomfort when teeth are subjected to temperature changes, osmotic gradients such as those caused by sweet or salty foods, or even tactile stimuli. The cervical area of teeth is the most common site of hypersensitivity. Cervical hypersensitivity may be caused not only by chemical erosion but also by mechanical abrasion or even occlusal stresses.[383,384]

Theories about the transmission of pain stimuli in dentin sensitivity suggest that pain is amplified when the dentinal tubules are open to the oral cavity.[385,386] Dentin hypersensitivity can be a major problem for periodontal patients who frequently have gingival recession and exposed root surfaces. The relationship between dentin hypersensitivity and the patency of dentin tubules in vivo has been established; occlusion of the tubules seems to decrease that sensitivity.[387]

The use of dentin adhesives to treat hypersensitive root surfaces has gained popularity.[27,28] Reductions in sensitivity can result from formation of resin tags and a hybrid layer[388] when a dentin adhesive is used. The precipitation of proteins from the dentinal fluid in the tubules may also account for the efficacy of desensitizing solutions.[389] Other factors may be involved in the action of dentin desensitizing solutions.[390] The primer of the multibottle adhesive system All-Bond 2 has a desensitizing effect, even without consistent resin tag formation.[391] In a clinical study using the primer of the original GLUMA adhesive system (an aqueous solution of 5% glutaraldehyde and 35% HEMA, currently marketed as GLUMA Desensitizer [Heraeus Kulzer GmbH]), the desensitizing solution was applied to crown preparations.[392] The authors concluded that GLUMA primer reduced dentin sensitivity through a protein denaturation process with concomitant changes in dentin permeability. Glutaraldehyde has long been used as a fixative that cross-links proteins.[393] This theory has been supported by studies using confocal microscopy, which found the formation of transversal septa occluding the dentinal tubules after application of GLUMA Desensitizer.[394] Another study evaluated dentin permeability in dogs up to 3 months. At the end of this period, GLUMA Desensitizer had the lowest permeability value, providing a longer lasting tubule-occluding effect.[395] Most desensitizing agents, however, are able to greatly decrease dentin permeability.[396]

The same glutaraldehyde-based desensitizing agent has been suggested as a rewetting agent on etched dentin to help prevent postoperative sensitivity under posterior composite restorations.[397,398] In spite of the favorable in vitro bond strengths, one clinical pilot study found that the operative technique might be more relevant to prevent postoperative sensitivity than the use of the glutaraldehyde-based desensitizer.[399] A randomized clinical trial of Class I restorations in molars and premolars included a glutaraldehyde-containing two-step etch-and-rinse adhesive, a glutaraldehyde-containing one-step SEA, and a glutaraldehyde-free two-step etch-and-rinse adhesive. There was no difference in postoperative sensitivity after 48 hours and after 7 days.[400]

The use of a dentin desensitizer before cementing full-coverage crowns is supported by studies that showed dentin-desensitizing solutions do not interfere with crown retention, regardless of the type of luting cement used.[401,402]

Adhesion to Root Canal Dentin

Adhesive strategies used in root dentin are similar to those used in coronal dentin. There are however differences in terms of bonding substrate and the restorative technique.

A. Substrate for Adhesion

Dentin located in the root walls of teeth that have been endodontically treated contains 9% less moisture than root dentin of vital teeth.[403] That is a positive feature for dentin adhesion. However, the area occupied by the more calcified transparent dentin in the root, also called sclerotic dentin,[404,405] widens with aging. Additionally the apical area of root dentin has fewer tubules than the occlusal part.[406]

The cutting instruments and cutting speed used for root dentin during endodontic therapy, as well as the irrigation methods (including chelating and deproteinizing solutions), are different from those used for coronal dentin, which results in different composition of the respective smear layers and dentin substrate.[407,408] Differently from the smear layer formed during a conventional coronal preparation, the morphology of the smear layer formed in the root canal walls includes two zones. The deepest part of endodontic smear layer is 1 to 2 μm thick and similar to that formed in coronal dentin. The most superficial zone forms smear plugs into the dentinal tubules to a depth of at least 10 μm,[409] which are not as accessible to dentin adhesives. Furthermore, there is a great variability in the composition of this deepest smear layer[407,410] aside from the presence of more organic tissue remnants and residual gutta-percha and endodontic sealer in some occasions.[410]

B. Restorative Technique

As discussed, stress relief within a three-dimensional bonded restoration is limited by its C-factor.[92] While the magnitude of the C-factor typically varies from 1 to 5 in direct coronal restorations, the estimated C-factor in the root canal may exceed 200, which is extremely unfavorable for restorative procedures that involve composite-based materials.[411] The polymerization shrinkage stress also depends on the degree of compliance (or deformation) of the substrate, which provides stress relief for luted restorations.[412] As this compliance is minimal in the root canal space, all root canal luting procedures that involve radical polymerization resins are challenging.

The concept of anatomic or relined fiber post (a glass fiber post relined with composite to reduce the volume of resin luting cement to retain the glass fiber post in the root canal)[413-415] has been recently advocated as a technique to increase the pushout bond strengths and decrease the polymerization stress associated with increased volume of resin cement. This concept however does not seem to take into account the slow chemical polymerization of resin luting cements used in the root canal. The use of chemically cured composites, as well as the utilization of hand-mixed resin materials, may partially compensate for the polymerization stresses that develop in the interface formed by root dentin and the composite material.[412,416] The polymerization stresses decrease and the development of the curing stress decreases with increasing of the layer thickness of chemically cured composites up to a thickness of 2.7 mm.[412] There is no strong evidence to recommend this technique over the use a nonrelined glass fiber post.

Although both the etch-and-rinse and the self-etch strategies are still often used to bond to root canal dentin, more recently the use of self-adhesive resin cements (i.e., no separate dentin conditioner or adhesive required) has gained popularity for their user-friendliness and better sealing ability than conventional adhesive systems (Fig. 5.24).[417,418] A systematic review of in vitro studies

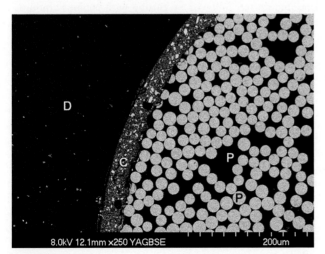

• **Fig. 5.24** Scanning electron micrograph (backscattered mode) of a dentin/self-adhesive resin cement/fiber post interface. *D*, Root dentin; *C*, self-adhesive resin cement; *P*, fiber post.

also suggested that self-adhesive resin cements may improve the retention of glass fiber posts into the root canal,[419] while being less technique sensitive.[420]

There is some controversy regarding the use of eugenol-containing sealers and their influence on the retention of luted posts, as eugenol is a phenolic component that can scavenge free radicals and delay or inhibit the polymerization of resin-based materials.[421] Some authors have reported lower bond strengths to root canal dentin when eugenol-based sealers were used with the root canal treatment.[422-424] Other authors have reported no significant differences in bond strengths to root canal dentin when eugenol-based sealers were used.[425,426]

Unfilled controls revealed significantly higher retentive post strengths compared to root-filled groups indicating that remnants of sealer might hamper adhesion inside the root canal.[425,427] When the post is luted 1 week after the completion of the root canal treatment, bond strengths to root canal dentin are not compromised regardless of the presence of eugenol in the endodontic sealer.[428,429]

Indirect Adhesive Restorations

Some current dentin adhesive systems bond to various substrates besides dentin.[7,418,430-433] Developments in adhesion technology have led to new indications for bonding to tooth structure, such as indirect ceramic and resin-based restorations (crowns, inlays, onlays, and veneers). The use of a dentin/enamel adhesive system in conjunction with a resin cement provides durable bonding of indirect restorations to tooth structure.[13,431]

A. Glass-Matrix Ceramics

Silica-based or glass-matrix ceramics[434] are still extensively used for porcelain veneers, inlays/onlays, and single crowns. Examples of glass-matrix ceramics are feldspathic porcelain, leucite-reinforced, and lithium disilicate–reinforced ceramics. Glass-matrix ceramic restorations must be etched internally with ~5% to ~10% hydrofluoric acid (HF) for 20 to 180 seconds [435-437] to create retentive microporosities (Fig. 5.25) analogous to those created in enamel by phosphoric acid etching.[438] HF must be rinsed off thoroughly with running water.[439] The adhesion of a resin luting cement to glass-matrix ceramics is achieved through a combination of mechanical retention from HF etching and chemical adhesion provided by the silane coupling agent to achieve durable adhesion.[13,431] Etched porcelain is an inorganic substrate, which silane makes more receptive to organic materials, the adhesive system, and resin cement.

Silane coupling agents were introduced in 1952 to bond organic with inorganic substances.[440] In 1962, this technology was transferred to dentistry to couple inorganic filler particles with Bis-GMA resin to form a composite resin.[441-444] After rinsing off the HF and air-drying, a silane coupling agent is applied on the etched glass-matrix ceramics intaglio surface and air-dried. The silane acts as a primer because it modifies the surface characteristics of etched glass-matrix ceramics. The application of a silane solution on HF-etched surfaces increases bond strengths between resin-based composite materials and glass-matrix ceramics up to 50% compared to HF alone, including bond strengths obtained with feldspathic porcelain and lithium disilicate–reinforced ceramic blocks.[437,442]

With the introduction of universal one-bottle adhesives and new silane solutions containing 10-MDP, some manufacturers do not recommend the application of a separate silane coupling agent to HF-etched glass-matrix ceramic surface. Clearfil Universal Bond and Scotchbond Universal Adhesive are examples of universal adhesives that contain a silane in their composition; however, the combination of resin monomers with a silane in the same solution

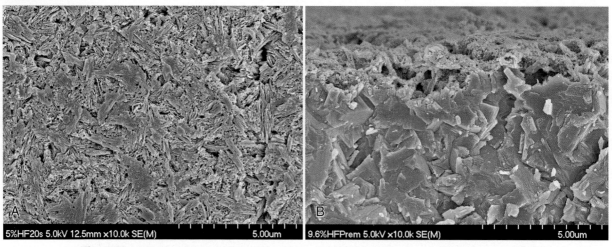

• **Fig. 5.25** Scanning electron micrograph of lithium disilicate–reinforced ceramics (IPS e.max CAD, Ivoclar Vivadent). A, Top view, etched with 5% hydrofluoric acid for 20 seconds. B, Lateral view, etched with 9.6% hydrofluoric acid for 20 seconds.

remains controversial.[378,445] Bond strengths to lithium disilicate–reinforced and leucite-reinforced ceramics are lower when a silane-containing universal adhesive is used compared to the application of a silane solution followed by a conventional multistep adhesive or a universal adhesive.[378,446] Contact angle and bond strength measurements have demonstrated that a silane primer may not be compatible mixed with resin monomers in the same solution.[445]

Some clinicians use sandblasting with aluminum oxide particles (airborne-particle abrasion) in the internal surface of glass-matrix ceramics restorations to roughen the intaglio surface. Mean bond strengths decrease however when hydrofluoric acid etching is not used.[437] Additionally airborne-particle abrasion of glass-matrix ceramics with alumina particles results in immediate lower intrinsic strength[447] triggered by the reduction in flexural strength of feldspathic porcelains[448] as well as of lithium disilicate–reinforced ceramics.[431]

B. Polycrystalline Ceramics

The discovery of a stress-induced transformation from the metastable tetragonal form to the stable monoclinic form $(t \rightarrow m)$[449-451] has led to a new class of strong, tough, dense, relatively flaw-tolerant oxide-based or polycrystalline ceramics known as zirconium oxide or zirconia.[449-451] This $t \rightarrow m$ phase transformation can occur in the vicinity of a propagating crack, causing an increase in volume, thereby closing the crack tip and preventing further crack propagation.[450,451] These high-strength ceramic materials have become extremely popular in dentistry, especially yttria-stabilized tetragonal zirconia polycrystal (Y-TZP) and ceria-stabilized tetragonal zirconia polycrystal/alumina (Ce-TZP/Al$_2$O$_3$).[452-454]

HF etching does not improve bond strengths to oxide-based or polycrystalline ceramics,[434,435,455-457] since these substrates do not contain a glass matrix. Accordingly, other surface conditioning methods have been used in the last two decades to improve bond strengths of resin luting cements to polycrystalline ceramics.[435,456,458,459] Some of the newest protocols include airborne-particle abrasion, tribochemical silica coating, and primers or silanes mixed with functional monomers such as the phosphate ester monomer 10-MDP.[430,459-461] Recent meta-analysis and systematic reviews of in vitro studies[430,458,459] concluded that the combination of mechanical and chemical pretreatment is recommended for bonding to

zirconia. Although the luting material may not be a determining factor after aging, as long as resin-based cement is used, adhesion to zirconia is increased after mechanical and chemical surface pretreatment and the use of a 10-MDP–based resin cement. The recommended chemical treatment of the Y-TZP intaglio is the application of a 10-MDP–based primer or a 10-MDP–based universal adhesive solution.[376,377,430,460,462] Chemical bonding between 10-MDP solutions and Y-TZP substrates was confirmed with time-of-flight secondary ion mass spectroscopy.[460] When dual-cure resin cements were used on Y-TZP surfaces that had not been air-abraded, higher bond strengths were achieved when a specific 10-MDP–containing zirconia primer was used,[462] confirming its chemical bonding ability. Nevertheless, micromechanical retention plays a more prominent role in adhesion to Y-TZP than chemical bonding.[463]

As surface contamination and aging in water have negative effects on adhesion to zirconia, the residual alumina particles and other surface contamination must be removed prior to adhesive luting.[459] The protocol for removing surface contaminants from intaglio surfaces of Y-TZP restorations includes cleaning the restoration in distilled water or ethanol for at least 3 minutes in an ultrasonic device, followed by rinsing with copious amounts of water spray and drying the surface with a strong stream of oil-free air.[464]

The durability of Y-TZP–based biomaterials has been questioned. In 1981 a phenomenon currently known as low-temperature degradation of Y-TZP was first described for applications near 250°C.[465] It was revealed that Y-TZP could undergo a slow superficial $t \rightarrow m$ transformation in a humid atmosphere followed by microcracking and loss in strength. In 1999 the $t \rightarrow m$ transformation of a 3Y-TZP from 70°C to 130°C in water and in steam was reported, confirming the susceptibility of Y-TZP to degradation in humid environments.[466] Stress corrosion by water molecules was also described as responsible for slow crack propagation in Y-TZP under cyclic loading.[467] This slow aging under humid environment was associated with roughening and microcracking, which led to increased wear and the release of wear debris in the body from hip replacement zirconia prostheses.[468]

Regarding the oral environment, Y-TZP–based materials may undergo fatigue and subcritical crack growth under functional loading with subsequent reduction in flexural strength.[469,470] New ceria-stabilized zirconia (Ce-TZP) materials do not undergo the same reduction in flexural strength compared to Y-TZP.[471] Significant decrease in bond strengths were noticed after aging through water storage at 37°C for 3 days or 150 days and 37,500 thermal cycles, regardless of the surface conditioning method (airborne-particle abrasion or tribochemical silica coating abrasion) and the luting system used.[376]

The clinical relevance of these structural changes in Y-TZP used in dentistry is not clear, as most in vitro studies have tested Y-TZP without a glaze coating.[472,473] The Y-TZP structure is not usually exposed directly to the oral environment except for zirconia abutments[474] and for glazed monolithic zirconia restorations that are adjusted prior to cementation.

C. Resin-Matrix Ceramics

Resin-based CAD/CAM materials for indirect restorations have become recently popular. Ambarino High-Glass (Creamed GmbH & Co. Produktions, Marburg, Germany), Brilliant Crios (Coltene), Ceramill COMP (Amann Girrbach AG, Herrschaftswiesen, Austria), Cerasmart (GC Corporation, Tokyo, Japan), and Lava Ultimate (3M Oral Care) are examples of CAD/CAM resin blocks currently available. These new resin-based CAD/CAM materials have a much lower modulus of elasticity compared to CAD/CAM ceramic materials.[446,447] It is recommended to treat the intaglio surface with airborne particle abrasion without any chemical etching.[475,476] Air abrasion with alumina particles improves fracture resistance of Lava Ultimate compared to polished specimens,[447] which may be a result of better mechanical interlocking of the bonding resins into the resin microporosities and better stress distribution at higher loads. Most universal adhesives also seem to bond effectively to air-abraded resin-based CAD/CAM materials.[380]

Hybrid resin-ceramic materials consisting of a polymer-infiltrated ceramic network (PICN) have been recently introduced with the goal to more closely mimic the physical properties of the natural tooth compared to other tooth-colored restorative materials.[477] Vita Enamic (VITA Zahnfabrik H. Rauter GmbH & Co. KG, Bad Säckingen, Germany) is a PICN containing an aluminum oxide–enriched feldspathic porcelain (86 wt%) into which 14 wt% urethane dimethacrylate and triethylene glycol dimethacrylate polymer material is injected.[478] The bond strengths obtained with HF-etched PICN materials are similar to those obtained with lithium disilicate–reinforced ceramics.[475]

Indirect tooth-colored restorations are luted with low-viscosity composite resin materials. Many of these resin cements are dual cured—that is, they polymerize both chemically and by light activation. Some materials marketed as "dual cure" may not polymerize efficiently in the absence of a curing light.[479-481] Self-adhesive cements, a recent category of resins, have become very popular to cement oxide–based ceramic restorations. Self-adhesive cements are dual-cured phosphate monomer-based resin cements (BisCem, Bisco Inc.; G-CEM LinkAce, GC Corporation; Maxcem Elite, Kerr Corporation; Panavia SA Cement Plus, Kuraray Noritake Dental Inc.; RelyX Unicem 2, 3M Oral Care; SmartCem2, DENTSPLY Sirona; Solocem, Coltene; SpeedCEM Plus, Ivoclar Vivadent) that do not require any pretreatment of the tooth substrate. The acidic phosphate groups react with the filler and simultaneously etch enamel or dentin in the same manner as do self-etch adhesives. A chemical interaction between self-adhesive cements and hydroxyapatite has been reported,[481,482] but this interaction depends of the activation mode and the specific self-adhesive resin cement tested.[482] The pH of some self-adhesive cements increases from 1 to 5 or 6 during their acid-base setting reaction.[483] The setting pH profiles of self-adhesive resin cements depend on the brand and mode of cure. In spite of their dual-curing ability, the physical properties improve significantly when light activated.[482,484] Self-adhesive resin cements result in lower bond strengths to etched glass-matrix ceramics than traditional resin cements.[437]

Summary

Reliable bonding of resins to enamel and dentin has revolutionized the practice of operative dentistry. Improvements in dentin bonding materials and techniques are likely to continue. Even as the materials themselves become better and easier to use however, proper attention to technique and a good understanding of the bonding process remain essential for clinical success, with emphasis in evidence-based dentistry.

References

1. Packham DE: Adhesion. In Packham DE, editor: *Handbook of adhesion*, Essex, UK, 1992, Longman Scientific & Technical, pp 18–20.
2. Akinmade AO, Nicholson JW: Glass-ionomer cements as adhesives: part I. Fundamental aspects and their clinical relevance. *J Mater Sci Mater Med* 4:95–101, 1993.
3. Allen KW: Theories of adhesion. In Packham DE, editor: *Handbook of adhesion*, Essex, UK, 1992, Longman Scientific & Technical, pp 473–475.
4. Söderholm K-JM: Correlation of in vivo and in vitro performance of adhesive restorative materials: a report of the ASC MD156 Task Group on test methods for the adhesion of restorative materials. *Dent Mater* 7:74–83, 1991.
5. Rueggeberg FA: Substrate for adhesion testing to tooth structure: review of the literature. *Dent Mater* 7:2–10, 1991.
6. Buonocore MG: A simple method of increasing the adhesion of acrylic filling materials to enamel surfaces. *J Dent Res* 34:849–853, 1955.
7. Van Meerbeek B, Perdigão J, Lambrechts P, et al: The clinical performance of adhesives. *J Dent* 26:1–20, 1998.
8. Black GV: *A work on operative dentistry in two volumes*, ed 3, Chicago, 1917, Medico-Dental Publishing Company.
9. Peumans M, Van Meerbeek B, Lambrechts P, et al: The 5-year clinical performance of direct composite additions to correct tooth form and position. I. Esthetic qualities. *Clin Oral Investig* 1:12–18, 1997.
10. Coelho-de-Souza FH, Gonçalves DS, Sales MP, et al: Direct anterior composite veneers in vital and non-vital teeth: a retrospective clinical evaluation. *J Dent* 43:1330–1336, 2015.
11. Christensen GJ: Cementing porcelain-fused-to-metal crowns. *J Am Dent Assoc* 128:1165–1167, 1997.
12. Jokstad A: A split-mouth randomized clinical trial of single crowns retained with resin-modified glass-ionomer and zinc phosphate luting cements. *Int J Prosthodont* 17:411–416, 2004.
13. Layton DM, Clarke M, Walton TR: A systematic review and meta-analysis of the survival of feldspathic porcelain veneers over 5 and 10 years. *Int J Prosthodont* 25:590–603, 2012.
14. Heintze SD, Rousson V: Fracture rates of IPS Empress all-ceramic crowns—a systematic review. *Int J Prosthodont* 23:129–133, 2010.

15. Feigal RJ, Musherure P, Gillespie B, et al: Improved sealant retention with bonding agents: a clinical study of two-bottle and single-bottle systems. *J Dent Res* 79:1850–1856, 2000.

16. Fleming PS, Johal A, Pandis N: Self-etch primers and conventional acid-etch technique for orthodontic bonding: a systematic review and meta-analysis. *Am J Orthod Dentofacial Orthop* 142:83–94, 2012.

17. Diangelis AJ, Andreasen JO, Ebeleseder KA, et al: International Association of Dental Traumatology: International Association of Dental Traumatology guidelines for the management of traumatic dental injuries: 1. Fractures and luxations of permanent teeth. *Dent Traumatol* 28:2–12, 2012.

18. Kumbuloglu O, Saracoglu A, Ozcan M: Pilot study of unidirectional E-glass fibre-reinforced composite resin splints: up to 4.5-year clinical follow-up. *J Dent* 39:871–877, 2011.

19. Gupta A, Yelluri RK, Munshi AK: Fiber-reinforced composite resin bridge: a treatment option in children. *Int J Clin Pediatr Dent* 8:62–65, 2015.

20. Liu X, Zhang Y, Zhou Z, et al: Retrospective study of combined splinting restorations in the aesthetic zone of periodontal patients. *Br Dent J* 220:241–247, 2016.

21. Opdam NJ, Bronkhorst EM, Loomans BA, et al: Longevity of repaired restorations: a practice based study. *J Dent* 40:829–835, 2012.

22. Hickel R, Brüshaver K, Ilie N: Repair of restorations–criteria for decision making and clinical recommendations. *Dent Mater* 29:28–50, 2013.

23. Baur V, Ilie N: Repair of dental resin-based composites. *Clin Oral Investig* 17:601–608, 2013.

24. Latta MA, Barkmeier WW: Approaches for intraoral repair of ceramic restorations. *Compend Contin Educ Dent* 21:635–639, 642-644, 2000.

25. Combe EC, Shaglouf AM, Watts DC, et al: Mechanical properties of direct core build-up materials. *Dent Mater* 15:158–165, 1999.

26. Hagge MS, Lindemuth JS: Shear bond strength of an autopolymerizing core buildup composite bonded to dentin with 9 dentin adhesive systems. *J Prosthet Dent* 86:620–623, 2001.

27. Calamia JR, Styner DL, Rattet AH: Effect of Amalgambond on cervical sensitivity. *Am J Dent* 8:283–284, 1996.

28. Ferrari M, Cagidiaco MC, Kugel G, et al: Clinical evaluation of a one-bottle bonding system for desensitizing exposed roots. *Am J Dent* 12:243–249, 1999.

29. Veitz-Keenan A, Barna JA, Strober B, et al: Treatments for hypersensitive noncarious cervical lesions: a Practitioners Engaged in Applied Research and Learning (PEARL) Network randomized clinical effectiveness study. *J Am Dent Assoc* 144:495–506, 2013.

30. Gibson M, Sharif MO, Smith A, et al: A practice-based randomised controlled trial of the efficacy of three interventions to reduce dentinal hypersensitivity. *J Dent* 41:668–674, 2013.

31. Robinson C, Hallsworth AS, Weatherell JA, et al: Arrest and control of carious lesions: a study based on preliminary experiments with resorcinol-formaldehyde resin. *J Dent Res* 55:812–818, 1976.

32. Zhang N, Melo MA, Chen C, et al: Development of a multifunctional adhesive system for prevention of root caries and secondary caries. *Dent Mater* 31:1119–1131, 2015.

33. Macedo GV, Diaz PI, De O, et al: Reattachment of anterior teeth fragments: a conservative approach. *J Esthet Restor Dent* 20:5–18, 2008.

34. Ree M, Schwartz RS: The endo-restorative interface: current concepts. *Dent Clin North Am* 54:345–374, 2010.

35. Goncalves LA, Vansan LP, Paulino SM, et al: Fracture resistance of weakened roots restored with a transilluminating post and adhesive restorative materials. *J Prosthet Dent* 96:339–344, 2006.

36. Schmitter M, Huy C, Ohlmann B, et al: Fracture resistance of upper and lower incisors restored with glass fiber reinforced posts. *J Endod* 32:328–330, 2006.

37. Doyle MD, Loushine RJ, Agee KA, et al: Improving the performance of EndoRez root canal sealer with a dual-cured two-step self-etch adhesive. I. Adhesive strength to dentin. *J Endod* 32:766–770, 2006.

38. Teixeira FB, Teixeira EC, Thompson J, et al: Dentinal bonding reaches the root canal system. *J Esthet Restor Dent* 16:348–354, 2004.

39. Wu MK, Kontakiotis EG, Wesselink PR: Long-term seal provided by some root-end filling materials. *J Endod* 24:557–560, 1998.

40. Murray MJ, Loushine RJ, Weller RN, et al: Use of self-etching adhesives to seal resected apices. *J Endod* 30:538–540, 2004.

41. Buonocore MG, Matsui A, Gwinnett AJ: Penetration of resin dental materials into enamel surfaces with reference to bonding. *Arch Oral Biol* 13:61–70, 1968.

42. Gwinnett AJ: Histologic changes in human enamel following treatment with acidic adhesive conditioning agents. *Arch Oral Biol* 16:731–738, 1971.

43. Gottlieb EW, Retief DH, Jamison HC: An optimal concentration of phosphoric acid as an etching agent: part I. tensile bond strength studies. *J Prosthet Dent* 48:48–51, 1982.

44. Gwinnett AJ, Kanca JA, 3rd: Micromorphology of the bonded dentin interface and its relationship to bond strength. *Am J Dent* 5:73–77, 1992.

45. Soetopo , Beech DR, Hardwick JL: Mechanism of adhesion of polymers to acid-etched enamel: effect of acid concentration and washing on bond strength. *J Oral Rehabil* 5:69–80, 1978.

46. Barkmeier WW, Shaffer SE, Gwinnett AJ: Effects of 15 vs 60 second enamel acid conditioning on adhesion and morphology. *Oper Dent* 11:111–116, 1986.

47. Mardaga WJ, Shannon IL: Decreasing the depth of etch for direct bonding in orthodontics. *J Clin Orthod* 16:130–132, 1982.

48. Barkmeier WW, Gwinnett AJ, Shaffer SE: Effects of enamel etching time on bond strength and morphology. *J Clin Orthod* 19:36–38, 1985.

49. Nordenvall K-J, Brännström M, Malmgren O: Etching of deciduous teeth and young and old permanent teeth: a comparison between 15 and 60 seconds of etching. *Am J Orthod* 78:99–108, 1980.

50. Bastos PAM, Retief DH, Bradley EL, et al: Effect of etch duration on the shear bond strength of a microfill composite resin to enamel. *Am J Dent* 1:151–157, 1988.

51. Crim GA, Shay JS: Effect of etchant time on microleakage. *J Dent Child* 54:339–340, 1987.

52. Gilpatrick RO, Ross JA, Simonsen RJ: Resin-to-enamel bond strengths with various etching times. *Quintessence Int* 22:47–49, 1991.

53. Shaffer SE, Barkmeier WW, Kelsey WP, 3rd: Effects of reduced acid conditioning time on enamel microleakage. *Gen Dent* 35:278–280, 1987.

54. Barkmeier WW, Erickson RL, Kimmes NS, et al: Effect of enamel etching time on roughness and bond strength. *Oper Dent* 34:217–222, 2009.

55. De Munck J, Van Meerbeek B, Satoshi I, et al: Microtensile bond strengths of one- and two-step self-etch adhesives to bur-cut enamel and dentin. *Am J Dent* 16:414–420, 2003.

56. Swift EJ, Jr, Perdigão J, Heymann HO: Enamel bond strengths of "one-bottle" adhesives. *Pediatr Dent* 20:259–262, 1998.

57. Senawongse P, Sattabanasuk V, Shimada Y, et al: Bond strengths of current adhesive systems on intact and ground enamel. *J Esthet Restor Dent* 16:107–115, 2004.

58. Barkmeier WW, Erickson RL, Latta MA: Fatigue limits of enamel bonds with moist and dry techniques. *Dent Mater* 25:1527–1531, 2009.

59. Gwinnett AJ, Matsui A: A study of enamel adhesives: the physical relationship between enamel and adhesive. *Arch Oral Biol* 12:1615–1620, 1967.

60. Asmussen E, Hansen EK, Peutzfeldt A: Influence of the solubility parameter of intermediary resin on the effectiveness of the Gluma bonding system. *J Dent Res* 70:1290–1293, 1991.

61. Nakabayashi N, Kojima K, Masuhara E: The promotion of adhesion by the infiltration of monomers into tooth substrates. *J Biomed Mater Res* 16:265–273, 1982.

62. Yoshida Y, Van Meerbeek B, Nakayama Y, et al: Evidence of chemical bonding at biomaterial-hard tissue interfaces. *J Dent Res* 79:709–714, 2000.

63. Fukuda R, Yoshida Y, Nakayama Y, et al: Bonding efficacy of polyalkenoic acids to hydroxyapatite, enamel and dentin. *Biomaterials* 24:1861–1867, 2003.

64. Fu B, Sun X, Qian W, et al: Evidence of chemical bonding to hydroxyapatite by phosphoric acid esters. *Biomaterials* 26:5104–5110, 2005.

65. Yoshihara K, Yoshida Y, Hayakawa S, et al: Nano-layering of phosphoric-acid ester monomer at enamel and dentin. *Acta Biomater* 7:3187–3195, 2011.

66. Mitra SB, Lee CY, Bui HT, et al: Long-term adhesion and mechanism of bonding of a paste-liquid resin-modified glass-ionomer. *Dent Mater* 25:459–466, 2009.

67. Van Meerbeek B, Ionkoshi S, Braem M, et al: Morphological aspects of the resin-dentin interdiffusion zone with different dentin adhesive systems. *J Dent Res* 71:1530–1540, 1992.

68. Tay FR, Gwinnett AJ, Wei SH: Ultrastructure of the resin-dentin interface following reversible and irreversible rewetting. *Am J Dent* 10:77–82, 1997.

69. Veis A: Mineral-matrix interactions in bone and dentin. *J Bone Miner Res* 8(Suppl 2):S493–S497, 1993.

70. Brännström M, Lindén LA, Johnson G: Movement of dentinal and pulpal fluid caused by clinical procedures. *J Dent Res* 47:679–682, 1968.

71. Terkla LG, Brown AC, Hainisch AP, et al: Testing sealing properties of restorative materials against moist dentin. *J Dent Res* 66:1758–1764, 1987.

72. Van Hassel HJ: Physiology of the human dental pulp. *Oral Surg Oral Med Oral Pathol* 32:126–134, 1971.

73. Garberoglio R, Brännström M: Scanning electron microscopic investigation of human dentinal tubules. *Arch Oral Biol* 21:355–362, 1976.

74. Pashley DH: Dentin: a dynamic substrate—a review. *Scanning Microsc* 3:161–176, 1989.

75. Marchetti C, Piacentini C, Menghini P: Morphometric computerized analysis on the dentinal tubules and the collagen fibers in the dentine of human permanent teeth. *Bull Group Int Rech Sci Stomatol Odontol* 35:125–129, 1992.

76. Suzuki T, Finger WJ: Dentin adhesives: site of dentin vs. bonding of composite resins. *Dent Mater* 4:379–383, 1988.

77. Rosales-Leal JI, Osorio R, Holgado-Terriza JA, et al: Dentin wetting by four adhesive systems. *Dent Mater* 17:526–532, 2001.

78. Sattabanasuk V, Shimada Y, Tagami J: The bond of resin to different dentin surface characteristics. *Oper Dent* 29:333–341, 2004.

79. Adebayo OA, Burrow MF, Tyas MJ: Bonding of one-step and two-step self-etching primer adhesives to dentin with different tubule orientations. *Acta Odontol Scand* 66:159–168, 2008.

80. Zhang L, Wang DY, Fan J, et al: Stability of bonds made to superficial vs. deep dentin, before and after thermocycling. *Dent Mater* 30:1245–1251, 2014.

81. Bowen RL, Eick JD, Henderson DA, et al: Smear layer: removal and bonding considerations. *Oper Dent* 3(Suppl):30–34, 1984.

82. Ishioka S, Caputo AA: Interaction between the dentinal smear layer and composite bond strengths. *J Prosthet Dent* 61:180–185, 1989.

83. Pashley DH, Livingston MJ, Greenhill JD: Regional resistances to fluid flow in human dentine in vitro. *Arch Oral Biol* 23:807–810, 1978.

84. Eick JD, Cobb CM, Chappell RP, et al: The dentinal surface: its influence on dentinal adhesion: part I. *Quintessence Int* 22:967–977, 1991.

85. Pashley DH: The effects of acid etching on the pulpodentin complex. *Oper Dent* 17:229–242, 1992.

86. Torney D: The retentive ability of acid-etched dentin. *J Prosthet Dent* 39:169–172, 1978.

87. Opdam NJ, Feilzer AJ, Roeters JJ, et al: Class I occlusal composite resin restorations: in vivo post-operative sensitivity, wall adaptation, and microleakage. *Am J Dent* 11:229–234, 1998.

88. Bowen RL, Nemoto K, Rapson JE: Adhesive bonding of various materials to hard tooth tissue: forces developing in composite materials during hardening. *J Am Dent Assoc* 106:475–477, 1983.

89. Davidson CL, Feilzer AJ: Polymerization shrinkage and polymerization shrinkage stress in polymer-based restoratives. *J Dent* 25:435–440, 1997.

90. Davidson CL, de Gee AJ, Feilzer A: The competition between the composite-dentin bond strength and the polymerization contraction stress. *J Dent Res* 63:1396–1399, 1984.

91. Hegdahl T, Gjerdet NR: Contraction stresses of composite filling materials. *Acta Odontol Scand* 35:191–195, 1977.

92. Feilzer A, De Gee AJ, Davidson CL: Setting stress in composite resin in relation to configuration of the restoration. *J Dent Res* 66:1636–1639, 1987.

93. Davidson CL, de Gee AJ: Relaxation of polymerization contraction stresses by flow in dental composites. *J Dent Res* 63:146–148, 1984.

94. Perdigão J, Lambrechts P, Van Meerbeek B, et al: The interaction of adhesive systems with human dentin. *Am J Dent* 9:167–173, 1996.

95. Yoshikawa T, Sano H, Burrow MF, et al: Effects of dentin depth and cavity configuration on bond strength. *J Dent Res* 78:898–905, 1999.

96. Carvalho RM, Pereira JC, Yoshiyama M, et al: A review of polymerization contraction: the influence of stress development versus stress relief. *Oper Dent* 21:17–24, 1996.

97. Mantri SP, Mantri SS: Management of shrinkage stresses in direct restorative light-cured composites: a review. *J Esthet Restor Dent* 25:305–313, 2013.

98. Masouras K, Silikas N, Watts DC: Correlation of filler content and elastic properties of resin-composites. *Dent Mater* 24:932–939, 2008.

99. Gonçalves F, Kawano Y, Braga RR: Contraction stress related to composite inorganic content. *Dent Mater* 26:704–709, 2010.

100. Son SA, Park JK, Seo DG, et al: How light attenuation and filler content affect the microhardness and polymerization shrinkage and translucency of bulk-fill composites? *Clin Oral Investig* 21:559–565, 2017.

101. Munksgaard EC, Irie M, Asmussen E: Dentin-polymer bond promoted by Gluma and various resins. *J Dent Res* 64:1409–1411, 1985.

102. Soares CJ, Bicalho AA, Tantbirojn D, et al: Polymerization shrinkage stresses in a premolar restored with different composite resins and different incremental techniques. *J Adhes Dent* 15:341–350, 2013.

103. Park JW, Ferracane JL: Water aging reverses residual stresses in hydrophilic dental composites. *J Dent Res* 93:195–200, 2014.

104. Sideridou ID, Karabela MM, Vouvoudi ECh: Volumetric dimensional changes of dental light-cured dimethacrylate resins after sorption of water or ethanol. *Dent Mater* 24:1131–1136, 2008.

105. Wei YJ, Silikas N, Zhang ZT, et al: The relationship between cyclic hygroscopic dimensional changes and water sorption/desorption of self-adhering and new resin-matrix composites. *Dent Mater* 29:e218–e226, 2013.

106. Uno S, Asmussen E: Marginal adaptation of a restorative resin polymerized at reduced. *Scand J Dent Res* 99:440–444, 1991.

107. Kanca J, 3rd, Suh BI: Pulse activation: reducing resin-based composite contraction stresses at the enamel cavosurface margins. *Am J Dent* 12:107–112, 1999.

108. Park J, Chang J, Ferracane J, et al: How should composite be layered to reduce shrinkage stress: incremental or bulk filling? *Dent Mater* 24:1501–1505, 2008.

109. Alomari QD, Reinhardt JW, Boyer DB: Effect of liners on cusp deflection and gap formation in composite restorations. *Oper Dent* 26:406–411, 2001.

110. Ferracane JL, Hilton TJ: Polymerization stress - Is it clinically meaningful? *Dent Mater* 32:1–10, 2016.
111. Kemp-Scholte CM, Davidson CL: Marginal integrity related to bond strength and strain capacity of composite resin restorative systems. *J Prosthet Dent* 64:658–664, 1990.
112. Finger WJ: Dentin bonding agents: relevance of in vitro investigations. *Am J Dent* 1:184–188, 1988.
113. Kemp-Scholte CM, Davidson CL: Complete marginal seal of Class V resin composite restorations effected by increased flexibility. *J Dent Res* 69:1240–1243, 1990.
114. Lindberg A, van Dijken JW, Hörstedt P: In vivo interfacial adaptation of Class II resin composite restorations with and without a flowable resin composite liner. *Clin Oral Investig* 9:77–83, 2005.
115. Reis A, Loguercio AD: A 24-month follow-up of flowable resin composite as an intermediate layer in non-carious cervical lesions. *Oper Dent* 31:523–529, 2006.
116. Efes BG, Dörter C, Gömeç Y, et al: Two-year clinical evaluation of ormocer and nanofill composite with and without a flowable liner. *J Adhes Dent* 8:119–126, 2006.
117. Celik C, Ozgünaltay G, Attar N: Clinical evaluation of flowable resins in non-carious cervical lesions: two-year results. *Oper Dent* 32:313–321, 2007.
118. van Dijken JWV, Pallesen U: Clinical performance of a hybrid resin composite with and without an intermediate layer of flowable resin composite: a 7-year evaluation. *Dent Mater* 27:150–156, 2011.
119. van de Sande FH, Rodolpho PA, Basso GR, et al: 18-year survival of posterior composite resin restorations with and without glass ionomer cement as base. *Dent Mater* 31:669–675, 2015.
120. Condon JR, Ferracane JL: Reduced polymerization stress through non-bonded nanofiller particles. *Biomaterials* 23:3807–3815, 2002.
121. Palin WM, Fleming GJ, Nathwani H, et al: In vitro cuspal deflection and microleakage of maxillary premolars restored with novel low-shrink dental composites. *Dent Mater* 21:324–335, 2005.
122. Braga RR, Ferracane JL: Alternatives in polymerization contraction stress management. *Crit Rev Oral Biol Med* 15:176–184, 2004.
123. Papadogiannis D, Kakaboura A, Palaghias G, et al: Setting characteristics and cavity adaptation of low-shrinking resin composites. *Dent Mater* 25:1509–1516, 2009.
124. Xu HC, Liu WY, Wang T: Measurement of thermal expansion coefficient of human teeth. *Aust Dent J* 34:530–535, 1989.
125. Sideridou I, Achilias DS, Kyrikou E: Thermal expansion characteristics of light-cured dental resins and resin composites. *Biomaterials* 25:3087–3097, 2004.
126. Versluis A, Douglas WH, Sakaguchi RL: Thermal expansion coefficient of dental composites measured with strain gauges. *Dent Mater* 12:290–294, 1996.
127. Bullard RH, Leinfelder KF, Russell CM: Effect of coefficient of thermal expansion on microleakage. *J Am Dent Assoc* 116:871–874, 1988.
128. Asmussen E: Clinical relevance of physical, chemical, and bonding properties of composite resins. *Oper Dent* 10:61–73, 1985.
129. Borges AL, Borges AB, Xavier TA, et al: Impact of quantity of resin, C-factor, and geometry on resin composite polymerization shrinkage stress in Class V restorations. *Oper Dent* 39:144–151, 2014.
130. Hansen EK: Effect of Scotchbond dependent on cavity cleaning, cavity diameter and cavosurface angle. *Scand J Dent Res* 92:141–147, 1984.
131. Schroeder M, Reis A, Luque-Martinez I, et al: Effect of enamel bevel on retention of cervical composite resin restorations: a systematic review and meta-analysis. *J Dent* 43:777–788, 2015.
132. Mahn E, Rousson V, Heintze S: Meta-analysis of the influence of bonding parameters on the clinical outcome of tooth-colored cervical restorations. *J Adhes Dent* 17:391–403, 2015.
133. Jørgensen KD, Matono R, Shimokobe H: Deformation of cavities and resin fillings in loaded teeth. *Scand J Dent Res* 84:46–50, 1976.
134. Tonami K, Takahashi H: Effects of aging on tensile fatigue strength of bovine dentin. *Dent Mater J* 16:156–169, 1997.
135. Qvist V: The effect of mastication on marginal adaptation of composite restorations in vivo. *J Dent Res* 62:904–906, 1983.
136. Nikaido T, Kunzelmann KH, Chen H, et al: Evaluation of thermal cycling and mechanical loading on bond strength of a self-etching primer system to dentin. *Dent Mater* 18:269–275, 2002.
137. Toledano M, Osorio R, Albaladejo A, et al: Effect of cyclic loading on the microtensile bond strengths of total-etch and self-etch adhesives. *Oper Dent* 31:25–32, 2006.
138. Brudevold F, Buonocore M, Wileman W: A report on a resin composition capable of bonding to human dentin surfaces. *J Dent Res* 35:846–851, 1956.
139. McLean JW: Bonding to enamel and dentin [letter]. *Quintessence Int* 26:334, 1995.
140. McLean JW, Kramer IRH: A clinical and pathological evaluation of a sulphinic acid activated resin for use in restorative dentistry. *Br Dent J* 93:255, 1952.
141. Bowen RL: Adhesive bonding of various materials to hard tooth tissues: II. Bonding to dentin promoted by a surface-active comonomer. *J Dent Res* 44:895–902, 1965.
142. Barkmeier WW, Cooley RL: Laboratory evaluation of adhesive systems. *Oper Dent* 5(Suppl):50–61, 1992.
143. Albers HF: Dentin-resin bonding. *ADEPT Report* 1:33–42, 1990.
144. Alexieva C: Character of the hard tooth tissue-polymer bond: II. Study of the interaction of human tooth enamel and dentin with N-phenylglycine-glycidyl methacrylate adduct. *J Dent Res* 58:1884–1886, 1979.
145. Retief DH, Denys FR: Adhesion to enamel and dentin. *Am J Dent* 2:133–144, 1989.
146. Jendresen MD: Clinical performance of a new composite resin for Class V erosion (abstract 1057). *J Dent Res* 57:339, 1978.
147. Eick JD: Smear layer—materials surface. *Proc Finn Dent Soc* 88:225–242, 1992.
148. Asmussen E, Munksgaard EC: Bonding of restorative materials to dentine: status of dentine adhesives and impact on cavity design and filling techniques. *Int Dent J* 38:97–104, 1988.
149. Baier RE: Principles of adhesion. *Oper Dent* 5(Suppl):1–9, 1992.
150. Causton BE: Improved bonding of composite restorative to dentine: a study in vitro of the use of a commercial halogenated phosphate ester. *Br Dent J* 156:93–95, 1984.
151. Huang GT, Söderholm K-JM: In vitro investigation of shear bond strength of a phosphate based dentinal bonding agent. *Scand J Dent Res* 97:84–92, 1989.
152. Eliades GC: Dentine bonding systems. In Vanherle G, et al, editors: *State of the art on direct posterior filling materials and dentine bonding*, Leuven, 1993, Van der Poorten, pp 49–74.
153. Tyas MJ, Burns GA, Byrne PF, et al: Clinical evaluation of Scotchbond: three-year results. *Aust Dent J* 34:277–279, 1989.
154. Van Meerbeek B, Peumans M, Verschueren M, et al: Clinical status of ten dentin adhesive systems. *J Dent Res* 73:1690–1702, 1994.
155. Fusayama T, Nakamura M, Kurosaki N, et al: Non-pressure adhesion of a new adhesive restorative resin. *J Dent Res* 58:1364–1370, 1979.
156. van Dijken JWV, Horstedt P: In vivo adaptation of restorative materials to dentin. *J Prosthet Dent* 56:677–681, 1986.
157. Retief DH, Austin JC, Fatti LP: Pulpal response to phosphoric acid. *J Oral Pathol* 3:114–122, 1974.
158. Stanley HR, Going RE, Chauncey HH: Human pulp response to acid pretreatment of dentin and to composite restoration. *J Am Dent Assoc* 91:817–825, 1975.
159. American Dental Association Council on Scientific Affairs: *Revised American Dental Association acceptance program guidelines: Dentin and enamel adhesives* (pp. 1–9), Chicago, 2001, American Dental Association.
160. Mine A, De Munck J, Vivan Cardoso M, et al: Enamel-smear compromises bonding by mild self-etch adhesives. *J Dent Res* 89:1505–1509, 2010.
161. Suyama Y, Lührs AK, De Munck J, et al: Potential smear layer interference with bonding of self-etching adhesives to dentin. *J Adhes Dent* 15:317–324, 2013.

162. Eliades G: Clinical relevance of the formulation and testing of dentine bonding systems. *J Dent* 22:73–81, 1994.

163. Barkmeier WW, Suh B, Cooley RL: Shear bond strength to dentin and Ni-Cr-Be alloy with the All-Bond universal adhesive system. *J Esthet Dent* 3:148–153, 1991.

164. Kanca J, 3rd: Effect of resin primer solvents and surface wetness on resin composite bond strength to dentin. *Am J Dent* 5:213–221, 1992.

165. Kanca J, 3rd: Resin bonding to wet substrate: I. Bonding to dentin. *Quintessence Int* 23:39–41, 1992.

166. Swift EJ, Triolo PT: Bond strengths of Scotchbond Multi-Purpose to moist dentin and enamel. *Am J Dent* 5:318–320, 1992.

167. Perdigão J, Lambrechts P, Van Meerbeek B, et al: Morphological field emission SEM study of the effect of six phosphoric acid etching agents on human dentin. *Dent Mater* 12:262–271, 1996.

168. Ermis RB, Kam O, Celik EU, et al: Clinical evaluation of a two-step etch & rinse and a two-step self-etch adhesive system in Class II restorations: two-year results. *Oper Dent* 34:656–663, 2009.

169. Wilder AD, Swift EJ, Jr, Heymann HO, et al: A 12-year clinical evaluation of a three-step dentin adhesive in noncarious cervical lesions. *J Am Dent Assoc* 140:526–535, 2009.

170. Peumans M, De Munck J, Van Landuyt KL, et al: A 13-year clinical evaluation of two three-step etch-and-rinse adhesives in non-carious Class-V lesions. *Clin Oral Investig* 16:129–137, 2012.

171. Erickson RL: Surface interactions of dentin adhesive materials. *Oper Dent* 5(Suppl):81–94, 1992.

172. Panighi M, G'Sell C: Influence of calcium concentration on the dentin wettability by an adhesive. *J Biomed Mater Res* 26:1081–1089, 1992.

173. Armstrong SR, Vargas MA, Fang Q, et al: Microtensile bond strength of a total-etch 3-step, total-etch 2-step, self-etch 2-step, and a self-etch 1-step dentin bonding system through 15-month water storage. *J Adhes Dent* 5:47–56, 2003.

174. Peumans M, De Munck J, Mine A, et al: Clinical effectiveness of contemporary adhesives for the restoration of non-carious cervical lesions. A systematic review. *Dent Mater* 30:1089–1103, 2014.

175. De Munck J, Mine A, Poitevin A, et al: Meta-analytical review of parameters involved in dentin bonding. *J Dent Res* 91:351–357, 2012.

176. Tay FR, Pashley DH: Have dentin adhesives become too hydrophilic? *J Can Dent Assoc* 69:726–731, 2003.

177. Loguercio AD, Raffo J, Bassani F, et al: 24-month clinical evaluation in non-carious cervical lesions of a two-step etch-and-rinse adhesive applied using a rubbing motion. *Clin Oral Investig* 15:589–596, 2011.

178. Reis A, Pellizzaro A, Dal-Bianco K, et al: Impact of adhesive application to wet and dry dentin on long-term resin-dentin bond strengths. *Oper Dent* 32:380–387, 2007.

179. Perdigão J, Lopes L, Lambrechts P, et al: Effects of a self-etching primer on enamel shear bond strengths and SEM morphology. *Am J Dent* 10:141–146, 1997.

180. Watanabe I, Nakabayashi N, Pashley DH: Bonding to ground dentin by a Phenyl-P self-etching primer. *J Dent Res* 73:1212–1220, 1994.

181. Tay FR, Pashley DH, Suh BI, et al: Single-step adhesives are permeable membranes. *J Dent* 30:371–382, 2002.

182. Fukuoka A, Koshiro K, Inoue S, et al: Hydrolytic stability of one-step self-etching adhesives bonded to dentin. *J Adhes Dent* 13:243–248, 2011.

183. Clinician's preferences 2001, *CRA Newsletter* 25, 2001.

184. Perdigão J, Gomes G, Gondo R, et al: In vitro bonding performance of all-in-one adhesives. Part I – microtensile bond strengths. *J Adhes Dent* 8:367–373, 2006.

185. Perdigão J, Lopes MM, Gomes G: In vitro bonding performance of self-etch adhesives: II–ultramorphological evaluation. *Oper Dent* 33:534–549, 2008.

186. Ferrari M, Mannocci F, Vichi A, et al: Effect of two etching times on the sealing ability of Clearfil Liner Bond 2 in Class V restorations. *Am J Dent* 10:66–70, 1997.

187. Opdam NJ, Roeters FJ, Feilzer AJ, et al: Marginal integrity and postoperative sensitivity in Class 2 resin composite restorations in vivo. *J Dent* 26:555–562, 1998.

188. Miyazaki M, Sato M, Onose H: Durability of enamel bond strength of simplified bonding systems. *Oper Dent* 25:75–80, 2000.

189. Akimoto N, Takamizu M, Momoi Y: 10-year clinical evaluation of a self-etching adhesive system. *Oper Dent* 32:3–10, 2007.

190. Tay FR, Sano H, Carvalho R, et al: An ultrastructural study of the influence of acidity of self-etching primers and smear layer thickness on bonding to intact dentin. *J Adhes Dent* 2:83–98, 2000.

191. Pashley DH, Tay FR: Aggressiveness of contemporary self-etching adhesives: part II: etching effects on unground enamel. *Dent Mater* 17:430–444, 2001.

192. Peumans M, De Munck J, Van Landuyt K, et al: Thirteen-year randomized controlled clinical trial of a two-step self-etch adhesive in non-carious cervical lesions. *Dent Mater* 31:308–314, 2015.

193. Yoshihara K, Yoshida Y, Nagaoka N, et al: Nano-controlled molecular interaction at adhesive interfaces for hard tissue reconstruction. *Acta Biomater* 6:3573–3582, 2010.

194. Anchieta RB, Machado LS, Sundfeld RH, et al: Effect of partially demineralized dentin beneath the hybrid layer on dentin-adhesive interface micromechanics. *J Biomech* 48:701–707, 2015.

195. Wang Y, Spencer P: Physiochemical interactions at the interfaces between self-etch adhesive systems and dentine. *J Dent* 32:567–579, 2004.

196. Wang Y, Spencer P: Continuing etching of an all-in-one adhesive in wet dentin tubules. *J Dent Res* 84:350–354, 2005.

197. Cao Y, Mei ML, Xu J, et al: Biomimetic mineralisation of phosphorylated dentine by CPP-ACP. *J Dent* 41:818–825, 2013.

198. Tay FR, Pashley DH: Guided tissue remineralisation of partially demineralised human dentine. *Biomaterials* 29:1127–1137, 2008.

199. Zhang W, Luo XJ, Niu LN, et al: Biomimetic intrafibrillar mineralization of type I collagen with intermediate precursors-loaded mesoporous carriers. *Sci Rep* 5:11199, 2015.

200. Niu LN, Zhang W, Pashley DH, et al: Biomimetic remineralization of dentin. *Dent Mater* 30:77–96, 2014.

201. Akpata ES, Behbehani J: Effect of bonding systems on post-operative sensitivity from posterior composites. *Am J Dent* 19:151–154, 2006.

202. Browning WD, Blalock JS, Callan RS, et al: Postoperative sensitivity: a comparison of two bonding agents. *Oper Dent* 32:112–117, 2007.

203. Casselli DS, Martins LR: Postoperative sensitivity in Class I composite resin restorations in vivo. *J Adhes Dent* 8:53–58, 2006.

204. Wegehaupt F, Betke H, Solloch N, et al: Influence of cavity lining and remaining dentin thickness on the occurrence of postoperative hypersensitivity of composite restorations. *J Adhes Dent* 11:137–141, 2009.

205. Burrow MF, Banomyong D, Harnirattisai C, et al: Effect of glass-ionomer cement lining on postoperative sensitivity in occlusal cavities restored with resin composite—A randomized clinical trial. *Oper Dent* 34:648–655, 2009.

206. Reis A, Dourado Loguercio A, Schroeder M, et al: Does the adhesive strategy influence the post-operative sensitivity in adult patients with posterior resin composite restorations?: a systematic review and meta-analysis. *Dent Mater* 31:1052–1067, 2015.

207. Perdigão J: Dentin bonding as a function of dentin structure. *Dent Clin North Am* 46:277–301, 2002.

208. Tay FR, Pashley DH, Peters MC: Adhesive permeability affects composite coupling to dentin treated with a self-etch adhesive. *Oper Dent* 28:610–621, 2003.

209. Tay FR, Pashley DH, Yiu CK, et al: Factors contributing to the incompatibility between simplified-step adhesives and chemically-cured or dual-cured composites: part I. Single-step self-etching adhesive. *J Adhes Dent* 5:27–40, 2003.

210. Tay FR, Pashley DH: Aggressiveness of contemporary self-etching adhesives: part I. Depth of penetration beyond dentin smear layers. *Dent Mater* 17:296–308, 2001.

211. Ito S, Tay FR, Hashimoto M, et al: Effects of multiple coatings of two all-in-one adhesives on dentin bonding. *J Adhes Dent* 7:133–141, 2005.

212. Reis A, Leite TM, Matte K, et al: Improving clinical retention of one-step self-etching adhesive systems with an additional hydrophobic adhesive layer. *J Am Dent Assoc* 140:877–885, 2009.

213. Reis A, Albuquerque M, Pegoraro M, et al: Can the durability of one-step self-etch adhesives be improved by double application or by an extra layer of hydrophobic resin? *J Dent* 36:309–315, 2008.

214. Van Landuyt KL, Peumans M, De Munck J, et al: Extension of a one-step self-etch adhesive into a multi-step adhesive. *Dent Mater* 22:533–544, 2006.

215. Tay FR, Frankenberger R, Krejci I, et al: Single-bottle adhesives behave as permeable membranes after polymerization. I. In vivo evidence. *J Dent* 32:611–621, 2004.

216. Hanabusa M, Mine A, Kuboki T, et al: Bonding effectiveness of a new 'multi-mode' adhesive to enamel and dentine. *J Dent* 40:475–484, 2012.

217. Perdigão J, Sezinando A, Monteiro PC: Laboratory bonding ability of a multi-purpose dentin adhesive. *Am J Dent* 25:153–158, 2012.

218. Chen C, Niu LN, Xie H, et al: Bonding of universal adhesives to dentine–Old wine in new bottles? *J Dent* 43:525–536, 2015.

219. Sezinando A, Luque-Martinez I, Muñoz MA, et al: Influence of a hydrophobic resin coating on the immediate and 6-month dentin bonding of three universal adhesives. *Dent Mater* 31:e236–e246, 2015.

220. Tian F, Zhou L, Zhang Z, et al: Paucity of nanolayering in resin-dentin interfaces of MDP-based adhesives. *J Dent Res* 95:380–387, 2016.

221. Van Meerbeek B, Yoshihara K, Yoshida Y, et al: State of the art of self-etch adhesives. *Dent Mater* 27:17–28, 2011.

222. Yoshida Y, Yoshihara K, Hayakawa S, et al: HEMA inhibits interfacial nano-layering of the functional monomer MDP. *J Dent Res* 91:1060–1065, 2012.

223. Loguercio AD, Muñoz MA, Luque-Martinez I, et al: Does active application of universal adhesives to enamel in self-etch mode improve their performance? *J Dent* 43:1060–1070, 2015.

224. Marchesi G, Frassetto A, Mazzoni A, et al: Adhesive performance of a multi-mode adhesive system: 1-year in vitro study. *J Dent* 42:603–612, 2014.

225. Kanca J, 3rd: Wet bonding: effect of drying time and distance. *Am J Dent* 9:273–276, 1996.

226. Eick JD, Gwinnett AJ, Pashley DH, et al: Current concepts on adhesion to dentin. *Crit Rev Oral Biol Med* 8:306–335, 1997.

227. Maciel KT, Carvalho RM, Ringle RD, et al: The effect of acetone, ethanol, HEMA, and air on the stiffness of human decalcified dentin matrix. *J Dent Res* 75:1851–1858, 1996.

228. Perdigão J, Swift EJ, Cloe BC: Effects of etchants, surface moisture, and resin composite on dentin bond strengths. *Am J Dent* 6:61–64, 1993.

229. Goes MF, Pachane GC, García-Godoy F: Resin bond strength with different methods to remove excess water from the dentin. *Am J Dent* 10:298–301, 1997.

230. Magne P, Mahallati R, Bazos P, et al: Direct dentin bonding technique sensitivity when using air/suction drying steps. *J Esthet Restor Dent* 20:130–138, 2008.

231. Carvalho RM, Yoshiyama M, Pashley EL, et al: In vitro study on the dimensional changes of dentine after demineralization. *Arch Oral Biol* 41:369–377, 1996.

232. Perdigão J, Van Meerbeek B, Lopes MM, et al: The effect of a re-wetting agent on dentin bonding. *Dent Mater* 15:282–295, 1999.

233. Tay FR, Gwinnett JA, Wei SH: Micromorphological spectrum from overdrying to overwetting acid-conditioned dentin in water-free acetone-based, single-bottle primer/adhesives. *Dent Mater* 12:236–244, 1996.

234. Sasaki N, Odajima S: Stress-strain curve and Young's modulus of a collagen molecule as determined by the x-ray diffraction technique. *J Biomech* 29:655–658, 1996.

235. Sasaki N, Shiwa S, Yagihara S, et al: X-ray diffraction studies on the structure of hydrated collagen. *Biopolymers* 22:2539–2547, 1983.

236. Van der Graaf ER, ten Bosch JJ: Changes in dimension and weight of human dentine after different drying procedures and during subsequent rehydration. *Arch Oral Biol* 38:97–99, 1993.

237. Eanes ED, Lundy DR, Martin GN: X-ray diffraction study of the mineralization of turkey leg tendon. *Calcif Tissue Res* 6:239–248, 1970.

238. Perdigão J, Frankenberger R: Effect of solvent and re-wetting time on dentin adhesion. *Quintessence Int* 32:385–390, 2001.

239. Tay FR, Gwinnett AJ, Pang KM, et al: Resin permeation into acid-conditioned, moist, and dry dentin: a paradigm using water-free adhesive primers. *J Dent Res* 75:1034–1044, 1996.

240. Swift EJ, Perdigao J, Heymann HO: Bonding to enamel and dentin: a brief history and state of the art, 1995. *Quintessence Int* 26:95–110, 1995.

241. Luque-Martinez IV, Perdigão J, Muñoz MA, et al: Effects of solvent evaporation time on immediate adhesive properties of universal adhesives to dentin. *Dent Mater* 30:1126–1135, 2014.

242. Perdigão J, Reis A, Loguercio AD: Dentin adhesion and MMPs: a comprehensive review. *J Esthet Restor Dent* 25:219–241, 2013.

243. Tay FR, Pashley SH, Kapur RR, et al: Bonding BisGMA to dentin—a proof of concept for hydrophobic dentin bonding. *J Dent Res* 86:1034–1039, 2007.

244. Hosaka K, Nishitani Y, Tagami J, et al: Durability of resin-dentin bonds to water- vs. ethanol-saturated dentin. *J Dent Res* 88:146–151, 2009.

245. Salz U, Zimmermann J, Zeuner F, et al: Hydrolytic stability of self-etching adhesive systems. *J Adhes Dent* 7:107–116, 2005.

246. Hiraishi N, Nishiyama N, Ikemura K, et al: Water concentration in self-etching primers affects their aggressiveness and bonding efficacy to dentin. *J Dent Res* 84:653–658, 2005.

247. Hosaka K, Nakajima M, Takahashi M, et al: Relationship between mechanical properties of one-step self-etch adhesives and water sorption. *Dent Mater* 26:360–367, 2010.

248. Ito S, Hoshino T, Iijima M, et al: Water sorption/solubility of self-etching dentin bonding agents. *Dent Mater* 26:617–626, 2010.

249. Hashimoto M, Ohno H, Sano H, et al: In vitro degradation of resin-dentin bonds analyzed by microtensile bond test, scanning and transmission electron microscopy. *Biomaterials* 24:3795–3803, 2003.

250. Tay FR, Pashley DH, Suh BI, et al: Water treeing in simplified dentin adhesives–déjà vu? *Oper Dent* 30:561–579, 2005.

251. Kato G, Nakabayashi N: Effect of phosphoric acid concentration on wet-bonding to etched dentin. *Dent Mater* 12:250–255, 1996.

252. Sano H, Shono T, Takatsu T, et al: Microporous dentin zone beneath resin-impregnated layer. *Oper Dent* 19:59–64, 1994.

253. Tatsumi T, Inokoshi S, Yamada T, et al: Remineralization of etched dentin. *J Prosthet Dent* 67:617–620, 1992.

254. Okamoto Y, Heeley JD, Dogon IL, et al: Effects of phosphoric acid and tannic acid on dentine collagen. *J Oral Rehabil* 18:507–512, 1991.

255. El Feninat F, Ellis TH, Sacher E, et al: Moisture-dependent renaturation of collagen in phosphoric acid etched human dentin. *J Biomed Mater Res* 42:549–553, 1998.

256. Klont B, Ten Cate JM: Denaturation and degradation of dentin collagen during dentinal caries: possible mechanisms. In Thylstrup A, Leach SA, Qvist V, editors: *Dentin and dentin reactions in the oral cavity*, Oxford, 1987, IRL Press, pp155–164.

257. Ritter AV, Swift EJ, Jr, Yamauchi M: Effects of phosphoric acid and glutaraldehyde-HEMA on dentin collagen. *Eur J Oral Sci* 109:348–353, 2001.

258. Breschi L, Perdigão J, Gobbi P, et al: Immunolocalization of type I collagen in etched dentin. *J Biomed Mater Res A* 66:764–769, 2003.

259. Landis WJ, Hodgens KJ, Arena J, et al: Structural relations between collagen and mineral in bone as determined by high voltage electron microscopic tomography. *Microsc Res Tech* 33:192–202, 1996.

260. Landis WJ, Silver FH: Mineral deposition in the extracellular matrices of vertebrate tissues: identification of possible apatite nucleation sites on type I collagen. *Cells Tissues Organs* 189:20–24, 2009.

261. Wainwright SA, Biggs WD, Currey JD, et al: *Mechanical design in organisms*, Princeton, 1982, Princeton Univ. Press.

262. Rivera EM, Yamauchi M: Site comparisons of dentine collagen cross-links from extracted human teeth. *Arch Oral Biol* 38:541–546, 1993.

263. Miguez PA, Pereira PN, Atsawasuwan P, et al: Collagen cross-linking and ultimate tensile strength in dentin. *J Dent Res* 83:807–810, 2004.

264. Yang W, Sherman VR, Gludovatz B, et al: On the tear resistance of skin. *Nat Commun* 6:6649, 2015.

265. Prasad M, Butler WT, Qin C: Dentin sialophosphoprotein in biomineralization. *Connect Tissue Res* 51:404–417, 2010.

266. Eanes ED: Amorphous calcium phosphate. *Monogr Oral Sci* 18:130–147, 2001.

267. Weiner S: Biomineralization: a structural perspective. *J Struct Biol* 163:229–234, 2008.

268. Weiner S, Sagi I, Addadi L: Structural biology. Choosing the crystallization path less traveled. *Science* 309:1027–1028, 2005.

269. Dahl T, Sabsay B, Veis A: Type I collagen-phosphophoryn interactions: specificity of the monomer-monomer binding. *J Struct Biol* 123:162–168, 1998.

270. Tay FR, Pashley DH: Biomimetic remineralization of resin-bonded acid-etched dentin. *J Dent Res* 88:719–724, 2009.

271. Mai S, Kim YK, Toledano M, et al: Phosphoric acid esters cannot replace polyvinylphosphonic acid as phosphoprotein analogs in biomimetic remineralization of resin-bonded dentin. *Dent Mater* 25:1230–1239, 2009.

272. Mai S, Kim YK, Kim J, et al: In vitro remineralization of severely compromised bonded dentin. *J Dent Res* 89:405–410, 2010.

273. Mazzoni A, Pashley DH, Nishitani Y, et al: Reactivation of inactivated endogenous proteolytic activities in phosphoric acid-etched dentine by etch-and-rinse adhesives. *Biomaterials* 27:4470–4476, 2006.

274. Sulkala M, Larmas M, Sorsa T, et al: The localization of matrix metalloproteinase-20 (MMP-20, enamelysin) in mature human teeth. *J Dent Res* 81:603–638, 2002.

275. Martin-De Las Heras S, Valenzuela A, Overall CM: The matrix metalloproteinase gelatinase A in human dentine. *Arch Oral Biol* 45:757–765, 2000.

276. Gendron R, Grenier D, Sorsa T, et al: Inhibition of the activities of matrix metalloproteinases 2, 8, and 9 by chlorhexidine. *Clin Diagn Lab Immunol* 6:437–443, 1999.

277. Perdigao J, Denehy GE, Swift EJ, Jr: Effects of chlorhexidine on dentin surfaces and shear bond strengths. *Am J Dent* 7:81–84, 1994.

278. Pashley DH, Tay FR, Yiu C, et al: Collagen degradation by host-derived enzymes during aging. *J Dent Res* 83:216–221, 2004.

279. Ricci HA, Sanabe ME, de Souza Costa CA, et al: Chlorhexidine increases the longevity of in vivo resin-dentin bonds. *Eur J Oral Sci* 118:411–416, 2010.

280. Carrilho MR, Carvalho RM, de Goes MF, et al: Chlorhexidine preserves dentin bond in vitro. *J Dent Res* 86:90–94, 2007.

281. Hebling J, Pashley DH, Tjäderhane L, et al: Chlorhexidine arrests subclinical degradation of dentin hybrid layers in vivo. *J Dent Res* 84:741–746, 2005.

282. Loguercio AD, Hass V, Gutierrez MF, et al: Five-year effects of chlorhexidine on the in vitro durability of resin/dentin interfaces. *J Adhes Dent* 18:35–42, 2016.

283. Boushell LW, Kaku M, Mochida Y, et al: Immunohistochemical localization of matrixmetalloproteinase-2 in human coronal dentin. *Arch Oral Biol* 53:109–116, 2008.

284. De Munck J, Mine A, Van den Steen PE, et al: Enzymatic degradation of adhesive-dentin interfaces produced by mild self-etch adhesives. *Eur J Oral Sci* 118:494–501, 2010.

285. Sadek FT, Castellan CS, Braga RR, et al: One-year stability of resin-dentin bonds created with a hydrophobic ethanol-wet bonding technique. *Dent Mater* 26:380–386, 2010.

286. Bergenholtz G, Cox CF, Loesche WJ, et al: Bacterial leakage around dental restorations its effect on the dental pulp. *J Oral Pathol* 11:439–450, 1982.

287. Brännström M, Nyborg H: Pulpal reaction to polycarboxylate and zinc phosphate cements used with inlays in deep cavity preparations. *J Am Dent Assoc* 94:308–310, 1977.

288. Brännström M, Vojinovic O, Nordenvall KJ: Bacteria and pulpal reactions under silicate cement restorations. *J Prosthet Dent* 41:290–295, 1979.

289. Torstenson B, Nordenvall KJ, Brännström M: Pulpal reaction and microorganisms under Clearfil Composite Resin in deep cavities with acid etched dentin. *Swed Dent J* 6:167–176, 1982.

290. Reference deleted in pages.

291. Brännström M, Nordenvall J: Bacterial penetration, pulpal reaction and the inner surface of Concise Enamel Bond: composite fillings in etched and unetched cavities. *J Dent Res* 57:3–10, 1978.

292. Brännström M, Nyborg H: Cavity treatment with a microbicidal fluoride solution: growth of bacteria and effect on the pulp. *J Prosthet Dent* 30:303–310, 1973.

293. Mejàre B, Mejàre I, Edwardsson S: Acid etching and composite resin restorations: a culturing and histologic study on bacterial penetration. *Acta Odontol Scand* 3:1–5, 1987.

294. Mejàre I, Mejàre B, Edwardsson S: Effect of a tight seal on survival of bacteria in saliva-contaminated cavities filled with composite resin. *Endod Dent Traumatol* 3:6–9, 1987.

295. Turkistani A, Nakashima S, Shimada Y, et al: Microgaps and demineralization progress around composite restorations. *J Dent Res* 94:1070–1077, 2015.

296. Heintze SD: Systematic reviews: I. The correlation between laboratory tests on marginal quality and bond strength. II. The correlation between marginal quality and clinical outcome. *J Adhes Dent* 9 Suppl 1:77–106, 2007.

297. Perdigão J, Lopes M: Dentin bonding—questions for the new millennium. *J Adhes Dent* 1:191–209, 1999.

298. De Munck J, Van Meerbeek B, Yoshida Y, et al: Four-year water degradation of total-etch adhesives bonded to dentin. *J Dent Res* 82:136–140, 2003.

299. Hashimoto M, Ohno H, Sano H, et al: Degradation patterns of different adhesives and bonding procedures. *J Biomed Mater Res* 66B:324–330, 2003.

300. Hashimoto M, Ohno H, Kaga M, et al: In vivo degradation of resin-dentin bonds in humans over 1 to 3 years. *J Dent Res* 79:1385–1391, 2000.

301. Sano H, Yoshiyama M, Ebisu S, et al: Comparative SEM and TEM observations of nanoleakage within the hybrid layer. *Oper Dent* 20:160–167, 1995.

302. Li HP, Burrow MF, Tyas MJ: The effect of long-term storage on nanoleakage. *Oper Dent* 26:609–616, 2001.

303. Tay FR, Pashley DH, Yoshiyama M: Two modes of nanoleakage expression in single-step adhesives. *J Dent Res* 81:472–476, 2002.

304. Van Meerbeek B: The "myth" of nanoleakage. *J Adhes Dent* 9:491–492, 2007.

305. Pashley DH, Ciucchi B, Sano H, et al: Permeability of dentin to adhesive agents. *Quintessence Int* 24:618–631, 1993.

306. Lee HL, Orlowski JA, Scheidt GC, et al: Effects of acid etchants on dentin. *J Dent Res* 52:1228–1233, 1973.

307. Marshall GW, Inai N, Wu-Magidi IC, et al: Dentin demineralization: effects of dentin depth, pH and different acids. *Dent Mater* 13:338–343, 1997.

308. Selvig KA: Ultrastructural changes in human dentine exposed to a weak acid. *Arch Oral Biol* 13:719–734, 1968.

309. Wang J-D, Hume WR: Diffusion of hydrogen ion and hydroxyl ion from various sources through dentine. *Int Endod J* 21:17–26, 1988.

310. Uno S, Finger WJ: Effects of acidic conditioners on dentine demineralization and dimension of hybrid layers. *J Dent* 24:211–216, 1996.

311. Macko DJ, Rutberg M, Langeland K: Pulpal response to the application of phosphoric acid to dentin. *Oral Surg Oral Med Oral Pathol* 6:930–946, 1978.

312. Cox CF, Suzuki S: Re-evaluating pulp protection: calcium hydroxide liners vs. cohesive hybridization. *J Am Dent Assoc* 125:823–831, 1994.

313. Cox CF, Keall CL, Keall HJ, et al: Biocompatibility of surface-sealed dental materials against exposed pulps. *J Prosthet Dent* 57:1–8, 1987.

314. Fuks AB, Funnell B, Cleaton-Jones P: Pulp response to a composite resin inserted in deep cavities with and without a surface seal. *J Prosthet Dent* 63:129–134, 1990.

315. Inokoshi S, Iwaku M, Fusayama T: Pulpal response to a new adhesive restorative resin. *J Dent Res* 61:1014–1019, 1982.

316. Qvist V, Stoltze K, Qvist J: Human pulp reactions to resin restorations performed with different acid-etched restorative procedures. *Acta Odontol Scand* 47:253–263, 1989.

317. Snuggs HM, Cox CF, Powell CS, et al: Pulpal healing and dentinal bridge formation in an acidic environment. *Quintessence Int* 24:501–509, 1993.

318. Tsuneda Y, Hayakawa T, Yamamoto H, et al: A histopathological study of direct pulp capping with adhesive resins. *Oper Dent* 20:223–229, 1995.

319. White KS, Cox CF, Kanca J, 3rd, et al: Pulp response to adhesive resin systems applied to acid-etched vital dentin: damp versus dry primer application. *Quintessence Int* 25:259–268, 1994.

320. Kanca J, 3rd: Replacement of a fractured incisor fragment over pulpal exposure: a long-term case report. *Quintessence Int* 27:829–832, 1996.

321. Heitman T, Unterbrink G: Direct pulp capping with a dentinal adhesive resin system: a pilot study. *Quintessence Int* 11:765–770, 1995.

322. Cox CF, Hafez AA, Akimoto N, et al: Biocompatibility of primer, adhesive and resin composite systems on non-exposed and exposed pulps of non-human primate teeth. *Am J Dent* 11:S55–S63, 1998.

323. Gwinnett AJ, Tay FR: Early and intermediate time response of the dental pulp to an acid etch technique in vivo. *Am J Dent* 11:S35–S44, 1998.

324. Hebling J, Giro EM, Costa CA: Biocompatibility of an adhesive system applied to exposed human dental pulp. *J Endod* 25:676–682, 1999.

325. Pameijer CH, Stanley HR: The disastrous effects of the "total etch" technique in vital pulp capping in primates. *Am J Dent* 11:S45–S54, 1998.

326. Costa CA, Hebling J, Hanks CT: Current status of pulp capping with dentin adhesive systems: a review. *Dent Mater* 16:188–197, 2000.

327. Bjørndal L, Darvann T: A light microscopic study of odontoblastic and non-odontoblastic cells involved in tertiary dentinogenesis in well-defined cavitated carious lesions. *Caries Res* 33:50–60, 1999.

328. Bergenholtz G: Iatrogenic injury to the pulp in dental procedures: aspects of pathogenesis, management and preventive measures. *Int Dent J* 41:99–110, 1991.

329. Brännström M: The effect of dentin desiccation and aspirated odontoblasts on the pulp. *J Prosthet Dent* 20:165–171, 1968.

330. Stanley HR, Weisman MI, Michanowicz AE, et al: Ischemic infarction of the pulp: sequential degenerative changes of the pulp after traumatic injury. *J Endod* 4:325–355, 1978.

331. Ravn JJ: Follow-up study of permanent incisors with enamel fractures as a result of an acute trauma. *Scand J Dent Res* 89:213–217, 1981.

332. Murray PE, Smith AJ, Garcia-Godoy F, et al: Comparison of operative procedure variables on pulpal viability in an ex vivo model. *Int Endod J* 41:389–400, 2008.

333. Hannig M, Bott B: In-vitro pulp chamber temperature rise during composite resin polymerization with various light-curing sources. *Dent Mater* 15:275–281, 1999.

334. Baroudi K, Silikas N, Watts DC: In vitro pulp chamber temperature rise from irradiation and exotherm of flowable composites. *Int J Paediatr Dent* 19:48–54, 2009.

335. Bergenholtz G: Evidence for bacterial causation of adverse pulpal responses in resin-based dental restorations. *Crit Rev Oral Biol Med* 11:467–480, 2000.

336. Knezevic A, Zeljezic D, Kopjar N, et al: Cytotoxicity of composite materials polymerized with LED curing units. *Oper Dent* 33:23–30, 2008.

337. Eren D, Bektaş ÖÖ, Siso SH: Three different adhesive systems; three different bond strength test methods. *Acta Odontol Scand* 71:978–983, 2013.

338. Heintze SD, Thunpithayakul C, Armstrong SR, et al: Correlation between microtensile bond strength data and clinical outcome of Class V restorations. *Dent Mater* 27:114–125, 2011.

339. Paul SJ, Welter DA, Ghazi M, et al: Nanoleakage at the dentin adhesive interface vs microtensile bond strength. *Oper Dent* 24:181–188, 1999.

340. Eick JD, Robinson SJ, Chappell RP, et al: The dentinal surface: its influence on dentinal adhesion: part III. *Quintessence Int* 24:571–582, 1993.

341. Tam LE, Pilliar RM: Fracture surface characterization of dentin-bonded interfacial fracture toughness specimens. *J Dent Res* 73:607–619, 1994.

342. Fortin D, Swift EJ, Jr, Denehy GE, et al: Bond strength and microleakage of current adhesive systems. *Dent Mater* 10:253–258, 1994.

343. Sano H, Shono T, Sonoda H, et al: Relationship between surface area for adhesion and tensile bond strength: evaluation of a microtensile bond test. *Dent Mater* 10:236–240, 1994.

344. Nakajima M, Sano H, Burrow MF, et al: Tensile bond strength and SEM evaluation of caries-affected dentin using dentin adhesives. *J Dent Res* 74:1679–1688, 1995.

345. Phrukkanon S, Burrow MF, Tyas MJ: The influence of cross-sectional shape and surface area on the microtensile bond test. *Dent Mater* 14:212–221, 1998.

346. Shono Y, Ogawa T, Terashita M, et al: Regional measurement of resin-dentin bonding as an array. *J Dent Res* 78:699–705, 1998.

347. Reis A, Rocha de Oliveira Carrilho M, Schroeder M, et al: The influence of storage time and cutting speed on microtensile bond strength. *J Adhes Dent* 6:7–11, 2004.

348. Poitevin A, De Munck J, Van Landuyt K, et al: Critical analysis of the influence of different parameters on the microtensile bond strength of adhesives to dentin. *J Adhes Dent* 10:7–16, 2008.

349. Van Meerbeek B, Peumans M, Poitevin A, et al: Relationship between bond-strength tests and clinical outcomes. *Dent Mater* 26:e100–e121, 2010.

350. Heintze SD, Bluck U, Göhring TN, et al: Marginal adaptation in vitro and clinical outcome of Class V restorations. *Dent Mater* 25:605–620, 2009.

351. Armstrong SR, Boyer DB, Keller JC: Microtensile bond strength testing and failure analysis of two dentin adhesives. *Dent Mater* 14:44–50, 1998.

352. Pashley DH: Dentin bonding: overview of the substrate with respect to adhesive material. *J Esthet Dent* 3:46–50, 1991.

353. Pameijer CH, Louw NP: Significance of pulpal pressure during clinical bonding procedures. *Am J Dent* 10:214–218, 1997.

354. Yoshiyama M, Carvaho RM, Sano H, et al: Regional bond strengths of resins to human root dentine. *J Dent* 24:435–442, 1996.

355. Yoshiyama M, Sano H, Ebisu S, et al: Regional strengths of bonding agents to cervical sclerotic root dentin. *J Dent Res* 75:1404–1413, 1996.

356. Perinka L, Sano H, Hosoda H: Dentin thickness, hardness and Ca-concentration vs bond strength of dentin adhesives. *Dent Mater* 8:229–233, 1992.

357. Brännström M, Lindén LA, Aström A: The hydrodynamics of the dental tubule and of pulp fluid. A discussion of its significance in relation to dentinal sensitivity. *Caries Res* 1:310–317, 1967.

358. Harnirattisai C, Inokoshi S, Shimada Y, et al: Adhesive interface between resin and etched dentin of cervical erosion/abrasion lesions. *Oper Dent* 18:138–143, 1993.

359. Kwong SM, Cheung GS, Kei LH, et al: Micro-tensile bond strengths to sclerotic dentin using a self-etching and a total-etching technique. *Dent Mater* 18:359–369, 2002.

360. Heymann HO, Sturdevant JR, Bayne S, et al: Examining tooth flexure effects on cervical restorations: a two-year clinical study. *J Am Dent Assoc* 122:41–47, 1991.

361. Van Meerbeek B, Braem M, Lambrechts P, et al: Morphological characterization of the interface between resin and sclerotic dentine. *J Dent* 22:141–146, 1994.

362. van Dijken JWV: Clinical evaluation of three adhesive systems in Class V non-carious lesions. *Dent Mater* 16:285–291, 2000.

363. Braem M, Lambrechts P, Vanherle G, et al: Stiffness increase during the setting of dental composite resins. *J Dent Res* 66:1713–1716, 1987.

364. Heymann HO, Sturdevant JR, Brunson WD, et al: Twelve-month clinical study of dentinal adhesives in Class V cervical lesions. *J Am Dent Assoc* 116:179–183, 1988.

365. Heintze SD, Rousson V: Clinical effectiveness of direct class II restorations - a meta-analysis. *J Adhes Dent* 14:407–431, 2012.

366. Gladys S, Van Meerbeek B, Braem M, et al: Comparative physico-mechanical characterization of new hybrid restorative materials with conventional glass-ionomer and resin composite restorative materials. *J Dent Res* 76:883–894, 1997.

367. Miyazaki M, Hinoura K, Onose H, et al: Effect of filler content of light-cured composites on bond strength to bovine dentine. *J Dent* 19:301–303, 1991.

368. Browning WD, Brackett WW, Gilpatrick RO: Two-year clinical comparison of a microfilled and a hybrid resin-based composite in non-carious Class V lesions. *Oper Dent* 25:46–50, 2000.

369. Peumans M, De Munck J, Van Landuyt KL, et al: Restoring cervical lesions with flexible composites. *Dent Mater* 23:749–754, 2007.

370. Peumans M, Kanumilli P, De Munck J, et al: Clinical effectiveness of contemporary adhesives: a systematic review of current clinical trials. *Dent Mater* 21:864–881, 2005.

371. Heintze SD, Ruffieux C, Rousson V: Clinical performance of cervical restorations–a meta-analysis. *Dent Mater* 26:993–1000, 2010.

372. Loguercio AD, De Paula EA, Hass V, et al: A new universal simplified adhesive: 36-month randomized double-blind clinical trial. *J Dent* 43:1083–1092, 2015.

373. Lawson NC, Robles A, Fu CC, et al: Two-year clinical trial of a universal adhesive in total-etch and self-etch mode in non-carious cervical lesions. *J Dent* 43:1229–1234, 2015.

374. Sanares AME, Itthagarun A, King NM, et al: Adverse surface interactions between one-bottle light-cured adhesives and chemical-cured composites. *Dent Mater* 17:542–556, 2001.

375. Swift EJ, Jr, Perdigão J, Combe EC, et al: Effects of restorative and adhesive curing methods on dentin bond strengths. *Am J Dent* 14:137–140, 2001.

376. Bömicke W, Schürz A, Krisam J, et al: Durability of resin-zirconia bonds produced using methods available in dental practice. *J Adhes Dent* 18:17–27, 2016.

377. Seabra B, Arantes-Oliveira S, Portugal J: Influence of multimode universal adhesives and zirconia primer application techniques on zirconia repair. *J Prosthet Dent* 112:182–187, 2014.

378. Kalavacharla VK, Lawson NC, Ramp LC, et al: Influence of etching protocol and silane treatment with a universal adhesive on lithium disilicate bond strength. *Oper Dent* 40:372–378, 2015.

379. Perdigão J, Swift EJ, Jr: Universal adhesives. *J Esthet Restor Dent* 27:331–334, 2015.

380. Siqueira F, Cardenas AM, Gutierrez MF, et al: Laboratory performance of universal adhesive systems for luting CAD/CAM restorative materials. *J Adhes Dent* 18:331–340, 2016.

381. Pashley DH, Matthews WG, Zhang Y, et al: Fluid shifts across human dentine in vitro in response to hydrodynamic stimuli. *Arch Oral Biol* 41:1065–1072, 1996.

382. Markowitz K: Pretty painful: Why does tooth bleaching hurt? *Med Hypotheses* 74:835–840, 2010.

383. Gray A, Ferguson MM, Wall JG: Wine tasting and dental erosion: case report. *Aust Dent J* 43:32–34, 1988.

384. Grippo JO: Abfractions: a new classification of hard tissue lesions of teeth. *J Esthet Dent* 3:14–19, 1991.

385. Cuenin MF, Scheidt MJ, O'Neal RB, et al: An in vivo study of dentin sensitivity: the relation of dentin sensitivity and the patency of dentin tubules. *J Periodontol* 62:668–673, 1991.

386. Reinhardt JW, Stephens NH, Fortin D: Effect of Gluma desensitization on dentin bond strength. *Am J Dent* 8:170–172, 1995.

387. Kerns DG, Scheidt MJ, Pashley DH, et al: Dentinal tubule occlusion and root hypersensitivity. *J Periodontol* 62:421–428, 1991.

388. Nakabayashi N, Nakamura M, Yasuda N: Hybrid layer as a dentin-bonding mechanism. *J Esthet Dent* 3:133–138, 1991.

389. Scherman A, Jacobsen PL: Managing dentin hypersensitivity: What treatment to recommend to patients. *J Am Dent Assoc* 123:57–61, 1992.

390. Nikaido T, Burrow MF, Tagami J, et al: Effect of pulpal pressure on adhesion of resin composite to dentin: bovine serum versus saline. *Quintessence Int* 26:221–226, 1995.

391. Swift EJ, Hammel SA, Perdigao J, et al: Prevention of root surface caries using a dental adhesive. *J Am Dent Assoc* 125:571–576, 1994.

392. Felton DA, Bergenholtz G, Kanoy BE: Evaluation of the desensitizing effect of Gluma dentin bond on teeth prepared for complete coverage restorations. *Int J Prosthodont* 4:292–298, 1991.

393. Bowes JH, Cater CW: The reaction of glutaraldehyde with proteins and other biological materials. *J Royal Microsc Soc* 85:193–200, 1966.

394. Schüpbach P, Lutz F, Finger WJ: Closing of dentinal tubules by Gluma desensitizer. *Eur J Oral Sci* 105:414–421, 1997.

395. Duran I, Sengun A, Yildirim T, et al: In vitro dentine permeability evaluation of HEMA-based (desensitizing) products using split-chamber model following in vivo application in the dog. *J Oral Rehabil* 32:34–38, 2005.

396. Camps J, About I, Van Meerbeek B, et al: Efficiency and cytotoxicity of resin-based desensitizing agents. *Am J Dent* 15:300–304, 2002.

397. Finger WJ, Balkenhol M: Rewetting strategies for bonding to dry dentin with an acetone-based adhesive. *J Adhes Dent* 2:51–56, 2000.

398. Ritter AV, Heymann HO, Swift EJ, Jr, et al: Effects of different re-wetting techniques on dentin shear bond strengths. *J Esthet Dent* 12:85–96, 2000.

399. Sobral MA, Garone-Netto N, Luz MA, et al: Prevention of postoperative tooth sensitivity: a preliminary clinical trial. *J Oral Rehabil* 32:661–668, 2005.

400. Chermont AB, Carneiro KK, Lobato MF, et al: Clinical evaluation of postoperative sensitivity using self-etching adhesives containing glutaraldehyde. *Braz Oral Res* 24:349–354, 2010.

401. Cobb DS, Reinhardt JW, Vargas MA: Effect of HEMA-containing dentin desensitizers on shear bond strength of a resin cement. *Am J Dent* 10:62–65, 1997.

402. Swift EJ, Jr, Lloyd AH, Felton DA, et al: The effect of resin desensitizing agents on crown retention. *J Am Dent Assoc* 128:195–200, 1997.

403. Helfer AR, Melnick S, Schilder H: Determination of the moisture content of vital and pulpless teeth. *Oral Surg Oral Med Oral Pathol* 34:661–670, 1972.

404. Nalbandian J, Gonzales F, Sognnaes RF: Sclerotic age changes in root dentin of human teeth as observed by optical, electron, and X-ray microscopy. *J Dent Res* 39:598–607, 1960.

405. Kinney JH, Nalla RK, Pople JA, et al: Age-related transparent root dentin: mineral concentration, crystallite size, and mechanical properties. *Biomaterials* 26:3363–3376, 2005.

406. Mjör IA, Smith MR, Ferrari M, et al: The structure of dentine in the apical region of human teeth. *Int Endod J* 34:346–353, 2001.

407. Violich DR, Chandler NP: The smear layer in endodontics - a review. *Int Endod J* 43:2–15, 2010.

408. McComb D, Smith DC: A preliminary scanning electron microscopic study of root canals after endodontic procedures. *J Endod* 1:238–242, 1975.

409. Mader CL, Baumgartner JC, Peters DD: Scanning electron microscopic investigation of the smeared layer on root canal walls. *J Endod* 10:477–483, 1984.

410. Reis A, Loguercio AD, Bitter K, et al: Adhesion to root dentin: A challenging task. In Perdigão J, editor: *Restoration of root canal-treated teeth - an adhesive dentistry perspective*, Switzerland, 2016, Springer International Publishing, pp 137–151.

411. Bouillaguet S, Troesch S, Wataha JC, et al: Microtensile bond strength between adhesive cements and root canal dentin. *Dent Mater* 19:199–205, 2003.

412. Alster D, Feilzer AJ, de Gee AJ, et al: Polymerization contraction stress in thin resin composite layers as a function of layer thickness. *Dent Mater* 13:146–150, 1997.

413. Santos-Filho PC, Veríssimo C, Raposo LH, et al: Influence of ferrule, post system, and length on stress distribution of weakened root-filled teeth. *J Endod* 40:1874–1878, 2014.

414. Gomes GM, Gomes OM, Gomes JC, et al: Evaluation of different restorative techniques for filling flared root canals: fracture resistance and bond strength after mechanical fatigue. *J Adhes Dent* 16:267–276, 2014.

415. Farina AP, Chiela H, Carlini-Junior B, et al: Influence of cement type and relining procedure on push-out bond strength of fiber posts after cyclic loading. *J Prosthodont* 25:54–60, 2016.

416. Feilzer AJ, de Gee AJ, Davidson CL: Setting stresses in composites for two different curing modes. *Dent Mater* 9:2–5, 1993.

417. Bitter K, Perdigão J, Hartwig C, et al: Nanoleakage of luting agents for bonding fiber posts after thermo-mechanical fatigue. *J Adhes Dent* 13:61–69, 2011.

418. Bitter K, Perdigão J, Exner M, et al: Reliability of fiber post bonding to root canal dentin after simulated clinical function in vitro. *Oper Dent* 37:397–405, 2012.

419. Sarkis-Onofre R, Skupien JA, Cenci MS, et al: The role of resin cement on bond strength of glass-fiber posts luted into root canals: a systematic review and meta-analysis of in vitro studies. *Oper Dent* 39:E31–E44, 2014.

420. Skupien JA, Sarkis-Onofre R, Cenci MS, et al: A systematic review of factors associated with the retention of glass fiber posts. *Braz Oral Res* 29:pii: S1806-83242015000100401, 2015.

421. Mayer T, Pioch T, Duschner H, et al: Dentinal adhesion and histomorphology of two dentinal bonding agents under the influence of eugenol. *Quintessence Int* 28:57–62, 1997.

422. AlEisa K, Al-Dwairi ZN, Lynch E, et al: In vitro evaluation of the effect of different endodontic sealers on retentive strength of fiber posts. *Oper Dent* 38:539–544, 2013.

423. Aleisa K, Alghabban R, Alwazzan K, et al: Effect of three endodontic sealers on the bond strength of prefabricated fiber posts luted with three resin cements. *J Prosthet Dent* 107:322–326, 2012.

424. Demiryurek EO, Kulunk S, Yuksel G, et al: Effects of three canal sealers on bond strength of a fiber post. *J Endod* 36:497–501, 2010.

425. Hagge MS, Wong RD, Lindemuth JS: Effect of three root canal sealers on the retentive strength of endodontic posts luted with a resin cement. *Int Endod J* 35:372–378, 2002.

426. Kurtz JS, Perdigao J, Geraldeli S, et al: Bond strengths of tooth-colored posts, effect of sealer, dentin adhesive, and root region. *Am J Dent* 16 Spec No:31A–36A, 2003.

427. Boone KJ, Murchison DF, Schindler WG, et al: Post retention: the effect of sequence of post-space preparation, cementation time, and different sealers. *J Endod* 27:768–771, 2001.

428. Mesquita GC, Verissimo C, Raposo LH, et al: Can the cure time of endodontic sealers affect bond strength to root dentin? *Braz Dent J* 24:340–343, 2013.

429. Vano M, Cury AH, Goracci C, et al: The effect of immediate versus delayed cementation on the retention of different types of fiber post in canals obturated using a eugenol sealer. *J Endod* 32:882–885, 2006.

430. Tzanakakis EG, Tzoutzas IG, Koidis PT: Is there a potential for durable adhesion to zirconia restorations? A systematic review. *J Prosthet Dent* 115:9–19, 2016.

431. Morimoto S, Albanesi RB, Sesma N, et al: Main clinical outcomes of feldspathic porcelain and glass-ceramic laminate veneers: a systematic review and meta-analysis of survival and complication rates. *Int J Prosthodont* 29:38–49, 2016.

432. Sterzenbach G, Franke A, Naumann M: Rigid versus flexible dentine-like endodontic posts–clinical testing of a biomechanical concept: seven-year results of a randomized controlled clinical pilot trial on endodontically treated abutment teeth with severe hard tissue loss. *J Endod* 38:1557–1563, 2012.

433. Esquivel-Upshaw J, Rose W, Oliveira E, et al: Randomized, controlled clinical trial of bilayer ceramic and metal-ceramic crown performance. *J Prosthodont* 22:166–173, 2013.

434. Gracis S, Thompson VP, Ferencz JL, et al: A new classification system for all-ceramic and ceramic-like restorative materials. *Int J Prosthodont* 28:227–235, 2015.

435. Ozcan M, Vallittu PK: Effect of surface conditioning methods on the bond strength of luting cement to ceramics. *Dent Mater* 19:725–731, 2003.

436. Addison O, Marquis PM, Fleming GJ: The impact of hydrofluoric acid surface treatments on the performance of a porcelain laminate restorative material. *Dent Mater* 23:461–468, 2007.

437. Peumans M, Valjakova EB, De Munck J, et al: Bonding effectiveness of luting composites to different CAD/CAM materials. *J Adhes Dent* 18:289–302, 2016.

438. al Edris A, al Jabr A, Cooley RL, et al: SEM evaluation of etch patterns by three etchants on three porcelains. *J Prosthet Dent* 64:734–739, 1990.

439. Calamia JR: Etched porcelain facial veneers: a new treatment modality based on scientific and clinical evidence. *N Y J Dent* 53:255–259, 1983.

440. Bjorksten J, Yaeger LL: Vinyl silane size for glass fabric. *Mod Plast* 29:124, 128, 1952.

441. Bowen RL, Rodriguez MS: Tensile strength and modulus of elasticity of tooth structure and several restorative materials. *J Am Dent Assoc* 64:378–387, 1962.

442. Diaz-Arnold AM, Schneider RL, Aquilino SA: Porcelain repairs: an evaluation of the shear strength of three porcelain repair systems (abstract 806). *J Dent Res* 66:207, 1987.

443. Newburg R, Pameijer CH: Composite resin bonded to porcelain with a silane solution. *J Am Dent Assoc* 96:288–291, 1978.

444. Sheth J, Jensen M, Tolliver D: Effect of surface treatment on etched porcelain and bond strength to enamel. *Dent Mater* 4:328–337, 1998.

445. Chen L, Shen H, Suh BI: Effect of incorporating BisGMA resin on the bonding properties of silane and zirconia primers. *J Prosthet Dent* 110:402–407, 2013.

446. Kim RJ, Woo JS, Lee IB, et al: Performance of universal adhesives on bonding to leucite-reinforced ceramic. *Biomater Res* 19:11, 2015.

447. Chen C, Trindade FZ, de Jager N, et al: The fracture resistance of a CAD/CAM Resin NanoCeramic (RNC) and a CAD ceramic at different thicknesses. *Dent Mater* 30:954–962, 2014.

448. Fleming GJ, Jandu HS, Nolan L, et al: The influence of alumina abrasion and cement lute on the strength of a porcelain laminate veneering material. *J Dent* 32:67–74, 2004.

449. Garvie RC, Hannink RH, Pascoe RT: Ceramic steel? *Nature* 258:703–704, 1975.
450. Heuer AH: Transformation toughening in ZrO₂-containing ceramics. *J Am Ceram Soc* 70:689–698, 1987.
451. Hannink RHJ, Kelly PM, Muddle BC: Transformation toughening in zirconia-containing ceramics. *J Am Ceram Soc* 83:461–487, 2000.
452. Piconi C, Maccauro G: Zirconia as a ceramic biomaterial. *Biomaterials* 20:1–25, 1999.
453. Tanaka K, Tamura J, Kawanabe K, et al: Phase stability after aging and its influence on pin-on-disk wear properties of Ce-TZP/Al₂O₃ nanocomposite and conventional Y-TZP. *J Biomed Mater Res A* 67:200–207, 2003.
454. Benzaid R, Chevalier J, Saâdaoui M, et al: Fracture toughness, strength and slow crack growth in a ceria stabilized zirconia-alumina nanocomposite for medical applications. *Biomaterials* 29:3636–3641, 2008.
455. Kern M, Wegner SM: Bonding to zirconia ceramic: adhesion methods and their durability. *Dent Mater* 14:64–71, 1998.
456. Borges GA, Spohr AM, de Goes MF, et al: Effect of etching and airborne particle abrasion on the microstructure of different dental ceramics. *J Prosthet Dent* 89:479–488, 2003.
457. Kern M, Barloi A, Yang B: Surface conditioning influences zirconia ceramic bonding. *J Dent Res* 88:817–822, 2009.
458. Inokoshi M, De Munck J, Minakuchi S, et al: Meta-analysis of bonding effectiveness to zirconia ceramics. *J Dent Res* 93:329–334, 2014.
459. Özcan M, Bernasconi M: Adhesion to zirconia used for dental restorations: a systematic review and meta-analysis. *J Adhes Dent* 17:7–26, 2015.
460. Chen L, Suh BI, Brown D, et al: Bonding of primed zirconia ceramics: evidence of chemical bonding and improved bond strengths. *Am J Dent* 25:103–108, 2012.
461. Yoshida K, Tsuo T, Atsuta M: Bonding of dual-cured resin cement to zirconia ceramic using phosphate acid ester monomer and zirconate coupler. *J Biomed Mater Res B Appl Biomater* 77:28–33, 2006.
462. Maeda FA, Bello-Silva MS, de Paula Eduardo C, et al: Association of different primers and resin cements for adhesive bonding to zirconia ceramics. *J Adhes Dent* 16:261–265, 2014.
463. Amaral M, Belli R, Cesar PF, et al: The potential of novel primers and universal adhesives to bond to zirconia. *J Dent* 42:90–98, 2014.
464. Özcan M, Bock T: Protocol for removal of clinically relevant contaminants from zirconium dioxide fixed dental prostheses. *J Adhes Dent* 17:576–577, 2015.
465. Kobayashi K, Kuwajima H, Masaki T: Phase change and mechanical properties of ZrO₂-Y₂O₃ solid electrolyte after ageing. *Solid State Ion* 3/4:489–493, 1981.
466. Chevalier J, Cales B, Drouin JM: Low-temperature aging of Y-TZP ceramics. *J Am Ceram Soc* 82:2150–2154, 1999.
467. Chevalier J, Olagnon C, Fantozzi G: Subcritical crack propagation in 3Y-TZP ceramics: static and cyclic fatigue. *J Am Ceram Soc* 82:3129–3138, 1999.
468. Chevalier J, Gremillard L, Deville S: Low-temperature degradation of zirconia and implications for biomedical implants. *Annu Rev Mater Res* 37:1–32, 2007.
469. Studart AR, Filser F, Kocher P, et al: Fatigue of zirconia under cyclic loading in water and its implications for the design of dental bridges. *Dent Mater* 23:106–114, 2007.
470. Kohorst P, Dittmer MP, Borchers L, et al: Influence of cyclic fatigue in water on the loadbearing capacity of dental bridges made of zirconia. *Acta Biomater* 4:1440–1447, 2008.
471. Kohorst P, Borchers L, Strempel J, et al: Low-temperature degradation of different zirconia ceramics for dental applications. *Acta Biomater* 8:1213–1220, 2012.
472. Perdigão J, Pinto AM, Monteiro RC, et al: Degradation of dental ZrO₂-based materials after hydrothermal fatigue. Part I: XRD, XRF, and FESEM analyses. *Dent Mater J* 31:256–265, 2012.
473. Bergamo E, da Silva WJ, Cesar PF, et al: Fracture load and phase transformation of monolithic zirconia crowns submitted to different aging protocols. *Oper Dent* 41:E118–E130, 2016.
474. Ângela Maziero Volpato C, Francisco Cesar P, Antônio Bottino M: Influence of accelerated aging on the color stability of dental zirconia. *J Esthet Restor Dent* 28:304–312, 2016.
475. Frankenberger R, Hartmann VE, Krech M, et al: Adhesive luting of new CAD/CAM materials. *Int J Comput Dent* 18:9–20, 2015.
476. Kassotakis EM, Stavridakis M, Bortolotto T, et al: Evaluation of the effect of different surface treatments on luting CAD/CAM composite resin overlay workpieces. *J Adhes Dent* 17:521–528, 2015.
477. Coldea A, Swain MV, Thiel N: Mechanical properties of polymer-infiltrated-ceramic-network materials. *Dent Mater* 29:419–426, 2013.
478. Özcan M, Volpato CÂ: Surface conditioning and bonding protocol for polymer-infiltrated ceramic: How and why? *J Adhes Dent* 18:174–175, 2016.
479. Darr AH, Jacobson PH: Conversion of dual-cure luting cements. *J Oral Rehabil* 22:43–47, 1995.
480. Lührs AK, De Munck J, Geurtsen W, et al: Composite cements benefit from light-curing. *Dent Mater* 30:292–301, 2014.
481. D'Alpino PH, Silva MS, Vismara MV, et al: The effect of polymerization mode on monomer conversion, free radical entrapment, and interaction with hydroxyapatite of commercial self-adhesive cements. *J Mech Behav Biomed Mater* 46:83–92, 2015.
482. Gerth HU, Dammaschke T, Züchner H, et al: Chemical analysis and bonding reaction of RelyX Unicem and Bifix composites–a comparative study. *Dent Mater* 22:934–941, 2006.
483. Saskalauskaite E, Tam LE, McComb D: Flexural strength, elastic modulus, and pH profile of self-etch resin luting cements. *J Prosthodont* 17:262–268, 2008.
484. Vrochari AD, Eliades G, Hellwig E, et al: Curing efficiency of four self-etching, self-adhesive resin cements. *Dent Mater* 25:1104–1108, 2009.

Disclosure

Dr. Perdigão has received compensation for speaking at events sponsored by 3M Oral Care and Coltene. This relationship has been reviewed and managed by the University of Minnesota in accordance with its conflict of interest policies.

6

Light Curing of Restorative Materials

RICHARD B. PRICE, FREDERICK A. RUEGGEBERG

The ability to light cure dental resins "on demand" has revolutionized the practice of restorative dentistry and the dental curing light has become an indispensable tool in almost every dental office.[1-3] Despite their ubiquitous presence and routine use, the interaction between curing lights and light-activated dental resins or resin cements is poorly understood.[4] At first glance, it appears that the process of light curing is simple and requires little attention. This misconception is concerning. Although the surface of the resin closest to the light polymerizes readily, giving the appearance that all the resin has been fully "light cured," this has not always occurred in the deeper layers of the restoration. This may result in bulk fracture of the restoration, increased wear, increased release of chemicals, a low bond strength to the tooth, and increased microleakage between the tooth and the resin.[5-15]

In most countries, dental curing lights are classified as medical devices that must pass stringent tests before they are approved for use. This chapter will review the background and discuss the current knowledge of dental curing light and its use in contemporary resin photopolymerization. The International System of Units (SI) terminology that should be used to describe the output from a curing light will also be presented (Table 6.1).

Methacrylate-Based, Free Radical Polymerization

Virtually all resin-based restorative materials used to directly restore teeth belong to the methacrylate family.[1] These methacrylate-based monomers are linked to form polymers by a process called free radical addition polymerization. Once the free radical species are formed, the polymerization process is the same for all types of methacrylate-based restorative materials that are in use today. The only difference is how the free radicals are generated, the rate at which they are generated, and the number of free radicals that are produced. This process consists of the following four steps: activation, initiation, propagation, and termination (Fig. 6.1).

Activation and Initiation

The first step involves activation of a free radical species. This is a compound with an unpaired electron that aggressively seeks another electron with which it can form a covalent bond. There are many types of free radical species, but to become activated they all require an external energy source such as heat, an amine reducing agent (used in "self-curing" or "cold-curing"), or electromagnetic radiation (ultraviolet [UV] light, visible blue light, or microwave energy). In dental resins, the activated, free radical species seek out the electron-rich carbon double bond that is present in methacrylate groups of a monomer molecule. This double bond gives up one electron to the newly initiated radical, and the other electron acts as the free radical agent. This process is called "initiation."

Propagation

This monomer-radical species then seeks another carbon double bond in an adjacent monomer molecule; it absconds one of the double bond electrons and forms a new covalent bond between the two monomer molecules. This newly attached monomer possesses the unpaired electron, and it brings along the entire polymer chain to find yet more electron-rich carbon double bonds with which it can react. With every additional methacrylate-based monomer that is added to the end, the polymer chain grows longer. This process is called "propagation."

Termination

As the chain length increases, its molecular weight grows, thus decreasing the ability of the polymer chain to move. Also, because the surrounding resin changes from a liquid to a gel, the mobility of the reacting molecules decreases. Further increases in the chain length become diffusion controlled and the inability of the growing polymer chains to readily find and join to additional unreacted methacrylate monomers causes the rate of polymerization to decrease. This phenomenon is termed auto-deceleration. Eventually the polymerized resin becomes a solid, thus further inhibiting linear chain growth. At this point, the probability increases that two free radical ends from two different polymer chains will meet and form a covalent bond. Once this occurs, further increase in the linear chain length becomes impossible. This phase is called "termination." Most direct resin restorative materials used intraorally also contain monomer units that have two or more carbon double bonds that also allow cross-linking between adjacent polymer chains. Cross-linking between chains is highly desirable because polymers that have little cross-linking tend to be weak and flexible, whereas those that are highly cross-linked have greater fracture resistance, are harder, are less flexible, and are more heat resistant.[16] Of note, the use of different curing lights or light exposure modes can result in polymers that have different amounts of cross-linking.[1,16,18] This phenomenon means that solvents, food substances, and enzymatic attack can have different effects on the same dental resin, depending on how it was light cured.[16-18]

TABLE 6.1	Radiometric Terminology Used to Describe the Emission From Dental Curing Lights		
Term	**Units**	**Symbol**	**Notes**
Radiant energy	Joule	J	Describes the energy emitted or received
Radiant exposure	Joule per square centimeter	J/cm^2	Describes the energy emitted or received
Radiant energy density	Joule per cubic centimeter	J/cm^3	The volumetric (cm^3) energy density Not to be confused with the energy density term that has been used in dentistry
Radiant power, or Radiant flux	Watt	W or J/s	Radiant energy per unit time
Radiant exitance, or Radiant emittance	Watt per square centimeter	W/cm^2	Radiant power (flux) emitted from a defined area (e.g., the tip of a light-curing unit)
Irradiance (incident irradiance)	Watt per square centimeter	W/cm^2	Radiant power (flux) incident on a known surface area An averaged value over this surface area
Spectral radiant power	Watt per nanometer	W/nm	Radiant power at each wavelength of light in nm
Spectral irradiance	Watt per square centimeter per nanometer	$W/cm^2/nm$	Irradiance per wavelength of light at each nm
Luminous efficacy	Lumens per watt	lm/W	The ratio of luminous flux to power A measure of how efficiently a light source can produce light in terms of the human eye response to light

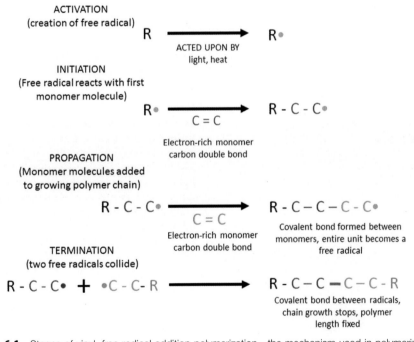

• Fig. 6.1 Stages of vinyl, free radical addition polymerization—the mechanism used in polymerization of all methacrylate-based dental resins.

Development of Polymerization Strategies for Dentistry

Self-Curing Direct Restorative Products

The first dental resins were "self-curing" or "cold-cure" acrylics. This reaction combined the same benzoyl peroxide free radical generator that is used in heat-cured resins with an aromatic amine. These components are packaged separately as a "catalyst" and a "base" because when mixed together at room temperature, they react together to form free radicals[19] (Fig. 6.2). The resin component was improved over the years to include dimethacrylate-based monomers and ground glass particles (to make a composite), but the same basic components were used in this self-curing polymerization reaction. Following mixing, the paste was packed into the cavity and held *in situ* for several minutes as the resin polymerized.[19] Additional material could be added to the original increment after it became hard. The material could be used in bulk increments because free radicals are produced throughout the resin as the benzoyl peroxide and the aromatic amine interact. The relatively slow chemical reaction of these self-curing resin-based restorative materials was a limitation and it was recommended to delay final polishing for 24 hours. Polymerization shrinkage still occurred and was an undesirable outcome.

Light-Cured Polymerization Reactions

A few years later, a faster and less complicated method of free radical polymerization was developed. This process used photons of radiant electromagnetic energy (light) to penetrate a mixture of polymerizable monomers that contained a photoinitiator to generate the free radicals. Only a single component was needed, but it had to be protected from excessive light exposure and inhibitors were included in the system; otherwise the resin would prematurely self-polymerize. After placing this light-curable resin into a tooth, the operator adjusted and contoured the material to achieve the correct shape. The resin restoration was then exposed to light at specific wavelengths and for the specified time to activate the photoinitiator and produce the necessary free radicals. The same sequence of free radical vinyl polymerization then occurred as in the self-curing resins and polymerization shrinkage still occurred.

Radiometric Terminology

To understand the basics of photochemistry and to be able to communicate with others, a background in the proper terminology

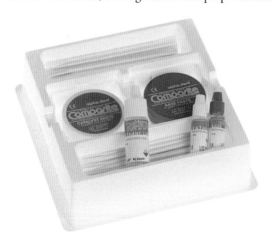

• **Fig. 6.2** Example of a self-curing, paste-paste, resin-based composite. (Courtesy Dental Technologies, Inc.)

used in this field is required. Commonly used terms to describe the output from a curing light such as *intensity, power density,* or *energy density* are not SI terms, they are confusing as to what they mean, and ideally they should not be used. The appropriate SI radiometric terms to better describe the output from a curing light are provided in Table 6.1.[3]

When measured at zero distance, such as when the curing light tip is in direct contact with the meter detector or the resin surface, the SI term *radiant exitance* is effectively the same as the SI term *incident irradiance* and is usually described in milliWatts per square centimeter (mW/cm^2). The radiant exitance (*irradiance at 0 mm distance*) is commonly used to describe the output from a curing light; however, this parameter provides limited information about how powerful (Watts) the curing light is, the effect of tip-to-target distance on the irradiance received, the spectral radiant power, or the beam uniformity. For example, if two curing lights deliver the same radiant power, but one has a 7-mm and the other has a 10-mm tip diameter, the smaller diameter tip will be half the area ($0.38~cm^2$) of the larger one ($0.79~cm^2$). This decrease in tip area will double the radiant exitance (irradiance) at the tip, even though both lights deliver the same radiant power. Such small tip diameters are often seen in budget curing lights that need only deliver a low radiant power from a small tip to deliver what appears to be an acceptably high irradiance.[20,21] For this reason, both the radiant power (watts) and the irradiance (mW/cm^2) should be reported; otherwise a curing light could deliver a high irradiance, but not be very powerful.

Electromagnetic Energy / Electromagnetic Spectrum

The radiant energy perceived by humans as "light" is electromagnetic (EM) radiation. The visible spectrum ranges from red, which is comprised of longer wavelengths of light (700 to 750 nm), through various colors, until reaching violet (comprised of shorter wavelengths between 390 and 400 nm). Fig. 6.3 shows the portion of EM spectrum associated with what humans perceive as visible light, as well as the colors corresponding to those wavelength ranges. EM radiation is delivered in packages of energy called photons and the energy carried by each photon is expressed in the following equation:

$$E = \frac{hc}{\lambda}$$

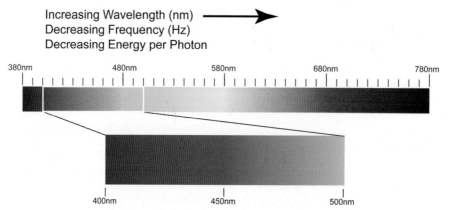

• **Fig. 6.3** Correlation between electromagnetic energy wavelength (in nanometers) and the human perception of color.

where E is the photon energy, h is Planck's constant, c is the speed of light in vacuum, and λ is the photon's wavelength. The energy carried by each photon changes in direct relation to wavelength λ because h and c are both constants and two photons of the same wavelength will carry the same energy, even if one photon was emitted from a dental curing light and the other from the Sun.

The relationship between the speed of light and wavelength is expressed as the frequency (*f*), where:

$$\frac{c}{\lambda} = f$$

The photon energy equation can be simplified to the Planck-Einstein relation as:

$$E = hf$$

For simplicity, dental terminology utilizes wavelength (in nanometers) rather than the frequency (Hz) to describe the properties of light, although both are directly related. Longer wavelength electromagnetic energy (lower frequency) than what the human eye can perceive as the color red is in the region of the EM spectrum known as infrared (IR) radiation. Photonic energy delivered in this region interacts with molecules of matter and increases their vibrational amplitudes. This interaction increases the probability that two molecules will collide with each other, producing friction and ultimately heat. In contrast, photons of shorter wavelengths (higher frequency) in the ultraviolet (UV) range contain more energy than those in the longer wavelength range (red color). Photons in the UV range are considered to be ionizing because they deliver sufficient energy to totally remove an electron from the outer shell of an atom, creating a negatively charged species: an ion.

Light Curing of Restorative Resins

The Photoinitiator Molecule and Free Radical Generation

The interaction between EM radiation and matter is used in the various curing mechanisms to create the free radicals that are required to polymerize dental resins. For a photochemical reaction to take place, the first law of photochemistry, the Grotthuss-Draper law, states that light must first be absorbed by the chemical substance. The second law of photochemistry, the Stark-Einstein law, states that, for each photon of light absorbed, only one molecule within the chemical system can be activated. These two laws, together with the Planck-Einstein relationship, explain why two curing lights that deliver the same radiant power, but at different wavelengths, may produce different results.

The photoinitiator molecules used in light-curable resin materials contain specific types of bonds that are only capable of absorbing EM radiation within certain wavelength ranges. The interactions of a photon with electrons present in the outermost orbital level of a photoinitiator atom are diagrammatically described in Fig. 6.4. When the photoinitiator atom is struck by a photon at the appropriate energy level (wavelength), an electron in the outermost orbital level absorbs the energy, thus quenching the photon (Fig. 6.5). This electron is then raised to the next higher orbital (quantum) level (E_2) and the excited atom now contains potential energy that can be transferred (Fig. 6.6) because in this excited state the electron is unstable and rapidly decays its ground state level. This causes chemical reactions to occur that create free radicals that initiate the free radical polymerization process. If no reaction occurs, the electron falls back to its ground state and returns the absorbed

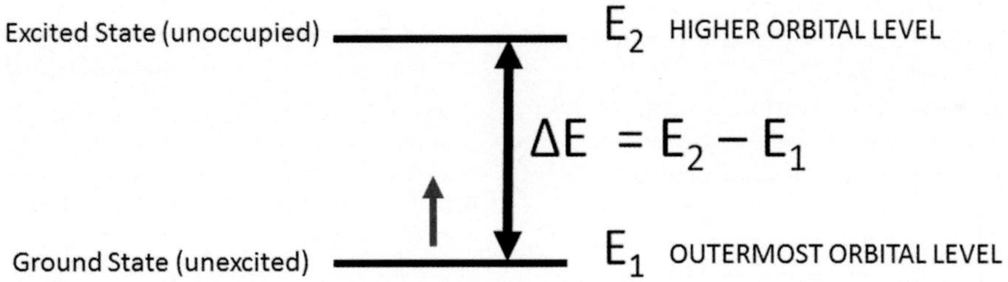

• **Fig. 6.4** Prior to absorbing a photon, an electron exists in an outer orbital shell at a specific quantum energy level—its "ground state" *(red arrow)*. A discrete amount of energy exists between this orbital level (E_1) and the higher level (E_2, designated as ΔE).

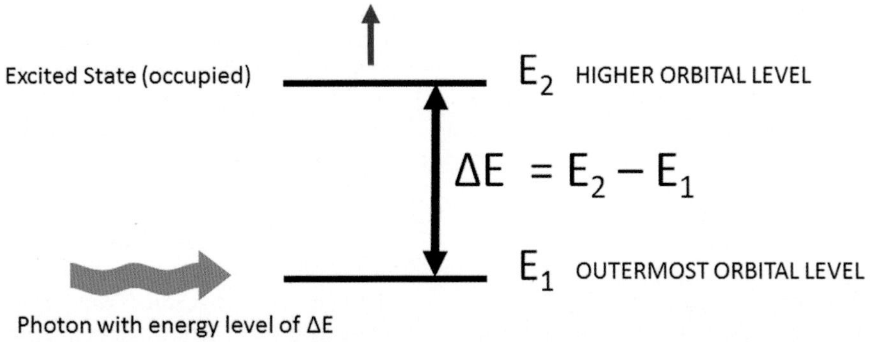

• **Fig. 6.5** When struck by a photon of light at the correct wavelength (frequency) and energy level (ΔE), the electron in the lower orbital shell absorbs this energy and is raised to a higher orbital level *(red arrow)* that is dependent on the energy difference.

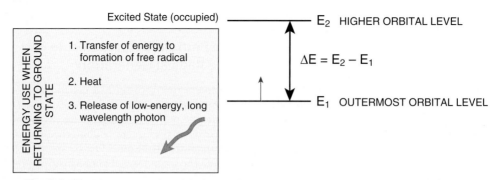

• **Fig. 6.6** Upon its return to the original ground state orbital level, the stored energy is released from the electron.

energy as heat as well as a longer wavelength photon. The ability of a photoinitiator to interact with electromagnetic energy is dependent on the frequency (wavelength) of the photon and the very specific electron configuration of the photoinitiator molecule. If these two needs do not match, then no radicals are formed. Thus in accordance with the first and second laws of photochemistry the critical parameter for effective photocuring is the *number of photons of the correct wavelength that are absorbed by the photoinitiator system(s)* within the resin composite.

Generally, two types of photoinitiators are used in dentistry: Type I photoinitiators have a high quantum yield, meaning they require fewer photons to generate a free radical than do Type II initiators.[22-24] Type II photoinitiators (e.g., camphorquinone [CQ] and 1-phenyl-1,2-propanedione [PPD]) also require an additional secondary electron transfer agent (this is typically an amine electron accepting agent) to generate a free radical.[22] Thus Type II photoinitiators are slower and less efficient than Type I initiators (e.g., Lucirin TPO, and derivatives of dibenzoyl germanium such as Ivocerin). These Type I initiators do not require additional co-initiators and break down directly into one or more free radicals when they absorb light at the correct wavelengths.

Fig. 6.7 indicates the spectral absorption profiles of four photoinitiators present at equivalent molar concentrations, and the relative ability of each photoinitiator to absorb radiant energy at each wavelength. It can be seen that CQ is best activated by light in the blue region close to 470 nm, whereas Lucirin TPO absorbs light only within the violet region below 420 nm, with a maximum absorption near 385 nm.[23,24] Initiators such as Ivocerin and PPD are reactive to a broader-spectrum of light because they are activated by EM radiation, both the violet and blue color ranges. For example, Ivocerin is most reactive near 410 nm but is still very sensitive to wavelengths of light between 400 and 430 nm.[24]

Ultraviolet vs. Blue Light

Initial attempts to light cure directly placed resin-based restorative materials used UV light at wavelengths shorter than 400 nm. Although the polymerization reaction was under the direct control of the clinician, the inability of these short UV wavelengths to penetrate deeply into the resin composite meant that the incremental layers of resin could be at most 1 mm thick. This limitation increased the chairside treatment time required to restore a tooth and did not save much time when compared to using a self-curing product.[25] Although some of the UV-cured materials were successful when placed by excellent clinicians,[26] concerns that the UV light could cause cataract formation or selective changes in the oral bioflora meant that the use of UV light was discontinued. Instead a different

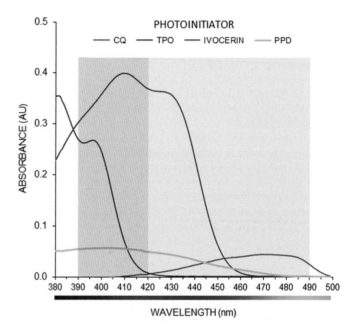

• **Fig. 6.7** Spectral absorption profiles of the most commonly used photoinitiators in dentistry, when all are at equivalent molar concentration. As a reference, the bandwidths associated with "violet light" (390 to 420 nm) and that of "blue light" (420 to 490 nm) are also provided to present the potential for interaction between these photoinitiators and the output from a dental curing light: For example, some LED units deliver no light below 420 nm.

light source and photoinitiator, camphorquinone (CQ), was used. CQ is very reactive both to EM radiation shorter than 320 nm and to blue light, with an absorption peak near 470 nm. The initial curing lights developed to activate CQ used a quartz-tungsten-halogen (QTH) filament-based light source, similar to a projector bulb. This QTH light source emitted a broad spectrum of radiant energy, from near UV through visible light and well into the infrared region. Aggressive optical filtering was used to eliminate IR wavelengths that might generate excessive heat, or UV wavelengths that deliver ionizing EM radiation. Thus the curing light delivered only blue light between approximately 400 and 500 nm. This blue light can penetrate deeper into the resin than UV or violet light, such that some "blue light–cured" restorations can now be adequately light cured in increments that are up to 5-mm thick. This enhancement reduced chairside treatment time and provided a "set-on-command" restorative product. However, polymerization shrinkage still occurred and remains a concern.

Factors Affecting the Ability to Polymerize a Resin-Based Composite

Depth of Cure

Within a composite, the degree of conversion (the extent to which resin monomer has been converted into polymer) and the depth to which the resin is cured are related to the radiant exposure (the number of photons) received by the resin (J/cm^2) (Table 6.1). Where insufficient light is delivered, the resin is inadequately polymerized and the boundary between what is considered the cured and uncured resin is called the *depth of cure*. Under optimum light curing conditions, this point is reached at a depth of 1.5 to 2 mm from the surface for a conventional resin composite and between 4 and 6 mm for a bulk-fill resin composite. In cases of poor access to the restoration, or when using more opaque shades, the depth of cure will be less.

Exposure Time

Under optimal conditions using a curing light that delivers 1000 mW/cm^2 from an 8- to 10-mm-diameter tip, many resin composites require a 20-second exposure time typically (delivering 20 J/cm^2) to adequately cure a 2-mm-thick increment of resin. Increasing the concentration of photoinitiator in the resin composite system, reducing the inhibitor concentration, matching the refractive indices of the resin and the filler, and, to a limited extent, increasing the irradiance can shorten this time. However, true reciprocity between the duration of exposure and the irradiance does not exist and short exposure times are not recommended.[14,27-31] If the manufacturer recommends delivering 500 mW/cm^2 for 40 seconds (delivering 20 J/cm^2), this does not mean that the same extent or type of resin polymerization would occur if 4000 mW/cm^2 was delivered for 5 seconds, even though both resins would receive an identical radiant exposure, 20 J/cm^2. However, it is possible to somewhat compensate for a lower irradiance (e.g., if a weaker light is used, or if the distance between the light tip and the top surface is increased) by following the instructions for use and increasing the exposure time.

Effect of Thickness of the Restorative Material

The number of photons of light that reach the depths of the resin depend on many factors, which include the thickness of the resin increment, the wavelengths of the light delivered, the refractive indices of the resin and filler components, the filler content and size, and the overall opacity of the material.[32,33] As the resin composite thickness increases, exponentially fewer and fewer photons reach to the bottom, thus potentially reducing the degree of conversion of the resin at the bottom.[34-37] Even small increases in resin thickness can have a large effect on the amount of transmitted light and resin polymerization such that doubling the exposure time cannot compensate for a doubling of the increment thickness (Fig. 6.8).

Interaction Between Wavelength of Light and Filler Particles

The influence of the Rayleigh scattering of light somewhat helps to explain why the shorter "violet" wavelengths of light do not penetrate as deeply as do longer wavelengths of "blue" light, into dental resins,[1,2] and it has been reported that light scattering is greater when the filler particle size is equal to or smaller than the wavelength of light (i.e., less than 460 nm or 0.46 microns) (Fig. 6.9).[32,38] Although the Beer-Lambert law plays a role in the amount of light penetrating through the resin, this law can only partly predict the amount of light transmitted through the resin material because there is a complex interaction between the filler particles scattering the light, the colorants that absorb the light, the photoinitiator(s) that use the light, and the differences between the refractive indices of the resin and the fillers.[38,39] Manufacturers will often adjust the type and concentration of photoinitiators, inhibitors, and fillers for different shades of the same product to compensate for this decreased light penetration and to optimize

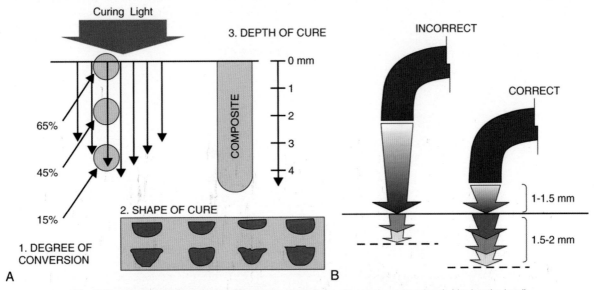

• **Fig. 6.8** Influence of irradiance on the polymerization zone in a resin composite. A, Varying the irradiance with width and depth affects the degree of monomer conversion, the shape of the cured material, and its depth. B, The proximity of the curing light tip to the restoration surface affects the number of photons reaching the top surface and thus the monomer conversion throughout the restoration.

the exposure time. Consequently, the resin manufacturer instructions should be followed because an opaque, but white, shade of composite may require a longer exposure time than a yellow, but more transparent, shade.

Matching Resin and Filler Refractive Indices

The closer the refractive indices of the resin and the filler are matched, the better will be the light transmission through the resin composite and the better the depth of cure.[32,38,39] If they are perfectly matched, the filler particles will optically disappear, but the increased translucency will mean that the resin composite will appear gray in the mouth. In the unpolymerized state, the refractive index of the resin is often lower than that of the filler. As

polymerization occurs, the refractive index of the resin component increases. Consequently, most, but not all, resin composites become more translucent after light curing. For this reason, shade selection of composite should not be performed using uncured resin composite paste, but instead using the light-cured product.

Development of Dental Curing Lights

There are four types of blue light sources that have been used to activate the photoinitiators in dental resins: quartz-tungsten-halogen (QTH), plasma-arc (PAC), argon-ion laser, and the light-emitting diode (LED). These sources produce light in different ways, and guidelines for the selection and use of curing lights have been proposed.[1-3,40-42] Examples of PAC, QTH, and LED curing lights are shown in Fig. 6.10.

Quartz-Tungsten-Halogen Lights

The first visible curing lights used QTH low-voltage 35- to 150-watt projector bulbs (one water-cooled unit used a 300-watt bulb).[1,42] The QTH source consists of a tungsten filament that is surrounded by a clear, crystalline quartz bulb containing a chlorine-based halogen gas. When electrical current passes through the filament, the tungsten wire becomes incandescent and atoms are vaporized from the filament surface. This vaporization releases a large amount of electromagnetic energy, most of which falls into the infrared region. When the current is turned off, the filament cools and the vaporized tungsten atoms are redeposited from the halogen gas back onto the filament surface in a process termed "the halogen cycle."

To prevent the QTH light from delivering significant amounts of unwanted EM radiation to the resin and tooth, the optical radiation from the QTH bulb must be filtered. The light is first directed toward a silverized parabolic reflector behind the bulb. The reflector acts as dichroic filter that allows some of the longer wavelengths of infrared light to pass through and not be reflected forward. The shorter wavelengths of visible light are reflected forward toward an infrared bandpass filter (see Fig. 6.10A) to block the remaining infrared wavelengths. The light then passes through a visible light bandpass filter (see Fig. 6.10B). Thus only light at

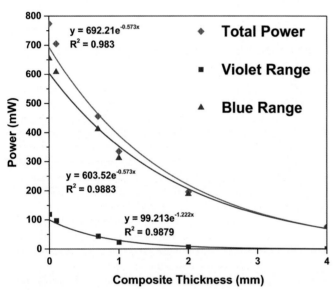

• **Fig. 6.9** Differences in the loss of "blue" (>420 nm) and "violet" (<420 nm) wavelengths of light when passing through a commercial resin-based composite. The light in both regions decreases exponentially with increasing composite thickness, and almost no violet light penetrates beyond 3.5 mm of resin composite.

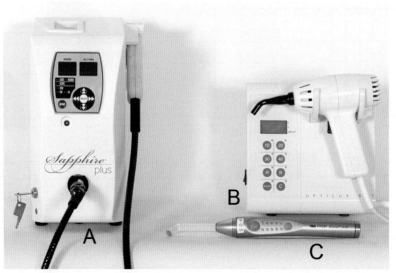

• **Fig. 6.10** Examples of a PAC (A), QTH (B), and LED (C) curing light.

wavelengths between 400 and 500 nm reaches the proximal surface of a multistranded, bundled, glass fiberoptic light guide, where it is transmitted through hundreds of small optical fibers to the tip end. QTH curing lights are very inefficient; it has been estimated that as much as 70% of the input power to the QTH bulb is converted to heat, with only 10% producing visible light, and only 0.5% to 2% of the total energy input is emitted as useful blue light.[42,43]

These QTH units were developed using a handheld, gun-style form factor, with the QTH bulb located within the body of the unit (Fig. 6.11). Although an internal fan dissipates some of the unwanted heat away from the bulb, filters, and reflector, the reflector surface and QTH bulb still become very hot when the light is on, and then cool down between uses. Vapors from bonding systems, solvents, cleaning agents, or even moisture in the operatory air can become deposited onto the reflector, thus dulling or clouding

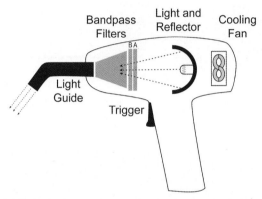

• **Fig. 6.11** Internal components of a quartz-tungsten-halogen (QTH) curing light, using a gun-style form factor and pistol-like trigger activation. A, Infrared light filter; B, band pass filter allowing only light between 400 and 500 nm to pass through.

its surface. If this occurs, the reflector or the lamp unit should ideally be replaced, but they can be carefully cleaned with alcohol or methyl ethyl ketone solvents on cotton swabs. Under ideal conditions, the QTH bulb should last for about 50 hours,[1,2] but the lifespan will be shortened if the operator immediately turns the power supply off after use to stop the noise from the fan. This action prevents the halogen cycle from occurring because if the bulb does not cool down at a controlled rate, the vaporized tungsten atoms are not properly deposited back onto the filament surface. This permanently darkens the inner surface of the quartz glass, thins the tungsten filament, and shortens the lifespan of the bulb. All these changes can occur without any outward sign to the dentist that the output from the curing light is decreasing.

The emission spectrum from a typical QTH light source developed is shown in Fig. 6.12.

Although QTH lights deliver a broad emission spectrum, most of these units were mains powered. The cooling fan was noisy, and the units delivered a relatively low radiant power and low irradiance. Consequently, they required an exposure duration between 30 and 60 seconds to adequately polymerize a 2-mm-thick increment of resin composite.

Plasma-Arc Lights

In an attempt to reduce light exposure times, high-power PAC lights were introduced. These lights were promoted to deliver a very high irradiance and the initial units claimed that exposure times between 3 and 5 seconds could successfully light cure a 2-mm-thick increment of resin composite. Instead of a filament, the PAC light source has two tungsten electrodes that are surrounded by xenon gas. When a high voltage is applied, a spark is formed that ionizes the gas.[1] This spark then acts as both a light emitter and an electrically conductive gaseous medium (a plasma) to maintain the spark. The gap between the electrodes is parallel to the long axis of a parabolic-shaped reflector that directs the emitted

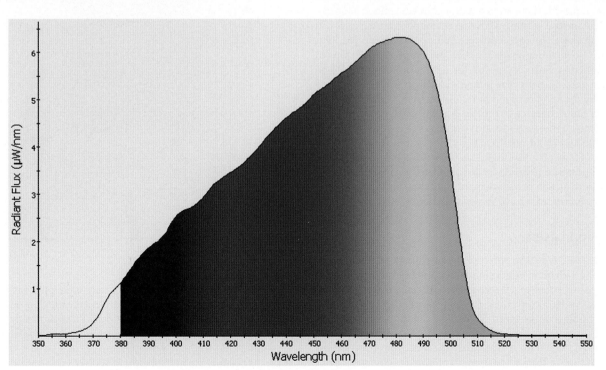

• **Fig. 6.12** Emission spectrum from a typical QTH curing light (Demetron 400, Kerr Dental).

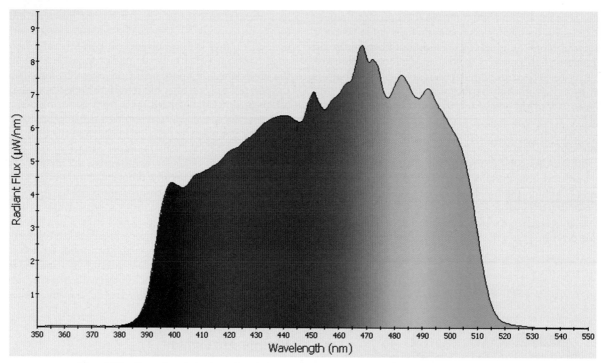

• **Fig. 6.13** Example of the broad emission spectrum from a PAC curing light (ARC Light II, Air Techniques).

light forward and through a sapphire window. Extreme optical filtering is used to prevent both the emission of unwanted ionizing radiation and infrared wavelengths of light that would overheat the tooth.

The emission spectrum of a typical broad-spectrum PAC curing light is shown in Fig. 6.13. Most PAC lights deliver a broad emission spectrum from 390 to 510 nm, a high radiant power, and a high irradiance. However, an early brand of PAC light used multiple light tips to provide different light outputs and outcomes: a bleaching tip (full spectral output), a 430-nm tip for photocuring materials containing the alternative initiators, and a 470-nm tip for light curing CQ-containing materials. This use of specific light tips to deliver different emission spectra for particular situations led to confusion and clinicians were unsure which light guide they should use to cure the specific brand of resin they were placing. Initially, this PAC light could only run for 3 s, but later generations of PAC lights used more sophisticated electronics to control the voltage to the bulb and could provide a high light output for 60 minutes or more.[1] However, PAC lights are expensive, noisy, large, not portable, cannot be battery operated, and have become less popular with the introduction of high-output LED curing lights. In addition, the xenon bulb is expensive to replace when it fails.

Argon-Ion Lasers

The term "laser" is an acronym for **l**ight **a**mplification by **s**timulated **e**mission of **r**adiation. Argon-ion laser curing lights also claimed short exposure times of 10 seconds or less compared with 40 to 60 seconds using a conventional QTH source.[1] An example of a laser curing light is shown in Fig. 6.14.

These curing lights work by delivering electrical energy to specific atoms present within the light emitter. These electrons then become excited and move from a low-energy orbit to a high-energy orbit around the atom's nucleus. When these excited electrons return

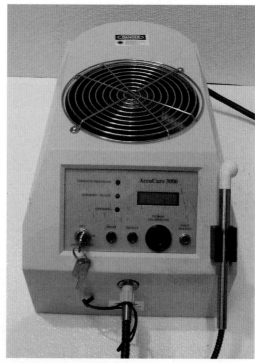

• **Fig. 6.14** Laser curing light (AccuCure 3000, LaserMed, Inc).

to their normal or "ground" state, they emit photons of light. These photons are all at the same wavelength, which is determined by the amount of energy released when the electron drops back to a lower orbit. The internally generated laser light is directed to an emitting tip through a thin fiberoptic cable, where the size of the light beam is expanded before it is directed toward the target. The argon-ion laser does not produce a broad spectrum of light

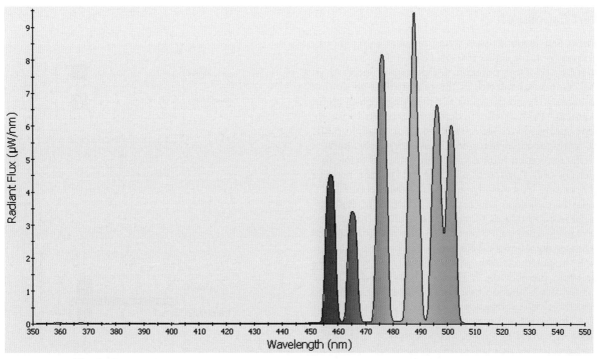

• **Fig. 6.15**   Emission spectrum from an argon-ion laser curing light (AccuCure 3000, LaserMed, Inc.).

but instead produces several intense and well-defined emission peaks in the blue spectral region. Thus argon-ion lasers were considered to be a viable option for a high irradiance curing light that could rapidly cure dental resins. Fig. 6.15 shows the narrow emission spectrum from a typical argon-ion laser curing light. With the introduction of LED curing lights, lasers have become less popular because they are expensive, not portable, have a narrow emission spectrum, and cannot be battery operated.

"Turbo" Light Guides

To reclaim some of the market from the PAC and laser curing lights, two features were added to QTH curing lights to boost their irradiance and thus attempt to reduce exposure times. The first was the so-called "turbo-tip." At that time, conventional glass-fibered light guides came in a variety of diameters, but the proximal entrance aperture and distal exit diameters of the light guide were the same size. To increase the irradiance (the number of photons emitted over the output area), the entrance to the turbo light guide was made larger than the exit diameter.[44,45] This enhancement was accomplished by using hundreds of glass fibers that were larger in diameter at the proximal end (nearest to the light source) than the opposite (distal) end, nearest to the exit tip. Thus many photons could enter the large entrance to the light guide, and the same number (assuming no loss) of photons were then emitted over a smaller area at the exit tip. This arrangement delivered the same radiant power (watts) as would come from a conventional light guide placed on the same device, but over a smaller tip area. This modification increased the irradiance (mW/cm²) to a value similar to that from PAC lights. Some QTH lights also included a special boost mode, where the voltage to the bulb was raised for a short time, thus increasing light output. By combining the increased irradiance from the small diameter turbo tip with the increased emission from a QTH bulb that was powered above its maximum voltage rating, a higher output was obtained from the QTH unit. Unfortunately, this procedure shortened the life expectancy of the QTH bulb and the optical design of the turbo tip increased the irradiance for only a few millimeters from the tip end. The irradiance from these turbo tips then declined rapidly as the distance from the tip increased and the light beam dispersed.[44,45] This dispersion adversely affected the extent of resin polymerization when the light tip was more than 5 mm away from the resin[46] and alerted researchers to the fact that it is not the light output at the light tip that matters, but it is what is received by the resin that is important.[45]

Stress Development During Polymerization

Fast polymerization of dental resin composites is thought to adversely affect the mechanical properties of the polymer network.[1,47,48] This phenomenon occurs because, when the reaction rate is very fast, the liquid monomer is quickly converted to a solid, and the polymerization reaction rapidly becomes diffusion limited.[49] Thus, in some contemporary dental resins, rapid photopolymerization produces undesirably short polymer chain lengths because there is simply insufficient time to form many long chains before resin solidification is reached.[47] In addition, the formation of the monomer-to-monomer bonds also causes the resin to shrink, thus decreasing the overall net volume of the system. As long as the system is in a liquid state, it can physically deform and no stress develops; however, beyond the gel point, the resin becomes a solid and further polymerization shrinkage creates strain both within the resin network and at the interfaces between the tooth and the resin. When the polymerization reaction occurs rapidly rather than slowly, the gel point is reached sooner, the resin becomes hard sooner, and these outcomes may result in increased stress,[50] bond failure, and increased gap formation between the tooth and restorative material.[51,52] Ultimately, these consequences can lead to premature restoration failure, cusp fracture, or increased tooth sensitivity.

Soft-Start Exposures

With dentists and manufacturers trying to achieve ever shorter exposure times by using lights that delivered a high irradiance, concerns arose about the potential for damaging increases in intrapulpal temperature as well as the potential for generating excessive internal stresses when using fast-shrinking, high-modulus resin composites.[1] In an attempt to decrease these effects, a variety of different curing modes were developed. An example is the "soft-start" curing mode, where a low irradiance value is initially applied to the restoration surface for a short time, and then either immediately, or over a period of time, the light output increases to its full operating level for the remainder of the exposure.[52,53,54] Theoretically this technique reduces the rate at which the photocurable material reacts, produces a more desirable polymer structure, allows the partially cured resin composite to deform at its unbonded surface, reduces the stresses developing at the bonded interface, and reduces the polymerization contraction stress.[50,55-58] Another type of soft-start method (the "pulse delay") delivered an initial low irradiance, short-duration exposure. After waiting some 3 to 5 minutes, the final exposure was provided at the full light output.[52,53] This technique may work *in vitro* for certain resin composites polymerized by specific curing lights.[52,57,59] However, some evidence suggests that soft-start polymerization can result in polymers that have different amounts of cross-linking and that solvents, food substances, and enzymatic attack can have different effects on the same dental resin, depending on how it was light cured.[16-18] It is thought that any potential correlation between enhanced marginal adaptation, reduced shrinkage, and lowered polymerization contraction stress using soft-start polymerization is probably due to the resin receiving less total energy and consequently reaching a lower degree of conversion.[1,60] None of these attempts to reduce the polymerization shrinkage rate and reduce stress development have yet been found to provide better clinical performance compared to continuous light exposure,[1,61] possibly because of the irradiance levels used or the different exposure times used by commercial curing lights to ramp up to full power. Some soft-start exposures in commercial curing lights can be as short as 2 s,[62] whereas in the encouraging *in vitro* tests there was up to a 5-minute delay between the initial light and the final light exposure.[52]

Light-Emitting Diode Technology

The next innovation in dental photocuring came in the 1990s, with the development of blue light-emitting diodes, or LEDs.[63,64] These LED curing lights have many advantages over their predecessors and they dominate the market.[2,42] The LED emitters are solid state, lightweight, battery driven, and more efficient; do not require any bandpass filters; and have emitting sources that can provide an extremely long working life when compared to any filament or spark-based light source.[1,2,63,64] LEDs are also very efficient at converting electrical energy to electromagnetic radiation. Their luminous efficacy (measured in lumens per watt) was initially at least twice that of a QTH bulb, but, with continued improvements, some are now 10 times more efficient.[2]

LEDs are semiconductor light sources that have been doped with impurities to create a p-n junction. Light is produced by interposing the electron-excessive (n) and electron-depleted (p) surfaces of two different semiconductor materials in an electrical circuit.[2] When a current is applied, this p-n junction emits light by a process called electroluminescence. The semiconductor substrate

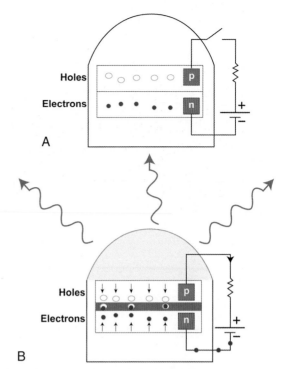

• **Fig. 6.16** Light is emitted from the p-n junction of a light-emitting diode (LED) when electrons from the n substrate pass into the holes from the p substrate, as electrical current flows through the circuit.

on the n side, or cathode, has an excess of electrons and will rise in potential when supplied with sufficient electrical energy. Electrons from the n substrate then pass through and "fall" into "holes" in the electron-deficient p side, or anode. When an electron meets a hole, it "falls" into a lower energy level and releases energy in the form of a photon of light, as illustrated in Fig. 6.16.

The color of the light emitted corresponds to the energy of the photon that is in turn determined by the composition of the two semiconductors and their resulting "band gap" potential.[2] The semiconductor material used in blue LEDs is composed of a mix of gallium nitride (GaN) and indium nitride (InN). This combination produces light in the blue spectral range that has a relatively narrow bandwidth with a full-width half maximum (FWHM) range of only about 20 nm (Fig. 6.17).

First-Generation LED Lights

The early versions of these energy-efficient, gallium nitride, blue light–emitting LED curing lights emitted blue light from an array of individual, but similar, low-power LED casings (cans). Although these first-generation blue LED curing lights (Fig. 6.18) delivered a low radiant power output, they generated great interest. They were portable, battery operated, and lightweight, and the blue wavelength output from these early LED chips was in the range of maximum absorption of CQ (470 nm).[1] This made these blue LED lights very efficient at producing the free radicals required to photocure CQ-containing dental resins.

When the first-generation LED lights were marketed, they were promoted as "cool" lights that produced less temperature rise in the pulp than did QTH lights,[65-67] and it was initially thought that all LED units would generate little heat—something that was becoming a concern. However, in retrospect, it is now recognized that the claims of low heat generation from the early LED lights

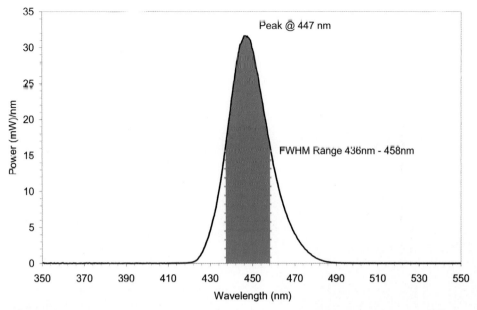

• **Fig. 6.17** Emission spectrum of a typical single-peak LED curing light showing a typical full-width half maximum (FWHM) bandwidth of about 22 nm of blue light.

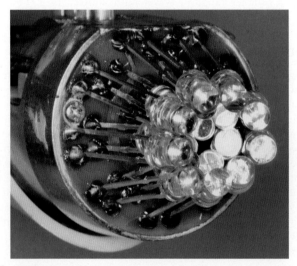

• **Fig. 6.18** Example of the internal configuration of a first-generation LED curing light that contained multiple, individual low-power LED "cans."

were due to their low radiant power output rather than to any property of the light they emitted.[68]

Second-Generation LED Lights

Advancements in LED chip design and increased radiant power output provided small, integrated packages containing surface area emitting LED pads instead of discrete LED casings. These new chips greatly increased the radiant power output of curing lights to the level that the number of photons emitted within the absorption range of CQ increased, and sometimes exceeded, what was delivered from high-output QTH or PAC lights.[1] Thus the recommended exposure times from some curing lights using the new high output blue LED chips became less than those for QTH lights, a feature that further increased the marketability of LED curing lights. However, with the increase in radiant power output, the need to cool the LED chip became critical; otherwise the LED

would overheat and destroy itself. Fig. 6.19 displays images of such damaged arrays. For this reason, internal cooling fans as well as large metal heat sinks were used within these units. Often the metal cladding of these devices also acted as a large heat sink. Fig. 6.20 shows an example of a LED chip assembly, heat sink, and cooling fan. The typical second-generation blue LED light still has a relatively narrow emission spectrum with a full-width half-maximum (FWHM) emission spectrum that is still only about 25 nm (Fig. 6.21).

These curing lights were more compact and more powerful than the "first generation" of LED lights and thus were termed the "second generation" products. However, neither the first- nor the second-generation LED curing lights delivered much light of wavelengths below 420 nm, and thus they were incompatible with some of the "alternative" photoinitiators, such as Lucirin TPO.

Third-Generation LED Lights: Multiwave, Multipeak, Polywave

As vital, intraoral tooth bleaching became popular, many dentists discovered that the shades of composites available at that time were too yellow and did not match the color of bleached teeth. This effect occurred because the CQ photoinitiator used in most dental resins is bright yellow. To overcome this problem, some manufacturers incorporated co-initiators to boost the effectiveness of CQ and thus reduce the amount of CQ required in the resin, while others started using resin compositions that contained alternative photoinitiators to reduce the CQ concentration.[1] These alternative initiators imparted less of a yellow color in the resin and allowed manufacturers to make translucent and bleaching (lighter) shades of their restorative resins. These photoinitiators still function within the visible spectrum, but they are activated by shorter wavelengths of light closer to violet (<420 nm) light and could be photocured using the broad emission spectrum from QTH and PAC curing lights. Unfortunately, the first- and second-generation LEDs that emitted only blue light above 420 nm could only activate the CQ component within these resins and were unable to activate the alternative initiators.

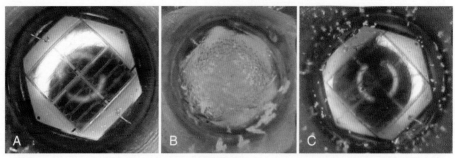

• **Fig. 6.19**   Undamaged LED chip (A) compared to overheated and damaged LED chips (B, C).

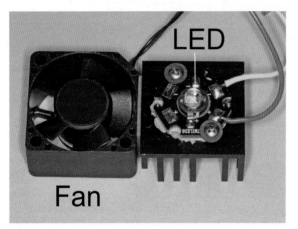

• **Fig. 6.20**   Example of the internal layout of a second-generation LED curing light having a single emitting LED chip. Note the heat sink and fan that help dissipate heat away from the LED chip.

To solve the problem caused by the narrow emission spectrum from the blue-only LED units, an additional color chip(s) was added to the blue LED array (Fig. 6.22). By incorporating different LED color chips into the curing light, the lights now emitted both the lower wavelengths of violet light, usually from 390 to 430 nm, as well as light from 440 to 500 nm[1,2] and could now activate all the different photoinitiators used in a dental resin.

These LED curing lights have been called the "third generation" units, meaning that they emit light of more than one wavelength range (or color). Curing lights of this generation have also been described as "multiwave," "multipeak," or *Polywave* curing lights. The term *Polywave* is a registered trademark of Ivoclar Vivadent, and applies to their current line of "Bluephase" curing lights. The emission spectrum from a typical third-generation LED light is shown in Fig. 6.23, where it can be seen that the emission spectrum from these units includes wavelengths that activate not only CQ but also the alternative initiators.[1,2] However, including radiant power in the lower wavelengths may not be ideal for photo-curing bulk-filled resin-based composites because of the limited ability of the shorter wavelengths of violet light to reach down to the bottom of 4 or 5 mm of resin composite. Here the resin will polymerize primarily due to the activation of the CQ photoinitiator by the longer wavelengths of blue light. Additionally, although these LED units produce a broader emission spectrum, in some lights, the location of the various different wavelength LED emitters in the LCU affects both the irradiance beam profile and the wavelength distribution of light from these curing lights.[69,70] This finding is concerning because a strong positive correlation has been reported between the irradiance beam profile values and localized microhardness values both across and through the resin composite.[69,71,72] For this reason, the internal optics of broad-spectrum, multiple peak LED curing lights that include multiple LED emitters must be carefully designed so that a homogeneous light output is produced.

To appreciate differences in the spectral distribution of photons emitted from different types of dental curing lights, Fig. 6.24 shows examples of the emission spectra from QTH, PAC, and LED curing lights. Note the relatively narrow emission spectrum from the LED units and the high spectral radiant power emitted by LED units in the 450-nm region compared to the broader range of wavelength emitted by QTH and PAC lights.

Batteries

Originally, LED curing lights were powered by nickel-cadmium (NiCad) batteries. These batteries can be damaged if they are discharged to below 75% of their rated voltage, or by being overcharged. Smaller, high-capacity, nickel-metal hydride or lithium-polymer batteries later replaced the NiCad sources, and these newer types should last between 2 to 3 years from the date of manufacture before needing to be replaced. Ultracapacitors are well-suited for applications such as a curing light, where high bursts of power are required for a short time. They are used in one curing light to deliver sufficient power for approximately 25 ten-second exposures before needing to be recharged. However, ultracapacitors can be fully recharged in as little as 40 seconds and they may last up to 10 years before needing to be replaced.

Budget Curing Lights

The dental profession can now purchase dental equipment, including curing lights, directly online and at low cost, without using an approved distributor. These "budget curing lights" may not have been approved for sale in the country of use, and often use small diameter (6 to 7 mm) light guides. As described previously in the chapter, by decreasing light tip diameter, budget curing lights can deliver the same irradiance values as more expensive lights from major manufacturers that use wider diameter tips (Fig. 6.25). The light beam profiles from these budget lights can also be inferior compared with those of the higher priced lights from major manufacturers,[20,21] and the electronics in these units may not compensate for the decrease in the output from the battery during use. Thus, without any warning to the user, the light output from battery-operated budget curing lights may not be stable during operation.[20] Dental curing lights are medical devices; thus it is recommended that you do not use curing lights that have not been approved for use in your country.

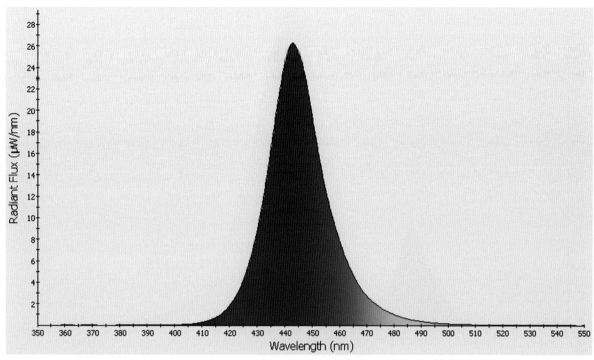

• **Fig. 6.21** Emission spectrum from a typical second-generation LED light (Bluephase 16i, Ivoclar Vivadent). Note the single emission peak in the blue wavelength range.

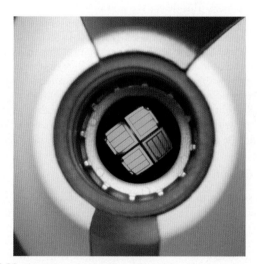

• **Fig. 6.22** Multiple wavelength emitting LED chip set in a commercial third-generation *Polywave* light (Bluephase G2, Ivoclar Vivadent) showing an array of three blue chips and one violet LED chip in the body of the light. Note the absence of any filter within the unit.

Evaluation of Light Output From a Curing Light

Radiant Power Measurement

The 2015 ISO 10650 standard for measuring the output from dental curing lights recommends using a laboratory-grade power meter to measure radiant power output and dividing this power by the tip area to produce an average irradiance value from the curing light.[73] An example of a laboratory-grade power sensor is a thermopile that converts thermal energy delivered by photons

into electrical energy. The sensor is composed of hundreds of interconnected thermocouples that generate an output voltage that is proportional to a local temperature difference. An alternative power sensor also suggested in the ISO 10650 standard is the PowerMax-Pro 150HD with a broadband detector (Coherent Inc., Santa Clara, CA). This detector differs from a thermopile (Fig. 6.26) because the sensor contains a stack of thin films to generate an electrical current when light hits the surface of the detector. In contrast to thermopiles that can take several seconds to respond, this type of sensor responds rapidly and can provide a radiant power reading within microseconds.[21,74]

Spectral Radiant Power Measurement

An optical spectrometer, or more accurately termed a spectrophotometer, measures the properties of a light source over a specific portion of the electromagnetic spectrum. Inside the spectrophotometer, light is broken down into its various wavelength components, and the signal is digitized as a function of wavelength and power (W/nm). The first step in this process is to direct light from a source being evaluated into a spectrophotometer through a narrow aperture known as an entrance slit. This slit vignettes the light and directs it onto a grating. The grating inside the spectrophotometer then disperses the various spectral components of the light, much like a prism, at slightly varying angles, onto a detector. These gratings can be ruled or holographic diffraction plates. Holographic gratings produce less stray light, while ruled gratings tend to be more reflective. The groove density on a grating determines the extent of light dispersion, and the optimum spectral range (bandwidth) is a function of the groove density. The greater the groove density, the better is the optical resolution, but the more truncated will be the spectral range. Thus, to produce the best response from the spectrophotometer, the correct slit dimensions

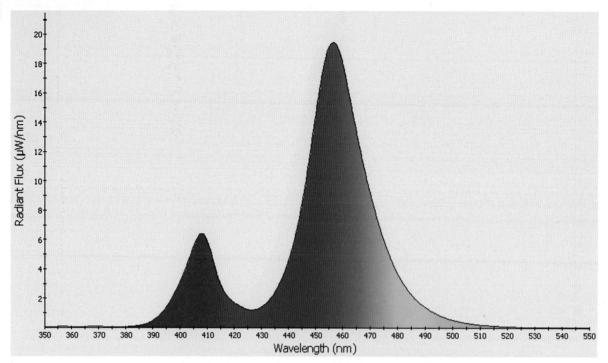

• **Fig. 6.23** Emission spectrum of a typical third-generation *Polywave* LED curing lights (Bluephase Style, Ivoclar Vivadent). Note the distinct emission peaks in the violet and blue wavelength ranges.

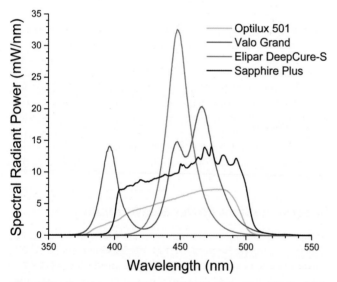

• **Fig. 6.24** Emission spectra from a PAC (*black line,* Sapphire DenMat), QTH (*green line,* Optilux 501, Kerr), and second-generation (*red line,* Deep Cure-S, 3M), and third-generation (*blue line,* Valo Grand, Ultradent) LED curing light.

and grating groove density must be carefully chosen to match the radiant power, the wavelength being examined, and the resolution required. A schematic of the internal components of a miniature spectrophotometer is shown in Fig. 6.27.

Integrating Sphere

The total radiant power (radiant flux) from a light source can be collected, without any influence of the directional characteristics from the source, using an integrating sphere (also known as an

Ulbricht sphere). This device is a hollow sphere that has a diffuse, white, reflective inner coating. Light enters the sphere through a port and strikes the sphere sides. The light is then scattered in a diffuse manner, called Lambertian reflectance, that minimizes the effects of the original direction of light. Thus only light that has been diffused within the sphere reaches the detector. This is usually via a fiberoptic cable that is connected to the entrance port of a spectrophotometer; however, the detector can also be attached directly to the sphere. Integrating spheres can be small and portable (Fig. 6.28) or they can be so large that a person can walk inside.

Light Beam Uniformity

Recognizing that the power and emission spectrum across the light tip cannot be adequately described by a single value, laser beam analyzers have been used to examine the homogeneity of power and the wavelengths of light emitted from curing lights. The charge couple detector (CCD) in a digital camera is used to record an image of the light as the light strikes a diffusing target screen. Since the type of screen or the use of a bandpass filter can affect the image, these components must be chosen carefully.[70] The radiant power received by each camera pixel in the CCD array is recorded and displayed as a color-coded, two- or three-dimensional image of the light output across the light tip end. A typical arrangement for using a beam analyzer to characterize the light distribution across the emitting end of a light-curing tip is shown in Fig. 6.29.

Several publications have shown that the irradiance from many dental curing lights is not evenly distributed across the emitting end of the light tip.[20,21,69,70,71,72,75,76] In addition, because of how the light is produced, the emission spectrum is not evenly distributed across the emitting end of the light tip of some broad-spectrum LED curing lights.[70] In contrast, although the local irradiance values may differ greatly, because of the light source used, the emission spectra are distributed evenly across the tip for QTH,

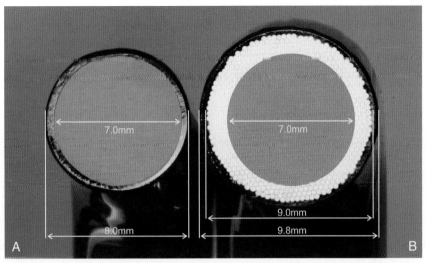

• **Fig. 6.25** By decreasing the internal tip diameter from 9 mm to 7 mm, the output area decreases. If the same radiant power is emitted, the irradiance will increase when using the 7 mm diameter light tip. 9 mm diameter = area of 63.6 mm², 400mW radiant power: irradiance = 629 mW/cm²; 7 mm diameter = area of 38.5 mm², 400mW radiant power: irradiance is now increased to 1039 mW/cm².

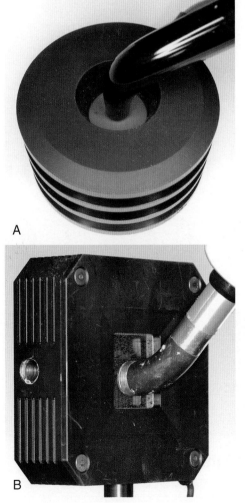

• **Fig. 6.26** Images of a conventional thermopile (A) and a PowerMax Pro 150HD with a high-speed broadband sensor (B).

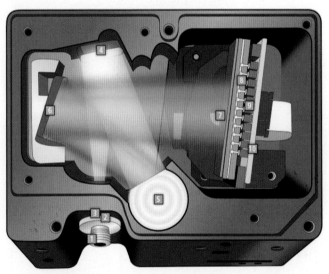

• **Fig. 6.27** Schematic diagram of a spectrometer. 1. Fiberoptic connector. 2. Interchangeable entrance slit. 3. Long pass filter. 4. Collimating mirror. 5. Grating. 6. Focusing mirror. 7. Collection lens. 8. Detector. 9. Variable long pass filter. 10. UV detector window. (Image courtesy Ocean Optics.)

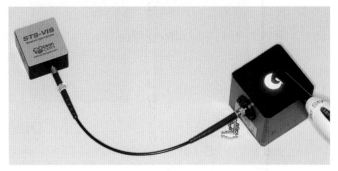

• **Fig. 6.28** A small integrating sphere attached to a miniature fiberoptic spectrometer (Ocean Optics).

PAC, and single peak LED units.[76] The localized inhomogeneity in the irradiance results in "hot spots" of high-intensity light and "cold spots" of lower values, where very little light, or different wavelengths of light, may be present. Examples of homogeneous and inhomogeneous distributions of light across the emitting tips of different dental curing lights are shown in Fig. 6.30.

The beam profile images illustrate that the irradiance across the light tip is a range of values and the irradiance homogeneity depends on the design of the curing light. Thus using a single irradiance value to describe the output from a curing light does not adequately describe the irradiance that is delivered across the entire light tip.[76] Instead, this commonly used value represents the average irradiance value that is emitted across the tip.

Fig. 6.31 shows how scaled images of the irradiance beam profile can be overlaid on an image of a tooth preparation to demonstrate the local irradiance values that are delivered to different locations of the preparation. These beam profile images show that, unless the operator is careful, the irradiance and radiant exposure received at the gingival margins of the proximal boxes from some curing lights may be inadequate to ensure adequate polymerization of the adhesive or the resin restoration in these regions.[20,21,69] These regions are also the most difficult to reach and are the furthest away from the light source.[45,77] Consequently, the resin at these locations may well be underpolymerized unless the operator pays careful attention and ensures that all areas of the resin receive an adequate amount of light.

Monitoring the Output From Curing Lights

When using a curing light, the intense blue light and the hardness of the topmost layer of resin provide a false sense of security that the curing light has adequately polymerized all of the restorative material that is underneath the top, exposed surface. Without warning the user, the light source inside the unit can degrade over

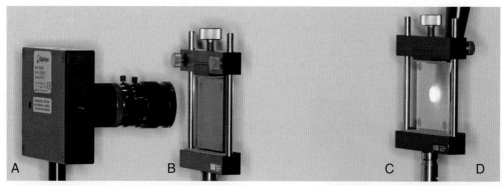

• **Fig. 6.29** Typical arrangement for using a beam analyzer to examine a dental curing light: (A) the CCD camera, and neutral density filter (B) and the diffusing screen (C) upon which the output of the curing light tip is directed (D).

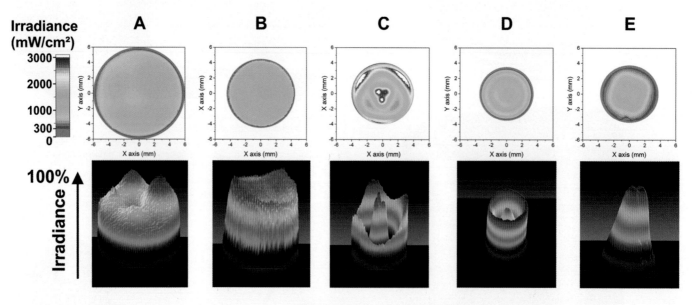

Diameter of Light Tip

• **Fig. 6.30** Images of beam profiles from five contemporary curing lights. The upper set of images are a scaled, two-dimensional representation of the irradiance distribution from 0 to 3,000 mW/cm². The lower view is a three-dimensional representation with all images scaled to their individual maximum irradiance value. Note the differences in the beam diameters and the inhomogeneous irradiance distribution across the light tips. Using a single irradiance value cannot fully describe the light output.

time[20,78] and thus decrease the light output. The light output can also be reduced due to the buildup of scale on the fiberoptic light probe after repeated autoclaving,[79] after breakage or fracture at the light tip,[80,81] or due to the presence of cured composite resin or debris on the light tip.[80,82] All these factors can significantly decrease the ability of the curing light to photocure the resin (Fig. 6.32). Thus it is important to use a dental radiometer to routinely measure the output from the curing light. The value should be recorded, as well as the condition of the curing light. Ideally, the value of the light/tip combination should be recorded when the unit is new and subsequent readings can be used to indicate the relative performance of the curing light as a function of time.

Handheld "Dental Radiometers"

Examples of seven handheld dental radiometers that can be used to monitor the output from dental curing lights are displayed in Fig. 6.33A. These radiometers usually have a bandpass filter in front of a silicon photodiode detector that converts the photons received from the curing light into electrical current and, when calibrated, into units of irradiance. However, the light is rarely emitted uniformly across the entire light tip, and because the entrance apertures on some dental radiometers are smaller than the light tip (see Fig. 6.33B), most dental radiometers do not

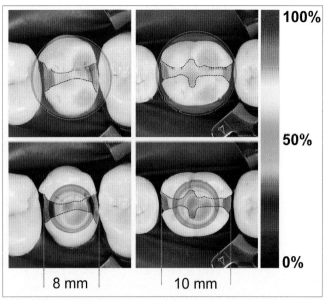

• **Fig. 6.31** Images of good *(top)* and poor *(bottom)* beam profiles, superimposed on images of premolar and molar tooth preparations. Each image is normalized and scaled to 100% of its individual, maximum irradiance value. (From Rueggeberg FA, Giannini M, Arrais CAG, Price RBT: Light curing in dentistry and clinical implications: a literature review, *Braz Oral Res* 31(suppl 1): e61, 2017. http://dx.doi.org/10.1590/1807-3107bor-2017.vol31.0061. Licensed under CC BY 2.0, https://creativecommons.org/licenses/by/2.0/.)

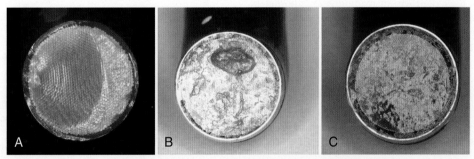

• **Fig. 6.32** Examples of damaged (A) and debris-contaminated light tips (B and C).

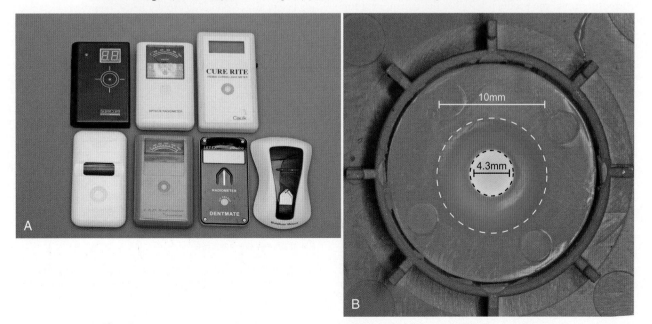

• **Fig. 6.33** Image of seven commercial dental radiometers (A), and an example of the difference between the 4.3-mm entrance aperture into the radiometer and the 10-mm tip of the curing light (B).

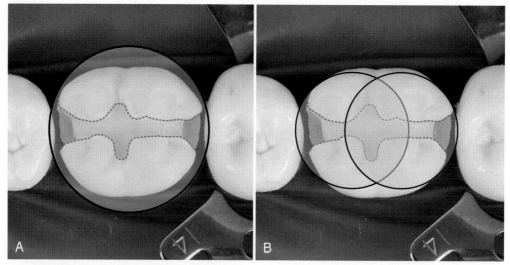

• **Fig. 6.34** A large diameter light tip (A) can cover an entire molar tooth, whereas smaller diameter light tips (B) require multiple exposures to cover an entire the surface of a molar MOD restoration.

capture all the light from the light emitting tip.[83] Thus, depending on where the light tip is positioned over the detector area, a region of high or low irradiance may be measured. This limitation helps to explain why several studies have reported that most dental radiometers are inaccurate.[83-86] In addition, because QTH, PAC, or LED dental curing lights all deliver different emission spectra, the type of bandpass filter used within many dental radiometers will affect the accuracy of the irradiance value reported.[83,85] Thus the radiometer manufactured by the maker of the curing light being tested should be the most accurate.

Practical Considerations for Light Curing Dental Resins in the Mouth

Factors Affecting Light Delivery to the Target

Table 6.1 shows that when the irradiance delivered is multiplied by the exposure time, the product describes the radiant exposure (in J/cm^2) delivered to the exposed surface of the resin. It has been recommended that a QTH curing light should deliver a minimum irradiance of 400 mW/cm^2 for 60 seconds to adequately polymerize a 1.5- to 2-mm-thick increment of resin.[87] It has also been recommended that most dental resins require a radiant exposure of approximately 16 J/cm^2 to adequately cure to a depth of 2 mm.[88] Thus this threshold could be reached in 40 seconds if the curing light delivers an average irradiance of 400 mW/cm^2 to the resin. However, different brands of resin require different exposure times, and the minimum radiant exposure may range from 6 to at least 24 J/cm^2 to achieve an adequate level of polymerization in the various shades and colors.[89,90]

Light Guide Tip Design

As discussed previously, the design of the light tip can have a significant impact on the irradiance delivered to the restoration[45,91] and can negatively affect the physical properties of the resin and its bond strength to the tooth.[7,92-94] Twenty years ago, most light tips had a 10 to 13 mm tip diameter, but recently this has changed and many light tips are now only 6 to 8 mm in diameter. Although a smaller diameter tip can increase irradiance, small light tips may

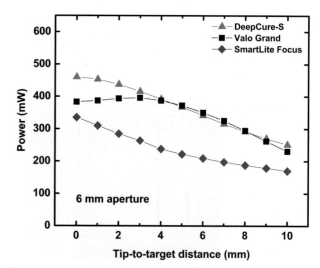

• **Fig. 6.35** Overlay graph indicating differences among three commercial curing lights with respect to the power received using tip-to-target distances from 0 to 10 mm.

not cover the entire restoration area. Since there is increased interest in bulk filling and bulk curing of large restorations, this decrease in tip diameter is now of concern. With the dimensions of a mandibular molar being approximately 11.0 mm mesiodistally and 10.5 mm buccolingually at the crown,[95] the clinician who wishes to reduce time spent light curing restorations should use a curing light with a tip that completely covers the entire restoration surface. Otherwise, as seen in Fig. 6.34, even when using a resin intended for bulk filling, multiple, sequential, overlapping exposures will be required to ensure that all areas of the restorative material have received an adequate amount of light.[21]

Distance to Target

Irradiance (radiant exitance) values stated by manufacturers are usually measured at the light tip end. Because the resin is usually 2 to 8 mm away from the light tip, this value does not reflect the irradiance values that are received by the restoration. Fig. 6.35 displays how the effect of increasing the tip-to-target distance differs

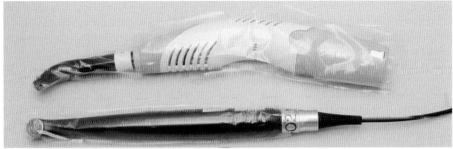

• **Fig. 6.36** Examples of different types of plastic barriers placed over the curing light to minimize contamination. Ideally, the plastic barrier should cover the entire unit instead of just the light tip.

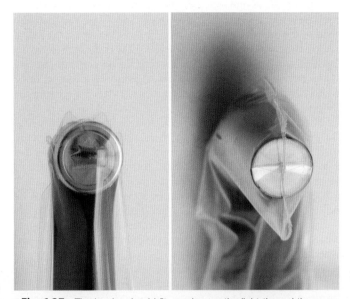

• **Fig. 6.37** The barrier should fit snugly over the light tip and the seam should be positioned so that it does not impede light output.

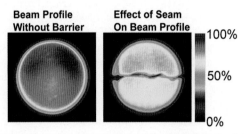

• **Fig. 6.38** If the seam of the barrier crosses the light tip, light output will be reduced.

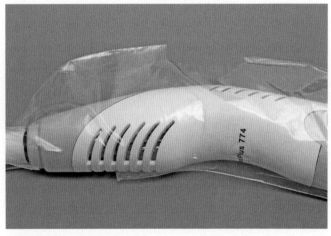

• **Fig. 6.39** Example of a curing light with air vents that should not be covered by the protective barrier.

among various brands of dental curing lights. Depending on their design, some curing lights deliver only 25% of the irradiance measured at the tip when they are 8 mm away from the resin surface.[7,45,96-98] This decrease occurs because the design and the optics of the light source and the light guide all affect the beam divergence angle from the distal tip end of the light guide. Some of the light from a curing light is delivered as a collimated beam, some is focused to a point, and some is immediately dispersed laterally from the tip. Thus curing lights do not act as a point source and depending on the unit's optical design, which sometimes includes a lens, the effect of changes in the tip to target distance on the irradiance received does not obey the inverse square law.

Infection Control

Although some fiberoptic light guides can be autoclaved, the body of the curing light itself cannot. Thus the use of infection control barriers, such as the plastic barriers presented in Figs. 6.36 and 6.37, that ideally should cover the entire curing light and light guides are recommended. The barrier should fit snugly over the light tip and the sleeve seam should not impede the light output. Fig. 6.38 illustrates the detrimental effect that occurs when the seam of a barrier traverses across the light tip and disrupts the light beam.

Unfortunately, the design of these preformed plastic sheaths that fit over a curing light is not standardized and they may not be designed to optimize light transmission (Fig. 6.39). Some barriers can reduce the radiant exitance by up to 40%, and latex-based barriers should be avoided as they have been reported to negatively affect resin polymerization.[75,99-101] For this reason, the output from curing lights should be tested on the radiometer with the barrier over the light tip. Clear, plastic food wrap stretched over the light tip in a single layer can also be an effective and inexpensive infection control barrier that has minimal effect on light output.[81,100,101]

When using cold sterilizing techniques, only approved cleaning solutions should be used. Disinfectant sprays can erode the O-rings used to stabilize light guides, and the residual fluid can bake onto the lens or reflectors inside the light housing, thus decreasing the light output.[102] Therefore, if it can be detached, the light guide should be removed from time to time and any lens, reflector, and filter inside the curing light should be checked to ensure that they, and both ends of the light guide, are clean and undamaged.

Health-Related Issues

Intrapulpal Temperature Considerations

An *in vivo* study involving the direct application of heat from a soldering iron to the facial surfaces of intact rhesus monkey teeth indicated that an increase in intrapulpal temperature of 5.5°C resulted in pulpal necrosis in 15% of the teeth tested.[103] This temperature value has been extrapolated to predict that similar pulpal temperature increases when light curing may cause pulpal necrosis to an already affected human dental pulp.

As the radiant power output from curing lights has increased, the potential for generating a damaging temperature increase in the pulp and oral tissues has also risen.[6,68,104-108] This increase in temperature is related to the amount of energy delivered (the product of irradiance delivered and exposure time) and the thermal properties (conductivity and diffusivity) of the tooth. Based on *in vitro* test results, it is suggested that curing lights that deliver an irradiance greater than 1,200 mW/cm² should be used for at most 15 seconds.[108]

However, this guideline has been questioned because recent human-based intrapulpal temperature studies have measured the baseline temperature of anesthetized, healthy human pulp tissue.[109] In that work, patients requiring extraction of bicuspids for orthodontic reasons volunteered as participants. Class I preparations were made, which intentionally exposed the most coronal portion of the buccal pulp horn. A sterile temperature probe was inserted directly into the pulp chamber and remained in place during temperature measurements, while the access opening was filled with temporary restorative material. The intrapulpal temperature rise in the teeth, when using a LED curing light, was then measured. The radiant exposure was determined, and the resulting increase in intrapulpal temperature is shown in Fig. 6.40.

As the radiant exposure increased, there was a corresponding increase in intrapulpal temperature. However, only when the radiant exposure levels approached 72 J/cm² did some *in vivo* temperature values meet or exceed the 5.5°C increase threshold, and thus potentially cause pulpal damage.[103]

Time-based profiles of *in vivo* temperature values inside the pulp of upper bicuspid teeth exposed using the same curing light, but with one tooth having an intact buccal enamel surface and another tooth having a Class V preparation with approximately 1-mm thickness of dentin remaining, are shown in Fig. 6.41.

Although both conditions demonstrate similar pulpal temperature prior to the 30-second exposure, the rate and extent of temperature increase is much greater in the tooth with the Class V preparation than in the intact tooth. In addition, it takes longer for the pulpal temperature to return to baseline levels at the end of the exposure. Such evidence supports the concept that the potential for causing temperature increase in pulpal tissue greatly increases as more tooth structure is removed and there is less dentin overlying the pulpal tissues.[110,111]

Where the pulp is at greater risk, such as in deep cavities with little overlying dentin, consideration should be given to the choice of LCU and light exposure program. It has been recommended that the tooth should be air-cooled during light exposure[112,113] from the opposite side (Fig. 6.42) of the exposure. Alternatively, a high-volume suction device can be used to cool the tooth by pulling air across the coronal portion of the tooth.

Fig. 6.43 illustrates the *in vivo* cooling effect of the air spray when it was applied 3 seconds prior to light exposure, and stopped when the light was turned off.

Although the pulpal temperature starts to rise shortly after light exposure, when air-cooled, the pulp temperature decreases both during and after light exposure. Consequently, it may be possible to use irradiance levels greater than 1200 mW/cm² for longer than 15 seconds if appropriate cooling measures are used.

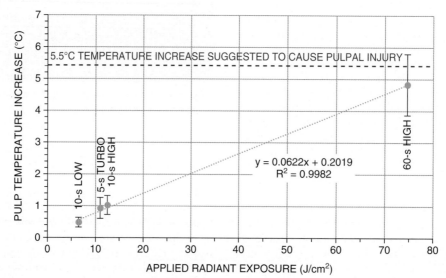

• **Fig. 6.40**   Relationship between delivering known radiant exposures to the facial surfaces of intact, upper bicuspid teeth and the resulting increase in human intrapulpal temperature rise when using a commercial *Polywave*® LED-based curing light. Exposure duration and output mode selection noted vertically for each group. N = 15 per test group. (Courtesy Dr. Cesar A.G. Arrais.)

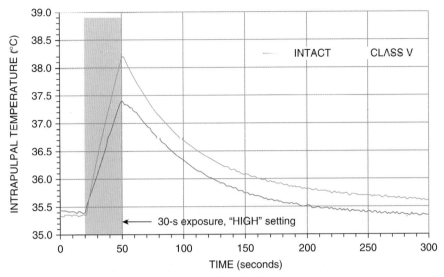

• **Fig. 6.41** Comparison of real-time temperature profiles inside the pulp of an intact bicuspid, and one having a Class V preparation with approximately 1-mm of dentin remaining when exposed to the same output time and curing mode from an LED-based curing light. (Courtesy Dr. Cesar A.G. Arrais.)

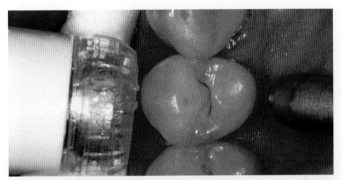

• **Fig. 6.42** Directing an air syringe at the opposite surface being light-exposed will help to lower the *in vivo* intrapulpal temperature. (Courtesy Professor Marcelo Giannini.)

Soft Tissue Damage

Current literature has reported several cases of soft tissue burns that were caused by excessive heat either from a hot light curing tip or from excessive amounts of light energy delivered to the oral tissues.[114] Soft tissue damage to oral tissues arising from photocuring restorations can arise from two sources: heat developed by the external housing of the curing light or from heat developed in tissues that are exposed to the high-intensity light. Often the light guide of the curing light is used to retract the cheek or tongue. For LED-based lights that contain the chip sets at the tip, heat generated by the chips is diffused to the outer surface of the curing light. In so doing, the surface temperature of areas on the curing light body opposite to where the chips are emitting may become hot and thus burn the soft tissues. Fig. 6.44 provides examples of how the distal portions of light guides are used to retract the soft tissue and illustrates the potential for causing soft tissue damage. However, the maximum acceptable external curing light temperature increases for curing lights is stipulated in the International Electrotechnical Commission specification, IEC 60601, that applies to dental curing lights.[115] Thus, if the curing light has passed this specification, the heat from the external housing of the unit should not be high enough to cause a burn.

When light-curing gingival areas, as in Class V situations, the gingival portions of veneers, and the margins of crowns, a portion of light output also reaches soft tissue that is often not protected by a rubber dam. Because of the translucent properties of the poorly keratinized oral epithelium, light easily penetrates and is absorbed by these tissues. This may result in a significant tissue burn if some protection is not provided. Even when using a rubber dam, the potential for elevated tissue temperatures may occur.[114] Fig. 6.45 displays a tissue burn resulting from a 30-second direct light exposure from a high-intensity LED curing light on the attached gingiva of a pig. Thus, especially when using contemporary high-power curing lights, clinicians must keep in mind the potential for causing both direct heat and radiant thermal damage to the soft tissues and the dental pulp. Clinicians should closely monitor the position of the light tip and not arbitrarily increase the exposure time in an attempt to ensure maximal polymerization without using strategies to minimize thermal damage from the curing light. One option is to place a small section of cotton gauze under the dam to protect the gingiva (Fig. 6.46). Another is to carefully position the light tip just over the resin and watch what you are doing when light curing so that the light tip does not wander over the lips or gingiva.

The Optical "Blue Light Hazard"

Dentists have a duty to protect both their patients and employees from harm. There has been concern that blue light from high-power curing lights can place dental personnel at risk for ocular damage.[116-120] Although this hazard can be prevented by using appropriate eye protection, these items are not universally used.[121]

This blue light hazard is related to the wavelength of light (Fig. 6.47). The hazard mostly occurs between about 415 nm and 480 nm and is greatest at 440 nm.[122] This wavelength range is well within the emission spectra from all dental curing lights[1] (Fig. 6.48). If eye protection is not used to eliminate the blue light, and instead the operator looks directly at the curing light, even for just 1 second during the curing cycle before averting his or her eyes, it may only take as few as seven curing cycles to exceed the recommended maximum daily exposure to blue light.[116]

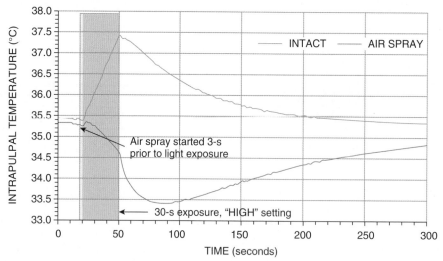

• **Fig. 6.43** Comparison of real-time, human pulpal temperature values between an intact facial surface, with no air-cooling during exposure *(blue profile)*, and when the lingual surface was air-cooled prior to and all throughout the light exposure *(orange profile)*. Air-cooling resulted in a 2°C pulp temperature decrease. (Courtesy Dr. Cesar A.G. Arrais.)

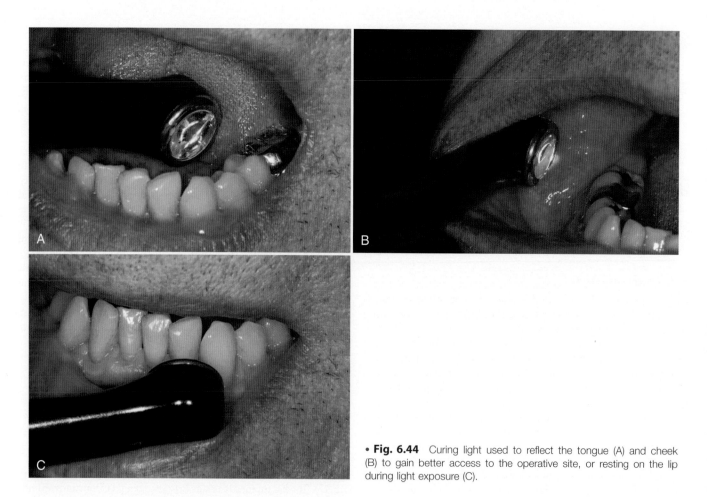

• **Fig. 6.44** Curing light used to reflect the tongue (A) and cheek (B) to gain better access to the operative site, or resting on the lip during light exposure (C).

Blue light is transmitted through the ocular media and absorbed by the retina. Although high levels of blue light can cause immediate and irreversible retinal burning, there are also concerns that repeated, chronic exposure to low levels of blue light will cause accelerated retinal degeneration and chronic photochemical injury to the retinal-pigmented epithelium and choroid. This chronic exposure is thought to accelerate age-related macular degeneration (ARMD).[123,124] Most countries follow international guidelines, such as those from the International Commission on Non-Ionizing Radiation Protection (ICNIRP) and the American Conference of Governmental Industrial Hygienists (ACGIH), when determining safe levels of exposure to blue light in all workplaces, not just

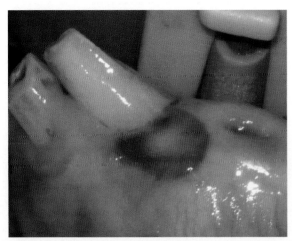

• **Fig. 6.45** Erythema resulting from exposure of pig gingiva to a high-intensity LED curing light. (Reprinted from Maucoski C, Zarpellon DC, Dos Santos FA, et al: Analysis of temperature increase in swine gingiva after exposure to a Polywave® LED light curing unit, *Dent Mater* 33(11): 1266-1273, 2017. With permission from The Academy of Dental Materials.)

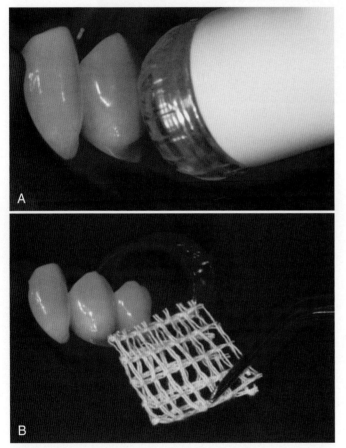

• **Fig. 6.46** Conventional positioning of a curing tip when exposing a Class V preparation (A). Such a position can cause a tissue burn even under the rubber dam. A small section of cotton gauze can be placed under the dam to protect the gingiva (B). (Courtesy Professor Marcelo Giannini.)

dental offices.[122,123] It should also be noted that these maximum recommended exposure times have been developed for individuals with normal photosensitivity. Patients or dental personnel who have had cataract surgery or who are taking photosensitizing medications will have a greater susceptibility for retinal damage.[122,123]

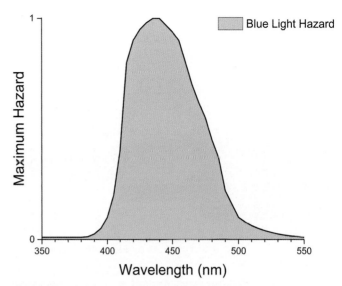

• **Fig. 6.47** Graphical depiction of the blue light hazard function related to wavelength. The maximum hazard values occur between 415 and 480 nm. (From Rueggeberg FA, Giannini M, Arrais CAG, Price RBT: Light curing in dentistry and clinical implications: a literature review, *Braz Oral Res* 31(suppl 1): e61, 2017. http://dx.doi.org/10.1590/1807-3107bor-2017.vol31.0061. Licensed under CC BY 2.0, https://creativecommons.org/licenses/by/2.0/.)

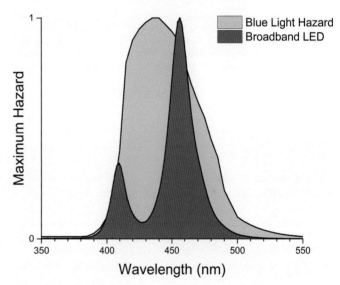

• **Fig. 6.48** Superimposition of the wavelengths of light that cause the blue light hazard *(light blue area)* and that of the emission spectrum from a multiwave LED dental curing light *(violet area)*. The blue light component from dental curing light is within the hazard range. (From Rueggeberg FA, Giannini M, Arrais CAG, Price RBT: Light curing in dentistry and clinical implications: a literature review, *Braz Oral Res* 31(suppl 1): e61, 2017. http://dx.doi.org/10.1590/1807-3107bor-2017.vol31.0061. Licensed under CC BY 2.0, https://creativecommons.org/licenses/by/2.0/.)

Blue Light Blocking Protection

Using appropriate ocular protection can completely prevent the blue light hazard and all LCU manufacturers supply and recommend the use of protective blue-blocking orange shields to protect the eyes from the bright blue light. These orange plastic shields are usually attached to the light tip and can be adjusted to provide eye protection to the operator. Other types of protective glasses and paddles are also available in various sizes, thickness, and designs (Fig. 6.49).

Most of the protective orange filters used in dentistry are designed to reduce the risks of exposure to wavelengths of blue light between

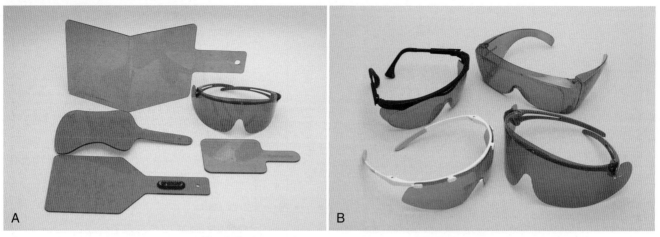

• **Fig. 6.49**   Various forms of "blue-blocker" eye protection.

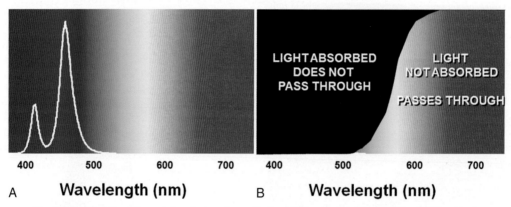

• **Fig. 6.50**   Depiction of spectral emission of a multiwave LED curing light (A) and how the blue-blocker shield filters harmful radiation while allowing light of longer wavelengths to pass (B).

420 and 500 nm. A schematic representation of how blue-blocking filters block the damaging radiation from curing lights is seen in Fig. 6.50.

The best blue light filtering glasses ("orange blue-blockers") have been shown to reduce the transmission of light below 500 nm by 99%.[125] When such blue light filtering glasses are used, instead of looking away from the bright blue light, the operator can safely watch what he or she is doing when light curing; thus they can keep the light tip directly over the resin they are trying to light cure. However, not all brands of protective filters are equally effective and some protective filters have been reported to be inadequate if they are used to protect the eye against a range of wavelengths other than the intended range.[125] Thus it is important to use the correct blue-blocking filter for the curing light being used.

Electromagnetic Risk From Curing Lights

There is some concern that the electrical circuitry in curing light can interact with implanted pacemakers.[126] Although there is a theoretical risk, the initial laboratory tests were performed under conditions where the investigators used physiologic saline baths and benchtop settings. Major companies are required to test for this hazard before selling their curing lights, and there should be no risk if the curing light has been purchased from a reputable manufacturer.[127,128] There may be a risk when using untested budget curing lights.

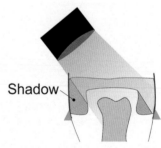

• **Fig. 6.51**   The position of the light tip can produce unwanted shadows and under-cured resin.

Teaching How to Light Cure

Much of the research on dental resins has been conducted in a laboratory setting, using a curing light held in a fixed position that is very close to the resin surface. Although this method makes the results more consistent, this is not a clinically relevant condition. When light curing a restoration in the mouth both the dentist and the patient often move, and access to the posterior teeth is often limited. Unless the operator is very careful, the position of the light tip can drift away from the restoration, or unwanted shadows may be produced that can have an adverse effect on the amount of energy delivered to the restoration and the subsequent level of resin polymerization (Fig. 6.51).[129,130]

It is known that the light-delivery technique used by the operator can have a significant effect on the radiant exposure delivered to the restorative material, especially when it is common practice not to watch the position of the curing light tip over the restoration when light curing. Not only can this practice negatively affect the amount of energy delivered to the restoration, it can also result in a tissue burn.[6,114,130-133] The operator variability in how much light is delivered can be reduced and the radiant exposure delivered to restorations increased if the operator has been trained using a device that shows, in real time, his or her ability to effectively deliver light energy to a simulated restoration. Such a clinical training simulator (MARC-Patient Simulator, BlueLight Analytics, Halifax, Canada) is seen in Fig. 6.52.

Individualized hands-on training on how to perform light curing of a restoration includes learning how to correctly position the patient to improve access and how to position the light guide throughout the light curing process.[129,131,133-135] By providing immediate feedback to the operator on how much irradiance and energy is being delivered, together with instructor coaching on how to avoid mistakes, the MARC-Patient Simulator has been shown to be an effective method to teach how to light cure a restoration. Examples of the real-time irradiance delivered to a specific restorative location by several operators during a 10-second exposure

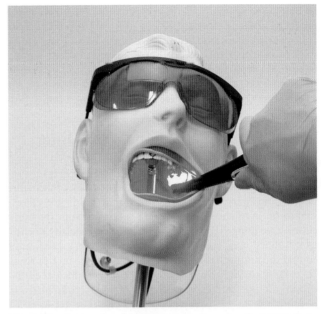

• **Fig. 6.52** Light curing a simulated restoration using the MARC-Patient Simulator (BlueLight Analytics, Halifax, Canada).

• **Fig. 6.53** Before and after images of irradiance levels delivered by several operators to a specific intraoral location during a 10-second light exposure, as monitored using the MARC-PS patient simulator. The after image shows great improvement in how consistently the light was delivered throughout the exposures. The operators also delivered more total energy after instruction.

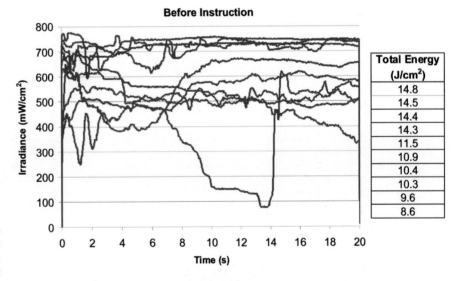

Before Instruction

Total Energy (J/cm²)
14.8
14.5
14.4
14.3
11.5
10.9
10.4
10.3
9.6
8.6

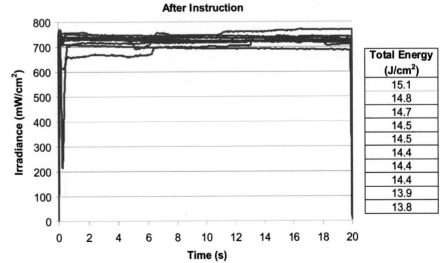

After Instruction

Total Energy (J/cm²)
15.1
14.8
14.7
14.5
14.5
14.4
14.4
14.4
13.9
13.8

and monitored using the MARC-PS patient simulator are seen in Fig. 6.53. The after-image shows a great improvement in the consistency in the irradiance that was delivered throughout the exposure. The operators also delivered a greater radiant exposure (amount of energy in J/cm^2) after instruction, thereby increasing the potential for achieving the intended properties and the promising *in vitro* results for the restorative material they are using.

General Recommendations When Using a Curing Light

As a general recommendation, users should be aware of the radiant power output, active emitting tip dimensions, irradiance, effect of distance on irradiance, and emission spectrum from the curing light they are using. Their light should be tested regularly to ensure that it is functioning according to the manufacturer's specifications and that the output has not changed significantly since purchase. When light curing, clinicians should deliver sufficient radiant exposure at the correct wavelengths of light required by the photoinitiator used in the resin composite they are using. To maximize the radiant exposure delivered, the light tip should be held both close to and perpendicular to the surface of the restoration. Operators should directly observe what they are doing throughout the entire light exposure, and to do so safely, they must also use appropriate eye protection. Precautions should be taken to avoid causing an unacceptable temperature increase in the tooth and the adjacent soft tissues.[41,102,136]

References

1. Rueggeberg FA: State-of-the-art: dental photocuring–a review. *Dent Mater* 27:39–52, 2011.
2. Jandt KD, Mills RW: A brief history of LED photopolymerization. *Dent Mater* 29:605–617, 2013.
3. Price RB, Ferracane JL, Shortall AC: Light-curing units: A review of what we need to know. *J Dent Res* 94:1179–1186, 2015.
4. Santini A, Turner S: General dental practitioners' knowledge of polymerisation of resin-based composite restorations and light curing unit technology. *Br Dent J* 211:E13, 2011.
5. Ferracane JL, Mitchem JC, Condon JR, et al: Wear and marginal breakdown of composites with various degrees of cure. *J Dent Res* 76:1508–1516, 1997.
6. Shortall A, El-Mahy W, Stewardson D, et al: Initial fracture resistance and curing temperature rise of ten contemporary resin-based composites with increasing radiant exposure. *J Dent* 41:455–463, 2013.
7. Xu X, Sandras DA, Burgess JO: Shear bond strength with increasing light-guide distance from dentin. *J Esthet Restor Dent* 18:19–27, discussion 28, 2006.
8. Vandewalle KS, Ferracane JL, Hilton TJ, et al: Effect of energy density on properties and marginal integrity of posterior resin composite restorations. *Dent Mater* 20:96–106, 2004.
9. Purushothaman D, Kailasam V, Chitharanjan AB: Bisphenol A release from orthodontic adhesives and its correlation with the degree of conversion. *Am J Orthod Dentofacial Orthop* 147:29–36, 2015.
10. Nocca G, Iori A, Rossini C, et al: Effects of barriers on chemical and biological properties of two dual resin cements. *Eur J Oral Sci* 123:208–214, 2015.
11. El-Damanhoury HM, Gaintantzopoulou M: Effect of thermocycling, degree of conversion, and cavity configuration on the bonding effectiveness of all-in-one adhesives. *Oper Dent* 40:480–491, 2015.
12. Bhalla M, Patel D, Shashikiran ND, et al: Effect of light-emitting diode and halogen light curing on the micro-hardness of dental composite and resin-modified glass ionomer cement: an in vitro study. *J Indian Soc Pedod Prev Dent* 30:201–205, 2012.
13. Sigusch BW, Pflaum T, Volpel A, et al: Resin-composite cytotoxicity varies with shade and irradiance. *Dent Mater* 28:312–319, 2012.
14. Durner J, Obermaier J, Draenert M, et al: Correlation of the degree of conversion with the amount of elutable substances in nano-hybrid dental composites. *Dent Mater* 28:1146–1153, 2012.
15. Salehi S, Gwinner F, Mitchell JC, et al: Cytotoxicity of resin composites containing bioactive glass fillers. *Dent Mater* 31:195–203, 2015.
16. Soh MS, Yap AU: Influence of curing modes on crosslink density in polymer structures. *J Dent* 32:321–326, 2004.
17. Asmussen E, Peutzfeldt A: Influence of pulse-delay curing on softening of polymer structures. *J Dent Res* 80:570–573, 2001.
18. Benetti AR, Peutzfeldt A, Asmussen E, et al: Influence of curing rate on softening in ethanol, degree of conversion, and wear of resin composite. *Am J Dent* 24:115–118, 2011.
19. Craig RG: Chemistry, composition, and properties of composite resins. *Dent Clin North Am* 25:219–239, 1981.
20. AlShaafi MM, Harlow JE, Price HL, et al: Emission characteristics and effect of battery drain in "budget" curing lights. *Oper Dent* 41:397–408, 2016.
21. Shimokawa CA, Turbino ML, Harlow JE, et al: Light output from six battery operated dental curing lights. *Mater Sci Eng C Mater Biol Appl* 69:1036–1042, 2016.
22. Stansbury JW: Curing dental resins and composites by photopolymerization. *J Esthet Dent* 12:300–308, 2000.
23. Neumann MG, Miranda WG, Jr, Schmitt CC, et al: Molar extinction coefficients and the photon absorption efficiency of dental photoinitiators and light curing units. *J Dent* 33:525–532, 2005.
24. Burtscher P: Ivocerin in comparison to camphorquinone. Ivoclar Vivadent Report, No. 19, July, 2013: 2013.
25. Tirtha R, Fan PL, Dennison JB, et al: In vitro depth of cure of photo-activated composites. *J Dent Res* 61:1184–1187, 1982.
26. Wilder AD, Jr, May KN, Jr, Bayne SC, et al: Seventeen-year clinical study of ultraviolet-cured posterior composite Class I and II restorations. *J Esthet Dent* 11:135–142, 1999.
27. Musanje L, Darvell BW: Polymerization of resin composite restorative materials: exposure reciprocity. *Dent Mater* 19:531–541, 2003.
28. Selig D, Haenel T, Hausnerova B, et al: Examining exposure reciprocity in a resin based composite using high irradiance levels and real-time degree of conversion values. *Dent Mater* 31:583–593, 2015.
29. Leprince JG, Hadis M, Shortall AC, et al: Photoinitiator type and applicability of exposure reciprocity law in filled and unfilled photoactive resins. *Dent Mater* 27:157–164, 2011.
30. Hadis M, Leprince JG, Shortall AC, et al: High irradiance curing and anomalies of exposure reciprocity law in resin-based materials. *J Dent* 39:549–557, 2011.
31. Wydra JW, Cramer NB, Stansbury JW, et al: The reciprocity law concerning light dose relationships applied to BisGMA/TEGDMA photopolymers: theoretical analysis and experimental characterization. *Dent Mater* 30:605–612, 2014.
32. Ruyter IE, Øysæd H: Conversion in different depths of ultraviolet and visible light activated composite materials. *Acta Odontol Scand* 40:179–192, 1982.
33. Harlow JE, Rueggeberg FA, Labrie D, et al: Transmission of violet and blue light through conventional (layered) and bulk cured resin-based composites. *J Dent* 53:44–50, 2016.
34. Cook WD, Standish PM: Cure of resin based restorative materials. II. White light photopolymerized resins. *Aust Dent J* 28:307–311, 1983.
35. Chen YC, Ferracane JL, Prahl SA: A pilot study of a simple photon migration model for predicting depth of cure in dental composite. *Dent Mater* 21:1075–1086, 2005.

36. dos Santos GB, Alto RV, Filho HR, et al: Light transmission on dental resin composites. *Dent Mater* 24:571–576, 2008.

37. Price RB, Murphy DG, Dérand T: Light energy transmission through cured resin composite and human dentin. *Quintessence Int* 31:659–667, 2000.

38. Taira M, Suzuki H, Toyooka H, et al: Refractive index of inorganic fillers in seven visible-light-cured dental composite resins. *J Mater Sci Lett* 13:68–70, 1994.

39. Shortall AC, Palin WM, Burtscher P: Refractive index mismatch and monomer reactivity influence composite curing depth. *J Dent Res* 87:84–88, 2008.

40. Price RB, Shortall AC, Palin WM: Contemporary issues in light curing. *Oper Dent* 39:4–14, 2014.

41. Shortall AC, Price RB, MacKenzie L, et al: Guidelines for the selection, use, and maintenance of LED light-curing units - Part II. *Br Dent J* 221:551–554, 2016.

42. Shortall AC, Price RB, MacKenzie L, et al: Guidelines for the selection, use, and maintenance of LED light-curing units - Part 1. *Br Dent J* 221:453–460, 2016.

43. Yaman BC, Efes BG, Dorter C, et al: The effects of halogen and light-emitting diode light curing on the depth of cure and surface microhardness of composite resins. *J Conserv Dent* 14:136–139, 2011.

44. Curtis JW, Jr, Rueggeberg FA, Lee AJ: Curing efficiency of the Turbo Tip. *Gen Dent* 43:428–433, 1995.

45. Price RB, Derand T, Sedarous M, et al: Effect of distance on the power density from two light guides. *J Esthet Dent* 12:320–327, 2000.

46. Busemann I, Lipke C, Schattenberg A, et al: Shortest exposure time possible with LED curing lights. *Am J Dent* 24:37–44, 2011.

47. Burdick JA, Lovestead TM, Anseth KS: Kinetic chain lengths in highly cross-linked networks formed by the photoinitiated polymerization of divinyl monomers: A gel permeation chromatography investigation. *Biomacromolecules* 4:149–156, 2003.

48. Feng L, Carvalho R, Suh BI: Insufficient cure under the condition of high irradiance and short irradiation time. *Dent Mater* 25:283–289, 2009.

49. Lovell LG, Newman SM, Bowman CN: The effects of light intensity, temperature, and comonomer composition on the polymerization behavior of dimethacrylate dental resins. *J Dent Res* 78:1469–1476, 1999.

50. Taubock TT, Feilzer AJ, Buchalla W, et al: Effect of modulated photo-activation on polymerization shrinkage behavior of dental restorative resin composites. *Eur J Oral Sci* 122:293–302, 2014.

51. Randolph LD, Palin WM, Watts DC, et al: The effect of ultra-fast photopolymerisation of experimental composites on shrinkage stress, network formation and pulpal temperature rise. *Dent Mater* 30:1280–1289, 2014.

52. Kanca J, 3rd, Suh BI: Pulse activation: reducing resin-based composite contraction stresses at the enamel cavosurface margins. *Am J Dent* 12:107–112, 1999.

53. Suh BI, Feng L, Wang Y, et al: The effect of the pulse-delay cure technique on residual strain in composites. *Compendium* 20:4–12, 1999.

54. Feng L, Suh BI: A mechanism on why slower polymerization of a dental composite produces lower contraction stress. *J Biomed Mater Res B Appl Biomater* 78:63–69, 2006.

55. Bouschlicher MR, Rueggeberg FA: Effect of ramped light intensity on polymerization force and conversion in a photoactivated composite. *J Esthet Dent* 12:328–339, 2000.

56. Chye CH, Yap AU, Laim YC, et al: Post-gel polymerization shrinkage associated with different light curing regimens. *Oper Dent* 30:474–480, 2005.

57. Lopes LG, Franco EB, Pereira JC, et al: Effect of light-curing units and activation mode on polymerization shrinkage and shrinkage stress of composite resins. *J Appl Oral Sci* 16:35–42, 2008.

58. Ilie N, Jelen E, Hickel R: Is the soft-start polymerisation concept still relevant for modern curing units? *Clin Oral Investig* 15:21–29, 2011.

59. Dall'Magro E, Correr AB, Costa AR, et al: Effect of different photoactivation techniques on the bond strength of a dental composite. *Braz Dent J* 21:220–224, 2010.

60. Inoue K, Howashi G, Kanetou T, et al: Effect of light intensity on linear shrinkage of photo-activated composite resins during setting. *J Oral Rehabil* 32:22–27, 2005.

61. van Dijken JW, Pallesen U: A 7-year randomized prospective study of a one-step self-etching adhesive in non-carious cervical lesions. The effect of curing modes and restorative material. *J Dent* 40:1060–1067, 2012.

62. Harlow JE, Sullivan B, Shortall AC, et al: Characterizing the output settings of dental curing lights. *J Dent* 44:20–26, 2016.

63. Fujibayashi K, Shimaru K, Takahashi N, et al: Newly developed curing unit using blue light-emitting diodes. *Dent Jpn (Tokyo)* 34:49–53, 1998.

64. Mills RW, Jandt KD, Ashworth SH: Dental composite depth of cure with halogen and blue light emitting diode technology. *Br Dent J* 186:388–391, 1999.

65. Hofmann N, Hugo B, Klaiber B: Effect of irradiation type (LED or QTH) on photo-activated composite shrinkage strain kinetics, temperature rise, and hardness. *Eur J Oral Sci* 110:471–479, 2002.

66. Weerakoon AT, Meyers IA, Symons AL, et al: Pulpal heat changes with newly developed resin photopolymerisation systems. *Aust Endod J* 28:108–111, 2002.

67. Ozturk AN, Usumez A: Influence of different light sources on microtensile bond strength and gap formation of resin cement under porcelain inlay restorations. *J Oral Rehabil* 31:905–910, 2004.

68. Andreatta LM, Furuse AY, Prakki A, et al: Pulp chamber heating: An in vitro study evaluating different light sources and resin composite layers. *Braz Dent J* 27:675–680, 2016.

69. Price RB, Labrie D, Rueggeberg FA, et al: Correlation between the beam profile from a curing light and the microhardness of four resins. *Dent Mater* 30:1345–1357, 2014.

70. Price RB, Labrie D, Rueggeberg FA, et al: Irradiance differences in the violet (405 nm) and blue (460 nm) spectral ranges among dental light-curing units. *J Esthet Restor Dent* 22:363–377, 2010.

71. Issa Y, Watts DC, Boyd D, et al: Effect of curing light emission spectrum on the nanohardness and elastic modulus of two bulk-fill resin composites. *Dent Mater* 32:535–550, 2016.

72. Magalhaes Filho TR, Weig KM, Costa MF, et al: Effect of LED-LCU light irradiance distribution on mechanical properties of resin based materials. *Mater Sci Eng C Mater Biol Appl* 63:301–307, 2016.

73. ISO 10650 Dentistry-Powered polymerization activators. Geneva, Switzerland: International Standards Organization: International Standards Organization; 2015. p. 14.

74. Coherent. White Paper: Novel Laser Power Sensor Improves Process Control. https://http://www.coherent.com/?fuseaction=form.required&download=8992&title=PowerMax-Pro-White-Paper-Novel-Laser-Power-Sensor-Improves-Process-Control: Coherent; (Cited 12 August 2016). 1-7.

75. Vandewalle KS, Roberts HW, Rueggeberg FA: Power distribution across the face of different light guides and its effect on composite surface microhardness. *J Esthet Restor Dent* 20:108–117, discussion 118, 2008.

76. Michaud PL, Price RB, Labrie D, et al: Localised irradiance distribution found in dental light curing units. *J Dent* 42:129–139, 2014.

77. Yearn JA: Factors affecting cure of visible light activated composites. *Int Dent J* 35:218–225, 1985.

78. Friedman J: Variability of lamp characteristics in dental curing lights. *J Esthet Dent* 1:189–190, 1989.

79. Rueggeberg FA, Caughman WF, Comer RW: The effect of autoclaving on energy transmission through light-curing tips. *J Am Dent Assoc* 127:1183–1187, 1996.

80. Poulos JG, Styner DL: Curing lights: changes in intensity output with use over time. *Gen Dent* 45:70–73, 1997.

81. McAndrew R, Lynch CD, Pavli M, et al: The effect of disposable infection control barriers and physical damage on the power output of light curing units and light curing tips. *Br Dent J* 210:E12, 2011.

82. Strydom C: Dental curing lights–maintenance of visible light curing units. *SADJ* 57:227–233, 2002.

83. Price RB, Labrie D, Kazmi S, et al: Intra- and inter-brand accuracy of four dental radiometers. *Clin Oral Investig* 16:707–717, 2012.

84. Leonard DL, Charlton DG, Hilton TJ: Effect of curing-tip diameter on the accuracy of dental radiometers. *Oper Dent* 24:31–37, 1999.

85. Roberts HW, Vandewalle KS, Berzins DW, et al: Accuracy of LED and halogen radiometers using different light sources. *J Esthet Restor Dent* 18:214–222, discussion 223-214, 2006.

86. Marovic D, Matic S, Kelic K, et al: Time dependent accuracy of dental radiometers. *Acta Clin Croat* 52:173–180, 2013.

87. Rueggeberg FA, Caughman WF, Curtis JW, Jr: Effect of light intensity and exposure duration on cure of resin composite. *Oper Dent* 19:26–32, 1994.

88. Anusavice KJ, Phillips RW, Shen C, et al: *Phillips' science of dental materials*, ed 12, St. Louis, Mo., 2013, Elsevier/Saunders, p 290, xiii. 571 p.

89. Calheiros FC, Daronch M, Rueggeberg FA, et al: Degree of conversion and mechanical properties of a BisGMA:TEGDMA composite as a function of the applied radiant exposure. *J Biomed Mater Res B Appl Biomater* 84:503–509, 2008.

90. Fan PL, Schumacher RM, Azzolin K, et al: Curing-light intensity and depth of cure of resin-based composites tested according to international standards. *J Am Dent Assoc* 133:429–434, 2002.

91. Nitta K: Effect of light guide tip diameter of LED-light curing unit on polymerization of light-cured composites. *Dent Mater* 21:217–223, 2005.

92. Leprince JG, Palin WM, Hadis MA, et al: Progress in dimethacrylate-based dental composite technology and curing efficiency. *Dent Mater* 29:139–156, 2013.

93. Shortall AC, Felix CJ, Watts DC: Robust spectrometer-based methods for characterizing radiant exitance of dental LED light curing units. *Dent Mater* 31:339–350, 2015.

94. D'Alpino PH, Wang L, Rueggeberg FA, et al: Bond strength of resin-based restorations polymerized with different light-curing sources. *J Adhes Dent* 8:293–298, 2006.

95. Ash MM, Nelson SJ, Ash MM: *Dental anatomy, physiology, and occlusion*, ed 8, Philadelphia, 2003, W.B. Saunders, p xiv. 523 p., 516 p. of col. plates p.

96. Price RB, Labrie D, Whalen JM, et al: Effect of distance on irradiance and beam homogeneity from 4 light-emitting diode curing units. *J Can Dent Assoc* 77:b9, 2011.

97. Corciolani G, Vichi A, Davidson CL, et al: The influence of tip geometry and distance on light-curing efficacy. *Oper Dent* 33:325–331, 2008.

98. Vandewalle KS, Roberts HW, Andrus JL, et al: Effect of light dispersion of LED curing lights on resin composite polymerization. *J Esthet Restor Dent* 17:244–254, discussion 254-245, 2005.

99. Coutinho M, Trevizam NC, Takayassu RN, et al: Distance and protective barrier effects on the composite resin degree of conversion. *Contemp Clin Dent* 4:152–155, 2013.

100. Scott BA, Felix CA, Price RB: Effect of disposable infection control barriers on light output from dental curing lights. *J Can Dent Assoc* 70:105–110, 2004.

101. Sword RJ, Do UN, Chang JH, et al: Effect of curing light barriers and light types on radiant exposure and composite conversion. *J Esthet Restor Dent* 28:29–42, 2016.

102. Strassler HE, Price RB: Understanding light curing, Part II. Delivering predictable and successful restorations. *Dent Today* 1–8, quiz 9, 2014.

103. Zach L, Cohen G: Pulp response to externally applied heat. *Oral Surg Oral Med Oral Pathol* 19:515–530, 1965.

104. Baroudi K, Silikas N, Watts DC: In vitro pulp chamber temperature rise from irradiation and exotherm of flowable composites. *Int J Paediatr Dent* 19:48–54, 2009.

105. Atai M, Motevasselian F: Temperature rise and degree of photopolymerization conversion of nanocomposites and conventional dental composites. *Clin Oral Investig* 13:309–316, 2009.

106. Gomes M, DeVito-Moraes A, Francci C, et al: Temperature increase at the light guide tip of 15 contemporary LED units and thermal variation at the pulpal floor of cavities: an infrared thermographic analysis. *Oper Dent* 38:324–333, 2013.

107. Mouhat M, Mercer J, Stangvaltaite L, et al: Light-curing units used in dentistry: factors associated with heat development—potential risk for patients. *Clin Oral Investig* 1–10, 2016.

108. Park SH, Roulet JF, Heintze SD: Parameters influencing increase in pulp chamber temperature with light-curing devices: curing lights and pulpal flow rates. *Oper Dent* 35:353–361, 2010.

109. Runnacles P, Arrais CA, Pochapski MT, et al: Direct measurement of time-dependent anesthetized in vivo human pulp temperature. *Dent Mater* 31:53–59, 2015.

110. Kodonas K, Gogos C, Tziafas D: Effect of simulated pulpal microcirculation on intrapulpal temperature changes following application of heat on tooth surfaces. *Int Endod J* 42:247–252, 2009.

111. Flávio Henrique Baggio A, Gisele Kanda Peres B, Débora Alves Nunes Leite L, et al: Effect of composite resin polymerization modes on temperature rise in human dentin of different thicknesses: an in vitro study. *Biomed Mater* 1:140, 2006.

112. Onisor I, Asmussen E, Krejci I: Temperature rise during photopolymerization for onlay luting. *Am J Dent* 24:250–256, 2011.

113. Strassler HE: Successful light curing- not as easy as it looks. *Oral Health* 103:18–26, 2013.

114. Spranley TJ, Winkler M, Dagate J, et al: Curing light burns. *Gen Dent* 60:e210–e214, 2012.

115. International Electrotechnical Commission: IEC 60601-1:2015 SER Series. Medical electrical equipment. Geneva, Switzerland. 2015.

116. Labrie D, Moe J, Price RB, et al: Evaluation of ocular hazards from 4 types of curing lights. *J Can Dent Assoc* 77:b116, 2011.

117. McCusker N, Lee SM, Robinson S, et al: Light curing in orthodontics; should we be concerned? *Dent Mater* 29:e85–e90, 2013.

118. Bruzell Roll EM, Jacobsen N, Hensten-Pettersen A: Health hazards associated with curing light in the dental clinic. *Clin Oral Investig* 8:113–117, 2004.

119. Price RB, Labrie D, Bruzell EM, et al: The dental curing light: A potential health risk. *J Occup Environ Hyg* 13:639–646, 2016.

120. Stamatacos C, Harrison JL: The possible ocular hazards of LED dental illumination applications. *J Tenn Dent Assoc* 93:25–29, quiz 30-21, 2013.

121. Hill EE: Eye safety practices in U.S. dental school restorative clinics, 2006. *J Dent Educ* 70:1294–1297, 2006.

122. American Conference of Governmental Industrial Hygienists (ACGIH): TLVs and BEIs Based on the Documentation for Threshold Limit Values for Chemical Substances and Physical Agents and Biological Exposure Indices. *ACGIH* Cincinnati, Ohio, 2015.

123. International Commission on non-ionizing radiation protection: Guidelines on limits of exposure to broad-band incoherent optical radiation (0.38 to 3 μm). *Health Phys* 73:539–554, 1997.

124. Ham WT, Jr, Ruffolo JJ, Jr, Mueller HA, et al: Histologic analysis of photochemical lesions produced in rhesus retina by short-wavelength light. *Invest Ophthalmol Vis Sci* 17:1029–1035, 1978.

125. Bruzell EM, Johnsen B, Aalerud TN, et al: Evaluation of eye protection filters for use with dental curing and bleaching lamps. *J Occup Environ Hyg* 4:432–439, 2007.

126. Miller CS, Leonelli FM, Latham E: Selective interference with pacemaker activity by electrical dental devices. *Oral Surg Oral Med Oral Pathol Oral Radiol Endod* 85:33–36, 1998.

127. Elayi CS, Lusher S, Meeks Nyquist JL, et al: Interference between dental electrical devices and pacemakers or defibrillators: results from a prospective clinical study. *J Am Dent Assoc* 146:121–128, 2015.

128. Roedig JJ, Shah J, Elayi CS, et al: Interference of cardiac pacemaker and implantable cardioverter-defibrillator activity during electronic dental device use. *J Am Dent Assoc* 141:521–526, 2010.

129. Price RB, McLeod ME, Felix CM: Quantifying light energy delivered to a Class I restoration. *J Can Dent Assoc* 76:a23, 2010.

130. Konerding KL, Heyder M, Kranz S, et al: Study of energy transfer by different light curing units into a class III restoration as a function of tilt angle and distance, using a MARC Patient Simulator (PS). *Dent Mater* 32:676–686, 2016.

131. Seth S, Lee CJ, Ayer CD: Effect of instruction on dental students' ability to light-cure a simulated restoration. *J Can Dent Assoc* 78:c123, 2012.

132. Price RB, Felix CM, Whalen JM: Factors affecting the energy delivered to simulated class I and class v preparations. *J Can Dent Assoc* 76:a94, 2010.

133. Federlin M, Price R: Improving light-curing instruction in dental school. *J Dent Educ* 77:764–772, 2013.

134. Mutluay MM, Rueggeberg FA, Price RB: Effect of using proper light-curing techniques on energy delivered to a Class 1 restoration. *Quintessence Int* 45:549–556, 2014.

135. Price RB, Strassler HE, Price HL, et al: The effectiveness of using a patient simulator to teach light-curing skills. *J Am Dent Assoc* 145:32–43, 2014.

136. Price RB: Light curing in dentistry. *Dent Clin North Am* 61:578–778, 2017.

7

Color and Shade Matching in Operative Dentistry

JOE C. ONTIVEROS, RADE D. PARAVINA

Color plays a critical role in the success or failure of esthetic dental restorations. Shade matching is as much an art as it is a science, and requires knowledge of color science principles and the implementation of adequate shade matching techniques. This chapter provides a working knowledge of the principles of color and perception relative to understanding the complex nature of tooth color and appearance. Shade matching methods and tools for achieving predictable esthetic outcomes will be discussed along with resources available for continued improvement.

Color and Perception

The Color Triplet (Observer Situation)

The human perception of color results from the interaction of three elements: light source, object, and observer (Fig. 7.1). Because all three of these elements can be modified, any change in one element will affect the final perception of color. The light source is a visible form of electromagnetic (EM) radiation that illuminates the object. When light strikes the object (tooth), a proportion of the energy is absorbed, transmitted, or reflected. Color perception is dependent upon the subjective ability of the human visual system to combine and interpret the physical interactions of light and object. The quantity of reflected light reaching the observer's eyes stimulates a subjective sensation in the brain that we experience as color. In other words, the perception of color ultimately resides in the brain and not merely in the property of the object. For this reason, color can be defined as a psychophysical sensation provoked in the eye by the visible light and interpreted by the brain.

Color Vision

Rods and Cones

The human eye and brain, which enable color vision, form an amazing and complex system. The visual system of a person with normal color vision can identify millions of different colors.[1,2] At the innermost retinal layer of the eye are two types of specialized neurons that function as photoreceptors, called rods and cones.

The more numerous of the two photoreceptors are the rods, which are sensitive to low levels of light. The rods are primarily responsible for our peripheral vision and are unable to detect color. In low levels of light, rods help us see objects in gray scale; as the light becomes brighter, the rods become inactive. On the other hand, the cones operate in bright light and provide high acuity color vision. Both photoreceptors transform light into chemical energies that stimulate millions of nerve endings. The neural signals are transported by the optic nerve to the brain, where color is interpreted. There are three types of cones in the retina that are sensitive to different wavelengths of light: blue, green, and red. The blue cones are most responsive to short wavelengths. The green and red cones are most responsive to medium and longer wavelengths, respectively, with some overlap.

Color Deficiency

Color vision deficiency is a weakness or absence in one or more of the three types of cones. The most common color deficiency in the population is an individual with a partial green defect known as *deuteranomaly*. Other deficiencies are *protanomaly*, which is caused by a reduced sensitivity to red light, and *tritanomaly*, which is someone lacking blue vision. Individuals with these color deficiencies still see color; however, their color vision is distorted (Fig. 7.2). Color blind individuals lack all three types of cones; this condition is called *monochromacy* or *achromatopsia*. Color deficiency poses a challenge for the clinician when performing visual shade matching. Popular general tests to check color vision are the *Ishihara Test* (Fig. 7.3) and the *Farnsworth-Munsell Test*.

Color Dimensions

There are numerous systems and theories for arranging color in some orderly fashion (i.e., color spaces). The most popular system for visual color matching in dentistry is based on the three-dimensional model devised by American artist Alfred H. Munsell in 1898.[2] Munsell's color system forms the basis for the classification of colored objects in the three dimensions: hue, value, and chroma. It is important to grasp the concepts of hue, value, and chroma to fully understand dental shade matching as described in this chapter.

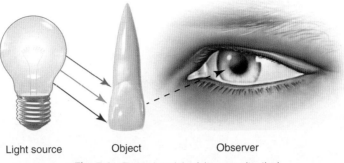

• **Fig. 7.1** The color triplet (observer situation).

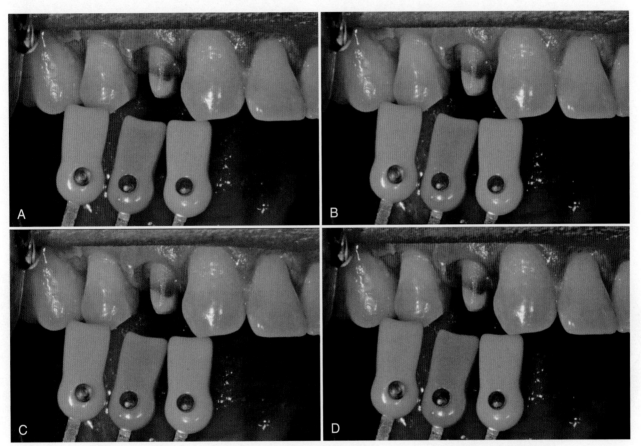

• **Fig 7.2** A, Unaltered digital image, corresponding to normal color vision and after color deficiency simulations. B, Protanomaly. C, Deuteranomaly. D, Tritanomaly. (The original image processed at http://www.color-blindness.com/coblis-color-blindness-simulator/.)

Hue

This color dimension is the attribute by which an object is judged to appear red, orange, yellow, green, blue, purple, etc. These are the "pure" colors found on a basic color wheel or a simple box of crayons. These hues, which appear on the visual spectrum, are placed on a continuous, circular scale as seen in Fig. 7.4. Compared to a standard, the hue of an object would be communicated in terms such as redder, yellower, greener, or bluer.

Value

The dimension of value refers to the lightness of a color. It is the achromatic vertical scale from black to white representing all shades of gray. It is usually communicated in terms of lighter or darker. A tooth that appears lighter, or "brighter," as a result of bleaching would display an increase in value.

Chroma

While hue enables the distinction and differentiation among different colors, chroma is related to variation in strength of the same color. The further away from the achromatic vertical axis, the higher the chroma (stronger, more intense). The closer the color is to the achromatic (value) axis, the lower the chroma (paler, weaker). Chroma is often described as more chromatic or less chromatic. A tooth with a redder and/or yellower appearance at

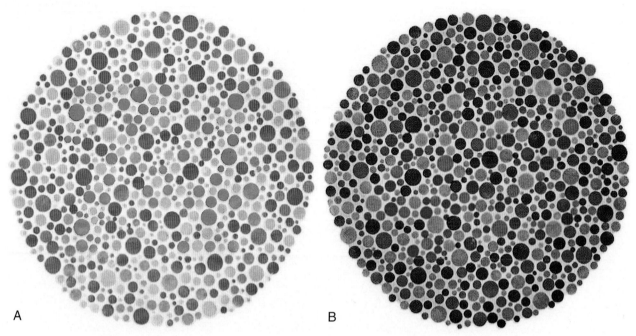

• **Fig. 7.3** Ishihara Test. Observer should see number 74 (A) and number 42 (B). (Reproduced from Ishihara's Tests for Colour Blindness. Tokyo: Kanehara & Co., but tests for color blindness cannot be conducted with this material. For accurate testing, the original plates should be used.)

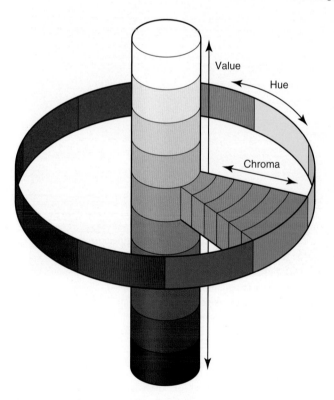

Munsell 1898

• **Fig 7.4** Munsell color system, with achromatic vertical value axis. Hues (*different* colors) are arranged in a 360-degree circle. Chroma is represented as the distance from the value axis—that is, the strength of the *same* color increases as it departs from the value axis.

the cervical region, as commonly seen on a canine, can be described as more chromatic at that region. As the chroma increases, the hue becomes more specific.

Other Optical Properties

When light waves strike the surface of an object, the change in refractive index can cause waves to be reflected, absorbed, or transmitted by the material. The combination of light speed and directional changes of the waves results in particular optical appearances of teeth as described later in the chapter.

Translucency

Translucency is the degree to which an object scatters light upon transmission, resulting in an appearance between complete opacity and complete transparency. Complete opacity will obscure the substrate beneath it by blocking the passage of light, while a completely transparent object will transmit light without scattering and will clearly show the substrate beneath it.

Iridescence

Iridescence is a rainbowlike effect caused by the diffraction of light that changes according to the angle from which it is viewed or the angle of incidence of the light source. Iridescence occurs when light is diffracted from a thin layer that lies between two mediums of different refractive index (e.g., air and water), as in a soap bubble or a thin film of oil on water. Teeth do not display the property of iridescence, which is often confused with opalescence.

Opalescence

Opalescence is a milky iridescence that resembles the internal play of colors of an opal. In a natural tooth, opalescence is caused by light scattering between two phases of enamel that have different indexes of refraction. Short wavelengths of light are reflected displaying a blue hue, whereas longer light wavelengths, such as the orange and red, are transmitted through the tooth.

Gloss

Gloss is an attribute of visual appearance that originates from the geometrical distribution of light reflected by surfaces.[3] Particularly, gloss is a term used to describe the relative amount of mirrorlike (specular) reflection from the surface of an object. Metals are usually distinguished by stronger specular reflection than that from other materials, and smooth surfaces will appear glossier than rough ones.

Fluorescence

Fluorescence is a form of luminescence, that is, a form of light emission by a substance as the result of some external stimuli. Following the excitation by light, usually ultraviolet (UV), a fluorescent substance will reemit some of the absorbed energy in the form of longer wavelengths. When the luminescence continues after the source of excitation has been removed, the "after-glow" is referred to as *phosphorescence*.

Surround Effects and Blending

Color not only is defined by its color dimensions and optical properties, but also depends on the surroundings in which the object appears, the adaptation of our eyes, and our recent visual experience.[3,4]

Chromatic Induction

When two objects of the same color are surrounded by different colored backgrounds, an illusory sensation of color can be created without direct stimulation of the corresponding cones. The two objects can be the same color when viewed in isolation, but when each is combined with different surroundings, the objects can have a perceived color difference in relation to each other. This is what color scientists call *chromatic induction*.

Contrast and Assimilation

Chromatic induction can generate either a contrast effect or an assimilation effect. When the object's color shifts toward the complementary color of its surroundings, this is known as *simultaneous color contrast* (Fig. 7.5A) (http://www.andrewkelsall.com/

color-effect-designers-should-see/). When the opposite occurs, that is, the perceived difference between the object's color and its surrounding is reduced, this is known as *chromatic assimilation*.

Blending Effect

Clinically, the perceptual phenomenon of assimilation occurs when a restorative material (object) takes on the color of the tooth (background/surround) and appears more similar combined than when viewed in isolation. In the dental literature, this visual blending of tooth and material is known as *blending effect* (BE).[5,6] The blending effect is commonly (and incorrectly) referred to as "chameleon effect."

Complementary Afterimage

Similar to contrast and assimilation effects, our eyes can adapt to a recent visual experience and provoke illusionary perceptions of color. When we stare at a solid color for approximately 30 seconds or more, our photoreceptors become sensitized (retinal fatigue) and can create illusionary images of the complementary color; this is known as *complementary afterimage*. If one concentrates on a solid color red target, for example, the red cones gradually respond less strongly to that reflected red signal. If one switches his or her gaze to a solid white target, now all colors are reflected to the retina and cones will send a strong green signal and a strong blue signal, but a weak red signal. One will see a cyan color afterimage, cyan being the complementary color of red (see Fig. 7.5B).

Color and Appearance of Teeth and Dental Materials

Tooth Color and Appearance

How various reflections and transmissions of light integrate to generate perceived colors in human teeth is a complex process that is not entirely understood. The polychromatic appearance of the tooth originates from the relative interactions of light signals and perceptions (Fig. 7.6).

The quantification of tooth color has been reported in the past by measuring the three regions of the tooth: cervical, middle, and incisal.[7-9] Describing tooth regions can help understand how they are related to overall tooth color and appearance. However, this approach is not necessarily sufficient to capture the polychromatic and complex tooth appearance (Fig. 7.7).

Dentin

In general, the color of the tooth is not uniform. Dentin contributes significantly to tooth color. This is particularly noticeable in the cervical region, where only a thin layer of enamel exists. This region is typically the most chromatic (Fig. 7.8), with the chroma progressively decreasing through the middle to the incisal third, displaying hues ranging from yellow to red.[7] Dentin is also the primary source of tooth fluorescence.[10]

Enamel

In a healthy unworn tooth, the incisal third is typically all enamel. If the enamel were isolated from the dentin, it would appear primarily achromatic like transparent or white frosted glass (Fig. 7.9). The translucency and value of the enamel can vary depending on many factors such as its thickness and age. Thick enamel generally appears higher in value relative to thin enamel. High-value white patterns, or white spots, also may demonstrate hypomineralized

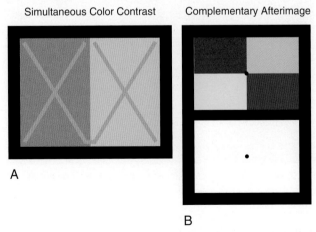

Simultaneous Color Contrast   Complementary Afterimage

A

B

• **Fig. 7.5** A, Simultaneous color contrast. The two Xs appear to be of different colors due to different backgrounds; however, when observed at their intersection at the middle base of the image it becomes obvious they are of the same color. B, Complementary afterimage. Stare for 30 seconds at the point where the four colors intersect; then switch gaze to the white target below the color images. Retinal fatigue results in the illusionary appearance of the complementary colors.

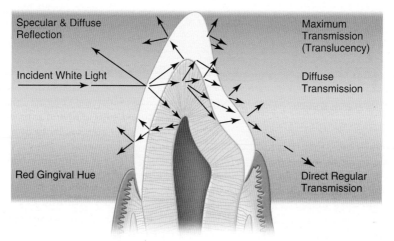

• **Fig. 7.6** Complex interactions of light and tooth appearance.

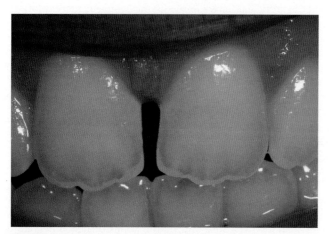

• **Fig. 7.7** Polychromatic appearance of natural teeth. Notice the progression of color from cervical to incisal on teeth #8 and #9—from chromatic to translucent, changes in hue and incisal opalescence.

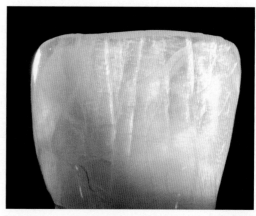

• **Fig. 7.9** Translucency of isolated enamel. (Courtesy Adam J. Mieleszko, CDT.)

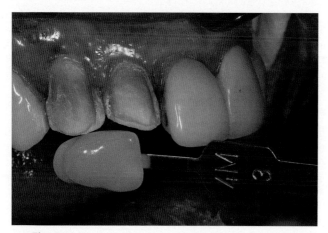

• **Fig. 7.8** The exposed dentin showing accentuated chroma.

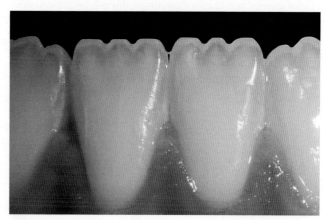

• **Fig. 7.10** The incisal halo: distinct line of opalescent reflection at incisal edge.

regions within the enamel. For anterior teeth, the enamel gets thinner toward the incisal and can appear gray to bluish against the dark background of the oral cavity. Depending on the transmission or reflection of light at the incisal edge, the incisal third may display an opalescent pattern with a distinct line of reflection described as the incisal halo (Fig. 7.10).

Color-Related Properties of Restorative Materials

Restorative materials should display color and optical properties similar to those of dentin and enamel. In this section, we will primarily focus on composite resin and ceramic dental materials as they relate to color compatibility, stability, and interactions.

Compatibility

When choosing dental materials such as composite resins or dental ceramics for restorative procedures, the shade selection of the material will be dependent on the brand or system in use. Most commonly a material is keyed to a commercially available shade guide. Shade guides will be further discussed under Color Matching Tools. At other times, a restorative material may be labeled with a shade descriptor, such as "universal dentin" or names like "milky white" or "pearl frost," without any reference to a shade guide. In either case, a material will be most compatible with a tooth when it has shades that mimic both dentin and enamel.

Stability

The color stability of dental materials is a significant concern for color and appearance in restorative dentistry. When comparing composite resins and dental ceramics, resins are less color stable after aging.[11] Over time, resins are susceptible to extrinsic staining from dietary exposures and intrinsic degradation of the inherent chemical components.[12] Resins also can shift color upon curing. Generally, microfill composite resins become lighter and less translucent upon curing while microhybrid composite resins become darker and more translucent.[13] Ceramic materials, while more stable in service, can vary by batch and still undergo color shifts upon firing and glazing.[14]

Interactions

An existing color difference between the restorative material and the tooth can be lessened with favorable color interaction properties, such as layering and blending.

Layering is the essence of tooth anatomy as layers of enamel and dentin of different thicknesses interact creating a polychromatic appearance. Color of both enamel and dentin can change over time due to dietary habits or aging, respectively. Given that the task is to mimic nature, layering is equally essential for creation of tooth colored restorations.

A blending effect or color shift of a dental material, such as composite resin or dental ceramic, toward the surrounding tooth color is a desirable property. This blending effect decreases the color difference between the tooth-material interface giving the restoration a more lifelike and natural appearance. The blending effect is predominantly related to smaller restorations, surrounded by hard dental tissues, such as composite restorations. It can reduce suboptimal shade matches due to operational error or lack of satisfactory match in the shade guide or restorative material. The veneers designed with "contact lens effect" margins before and after cementation are another example of blending effect (Fig. 7.11).[15]

Color Matching Tools—Dental Shade Guides

Dental Shade Guides

The standard color matching tool used in dentistry for visual shade matching is the dental shade guide. Dental shade guides are tab-based tools fabricated from ceramic, resin, or some other form of plastic or acrylic material. The shade tabs are typically arranged according to some dimension of color, but because of the complex polychromatic nature of natural teeth, a given shade guide system will only serve as a guide and not as an exact color matcher. While dental shade guides exist for oral soft tissues and facial skin, the focus of this section will be on guides designed for shade matching a tooth during the dental restorative procedure.

Commercial Shade Guides

Ceramic Based

For direct restorative procedures, there are many shortcomings associated with the use of a ceramic-based tooth shade guide for dental shade matching, but it is the most logical starting point for shade matching as most composite resins are keyed to a commercially available ceramic-based system. The most popular of the ceramic-based commercial guides is the Vita classical A1-D4 shade guide (VITA Zahnfabrik). This 16-tab shade guide can be arranged according to the hue order ("A-D arrangement" [Fig. 7.12A]) or according to an apparent light to dark arrangement ("Value Scale" [see Fig. 7.12B]).

Each tab has a number and a letter. According to the manufacturer, the letters represent one of the following hue groups:

A = Reddish-brown
B = Reddish-yellow
C = Grey
D = Reddish-grey

The number next to the letter on the tab label represents the chroma and value within each of the A to D groups: 1 = lowest chroma, lightest, 4 = highest chroma, darkest. Within this system, shade B1 is the least chromatic and lightest of the reddish-yellow shades, whereas B4 is the most chromatic and darkest of the reddish-yellow shades. One way to use this shade guide is to observe the most chromatic portion of the patient's tooth, usually the cervical region of the canine and select the best hue group. Next, the best shade within that hue group should be selected based on the closest chroma number. A second way to use this shade guide

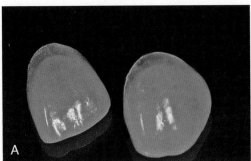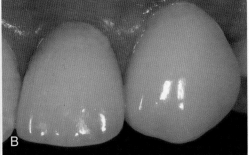

• **Fig. 7.11** A, Laminate veneers designed with "contact lens effect" margins. B, The blending effect of indistinguishable translucent margins of laminate veneers.

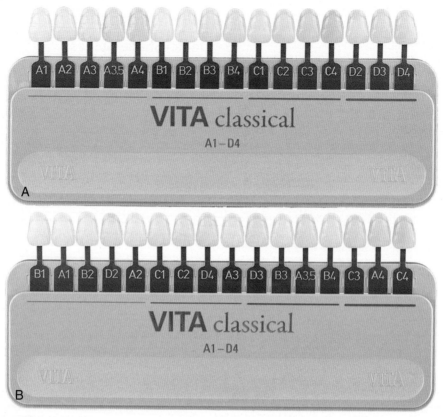

• **Fig. 7.12** A, Vita classical shade guide: A–D arrangement. B, "Value Scale" arrangement of same shade guide.

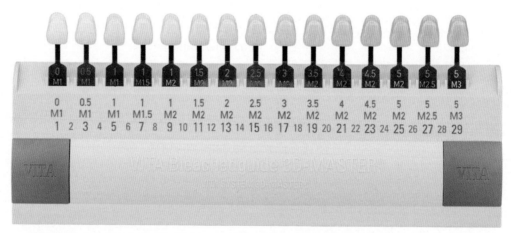

• **Fig. 7.13** Vita Bleachedguide 3D-Master. Shade tabs are getting lighter and less chromatic *(right to left)*, matching the changes that occur of natural teeth when exposed to whitening agents.

is to arrange the shade tabs from light to dark according to the so-called "Value Scale." With the most contrasted end of the shade guide against the teeth, one would slide down or up the scale and stop on the best match. The "Value Scale" is helpful when monitoring changes in color after bleaching. However, the change from one tab to the next varies and with inconsistent value shift. For this reason, the same company released a shade guide in 2007 specifically designed for bleach monitoring—Vita Bleachedguide 3D-Master (Fig. 7.13). It has many advantages over the "Value Scale," from much wider range and more uniform color differences between the adjacent tabs, to the inclusion of very light shades

that enable monitoring of whitening efficacy of initially light teeth (e.g., shade B1 before bleaching).[16,17] This scale includes 29 shades (15 tabs with 14 interpolations) with color evenly distributed between tabs.

Other ceramic shade guides of the 3D-Master system include the Vita Toothguide 3D-Master and Vita Linearguide 3D-Master (Fig. 7.14). The latter one is user friendly, simplifying the shade matching method. Tabs are marked using a number-letter-number code that correspond to value-hue-chroma, respectively. There are five light gray holders, containing tabs from groups 0 to 5 (created based on decreasing lightness), with groups 0 and 1 on the same

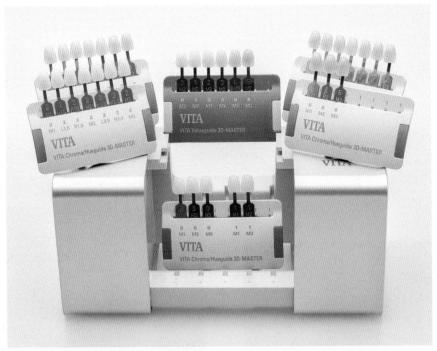

• **Fig. 7.14** Vita Linearguide 3D-Master. Primary division into groups is made according to value (0–5); within the groups the chroma (1 = least; 3 = most) and hue (M = "neutral" middle hue; L = less red; R = more red) vary.

holder. Group selection is facilitated by having the middle tab of each group (M2) in a dark gray holder for initial shade matching. No more than 7 tabs, arranged in linear order, are viewed at once with the Linearguide. Furthermore, the 3D-Master system has the smallest "coverage error" (it covers the color of natural teeth the best).[18] Consequently, it has been reported that this shade guide was preferred and outperformed others.[19]

A major concern with using the ceramic-based shade guides such as the Vita classical A1-D4 for selecting a composite resin shade keyed to this system is that the actual composite shade may or may not match the original classical tabs. It should be noted that large color differences exist among the composite materials of the same shade designations.[20] If a restorative system is not supplied with a shade guide, then a ceramic shade guide may be used as a starting reference.

Polymer Resin Based

Proprietary shade guides supplied with a restorative composite resin system are often fabricated using the same restorative material. In other words, they are resin-based tooth shade guides. Initially, this is a good option because they will have the same optical properties as the restorative material. However, color stability of the tabs may become problematic over time as the tabs are disinfected and get darker.

Other Materials (Plastics/Acrylics)

Shade guides are sometimes supplied with a restorative system fabricated from materials other than ceramics or resin-based materials, such as plastics or acrylics. These shade guides are generally inferior in comparison and are not good tools for shade matching teeth.

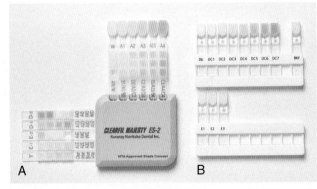

• **Fig. 7.15** Proprietary composite shade guides supplied by manufacturers and made of monochromatic single-layered composites. A, Kuraray shade guide. B, SDI shade guide.

Custom Shade Guides

Using the shade guide supplied with the restorative system in many cases would be advantageous over using a ceramic-based system. Yet, depending on the accuracy of the shade guide supplied with the system, it may be more accurate to use the actual composite cured on the tooth. It is important to fully cure the composite material when performing this evaluation as it has been shown that a shift in color will occur. In general, restorative composites will shift upon curing to become less saturated. A more advanced alternative would be to periodically fabricate custom shade tabs from the actual restorative material using proprietary composite shade guides supplied by manufacturers (Fig. 7.15),

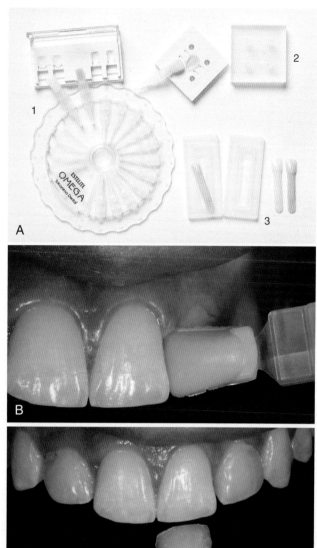

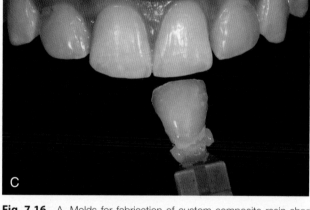

• **Fig. 7.16** A, Molds for fabrication of custom composite resin shade tabs: *(1)* Tokuyama dentin and enamel molds, tab holders, and custom made tabs; *(2)* Style Italiano mold for layered enamel and dentin, the enamel shell, and a layered tab; *(3)* Ultradent molds for dentin, enamel, or layered enamel-dentin, with respective tabs. B, Dentin custom shade tab—clinical application. C, Enamel custom shade tab—clinical application.

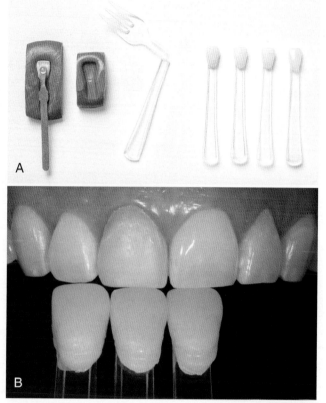

• **Fig. 7.17** A, Custom shade tabs from the actual restorative material made using a silicone index impression of a tab from a commercially available shade guide. B, Clinical application: enamel shades UE1, UE2, and UE3 *(left to right).*

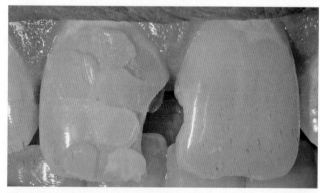

• **Fig. 7.18** Cured pieces of composite placed on respective areas of the tooth to be restored can be helpful in shade matching.

molds for fabrication of custom shade tabs (Fig. 7.16), a silicone index of a standard shade guide (Fig. 7.17), or cured pieces of composite placed onto respective areas of the tooth to be restored (Fig. 7.18).

Color Matching Instruments

Color differences can be difficult to verbally communicate between a tooth and a dental material. For example, what do we mean when we say a shade is too bright or too yellow? Digital instruments can be used to numerically quantify color differences and to help arrive at an objective standard color. Color matching instruments are designed to replicate how the human eye receives color, yet without the subjectivity of the human visual system. Various devices have been used in dentistry, including digital cameras, scanners, spectrophotometers, and colorimeters. Regardless of the device, the basis for all instrumental color measurement is the hypothetical standard observer. Colorimeters, for example, receive and reduce light to its RGB (red-green-blue) components similar to that of the three color receptors (cones) in the retina. The colorimeter expresses this information in terms of three values, converting the numeric information to a standard target color. Similarly, spectrophotometers measure light reflected from the target relative to the total light. The amount of reflected light at each wavelength along the visible spectrum is calculated and translated into shade terminology that makes sense to the dental professional. Historically, dentistry has not been a large market for color measuring devices. Many devices have come and gone without widespread adoption. The one instrument that has remained on the market over many generations is the Easyshade device manufactured by VITA. The latest generation of this spectrophotometer is the Vita Easyshade V (Fig. 7.19A). This instrument provides shade information correlated to the Vita classical A1–D4 and Vita System 3D-Master shade guides. Its proprietary software, Vita Assist, and smartphone application, Vita mobileAssist, allow Bluetooth transfer of the color information and digital images to a computer for patient and laboratory communication (see Fig. 7.19B). An advanced method used in research where repeatable measurements are necessary to monitor color changes involves using a custom jig to avoid angulation of the probe and ensure precise measurements (Fig. 7.20).[21]

While color measuring instruments continue to improve, they still do not replace the operator. Instead, color matching instruments provide the dental professional with an objective tool to confirm a "best match" among various shade guides. Ultimately, the best color matching tool would be the one whose results correspond to a clinician's normal color vision.

Dental Photography

The use of photography is integral to a complete analysis of tooth color and appearance. Digital single-lens reflex (DSLR, recommended) cameras, portable cameras, and cell phones are used for digital photography. A DSLR camera can be used with a general-purpose lens or dedicated macro lens, and a variety of flashes: single-point, ring, dual-point, and twin tube flash. Digital images can be captured and saved, probably most frequently in JPG format (with an adjustable degree of compression and consequently image quality), while advanced users typically prefer RAW format (with minimally processed data). Recommendations for basic settings of DSLR cameras for dental photography are provided in Table 7.1.[20] Mirrors and retractors are important accessories for digital photography.

Photography enables the use of a color monitor to both magnify a tooth image and discriminate subtle transitions of color and use black-and-white contrast adjustments to study translucency patterns, and is an essential tool for communicating color to the dental laboratory technician for indirect restorations. Today, a photo can be taken of a tooth with a shade tab held on the same plane, along with a standard black/white/gray standard card, and software can provide a "Color Map" of the target tooth. One example of this type of dental shade matching software is Shade Wave (Issaquah, WA). An attachment arm (Shade Arm) is available for fixing the distance, angle, and position of the color reference in the photo. The software will mathematically normalize, or color correct, the image to compensate for color imbalances that occur when the image is taken and will cross-reference the standard card to generate a "Shade Map," "Value Map," and "Translucency Map." The value of this type of system is that it does not rely on any specific camera or camera settings, nor is it influenced by surrounding colors or light. Digital photography is frequently used in conjunction with general software programs (such as Adobe Photoshop and Corel

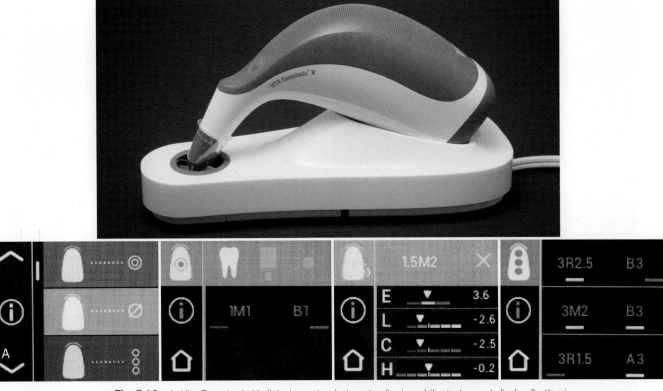

• **Fig. 7.19** A, Vita Easyshade V clinical spectrophotometer *(top)*, and the instrument display *(bottom)*. First, to measure color of natural teeth, the tooth symbol *(the upper icon)* should be selected; then best matches in Vita 3D-Master *(left)* and Vita classical A1–D4 shade guide *(right)*; next, color difference (ΔE*) and value, chroma, and hue differences compared to selected shade; and last, best matching tabs from Vita 3D-Master *(left)* and Vita classical A1–D4 *(right)* shade guides in cervical, middle, and incisal third.

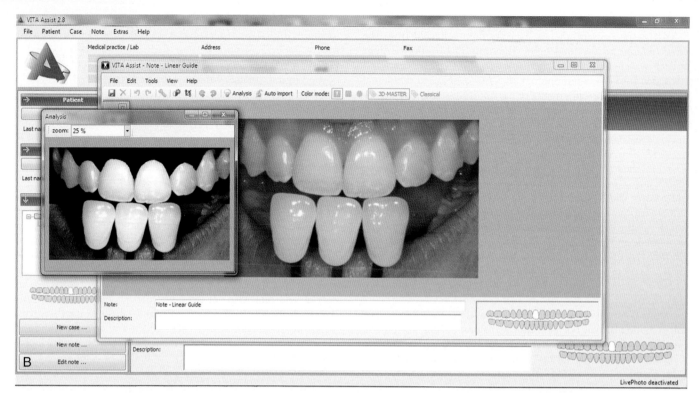

• **Fig. 7.19, cont'd** B, Vita Assist is software for Easyshade V that enables recording, storage, editing, and commenting of patient data and images. It facilitates communication on tooth shade and translucency between dentist and patient and between dentist and dental technician, including the communication via smartphone (Vita mobileAssist app).

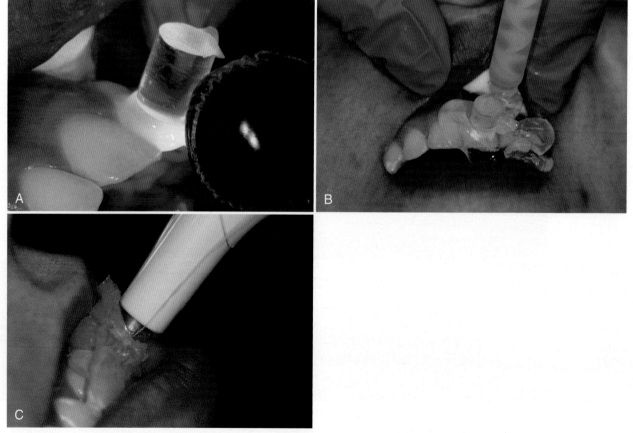

• **Fig. 7.20** Fabrication of clear silicone individual positioning jig for repeated spectrophotometer measurements. A, Acrylic rod cured to the tooth. B, Injection of clear silicone material. C, Measurement through the cylindrical tunnel created upon the removal of the acrylic rod.

TABLE 7.1	Basic Setting of DSLR Camera for Dental Photography[20]
Manual mode	M (Manual)
Focusing	Manual
Aperture	f22
Shutter speed	1.125 s
ISO	100
Image size	Maximum
Image format	JPG fine
White balance	Flash or 5300°K
Image optimization	Set to neutral
Flash output	One-half or one-quarter power (non-TTL flash)
Gridlines	On (for easier orientation)

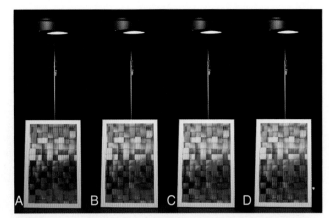

• **Fig. 7.21** Influence of lights of different color temperature on color perception of the same object. A, 3000°K. B, 4000°K. C, 5000°K. D, 6500°K.

Photo-Paint). Mobile apps are becoming increasingly popular for color management.

Visual Shade Matching Method

Color matching is dependent on controlling subjective variables such as color vision deficiencies and eye fatigue, while at the same time controlling the proper viewing conditions and selecting the correct light sources. The following order of three pre–shade matching steps and five shade matching steps will provide a predictable method for visual shade matching.

Three Pre–Shade Matching Steps

1. Check Color Vision

Prior to performing a shade matching trial, it is imperative to screen the vision of the clinician for any color deficiencies. A common myth about shade matching is that females are better color matchers than males. While statistics show that up to 8% of males and 0.5% of women have a color deficiency,[3] this does not equate to a gender superiority if both are trichromats, that is, have normal color vision.[22]

Test for color discrimination competency in dentistry consists of creating pairs of shade tabs from two identical shade guides (at least one set should not have original markings, such as A1 to D4 of classical, visible).[23] Under controlled conditions, this test is an accepted standard for dental color research but also could be implemented for everyday practice.

2. Use Color Corrected Lighting

The way we perceive color is greatly influenced by the light source used to illuminate the object. In shade matching, we want to use an illuminant that best matches the white light of natural daylight. White light is a creation of our minds as a result of interpreting the spectral colors present in a particular illuminate; there is no "color white" on the visible light spectrum. White light is actually a mixture of all the colors of light. To understand correct lighting for shade matching we first should consider the issue of *correlated color temperature (CCT)*. It is based on early 20th-century German Nobel Laureate Max Planck's experiments in quantum physics. He developed a mathematical standard that correlates to a theoretical

"black body" whose spectral color changes with temperature. The perfect black body emits the exact amount of electromagnetic radiation (light) as is absorbed. As the temperature increases, the object begins to glow a particular color, turning "red hot" near 1500°K. As the object gets hotter, it changes to a reddish-yellow around 3000°K (household incandescent lamp) and becomes "white hot" near 5000°K as it moves throughout the visible spectrum, eventually turning blue-white. For shade matching, light sources with a CCT of 5500°K and 6500°K are recommended; the colors are correlated to standard phases of natural daylight.

The CCT of a light source alone is not the only specification important for correct lighting for shade matching. The *color rendering index (CRI)* and intensity of the light source should be considered. The CRI is an average performance rating score for a light source based on comparisons to reference colors. The maximum score is 100 representing a full-spectrum light source (like the sun) that affects our color judgment as natural daylight. For best color rendering results, light sources with CRI of 90 or higher are recommended. The intensity of the light source, or *illuminance*, is measured in lux (lx) and should be between 1000 and 2000 lx. If the illuminance is too low, colors cannot be discerned; if the illuminance is too high, colors will be washed out. Despite using quality light sources with the correct CRI, CCT, and intensity, some dental materials may have spectral properties that appear to match under a given set of viewing conditions and not match under another. This phenomenon known as *illuminant metamerism* at times is unavoidable due to the inherent properties of the dental material relative to the complex nature of natural teeth. It is advisable to use lights with different CCT to verify the existence of metamerism (Fig. 7.21).

There are a variety of lights that exhibit the recommended color characteristics either as ceiling light, floor and table lamps, or handheld lights. Handheld lights, such as Rite-Lite 2 HI CRI (http://www.addent.com/rite-lite-2/) and Smile Lite (http://www.smileline-by-styleitaliano.com/en/shade-taking-dental-photography/5-smile-lite-style-lense.html), are becoming increasingly popular for visual shade matching. They can be used with or without (standard) polarizing filters (Fig. 7.22). Polarizing filters are intended to reduce glare, thus enabling better comparison of "pure color" and better visualization of color transitions. However, no one normally observes a restoration and/or teeth through a polarizing filter, and the filters were not found advantageous in terms of improving shade matching quality.[24] In addition, the

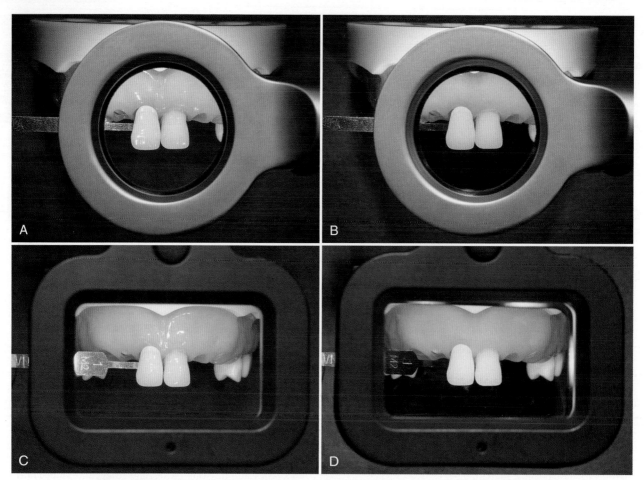

• **Fig. 7.22** Handheld shade matching lights. A, Rite-Lite 2 HI CRI without polarizing filter. B, Rite-Lite 2 HI CRI with polarizing filter. C, Smile Lite without polarizing filter. D, Smile lite with polarizing filter. (Photos from Clary JA, Ontiveros JC, Cron SG, et al: Influence of light source, polarization, education, and training on shade matching quality. *J Prosthet Dent* 116:91-97, 2016.)

Rite-Lite 2 HI CRI has three light options for shade matching: with CCT of 5500°K, 3200°K, and their combination, which enables better visualization of metamerism.

3. Control Surround/Viewing Conditions

As discussed earlier in this chapter (see Color and Perception) the surrounding conditions can change the overall color perception of an object. Any surround conditions that may influence color perception should be addressed prior to shade matching. Distracting color should be eliminated from the trial room with walls preferably painted a neutral gray color. Any bold colors on the patient should be eliminated. Start by placing a neutral color patient napkin over sparkling jewelry or bright clothes and having the patient remove reflective glasses and colored lipstick (Fig. 7.23).

Five Shade Matching Steps

Once the pre–shade matching steps have been addressed, the following shade matching steps can be implemented to further improve visual shade matching performance.

1. Perform at the Beginning

The issue of timing is important to visual shade matching and should be performed at the beginning of the appointment. *Tooth*

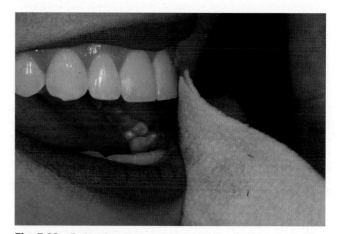

• **Fig. 7.23** Patient is asked to remove intense lipstick prior to shade matching (note the lipstick on canine and premolar).

dehydration occurs during restorative field isolation and alters the tooth color.[25] As teeth dehydrate, they will appear lighter, less chromatic, and more opaque. Performing shade matching at the start of the appointment will also help prevent eye fatigue and strain on the visual system as time progresses.

2. Set Light and Observer

This step involves using the correct viewing distance and position (Fig. 7.24). The correct viewing distance for shade matching will vary based on the clinician's visual acuity. Generally, the ideal distance should correspond to the best reading distance and *visual angle of subtense* (>2 degrees). For most, this distance will fall in the range of 25 to 35 cm (10–14 in). The angle of illumination and person performing shade matching relative to the shade tab is also an important factor, known as the *optical geometry*. The optical geometry of 45/0 degrees (light at 45 degrees, unidirectional, bidirectional, or circumferential; observing at 0 degrees,

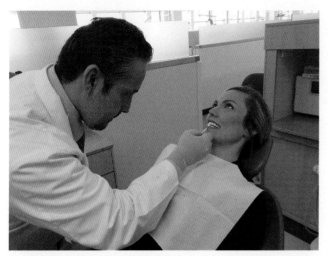

• **Fig. 7.24** Shade matching should be performed at the distance of 25 to 35 cm (10–14 in), with tooth being observed perpendicularly to its labial surface and with the 45-degree angle of illumination.

perpendicular to tooth surface) or diffuse/0 degrees is typically used for clinical evaluation. The viewer's eyes should be on the same level as the shade tab.

3. Use Appropriate Technique

The shade matching technique includes selection of the appropriate shade guide for the task (see *Color Matching Tools—Dental Shade Guides* earlier in the chapter), appropriate shade tab positioning, technique, and duration.

Shade Tab Positioning

After the position of the clinician is set, attention should be focused on the positioning of the shade tab. The tab should be placed in accordance with the clinical situation and the goal (overall tooth color or color in different regions). The ideal position of the tab is on the same plane and the same vertical (cervical to incisal) orientation (Fig. 7.25). This is easy to achieve if the adjacent tooth is missing. However, this is most often not the case, so the shade tab can be placed in between upper and lower teeth, vertically or horizontally (see Fig. 7.25) to the longitudinal axes of the natural teeth. Shade tabs should not be positioned in front or behind the natural teeth (Fig. 7.26).

The shade tab is sometimes placed in front of the adjacent tooth, but the shade tab will appear lighter solely for being physically closer to the eye of the clinician. One way to avoid this is to incline the shade tab to approximately 120 degrees relative to the natural tooth and observe both from a symmetrical angle (see Fig. 7.25B). Attention should be given that the tab carrier is opposite the incisal edge as not to influence the evaluation of translucency.

As the middle portion of shade tabs, both cervical to incisal and mesial to distal, is the most accurate representation of the tab color, tabs can be modified by reducing the cervical third or keeping

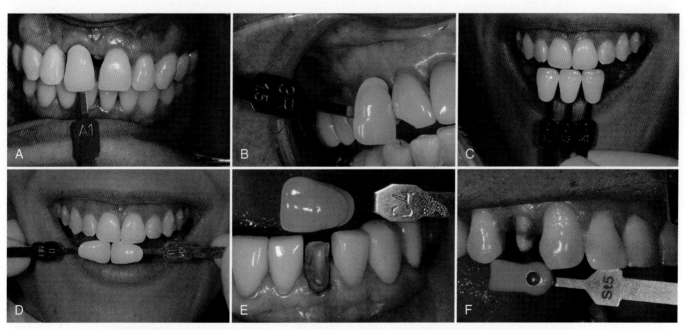

• **Fig. 7.25** Suggested shade tab positions. Vertical positioning: A, When the adjacent tooth is missing, the ideal position of the tab is on the same plane and the same vertical orientation (cervical to incisal); B, When the adjacent tooth is present, the ideal position of the tab is inclined at approximately 120 degrees relative to the tooth, with both observed from the angle symmetrical and with the same vertical orientation (cervical to incisal); C, On the same plane, incisal to incisal orientation. Horizontal positioning on the same plane, but at 90 degrees to tooth cervical to incisal orientation: D, Tooth shade matching; E, Stump shade matching with tooth shade tab; F, Stump shade matching with stump shade tab.

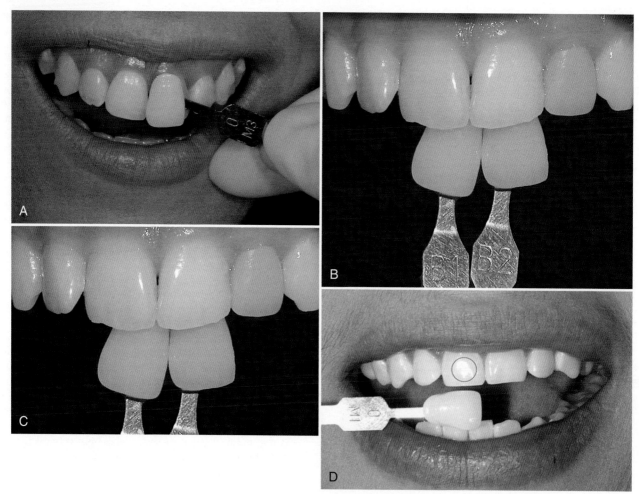

• **Fig. 7.26** Suboptimal shade tab positioning and/or image capturing. A, Tab in front of tooth appears lighter. B, Tab behind tooth appears darker. C, Shade designation not captured in image. D, Light reflection of tab washes out shade.

only the middle third, as shown on Fig. 7.27. The tab ledges enable tab positioning at the same anterior-posterior plane with the tooth.

Macro-Mini-Micro Shade Matching Technique

Macro Phase. Shade matching typically begins with a quick glance and selection of potentially adequate tabs. The entire shade guide is used, positioned close to the tooth whose color is being matched, and moved laterally to facilitate this selection (Fig. 7.28A).

Mini Phase. After this, the potentially adequate tabs are clustered together (in or outside the shade guide holder), and the best matches for incisal, middle, and cervical third are identified (see Fig. 7.28B).

Micro Phase. Once the best match or matches have been selected in the final micro phase, one needs to determine and describe differences in hue, value, and chroma between the regions of natural tooth and selected shades. Local color characteristics such as white spots, amber stains, striation patterns, and any other appearance attributes or details, including translucency, enamel cracks, and craze lines, should be documented and described (see Fig. 7.28C).

The same process is followed when using the Vita classical shade guide (see Fig. 7.28D-F)

Shade Matching Duration

A key to discerning the difference in shade between two colors, especially if the color difference is small, is to use very short glances for visual shade matching. This will help avoid illusory sensations of color (chromatic induction, complementary afterimage) due to saturation of the rods and cones. It is not advisable to stare at any color during shade matching. Staring at blue for example will create the illusion that the teeth are more yellow than they actually are in reality. It is preferable to see the true color, not a complementary afterimage. To avoid staring at the target, it is best to gaze at a neutral gray card in between shade matching trials (Fig. 7.29). Ideally the glances at the target shade should last only between 5 and 7 seconds.

4. Communicate

The next step in the shade matching process is to capture, record, and communicate the selected tooth shades. The shades observed for direct restorations should be mapped out to assist in material selection during the restorative procedure. A simple sketch of the tooth illustrating the cervical, middle, and incisal shades can help document the selected shades even through color shifts after field isolation.[3] The aid of digital photography, software, or data from a shade matching instrument can nicely supplement visual shade matching in color documentation and communication.

5. Verify

The final step is to verify the color of restoration (direct/indirect) visually, using several different lights, shade matching distances,

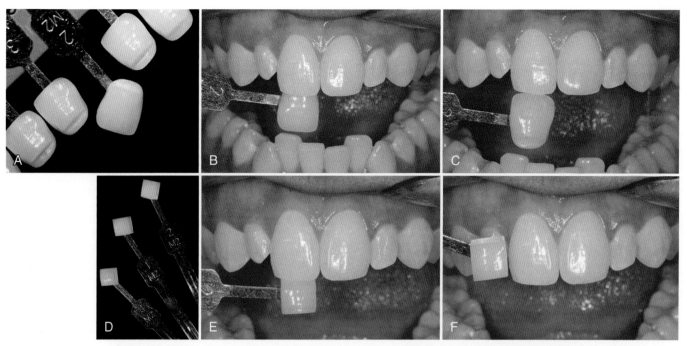

• **Fig. 7.27**   As the middle portion of shade tabs, both cervical to incisal and mesial to distal, is the most accurate representation of the tab color, tabs can be modified as follows: First, by reducing the cervical third: A, Shade tabs; B, Modified shade tab positioned on the same plane, cervical (tab) to incisal (tooth); C, Modified shade tab positioned on the same plane, incisal (tab) to incisal (tooth). Second, by keeping only the middle third: D, Shade tabs; E, Tab on the same plane, underneath the natural tooth; F, Tab at 120 degrees relative to the natural tooth, observed/photographed from a symmetrical angle.

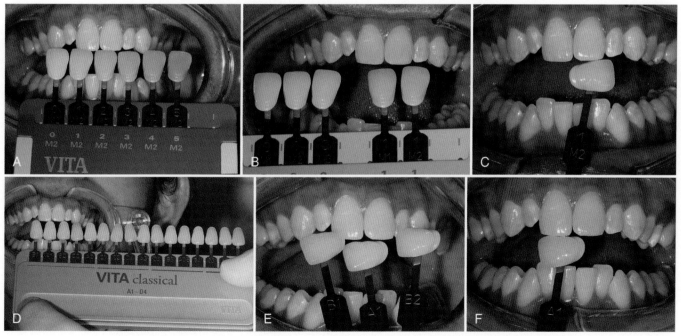

• **Fig. 7.28**   Macro-mini-micro shade matching technique. With Linearguide 3D-Master: A, *Macro phase*. Start with the entire shade guide and a quick glance and selection of potentially adequate tabs (in this case, the group selection, 0–5); B, *Mini phase*. The potentially adequate tabs are clustered together (in this case into groups) and the best matches for incisal, middle, and cervical third are identified; C, *Micro phase*. In the final phase, determine and describe differences in hue, value, and chroma between the regions of natural tooth and selected shades. Local color characteristics and other appearance attributes or details should be documented and described. The same also applies with Vita classical A1–D4, arranged according to "Value Scale"; D, *Macro phase*. Selection of potentially adequate tabs; E, *Mini phase*. These tabs are clustered and the best matches by thirds are identified; F, *Micro phase*. Determining and describing differences in hue, value, and chroma between the regions of natural tooth and selected tabs.

TABLE 7.2	Available Color Education and Training Programs		
Name	Type	Publisher	Available at
Color Matching Curriculum (CMC)	Didactic and hands-on CE program	Society for Color and Appearance in Dentistry (SCAD)	www.scadent.org
Dental Color Matcher (DCM)	Color education and training software	SCAD	www.scadent.org
A Contemporary Guide to Color and Shade Selection for Prosthodontics	Educational DVD	American College of Prosthodontists	http://dentistry.llu.edu/continuing-education/
Toothguide Trainer (TT)	Color training software	VITA Zahnfabrik	www.toothguide.com

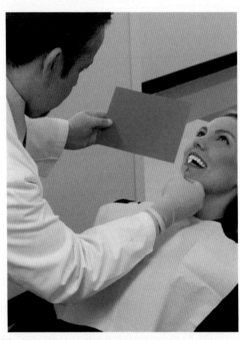

• **Fig. 7.29** The clinician glances at a neutral gray card to rest his eyes in between shade matching trials (lasting 5–7 seconds).

observation angles, and/or observers. The same is true for verification using shade matching instruments. The findings before the restoration is fabricated can supplement communication and case documentation. For direct composite resin restorations, the verification step can be made with a mockup restoration or by simply applying (and light-curing) a small increment of the selected composite material to the area(s) of the tooth corresponding to the selected shade. The selection can then be fine-tuned accordingly. If this approach is used, the operator should consider variables such as viewing angle, proximity, and others that may influence the results.

Improving Shade Matching Skills

Shade matching is a skill that can be learned and improved upon with implementation of sound color principles. Like any skill worth mastering, it will require consistent and intentional practice of the methods covered in this chapter. The amount of time devoted to color education and training in dental curriculums has been lacking in the past.[26] While up-to-date content is still lacking among educational institutions, significant advances have been made and greater resources are currently available for further study on the topic (Table 7.2).

The Color Matching Curriculum (CMC) is the newest and most comprehensive color education and training program for dental professionals and dental students.[27] This half-day continuing education program consists of didactic (color concepts and resources, color matching conditions, methods, tools, and communication) and hands-on (visual and instrumental color matching) portions.

Appendix

The Curious Case of a "Bleaching Mishap"

A 22-year-old woman with "Hollywood White" expectations presented with a chief complaint of "two dark front crowns" (Fig. 7.30A). Her dental history reveals gingival recession and overbleaching of her natural teeth with at-home whitening products resulting in a mismatch of all-ceramic crowns on the upper right central incisor and upper left lateral incisor (see Fig. 7.30B). The patient declined treatment for gingival recession while accepting treatment to replace mismatched crowns. A ceramic-based shade tab (Vita Linearguide, 0M3) is used with a black-and-white standard card held on the same plane as the teeth to be restored. In conjunction with digital photography and the standard reference card, digital shade mapping with computer software can be performed for effective laboratory communication (see Fig. 7.30C). The mismatched crowns were removed to reveal the natural high chromaticity of the dentinal preparations. The color of the preparations, "stump shade," is photographed for further laboratory communication with a reference shade tab (Vita Linearguide 3D-Master, 2M2) held in a horizontal position with the most chromatic portion of the tab (cervical) in contact with the tooth reference (see Fig. 7.30D). All-ceramic crowns were delivered with improved color matching to bleached natural teeth (see Fig. 7.30E).

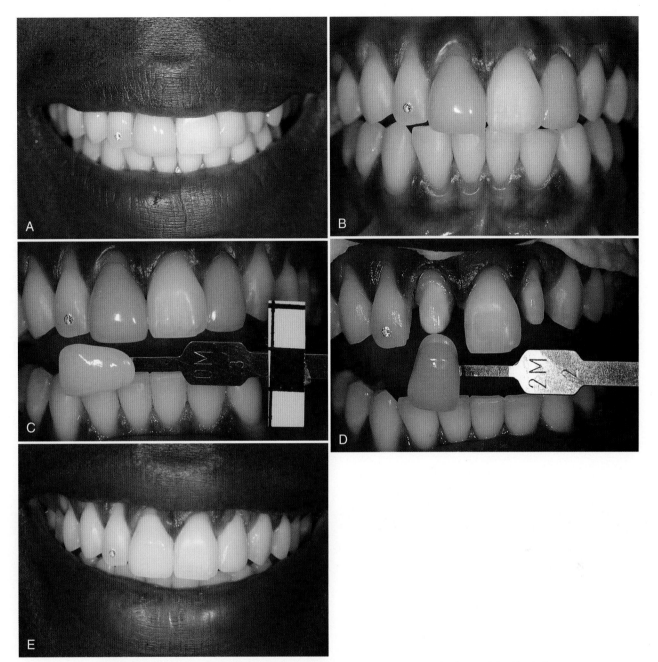

• **Fig. 7.30** A patient with "Hollywood White" expectations. The crowns matched natural dentition before at-home whitening, which appeared "dark" upon whitening. A, Preoperative smile. B, Preoperative smile, retracted. C, Shade tab 0M3 with black-and-white standardized card. D, Shade tab 2M2 (stump shade) of prepared teeth. E, Postoperative smile with all ceramic crowns on the upper right central incisor and upper left lateral incisor.

References

1. Hunter RS, Harold RW: *Measurement of appearance*, ed 2, New York, 1987, Wiley-Interscience.
2. Berns RS: *Billmeyer and Saltzman's principles of color technology*, ed 3, New York, 2000, John Wiley.
3. Paravina RD, Powers JM: *Esthetic color training in dentistry*, St. Louis, 2004, Elsevier Mosby.
4. Brown RO, MacLeod DI: Color appearance depends on the variance of surround colors. *Curr Biol* 7:844–849, 1997.
5. Paravina RD, Westland S, Johnston WM, et al: Color adjustment potential of resin composites. *J Dent Res* 87:499–503, 2008.
6. Paravina RD, Westland S, Imai FH, et al: Evaluation of blending effect of composites related to restoration size. *Dent Mater* 22:299–307, 2006.
7. O'Brien WJ, Hemmendinger H, Boenke KM, et al: Color distribution of three regions of extracted human teeth. *Dent Mater* 13:179–185, 1997.
8. Goodkind RJ, Schwabacher WB: Use of a fiberoptic colorimeter for in vivo color measurements of 2830 anterior teeth. *J Prosthet Dent* 58:535–542, 1987.
9. Ishikawa T, Ishiyama T, Ohsone M, et al: Trial manufacture of photoelectric colorimeter using optical fibers. *Bull Tokyo Dent Coll* 10:191–197, 1969.

10. Meller C, Klein C: Fluorescence properties of commercial composite resin restorative materials in dentistry. *Dent Mater J* 31:916–923, 2012.

11. Paravina RD, Ontiveros JC, Powers JM: Accelerated aging effects on color and translucency of bleaching-shade composites. *J Esthet Restor Dent* 16:117–126, 2004.

12. Dede DÖ, Şahin O, Koroglu A, et al: Effect of sealant agents on the color stability and surface roughness of nanohybrid composite resins. *J Prosthet Dent* 116:119–128, 2016.

13. Paravina RD, Ontiveros JC, Powers JM: Curing-dependent changes in color and translucency parameter of composite bleach shades. *J Esthet Restor Dent* 14:158–166, 2002.

14. Barghi N, Pedrero JA, Bosch RR: Effects of batch variation on shade of dental porcelain. *J Prosthet Dent* 54:625–627, 1985.

15. Paravina RD, Westland S, Johnston WM, et al: Color adjustment potential of resin composites. *J Dent Res* 87:499–503, 2008.

16. Paravina RD: New shade guide for tooth whitening monitoring: visual assessment. *J Prosthet Dent* 99:178–184, 2008.

17. Paravina RD, Johnston WM, Powers JM: New shade guide for evaluation of tooth whitening—colorimetric study. *J Esthet Restor Dent* 19:276–278, 2007.

18. Li Q, Yu H, Wang YN: In vivo spectroradiometric evaluation of color matching errors among five shade guides. *J Oral Rehabil* 36:65–70, 2009.

19. Paravina RD: Performance assessment of dental shade guides. *J Dent* 37 Suppl 1:e15–e20, 2009.

20. Paravina RD, Kimura M, Powers JM: Color compatibility of resin composites of identical shade designation. *Quintessence Int* 37:713–719, 2006.

21. Ontiveros JC, Paravina RD: Color change of vital teeth exposed to bleaching performed with and without supplementary light. *J Dent* 37:840–847, 2009.

22. Chu SJ, Devigus A, Paravina RD, et al: *Fundamentals of color: shade matching and communication in esthetic dentistry*, ed 2, Hanover Park, 2011, Quintessence.

23. International Organization for Standardization: ISO/TR 28642 dentistry—guidance on color measurement. Geneva: International Organization for Standardization, 2011.

24. Clary JA, Ontiveros JC, Cron SG, et al: Influence of light source, polarization, education, and training on shade matching quality. *J Prosthet Dent* 116:91–97, 2016.

25. Sneed WD, Nuckles DB: Shade determination prior to field isolation. *Dent Surv* 54:32, 1978.

26. Paravina RD, O'Neill PN, Swift EJ, Jr, et al: Teaching of color in predoctoral and postdoctoral dental education in 2009. *J Dent* 38 Suppl 2:e34–e40, 2010.

27. SCAD: Color matching curriculum. www.scadent.org. Society for Color and Appearance in Dentistry. (Assessed 1 March 2017).

8

Clinical Technique for Direct Composite Resin and Glass Ionomer Restorations

ANDRÉ V. RITTER, RICARDO WALTER, LEE W. BOUSHELL, SUMITHA N. AHMED

The search for an ideal esthetic material for restoring teeth has resulted in significant improvements in resin-based composite materials.[1-4] Although these materials are referred to as resin-based composites, composite resins, and other terms, this book refers to most direct esthetic restorations as composites. Chapter 13 presents information about composite development, types, classification, material properties, and so forth. This chapter presents many of the specific clinical applications of these materials in both anterior and posterior teeth (Fig. 8.1). This chapter also presents the clinical technique for glass ionomer restorations.

The choice of a material to restore caries lesions and other defects in teeth is not always simple. Tooth-colored materials, such as composite, are used in almost all types and sizes of restorations. Such restorations are accomplished with minimal loss of tooth structure, little or no discomfort, relatively short operating time, and modest expense to the patient compared with indirect restorations. When a tooth is significantly weakened by extensive defects, however, and esthetics is of primary concern, the best treatment may involve the use of a ceramic onlay or crown.

The lifespan of a direct esthetic restoration depends on many factors, including the nature and extent of the initial caries lesion or defect; the treatment procedure; the restorative material and technique used; operator skill; and patient factors such as oral hygiene, occlusion, caries risk, and adverse habits.[5-9] Because all direct esthetic restorations are bonded to tooth structure, the effectiveness of generating the bond is paramount for the success and longevity of such restorations. Failures can result from numerous causes, including trauma, improper tooth preparation, inferior materials, poor material selection, and patient-related risk factors.

Composites can be used in almost any tooth surface. Naturally, factors must be considered for each specific application. The reasons for such expanded usage of these materials relate to improvements in their ability to bond to tooth structure (enamel and dentin) and in their physical and mechanical properties. The ability to bond a relatively strong material to tooth structure results in a restored tooth that is well sealed and regains a portion of its strength.[10,11]

General Considerations for Composite Restorations

This section summarizes general considerations about all composite restorations. A successful composite restoration requires careful attention to technique detail, so as to gain the maximum benefit of the material's properties. In selecting a direct restorative material, clinicians usually choose between composite and amalgam. Consequently, some of the following information provides comparative analyses between those two materials.

Indications and Contraindications

The *indications* for direct composites are:
1. Class I, II, III, IV, V, and VI restorations
2. Foundations and core buildups
3. Sealants and preventive resin restorations (conservative composite restorations)
4. Esthetic enhancement procedures:
   Partial veneers
   Full veneers
   Tooth contour modifications
   Diastema closures
5. Temporary or provisional restorations
6. Periodontal splinting
7. Luting of indirect esthetic restorations (when used in flowable form, or when heated to increase flow)

The primary *contraindications* for use of direct composites relate to:
1. Inability to obtain adequate isolation
2. Occlusal considerations related to wear and fracture of the composite material
3. Extension of the restoration on root surface
4. Operator factors

If the operating site cannot be isolated from contamination by oral fluids, composite (or any other bonded material) should not be used. If all of the occlusion is on the restorative material, composite may not be the choice for use particularly in patients with heavy occlusal function; however, the need to strengthen remaining weakened unprepared tooth structure with an economical composite restoration procedure (compared with an indirect restoration) and the commitment to recall the patient routinely and in a timely manner may override any concern about excessive wear potential. Any restoration that extends onto the root surface may result in less than ideal marginal integrity. Lastly, the operator must be committed to pursuing procedures, such as tooth isolation, that make bonded restorations successful. These additional procedures may make successful

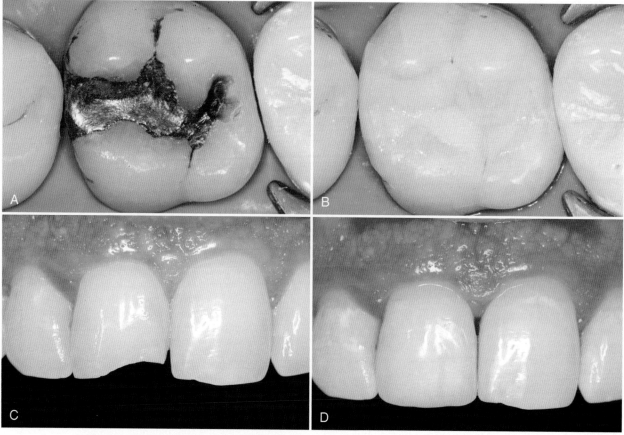

• **Fig. 8.1** Composite restorations. A and B, Class II composite restoration, before and after. C and D, Class IV composite restoration, before and after.

bonded restorations more difficult and time consuming to achieve.

Advantages and Disadvantages

The following are *advantages* of composite restorations:
1. Esthetics
2. Conservative tooth preparation (less extension, minimum depth not necessary, mechanical retention usually not necessary)
3. Low thermal conductivity
4. Universal use
5. Adhesion to the tooth
6. Repairability

The primary *disadvantages* of composite restorations relate to their dependence on adequate adhesion and polymerization protocols and procedural difficulties. Composite restorations:
1. May have poor marginal and internal cavity adaptation, usually occurring on root surfaces as a result of polymerization shrinkage stresses or improper insertion of the composite
2. May exhibit marginal deterioration over time in areas where no marginal enamel is available for bonding
3. Are more difficult and time consuming to place, and more costly (compared with amalgam restorations) because bonding usually requires multiple steps; insertion is more difficult; establishing proximal contacts, axial contours, embrasures, and occlusal contacts may be more difficult; and finishing and polishing procedures are more difficult

4. Are more technique sensitive because the operating site must be appropriately isolated, incremental placement technique must be used for most materials, and proper adhesive technique is absolutely mandatory
5. May exhibit greater occlusal wear in areas of high occlusal stress or when all of the tooth's occlusal contacts are on the composite material

Clinical Technique for Pit-and-Fissure Sealants

Pits and fissures typically result from an incomplete coalescence of enamel and are particularly prone to caries. These areas can be sealed with a low-viscosity fluid resin after acid etching. Long-term clinical studies indicate that pit-and-fissure sealants provide a safe and effective method of preventing caries.[12-14] In children, sealants are most effective when applied to the pits and fissures of permanent posterior teeth immediately on eruption of the clinical crowns, provided proper isolation can be achieved. Adults also can benefit from the use of sealants if the individual experiences an increase in caries susceptibility because of a change in diet, lack of adequate saliva, or a particular medical condition.

Sealants are indicated, regardless of the patient's age, for either preventive or therapeutic uses, depending on the patient's caries risk, tooth morphology, or presence of incipient enamel caries. In assessing the occlusal surfaces of posterior teeth as potential candidates for a sealant procedure, the primary decision is based on whether a cavitated lesion exists. This decision is based primarily on radiographic and clinical examinations, although other adjunctive technologies for occlusal caries detection are available. Explorers must be used judiciously in the detection of caries, as a sharp explorer tine may cause a cavitation. The clinical examination should be primarily focused on visual assessments of a clean, dry tooth surface preferably under adequate light and magnification. The patient's caries risk also should be a factor when considering treatment options. See Chapter 2 for a discussion of emerging technologies for occlusal caries detection and monitoring.

When no cavitated caries lesion is diagnosed, the treatment decision is either to pursue no treatment or to place a pit-and-fissure sealant, particularly if the surface is at high risk for future caries. If a small caries lesion is detected, and the adjacent grooves and pits, although sound at the present time, are at risk for caries in the future, a preventive resin restoration or conservative composite restoration of the active cavitated lesion and placement of a sealant to include any radiating noncarious fissure or pits is recommended.

Although studies show that sealants can be applied over small, cavitated lesions, with no subsequent progression of the caries lesion, sealants should be used primarily for the prevention of caries rather than for the treatment of existing caries lesions.[15,16] A bitewing radiograph should be obtained and evaluated before sealant placement to ensure that no dentinal or proximal caries lesion is evident. Only caries-free pits and fissures or incipient lesions in enamel not extending to the dentinoenamel junction (DEJ) currently are recommended for treatment with pit-and-fissure sealants.[17]

Because materials and techniques vary, it is important to follow the manufacturer's instructions for the sealant material being used. A standard method for applying sealants to posterior teeth is presented here. Each quadrant is treated separately and one or more teeth may be sealed, as indicated. The following presentation relates to an occlusal surface of a mandibular first permanent molar (Fig. 8.2A). The tooth is isolated with a rubber dam (or another effective isolation method such as cotton rolls or Isolite). If proper isolation cannot be obtained, the bond of the sealant material to the tooth surface will be compromised, resulting in either loss of the sealant or caries under the inadequately bonded sealant. The area is cleaned with a slurry of pumice on a bristle brush and the tooth is rinsed thoroughly, while the explorer tip is used carefully to remove residual pumice or additional debris. The tooth surface is dried, and etched with 35% to 40% phosphoric acid for 15 to 30 seconds. Airborne particle abrasion techniques have been advocated for preparing pits and grooves before sealant placement, but their effectiveness has not been fully investigated.[18]

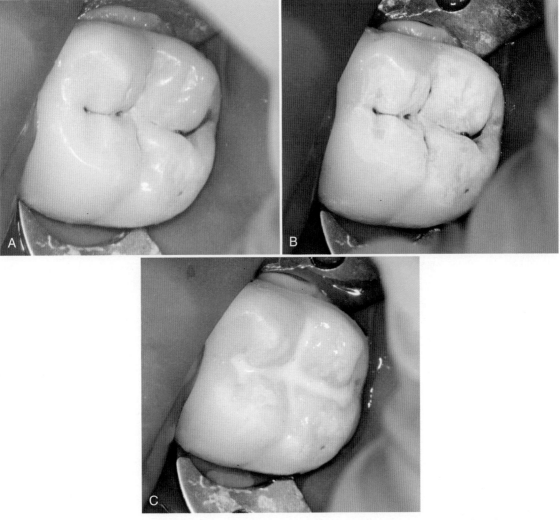

• **Fig. 8.2** Steps in application of pit-and-fissure sealant. A, After isolation and thorough cleaning of the occlusal surface to be sealed. B, After acid etching, rinsing, and drying. C, With sealant applied.

Properly acid-etched enamel surface has a lightly frosted (matte) appearance (see Fig. 8.2B). Any brown stains that originally may have been in the pits and fissures still may be present and should be allowed to remain. The sealant material is then applied and gently teased into place, to avoid entrapping air, and it should overfill slightly all pits and fissures, not extending onto unetched surfaces (see Fig. 8.2C). If too much sealant is applied, excess may be removed with a dry microbrush prior to light curing. After light curing and removal of the rubber dam, if used, the occlusion is evaluated by using articulating paper. If necessary, a round carbide finishing bur or white stone is used to remove any excess sealant. The surface usually does not require further polishing.

Clinical Technique for Preventive Resin and Conservative Composite Restorations

When restoring minimally carious pits and fissures on a previously unrestored tooth, an ultraconservative preparation design is recommended. This design allows for restoration of the caries lesion or defect with minimal removal of the tooth structure and often may be combined with the use of flowable composite or sealant to seal radiating noncarious fissures or pits that are at high risk for subsequent caries activity (Fig. 8.3). Originally referred to as a preventive resin restoration,[19-21] this type of ultraconservative restoration is now termed *conservative composite restoration* at the University of North Carolina.

An accurate diagnosis is essential before restoring the occlusal surface of a posterior tooth. The crucial factor in this clinical assessment is whether the suspicious pit or fissure has active caries that requires restorative intervention. Usually, a conservative composite restoration is the treatment of choice for the primary occlusal caries lesion as the tooth preparation can be minimally invasive.

If a definitive diagnosis of caries cannot be made for the entire occlusal surface, a conservative preparation of the suspicious area is performed with a small bur or diamond to determine the extent of the suspected fault without extending onto noncompromised fissures (Fig. 8.4). This approach is particularly indicated in patients with high caries activity and/or risk. As the tooth preparation is deepened, an assessment is made in the suspicious areas to determine whether to continue the preparation toward the DEJ (see Fig. 8.4C). If the suspicious fault is removed or found to be sound at a shallow preparation depth (minimal dentin caries), the conservative preparation and adjacent pits and fissures are etched with 35% to 40% phosphoric acid for 15 to 30 seconds, rinsed thoroughly, and lightly dried. The etched surfaces then are treated with an adhesive and restored with a flowable composite, which is placed and light cured according to manufacturer's instructions. The adjacent etched pits and fissures, if judged to be at risk, can be

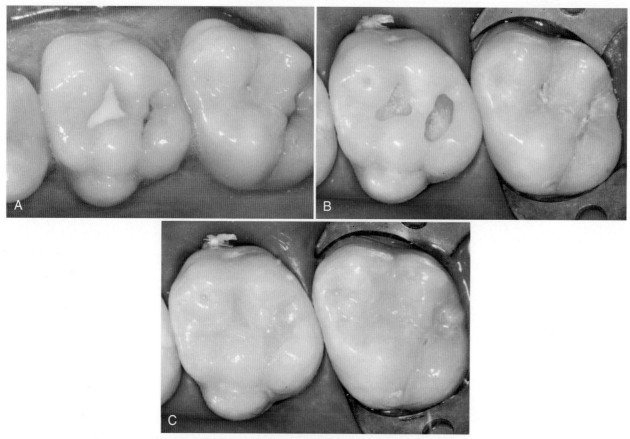

• **Fig. 8.3**　Conservative composite restoration. A, Occlusal view of the maxillary first and second molars. The first molar has caries on the distal occlusal pit and the second molar has suspicious pit on the disto-occlusal aspect. B, Caries was excavated from the first molar, and the second molar was minimally prepared. C, The first molar was restored with composite and the second molar received a conservative composite restoration with flowable composite.

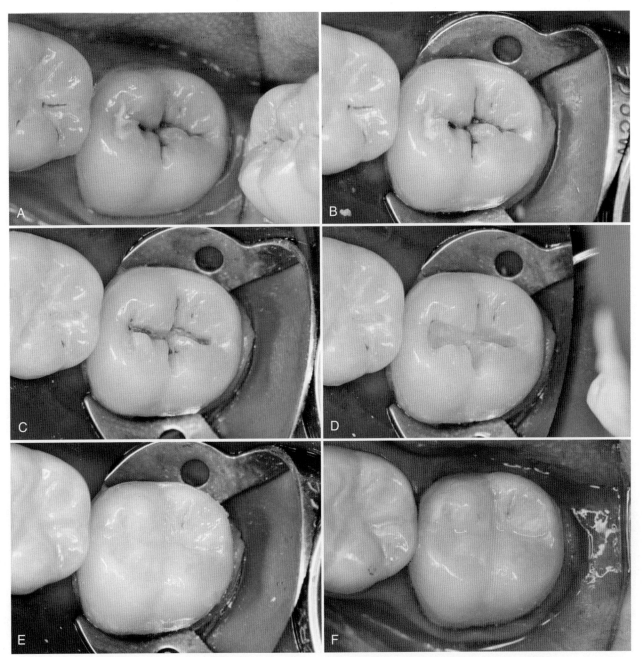

• **Fig. 8.4**   Class I direct composite restoration and conservative composite restoration. A, Mandibular second molar with suspicious occlusal pits; mandibular first molar with questionable sealant. B, After rubber dam isolation. C, Initial exploratory preparation reveals caries extending toward the dentinoenamel junction (DEJ). D, Conservative preparation on the second molar; the first molar was minimally prepared. E, Complete Class I direct composite restoration on the second molar; the first molar received a conservative composite restoration with flowable composite. F, Final restorations after the rubber dam was removed and the occlusion was checked.

sealed using a pit-and-fissure sealant or the same flowable composite following the technique described previously.

If the suspicious area is found to be carious, the preparation depth is extended until all of the soft carious dentin is removed (see Chapter 2 for a description of dentin caries zones), the prepared area is then restored with composite as described later in this chapter (Class I direct composite restoration), and unprepared pits and fissures are sealed. In the example presented in Fig. 8.4, the preparation was restored with composite.

Clinical Technique for Class I Direct Composite Restorations

Initial Clinical Procedures

A complete examination, diagnosis (including caries risk assessment), treatment plan, and informed consent should be finalized and obtained before the patient is scheduled for operative appointments (emergencies excepted). A brief review of the patient's record (including medical factors), treatment plan, radiographs, and current caries risk should precede each restorative procedure.

Local Anesthesia

Local anesthesia is required for many operative procedures. Profound anesthesia contributes to a more comfortable and uninterrupted procedure and may result in reduction in salivation. These effects of local anesthesia contribute to better operative dentistry, especially when placing bonded restorations.

Preparation of the Operating Site

Prior to beginning any composite restoration, it may be necessary to clean the operating site with a slurry of pumice to remove plaque biofilm and superficial stains. Calculus removal with appropriate instruments also may be needed, although it would be preferable to see the patient after a thorough hygiene visit has been completed in this case. Prophy pastes containing flavoring agents, glycerin, or fluorides act as contaminants and must not be used as they will compromise the adhesive procedure.

Shade Selection

Although not as important for posterior when compared to anterior, more visible restorations, proper shade selection should be accomplished for all direct composite restorations. The shade of the tooth should be determined before teeth are subjected to any prolonged drying. Dehydrated teeth become lighter in shade as a result of a decrease in translucency secondary to water loss from the naturally porous tooth structure. A more comprehensive review of factors affecting shade selection is presented in Chapter 7, while esthetic considerations of tooth restoration are presented in Chapter 9.

Isolation of the Operating Site

Isolation for tooth-colored restorations is critical and can be accomplished with a rubber dam, an isolation device (e.g., Isolite), or cotton rolls/dry angles. Regardless of the method, isolation of the area is imperative if a successful bond is to be obtained. Contamination of etched enamel or dentin by saliva results in a significantly decreased bond; likewise, contamination of the composite material during insertion results in degradation of physical and mechanical properties.

Other Preoperative Considerations

When restoring posterior occlusal surfaces, a preoperative assessment of the occlusion should be made. This assessment should identify not only the occlusal contacts of the tooth or teeth to be restored but also the occlusal contacts on adjacent teeth. Knowing the preoperative location of occlusal contacts is important in planning the restoration outline form (so as to prevent an area of occlusal contact directly at a cavosurface/restoration interface) and establishing the proper occlusal contact on the restoration. Remembering where the contacts are located on adjacent teeth provides guidance in knowing when the restoration contacts are correctly adjusted.

Tooth Preparation

As a general rule, the tooth preparation for direct posterior composites involves (1) creating access to the faulty structure, (2) removal of faulty structures (caries lesion, defective restoration, and base material, if present), and (3) creating convenience form for the restoration. When placing most posterior composites, it is not necessary to incorporate mechanical retention features in the tooth preparation.

Small to moderate Class I direct composite restorations may use minimally invasive tooth preparations and do not require typical resistance and retention form features. Instead, these conservative preparations typically result in more flared cavosurface forms without uniform or flat pulpal or axial walls. The initial pulpal depth is determined only by the selective removal of carious tooth structure, and there is no minimal thickness of restorative material requirement to limit bulk fracture.

These conservative preparations are prepared with a small round or elongated pear-shaped diamond or bur with round features, in an attempt to be as conservative as possible in the removal of the tooth structure. The size and shape of the instrument generally are dictated by the size of the lesion or other defect or by the type of defective restoration being replaced. If a round instrument is used, the resulting cavosurface margin angle may be more flared (obtuse) than if an elongated pear-shaped instrument is used (Fig. 8.5). Both carbide and diamond instruments can be used effectively. Although diamond instruments have been shown to create a thicker smear layer, thus raising concerns about the ability of self-etch adhesive systems to adequately reach and etch the underlying tooth structure, clinical trials have revealed excellent performance of mild self-etch adhesive systems suggesting this may not be a clinically relevant concern.[22-25]

Moderate to large Class I direct composite restorations, especially when used for larger caries lesions or to replace amalgam restorations, will typically feature flat walls that are perpendicular to occlusal forces, as well as strong tooth and restoration marginal configurations. All of these features help resist potential fracture in less conservative tooth preparations. However, the preparation should never be excessively extended beyond removal of faulty structures to justify resistance and retention forms, as this will further weaken the tooth structure and can ultimately lead to failure of the tooth-restoration unit. If the occlusal portion of the restoration is expected to be extensive, elongated pear-shaped cutting instruments with round features are preferred because they result in strong, 90-degree cavosurface margins without creating sharp internal line angles. However, this boxlike preparation form may increase the negative effects of the cavity configuration factor, or C-factor (see discussion in the next section). The objective of the tooth preparation is to remove all of the carious tissues or fault as conservatively as possible. Because the composite is bonded to the tooth structure, other less involved or at-risk areas can be sealed as part of the conservative

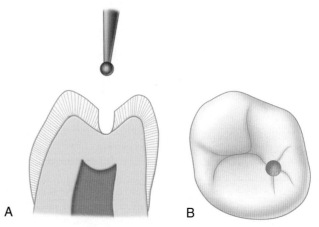

• Fig. 8.5 Faciolingual cross section of small Class I tooth preparation using round diamond.

preparation techniques. Sealants may be combined with the Class I composite restoration, as described previously.

In moderate to large composite restorations, the tooth is entered in the area most affected by the caries lesion, with the elongated pear-shaped diamond or bur positioned parallel to the long axis of the tooth crown. When it is anticipated that the entire mesiodistal length of a central groove will be prepared, it is easier to enter the distal portion first and then transverse mesially to permit better operator visibility during the preparation. The pulpal floor is prepared to an initial depth that is approximately 0.2 mm internal to the carious DEJ (Fig. 8.6). Ideally the instrument is moved mesially, along the central groove in a controlled manner, to follow the rise and fall of the DEJ. The preparation is then carefully extended facially, lingually, mesially, and distally as indicated at

the depth of the carious DEJ until a caries-free DEJ is identified around the whole periphery of the preparation. However, a flat pulpal floor with an initial preparation depth of 1.5 to 2 mm may also be acceptable (see Fig. 8.6B). Mesial, distal, facial, and lingual extensions are dictated by the caries lesion, old restorative material, or defect, always using the DEJ as a reference for both extensions and pulpal depth. Unnecessary extension into cuspal and marginal ridge areas should be avoided as much as possible as this compromises the strength of the tooth. Although the final bonded composite restoration may help restore some of the strength of weakened, unprepared tooth structure, the outline form should be as conservative as possible. Extensions into marginal ridges should result in at least 1.5 mm of remaining tooth structure (measured from the internal extension to the proximal height of contour) for premolars and approximately 2 mm for molars (Fig. 8.7). These limited extensions help preserve the dentinal support of the marginal ridge enamel and cusp tips and thus the overall ability of the tooth to resist occlusal forces.

As the instrument is moved along the central groove, the resulting pulpal floor is usually moderately flat and follows the rise and fall of the DEJ (Fig. 8.8A). If extension is required toward the cusp tips, the same depth that is approximately 0.2 mm inside the DEJ

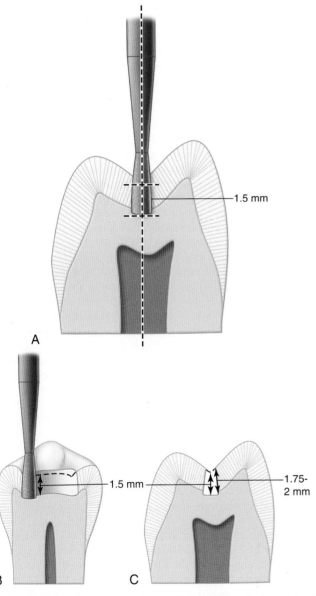

A

B

C

• **Fig. 8.6**   A, Entry cut. Diamond or bur held parallel to the long axis of the crown. Initial pulpal depth is 1.5 mm from the central groove. When the central groove is removed, facial and lingual wall measurements usually are greater than 1.5 mm. (The steeper the wall, the greater is the height.) B, 1.5-mm depth from the central groove. C, Approximately 1.75- to 2-mm facial or lingual wall heights.

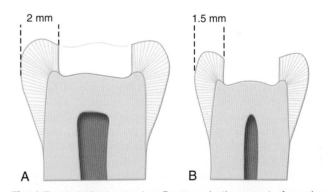

A

B

• **Fig. 8.7**   Mesiodistal extension. Preserve dentin support of marginal ridge enamel. A, Molar. B, Premolar.

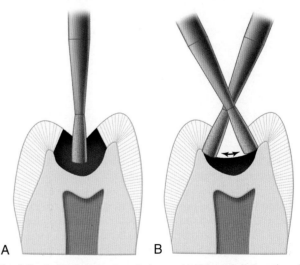

A

B

• **Fig. 8.8**   A, After initial entry cut at correct initial depth (1.5 mm), caries remains facially and lingually. B, Orientation of diamond or bur must be tilted as the instrument is extended facially or lingually to maintain a 1.5-mm depth.

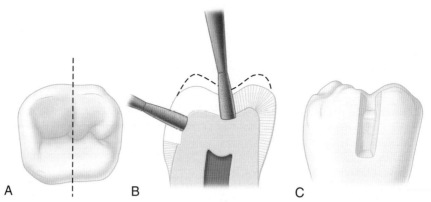

• **Fig. 8.9** Groove extension. A, Cross section through the faciolingual groove area. B, Extension through cusp ridge at 1.5-mm initial pulpal depth; the facial wall depth is 0.2 mm inside the dentinoenamel junction (DEJ). C, Facial view.

is maintained, usually resulting in the pulpal floor rising occlusally (see Fig. 8.8B). The same uniform depth concept also is appropriate when extending a facial or lingual groove radiating from the occlusal surface. When a groove extension is through the cusp ridge, the instrument prepares the facial (or lingual) portion of the faulty groove at an axial depth of 0.2 mm inside the DEJ and gingivally to include all caries and other defects (Fig. 8.9).

After extending the outline form to sound tooth structure, if any caries or old restorative material remains on the pulpal floor, it should be removed with the appropriately sized round bur or hand instrument. The occlusal margin is left as prepared. No attempt is made to bevel the occlusal margin because it may result in enlarging the occlusal isthmus of the preparation. Because of the occlusal surface enamel rod direction, the ends of the enamel rods already are exposed by the preparation, which further reduces the need for occlusal bevels.

Although large, extensive posterior composite restorations may have some potential disadvantages when used routinely, "real world" dentistry sometimes necessitates esthetic treatment alternatives that may provide a needed service to the patient. Often, patients simply cannot afford a more expensive esthetic restoration, or they may have dental or medical conditions that preclude their placement. In such instances, large posterior composite restorations sometimes may be used as a reasonable alternative when more definitive indirect options are not possible or realistic.

Restorative Technique

Placement of the Adhesive

See Chapter 5 for a more extensive discussion on adhesives. The dental adhesive is applied to the entire preparation with a microbrush, in accordance with the manufacturer's instructions. After application, the adhesive is polymerized with a light-curing unit, as recommended by the manufacturer.

When the final tooth preparation is judged to be near the pulp in vital teeth, the operator may elect to use a base material prior to placing the adhesive and the composite. If the remaining dentin thickness (RDT) is clinically judged to be between 0.5 and 1.5 mm, a resin-modified glass ionomer (RMGI) base is used; if the RDT is judged to be less than 0.5 mm, a calcium hydroxide liner should be applied to the deepest aspect of the preparation, then protected with an RMGI base prior to adhesive placement.[26] In cases of mechanical pulp exposure, calcium hydroxide or, increasingly,

mineral trioxide aggregate (MTA) can be used as a direct pulp-capping material.[26-28] If used, the calcium hydroxide or MTA liners should always be covered with a RMGI base, sealing the area and preventing the etchant (applied later) from dissolving the liner.[26,29]

Insertion and Light Curing of the Composite

A matrix is usually not necessary for Class I direct composite restorations, even when facial and lingual surface grooves are included. Composite insertion hand instruments or a compule may be used to place the composite material incrementally (Fig. 8.10). It is important to place (and light cure) the composite incrementally to ensure maximum polymerization and possibly to reduce the negative effects of polymerization shrinkage. Large increments or attempts at filling a preparation in bulk may compromise polymerization of the restoration secondary to inadequate depth of cure.

As mentioned, the term "C-factor" has been used to describe the ratio of bonded to unbonded surfaces in a tooth preparation and restoration. A typical Class I tooth preparation will have a high C-factor of 5/1 (i.e., five bonded surfaces—pulpal, facial, lingual, mesial, and distal—versus one unbonded surface—occlusal). The higher the C-factor of a tooth preparation, the higher the potential for composite polymerization shrinkage stress, as the composite shrinkage deformation is restricted by the bonded surfaces. The interface most likely to be adversely affected by high C-factor stresses is at the pulpal wall as the anatomy of dentin in this area makes establishment of a durable interface more difficult. Incremental insertion and light curing of the composite may reduce the negative C-factor effects for Class I composite restorations.[30-33]

The use of an RMGI liner or a flowable composite liner were thought to reduce the effects of polymerization shrinkage stress because of their favorable elastic modulus (a more elastic material would more effectively absorb polymerization stresses),[34,35] but those claims are not supported by current clinical evidence.[36] When composite is placed over an RMGI material, this technique is often referred to as a "sandwich" technique. The potential advantages of this technique are (1) the RMGI material bonds to the dentin without the need for a dental adhesive[37]; (2) the RMGI material, because of its bond to dentin and potential for fluoride release (potential anticariogenicity), may provide a better seal when used in cases where the preparation extends gingivally onto root structure[38]; and (3) the favorable elastic modulus of the RMGI may reduce the effects of polymerization shrinkage stresses. These suggested advantages are considered controversial, as no conclusive

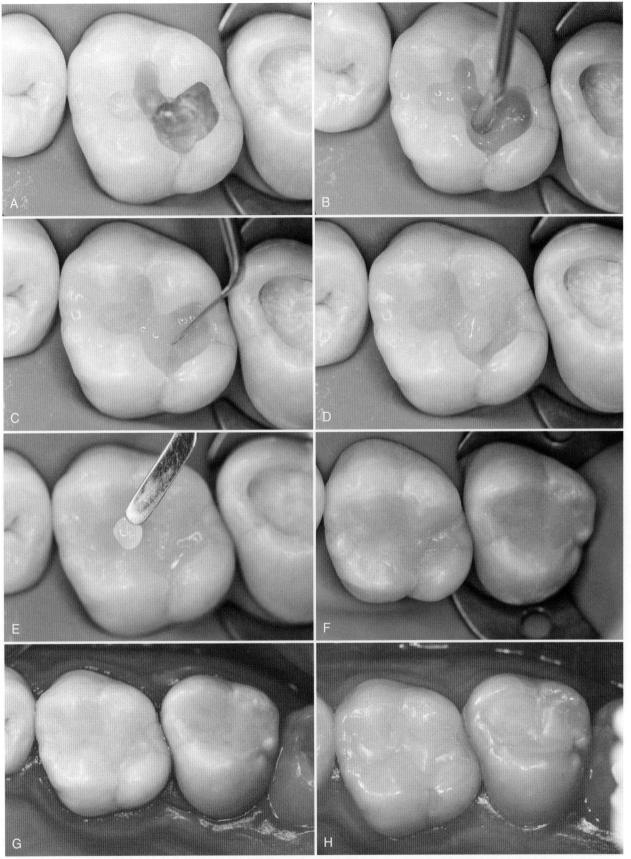

• **Fig. 8.10** Class I composite incremental insertion. A, Tooth preparation for Class I direct composite restoration. B, After a resin-modified glass ionomer base is placed, the first composite increment is inserted and light cured. C–F, Composite is inserted and light cured incrementally, using cusp inclines as anatomic references to sculpt the composite before light curing. G, Completed restorations. H, At 5-year follow-up.

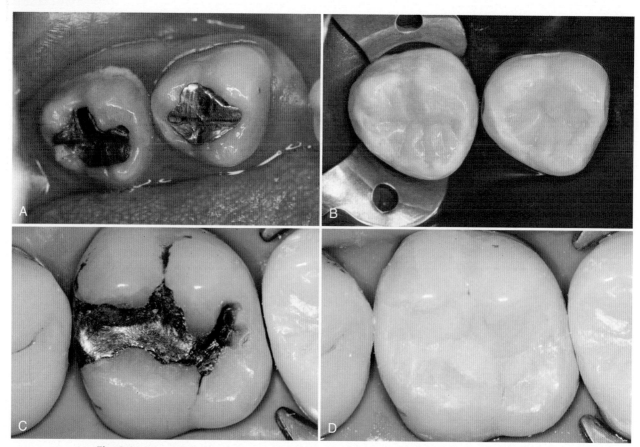

• **Fig. 8.11** Composite restorations. A and B, Class I composite, before and after. C and D, Class II composite, before and after.

published research based on longitudinal clinical trials evaluating the technique is available.

Regardless of the effect of incremental placement on shrinkage stress, posterior composites should be placed incrementally to facilitate proper light curing and development of correct anatomy. Especially in Class I direct composite restorations, the anatomic references of the occlusal unprepared tooth structure should guide the placement and shaping of the composite increments (Fig. 8.11; see Figs. 8.10G and 8.12I). If needed, very deep portions of the tooth preparation are restored first, with increments of no more than 2 mm in thickness (see Fig. 8.10B). The "enamel layer" of the restoration, that is, the occlusal increment(s), should be placed using an anatomic layering technique.[39] The operator places and shapes the composite before it is light cured so that the composite restores the occlusal anatomy of the tooth. Typically, the operator places and light cures one increment per cusp at a time and continues to place subsequent increments until the preparation is filled and the occlusal anatomy is fully developed (see Fig. 8.10C–F). The uncured composite can be shaped against the unprepared cusp inclines as visual guides, which will result in a very natural anatomic contour. Sculpture of the occlusal elements of the restoration following the anatomic references of the tooth respects the tooth's anatomy and occlusion and minimizes the need for contouring and finishing after the composite is polymerized. Furthermore, this technique prevents potential damage to the enamel adjacent to the restoration margins because it minimizes the need to use rotary instruments to remove excess composite extending beyond those margins. Any suitable composite hand instruments can be used with the anatomic layering technique. Fine

composite spatulas and the tine of an explorer can be used to further develop or refine the anatomy of uncured composite increments. Microbrushes also can be used to smooth uncured composite against the preparation margin, but these should never be saturated with adhesives. Once the composite is fully cured, if additional contouring is needed, the restoration can be finished immediately after the last increment is cured using appropriate finishing instruments.

"Bulk-fill composites" have gained increased interest in recent years. These materials are available as *flowable base bulk-fill composites* and *full-body bulk-fill composites*.[40] Flowable base bulk-fill composites require a conventional composite as the occlusal increment and therefore are used for dentin replacement only, whereas full-body bulk-fill composites can replace dentin and enamel in a single increment. Their use can expedite the restorative procedure as increments of up to 4 mm in thickness are often suggested.[41] However, in vitro studies have raised concerns about a possible compromised internal adaptation and increased wear when these techniques are used.[42,43] Although this technique may present advantages, namely more expediency during composite placement, bulk-fill composites should be used with caution due to the lack of long-term clinical performance information at this time.[44] Bulk filling may also limit the operator's ability to carve the occlusal anatomy of the restoration before light curing.

Finishing and Polishing of the Composite

If the composite is carefully placed and shaped before light curing, as described in the previous section, additional finishing with burs is substantially minimized. However, in many cases, refined finishing may be needed, especially when occlusion adjustments are necessary. The occlusal surface is shaped with a round or oval carbide finishing bur or similarly shaped finishing diamond. Polishing is accomplished with appropriate polishing cups, points, or both after the occlusion is adjusted as necessary (Fig. 8.12).

Clinical Technique for Class II Direct Composite Restorations

Initial Clinical Procedures

The same general procedures as described previously are necessary before beginning a Class II composite restoration. Several aspects of those activities, however, need emphasis. First, an assessment of the expected tooth preparation extensions (outline form) should be made and a decision rendered on whether or not an enamel periphery will exist on the tooth preparation, especially at the gingival margin. The expected presence of an enamel periphery strengthens the choice of composite as the restorative material because bonding to enamel is more predictable than bonding to dentin, especially along the gingival wall of the proximal preparation. If the preparation is expected to extend onto the root surface, potential problems with isolation of the operating area, adequate adhesion to the root dentin, and adequate composite polymerization exist. Good technique and proper use of the material may reduce these potential problems, but deep subgingival extension onto the

root surface may be a contraindication for using composite resin as a posterior teeth restorative material.

The preoperative occlusal relationship of the tooth to be restored must also be assessed. The presence of heavy occlusal contacts may indicate that wear may be more of a consideration. Also, preoperative wedging in the gingival embrasure of the proximal surfaces to be restored should occur. Placing wedges, bitine rings, or both before tooth preparation begins the separation of teeth, which may be beneficial in reestablishing the proximal contact with the composite restoration.

Tooth Preparation

Similar to the tooth preparation for Class I direct composite restorations, the tooth preparation for Class II direct composites involves (1) creating access to the faulty structure, (2) removal of faulty structures (the caries lesion, defective restoration, and base material, if present), and (3) creating the convenience form for the restoration. Retention, as with Class I restorations, is primarily obtained by bonding, so it is not necessary to use mechanical retention features in the tooth preparation for Class II composite restorations. Obtaining access to the defect may include removal of sound enamel to access the caries lesion. The extension of the preparation is therefore ultimately dictated by the extension of the fault or defect. It is usually not necessary to reduce sound tooth structure to provide "bulk for strength" or to provide conventional retention and resistance forms.

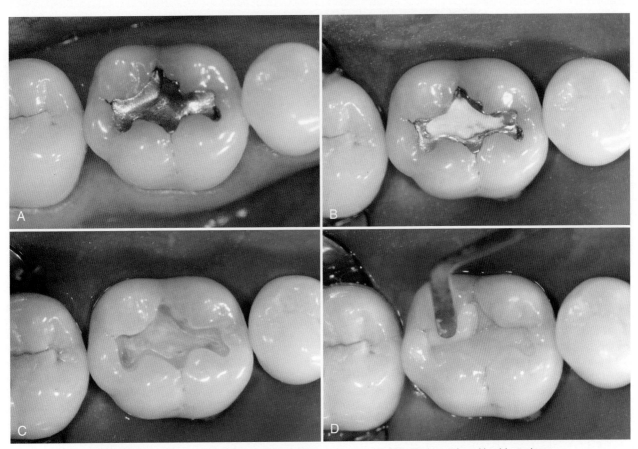

• **Fig. 8.12**   Contouring and polishing of Class I composite. A, Mandibular molar with old amalgam restoration. B, Rubber dam isolation; old restoration is carefully removed to minimize increasing preparation size. C, Final tooth preparation. D, Incremental placement of composite.   *Coutinued*

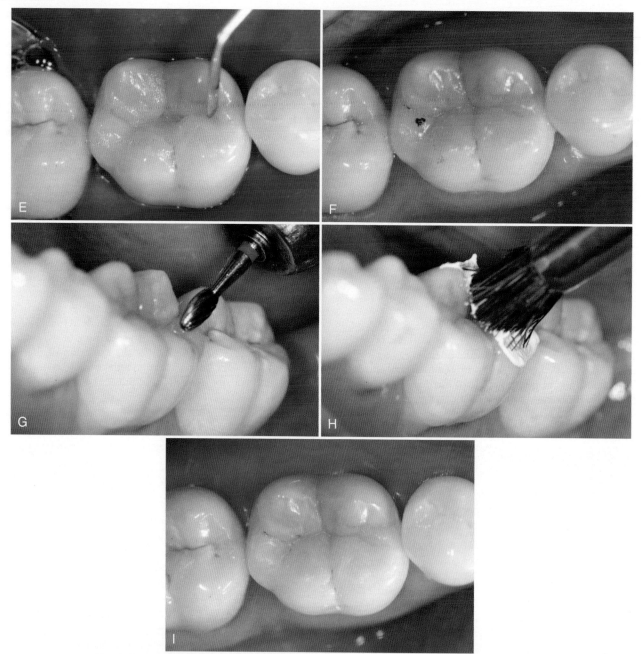

• **Fig. 8.12, cont'd** E, Incremental placement of composite. F, Rubber dam is removed and occlusion checked. G, Buccal view, a finishing fluted bur is used to selectively adjust the occlusion. H, Polishing with brush and diamond paste. I, Completed restoration.

Small Class II direct composite restorations are often used for primary caries lesions, that is, initial restorations. A small round or elongated pear-shaped diamond or bur with round features may be used for this preparation to remove the carious tissue or faulty material from the occlusal and proximal surfaces. To help prevent damage to the adjacent teeth and promote initial interproximal separation, wedges with or without stainless steel barriers may be utilized. The initial separation provided by wooden wedges will facilitate matrix placement in conservative preparations as well as result in tighter interproximal contacts. The pulpal and axial depths are dictated only by the depth of the lesion and are not necessarily uniform. The proximal extensions likewise are dictated only by the extent of the lesion but may require the use of another instrument with straight sides to prepare walls that are 90 degrees or greater (Fig. 8.13). The objective is to remove the caries lesion or defect conservatively, as well as any friable tooth structure.

Another conservative design for small Class II composites is the box-only tooth preparation (Fig. 8.14). This design is indicated when only the proximal surface is defective, with no lesions on the occlusal surface. A proximal box is prepared with a small, elongated pear-shaped or round instrument, held parallel to the long axis of the tooth crown. The instrument is extended through the marginal ridge in a gingival direction aiming at the center of the proximal caries lesion or defect. The axial depth is dictated by the extent of the caries lesion or fault. The form of the box depends on which instrument shape is used. The facial, lingual,

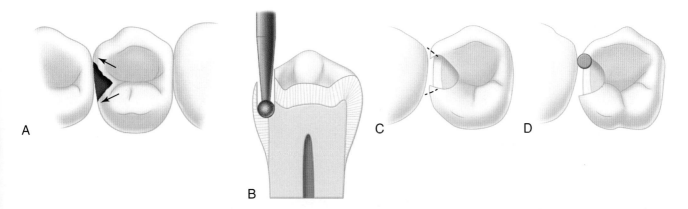

• **Fig. 8.13**   Class II direct composite tooth preparation. A, Preoperative visualization of faciolingual proximal box extensions. Arrows indicate desired extensions. B, Round or oval, small elongated pearl instrument used. C and D, Facial, lingual, and gingival margins may need undermined cavosurface enamel (indicated by dotted lines) removed with straight-sided thin and flat-tipped rotary instrument or hand instrument.

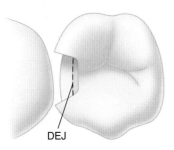

DEJ

• **Fig. 8.14**   Box-only Class II composite preparation.

and gingival extensions are dictated by the extension of the caries lesion or defect. No beveling or secondary retention is indicated.

A third conservative design for restoring proximal lesions on posterior teeth is the facial or lingual slot preparation (Fig. 8.15). Here, a lesion is detected on the proximal surface, but the operator believes that access to the lesion can be obtained from either a facial direction or a lingual direction, rather than through the marginal ridge in a gingival direction. Usually, a small round diamond or bur is used to gain access to the lesion. The instrument is oriented at the correct occlusogingival position, and the entry is made with the instrument as close to the adjacent tooth as possible, preserving as much of the facial or lingual surface as possible. The preparation is extended occlusally, facially, and gingivally enough to remove the lesion. The axial depth is determined by the extent of the lesion. The occlusal, facial, and gingival cavosurface margins are 90 degrees or greater. Care should be taken not to undermine the marginal ridge during the preparation. If the defect extends occlusally to the point of undermining the marginal ridge, a more conventional Class II preparation, with an occlusal access component, should be used.

The tooth preparation for *moderate to large Class II direct composite restorations* has features that resemble a more traditional Class II amalgam tooth preparation and may include an occlusal step and a proximal box depending on the location, extension, and depth of the caries lesion.

The occlusal portion of the Class II preparation is prepared similarly as described for the Class I preparation. The primary

differences are related to technique of incorporating the faulty proximal surface. Preoperatively, the proposed facial and lingual proximal extensions should be visualized (see Fig. 8.13A). Initial occlusal extension toward the involved proximal surface should go through the marginal ridge area at initial pulpal floor depth, exposing the DEJ. The DEJ serves as a guide for preparing the proximal box portion of the preparation.

A No. 330 or No. 245 shaped diamond or bur is used to enter the pit next to the carious proximal surface. The instrument is positioned parallel with the long axis of the tooth crown. If only one proximal surface is being restored, the opposite marginal ridge dentinal support should be maintained (Fig. 8.16).

The pulpal floor is initially prepared with the instrument to a depth that is approximately 0.2 mm inside the DEJ. The instrument is moved to include the caries lesion and all defects facially or lingually, or both, as it transverses the central groove. Every effort should be made, however, to keep the faciolingual width of the preparation as narrow as possible. The initial depth is maintained during the mesiodistal movement, but follows the rise and fall of the underlying DEJ. The pulpal floor is relatively flat in a faciolingual plane but may rise and fall slightly in a mesiodistal plane (Fig. 8.17). If more of the caries lesion remains in dentin, it is removed after the preparation outline, including the proximal box extensions, has been established.

Because the facial and lingual proximal extensions of the faulty proximal surface were visualized preoperatively, the occlusal extension toward that proximal surface begins to widen facially and lingually to begin to outline those extensions as conservatively as possible. Care is taken to preserve cuspal areas as much as possible during these extensions. At the same time, the instrument extends through the marginal ridge to within 0.5 mm of the outer contour of the marginal ridge. This extension exposes the proximal DEJ and protects the adjacent tooth (see Fig. 8.17). At this time, the occlusal portion of the preparation is complete except for possible additional pulpal floor caries lesion excavation. The occlusal walls generally converge occlusally because of the inverted shape of the instrument.

Typically, caries develops on a proximal surface immediately gingival to the proximal contact. The extent of the caries lesion and amount of old restorative material dictate the facial, lingual,

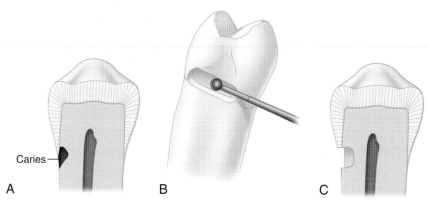

• **Fig. 8.15** Facial or lingual slot preparation. A, Cervical caries on the proximal surface. B, The round diamond or bur enters the tooth from the accessible embrasure, oriented to the occlusogingival middle of the lesion. C, Slot preparation.

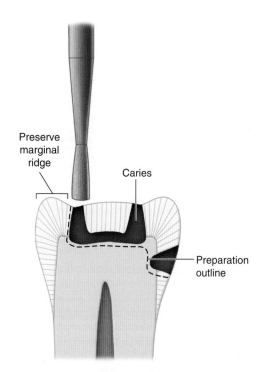

• **Fig. 8.16** When only one proximal surface is affected, the opposite marginal ridge should be maintained.

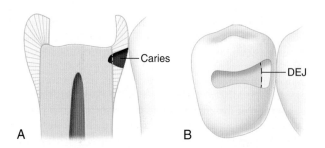

• **Fig. 8.17** Occlusal extension into faulty proximal surface. A and B, Extension exposes the dentinoenamel junction (DEJ) but does not hit the adjacent tooth. Facial and lingual extensions as preoperatively visualized (see Fig. 10.9 for initial pulpal floor depth).

and gingival extensions of the proximal box of the preparation. Although it is not required to extend the proximal box beyond contact with the adjacent tooth (i.e., provide clearance with the adjacent tooth), it may simplify the preparation, matrix placement, and contouring procedures. If all of the defect can be removed without extending the proximal preparation beyond the contact, however, the restoration of the proximal contact with the composite is simplified (Fig. 8.18D).

Before the instrument is extended through the marginal ridge, the proximal ditch cut is initiated. The operator holds the instrument over the DEJ with the tip of the instrument positioned to create a gingivally directed cut that is 0.2 mm inside the DEJ (see Fig. 8.18B–D). For a No. 245 instrument with a tip diameter of 0.8 mm, this would require one fourth of the instrument's tip positioned over the dentin side of the DEJ (the other three fourths of the tip over the enamel side). The instrument is extended facially, lingually, and gingivally to include all of the caries lesion or old material, or both. The faciolingual cutting motion follows the DEJ and therefore is usually in a slightly convex arc outward (see Fig. 8.18C). During this entire cutting, the instrument is held parallel to the long axis of the tooth crown. The facial and lingual margins are extended as necessary and should result in at least a 90-degree margin (indicating enamel that is supported by dentin), more obtuse being acceptable as well. If the preparation is conservative, then a smaller, thinner instrument is used to complete the facio-lingual wall formation, avoiding the creation of iatrogenic damage to the adjacent tooth (Fig. 8.19). Alternatively, a sharp hand instrument such as a chisel, hatchet, or a gingival margin trimmer can be used to finish the enamel wall. At this point, the remaining proximal enamel that was initially maintained to prevent damage to the adjacent tooth has been removed. The gingival floor is prepared flat with an approximately 90-degree cavosurface margin. Gingival extension should be as minimal as possible, to preserve marginal enamel. The axial wall should be 0.2 mm inside the DEJ and have a slight outward convexity. For large caries lesions, additional axial wall caries excavation may be necessary later (Fig. 8.20).

If no caries lesion in the dentin or other defect remains, the preparation is considered complete at this time (Fig. 8.21). However, if carious dentin or faulty restorative material/base remain on the axial and pulpal aspects of the preparation, which is typically the case for moderate to large Class II restorations, these areas should be selectively excavated to firm dentin. Often the initial preparation

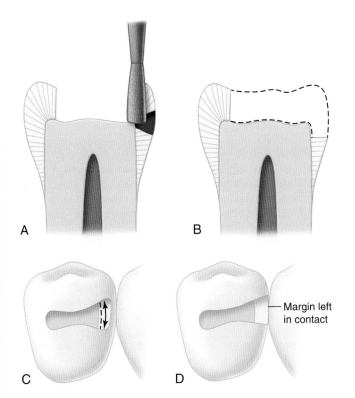

• **Fig. 8.18** A, The proximal wall may be left in contact with the adjacent tooth. B, Proximal ditch cut. The instrument is positioned such that a gingivally directed cut creates the axial wall 0.2 mm inside the dentinoenamel junction (DEJ). C, Faciolingual direction of axial wall preparation follows the DEJ. D, Axial wall 0.2 mm inside the DEJ.

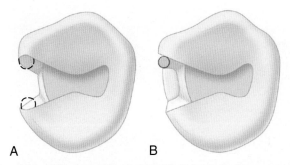

• **Fig. 8.19** Using a smaller instrument to prepare the cavosurface margin areas of facial and lingual proximal walls. A, Facial and lingual proximal margins undermined. B, Using a smaller instrument.

outline will have to be enlarged to allow access at this stage of the preparation. Once selective removal of any remaining carious tissue or removal of faulty existing restorative/base materials is accomplished, consideration should be given for pulp protection as described previously in the Class I restorative technique section of this chapter. When treating a tooth with very extensive and deep caries on a vital, asymptomatic tooth, care should be exercised to avoid a pulp exposure, which would considerably compromise the prognosis for the tooth. See Chapter 2 for considerations on selective removal of carious dentin.

Because the composite is retained in the preparation by adhesion, no secondary preparation retention features are necessary. No bevels are placed on the occlusal cavosurface margins because these walls already have exposed enamel rod ends. Beveled composite margins

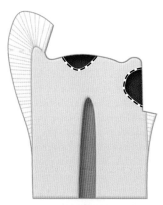

• **Fig. 8.20** Proximal extension. The enamel margin on the gingival floor is critical for bonding, so it should be preserved, if not compromised. Any remaining soft dentin on the axial wall (or the pulpal floor) is excavated as part of the final tooth preparation (as indicated by dotted lines).

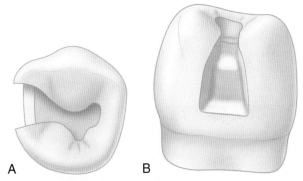

• **Fig. 8.21** Final Class II composite tooth preparation. A, Occlusal view. B, Proximal view.

also may be more difficult to finish. Bevels are rarely used on any of the proximal box walls because of the difficulty in restoring these areas, particularly when using inherently viscous composites. Bevels also are not recommended along the gingival margins of the proximal box; however, it is still necessary to remove brittle unsupported enamel rods along the margins because of the gingival orientation of the enamel rods. For most Class II preparations, this margin already is approaching the cementoenamel junction (CEJ), and the enamel is thin. Care is taken to maintain any enamel in this area to achieve a preparation with all-enamel margins. If the preparation extends onto the root surface, more attention must be focused on keeping the area isolated during the bonding technique, but no differences in tooth preparation are required. Usually, the only remaining final tooth preparation procedure that might be necessary is additional removal of the caries lesion associated with the dentin on either the pulpal floor or the axial wall. If necessary, a round bur or appropriate spoon excavator is used for selective removal of any remaining carious tissue.

Restorative Technique

Matrix Application

One of the most important steps in restoring Class II preparations with direct composites is proper matrix selection and setup. As with most restorative procedures involving a proximal surface, a matrix is necessary to (1) confine the restorative material excess and (2) assist in the development of the appropriate axial tooth contours. In contrast to amalgam, which can be condensed against the matrix and thereby improve the proximal contact, Class II composites are almost totally dependent on the contour and position of the matrix for establishing appropriate proximal contacts. Early wedging and retightening of the wedge during tooth preparation aid in achieving sufficient separation of teeth to compensate for the thickness of the matrix material. Before placing the composite material, the matrix material must be in absolute contact with (i.e., touching) the adjacent contact area.

Generally, the matrix is applied before adhesive placement. An ultrathin metal matrix band generally is preferred for the restoration of a Class II composite because it is thinner than a typical metal band and can be contoured better than a clear polyester matrix. No significant problems are experienced in placing and light curing composite material when using a metal matrix as long as an incremental technique is used.

Although a Tofflemire-type matrix band can be used for restoring a two-surface tooth preparation, precontoured sectional metallic matrices are preferable (Fig. 8.22), because only one thickness of metal matrix material is encountered instead of two, making contact generation easier. These sectional matrices are relatively easy to use, very thin, and come in different sizes so as to accommodate for varied occlusogingival heights of the proximal box. There are several systems available, and selection is based on operator preference. These systems may use a bitine ring to (1) aid in stabilizing the sectional matrix and (2) provide additional tooth separation while the composite is inserted. The primary benefit of these systems is a simpler method for establishing an appropriate composite proximal contour and contact.[45] Use of these systems for restoring wide faciolingual proximal preparations requires careful application; otherwise the bitine ring prongs may cause deformation of the matrix band, resulting in poor restoration contour.

When both proximal surfaces are involved, a Tofflemire retainer with an ultrathin (0.025 mm or 0.001 inch) and burnishable matrix band is used. The band is contoured, positioned, wedged, and shaped, as needed, for proper proximal contacts and embrasures. Before placement, the metal matrix band for posterior composites should be burnished on a paper pad to impart proper proximal contour to the band. Alternatively, an ultrathin precontoured metal matrix band may be used in the Tofflemire retainer.

Regardless of the type of matrix system used, the matrix material should extend at least 1 mm beyond the gingival margin (gingivally) and the area corresponding to the marginal ridge of the restoration (occlusally). The matrix should not extend further subgingivally or occlusally so as not to interfere with the restorative procedure. If a wedge was used during the tooth preparation procedures, it is removed so that the matrix band can be installed, and immediately reinserted. A wedge is needed at the gingival margin to (1) hold

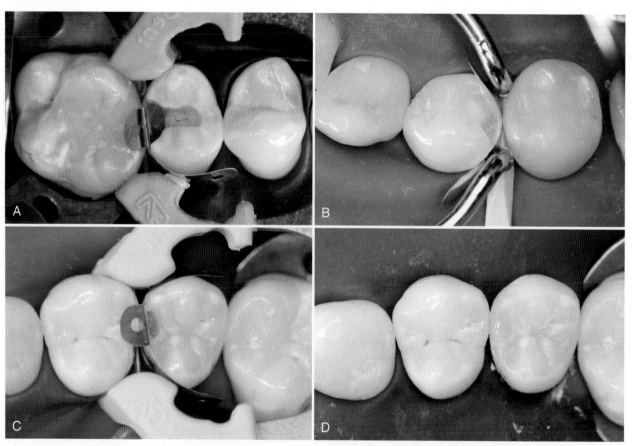

• **Fig. 8.22** Sectional matrix systems for posterior composites. A, Sectional matrix system in place with plastic wedge and bitine ring to restore the maxillary premolar with direct composite. B, Sectional matrix system in place with wooden wedge and bitine ring to restore the mandibular premolar with direct composite. C, Sectional matrix system in place with plastic wedge and bitine ring to restore the maxillary premolar with direct composite. D, Case presented in C after placement and light curing of the composite, and matrix removal, before any contouring. Note minimal excess composite as a result of good matrix adaptation to facial and lingual embrasures.

the matrix in position, (2) provide slight separation of the teeth, and (3) prevent a gingival overhang of the composite material. A wedge must be used to separate teeth sufficiently to compensate for the thickness of the matrix if the completed restoration is to have appropriate proximal contacts.

Several types of commercial wedges are available in assorted sizes. An anatomical (triangle-shaped) wedge of compatible size is indicated for most preparations. The wedge is kept as short as possible so as not to limit operator access to the preparation during insertion of the restorative material, and should also not push the matrix onto the preparation space.

For posterior restorations, the wedge is placed from the larger to the smaller interproximal gingival embrasure, typically from a lingual approach, just apical to the gingival margin. The wedge should engage (stabilize) the matrix band. When a rubber dam is used, wedge placement may be aided by a small amount of water-soluble lubricant on the tip of the wedge. The rubber dam is first stretched gingivally (on the side from which the wedge is inserted), then released gradually during wedge insertion.

Placement of the Adhesive

The technique for adhesive placement is as described previously for the Class I direct composite restoration. Care should be exercised to avoid adhesive pooling along the matrix and preparation margins gingivally, facially, and lingually.

Insertion and Light Curing of the Composite

The technique for insertion of Class II posterior composites is illustrated in Fig. 8.23. It is best to restore the proximal box portion of the preparation first. Hand instruments or a "composite gun" may be used to insert the composite material. It is important to place and light cure the composite incrementally to maximize the curing potential and to reduce the negative effects of polymerization shrinkage as discussed earlier in this chapter. Many techniques have been described for the restoration of the proximal box. Research comparing different insertion and light-curing techniques is not conclusive and no single technique has been universally accepted. The number of increments will depend on the size of the proximal box. At the University of North Carolina, we recommend an oblique incremental technique: The first increment(s) should be placed

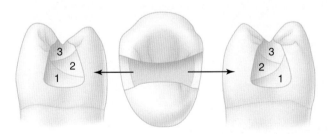

• **Fig. 8.23** Oblique incremental technique to restore proximal boxes in Class II direct composite restorations. The number of increments will depend on the size of the proximal box. The first increment(s) *(1)* should be placed along the gingival floor and should extend slightly up the facial wall. This increment should be only approximately 1 to 2 mm thick because it is the farthest increment from the curing light and the most critical in establishing a proper gingival seal. A second increment *(2)* is then placed against the lingual wall, to restore about two thirds of the box. The final increment *(3)* is then placed to complete the proximal box and develop the marginal ridge. Subsequent additions, if needed, are made and light cured (usually not exceeding 2 mm in thickness at a time) until the proximal box is filled.

along the gingival floor and should extend slightly up the facial (or lingual) wall (see Fig. 8.23). This increment (or increments for a large box) should be no more than 2 mm thick because it is the farthest increment from the curing light and the most critical in establishing a proper gingival seal. A second increment is then placed against the lingual (or facial) wall to restore about two thirds of the box. The final increment is then placed to complete the proximal box and develop the marginal ridge. Subsequent additions, if needed, are made and light cured (usually not exceeding 2 mm in thickness at a time) until the proximal box is fully restored (see Fig. 8.23). Increments should be light cured for as long as needed, depending on the shade and opacity of the composite used, the distance of the composite from the light tip, and the power of the light-curing unit. Regardless of the number of increments needed, when restoring the proximal box, an effort should be made to develop the anatomy of marginal ridge without excessive composite, to reduce the amount of rotary instrumentation required during finishing.

When the proximal box is completed, the occlusal step of the preparation is restored exactly as it was described for the Class I direct composite restoration—that is, using an anatomic layering technique.

The incremental insertion and light-curing technique described provides enhanced control over the application and polymerization of individual increments of composite. The incremental technique also allows for (1) orientation of the polymerization light beam according to the position of each increment of composite, thus enhancing the polymerization potential; (2) intrinsic restoration characterization with darker or pigmented composites; and (3) sculpture of the restoration occlusal stratum with a more translucent material simulating the natural enamel. Appropriate proximal contact intensity can also be better achieved when composite is applied in increments. The matrix can be held in physical contact with the adjacent proximal surface while the contact-related increment of composite is light cured. A hand instrument with a large surface area (e.g., a small football-shaped or round burnisher) is well suited for that purpose. Once this increment is cured, the proximal contact is established, and remaining increments can be inserted and light cured. The matrix is removed and the restoration is light cured from the facial and lingual directions. The restoration is finished and polished immediately after the last increment is cured.

Composite resin placement may be made more difficult by the stiffness and stickiness of some composite materials. Heating the composite material prior to insertion in the preparation may help overcome these problems. Commercial "composite warmers" are available (e.g., Calset, AdDent Inc., Danbury, CT) to preheat the composite resin to preset temperatures up to 68°C (155°F). The increased temperature lowers the viscosity of the composite resin, potentially resulting in better marginal adaptation and reduced microleakage, although some of these results have been shown to be composite specific.[46-49] The elevated composite temperatures have been shown to be safe for clinical use.[50,51]

When a stiffer or "packable" high-viscosity composite is used for the restoration of the proximal box, a very small increment of a flowable composite may be first placed in close proximity to the external margins of the proximal box so as to improve marginal adaptation of the restoration.[52,53]

Finishing and Polishing of the Composite

Finishing can be initiated immediately after the composite material has been fully light cured (Fig. 8.24). If the occlusal anatomy

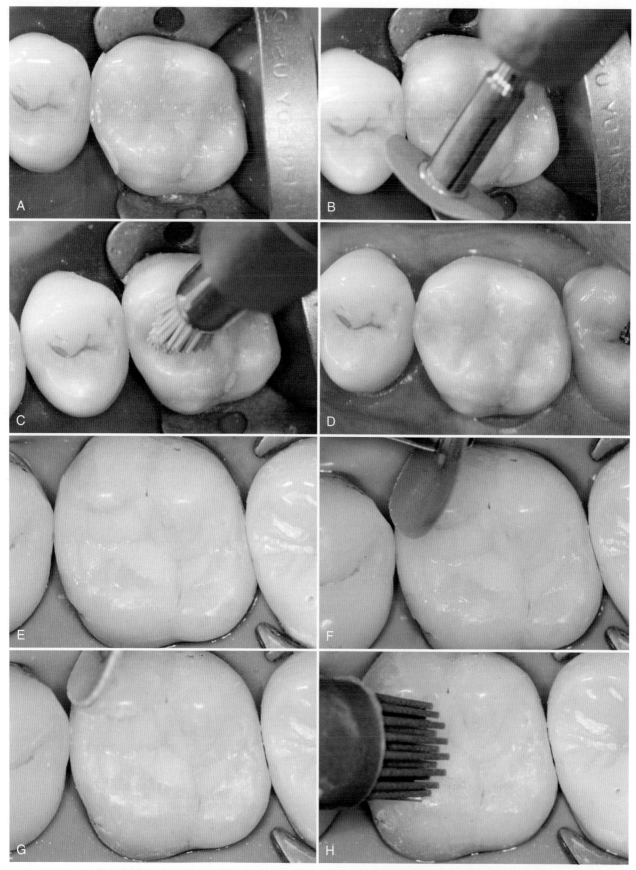

• **Fig. 8.24**   Contouring and finishing of posterior composite restorations. A, After sectional matrix removal, excess composite is noted on facial and lingual proximal embrasures. B, Contouring lingual embrasure with finishing disk. C, Polishing the occlusal surface with finishing brush. D, Completed restoration. E, Note minimal excess composite after removal of sectional matrix because of good matrix adaptation to facial and lingual embrasures and careful incremental insertion of the composite. F–H, Contouring and polishing with disks and brush.

was developed as described in the previous sections, the need for additional contouring is greatly minimized. If finishing is needed, the occlusal surface is shaped with a round or oval, 12-bladed carbide finishing bur or finishing diamond. Excess composite is removed at the proximal margins and embrasures with a flame-shaped, 12-bladed carbide finishing bur or finishing diamond and abrasive discs (see Fig. 8.24B). Any overhangs at the gingival area are removed with a No. 12 surgical blade mounted in a Bard-Parker handle with light shaving strokes to remove the excess. Narrow finishing strips may be used to smooth the gingival proximal surface. Care must be exercised in maintaining the position of the finishing strips gingival to the proximal contact area to avoid inadvertent removal of the composite contact with the adjacent proximal surface. The rubber dam (or other means of isolation) is removed, and the occlusion is evaluated for proper contact. Further adjustments are made, if needed, and the restorations are polished with appropriate polishing points, cups, brushes, or discs (see Fig. 8.24C, F–H).

Extensive Class II Direct Composite Restorations and Foundations

Direct composite is not usually indicated for extensive posterior restorations but may be used as such when economic factors prevent the patient from selecting a more ideal (and more costly) indirect restoration, or as a semipermanent restoration in teeth with questionable prognosis. The 12-year survival rate of large posterior composite restorations has been shown to be similar to that of large amalgam restorations, although amalgam performed better in patients with high caries risk.[54] In addition to being used in selected cases for extensive restorations, composites also may be considered for use as a foundation for indirect restorations (crowns and onlays) when the operator determines that insufficient natural tooth structure remains to provide adequate retention and resistance form for the crown. The tooth first is restored with a large restoration and is then prepared for the indirect restoration.

In addition to the tooth preparation form, the primary retention form for a very large Class II composite restoration is the micromechanical bonding of the composite to enamel and dentin. When a full-coverage preparation is anticipated, secondary retention features must be incorporated, however, because of (1) the decreased amount of tooth structure available for bonding and (2) the increased concern for retaining the composite in the tooth. These features may include grooves, coves, and slots.

The primary differences for these very large preparations include the following: (1) Some or all of the cusps may be reduced and covered with composite ("capped"), (2) extensions in most directions are greater than in more conservative preparations, (3) secondary retention features are used, and (4) additional resistance form features are used. A cusp must be reduced and covered with composite if loss of supporting dentin is severe enough to leave the cusp in a weakened, fracture prone state. Reducing and covering a cusp with composite usually is indicated when the occlusal outline form extends more than two thirds the distance from a primary groove to a cusp tip. An operator sometimes may choose to ignore this general rule when using a bonded restoration if that weakened cusp will be covered and reinforced as part of the preparation design for the subsequent indirect restoration.

If the tooth has had endodontic treatment, the pulp chamber can be opened and extensions can be made several millimeters into each treated canal. Because of the increased surface area for bonding and the mechanical retention from extensions into the canals, usually fewer secondary retention features are incorporated into the remaining tooth preparation.

The elongated pear-shaped diamond or bur is used to prepare the occlusal step. As already noted, the occlusal outline form is usually extensive. When moving the instrument from the central groove area toward a cuspal prominence, the pulpal depth that is approximately 0.2 mm inside the DEJ should be maintained, if possible. This creates a pulpal floor, which rises occlusally as it is extended either facially or lingually (see Fig. 8.8). If a cusp must be reduced and covered, the side of the rotary instrument can be used first to make several depth cuts in the remaining cuspal form to serve as a guide for cusp reduction. Cusps should be reduced as early in the tooth preparation procedure as possible, providing more access and visibility for the preparation. The depth cut is made with the instrument held parallel to the cuspal incline (from cusp tip to central groove) and approximately 1.5 to 2 mm deep. For a large cusp, multiple depth cuts can be made. Then, the instrument is used to join the depth cuts and extend to the remainder of the cuspal form (Fig. 8.25). The reduced cusp has a relatively flat surface that may rise and fall with the normal mesial and distal inclines of the cusp. It also should provide enough clearance with the opposing tooth to result in approximately 1.5 to 2 mm of composite material to restore form and function. The cusp reduction should be blended in with the rest of the occlusal step portion of the preparation.

The proximal boxes are prepared as described previously. The primary difference is that they may be much larger, that is, extend farther in every direction. The extent of the caries lesion may dictate that a proximal box extend around the line angle of the tooth to include the caries lesion or faulty facial or lingual tooth structure. When the outline form has been established (the margins extended to sound tooth structure), carious tissue at the pulpal and axial walls is selectively removed and the preparation is assessed carefully for additional retention form needs.

Retention form can be enhanced by the placement of grooves, coves, or slots. All such retention form features must be strategically placed in dentin so as to maintain dentinal support of remaining enamel while avoiding areas that increase the risk of pulpal involvement. At times, bevels may be placed on available enamel margins to enhance retention form, even on occlusal areas. Retention form for foundations must be placed far enough inside the DEJ (at least 1 mm) to remain after the crown preparation is subsequently accomplished. Otherwise, essential secondary features that are retaining the foundation may potentially be lost (Fig. 8.26).

Matrix placement is more demanding for these large restorations because more tooth structure is missing, and more margins may be subgingival. Proper burnishing of the matrix band to achieve appropriate axial contours is important, unless immediate full coverage of the tooth is planned. It also may be necessary to modify the matrix band to provide more subgingival extension in some areas and prevent extrusion of the composite at the matrix band–retainer tooth junction.

Typical adhesive placement techniques are followed. Because much of the composite bond is to dentin, proper technique is crucial. Placement of the adhesive is accomplished as previously described.

When a light-cured composite is used, first it is placed in 1- to 2-mm increments into the most gingival areas of the proximal boxes. Each increment is cured, as directed. It may be helpful to use a hand instrument to hold the matrix against the adjacent tooth while light curing the composite. This may assist in restoring the proximal contact.

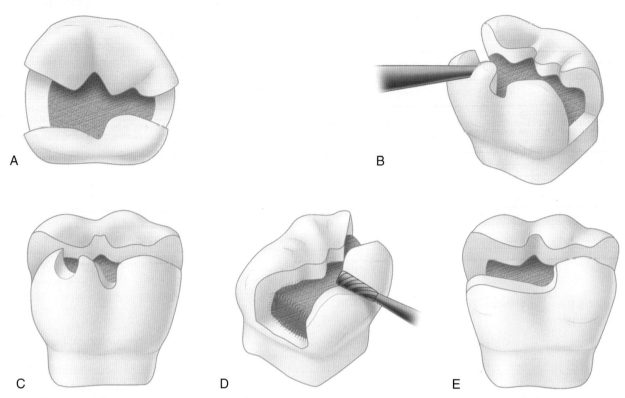

• **Fig. 8.25** Cusp reduction. A, The initial outline form weakens the mesiolingual cusp enough to necessitate capping. B, Depth cuts made. C, Depth cuts. D, Cusp reduction prepared. E, Vertical wall maintained between reduced and unreduced cusps.

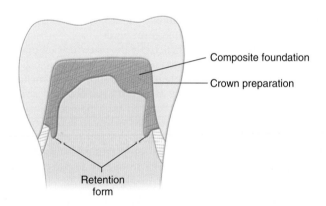

• **Fig. 8.26** The retention form for foundations must be internal to eventual crown preparation.

Self-cured and dual-cured composite resin materials are frequently used for large *composite foundations* because these can be injected in the preparation in a single increment. However, it is recommended that even when dual-cured composites are used, they be carefully light cured during and after the final placement. When this technique is used, the operator should carefully select the adhesive system, as some simplified adhesives have been shown to be incompatible with some self-cured composite foundation materials. Acidic monomers in these adhesives scavenge the activators (tertiary amines) in the self-cure composite.[55,56] If the activator does not function properly, then the composite at the adhesive interface does not polymerize thoroughly and does not polymerize with the previously placed adhesive. Some manufacturers have introduced optional chemical catalysts that can be mixed with the light-cured adhesive to reduce or prevent this problem.

Contouring the large composite also is more difficult because of the number of surfaces that may be involved and the amount of composite present. Anatomically correct contours and contacts are necessary for restorations, but they are less important for foundations that will be present only for a short time before the crown preparation is accomplished and the tooth is stabilized. Because of the extensiveness of these restorations, a careful assessment of the contours should be made from all angles. When finishing has been completed, the occlusion is adjusted as necessary, and the restoration is polished. Because these very large restorations may stretch the limits of composite restorations, the patient should be on a frequent recall regimen.

Clinical Technique for Class III Direct Composite Restorations

Initial Clinical Procedures

These are similar to those already described: (1) Anesthesia is usually necessary for patient comfort and may help decrease salivary flow during the procedure; (2) occlusal assessments should be made to determine the tooth preparation design and to properly adjust the restoration's function; (3) the composite shade must be selected before the tooth dehydrates and concomitantly lightens; (4) the area must be isolated to facilitate access and permit effective bonding;

and (5) if the restoration involves the proximal contact, inserting a wedge in the area beforehand may assist in the reestablishment of the proximal contact with composite.

Tooth Preparation

In general, the tooth preparation for a Class III direct composite restoration involves (1) obtaining access to the defect (caries lesion, fracture, noncarious defect), (2) removing faulty structures (carious tissue, defective dentin and enamel, defective restoration, base material), and (3) creating the convenience form for the restoration (Fig. 8.27). In most cases, an enamel bevel is used on the facial cavosurface margin to provide a gradual color transition from the restoration to the surrounding tooth structure for esthetics. If unsupported enamel is intentionally left on the facial aspect of the preparation, a facial cavosurface bevel may not be indicated as it can unnecessarily extend the facial display of the restoration. Obtaining access to the defect may include removal of sound enamel to access the caries lesion. The extension of the preparation is therefore ultimately dictated by the extension of the fault or defect. It is usually not necessary to reduce sound tooth structure to provide either "bulk for strength" or conventional retention and resistance forms.

Because of the adequate bond of composite to enamel and dentin, most Class III composite restorations are retained almost exclusively by bonding, and no additional preparation retention form is necessary. In the rare cases when additional retention form is needed, it can be achieved either by increasing the surface area with a wider enamel bevel or by adding retentive features in the preparation internal dentin walls.

When a proximal surface of an anterior tooth is to be restored, and a choice between facial or lingual entry into the tooth is available, the lingual approach is always preferable unless such an approach would necessitate excessive removal of the tooth structure, such as in instances of irregular alignment of teeth or facial positioning of the lesion. The advantages of restoring the proximal lesion using a *lingual approach* are:

1. The facial enamel is conserved for enhanced esthetics. (Some unsupported, but nonfriable, enamel may be left on the facial wall of the preparation.)
2. Shade matching of the composite is less critical.
3. Discoloration or deterioration of the restoration is less visible.

Indications for a *facial approach* include:

1. The caries lesion is positioned facially, and facial access would significantly conserve the tooth structure.
2. Teeth are irregularly aligned, and facial access would significantly conserve the tooth structure.
3. An extensive caries lesion extends onto the facial surface.
4. A faulty restoration that originally was placed from the facial approach needs to be replaced.

When the facial and the lingual surfaces are involved, the approach that provides the best access for instrumentation should be used.

The preparation is initiated from a lingual approach (if possible) by using a round carbide bur or diamond instrument of a size compatible with the extent of the lesion. The point of entry is located within the incisogingival dimension of the lesion or defect and as close to the adjacent tooth as possible without contacting it (Fig. 8.28A). The initial opening is made by holding the cutting instrument perpendicular to the enamel surface but at an entry angle that places the neck portion of the bur or diamond instrument as far into the embrasure (next to the adjacent tooth) as possible;

light pressure and intermittent cutting (brush stroke) are used to gain access into the preparation. Incorrect entry overextends the lingual outline and unnecessarily weakens the tooth (see Fig. 8.28B and C).

The same instrument may be used to enlarge the initial access opening sufficiently to permit, in subsequent steps, carious tissue removal, completion of the preparation, and insertion of the restorative material (see Fig. 8.28D). No effort is made to prepare the walls that are perpendicular to the enamel surface; for small preparations, the walls may diverge externally from the axial depth resulting in a beveled marginal design and conservation of internal tooth structure (Fig. 8.29). For larger preparations, the initial tooth preparation still is as conservative as possible, but the preparation walls may not be as divergent from the axial wall. Subsequent beveling or flaring of accessible enamel areas may be required. Despite the size of the lesion, the objective of the initial tooth preparation is the same: to prepare the tooth as conservatively as possible by extending the outline form just enough to include the peripheral extent of the lesion. Sometimes, the incorporation of an enamel bevel also may be used to extend the final outline form to include the caries lesion. If possible, the outline form should not (1) include the entire proximal contact area, (2) extend onto the facial surface, or (3) extend subgingivally. Extensions should be minimal, including only the tooth structure that is compromised by the extent of the caries lesion or defect. Some undermined enamel can be left in nonocclusal stress areas, but very friable enamel at the margins should be removed.

The extension axially also is dictated by the extent of the fault or caries lesion and usually is not uniform in depth. As noted earlier, most initial composite restorations (primary caries) use an ultraconservative preparation design (Fig. 8.30A and B). Because a caries lesion that requires a restoration usually extends into dentin, many Class III preparations extend to an initial axial wall depth of 0.2 mm into dentin and are widened such that peripheral enamel has dentinal support (Fig. 8.31). No attempt is made however to prepare distinct or uniform axial preparation walls; rather, the objective is to selectively remove carious tissue as conservatively as possible. Additional marginal refinement may be necessary later.

If the preparation outline extends gingivally onto the root surface, the gingival floor should form a cavosurface margin of 90 degrees, and the depth of the gingivoaxial line angle should be not more than 0.75 mm at this initial stage of tooth preparation. The external walls are prepared perpendicular to the root surface. In this area of the tooth, apical of the cementoenamel junction (CEJ), the external walls are composed entirely of dentin and cementum.

When completed, the initial tooth preparation extends the outline form to include the entire fault unless it is anticipated that the incorporation of an additional enamel bevel would enhance retention form or improve the potential for an optimal esthetic result. Small preparations typically have a beveled marginal configuration from the initial tooth preparation.

Little may need to be done in the final tooth preparation stage for these preparations. Final tooth preparation steps for a Class III direct composite restoration are, when indicated, (1) selective removal of carious dentin; (2) pulp protection; (3) bevel placement on accessible enamel margins; and (4) final procedures of cleaning and inspecting. The selective removal of carious dentin is accomplished using round burs, small spoon excavators, or both. Particular care must be exercised not to weaken the walls or incisal angles that are subject to masticatory forces.

Larger preparations may require additional beveling of the accessible enamel walls to enhance retention by bonding (Fig.

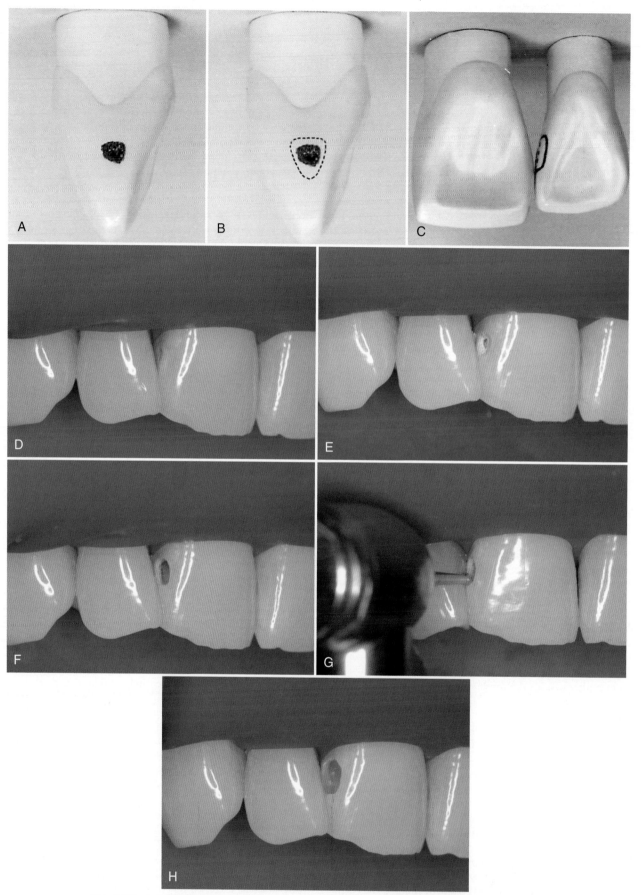

• **Fig. 8.27** A, Small proximal caries lesion on the mesial surface of a maxillary lateral incisor. B, Dotted line indicates normal outline form dictated by shape of the caries lesion. C, Extension (convenience form) required for preparing and restoring preparation from lingual approach when teeth are in normal alignment. D–H, Clinical case showing conservative Class III preparation, facial approach. D, Facial view of a caries lesion on the distal surface of the maxillary central incisor. E and F, Obtaining access to carious dentin. G, Infected dentin is removed with round bur. H, Completed caries excavation.

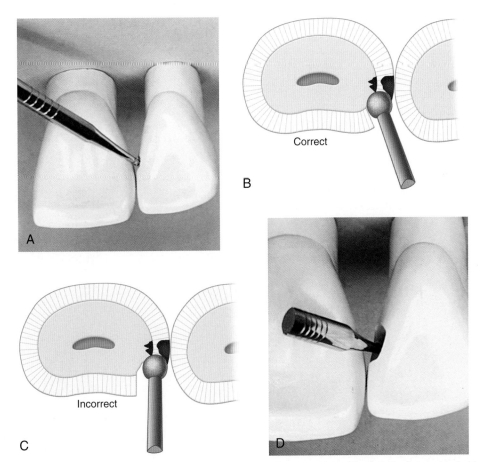

• **Fig. 8.28** Beginning Class III tooth preparation (lingual approach). A, The bur or diamond is held perpendicular to the enamel surface, and an initial opening is made close to the adjacent tooth at the incisogingival level of the caries. B, The correct angle of entry is parallel to the enamel rods on the mesio-lingual angle of the tooth. C, Incorrect entry overextends the lingual outline. D, The same bur or diamond is used to enlarge opening for caries removal and convenience form while establishing the initial axial wall depth.

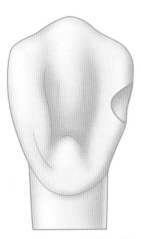

• **Fig. 8.29** A small, scoop-shaped Class III tooth preparation.

8.32; see Fig. 8.30C and D). These enamel margins are beveled with a flame-shaped or round diamond instrument. The bevel is prepared by creating a 45-degree angle to the external surface and to a width of 0.5 to 2 mm, depending on the size of the preparation, location of the margin, and esthetic requirements of the restoration (Fig. 8.33; see Fig. 8.32). If the gingival floor has been extended

gingivally to a position where the remaining enamel thickness is minimal or nonexistent, the bevel is omitted from this area to preserve the remaining enamel margin or maintain a 90-degree cavosurface margin in dentin. Likewise, a bevel on the lingual enamel margin of a maxillary incisor may be contraindicated if it would result in the creation of a restoration marginal interface at the area of occlusal contact.

Remaining old restorative material on the axial wall should be removed if any of the following conditions are present: (1) The old material is amalgam, and its color would negatively affect the color of the new restoration; (2) clinical or radiographic evidence of a caries lesion under the old material is present; (3) the tooth pulp was symptomatic preoperatively; (4) the periphery of the remaining restorative material is not intact; (5) there is noticeable deterioration of the bonding of the remaining restorative material; or (6) the use of the underlying dentin is necessary to effect a stronger bond for retention purposes. If none of these conditions is present, the operator may elect to leave the remaining restorative material rather than risk unnecessary excavation nearer to the pulp and subsequent irritation or exposure of the pulp. A RMGI base is applied only if the remaining dentin thickness is judged to be less than 1.5 mm and in the deepest portions of the preparation.[26] Calcium hydroxide liners are used only in cases when the remaining dentin thickness is 0.5 mm or less as an indirect pulp-capping

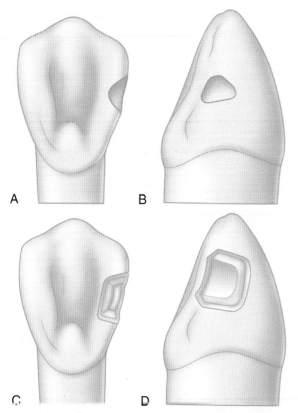

• **Fig. 8.30** Preparation designs for Class III (A and B); larger preparation designs for Class III (C and D).

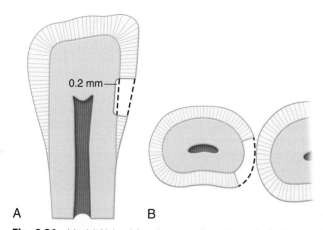

• **Fig. 8.31** Ideal initial axial wall preparation depth. A, Incisogingival section showing axial wall 0.2 mm into dentin. B, Faciolingual section showing facial extension and axial wall following the contour of the tooth.

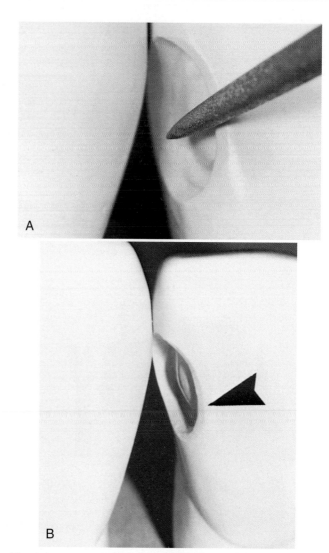

• **Fig. 8.32** Large Class III tooth preparation. A, Beveling. The cavosurface bevel is prepared with a flame-shaped or round diamond, resulting in an angle approximately 45 degrees to the external tooth surface. B, Completed cavosurface bevel *(arrowhead)*.

material; in cases of pulp exposures calcium hydroxide or, increasingly, MTA can be used as a direct pulp-capping material.[26-28] If used, the calcium hydroxide or MTA liners should always be covered with a RMGI base, sealing the area and preventing the etchant (applied later) from dissolving the liner.[26,29]

When replacing a large restoration or restoring a large Class III lesion, the operator may decide that retention form should be enhanced by placing groove (at gingival) or cove (at incisal) retention features in addition to bonding.

For Class III direct composite preparations with *facial access*, with a few exceptions, the same stages and steps of tooth preparation are followed as for lingual access. The ability to use direct vision simplifies the procedure (Fig. 8.34).

It is expeditious to prepare and restore approximating caries lesions or faulty restorations on adjacent teeth at the same appointment. If one of the lesions is larger (more extended outline form) than the other, then the larger outline form is developed first. The second preparation usually can be more conservative because of the improved access provided by the larger preparation. The reverse order would be followed when the restorative material is inserted.

A Class III lesion on the distal surface of a maxillary right central incisor is shown in Fig. 8.35A. The rubber dam is placed after the anesthetic has been administered and the shade has been selected. A wedge is inserted in the gingival embrasure to depress the rubber dam and underlying soft tissue, improving gingival access (see Fig. 8.35B). Using a carbide bur or diamond instrument rotating at high speed and with air-water spray, the outline form is prepared with appropriate extension and the initial, limited pulpal depth as previously described in the lingual approach preparation (see Fig. 8.35C). Carious tissue is removed with a

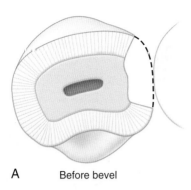

A   Before bevel

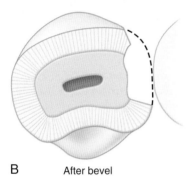

B   After bevel

• **Fig. 8.33** Cross section of facial approach Class III before (A) and after (B) 45-degree cavosurface bevel on the facial margin.

spoon excavator (see Fig. 8.35D). Some undermined enamel may be left if it is not in a high-stress area.

When a proximal caries lesion or defective restoration extends onto the facial *and* the lingual surfaces, access may be accomplished from either a facial approach or a lingual approach. An example of an extensive Class III initial tooth preparation that allows such choice is illustrated in Fig. 8.36.

Restorative Technique

Matrix Application

A matrix is a device that is applied to a prepared tooth before the insertion of the restorative material to (1) confine the restorative

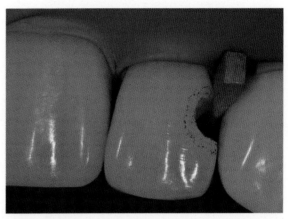

• **Fig. 8.34** Completed Class III tooth preparation (facial approach), with the bevel marked.

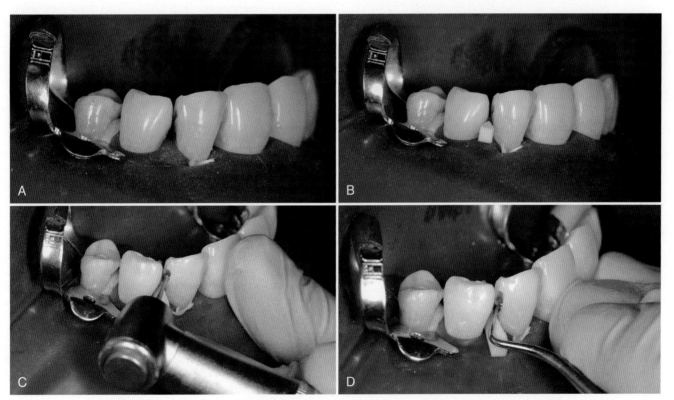

• **Fig. 8.35** Class III initial preparation (facial approach). A, Large proximal caries with facial involvement. B, Isolated area of operation. C, Entry and extension with No. 2 bur or diamond. D, Caries removal with spoon excavator. (Courtesy Vilhelm G. Ólafsson.)

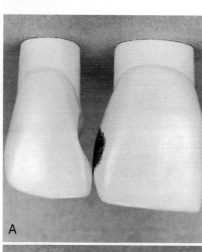

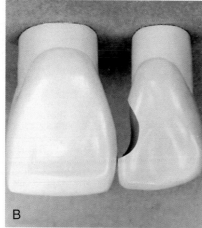

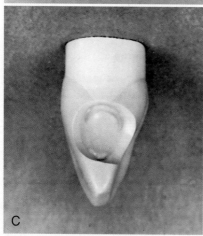

• **Fig. 8.36** Large Class III tooth preparation extending onto root surface. A, Facial view. B, Lingual view. C, Mesial view showing gingival and incisal retention, which is only used when deemed necessary to increase retention. The tooth preparation is now ready for beveling of the enamel walls.

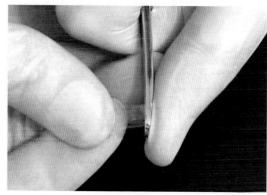

• **Fig. 8.37** Contouring Mylar strip matrix. (Courtesy Aldridge D. Wilder, DDS.)

completed by direct placement of the composite. When correctly used, not only would a matrix aid in placing and contouring the composite restorative material, but it may also reduce the amount of excess material, thus minimizing the finishing time.

A properly contoured section of Mylar matrix material is used for most Class III and IV preparations. Because the proximal surface of a tooth is usually convex incisogingivally and the matrix material may be flat, it is necessary to shape the matrix to conform to the desired tooth contour. One way to contour a Mylar matrix is by drawing it along a hard, rounded object (Fig. 8.37). The amount of convexity placed in the matrix depends on the size and contour of the anticipated restoration. Several pulls of the matrix, with heavy pressure, across the rounded end of the operating pliers may be required to obtain enough convexity. The contoured matrix is positioned between teeth so that the convex area conforms to the desired tooth contour (Fig. 8.38A). The matrix is extended at least 1 mm beyond the prepared gingival and incisal margins. Sometimes, the matrix does not slide through or is distorted by a tight contact or preparation margin. In such instances, a wedge is lightly positioned in the gingival embrasure before the matrix is inserted. Care must be taken not to injure the interproximal tissues and induce bleeding. When the matrix is past the binding area, it may be necessary to loosen the wedge to place the strip past the gingival margin (between the wedge and margin). Then the wedge is reinserted tightly (see Fig. 8.38B).

A wedge is needed at the gingival margin to (1) hold the Mylar matrix in position, (2) provide slight separation of the teeth, and (3) prevent a gingival overhang of the composite material. A wedge must be used to separate teeth sufficiently to compensate for the thickness of the matrix if the completed restoration is to contact the adjacent tooth properly.

Several types of commercial wedges are available in assorted sizes. A triangular-shaped wedge (in cross section) is indicated for preparations with margins that are deep in the gingival sulcus. The end of a round wooden toothpick usually is an excellent wedge for preparations with margins coronal to the gingival sulcus. The wedge is kept as short as possible so as not to limit operator access to the preparation during insertion of the restorative material.

The wedge is placed, using No. 110 pliers, from the facial approach for lingual access preparations, and vice versa for facial access, just apical to the gingival margin. When isolation is accomplished with the rubber dam, wedge placement may be aided by a small amount of water-soluble lubricant on the tip of the wedge. The rubber dam is first stretched gingivally (on the side from which the wedge is inserted), then released gradually

material excess and (2) assist in the development of the appropriate axial tooth contours. The matrix usually is applied and stabilized with a wedge before application of the adhesive because it helps contain the adhesive components to the prepared tooth. Care must be taken, however, to avoid pooling of adhesive adjacent to the matrix.

A properly contoured and wedged matrix is a prerequisite for a restoration involving the entire proximal contact area, unless the adjacent tooth is missing in which case the restoration may be

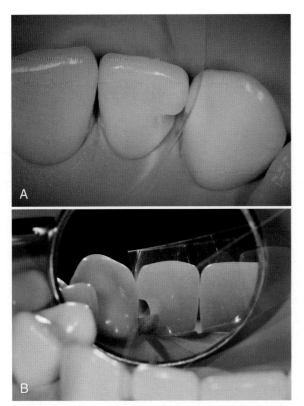

• **Fig. 8.38** Inserting and wedging Mylar strip matrix. A, Strip with concave area next to the preparation is positioned between teeth. B, Strip in position and wedge inserted. The length of the Mylar strip can be reduced as needed.

during wedge insertion (Fig. 8.39). Subsequently, a trial opening and closing of the Mylar matrix is helpful. It must open enough for access to insert the adhesive and composite and close sufficiently to ensure a proper contour. It may be necessary to shorten the wedge or insert it from the opposite embrasure to optimize access.

Placement of the Adhesive

Adhesive placement steps are accomplished with strict adherence to the manufacturer's directions for the particular adhesive system being used.

Insertion and Light Curing of the Composite

The mesial surface of a maxillary left lateral incisor is used to illustrate facial insertion of a light-cured composite (Fig. 8.40). The matrix is contoured, placed interproximally, and wedged at the gingival margin. The lingual aspect of the matrix is secured with the index finger, while the thumb reflects the facial portion out of the way (see Fig. 8.40). Light-cured materials are not dispensed until ready for use. The composite should be protected from ambient light to prevent premature polymerization. Likewise, the compule tip (when used) should be recapped immediately to prevent setting of the composite at the end of the syringe.

The composite is inserted by a hand instrument or syringe and pressed into the preparation. Most modern composites will not stick to a clean instrument, but if stickiness is perceived, the hand instrument should be thoroughly cleaned and dried. Once the desired aspect of the preparation is adequately restored, the material is polymerized. A second increment of composite is applied, if needed, to fill the preparation completely and provide a slight

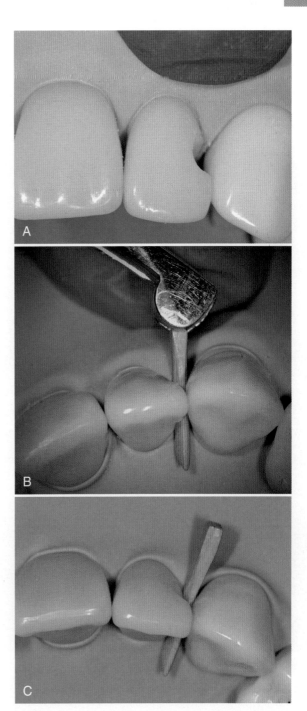

• **Fig. 8.39** Using a triangular wood wedge to expose gingival margin of large proximal preparation. A, The dam is stretched facially and gingivally with the fingertip. B, Insertion of wedge (the dam is released during wedge insertion). C, Wedge in place.

excess so that positive pressure can be applied with the matrix strip when closed. Any gross excess is removed quickly with the blade of the insertion instrument or an explorer tine before closing the matrix.

The operator closes the lingual end of the matrix over the composite and holds it with the index finger. Next, the operator pulls the matrix toward the facial direction to ensure excellent adaptation of the composite with the facial margin. Before light curing the composite, the operator closes the facial end of the matrix over the tooth with the thumb and index finger of the

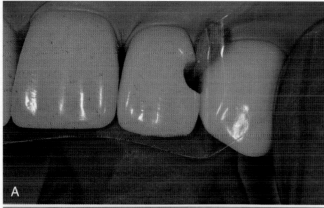

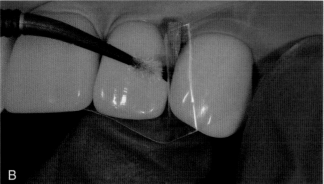

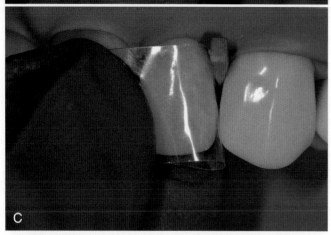

• **Fig. 8.40** Insertion of light-cured composite. A, Bonding adhesive is applied and light cured. B, The lingual aspect of the strip is secured with the index finger, while the facial portion is reflected away for access. C, After insertion of the composite, the matrix strip is closed and the material is cured through the strip.

other hand, tightening the gingival aspect of the matrix ahead of the incisal portion. The closed matrix is manually shifted so as to provide proximal contours that allow normal embrasure form and contact with the adjacent tooth, and the composite is light cured.

The composite is light cured through the matrix as directed (see Fig. 8.40C). The matrix should not be touched with the tip of the light initially because it could distort the contour of the restoration. The operator removes the index finger and light cures the lingual surface. Longer light exposures usually are required for the polymerization of dark and opaque shades. If the restoration is undercontoured, more composite can be added to the previously placed composite and light cured. No etching or adhesive is required

between layers if the surface has not been contaminated, and the oxygen-inhibited layer remains.

With large restorations, it is better to add and light cure the composite in several increments to reduce the effects of polymerization shrinkage and to ensure complete light curing in remote regions. If two adjacent preparations are present, the preparation with the least access (usually the one prepared second) is restored first. Contouring of the proximal surface of the first restoration should be completed before the second restoration is started. Because the second tooth preparation has been contaminated, it must be cleaned (usually by use of the adhesive system etchant) before bonding materials and composite are applied. During these procedures, a Mylar matrix or piece of Teflon tape should be in place to protect adjacent surfaces.

Finishing and Polishing of the Composite

Good technique and experience in inserting composites significantly reduce the amount of finishing required. Usually a slight excess of material will need to be removed so as to provide correct contours. Similar to tooth preparation rotary instruments, finishing and polishing instruments should be used according to the specific surface being finished and polished. For example, flexible discs and finishing strips are suitable for convex and flat surfaces; oval-shaped finishing burs and polishing points are more suitable for concave surfaces; and polishing cups can be used in both convex and concave surfaces.

Coarse diamond instruments may be used to efficiently remove gross excess, but leave a rough surface on the restoration and the tooth. A flame-shaped carbide finishing bur or diamond is recommended for removing excess composite on facial surfaces. Medium speed with light intermittent brush strokes and air coolant are used to create correct contours. Special fine diamond finishing instruments, 12-bladed carbide finishing burs, and abrasive finishing disks may then be used to obtain excellent surface smoothness if the manufacturers' instructions are followed. Care must be exercised with all rotary instruments so as to prevent damage to the tooth structure, especially at the gingival marginal areas.

Abrasive discs (the degree of abrasiveness depends on the amount of excess to be removed) mounted on a mandrel specific to the disc type, in a contra-angle handpiece at low speed, can be used instead of or after the finishing bur or diamond in facial surfaces and some interproximal and incisal embrasures (Fig. 8.41A). Several brands of abrasive discs are available, and most are effective when used correctly. These discs are flexible and are produced in different diameters, thicknesses, and abrasive textures. Thin discs with small diameters fit into embrasure areas easily and are especially useful in finishing and polishing accessible embrasure areas. Regardless of the type of disc chosen, discs are used sequentially from coarse to very fine grit so as to generate a smooth, final surface. The external enamel surface should act as a guide for proper contour and surface texture. A constant shifting motion aids in contouring and preventing the development of a flat surface. Final polishing is initiated after correct contours and surface texture have been achieved and is accomplished with rubber or silicone polishing instruments, diamond-impregnated polishers, polishing discs, and polishing pastes.

Excess lingual composite is removed using a round or oval-shaped, 12-bladed carbide finishing bur or finishing diamond. A smoother surface is produced using a finer round or oval carbide finishing bur (with 18–24 or 30–40 blades) or fine diamond at medium speed with air coolant and light intermittent pressure

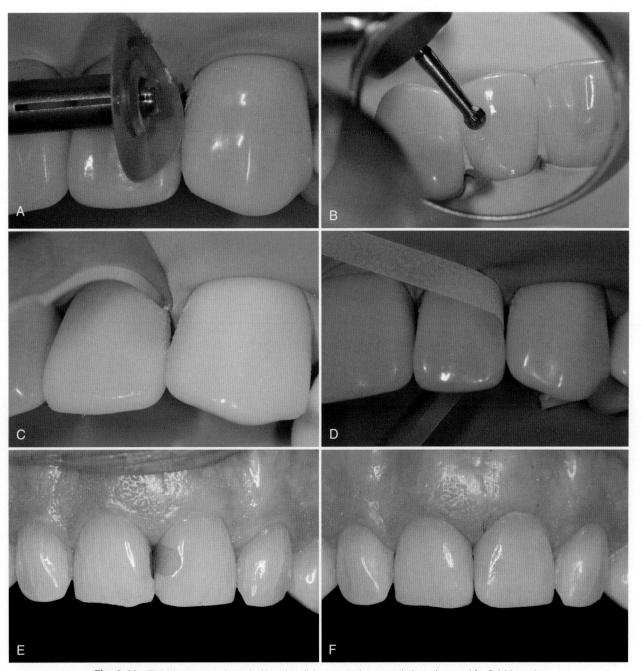

• **Fig. 8.41** Finishing composites. A, Abrasive disk mounted on mandrel can be used for finishing when access permits. B, The round carbide finishing bur is well suited for finishing lingual surfaces. C, The No. 12 surgical blade in Bard-Parker handle can be used for removing interproximal excess. D, The abrasive strip should be curved over the area to be finished. E and F, Replacement of old composite restoration, before (E) and after (F).

(see Fig. 8.41B). The appropriate size and shape depend on the amount of excess and shape of the lingual surface. Polishing is achieved with rubber polishing instruments and diamond-impregnated polishers.

Proximal surface contours and margins should be assessed visually and tactilely with an explorer and unwaxed, ultrathin dental floss. The floss is positioned apical to the gingival margin, adapted to the convex tooth surface, and slowly moved in an occlusal direction across the gingival tooth-restoration interface. The floss will begin to separate (catch, fray) as an indication of excess adhesive, composite, or other marginal defect. A No. 12 surgical blade mounted in a Bard-Parker handle (see Fig. 8.41C) is well suited for removing excess material from the gingival proximal area as it is thin and has a curved shape consistent with natural embrasure contours. The instrument should be moved from the tooth to the restoration or along the margins, using light shaving strokes, keeping a portion of the cutting edge on the external enamel surface as a guide to prevent overreduction. If a large amount of composite is removed with one stroke or in the wrong direction, it may compromise the restoration interface resulting in a marginal defect or void. Immediate correction of this area is indicated so as to limit the potential for plaque/debris accumulation resulting in additional caries and/or discoloration. Rotary instruments especially designed for this task are also available and can be used for removing excess and the creation of correct embrasure contours. Careless use of rotary instrumentation increases the risk of producing an undercontoured ("ledged") area just adjacent to the contact. All carbide instruments are made of carbon steel and may leave gray marks on the restoration. This discoloration is superficial and is removed easily during the final finishing by abrasive strips or discs (see Fig. 8.41D).

Further contouring of proximal surfaces may be completed with abrasive materials such as Sof-Lex Finishing Strips. These finishing strips have two different sizes of abrasive particles (e.g., medium and fine) impregnated on opposing ends of a polyester strip, with a small in-between area where no abrasive is present. The centrally located, nonabrasive area allows easy and safe passage of the strip through the contact area and apically to the gingival area in need of additional contouring. If the intensity of the contact is too great, then the finishing strip may need to be passed under the contact so as to position it for finishing the gingival/proximal contours. In addition, thin diamond-coated metal strips also are commercially available in various grits. Different widths of strips are available and the size of the strip must be selected based on the contouring needs of the particular situation. The strip should be curved over the restoration and tooth surface in a fashion similar to that used with a shoeshine cloth, concentrating on areas that need attention (see Fig. 8.41D). To open the lingual embrasure or round the marginal ridge, the lingual part of the strip is held against the composite with the index finger of one hand, while the other end of the strip is pulled facially with the other hand. Caution must be used so as to prevent gingival damage and/or excessive removal of the carefully created composite contours.

Finally, occlusion should be carefully checked after the rubber dam is removed, if one was used. The operator evaluates the occlusion in maximum intercuspation and eccentric movements by having the patient close on a piece of articulating paper and slide mandibular teeth over the restored area. If excess composite is present, the operator removes only a small amount at a time and rechecks with articulating paper. Usually, occlusion is adjusted until it does not differ from the original occlusion.

Instead of working sequentially by surface as previously described (facial, lingual, proximal, and occlusal), the operator may elect to work by instrument sequence—that is, contour all surfaces of the restoration by using finishing instruments first and then proceed to polish all surfaces by using the polishing instruments described. This approach improves efficiency of the overall procedure by limiting the number of times a finishing or polishing instrument is changed. Fig. 8.41E and F show before and after replacement of a Class III composite restoration.

Clinical Technique for Class IV Direct Composite Restorations

Initial Clinical Procedures

The same initial procedure considerations presented earlier are appropriate for Class IV direct composite restorations. The preoperative assessment of the occlusion is even more important for Class IV restorations because it might influence the tooth preparation extension (placing margins in noncontact areas) and retention and resistance form features (heavy occlusion requires increased retention and resistance form).

Also, proper shade selection can be more difficult for large Class IV restorations. Use of separate translucent and opaque shades of composite is often necessary. Specific information for esthetic considerations is presented in Chapters 7 and 9.

For large Class IV lesions or fractures, a preoperative impression may be taken to be used as a template for developing the restoration contours. This technique is described later in the chapter.

Tooth Preparation

Similar to the Class III preparation, the tooth preparation for a Class IV direct composite restoration involves (1) creating access to the defective structure (caries lesion, fracture, noncarious defect), (2) removing faulty structures (carious tissue removals, defective dentin and enamel, defective restoration, and base material), and (3) creating the convenience form for the restoration (Fig. 8.42A and B). The tooth preparation for large incisoproximal areas requires more attention to the retention form than that for a small Class IV defect (see Fig. 8.42C and D). If a large amount of tooth structure is missing and the restoration is in a high occlusal stress area, groove retention form may be indicated even when the preparation periphery is entirely in enamel. Also, enamel bevels can be increased in width to provide greater surface area for etching, resulting in a stronger bond between the composite and the tooth, and potentially a better esthetic result. Fig. 8.42E and F show a direct composite restoration of a Class IV defect.

The treatment of teeth with minor coronal fractures requires minimal preparation. If the fracture is confined to enamel, adequate retention usually can be attained by simply beveling the sharp cavosurface margins in the fractured area with a flame-shaped diamond instrument followed by bonding (Fig. 8.43). Regardless of its size, the extensions of the Class IV direct composite preparation are ultimately dictated by the extension of the caries lesion, fracture, or failed restoration being replaced. The outline form is prepared to include weakened, friable enamel.

Preparation of a maxillary right central incisor with a large Class IV defect and fractured mesioincisal corner, which necessitates a Class IV restoration, is illustrated in Fig. 8.44. The outline form is prepared using a round carbide bur or diamond instrument of

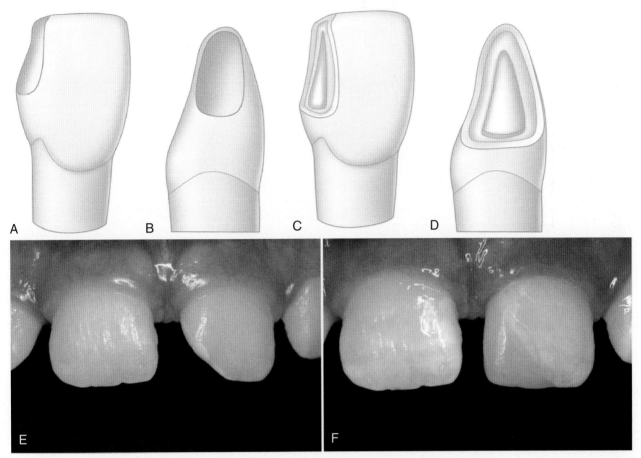

• **Fig. 8.42**   Preparation designs for Class IV (A and B), and larger preparation designs for Class IV (C and D). E and F, Direct composite restoration of a Class IV defect, before (E) and after (F).

appropriate size at high speed with air-water coolant. All weakened enamel is removed, and the initial axial wall depth is established. As with the Class III tooth preparation, the final tooth preparation steps for a Class IV tooth preparation are, when indicated, (1) selective carious tissue removal (if present), (2) pulp protection (if needed), (3) bevel placement on accessible enamel margins, and (4) final procedures of cleaning and inspecting. The operator bevels the cavosurface margin of all accessible enamel margins of the preparation. The bevel is prepared at a 45-degree angle to the external tooth surface with a flame-shaped or round diamond instrument (see Fig. 8.44A). The width of the bevel should be 0.5 to 2 mm, depending on the amount of tooth structure missing and the retention perceived necessary. The use of a scalloped, nonlinear bevel sometimes helps in masking the restoration margin.

Although retention for most Class IV direct composite restorations is provided primarily by bonding of the composite to enamel and dentin, when large incisoproximal areas are being restored, additional mechanical retention may be obtained by groove-shaped or other forms of undercuts, dovetail extensions, or a combination of these. If retention undercuts are deemed necessary, a gingival retention groove is prepared using a No. $\frac{1}{4}$ round bur. It is prepared 0.2 mm inside the DEJ at a depth of 0.25 mm (half the diameter of the No. $\frac{1}{4}$ round bur). This groove should extend the length of the gingival floor and slightly up the facioaxial and linguoaxial line angles (see Fig. 8.44B). No retentive undercut is usually needed at the incisal area, where mostly enamel exists. Fig. 8.44C illustrates the completed large Class IV tooth preparation.

Restorative Technique

Matrix Application

Most Class IV composite restorations require a matrix to confine the restorative material and to assist in the development of the appropriate axial tooth contours, except for very small incisal edge enamel fractures, which can be restored using a free-hand technique. The Mylar matrix, described previously, also can be used for most Class IV preparations, although matrix flexibility makes control difficult. This difficulty may result in an overcontoured or under-contoured restoration, open contact, or both. Also, composite material extrudes incisally, but this excess can be easily removed when contouring and finishing.

Creasing (folding) the matrix at the position of the lingual line angle helps reduce the potential undercontouring (rounding) of that area of the restoration. The matrix is positioned and wedged as described for the Class III composite technique. Gingival overhangs and open contacts are common with any matrix technique that does not employ gingival wedging. A commercially available preformed plastic or celluloid crown form is usually too thick and is not recommended as a matrix. Alternatively, a custom lingual matrix may be used for large Class IV preparations.[57] Fig. 8.45A illustrates a large defective distofacial Class IV that needs to be replaced. The shade should be selected before isolating the area and removing the restorative material (see Fig. 8.45B). Fig. 8.45C shows a lingual view of the defective restoration after a rubber dam has been placed. Before the existing restoration is removed, the lingual matrix is prepared with either a polyvinyl siloxane

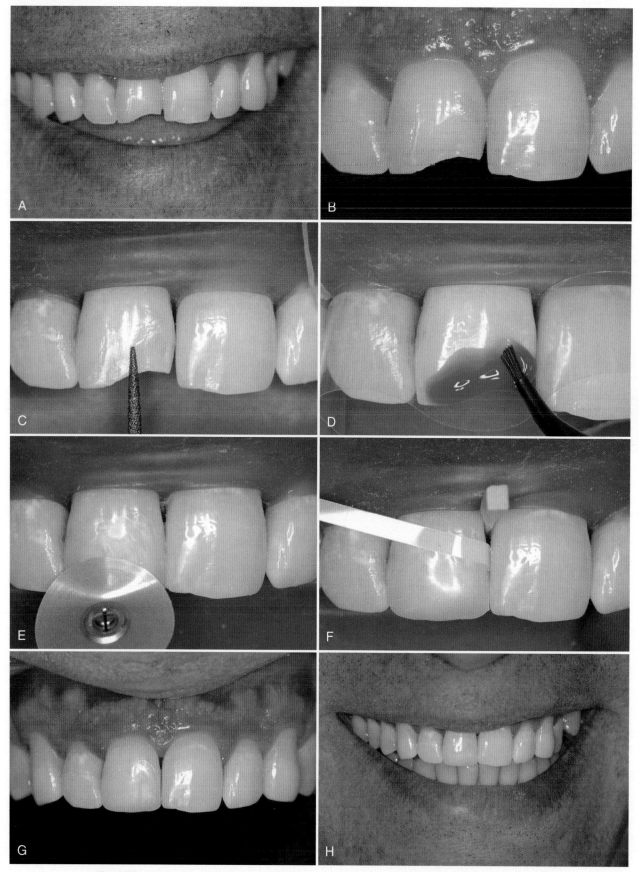

• **Fig. 8.43** Class IV tooth preparation and restoration. A, Extraoral view, minor traumatic fracture. B, Intraoral view. C, Fractured enamel is roughened with a flame-shaped diamond instrument. D, The conservative preparation is etched, while adjacent teeth are protected with Mylar strip. E and F, Contouring and polishing the composite. G, Intraoral view of the completed restoration. H, Extraoral view.

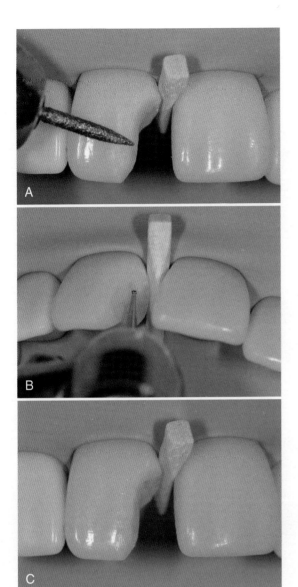

• **Fig. 8.44**   Class IV tooth preparation. A, Beveling cavosurface margin of a large Class IV preparation. B, Gingival retention groove. C, Completed Class IV tooth preparation.

impression putty or a fast-set silicone matrix material. The operator records the lingual and incisal contours of the existing restoration by using a small amount of the silicone material, thus creating a guide or index with which the new restoration will be formed. The lingual matrix also can be fabricated from a quickly inserted mockup restoration or waxed study model for more complex cases when tooth structure is missing preoperatively. When obtained, the lingual matrix is set aside until it is time to insert the composite. Fig. 8.45D-E illustrate how the lingual matrix fits with the tooth preparation.

Placement of the Adhesive

Steps for placing the adhesive are the same as previously described for the Class III composite restoration. Also, the same considerations presented previously are appropriate for whether or not the matrix is placed before or after adhesive placement. When the lingual

matrix technique is used, adhesive placement should occur before seating the matrix.

Insertion and Light Curing of Composite

After application of the adhesive, the operator inserts the composite with a hand instrument or a syringe as described earlier for Class III restorations. The composite is inserted in increments less than 2 mm thick. It is usually helpful to develop the lingual surface of the restoration first, then its body, and finally the facial surface. This approach facilitates the development of adequate anatomy with less potential for resultant excess composite material. This anatomic incremental layering also facilitates the development of adequate shade characterization, as dentin and enamel composite shades can be applied according to the structure they are replacing.

When using a properly contoured Mylar matrix, care must be taken when closing the matrix not to pull with excessive force because the soft material is extruded incisally and results in an undercontoured restoration. When this happens, composite should be added to restore proper contour and contact.

When a custom lingual matrix is used, the operator positions the lingual matrix and inserts the initial composite increment against the matrix in the lingual part of the preparation (see Fig. 8.45E). This initial increment, when polymerized, generally establishes the lingual, proximal, and incisal contours of the final restoration (see Fig. 8.45F). The operator continues to place and light cure additional increments until the desired form is obtained (see Fig. 8.45G). During these additions, color modifiers or tints may be incorporated to enhance the natural blue opalescence between tooth lobes or other subtle esthetic effects (see Fig. 8.45H). Because light-cured composites possess the advantage of an extended working time, the material can be manipulated and shaped to a considerable degree before light curing. Incremental insertion of light-cured composites also enables the clinician to layer composites with different optical properties (more opaque, darker in color, or both, to mimic dentin; and more translucent, lighter in color, or both, to mimic enamel), which can result in natural-looking composite restorations. After polymerization, the lingual matrix is removed. To ensure optimal polymerization, the operator light cures the restoration from facial and lingual directions. The final restoration is illustrated in Fig. 8.45I and J. This technique is particularly useful when the lingual contour of an existing composite restoration is to be duplicated in a new composite restoration, such as the case described. The technique facilitates the development of proper lingual, incisal, and proximal forms, reducing the need for contouring of the restoration.

Finishing and Polishing of the Composite

Finishing and polishing the Class IV composite are similar to the technique described for a Class III composite but usually more difficult. The primary differences are the involvement of the incisal angle and incisal edge of the tooth and an extended facial surface in large Class IV restorations. Finishing and polishing these sections of the restoration require similar procedural steps but close assessment of the incisal edge length and thickness, as well as of the facial macroanatomy and microanatomy of the tooth being restored. The functional demands of anterior guidance will have a direct influence on the final position and contours of the lingual surface and incisal edge. Careful adjustment and refinement will prevent excessive occlusal loading of the restoration and limit the potential for premature clinical failure. The facial, lingual, and proximal areas are finished and polished as described previously.

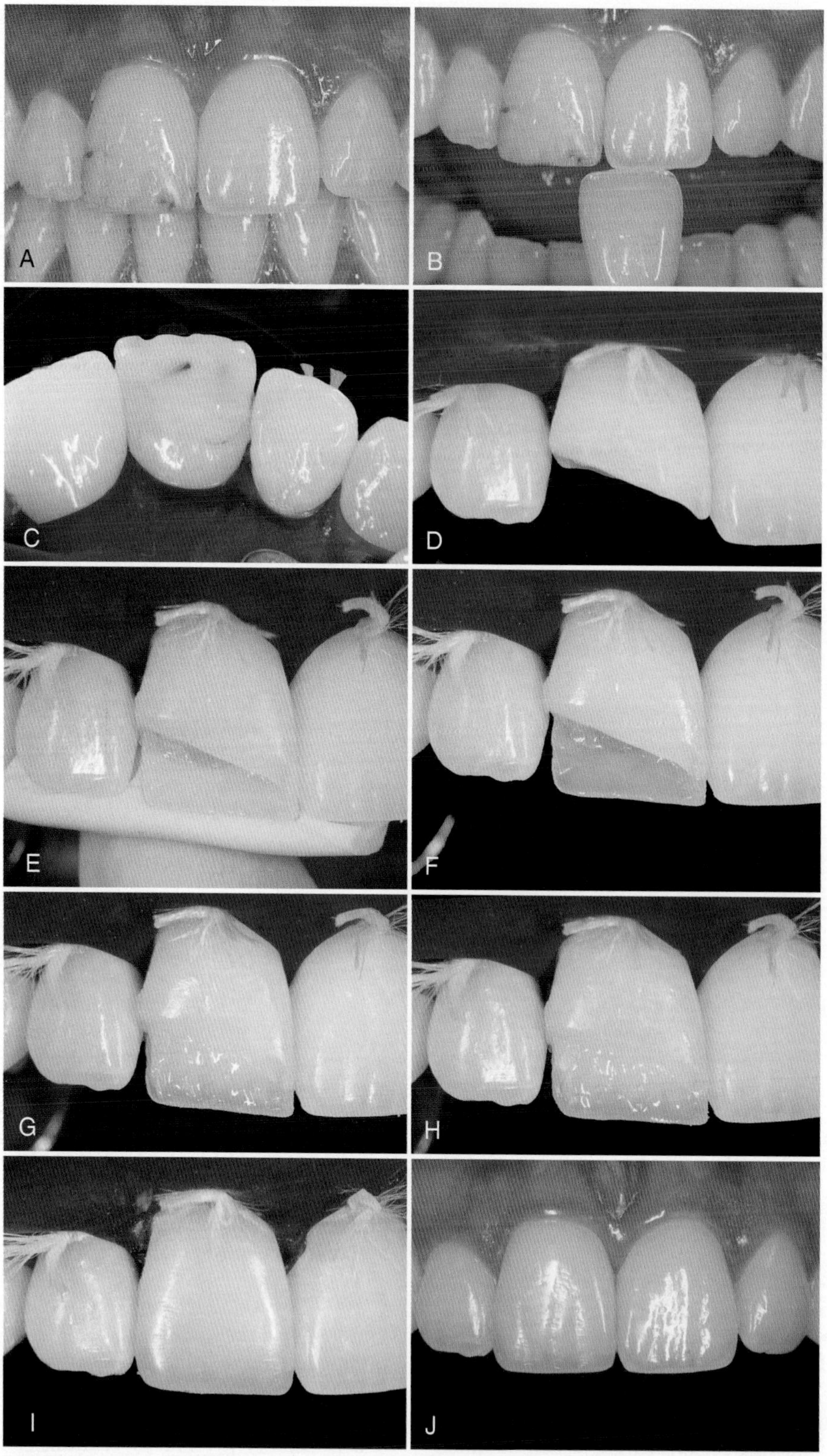

• **Fig. 8.45** Custom lingual matrix. A, Facial preoperative view. B, Preoperative shade determination. C, Lingual preoperative view after placement of the rubber dam. D, The old composite material is removed, and a conservative enamel bevel is placed. E, The lingual matrix obtained before tooth preparation is positioned and guides the application of the first lingual composite layer. F, The lingual composite layer determines the future contours of the restoration; note the intrinsic material translucency. Custom lingual matrix. G, The dentin buildup can be made directly against the lingual enamel; the clinician can visualize the whole tooth shape and place dentin with appropriate thickness and relation to the incisal edge. H, Color modifier or tint blue material is applied between the dentin lobes and slightly below the incisal edge to simulate the blue natural opalescence. I, View of the completed restoration (with second enamel layer placed on the buccal surface), after finishing. J, Facial postoperative view. (Courtesy of Dr. Didier Dietschi.)

Clinical Technique for Class V Direct Composite Restorations

Initial Clinical Procedures

The same initial procedure considerations presented for Class III restorations apply for Class V restorations, except for occlusal evaluation, which is not required for Class V restorations unless there are concerns about occlusal factors as an etiology for noncarious cervical lesions. During shade selection, it should be noted that the tooth is typically darker and more opaque in the cervical third. Isolation may be achieved by a rubber dam and No. 212 retainer or with a cotton roll and retraction cord.

Tooth Preparation

Class V tooth preparations, by definition, are located in the gingival one third of the facial and lingual tooth surfaces. Because of esthetic considerations, composites most frequently are used for the restoration of cervical caries lesions in anterior and premolar teeth. Numerous factors, including esthetics, nature of lesion and substrate characteristics, caries activity, caries risk, access to the lesion, and moisture control must be taken into consideration in material selection.

Because many Class V restorations involve root surfaces, at least on their cervical margins, careful consideration should be given to the choice of restorative material. The use of materials other than composite (i.e., that do not require adhesive placement) should be considered when factors that may compromise the performance of composite restorations are present. These factors include decreased salivary function, decreased patient motivation or ability for home care, increased difficulty in adequately isolating the operating area, and increased difficulty in performing the operative procedure because of the patient's physical or medical problems. Despite these concerns, the use of composite as a restorative material for cervical caries lesions predominates in areas of esthetic concern.

Similar to the Class III and IV preparations, tooth preparation for a Class V direct composite restoration involves (1) creating access to the defect (caries lesion, noncarious defect), (2) removing the defect (caries lesion, defective dentin and enamel, defective restoration and base material), and (3) creating the convenience form for the restoration. The tooth preparation for large Class V lesions or defects may require more attention to retention form than for conservative Class V defects, especially when little enamel is available for bonding. Areas of hypermineralized (sclerotic) dentin also may require special attention, as these respond differently to bonding than areas with normal dentin.[58-60] Enamel bevels are typically used on the occlusal/incisal margins of the preparation, while at the cervical margin, bevels are usually not recommended because of the absence of enamel in this area. Class V tooth preparations will vary slightly, depending on the type and extension of the defect being restored.

The objective of the *Class V tooth preparation for small or moderate lesions or defects that do not extend onto the root surface* is to restore the lesion or defect as conservatively as possible. No effort is made to prepare the walls as butt joints, and usually no secondary retentive features are incorporated. The lesion or defect is conservatively prepared resulting in a form that may have a divergent wall configuration and an axial surface that usually is not uniform in depth (Fig. 8.46A and B). Small or moderate Class V tooth preparations are ideal for small enamel defects or small primary caries lesions (Fig. 8.47A). These include decalcified and hypoplastic areas located in the cervical third of the teeth, which may be restored for esthetic reasons. The typical outline form for a Class V lesion in enamel is shown in Fig. 8.48.

After the usual preliminary procedures, the initial tooth preparation is accomplished with a round diamond or carbide bur, eliminating the entire enamel lesion or defect. The preparation is extended into dentin only when the defect warrants such extension. No effort is made to prepare 90-degree cavosurface margins. If carious tissue remains in dentin, it is selectively removed with a round bur or spoon excavator. Usually, this preparation technique will result in a slightly beveled enamel margin. If deemed necessary, the enamel margin can be further beveled. The completed restoration is shown in Fig. 8.47B.

An example of a small cervical caries lesion was presented in Fig. 8.49A, which illustrates a path of a decalcified enamel lesion (in enamel only) having a broken, rough surface that extends mesially or distally from the cavitated lesion (or failing existing restoration). After preparation of the cavitated lesion (or failing restoration), the margins of the preparation are extended to include these areas of decalcification by using a round diamond or bur to prepare the cavosurface margin in the form of a chamfer, extended in the enamel only to a depth that removes the defect. A completed preparation of this type was illustrated in Fig. 8.49B.

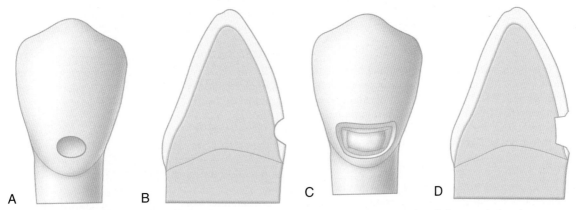

A   B   C   D

• **Fig. 8.46**   Preparation designs for Class V (A and B) initial composite restorations (primary caries) and larger preparation designs for Class V (C and D) restorations.

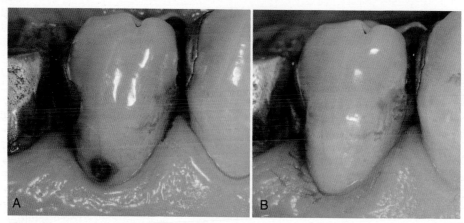

• **Fig. 8.47** Class V tooth preparation. A, Small cavitated Class V lesion. B, Restored with composite resin. (Courtesy Vilhelm G. Ólafsson.)

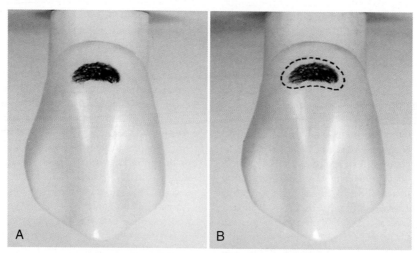

• **Fig. 8.48** A, Class V caries. B, Typical outline form.

Small or moderate Class V tooth preparations also are used to restore noncarious cervical lesions (NCCLs). As noted elsewhere in this textbook, NCCLs have a multifactorial etiology in which contributing factors include intrinsic and/or extrinsic erosion, abrasion, abfraction, and/or biocorrosion.[61] If the causative factors are not eliminated, these lesions tend to progress and enlarge with time. When they are detected (Fig. 8.50A), the operator first must decide, with input from the patient, whether the area needs to be restored. This decision is based on the following considerations.

Caries

If active caries is present, caries management should be initiated. For the incipient lesion, treatment may consist of application of a topical fluoride or resin-based materials including adhesives and resin infiltration materials. Inactive lesions may be monitored and kept unrestored indefinitely, but sometimes these can be esthetically unsatisfactory. (Most NCCLs are not carious.)

Gingival Health

If the defect is determined to be contributing to the development of gingival inflammation and/or gingival recession (i.e., plaque retention, mechanical trauma due to poor tooth contours), the defect should be restored.

Esthetics

If the defect is in an esthetically critical position, the patient may elect to have the area restored with a tooth-colored restoration.

Sensitivity

If the defect is very sensitive, application of an adhesive or desensitizing agent may reduce or eliminate the sensitivity, at least temporarily. Continuing sensitivity may require restoration of the area.

Pulp Protection

If the defect is very large and deep pulpally, its restoration may be indicated to avoid further defect development that may cause a pulpal exposure.

Tooth Strength

If the defect is very large or deep, the strength of the tooth at the cervical area may be compromised. Placement of a bonded restoration reduces the potential for further progression of the defect and may restore some of the lost strength.

Periodontal therapy with gingival grafts also may be considered as a treatment option for these exposed root surfaces being used solo or combined with the restorative therapy.

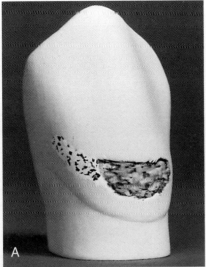

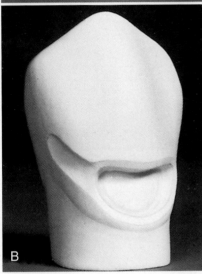

• **Fig. 8.49** A, Decalcified area extending mesially from cavitated Class V lesion. B, Completed Class V preparation with conservative mesial extension.

The tooth preparation for a *Class V NCCL* usually requires only surface debridement of any exposed dentin and roughening/beveling all enamel margins with a diamond instrument[22] (see Fig. 8.50B). Often, because of the inherent form of an abraded or eroded lesion, further preparation of root surface cavosurface margins is not needed. The completed preparation with etched enamel is shown in Fig. 8.50C.

In *Class V tooth preparation for large lesions or defects that extend onto the root surface* (Fig. 8.51A), the gingival aspect of the preparation form is similar to that described in Chapter 10 for a Class V amalgam restoration. The features of the preparation include a 90-degree cavosurface margin. Groove retention form usually is not necessary but may be used if retention of the restoration is a concern. The enamel margins are prepared using the same design described for small or moderate Class V tooth preparations, that is, with a conservative enamel bevel. This preparation design is indicated for the replacement of an existing, defective Class V restoration that initially used a conventional preparation or for a large, new caries lesion. The large Class V preparation initially exhibits 90-degree cavosurface margins (that subsequently can be beveled when in enamel) and an axial wall that may or may not

be uniform in depth (see Fig. 8.47C and D). The axial depth into dentin is determined by the selective removal of the carious tissue. Many of these larger preparations are a combination of beveled enamel margins and 90 degree root surface cavosurface margins. A completed large Class V preparation extending onto the root surface is illustrated in Fig. 8.52.

To initiate the preparation, a tapered fissure carbide bur (No. 271) or similarly shaped diamond is used at high speed with air-water spray. If interproximal or gingival access is limited, an appropriately sized round bur or diamond may be used. When a tapered fissure bur or diamond is used, the handpiece is maneuvered to maintain the bur's long axis perpendicular to the external surface of the tooth during preparation of the outline form, which should result in 90-degree cavosurface margins. At this initial tooth preparation stage, the extensions in every direction are to sound tooth structure. Deeper areas of the caries lesion or old restoration may still remain in the axial wall at this point in the procedure (see Fig. 8.51B). Carious tissue remaining on this initial axial wall is selectively removed during the final stage of tooth preparation (see Fig. 8.51C). Old restorative material remaining may or may not be removed according to the concepts stated previously. When the desired distal extension is obtained, the instrument is moved mesially, incisally (occlusally), and gingivally for indicated extensions, while maintaining proper depth and the instrument's long axis perpendicular to the external surface. The axial wall should follow the original contour of the facial or lingual surface, which is convex outward mesiodistally and sometimes occlusogingivally. The outline form extension of the mesial, distal, occlusal (incisal), and gingival walls is dictated by the extent of the caries lesion, defect, or old restorative material indicated for replacement (sometimes the new material abuts a still satisfactory old restoration).

All of the external preparation walls of a Class V tooth preparation are visible when viewed from a facial position (outwardly divergent walls). Final tooth preparation consists of the following steps: (1) removing the remaining carious dentin or old restorative material (if indicated) on the axial wall; (2) applying a base, only if necessary, as discussed previously in this chapter; and (3) beveling the enamel margins and adding groove retention, if indicated. The bevel on the enamel margin is accomplished with a flame-shaped or round diamond instrument, resulting in an angle approximately 45 degrees to the external tooth surface, and prepared to a width of at least 0.5 mm depending on the preparation size and esthetic considerations. A completed Class V preparation is shown in Fig. 8.53.

Occasionally, a tooth surface that normally is smooth has a pit in the enamel (Fig. 8.54A). Most unusual pit faults in enamel are restored best with the preparation design described for small or moderate Class V defects. For such a preparation for an unusual pit fault, the outline form (extensions and depth) is dictated by the extent of the fault or caries lesion. Faults existing entirely in enamel are prepared with an appropriately sized round diamond instrument by merely eliminating the defect leaving a flared enamel margin (see Fig. 8.54B). Adequate retention is obtained by bonding. When the defect includes carious dentin, the tissue is selectively removed as indicated.

Restorative Technique

In most cases no matrix is needed for Class V restorations because the contour can be controlled as the composite restorative material is being inserted. However, clear precontoured Class V matrix materials are available if the operator prefers a matrix-assisted technique.

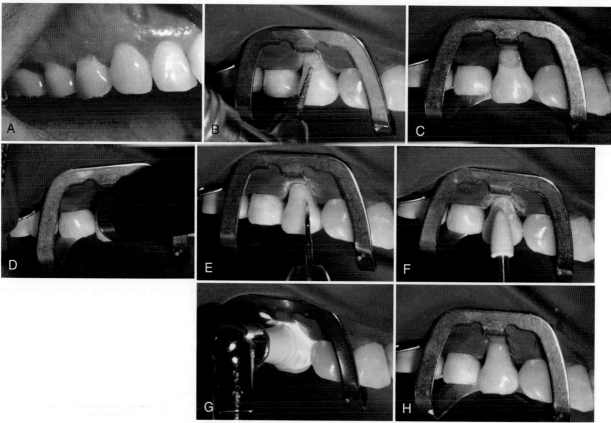

• **Fig. 8.50** Class V tooth preparation for abrasion and erosion lesions. A, Preoperative notched lesion. B, Beveling the enamel margin. C, Completed preparation with etched enamel. Restoration of a noncarious cervical lesion. D, After application of bonding adhesive, composite resin is inserted incrementally and the restorative material is light cured. Finishing and polishing. E, Flame-shaped finishing bur removing excess and contouring. F and G, Rubber polishing point (F) and aluminum oxide polishing paste (G) used for final polishing. H, Completed restoration.

Placement of the Adhesive

The techniques for acid etching of the involved tooth structure and placement of the adhesive are the same as previously described in this chapter.

Insertion and Light Curing of the Composite

The composite can be inserted with a hand instrument or syringe. Composites and RMGIs are recommended for Class V restorations. A light-cured material is recommended for most Class V preparations because of the extended working time and control of contour before polymerization. Careful placement allows for minimal need of rotary finishing. These features are particularly valuable when restoring large preparations or preparations with margins located on cementum because rotary instrumentation can easily damage the contiguous tooth structure and/or compromise the marginal integrity of the restoration.

After bonding procedures (according to manufacturer's instructions), it is recommended to insert the composite incrementally with a hand instrument or syringe. The number and position of the increments depend on the size and depth of the preparation. For large and deep preparations, an incremental technique is recommended. Deep preparations with retentive undercuts are usually filled with at least two axially placed increments with minimal contact on the occlusal/incisal and gingival walls. The operator should avoid placing increments that connect to both occlusal/incisal walls and gingival walls, or mesial and distal walls, simultaneously, so as to minimize polymerization shrinkage stresses. Regardless of the technique used, before light curing the last increment that defines the contour of the restoration, the material is shaped as close to the final contour as possible. An explorer or blade of a composite instrument, or a flat No. 2 sable brush, is useful in removing excess material from the cervical margin and obtaining the final contour. As noted earlier, clear plastic matrices are available for Class V composite restorations and can be used if the operator prefers a matrix-assisted approach rather than a free-hand technique. The light source is applied for polymerization (see Fig. 8.50D). The restoration should require very little finishing.

Finishing and Polishing of the Composite

When excess composite is present, a flame-shaped carbide finishing bur or diamond is recommended for removing excess composite on the facial surface (see Fig. 8.50E). Medium speed with light intermittent brush strokes and an air coolant are used for finishing the restoration to the correct contours. Final polishing is achieved with a rubber polishing point (see Fig. 8.50F) or cup, diamond-impregnated polisher, and sometimes a polishing paste (see Fig. 8.50G and H).

For some locations, abrasive discs, as stated earlier, mounted on an appropriate mandrel in an angled handpiece at low speed can be used (see Fig. 8.41A). The degree of abrasiveness depends

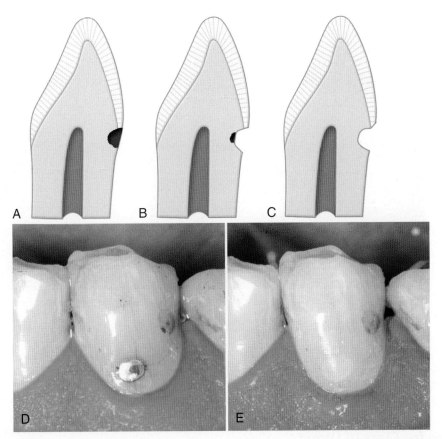

• **Fig. 8.51**   Class V tooth preparation. A, Lesion extending onto root surface. B, Initial tooth preparation with 90-degree cavosurface margins and axial wall depth of 0.75 mm. C, Remaining infected dentin excavated, and incisal enamel margin beveled. D and E, Direct composite restoration of three Class V lesions with composite resin, before (D) and after (E). (D and E, Courtesy Vilhelm G. Ólafsson.)

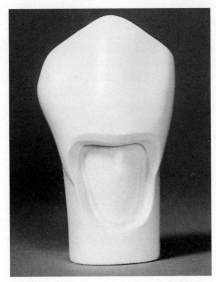

• **Fig. 8.52**   Completed Class V tooth preparation extending onto the root; the incisal margin is beveled; the root portion has a retention groove for increased retention. Retention grooves on the incisal aspect are rarely required and are shown here for illustration purposes only.

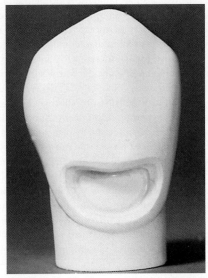

• **Fig. 8.53**   Completed large Class V preparation. A retention groove on the incisal aspect is rarely required and is shown here for illustration purposes only.

on the amount of excess to be removed. The external enamel surface should act as a guide for a proper contour, preventing the development of a flat surface contour.

Rotary instruments should be used carefully in gingival locations (especially on margins adjacent to the root surface) to prevent inadvertent and undesirable damage to tooth structure and periodontal tissues. Finely pointed rotary instruments (finishing burs or diamonds) are difficult to use to remove gingival margin excess. Because of the convexity that typically exists in this area, a more rounded rotary instrument (a fine diamond) may remove the excess

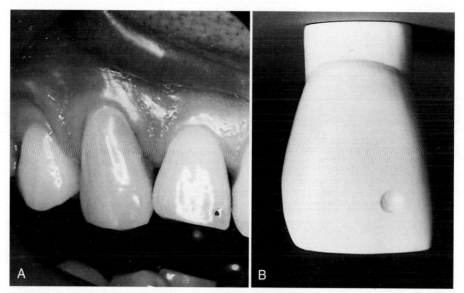

• **Fig. 8.54** A, Faulty pit on the facial surface of the maxillary incisor. B, Tooth preparation for an enamel pit defect.

with less potential to damage the unprepared root surface. Likewise, abrasive discs used on the root surface may cause ditching of the cementum, if not used correctly. Fig. 8.51D and E show restoration of a Class V lesion with composite resin.

Clinical Technique for Class VI Direct Composite Restorations

One of the most conservative indications for a directly placed posterior composite is a small faulty developmental pit located on a cusp tip. Fig. 8.55A is an example of a Class VI defect on the facial cusp tip of a maxillary premolar. The typical Class VI tooth preparation should be as small in diameter and as shallow in depth as possible. The faulty pit is entered with an appropriate round bur or diamond oriented perpendicular to the surface and extended pulpally to eliminate the lesion (see Fig. 8.55B). Visual examination and probing with an explorer often reveal that the fault is limited to enamel because the enamel in this area is quite thick. If a faulty restoration or extensive caries lesion is present on the cusp tip, a round bur of appropriate size is used to remove the faulty restoration or any remaining carious tissue. Stains that appear through the translucent enamel should be removed; otherwise they may be seen after the composite restoration is completed. Some undermined, but not friable, enamel may be left and bonded to the composite in areas that are not associated with a functional occlusal contact.

The conservative preparation is restored with composite following adhesion protocols, incremental placement and light curing of the composite material, and finishing and polishing. The final Class VI restoration should, as with any other type of restoration, restore the tooth to its ideal anatomy relative to tooth contours, occlusion, esthetics, and surface characteristics (Fig. 8.55C).

Clinical Technique for Glass Ionomer Restorations

Glass ionomers possess the favorable quality of releasing fluoride when exposed to the oral environment.[62,63] These materials also have been shown to "recharge" with fluoride when exposed to fluoride from various sources.[64] These properties theoretically may indicate the use of glass ionomer restorations in patients with high caries risk especially when esthetic demands are minimal. (See Chapter 13 for types of glass ionomers.)

Because of their limited strength and wear resistance, glass ionomers are indicated generally for the restoration of low-stress areas (not for typical Class I, II, or IV restorations), where caries activity potential is of significant concern. In addition to being indicated for root-surface caries lesions in Class V locations, slotlike preparations in Class II or III cervical locations (not involving the proximal contact) may be restored with glass ionomers, if access permits.

The restoration of caries lesions on the roots of patients with active caries is the primary indication for the use of a glass ionomer as a restorative material. Cervical defects of idiopathic erosion or abrasion origin (or any combination) also may be indications for restoration with glass ionomers, if esthetic demands are not critical. The tooth preparations for either of these clinical indications are the same as previously described for composite restorations (see Figs. 8.50, 8.51, and 8.52), except bevels are rarely used. Gingival recession and interproximal gingival inflammation also increase the risk of developing caries on proximal root surfaces. Gingival recession sometimes provides access to this type of caries lesion from the facial or lingual direction, allowing a slot preparation to be used. The same slot preparation design used for amalgam is used for glass ionomers. (The reader is referred to the sections on slot preparations in Chapter 10 and to Fig. 8.56 for specific details.) With the exception of the matrix used (if needed), slot preparations for Class II and III restorations are restored in a single increment and in a similar manner to a Class V preparation.

Most conventional glass ionomer systems require mild dentin conditioning to remove the smear layer, effecting improved adhesion of the glass ionomer to dentin. To condition dentin, a mild acid, such as 10% polyacrylic acid, is applied to the preparation according to manufacturer's instructions, followed by rinsing and removal of excess water, leaving dentin slightly moist. Some modified glass ionomer materials may have a substantial resin component

Most current restorative GICs and RMGIs available may be finished and polished immediately after light or complete chemical/dual curing. When the material has set, the matrix, if used, is removed and the gross excess is shaved away with a No. 12 surgical blade. Finishing should be accomplished as much as possible with hand instruments, while striving to preserve the smooth surface that occurs on setting. If rotary instrumentation is needed, care must be taken not to dehydrate the surface of the restoration. Also, flexible abrasive discs used with a lubricant can be effective. A fine-grit aluminum oxide polishing paste applied with a prophy cup is used to impart a smooth surface. Fig. 8.57 shows a conventional glass ionomer restoration with a modified matrix band. The Tofflemire matrix band was adapted around the tooth and an access hole was created using a No. 2 round bur. The conventional glass ionomer material was then injected into the preparation through the access hole until the material filled into the preparation space and excess material extruded through the access. Sufficient time was allowed for the material to set before finishing the surface with a No. 12 blade.

Repairing Composite Restorations

If a patient presents with a composite restoration that has a localized defect, a repair usually can be made.[65,66] Easily accessible areas may be roughened with a diamond; the area is etched; an appropriate adhesive is applied; and the composite is inserted, finished, and polished. If the defect is not easily accessible, a tooth preparation must be created that exposes the defective area, and a matrix may be necessary; the adhesive and the composite are then placed.

If a void is detected immediately after insertion of a composite restoration, but before contouring is initiated, more composite may be added directly to the void area. These materials bond because the void area has an oxygen-inhibited surface layer that permits composite additions. If any contouring has occurred, however, the oxygen-inhibited layer may have been removed or contaminated, and the area must be "refreshed" by a brief etch/rinse cycle and reapplication of the adhesive prior to the addition of more composite.

Common Problems: Causes and Potential Solutions

This section lists the causes of common problems associated with some composite restorations and potential solutions to those problems.

White Line Adjacent to the Enamel Margin

A white line adjacent to the enamel margin of a direct composite restoration is usually caused by a microseparation (space) between the composite and the tooth or a microfracture within the marginal enamel, either of which is typically caused by:
- Inadequate etching and bonding of the affected area
- High-intensity, fast light curing resulting in excessive polymerization stresses
- Traumatic finishing techniques
  Potential solutions are as follows:
- Use atraumatic finishing techniques (e.g., light intermittent pressure)
- Use proper polymerization techniques (see Chapter 6)

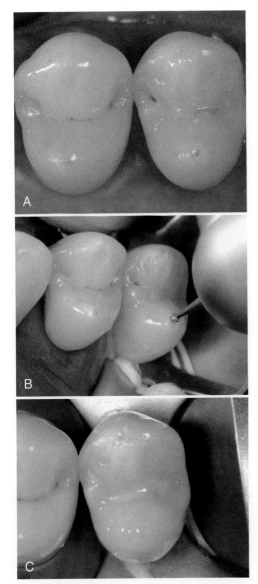

• **Fig. 8.55** Class VI tooth preparation for composite restoration. A, Class VI preparation on the lingual cusp tip of the maxillary premolar. B, Entry with small round bur or diamond. C, Final composite restoration and sealant placed in the occlusal groove. (Courtesy Vilhelm G. Ólafsson.)

and require a special primer to facilitate bonding. Each system should be used strictly according to the manufacturer's specific instructions.

Encapsulated glass ionomers, for triturator mixing, or paste–paste materials are greatly preferred to powder and liquid materials. Such systems optimize and simplify the mixing procedure. Glass ionomer material should be placed into the preparation in slight excess and quickly shaped with a composite instrument. Clear plastic cervical matrices also are available for providing contour to the restoration. If a conventional glass ionomer is used, a thin coat of light-cured, resin-based coating is placed on the surface immediately after placement to limit dehydration and resultant disintegration ("cracking") of the restoration during the initial setting phase. Newer glass ionomers may be more resistant to dehydration; however, careful attention to manufacturer's instructions for restoration placement is paramount.

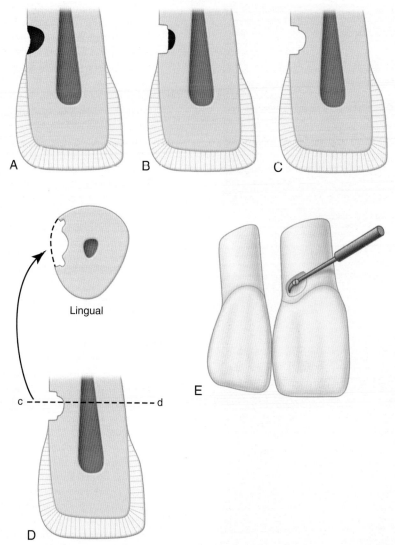

• **Fig. 8.56** Class III tooth preparation for a lesion entirely on the root surface. A, Mesiodistal longitudinal section illustrating a caries lesion. B, Initial tooth preparation. C, Tooth preparation with infected caries dentin removed. D, Retention grooves shown in longitudinal section. Transverse section through plane *cd* illustrates the contour of the axial wall and the direction of the facial and lingual walls. E, Preparing the retention form to complete the tooth preparation.

Some of these small defects may not be clinically relevant and can be monitored over time for signs of marginal deterioration. However, often they need to be managed, as follows:
- Seal the gap with adhesive
- Conservatively remove the defect and re-restore

Voids

Causes of voids include the following:
- Spaces left between increments during insertion (lamination defects)
- Adherence of composite to hand instruments during placement in the preparation, which is related to the previous item
  Potential solutions are as follows:
- Use a more careful restorative technique
- Repair marginal voids by preparing the area and re-restoring

Weak or Missing Proximal Contacts (Class II, III, and IV)

Causes of weak and missing proximal contacts are as follows:
- Inadequately contoured matrix band
- Inadequate wedging, preoperatively and during the composite insertion
- Matrix band movement during composite insertion or matrix band not in direct contact with the adjacent proximal surface
- A circumferential matrix being used when restoring only one contact
- Adherence of composite to hand instruments during insertion and resultant pulling away from matrix contact area
- Matrix band too thick
  Potential solutions include the following:
- Contour the matrix material properly
- Have the matrix in contact with the adjacent tooth

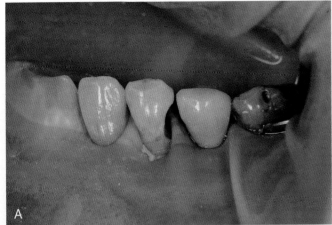

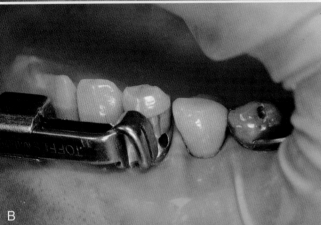

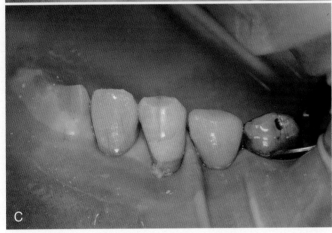

• **Fig. 8.57** Conventional glass ionomer restoration with a modified matrix band is shown before (A), matrix band adapted with access hole prepared into the band (B), and immediately postop (C). (Courtesy Vilhelm G. Ólafsson.)

• Use adequate preoperative and insertion wedging technique
• Use a matrix system that places the matrix only around the proximal surface to be restored
• Use a hand instrument to hold the matrix against the adjacent tooth while curing incremental placements of composite
• Be careful with insertion technique

Inaccurate Shade

Causes of an incorrect shade matching include the following:
• Inappropriate operatory lighting while selecting the shade
• Selection of shade after the tooth has dehydrated
• Shade tab not matching the actual composite shade
• Wrong shade utilized
  Potential solutions are as follows:
• Use natural light when selecting shade, if possible
• Select the shade before isolating the tooth
• Place some of the selected shade on the tooth and cure preoperatively to verify shade selection
• Do not shine the operator light (overhead or attached to operator loupes) directly on the area during shade selection
• Understand the typical zones of different shades for natural teeth

Contouring and Finishing Problems

Causes of contouring and/or finishing problems are as follows:
• Inadequate anatomic tooth form (overcontour or undercontour of the restoration)
• Improper selection of finishing instrument and improper composite placement
• Iatrogenic damage to adjacent unprepared tooth structure
  Potential solutions include the following:
• Have a proper matrix with appropriate axial and line angle contours
• Create embrasures to match the adjacent tooth embrasure form
• Remember the outline form of the preparation
• Use a properly shaped finishing instrument for the area being contoured
• Be careful with the use of rotary instruments to avoid adversely affecting the structure of the adjacent tooth or teeth
• Do not use rotary instruments that leave roughened surfaces

Postoperative Sensitivity

Postoperative sensitivity can result from the following:
• Aggressive tooth preparation (inadequate use of coolant systems, inefficient cutting instruments)
• Incorrect use of adhesive systems
• Not using a liner/base when indicated
• Formation of microgaps secondary to excessive polymerization shrinkage stress, particularly in situations of high C-factor
• Aggressive finishing of the restoration
  Potential solutions include the following:
• Use careful tooth preparation technique
• Use liners/bases properly
• Use adhesive systems properly
• Use a desensitizer solution after dentin acid etching
• Insert and polymerize the composite material properly
• Finish the composite restoration properly

Summary

Direct composite restorations are increasingly used because of the benefits accrued from adhesive bonding to tooth structure, esthetic qualities, and almost universal clinical use. When accomplished properly, a composite restoration is able to provide excellent service for many years. Composite is the material of choice for most Class III and IV restorations and most esthetically demanding Class V restorations. When used in Class I and II restorations, however, composites are more difficult and sensitive to the operator's technique than are amalgam restorations. To achieve optimal clinical results, the operating site must be free from contamination, and the bonding technique and composite handling must be meticulous in every way.

References

1. Bowen RL, inventor: Dental filling material comprising vinyl-silane treated fused silica and a binder consisting of the reaction product of bis-phenol and glycidyl acrylate. US patent 3,06,112. 1962 11/27/1962.

2. Bowen RL: Adhesive bonding of various materials to hard tooth tissues. 3. Bonding to dentin improved by pre-treatment and the use of surface-active comonomer. *J Dent Res* 44(5):903–905, 1965.

3. Bowen RL: Adhesive bonding of various materials to hard tooth tissues. II. Bonding to dentin promoted by a surface-active comonomer. *J Dent Res* 44(5):895–902, 1965.

4. Brudevold F, Buonocore M, Wileman W: A report on a resin composition capable of bonding to human dentin surfaces. *J Dent Res* 35(6):846–851, 1956.

5. Casagrande L, Seminario AT, Correa MB, et al: Longevity and associated risk factors in adhesive restorations of young permanent teeth after complete and selective caries removal: a retrospective study. *Clin Oral Investig* 2016.

6. Demarco FF, Correa MB, Cenci MS, et al: Longevity of posterior composite restorations: not only a matter of materials. *Dent Mater* 28(1):87–101, 2012.

7. Opdam N: Clinical trials: Randomization, completeness of data and restoration longevity. *Dent Mater* 32(4):489–491, 2016.

8. Opdam NJ, van de Sande FH, Bronkhorst E, et al: Longevity of posterior composite restorations: a systematic review and meta-analysis. *J Dent Res* 93(10):943–949, 2014.

9. Opdam NJ, Bronkhorst EM, Cenci MS, et al: Age of failed restorations: A deceptive longevity parameter. *J Dent* 39(3):225–230, 2011.

10. Ausiello P, De Gee AJ, Rengo S, et al: Fracture resistance of endodontically-treated premolars adhesively restored. *Am J Dent* 10(5):237–241, 1997.

11. Liberman R, Ben-Amar A, Gontar G, et al: The effect of posterior composite restorations on the resistance of cavity walls to vertically applied occlusal loads. *J Oral Rehabil* 17(1):99–105, 1990.

12. Ahovuo-Saloranta A, Hiiri A, Nordblad A, et al: Pit and fissure sealants for preventing dental decay in the permanent teeth of children and adolescents. *Cochrane Database Syst Rev* (3):CD001830, 2004.

13. Simonsen RJ: Retention and effectiveness of a single application of white sealant after 10 years. *J Am Dent Assoc* 115(1):31–36, 1987.

14. Swift EJ, Jr: The effect of sealants on dental caries: a review. *J Am Dent Assoc* 116(6):700–704, 1988.

15. Handelman SL, Leverett DH, Espeland MA, et al: Clinical radiographic evaluation of sealed carious and sound tooth surfaces. *J Am Dent Assoc* 113(5):751–754, 1986.

16. Mertz-Fairhurst EJ, Smith CD, Williams JE, et al: Cariostatic and ultraconservative sealed restorations: six-year results. *Quintessence Int (Berl)* 23(12):827–838, 1992.

17. Beauchamp J, Caufield PW, Crall JJ, et al: Evidence-based clinical recommendations for the use of pit-and-fissure sealants: a report of the American Dental Association Council on Scientific Affairs. *J Am Dent Assoc* 139(3):257–268, 2008.

18. Bendinskaite R, Peciuliene V, Brukiene V: A five years clinical evaluation of sealed occlusal surfaces of molars. *Stomatologija* 12(3):87–92, 2010.

19. Simonsen RJ: Preventive resin restorations (II). *Quintessence Int Dent Dig* 9(2):95–102, 1978.

20. Simonsen RJ: Preventive resin restorations (I). *Quintessence Int Dent Dig* 9(1):69–76, 1978.

21. Simonsen RJ: Preventive resin restorations: three-year results. *J Am Dent Assoc* 100(4):535–539, 1980.

22. Perdigao J: Dentin bonding-variables related to the clinical situation and the substrate treatment. *Dent Mater* 26(2):e24–e37, 2010.

23. Peumans M, De Munck J, Mine A, et al: Clinical effectiveness of contemporary adhesives for the restoration of non-carious cervical lesions. A systematic review. *Dent Mater* 30(10):1089–1103, 2014.

24. Peumans M, De Munck J, Van Landuyt KL, et al: Eight-year clinical evaluation of a 2-step self-etch adhesive with and without selective enamel etching. *Dent Mater* 26(12):1176–1184, 2010.

25. Van Meerbeek B, Yoshihara K, Yoshida Y, et al: State of the art of self-etch adhesives. *Dent Mater* 27(1):17–28, 2011.

26. Ritter AV, Swift EJ, Jr: Current restorative concepts of pulp protection. *Endod Topics* 5(1):41–48, 2003.

27. Hilton TJ, Ferracane JL, Mancl L: Comparison of CaOH with MTA for direct pulp capping: a PBRN randomized clinical trial. *J Dent Res* 92(7 Suppl):16S–22S, 2013.

28. Nair PN, Duncan HF, Pitt Ford TR, et al: Histological, ultrastructural and quantitative investigations on the response of healthy human pulps to experimental capping with Mineral Trioxide Aggregate: a randomized controlled trial. 2008. *Int Endod J* 42(5):422–444, 2009.

29. Goracci G, Mori G: Scanning electron microscopic evaluation of resin-dentin and calcium hydroxide-dentin interface with resin composite restorations. *Quintessence Int (Berl)* 27(2):129–135, 1996.

30. Tantbirojn D, Pfeifer CS, Braga RR, et al: Do low-shrink composites reduce polymerization shrinkage effects? *J Dent Res* 90(5):596–601, 2011.

31. Versluis A, Douglas WH, Cross M, et al: Does an incremental filling technique reduce polymerization shrinkage stresses? *J Dent Res* 75(3):871–878, 1996.

32. Versluis A, Tantbirojn D: Theoretical considerations of contraction stress. *Compend Contin Educ Dent Suppl* 25:S24–S32, quiz S73, 1999.

33. Versluis A, Tantbirojn D, Pintado MR, et al: Residual shrinkage stress distributions in molars after composite restoration. *Dent Mater* 20(6):554–564, 2004.

34. Ikemi T, Nemoto K: Effects of lining materials on the composite resins shrinkage stresses. *Dent Mater J* 13(1):1–8, 1994.

35. Tolidis K, Nobecourt A, Randall RC: Effect of a resin-modified glass ionomer liner on volumetric polymerization shrinkage of various composites. *Dent Mater* 14(6):417–423, 1998.

36. van Dijken JW, Pallesen U: Clinical performance of a hybrid resin composite with and without an intermediate layer of flowable resin composite: a 7-year evaluation. *Dent Mater* 27(2):150–156, 2011.

37. Browning WD: The benefits of glass ionomer self-adhesive materials in restorative dentistry. *Compend Contin Educ Dent Suppl* 27(5):308–314, quiz 15-6, 2006.

38. Loguercio AD, Alessandra R, Mazzocco KC, et al: Microleakage in class II composite resin restorations: total bonding and open sandwich technique. *J Adhes Dent* 4(2):137–144, 2002.

39. Ritter AV: Posterior composites revisited. *J Esthet Restor Dent* 20(1):57–67, 2008.

40. Van Ende A, De Munck J, Van Landuyt K, et al: Effect of bulk-filling on the bonding efficacy in occlusal class I cavities. *J Adhes Dent* 18(2):119–124, 2016.

41. Francis AV, Braxton AD, Ahmad W, et al: Cuspal flexure and extent of cure of a bulk-fill flowable base composite. *Oper Dent* 40(5):515–523, 2015.

42. Fronza BM, Rueggeberg FA, Braga RR, et al: Monomer conversion, microhardness, internal marginal adaptation, and shrinkage stress of bulk-fill resin composites. *Dent Mater* 31(12):1542–1551, 2015.

43. Leprince JG, Palin WM, Vanacker J, et al: Physico-mechanical characteristics of commercially available bulk-fill composites. *J Dent* 42(8):993–1000, 2014.

44. van Dijken JW, Pallesen U: A randomized controlled three year evaluation of "bulk-filled" posterior resin restorations based on stress decreasing resin technology. *Dent Mater* 30(9):e245–e251, 2014.

45. Wirsching E, Loomans BA, Klaiber B, et al: Influence of matrix systems on proximal contact tightness of 2- and 3-surface posterior composite restorations in vivo. *J Dent* 39(5):386–390, 2011.

46. da Costa J, McPharlin R, Hilton T, et al: Effect of heat on the flow of commercial composites. *Am J Dent* 22(2):92–96, 2009.

47. Elsayad I: Cuspal movement and gap formation in premolars restored with preheated resin composite. *Oper Dent* 34(6):725–731, 2009.

48. Froes-Salgado NR, Silva LM, Kawano Y, et al: Composite pre-heating: effects on marginal adaptation, degree of conversion and mechanical properties. *Dent Mater* 26(9):908–914, 2010.

49. Wagner WC, Aksu MN, Neme AM, et al: Effect of pre-heating resin composite on restoration microleakage. *Oper Dent* 33(1):72–78, 2008.

50. Daronch M, Rueggeberg FA, Hall G, et al: Effect of composite temperature on in vitro intrapulpal temperature rise. *Dent Mater* 23(10):1283–1288, 2007.

51. Rueggeberg FA, Daronch M, Browning WD, et al: In vivo temperature measurement: tooth preparation and restoration with preheated resin composite. *J Esthet Restor Dent* 22(5):314–322, 2010.

52. Chuang SF, Jin YT, Liu JK, et al: Influence of flowable composite lining thickness on Class II composite restorations. *Oper Dent* 29(3):301–308, 2004.

53. Olmez A, Oztas N, Bodur H: The effect of flowable resin composite on microleakage and internal voids in class II composite restorations. *Oper Dent* 29(6):713–719, 2004.

54. Opdam NJ, Bronkhorst EM, Loomans BA, et al: 12-year survival of composite vs. amalgam restorations. *J Dent Res* 89(10):1063–1067, 2010.

55. Sanares AM, Itthagarun A, King NM, et al: Adverse surface interactions between one-bottle light-cured adhesives and chemical-cured composites. *Dent Mater* 17(6):542–556, 2001.

56. Swift EJ, Jr, May KN, Jr, Wilder AD, Jr: Effect of polymerization mode on bond strengths of resin adhesive/cement systems. *J Prosthodont* 7(4):256–260, 1998.

57. Dietschi D: Free-hand bonding in the esthetic treatment of anterior teeth: creating the illusion. *J Esthet Dent* 9(4):156–164, 1997.

58. Ritter AV, Heymann HO, Swift EJ, Jr, et al: Clinical evaluation of an all-in-one adhesive in non-carious cervical lesions with different degrees of dentin sclerosis. *Oper Dent* 33(4):370–378, 2008.

59. Tay FR, Pashley DH: Resin bonding to cervical sclerotic dentin: a review. *J Dent* 32(3):173–196, 2004.

60. Yoshiyama M, Sano H, Ebisu S, et al: Regional strengths of bonding agents to cervical sclerotic root dentin. *J Dent Res* 75(6):1404–1413, 1996.

61. Grippo JO, Simring M, Coleman TA: Abfraction, abrasion, biocorrosion, and the enigma of noncarious cervical lesions: a 20-year perspective. *J Esthet Restor Dent* 24(1):10–23, 2012.

62. Mount GJ: Adhesion of glass-ionomer cement in the clinical environment. *Oper Dent* 16(4):141–148, 1991.

63. Swift EJ, Jr: Effects of glass ionomers on recurrent caries. *Oper Dent* 14(1):40–43, 1989.

64. Markovic D, Petrovic BB, Peric TO: Fluoride content and recharge ability of five glass-ionomer dental materials. *BMC Oral Health* 8:21, 2008.

65. Dias WR, Ritter AV, Swift EJ, Jr: Repairability of a packable resin-based composite using different adhesives. *Am J Dent* 16(3):181–185, 2003.

66. Teixeira EC, Bayne SC, Thompson JY, et al: Shear bond strength of self-etching bonding systems in combination with various composites used for repairing aged composites. *J Adhes Dent* 7(2):159–164, 2005.

9

Additional Conservative Esthetic Procedures

HARALD O. HEYMANN, ANDRÉ V. RITTER

Significant improvements in tooth-colored restorative materials and adhesive techniques have resulted in numerous conservative esthetic treatment possibilities. Although restorative dentistry is a blend of art and science, conservative esthetic dentistry truly emphasizes the artistic component. As Goldstein stated, "Esthetic dentistry is the art of dentistry in its purest form."[1] As with many forms of art, conservative esthetic dentistry provides a means of artistic expression that feeds on creativity and imagination. Dentists find performing conservative esthetic procedures enjoyable, and patients appreciate the immediate esthetic improvements rendered, often without the need for local anesthesia.

One of the greatest assets a person can have is a smile that shows beautiful, natural teeth (Fig. 9.1). Children and teenagers are especially sensitive about unattractive teeth. When teeth are discolored, malformed, crooked, or missing, often the person makes a conscious effort to avoid smiling and tries to "cover up" his or her teeth. Correction of these types of dental problems can produce dramatic changes in appearance, which often result in improved confidence, personality, and social life. The restoration of a smile is one of the most appreciated and gratifying services a dentist can render. The positive psychologic effects of improving a patient's smile often contribute to an improved self-image and enhanced self-esteem. These improvements make conservative esthetic dentistry particularly gratifying for the dentist and represent a new dimension of dental treatment for patients.

This chapter presents conservative esthetic procedures in the context of their clinical applications. The principles and clinical steps involved in adhesive bonding for the treatment alternatives discussed in this chapter are similar to those described in other chapters in this textbook. Only specific conservative esthetic clinical procedures or variations from previously described techniques are presented in this chapter.

Artistic Elements

Regardless of the result desired, certain basic artistic elements must be considered to ensure an optimal esthetic result. In conservative esthetic dentistry, these elements include the following:
- Shape or form
- Symmetry and proportionality
- Position and alignment
- Surface texture

- Color
- Translucency

Some or all of these elements are common to virtually every conservative esthetic dental procedure; a basic knowledge and understanding of these artistic elements is required to attain esthetic results consistently.

Shape or Form

The shape of teeth largely determines their esthetic appearance. To achieve optimal dental esthetics, it is imperative that natural anatomic forms be achieved. A basic knowledge of normal tooth anatomy is fundamental to the success of any conservative esthetic dental procedure.

When viewing the clinical crown of an incisor from a facial (or lingual) position, the crown outline is trapezoidal. Subtle variations in shape and contour produce very different appearances, however. Rounded incisal angles, open incisal and facial embrasures, and softened facial line angles typically characterize a youthful smile. A smile characteristic of an older individual having experienced attrition secondary to aging typically exhibits incisal embrasures that are more closed and incisal angles that are more prominent (i.e., less rounded). Frequently, minor modification of existing tooth contours, sometimes referred to as *cosmetic contouring*, can effect a significant esthetic change (see section Alterations of Shape of Natural Teeth). Reshaping enamel by rounding incisal angles, opening incisal embrasures, and reducing prominent facial line angles can produce a more youthful appearance (Fig. 9.2).

Significant generalized esthetic changes are possible when treating all anterior teeth (and occasionally the first premolars) visible in the patient's smile. This fact is particularly true when placing full-coverage facial restorations such as veneers (see section Veneers). With this treatment method, the dentist can produce significant changes in tooth shapes and forms to yield a variety of different appearances.

Although less extensive, restoring an individual tooth rather than all anterior teeth simultaneously may require greater artistic ability. Generalized restoration of all anterior teeth with full facial veneers affords the dentist significant control of the contours generated. When treating an isolated tooth, however, the success of the result is determined largely by how well the restored tooth esthetically matches the surrounding natural teeth. The contralateral tooth to the one being restored should be examined closely for subtle characterizing features such as developmental depressions, embrasure form, prominences, or other distinguishing characteristics of form. A high degree of realism must be reproduced artfully to achieve optimal esthetics when restoring isolated teeth or areas.

Illusions of shape also play a significant role in dental esthetics. The border outline of an anterior tooth (i.e., facial view) is primarily two dimensional (i.e., length and width). The third dimension of depth is crucial, however, in creating illusions, especially those of apparent width and length.

Prominent areas of contour on a tooth typically are highlighted with direct illumination, making them more noticeable, whereas areas of depression or diminishing contour are shadowed and less conspicuous. By controlling the areas of light reflection and shadowing, full facial coverage restorations (in particular) can be esthetically contoured to achieve various desired illusions of form.

The apparent size of a tooth can be changed by altering the position of facial prominences or heights of contour without changing the actual dimension of the tooth. Compared with normal tooth contours (Fig. 9.3A), a tooth can be made to appear narrower by positioning the mesiofacial and distofacial line angles closer together (see Fig. 9.3B). Developmental depressions also can be positioned closer together to enhance the illusion of narrowness. Similarly, greater apparent width can be achieved by positioning the line angles and developmental depressions further apart (see Fig. 9.3C).

Although more difficult, the apparent length of teeth also can be changed by illusion. Compared with normal tooth contours (Fig. 9.4A), a tooth can be made to appear shorter by emphasizing the horizontal elements such as gingival perikymata and by positioning the gingival height of contour further incisally (see Fig. 9.4B). Slight modification of the incisal area, achieved by moving the incisal height of contour further gingivally, also enhances the illusion of a shorter tooth. The opposite tenets are true for increasing the apparent length of a tooth. The heights of contour are moved farther apart incisogingivally, and vertical elements such as developmental depressions are emphasized (see Fig. 9.4C).

Used in combination, these illusionary techniques are particularly valuable for controlling the apparent dimension of teeth in procedures that result in an actual increased width of teeth, such as in diastema (i.e., space) closure (see section Correction of Diastemas). By contouring the composite additions in such a way that the original positions of the line angles are maintained, the increased widths of the restored teeth are less noticeable (Fig. 9.5). If full facial coverage restorations are placed in conjunction with a diastema

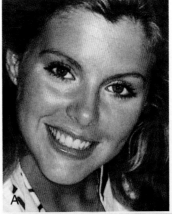
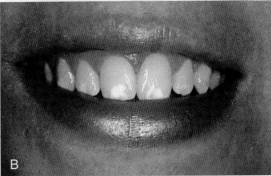
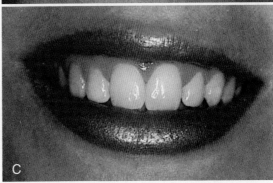

• **Fig. 9.1** Examples of conservative esthetic procedures. A, A beautiful radiant smile is one of the greatest assets a person can have. B, The appearance of this aspiring young model was marred by hypocalcified areas of maxillary anterior teeth. C, A simple treatment consisted of removing part of the discolored enamel, acid etching the preparations, and restoring with direct-composite partial veneers. (Courtesy Dr. C.L. Sockwell.)

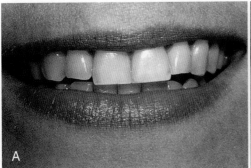
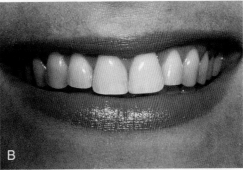

• **Fig. 9.2** Cosmetic contouring. A, Anterior teeth before treatment. B, By reshaping teeth, a more youthful appearance is produced.

closure, vertical elements can be enhanced and horizontal features deemphasized to control further the apparent dimension of teeth.

Symmetry and Proportionality

The overall esthetic appearance of a human smile is governed largely by the symmetry and proportionality of the teeth that constitute the smile. Asymmetric teeth or teeth that are out of proportion to the surrounding teeth disrupt the sense of balance and harmony essential for optimal esthetics. Assuming that the patient's teeth are aligned normally (i.e., rotations or faciolingual

positional defects are not present), dental symmetry can be maintained if the sizes of contralateral teeth are equivalent. A dental caliper should be used in conjunction with any conservative esthetic dental procedure that would alter the mesiodistal dimension of teeth. This recommendation is particularly true for procedures such as diastema closure or other procedures involving augmentation of proximal surfaces with composite. By first measuring and recording the widths of the interdental space and the teeth to be augmented, the appropriate amount of contour to be generated with composite resin addition can be determined (Fig. 9.6). In this manner, symmetric and equal tooth contours can be generated (see section Correction of Diastemas). When dealing with restorations involving the midline, particular attention also must be paid to the incisal and gingival embrasure forms; the mesial contours of both central incisors must be mirror images of one another to ensure an optimally symmetric and esthetic result.

In addition to being symmetric, anterior teeth must be in proper proportion to one another to achieve maximum esthetics. The quality of proportionality is relative and varies greatly, depending on other factors (e.g., tooth position, tooth alignment, arch form, configuration of the smile). One long-accepted theorem of the relative proportionality of maxillary anterior teeth typically visible in a smile involves the concept of *the golden proportion*.[2] Originally formulated as one of Euclid's elements, this theorem has been relied on through the ages as a geometric basis for proportionality in the beauty of art and nature.[3] On the basis of this formula, a smile, when viewed from the front, is considered to be esthetically pleasing if each tooth in that smile (starting from the midline) is approximately 60% of the *apparent* mesiodistal width of the tooth immediately mesial to it. The exact proportion of the distal tooth to the mesial tooth is 0.618 (Fig. 9.7A). These recurring esthetic dental proportions are based on the *apparent* mesiodistal

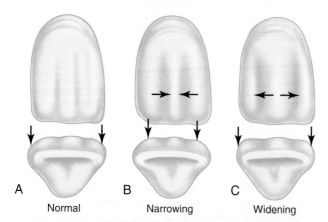

• **Fig. 9.3** Creating illusions of width. A, Normal width. B, A tooth can be made to appear narrower by positioning mesial and distal line angles closer together and by more closely approximating developmental depressions. C, Greater apparent width is achieved by positioning line angles and developmental depressions farther apart.

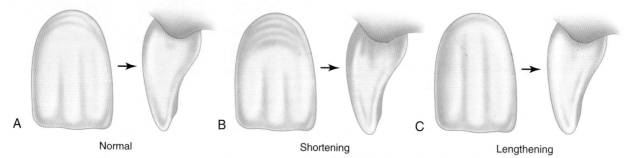

• **Fig. 9.4** Creating illusions of length. A, Normal length. B, A tooth can be made to appear shorter by emphasizing horizontal elements and by positioning the gingival height of contour farther incisally. C, The illusion of length is achieved by moving the gingival height of contour gingivally and by emphasizing vertical elements, such as developmental depressions.

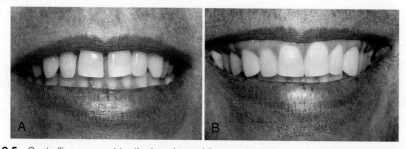

• **Fig. 9.5** Controlling apparent tooth size when adding proximal dimension. A, Teeth before treatment. B, By maintaining original positions of the facial line angles (see areas of light reflection), increased widths of teeth after composite augmentations are less noticeable.

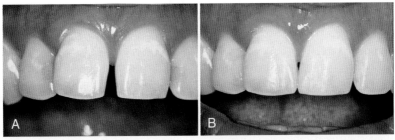

• **Fig. 9.6** Diastema closure. A, Teeth before composite additions. B, Symmetrical and equal contours are achieved in the final restorations.

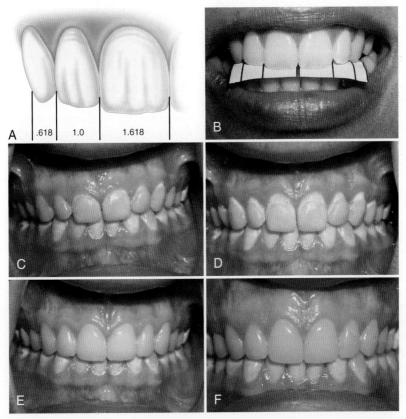

• **Fig. 9.7** Tooth proportions. A, The rule of the golden proportion. The exact ratios of proportionality. B, The anterior teeth of this patient are in golden proportion to one another. C, Width-to-length ratios. Preoperative view reveals width-to-length ratio of 1 to 1. D, Following a periodontal surgical crown lengthening procedure, a more esthetic width-to-length ratio of 0.80 exists. E, Final result with etched porcelain veneers. A width-to-length ratio of 0.80 is maintained. F, A 7-year postoperative view reveals a stable and esthetic long-term result.

width of teeth when viewed straight on and not the *actual* mesiodistal width of individual teeth. An example of an esthetically pleasing smile that meets the golden proportion can be seen in Fig. 9.7B.

Although the golden proportion is not the absolute determinant of dental esthetics, it does provide a practical and proven guide for establishing proportionality when restoring anterior teeth, especially if these teeth are considered long. However, according to a study by Preston, only 17% of the population naturally exhibits smiles that meet the golden proportion as the recurring esthetic dental proportion.[4] According to a survey of dentists by Ward, a recurring esthetic dental proportion of 70% (as opposed to 61.8% as with the golden proportion) is preferred when teeth are of normal dimension.[5]

Little scientific information is available regarding the proper proportions of individual anterior teeth. A study by Sterrett et al. revealed that the average width-to-length ratio for a maxillary central incisor in men was 0.85 and in women was 0.86.[6] The actual width-to-length ratios found in this same study for maxillary lateral incisors in men and women were 0.76 and 0.79, respectively. Another study by Magne et al. reported average width-to-length ratios of 0.87 for worn maxillary central incisors and 0.78 for unworn maxillary central incisors.[7] An accepted theorem for achieving esthetically pleasing central incisors maintains that the ideal width-to-length ratio should be 0.75 to 0.80.[8] This ratio represents the ideal proportions needed to optimize the esthetic result and can help guide the treatment planning process. Considering the range of recommended width-to-length ratios, 0.80 seems to be a good benchmark for achieving optimally esthetic results when restoring maxillary central incisors and 0.75 for maxillary lateral incisors.

A good example can be seen in Fig. 9.7C–F. Because of altered passive eruption, this teenaged patient exhibited a preoperative width-to-length ratio of 1 to 1 for her maxillary central incisors (see Fig. 9.7C). She revealed excessive gingival tissues relative to the display of her anterior teeth. To achieve a more esthetic appearance, it was determined that a width-to-length ratio of 0.80 would be desirable. After a periodontal surgical crown-lengthening procedure, a more esthetic width-to-length ratio of 0.80 was attained (see Fig. 9.7D). After placement of eight porcelain veneers for the treatment of fluorosis discoloration, the same 0.80 width-to-length ratio can be seen (see Fig. 9.7E). A 7-year postoperative photograph reveals the long-term esthetic result (see Fig. 9.7F).

Because central incisors are the dominant focal point in dental composition, the dentist must avoid narrow, elongated, or short-and-wide contours. Adequate treatment planning and a fundamental knowledge of the importance of the ideal width-to-length ratios can optimize the final esthetic outcome. The importance of interdisciplinary treatment involving orthodontics, periodontics, or both cannot be underestimated.

Position and Alignment

The overall harmony and balance of a smile depend largely on proper position of teeth and their alignment in the arch. Malposed or rotated teeth disrupt the arch form and may interfere with the apparent relative proportions of teeth. Orthodontic treatment of such defects always should be considered, especially if other positional or malocclusion problems exist in the mouth. If orthodontic treatment is either impractical or unaffordable, however, minor positional defects often can be treated with composite augmentation or full facial veneers indirectly made from composite or porcelain. Only problems that can be treated conservatively without significant alteration of the occlusion or gingival contours of teeth should be treated in this manner.

Minor rotations can be corrected by reducing the enamel in the area of prominence and augmenting the deficient area with composite resin (Fig. 9.8A and B). Care must be taken to restrict all recontouring of prominent areas to enamel. If the rotation is to be treated with an indirectly fabricated composite or porcelain veneer, an intraenamel preparation is recommended, with greater reduction provided in the area of prominence. This preparation allows subsequent restoration to appropriate physiologic contours.

Malposed teeth are treated in a similar manner. Teeth in mild linguoversion can be treated by augmentation with full facial veneers placed directly with composite or made indirectly from processed composite or porcelain (see Fig. 9.8C and D). Care must be exercised in maintaining physiologic gingival contours that do not impinge on tissue or result in an emergence profile of the restoration that is detrimental to gingival health. A functional incisal edge should be maintained by appropriate contouring of the restoration (an excessively thick incisal edge should be avoided). If the occlusion allows, limited reduction of enamel on the lingual aspect can be accomplished to reduce the faciolingual dimension of the incisal portion of the tooth. Lingual areas participating in protrusive functional contact should not be altered, however. Individual teeth that are significantly displaced facially (i.e., facioversion) are best treated orthodontically.

Surface Texture

The character and individuality of teeth are determined largely by their surface texture and existing characteristics. Realistic restorations closely mimic the subtle areas of stippling, concavity, and convexity that are typically present on natural teeth. Teeth in young individuals characteristically exhibit significant surface characterization, whereas teeth in older individuals tend to possess a smoother surface texture caused by abrasional wear. Even in older patients, however, restorations that are devoid of surface characterizations are rarely indicated.

The surfaces of natural teeth typically break up light and reflect it in many directions. Consequently, anatomic features (e.g., developmental depressions, prominences, facets, perikymata) should be examined closely and reproduced to the extent that they are present on the surrounding surfaces. The restored areas of teeth should reflect light as in the unrestored adjacent surfaces. In addition, as alluded to earlier, by controlling areas of light reflection and shadowing, various desired illusions also can be created.

Color

Color is the most complex and least understood artistic element. It is an area in which numerous interdependent factors exist, all of which contribute to the final esthetic outcome of the restoration. Although complex, a basic knowledge of color is imperative to producing consistently esthetic restorations (see Chapter 7).

Three fundamental elements of color are *hue, value,* and *chroma.* Hue is the intrinsic quality or shade of the color. Value refers to the relative lightness or darkness of a hue. It is determined by the amount of white or black in a hue. Chroma is the intensity of any

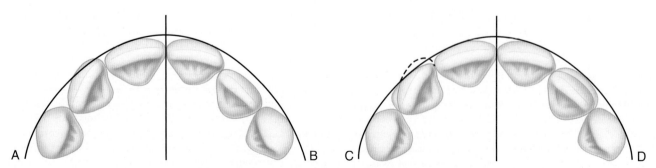

• **Fig. 9.8** Position and alignment. A, A minor rotation is first treated by reducing enamel in the area of prominence. B, The deficient area is restored to proper contour with composite. C, Maxillary lateral incisor is in slight linguoversion. D, Restorative augmentation of facial surface corrects malposition.

particular hue. Some current shade guides are based first on value because of the importance of this element of color.

Dentists also must understand the coloration of natural teeth to select the appropriate shades of restorative materials accurately and consistently. Teeth typically are composed of a multitude of colors. A gradation of color usually occurs from the gingival region to the incisal region, with the gingival region being typically darker because of thinner enamel. Use of several different shades of restorative material may be required to restore a tooth esthetically. Exposed root surfaces are particularly darker (i.e., dentin colored) because of the absence of overlying enamel. In most individuals, canines are slightly darker than are incisors.

Young individuals with thick enamel characteristically exhibit lighter teeth. Individuals with darker complexions usually appear to have lighter teeth because of the contrast that exists between teeth and the surrounding facial structures. Women can enhance the apparent lightness of their teeth simply by using a darker shade of makeup or lipstick. By increasing the contrast between teeth and the surrounding facial tissue, the illusion of lighter teeth can be created.

Color changes associated with aging also occur, primarily owing to wear. As the facial enamel is worn away, the underlying dentin becomes more apparent, resulting in a darker tooth. Incisal edges are often darker because of the thinning of enamel or the exposure of dentin because of normal attrition. Cervical areas also tend to darken because of abrasion.

An understanding of normal tooth coloration enhances the dentist's ability to create a restoration that appears natural. Several clinical factors also must be considered, however, to enhance the color-matching quality of the restoration. Many shade guides for composite materials are inaccurate. Not only are they often composed of a material dissimilar to that of the composite, but they also do not take into consideration color changes that occur from batch to batch or changes caused by aging of the composite. Accurate shade selection is best attained by applying and curing a small amount of the composite restorative material in the area of the tooth that may need restoration. Shade selection should be determined before isolating teeth so that color variations that can occur as a result of drying and dehydration of teeth are avoided.

Problems in color perception also complicate selection of the appropriate shade of restorative material. Various light sources produce different perceptions of color. This phenomenon is referred to as *metamerism*.[9] The color of the surrounding environment influences what is seen in the patient's mouth. Color perception also is influenced by the physiologic limitations of the dentist's eye. On extended viewing of a particular tooth site, eyes experience color fatigue, resulting in a loss of sensitivity to yellow-orange shades.[7] By looking away at a blue object or background (i.e., the complementary color), the dentist's eyes quickly recover and are able to distinguish subtle variations in yellow-orange hues again. Because of the many indirect factors that influence color perception, it is recommended that the dentist, the assistant, and especially the patient all be involved in shade selection.

Translucency

Translucency is another factor that affects the esthetic quality of the restoration. The degree of translucency is related to how deeply light penetrates into the tooth or restoration before it is reflected outward. Normally, light penetrates through enamel into dentin before being reflected outward (Fig. 9.9A); this affords the realistic esthetic vitality characteristic of normal, unrestored teeth. Shallow penetration of light often results in loss of esthetic vitality. This phenomenon is a common problem encountered when treating severely intrinsically stained teeth such as teeth affected by tetracycline with direct or indirect veneers. Although opaque resin media can mask the underlying stain, esthetic vitality is usually lost because of reduced light penetration (see Fig. 9.9B). Indirect veneers of processed composite or porcelain fabricated to include inherent opacity also may have this problem.

Illusions of translucency also can be created to enhance the realism of a restoration. Color modifiers (also referred to as *tints*) can be used to achieve apparent translucency and tone down bright stains or to characterize a restoration. Fig. 9.10 shows a case in which the maxillary right central incisor with intrinsic yellow staining caused by trauma to the tooth warranted restoration. When bleaching treatments were unsuccessful because of calcific metamorphosis, a direct composite veneer was used in this patient. After an intraenamel preparation and acid etching, a violet color modifier (the complementary color of yellow) was applied to the prepared facial surface to reduce the brightness and intensity of the underlying yellow tooth. Additionally, a mixture of gray and violet color modifiers was used to simulate vertical areas of translucency. The final restoration is shown in Fig. 9.10B. Color modifiers also can be incorporated in the restoration to simulate maverick colors, to check lines, or to surface spots for further characterization. Color modifiers always should be placed within a composite restoration, not on its surface.

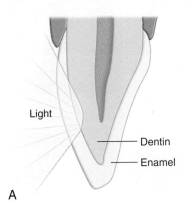

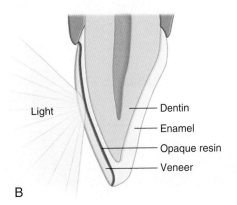

A

B

• **Fig. 9.9** Translucency and light penetration. A, Light normally penetrates deeply through enamel and into dentin before being reflected outward. This affords realistic esthetic vitality. B, Light penetration is limited by opaquing resin media under veneers. Esthetic vitality is compromised.

Clinical Considerations

Although an understanding of basic artistic elements is imperative to successfully placing esthetic restorations, certain clinical considerations must be addressed concomitantly to ensure the overall quality of the restoration. In addition to being esthetic, restorations must be functional. Dawson stated, "Esthetics and function go hand in hand. The better the esthetics, the better the function is likely to be and vice versa."[10]

The occlusion always must be assessed before any conservative esthetic procedure. Anterior guidance, in particular, must be maintained and occlusal harmony ensured when treating areas involved in occlusion. Another requirement of all conservative esthetic restorations is that they possess physiologic contours that promote good gingival health. Particular care must be taken in all treatments to finish the gingival areas of the restoration adequately and to remove any gingival excess of material. Emergence angles of the restorations must be physiologic and not impinge on gingival tissue.

Conservative Alterations of Tooth Contours and Contacts

Many unsightly tooth contours and diastemas can be corrected or the appearance greatly improved by several conservative methods.

Often these procedures can be incorporated into routine restorative treatment. The objective is to improve esthetics and yet preserve as much healthy tooth structure as possible, consistent with the acceptable occlusion and health of surrounding tissue. These procedures include reshaping natural teeth, correcting embrasures, and closing diastemas.

Alterations of Shape of Natural Teeth

Some esthetic problems can be corrected conservatively without the need for tooth preparation and restoration. Consideration always should be given to reshaping and polishing natural teeth to improve their appearance and function (Fig. 9.11). In addition, the rounding of sharp angles can be considered a prophylactic measure to reduce stress and to prevent chipping and fractures of the incisal edges.

Etiology

Attrition of the incisal edges often results in closed incisal embrasures and angular incisal edges (see Fig. 9.11A). Anterior teeth, especially maxillary central incisors, often are fractured in accidents. Other esthetic problems, including attrition and abnormal wear from poor dental habits (e.g., biting fingernails, holding objects with teeth), often can be corrected or the appearance improved by reshaping natural teeth.

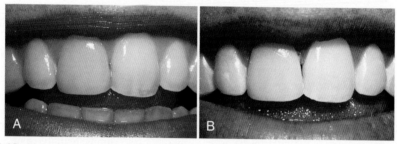

• **Fig. 9.10**   Use of internally placed color modifiers. A, The maxillary right central incisor exhibits bright intrinsic yellow staining as a result of calcific metamorphosis. B, Color modifiers under direct-composite veneer reduce brightness and intensity of stain and simulate vertical areas of translucency.

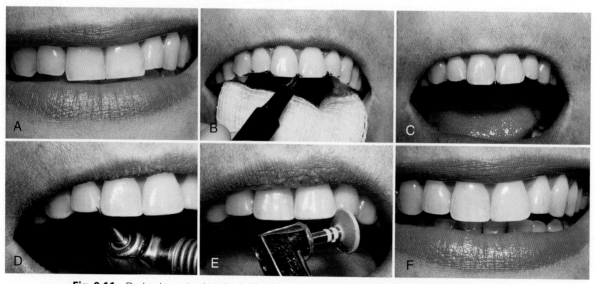

• **Fig. 9.11**   Reshaping natural teeth. A, Maxillary anterior teeth with worn incisal edges. B, Areas to be reshaped are outlined. C, Outlined areas give the patient an idea of what the final result will look like. D, A diamond instrument is used to reshape the incisal edges. E, A rubber abrasive disk is used to polish the incisal edges. F, Reshaping results in a more youthful smile.

Treatment

Consultation and examination are necessary before any changes are made to the shapes of teeth. Photographs, study models, line drawings, and esthetic imaging devices enable the patient to envision the potential improvement before any changes are made.

As noted earlier, cosmetic contouring to achieve youthful characteristics often includes rounding incisal angles, reducing facial line angles, and opening incisal embrasures. The opposite characteristics typically are considered more mature features. Cosmetic reshaping to smooth rough incisal edges and improve symmetry is equally beneficial to women and men.

The patient must understand what is involved and must want to have the alteration made. If reshaping is desired, it is helpful to mark, by using a pencil or alcohol-marking pen, an outline of the areas of the teeth to be reshaped (see Fig. 9.11B). By marking the anticipated areas for enamel reshaping, the patient is provided some indication of what the postoperative result may look like (see Fig. 9.11C). If available, esthetic computer imaging also can be used to illustrate the possible result before treatment.

Because all reshaping is restricted to enamel, anesthesia is not required. A cotton roll is recommended for isolation. Diamond instruments and abrasive disks and points are used for contouring, finishing, and polishing (see Fig. 9.11D and E). Through careful reshaping of appropriate enamel surfaces, a more esthetic smile (characterized by youthful features) is attained. Rounded incisal edges also are less likely to chip or fracture (see Fig. 9.11F).

A second example involves the irregular, fractured incisal surfaces of maxillary central incisors (Fig. 9.12A). An esthetic result can be accomplished by slightly shortening the incisal edges and reshaping both teeth to a symmetrical form. Photographs, line drawings, esthetic imaging, or marking the outline on the patient's teeth enables the patient to envision the potential improvement before any changes are made. Protrusive function always should be evaluated to prevent inadvertent elimination of this occlusal contact. Conservative treatment consists of using diamond instruments and abrasive disks and points for contouring and polishing the central incisors. The finished result is illustrated in Fig. 9.12B.

As some patients grow older or have the habit of bruxism, the incisal surfaces often wear away, leaving sharp edges that chip easily. This is also accompanied by loss of the incisal embrasures (Fig. 9.13A). To lessen the chance of more fractures and to create a more youthful smile, the incisal embrasures are opened and the incisal angles of teeth are rounded (see Fig. 9.13B).

Alterations of Embrasures

Etiology

Anterior teeth can have embrasures that are too open as a result of the shape or position of teeth in the arch. When the permanent lateral incisors are congenitally missing, canines and posterior teeth may drift mesially or the space may be closed orthodontically. The facial surface and cusp angle of some canines can be reshaped to appear like lateral incisors. In many instances, the mesioincisal embrasures remain too open (Fig. 9.14A).

Treatment

Composite can be added to establish an esthetic contour and correct the open embrasures. Evaluation of the occlusion before restoration determines if the addition would be compatible with functional movements. The patient should understand the procedures involved and should want to have the change made. Line drawings, esthetic imaging, or photographs of similar examples are often helpful in explaining the procedure and allaying patient concerns. Another patient aid involves adding composite to teeth (unetched/unbonded) to fill the embrasure temporarily to simulate the final result, which is known as a composite mockup.

Preliminary procedures include cleaning the involved teeth, selecting the shade, and isolating the area. Local anesthesia usually is not required because the preparation does not extend subgingivally and involves only enamel. A coarse, flame-shaped diamond

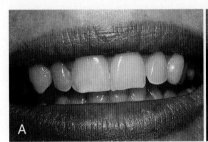
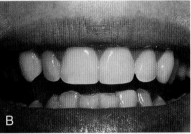

• **Fig. 9.12** Irregular incisal edges. A, Central incisors have rough, fractured incisal edges. B, Esthetic result is obtained by recontouring incisal edges.

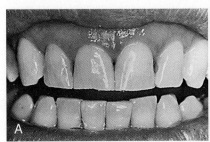
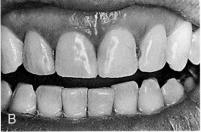

• **Fig. 9.13** Loss of incisal embrasures from attrition. Before (A) and after (B) recontouring teeth to produce a more youthful appearance and improve resistance to fracture.

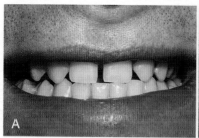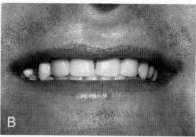

• **Fig. 9.14** Closing incisal embrasures. A, Maxillary canines moved to close spaces left by missing lateral incisors. The mesial incisal embrasures are too open. B, Canines reshaped to appear like lateral incisors.

instrument is used to remove overly convex enamel surfaces (if present) and to roughen the enamel surface area to be augmented with composite material. It may be necessary to place a wedge and use an abrasive strip to prepare the proximal surface. The final contour of the restoration should be envisioned before the preparation is made so that all areas to be bonded are adequately roughened.

A polyester strip or a Teflon tape is inserted to protect the adjacent tooth during acid etching. After etching, rinsing, and drying, the contoured strip is positioned. A light-cured composite material is inserted, and the strip is closed during polymerization. The incisal embrasures of both canines are corrected, and both restorations are finished by routine procedures (see Fig. 9.14B). The occlusion should be evaluated to assess centric contacts and functional movements, and any adjustments or corrections should be made, if indicated.

Correction of Diastemas

Etiology

The presence of diastemas between anterior teeth is an esthetic problem for some patients (Fig. 9.15A). Before treatment, a diagnosis of the cause is made, including an evaluation of the occlusion. A frequent site of a diastema is between maxillary central incisors. A prominent labial frenum with nonelastic fibers extending proximally often prevents the normal approximation of erupting central incisors.[11] Other causative factors include congenitally missing teeth, undersized or malformed teeth, interarch tooth size discrepancies (i.e., Bolton discrepancy), supernumerary teeth, and heredity. Diastemas also may result from other problems such as tongue thrusting, periodontal disease, or posterior bite collapse. Diastemas should not be closed without first recognizing and treating the underlying cause, as merely treating the cause may correct the diastema.

Treatment

Traditionally, diastemas have been treated by surgical, periodontal, orthodontic, and prosthetic procedures. These types of corrections can be impractical or unaffordable and often do not result in permanent closure of the diastema. In carefully selected cases, a more practical alternative is to use composite augmentation of proximal surfaces via adhesive procedures (see Figs. 9.5 and 9.6). All treatment options (including no treatment) should be considered before resorting immediately to composite augmentation. Line drawings, photographs, computer imaging, models with spaces filled, and direct temporary additions of ivory-colored wax or composite material on natural teeth (unetched) are important preliminary procedures.

The correction of a diastema between maxillary central incisors is described and illustrated in Fig. 9.15. After the teeth are cleaned and the shade selected, a Boley gauge or other suitable caliper is used to measure the width of the diastema and the individual teeth (see Fig. 9.15B and C). Occasionally, one central incisor is wider, requiring a greater addition to the narrower tooth. Assuming the incisors are of equal width, symmetrical additions can be ensured by using half of the total measurement of the diastema to gauge the width of the first tooth restored. Cotton rolls, instead of a rubber dam, are recommended for isolation because of the importance of relating the contour of the restoration directly to the proximal tissue. Usually the restoration must begin slightly below the gingival crest to appear natural and to be confluent with the tooth contours.

With cotton rolls in place, a gingival retraction cord of an appropriate size is tucked in the gingival crevice of each tooth from midfacial mesially to midlingual (see Fig. 9.15D). The cord retracts the soft tissue and prevents seepage from the crevice. In some instances, the retraction cord may need to be inserted for one tooth at a time to prevent strangulation of interproximal tissue during preparation and restorative procedures. To enhance retention of the composite, a coarse, flame-shaped diamond instrument is used to roughen the proximal surfaces, extending from the facial line angle to the lingual line angle (see Fig. 9.15E). More extension may be needed to correct the facial or lingual contours, depending on the anatomy and position of the individual tooth. The enamel is acid etched approximately 0.5 mm past the prepared, roughened surface. The acid should be applied gingivally only to the extent of the anticipated restoration. After rinsing and drying, the etched enamel should display a lightly frosted appearance (see Fig. 9.15F). A 5-cm by 5-cm (2-inch by 2-inch) gauze is draped across the mouth and tongue to prevent inadvertent contamination of the etched preparations by the patient. After both preparations are completed, the teeth are restored one at a time.

A polyester strip is contoured and placed proximally, with the gingival aspect of the strip extending below the gingival crest. Additional contouring may be required to produce enough convexity in the strip. In most cases, a wedge cannot be used. The strip is held (with the index finger) on the lingual aspect of the tooth to be restored, while the facial end is reflected for access. A light-cured composite is used for the restoration. After the bonding agent is applied, the composite material is inserted with a hand instrument (see Fig. 9.15G). Careful attention is given to pressing the material lingually to ensure confluence with the lingual surface. The matrix is gently closed facially, beginning with the gingival aspect (see Fig. 9.15H). Care must be taken not to pull the strip too tightly because the resulting restoration may be undercontoured faciolingually, mesiodistally, or both. The light-cured composite material

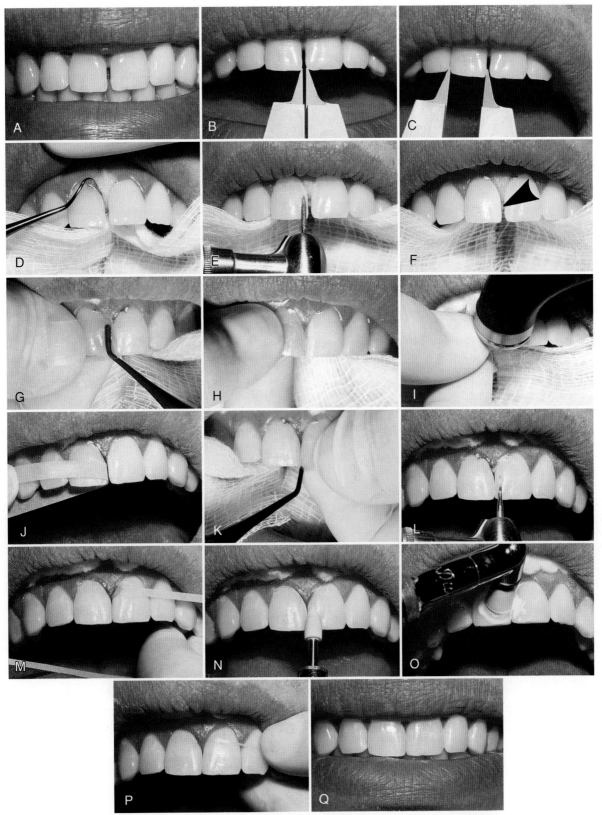

• **Fig. 9.15** Diastema closure. A, Esthetic problem created by space between central incisors. B and C, Interdental space and size of central incisors measured with caliper. D, Teeth isolated with cotton rolls and retraction cord tucked into the gingival crevice. E, A diamond instrument is used to roughen enamel surfaces. F, Etched enamel surface indicated *(arrow)*. G, Composite inserted with composite instrument. H, Matrix strip closed with thumb and forefinger. I, Composite addition is cured. J, Finishing strip used to finalize contour of first addition. K, A tight contact is attained by displacing the second tooth being restored in a distal direction with thumb and forefinger, while holding matrix in contact with adjacent restoration. L, Flame-shaped finishing bur used to contour restoration. M, Finishing strip used to smooth the subgingival areas. N, The restoration is polished with a rubber abrasive point. O, Final luster attained with polishing paste applied with Prophy cup. P, Unwaxed floss used to detect any excess composite. Q, Diastema closed with symmetrical and equal additions of composite.

is polymerized with the light directed from the facial and lingual directions for an appropriate amount of time. Note that curing times may vary according to the type of light source, the composite used, and the thickness of the material (see Fig. 9.15I). Initially, it is better to overcontour the first restoration slightly to facilitate finishing it to an ideal contour.

When polymerization is complete, the strip is removed. Contouring and finishing are achieved with appropriate carbide finishing burs, fine diamonds, or abrasive disks (see Fig. 9.15L). Finishing strips are invaluable for finalizing the proximal contours (see Fig. 9.15J and M). When composite is being added to two adjoining surfaces, which is often the case, final polishing is deferred until the contralateral restoration is completed. However, it is sometimes necessary to utilize finishing discs to contour the first composite addition to achieve the correct mesiodistal dimension of the first tooth before the second tooth is restored. It is imperative for good gingival health that the cervical aspect of the composite addition be immaculately smooth and continuous with the tooth structure. Overhangs must not be present. Removal of the gingival retraction cord facilitates inspection and smoothing of this area. Flossing with a length of unwaxed floss verifies that the gingival margin is correct and smooth if no fraying of the floss occurs (see Fig. 9.15P).

After etching, rinsing, and drying, the second restoration is completed. A tight proximal contact can be attained by displacing the second tooth being restored in a distal direction (with the thumb and the index finger) while holding the matrix in contact with the adjacent restoration (see Fig. 9.15K). Contouring is accomplished with a 12-fluted carbide bur and finishing strips (see Fig. 9.15L and M). Articulating paper should be used to evaluate the patient's occlusion to ensure that the restorations are not offensive in centric or functional movements; adjustments can be made with a carbide finishing bur or abrasive disks. Final polishing is achieved with rubber polishing points or polishing paste applied with a prophy cup in a low-speed handpiece (see Fig. 9.15N and O). Unwaxed floss is used to detect any excess material

or overhang (see Fig. 9.15P). The final esthetic result is seen in Fig. 9.15Q.

Multiple diastemas among the maxillary anterior teeth are shown in Fig. 9.16A. Closing the spaces by orthodontic movement was considered in this patient; however, because the patient's teeth were undercontoured mesiodistally, the diastemas were closed by bonding composite to the proximal surfaces. The teeth after treatment are shown in Fig. 9.16B. In the presence of defective Class III restorations or proximal caries, it is recommended that the teeth be restored with the same composite used for closing the diastema. Often these restorations can be performed at the same time the diastema is closed with composite additions (Fig. 9.17).

Occasionally, diastemas are simply too large to close esthetically with composite augmentation alone (Fig. 9.18A). Closing a large space of this magnitude with composite would merely create an alternative esthetic problem—that is, excessively large central incisors, which would further exacerbate the existing discrepancy in proportionality among anterior teeth. In such cases, large spaces are best redistributed orthodontically among anterior teeth so that symmetric and equal composite additions can be made to the central and lateral incisors (see Fig. 9.18B and C). This approach that involves space distribution results in improved proportionality among anterior teeth (see earlier section Artistic Elements). The final result, immediately after completion, is shown in Fig. 9.18D.

Conservative Treatments for Discolored Teeth

One of the most frequent reasons patients seek dental care is discolored anterior teeth. Even patients with teeth of normal color request whitening procedures. Treatment options include removal of surface stains, bleaching, microabrasion or macroabrasion, veneering, and placement of porcelain crowns. Many dentists recommend porcelain crowns as the best solution for badly

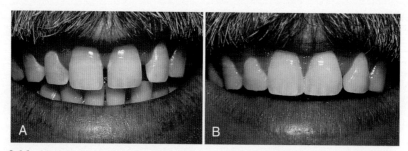

• **Fig. 9.16** Multiple diastemas occurring among maxillary anterior teeth. A, Before correction. B, Appearance after diastemas are closed with composite augmentation.

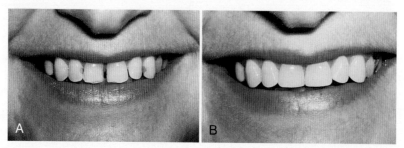

• **Fig. 9.17** A, Diastema closure and cosmetic contouring. B, Significant esthetic improvement is achieved by replacing defective Class III restorations and closing diastemas with conservative composite additions and cosmetically reshaping teeth.

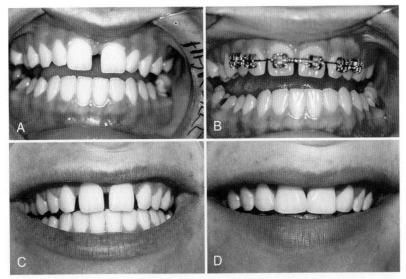

• **Fig. 9.18** Space distribution. A, Midline diastema too large for simple closure with composite additions. B and C, Space distributed among four incisors with orthodontic treatment. D, Final result after composite additions.

discolored teeth. If crowns are done properly with the highly esthetic ceramic materials currently available, they have great potential for being esthetic and long lasting. However, increasing numbers of patients do not want their teeth "cut down" for crowns and choose an alternative, conservative approach such as veneers (see section Veneers) that preserves as much of the natural tooth as possible. This treatment is performed with the understanding that the corrective measures may be less permanent.

Discolorations are classified as extrinsic or intrinsic. Extrinsic stains are located on the outer surfaces of teeth, whereas intrinsic stains are internal. The etiology and treatment of extrinsic and intrinsic stains are discussed in the following sections.

Extrinsic Discolorations

Etiology

Stains on the external surfaces of teeth (referred to as *extrinsic discolorations*) are common and may be the result of numerous factors. In young patients, stains of almost any color can be found and are usually more prominent in the cervical areas of teeth (Fig. 9.19A). These stains may be related to remnants of Nasmyth membrane, poor oral hygiene, existing restorations, gingival bleeding, plaque accumulation, eating habits, or the presence of chromogenic microorganisms.[12] In older patients, stains on the surfaces of teeth are more likely to be brown, black, or gray and occur on areas adjacent to gingival tissue. Poor oral hygiene is a contributing factor, but coffee, tea, and other types of chromogenic foods or medications can produce stains (even on plaque-free surfaces). Tobacco stains also are observed frequently. Existing restorations may be discolored for the same reasons.

An example of one of the most interesting and unusual types of external staining is illustrated in Fig. 9.19B. In Southeast Asia, some women traditionally dye their teeth with betel nut juice to match their hair and eyes as a sign of beauty.[13] Slices of lemon are held in contact with the teeth before applying the betel nut juice to make the staining process more effective. This example was probably one of the first applications of the acid-etch technique.

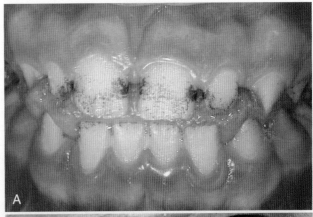

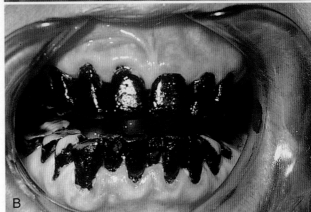

• **Fig. 9.19** Extrinsic stains. A, Surface stains on facial surfaces in a young patient. B, Exotic decoration of anterior teeth by etching with citrus fruit juice and applying black pigment (betel nut stain). (A, Courtesy Dr. Tim Wright. B, From Daniel SJ, Harfst SA, Wilder RS: *Mosby's dental hygiene: Concepts, cases, and competencies,* ed 2, St. Louis, 2008, Mosby. Courtesy Dr. George Taybos, Jackson, MS.)

A weak acid, such as that found in citrus fruits, is known to cause rapid decalcification of enamel.

Treatment

Most surface stains can be removed by routine prophylactic procedures (Fig. 9.20); however, some superficial discolorations on tooth-colored restorations and decalcified areas on teeth cannot be corrected by such cleaning. Conservative correction may be accomplished by mild microabrasion or by surfacing the thin, outer, discolored layer with a flame-shaped, carbide finishing bur or diamond instrument (i.e., macroabrasion), followed by polishing with abrasive disks or points to obtain an acceptable result. (See section Microabrasion and Macroabrasion for details of clinical technique.)

Intrinsic Discolorations

Etiology

Intrinsic discolorations are caused by deeper (not superficial) internal stains or enamel defects, and are more complex to treat than are external discolorations. Teeth with vital or nonvital pulps as well as endodontically treated teeth can be affected. Vital teeth may be discolored at the time the crowns are forming, and the abnormal condition usually involves several teeth. Causative factors include hereditary disorders, medications (particularly tetracycline preparations), excess fluoride, high fevers associated with early childhood illnesses, and other types of trauma.[12] The staining may be located in enamel or dentin. Discolorations restricted to dentin still may show through enamel. Discoloration also may be localized or generalized, involving the entire tooth.

Various preparations of the antibiotic drug tetracycline can cause the most distracting, generalized type of intrinsic discoloration (Fig. 9.21A).[14] The severity of the staining depends on the dose, the duration of exposure to the drug, and the type of tetracycline analogue used. Different types of tetracyclines induce different types of discoloration, varying from yellow-orange to dark blue-gray.

Dark blue-gray, tetracycline-stained teeth are considerably more difficult to treat than are teeth with mild yellow-orange discolorations. Staining from tetracycline-type drugs most frequently occurs at an early age and is caused by ingestion of the drug concomitant with the development of permanent teeth. Studies indicate that permanent teeth in adults also can experience a graying discoloration, however, as a result of long-term exposure to minocycline, a tetracycline analogue.[14]

The presence of excessive fluoride in drinking water and other sources at the time of teeth formation can result in another type of intrinsic stain called *fluorosis*. The staining usually is generalized. Localized areas of discoloration may occur on individual teeth because of enamel or dentin defects induced during tooth development. High fevers and other forms of trauma can damage the tooth during its development, resulting in unesthetic hypoplastic defects. Additionally, localized areas of dysmineralization, or the failure of the enamel to calcify properly, can result in hypocalcified white spots. After eruption, poor oral hygiene also can result in decalcified white spots. Poor oral hygiene during orthodontic treatment frequently results in these types of decalcified defects. White or discolored spots with intact enamel surface (i.e., surface not soft) are often evidence of intraoral remineralization, however, and such spots are not indications for invasive treatment (unless for esthetic concerns). Additionally, caries, metallic restorations, corroded pins, and leakage or secondary caries around existing restorations can result in various types of intrinsic discoloration.

As noted earlier, aging effects also can result in yellowed teeth. As patients grow older, the tooth enamel becomes thinner because of wear and allows underlying dentin to become more apparent. Also, often continuing deposition of secondary dentin occurs in older individuals, resulting in greater dentin thickness. This deposition results in a yellowing effect, depending on the intrinsic color of dentin. Additionally, the permeability of teeth usually allows the infusion (over time) of significant organic pigments (from chromogenic foods, drinks, and tobacco products) that produce a yellowing effect.

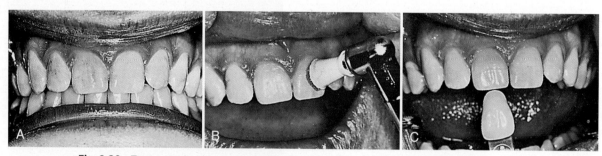

• **Fig. 9.20** Treatment of surface stains. A, Tobacco stains. B, Pumicing teeth with rubber cup. C, Shade guide used to confirm normal color of natural teeth.

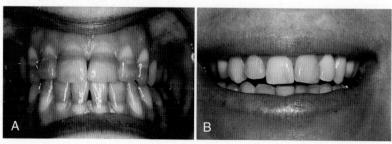

• **Fig. 9.21** Intrinsic stains. A, Staining by tetracycline drugs. B, Staining of the maxillary left central incisor from tooth trauma and degeneration of the pulp.

Nonvital teeth also can become discolored intrinsically. These stains usually occur in individual teeth after eruption has taken place. The pulp may become infected or degenerate as a result of trauma, deep caries, or irritation from restorative procedures. If these teeth are properly treated by endodontic therapy, they usually retain their normal color. If treatment is delayed, discoloration of the crown is more likely to occur. The degenerative products from the pulp tissue stain dentin, and this is readily apparent because of the translucency of enamel (see Fig. 9.21B). Trauma resulting in calcific metamorphosis (i.e., calcification of the pulp chamber, root canal, or both) also can produce significant yellowing of the tooth. This condition is extremely difficult to treat (see Fig. 9.10).

Treatment

Some people definitely have esthetic problems because of intrinsic stains, but others worry needlessly about the overall color of their teeth. In the latter instance, the dentist must decide if the color of teeth can be improved enough to justify treatment, even though the patient insists on having something done. Individuals with light complexions may believe that their teeth are too dark, when actually they are normal in color (Fig. 9.22A). Positioning a shade tab from a shade guide of tooth colors next to such teeth often shows these patients that the color of their teeth is well within the normal range of shades. As stated earlier, tanned skin, darker makeup, or darker lipstick usually make teeth appear much whiter by increasing the contrast between teeth and the surrounding facial features (see Fig. 9.22B).

The patient should be told that many discolorations can be corrected or the appearance of teeth greatly improved through conservative methods such as bleaching, microabrasion or macroabrasion, and veneering. Mild discolorations are best left untreated, are bleached, or are treated conservatively with microabrasion or macroabrasion because no restorative material is as good as the healthy, natural tooth structure. The patient should be informed that the gingival tissue adjacent to restorative material will never be as healthy as that next to normal tooth structure.

Color photographs of previously treated teeth with intrinsic staining (i.e., before and after treatment) are excellent adjuncts to help the patient make an informed decision. Esthetic imaging with modern computer simulation of the postoperative result also can be an effective educational tool. Patients appreciate knowing what the cause of the problem is, how it can be corrected, how much time is involved, and what the cost will be. They also should be informed of the life expectancy of the various treatment alternatives suggested. Vital bleaching usually results in tooth lightening for only 1 to 3 years, whereas an etched porcelain veneer should last 10 to 15 years or longer. With continuous improvements in materials and techniques, a much longer lifespan may be possible with any of these procedures. The clinical longevity of esthetic restorations also is enhanced in patients with good oral hygiene, proper diet, a favorable bite relationship, and little or no contact with agents that cause discoloration or deterioration.

Correction of intrinsic discolorations caused by failing restorations entails replacement of the faulty portion or the entire restoration. Correction of discolorations caused by caries lesions requires appropriate restorative treatment. Esthetic inserts for metal restorations are described later in this chapter. For the other types of intrinsic discolorations previously discussed, detailed treatment options are presented in the following three sections.

Bleaching Treatments

The lightening of the color of a tooth through the application of a chemical agent to oxidize the organic pigmentation in the tooth is referred to as *bleaching*. In keeping with the overall conservative philosophy of tooth restoration, consideration should be given first to bleaching anterior teeth when intrinsic discolorations are encountered. Bleaching techniques may be classified as to whether they involve vital or nonvital teeth and whether the procedure is performed in the office or outside the office. Bleaching of nonvital teeth was first reported in 1848; in-office bleaching of vital teeth was first reported in 1868.[15] By the early 1900s, in-office vital bleaching had evolved to include the use of heat and light for activation of the process. Although a 3% ether and peroxide mouthwash used for bleaching in 1893 has been reported in the literature, the "dentist-prescribed, home-applied" technique (also referred to as *nightguard vital bleaching* or *at-home bleaching*) for bleaching vital teeth outside the office began around 1968, although it was not commonly known until the late 1980s.[16]

Most bleaching techniques use some form or derivative of hydrogen peroxide in different concentrations and application techniques. The mechanism of action of bleaching teeth with hydrogen peroxide is considered to be oxidation of organic pigments, although the chemistry is not well understood. Bleaching generally has an approximate lifespan of 1 to 3 years, although the change may be permanent in some situations.

With all bleaching techniques, a transitory decrease occurs in the potential bond strength of composite when it is applied to bleached enamel and dentin. This reduction in bond strength results from residual oxygen or peroxide residue in the tooth that inhibits the setting of the bonding resin, precluding adequate resin

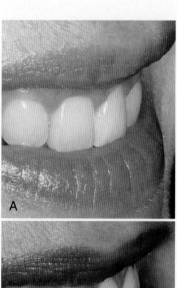
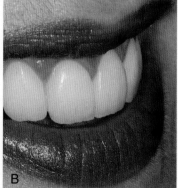

• **Fig. 9.22**　Illusion of a lighter appearance of teeth by use of darker makeup. A, Before. B, After. (From Freedman G: *Contemporary esthetic dentistry*, St. Louis, 2012, Mosby.)

tag formation in the etched enamel. No loss of bond strength is noted if the composite restorative treatment is delayed at least 1 week after cessation of any bleaching.[17]

Nonvital Bleaching Procedures

The primary indication for nonvital bleaching is to lighten teeth that have undergone endodontic therapy. Discoloration may be a result of bleeding into dentin from trauma before root canal therapy, degradation of pulp tissue left in the chamber after such therapy, or staining from restorative materials and cements placed in the tooth as a part of the endodontic treatment. Most posterior teeth that have received endodontic therapy require full-coverage restorations that encompass the tooth to prevent subsequent fracture. Anterior teeth needing restorative treatment and that are largely intact may be restored with composite rather than with partial-coverage or full-coverage restorations without significantly compromising the strength of the tooth.[18] This knowledge has resulted in a resurgence in the use of nonvital bleaching techniques. Nonvital bleaching techniques include an in-office technique and an out-of-office procedure referred to as *walking bleach*. (See the following sections for details of these two techniques.)

Although nonvital bleaching is effective, a slight potential (i.e., 1%) exists for a deleterious side effect termed *external cervical resorption* (Fig. 9.23).[19] This sequela requires prompt and aggressive treatment. In animal models, cervical resorption has been observed most when using a thermocatalytic technique with high heat.[20] The walking bleach technique or an in-office technique that does not require the use of heat is preferred for nonvital bleaching. To reduce the possibility of resorption, immediately after bleaching, a paste of calcium hydroxide powder and sterile water is placed in the pulp chamber as described in the following sections.[21] Also, sodium perborate alone, rather than in conjunction with hydrogen peroxide, should be used as the primary bleaching agent. Although sodium perborate may bleach more slowly, it is safer and less aggressive to the tooth.[22] Periodic radiographs should be obtained after bleaching to screen for cervical resorption, which generally has its onset in 1 to 7 years.[23]

In-Office Nonvital Bleaching Technique

The in-office bleaching for nonvital teeth historically has involved a thermocatalytic technique consisting of the placement of 35% hydrogen peroxide liquid into the debrided pulp chamber and acceleration of the oxidation process by placement of a heating

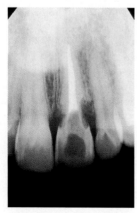

• **Fig. 9.23** Radiograph revealing the presence of extensive cervical resorption.

instrument into the pulp chamber. The thermocatalytic technique is not recommended, however, because of the potential for cervical resorption.[19] A more current technique uses 30% to 35% hydrogen peroxide pastes or gels that require no heat. This technique is frequently the preferred in-office technique for bleaching nonvital teeth. In both techniques, it is imperative that a sealing cement (resin-modified glass ionomer [RMGI] cement is recommended) be placed over the exposed endodontic filling before application of the bleaching agent to prevent leakage and penetration of the bleaching material in an apical direction. It is also recommended that the bleaching agent be applied in the coronal portion of the tooth incisal to the level of the periodontal ligament (not down into the root canal space) to prevent unwanted leakage of the bleaching agent through the lateral canals or canaliculi to the periodontal ligament.

Walking Bleach Technique

Before beginning the walking bleach technique, the dentist needs to evaluate the potential for occlusal contact on the area of the root canal access opening. The dentist places a rubber dam to isolate the discolored tooth and removes all materials in the coronal portion of the tooth (i.e., access opening). The dentist removes gutta-percha (to approximately 1–2 mm apical of the clinical crown) and enlarges the endodontic access opening sufficiently to ensure complete debridement of the pulp chamber. Next, the dentist places an RMGI liner to seal the gutta-percha of the root canal, filling from the coronal portion of the pulp chamber. After this seal has hardened, the dentist trims any excess material from the seal so that the discolored dentin is exposed peripherally.

Sodium perborate is used with this technique because it is deemed extremely safe.[24] Using a cement spatula, with heavy pressure on a glass slab, one drop of saline or sterile anesthetic solution is blended with enough sodium perborate to form a creamy paste. A spoon excavator or similar instrument is used to fill the pulp chamber (with the bleaching mixture) to within 2 mm of the cavosurface margin, avoiding contact with the enamel cavosurface margins of the access opening. The dentist uses a cotton pellet to blot the mixture and places a temporary sealing material (e.g., Cavit [3M ESPE, St. Paul, MN] or Fuji IX [GC America, Alsip, IL]) to seal the access opening. The area should remain isolated for approximately 5 minutes after closure to evaluate the adequacy of the seal of the temporary restoration. If bubbles appear around the margins of the temporary material indicating leakage, the temporary restoration must be replaced. If no bubbles appear, the dentist removes the rubber dam and checks the occlusion to assess the presence or absence of contact on the temporary restoration.

The sodium perborate should be changed weekly. On successful bleaching of the tooth, the chamber is rinsed and filled to within 2 mm of the cavosurface margin with a paste consisting of calcium hydroxide powder in sterile saline. (The enamel walls and margins are kept clean and free of the calcium hydroxide paste.) As noted earlier, a paste of calcium hydroxide powder and sterile water is placed immediately after bleaching in the pulp chamber to reduce the possibility of resorption.[21] The dentist reseals the access opening with a temporary restorative material, as previously described, and allows the calcium hydroxide material to remain in the pulp chamber for 2 weeks. Subsequently, the dentist removes the temporary restorative material, rinses away the calcium hydroxide, and dries the pulp chamber. Next, the dentist restores the tooth with a light-cured composite (Fig. 9.24).

Occasionally, a tooth that has been bleached by using the walking bleach technique and sealed with a composite restoration may

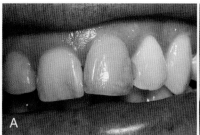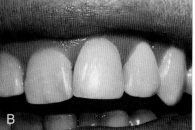

• **Fig. 9.24** Indication for bleaching root canal–filled tooth. A, Before. B, After intracoronal, nonvital bleaching.

subsequently become discolored. In this instance, the alternative treatment option should be an attempt to bleach the tooth externally with one of the external bleaching techniques (see next section).

Vital Bleaching Procedures

Generally the indications for the different vital bleaching techniques are similar, with patient preference, cost, compliance, and difficulty in the removal of certain discolorations dictating the choice of treatment or combination of treatments. Indications for vital bleaching include teeth intrinsically discolored because of aging, trauma, or certain medications. External vital bleaching techniques are alternative treatment options for a failed, nonvital, walking bleach procedure. Vital bleaching also is often indicated before and after restorative treatments to harmonize the shades of the restorative materials with those of natural teeth.

Teeth exhibiting yellow or orange intrinsic discoloration seem to respond best to vital bleaching, whereas teeth exhibiting bluish gray discolorations often are considerably more difficult to treat in this manner. Other indications for external bleaching include teeth that have been darkened by trauma but are still vital or teeth that have a poor endodontic prognosis because of the absence of a radiographically visible canal (i.e., calcific metamorphosis). Brown fluorosis stains also are often responsive to treatment, but white fluorosis stains may not be resolved effectively (although they can be made less obvious if the surrounding tooth structure can be significantly whitened).

Vital bleaching techniques include an in-office technique referred to as *power bleaching* and an out-of-office alternative that is a "dentist-prescribed, home-applied" technique (i.e., nightguard vital bleaching, or simply "at-home bleaching").[25,26] These techniques may be used separately or in combination with one another. (Details are provided in subsequent sections.) Some over-the-counter bleaching materials, particularly products involving a trayless strip delivery system, also are effective for whitening teeth, but these are not discussed in this chapter.[27]

Overall, vital bleaching has been proven to be safe and effective when performed by or under the supervision of a dentist. With short-term treatment, no appreciable effect has been observed on existing restorative materials, either in loss of material integrity or in color change, with one exception: Polymethyl methacrylate restorations exhibit a yellow-orange discoloration on exposure to carbamide peroxide. For this reason, temporary crowns should be made from bis-acryl materials, rather than polymethyl methacrylate crown and bridge resin, if exposure to carbamide peroxide is anticipated.

Because hydrogen peroxide has such a low molecular weight, it easily passes through enamel and dentin. This characteristic is thought to account for the mild tooth sensitivity occasionally experienced during treatment. This effect is transient, however, and no long-term harm to the pulp has been reported.

Often the dentist has to decide whether to use an in-office bleaching technique or prescribe a home-applied technique. The advantages of the in-office vital bleaching technique are that (although it uses very aggressive chemicals) it is totally under the dentist's control, soft tissue is generally protected from the process, and the technique has the potential for bleaching teeth more rapidly. Disadvantages primarily relate to the cost, the unpredictable outcome, and the unknown duration of the treatment. The features that warrant concern and caution include the potential for soft tissue damage to both patient and provider, discomfort caused by the rubber dam or other isolation devices, and the potential for posttreatment sensitivity. The advantages of the dentist-prescribed, home-applied technique are the use of a lower concentration of peroxide (generally 10% to 15% carbamide peroxide), ease of application, minimal side effects, and lower cost because of the reduced chair time required for treatment. The disadvantages are reliance on patient compliance, longer treatment time, and the (unknown) potential for soft tissue changes with excessively extended use.

In-Office Vital Bleaching Technique

In-office vital bleaching requires an excellent rubber dam technique and careful patient management. Vaseline or cocoa butter may be placed on the patient's lips and gingival tissue before application of the rubber dam to help protect these soft tissues from any inadvertent exposure to the bleaching agent. Anterior teeth (and sometimes the first premolars) are isolated with a heavy rubber dam to provide maximum retraction of tissue and an optimal seal around teeth. A good seal of the dam is ensured by ligation of the dam with waxed dental tape or the use of a sealing putty or varnish. Light-cured, resin-based "paint-on" rubber dam isolation media are available for use with in-office bleaching materials but cannot provide the same degree of protection and isolation as a conventionally applied rubber dam. Etching of teeth with 37% phosphoric acid, once considered a required part of this technique, is unnecessary.[28]

Numerous commercially available bleaching agents are available for in-office bleaching procedures. Most consist of paste or gel compositions that most commonly contain 30% to 35% hydrogen peroxide. Other additives, such as metallic ion–producing materials or alkalinizing agents that can speed up the oxidation reaction, also are commonly found in these commercially available whitening products. The dentist places the hydrogen peroxide–containing paste or gel on teeth. The patient is instructed to report any sensations of burning of the lips or gingiva that would indicate a leaking dam and the need to terminate treatment.

Most of the credible research indicates that the addition of light during the bleaching procedure does not improve the whitening result beyond what the bleach alone can achieve.[29] Use of a light to generate heat may accelerate the oxidation reaction of the hydrogen peroxide and expedite treatment through a thermocatalytic effect. PAC lights and high-output quartz halogen lights have been commonly used for this purpose. Use of lights to heat the bleaching agent, however, causes a greater level of tooth dehydration. This effect not only can increase tooth sensitivity but also results in an immediate apparent whitening of the tooth owing to dehydration that makes the actual whitening result more difficult to assess. Use of carbon dioxide laser to heat the bleaching mixture and accelerate the bleaching treatment has not been recommended, according to a report of the American Dental Association (ADA) because of the potential for hard or soft tissue damage.[30] On completion of the treatment, the dentist rinses the patient's teeth, removes the rubber dam or isolation medium, and cautions the patient about postoperative sensitivity. A nonsteroidal analgesic and antiinflammatory drug may be administered if sensitivity is anticipated.

Contrary to the claims of some manufacturers, optimal whitening typically requires more than one bleaching treatment.[31] Bleaching treatments generally are rendered weekly for two to six treatments, with each treatment lasting 30 to 45 minutes. Patients may experience transient tooth sensitivity between appointments, but no long-term adverse effects of bleaching teeth with otherwise healthy pulps have been reported in the literature. Because the enamel is not acid etched, it is not necessary to polish the teeth after they have been bleached, and it is not essential to provide any fluoride treatment.

Dentist-Prescribed, Home-Applied Technique

The dentist-prescribed, home-applied technique (i.e., nightguard vital bleaching) is much less labor intensive and requires substantially less in-office time. An impression of the arch to be treated is made and poured in cast stone. It should be ensured that the impression is free of bubbles on or around teeth by wiping the impression material onto teeth and the adjacent gingival areas before inserting the impression. After appropriate infection control procedures, the dentist rinses the impression vigorously and pours with cast stone. Incomplete rinsing of the impression may cause a softened surface on the stone, which may result in a nightguard (bleaching tray) that is slightly too small and that may irritate tissue. The dentist trims the cast around the periphery to eliminate the vestibule and thin out the base of the cast palatally (until a hole is produced). Generally, the cast must be lifted from the table of the cast-trimming machine to remove the vestibule successfully without damaging teeth. The dentist allows the cast to dry and blocks out any significant undercuts by using a blockout material (e.g., putty, clay, light-activated spacer material).

The nightguard is formed on the cast with the use of a heated vacuum-forming machine. After the machine has warmed up for 10 minutes, a sheet of 0.75- to 1.5-mm (0.020- to 0.040-inch) soft vinyl nightguard material is inserted and allowed to be softened by heat until the material sags approximately by 25 mm (1 inch). The top portion of the machine is closed slowly and gently, and the vacuum is allowed to form the heat-softened material around the cast. After sufficient time has been allowed for adaptation of the material, the dentist turns off the machine and allows the material to cool.

Next, the dentist uses scissors or a No. 11 surgical blade in a Bard-Parker handle to trim in a smooth, straight cut about 3 to

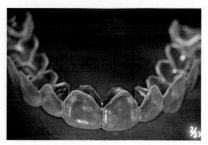

• **Fig. 9.25**   Vacuum-formed, clear plastic nightguard used for vital bleaching (i.e., scalloped version).

5 mm from the most apical portion of the gingival crest of teeth (facially and lingually). This excess material is removed first. The horseshoe-shaped nightguard is removed from the cast. The dentist trims the facial edges of the nightguard in a scalloped design, following the outline of the free gingival crest and using sharp, curved scissors. Scalloping of the lingual surface is optional because the bleaching material is applied primarily to the facial aspects of teeth. Alternatively (on the lingual aspect), the nightguard may be trimmed apically to within 2 mm of the free gingival crest in a smooth, horseshoe-shaped configuration. This scalloped design is preferred because it allows the tray to cover only teeth and prevents entrapment of the bleaching material between gingival tissue and the nightguard. The nightguard is completed and is ready for delivery to the patient (Fig. 9.25).

The dentist inserts the nightguard into the patient's mouth and evaluates it for adaptation, rough edges, or blanching of tissue. A properly fitting nightguard is shown in Fig. 9.26. Further shortening (i.e., trimming) may be indicated in problem areas. The dentist evaluates the occlusion on the nightguard with the patient in maximum intercuspation. If the patient is unable to obtain a comfortable occlusion because of premature posterior tooth contacts, the nightguard is trimmed to exclude coverage of the terminal posterior teeth, as needed (to allow optimal tooth contact in maximum intercuspation). In addition, if no lingual scalloping is done, the edges of the guard on the palate should terminate in grooves or valleys, where possible, rather than on the heights of soft tissue contours (e.g., in the area of the incisive papilla).

A 10% to 15% carbamide peroxide bleaching material generally is recommended for this bleaching technique. Commercial bleaching products are available as clear gels and white pastes. Carbamide peroxide degrades into 3% hydrogen peroxide (active ingredient) and 7% urea. Bleaching materials containing Carbopol are recommended because Carbopol thickens the bleaching solution and extends the oxidation process. On the basis of numerous research studies, carbamide peroxide bleaching materials seem to be safe and effective when administered by or under the supervision of a dentist.[22]

The patient is instructed in the application of the bleaching gel or paste into the nightguard. A thin bead of material is extruded into the nightguard along the facial aspects corresponding to the area of each tooth to be bleached. Usually, only the anterior six to eight teeth are bleached. The clinician should review proper insertion of the nightguard with the patient. After inserting the nightguard, excess material is wiped from the soft tissue along the edge with a soft-bristled toothbrush. No excess material should be allowed to remain on soft tissue because of the potential for gingival irritation. The patient should be informed not to drink liquids or rinse during treatment and to remove the nightguard for meals and oral hygiene.

Although no single treatment regimen is best for all patients, most patients prefer an overnight treatment approach because of the convenience. If the nightguard is worn at night, a single application of bleaching material at bedtime is indicated. In the morning, the patient should remove the nightguard, clean it under running water with a toothbrush, and store it in the container provided. Total treatment time using an overnight approach is usually 1 to 2 weeks. If patients cannot tolerate overnight bleaching, the bleaching time and frequency can be adjusted to accommodate the patient's comfort level. In addition, in these cases, tolerance to the nightguard and bleaching material generally are improved if the patient gradually increases the wearing time each day.

If either of the two primary adverse effects occurs (i.e., sensitive teeth or irritated gingiva), the patient should reduce or discontinue treatment immediately and contact the dentist so that the cause of the problem can be determined and the treatment approach modified. The dentist may prescribe desensitizing agents to help alleviate sensitivity associated with bleaching.

It is recommended that only one arch be bleached at a time, beginning with the maxillary arch. Bleaching the maxillary arch first allows the untreated mandibular arch to serve as a constant standard for comparison. Restricting the bleaching to one arch at a time reduces the potential for occlusal problems that could occur if the thicknesses of two mouthguards were interposed

simultaneously. Fig. 9.27 illustrates a typical case before and after treatment with nightguard vital bleaching.

Tetracycline-stained teeth typically are much more resistant to bleaching. Teeth stained with tetracycline require prolonged treatment durations of several months before any results are observed. Often, tetracycline-stained teeth are unresponsive to the procedure, especially if the stains are blue-gray in color. Tetracycline-stained teeth may approach but never seem to achieve the appearance of normal teeth. A single tetracycline-stained tooth with previous endodontic therapy or a different pulp size may respond differently from other teeth in the arch to the bleaching technique.

Because bleaching tetracycline-stained teeth is difficult, some clinicians advocate intentional endodontic therapy along with the use of an intracoronal nonvital bleaching technique to overcome this problem (Fig. 9.28). Although the esthetic result appears much better than that obtained from external bleaching, this approach involves all the inherent risks otherwise associated with endodontic treatment. External bleaching techniques offer a safer alternative, although they may not be as rapid or effective. Veneers or full crowns are alternative esthetic treatment methods for difficult tetracycline-stained teeth but involve irreversible restorative techniques (see section Indirect Veneer Techniques). No one bleaching technique is effective in all cases, and all successes are not equal. Often, with vital bleaching, a combination of the in-office

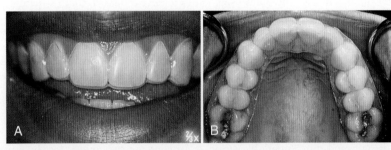

• **Fig. 9.26** Nightguard for vital bleaching. A and B, Clear plastic nightguard properly seated and positioned in the mouth (scalloped on facial, unscalloped on lingual).

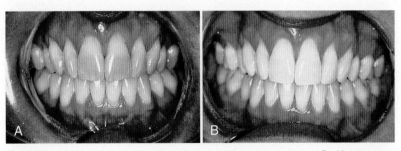

• **Fig. 9.27** Nightguard vital bleaching. A, Before bleaching treatment. B, After treatment.

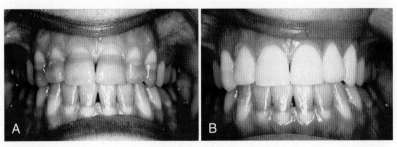

• **Fig. 9.28** Bleaching tetracycline-stained teeth. A, Before nonvital bleaching. B, After treatment. (Courtesy Dr. Wayne Mohorn.)

technique and the dentist-prescribed, home-applied technique has better results than either technique used alone.

Microabrasion and Macroabrasion

Microabrasion and *macroabrasion* represent conservative alternatives for the reduction or elimination of superficial discolorations. As the terms imply, the stained areas or defects are abraded away. These techniques result in the physical removal of the tooth structure and are indicated only for stains or enamel defects that do not extend beyond a few tenths of a millimeter in depth. If the defect or discoloration remains even after treatment with microabrasion or macroabrasion, a restorative alternative is indicated.

Microabrasion

In 1984, McCloskey reported the use of 18% hydrochloric acid swabbed on teeth for the removal of superficial fluorosis stains.[32] Subsequently, in 1986, Croll and Cavanaugh modified the technique to include the use of pumice with hydrochloric acid to form a paste applied with a tongue blade.[33] This technique is called *microabrasion* and involves the surface dissolution of the enamel by acid along with the abrasiveness of the pumice to remove superficial stains or defects. Since that time, Croll further modified the technique, reducing the concentration of the acid to approximately 11% and increasing the abrasiveness of the paste using silicon carbide particles (in a water-soluble gel paste) instead of pumice.[34] This product, marketed as Prema compound (Premier Dental Products Co., Plymouth Meeting, PA) or Opalustre (Ultradent Products, Inc., South Jordan, UT), represents an improved and safer means for the removal of superficial stains or defects. This technique involves the physical removal of tooth structure and does not remove stains or defects through any bleaching phenomena.

Before treatment, the clinician should evaluate the nature and extent of the enamel defect or stain and differentiate between nonhereditary developmental dysmineralization (i.e., abnormal mineralization) defects (e.g., white or light brown fluorotic enamel and the idiopathic white or light brown spot) versus incipient caries lesions. Incipient caries lesions usually are located near the gingival margin. These lesions have a smooth surface and appear opaque or chalky white when dried but are less visible when hydrated.

Incipient caries is reversible if treated immediately. Changing the oral environment through oral hygiene practices and dietary adjustments allows remineralization to occur. If the caries lesion has progressed to have a slightly roughened surface, however, microabrasion coupled with a remineralization program is an initial option. If this approach is unsuccessful, it can be followed by a restoration. Cavitation of the enamel surface is an indication for restorative intervention. As the location of smooth-surface enamel caries nears the cementoenamel junction (CEJ), then enamel is too thin to permit microabrasion or macroabrasion as a treatment option.

A developmental discolored spot (opaque white or light brown) is the result of an unknown, local traumatic event during amelogenesis and is termed *idiopathic*. Its surface is intact, smooth, and hard. It usually is located in the incisal (occlusal) half of enamel, which contributes to the unsightly appearance. The patient (or the patient's parents in the case of a child) must be informed that an accurate prognosis for microabrasion cannot be given but that microabrasion will be applied first. If microabrasion is unsuccessful

because of the depth of the defect exceeding 0.2 to 0.3 mm, the tooth will be restored with a tooth-colored restoration. Surface discolorations resulting from fluorosis also can be removed by microabrasion if the discoloration is within the 0.2- to 0.3-mm removal depth limit.

Fig. 9.29A shows a young patient with fluorosis stains on teeth Nos. 8 and 9. A rubber dam is placed to isolate the teeth to be treated and to protect the gingival tissues from the acid in the Prema paste or compound (Premier Dental Products). Protective glasses should be worn by the patient to shield the eyes from any spatter. The Prema paste is applied to the defective area of the tooth with a special rubber cup that has fluted edges (see Fig. 9.29B and C). The abrasive compound can be applied with either the side or the end of the rubber cup. A 10× gear reduction, low-speed handpiece (similar to that used for placing pins) is recommended for the application of the Prema compound to reduce the possibility of removing too much tooth structure and to prevent spatter. Moderately firm pressure is used in applying the compound.

For small, localized, idiopathic white or light brown areas, a hand application device also is available for use with the Prema compound (see Fig. 9.29D). Periodically, the paste is rinsed away to assess the extent of defect removal. The facial surface also is viewed with a mirror from the incisal aspect to determine how much tooth structure has been removed. Care must be taken not to remove too much tooth structure. The procedure is continued until the defect is removed or until it is deemed imprudent to continue further (see Fig. 9.29E). The treated areas are polished with a fluoride-containing prophy paste to restore surface luster (see Fig. 9.29F). Immediately after treatment, a topical fluoride is applied to teeth to enhance remineralization (see Fig. 9.29G). Results are shown in Fig. 9.29H.

Macroabrasion

An alternative technique for the removal of localized, superficial white spots (not subject to conservative, remineralization therapy) and other surface stains or defects is called *macroabrasion*. Macroabrasion simply uses a 12-fluted composite finishing bur or a fine-grit finishing diamond in a high-speed handpiece to remove the defect (Fig. 9.30A and B). Care must be taken to use light, intermittent pressure and to monitor the removal of tooth structure carefully to avoid irreversible damage to the tooth. Air-water spray is recommended, not only as a coolant but also to maintain the tooth in a hydrated state to facilitate the assessment of defect removal. Teeth that have white spot defects are particularly susceptible to dehydration resulting in other apparent white spots that are not normally seen when the tooth is hydrated. Dehydration exaggerates the appearance of white spots and makes defect removal difficult to assess. After removal of the defect or on termination of any further removal of tooth structure, a 30-fluted finishing bur is used to remove any facets or striations created by the previous instruments. Final polishing is accomplished with an abrasive rubber point (see Fig. 9.30C). The results are shown in Fig. 9.30D.

Comparable results can be achieved with microabrasion and macroabrasion. Both treatments have advantages as well as disadvantages. Microabrasion has the advantage of ensuring better control of the removal of tooth structure. High-speed instrumentation used in macroabrasion is technique sensitive and can have catastrophic results if the clinician fails to use extreme caution. Macroabrasion is considerably faster and does not require the use of a rubber dam or special instrumentation. Defect removal also

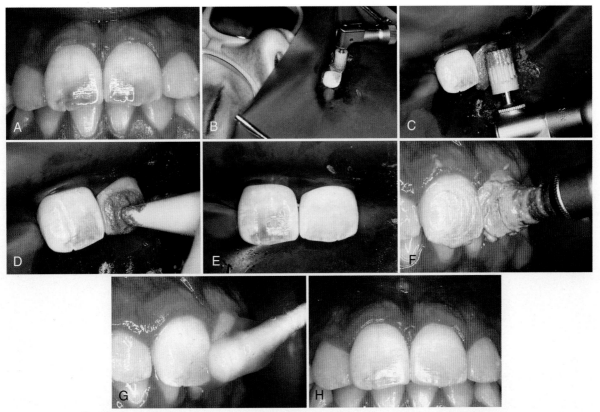

• **Fig. 9.29** Microabrasion. A, Young patient with unesthetic fluorosis stains on central incisors. B and C, Prema compound applied with special rubber cup with fluted edges. Protective glasses and rubber dam are needed for the safety of the patient. D, Hand applicator for applying Prema compound. E, Stain removed from the left central incisor after microabrasion. F, Treated enamel surfaces polished with pro-phylactic paste. G, Topical fluoride applied to treated enamel surfaces. H, Final esthetic result. (Courtesy Dr. Ted Croll.)

is easier with macroabrasion compared with microabrasion if an air-water spray is used during treatment to maintain hydration of teeth. Nonetheless, microabrasion is recommended over macroabrasion for the treatment of superficial defects in children because of better operator control and superior patient acceptance. To accelerate the process, a combination of macroabrasion and microabrasion also may be considered. Gross removal of the defect is accomplished with macroabrasion, followed by final treatment with microabrasion.

Veneers

A veneer is a layer of tooth-colored material that is applied to a tooth to restore localized or generalized defects and intrinsic discolorations (for examples, see Figs. 9.7, 9.33, 9.34, 9.35, and 9.41). Typically, veneers are made of directly applied composite, processed composite, porcelain, or pressed ceramic materials. Common indications for veneers include teeth with facial surfaces that are malformed, discolored, abraded, or eroded or have faulty restorations (Fig. 9.31).

Two types of esthetic veneers exist: (1) partial veneers and (2) full veneers (Fig. 9.32). Partial veneers are indicated for the restoration of localized defects or areas of intrinsic discoloration (Fig. 9.33; see also Fig. 9.1). Full veneers are indicated for the restoration of generalized defects or areas of intrinsic staining involving most of the facial surface of the tooth (for examples, see Figs. 9.7, 9.35, 9.36, 9.37, and 9.41). Several important factors including patient

age, occlusion, tissue health, position and alignment of teeth, and oral hygiene must be evaluated before pursuing full veneers as a treatment option. If full veneers are done, care must be taken to provide proper physiologic contours, particularly in the gingival area, to ensure good gingival health. An example of poorly contoured veneers is shown in Fig. 9.31D; severe gingival irritation exists around the overcontoured veneers, and a purulent exudate is evident on probing the margins with an explorer.

Full veneers can be accomplished by the direct or indirect technique. When only a few teeth are involved or when the entire facial surface is not faulty (i.e., partial veneers), directly applied composite veneers can be completed chairside in one appointment for the patient. Placing direct composite full veneers is time consuming and labor intensive. For cases involving young children or a single discolored tooth, or when the patient's time or money is limited, precluding a laboratory-fabricated veneer, the direct technique is a viable option. Indirect veneers require two appointments but typically offer three advantages over directly placed full veneers:

1. Indirectly fabricated veneers are much less sensitive to operator technique. Considerable artistic expertise and attention to detail are required to consistently achieve esthetically pleasing and physiologically sound direct veneers. Indirect veneers are made by a laboratory technician and are typically more esthetic.
2. If multiple teeth are to be veneered, indirect veneers usually can be placed much more expeditiously.

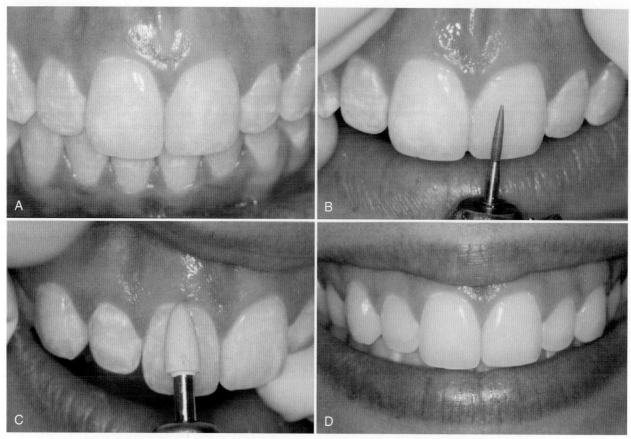

• **Fig. 9.30** Macroabrasion. A, Outer surfaces of maxillary anterior teeth are unesthetic because of superficial enamel defects. B and C, Removal of discoloration by abrasive surfacing and polishing procedures. D, Completed treatment revealing conservative esthetic outcome.

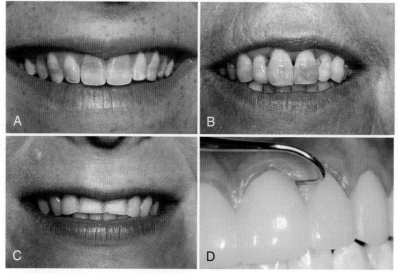

• **Fig. 9.31** Clinical examples of indications for treatment with veneers include teeth affected by tetracycline drug staining (A), fluorosis or enamel hypoplasia (B), acid-induced erosion (e.g., lemon-sucking habit) (C), and defective or improperly done existing veneers (note significant gingival overhang with associated purulent exudate) (D).

3. Indirect veneers typically last much longer than do direct veneers, especially if they are made of porcelain or pressed ceramic.

Some controversy exists regarding the extent of tooth preparation that is necessary and the amount of coverage for both direct and indirect fabricated veneers (see Fig. 9.32). Some operators prefer to etch the existing enamel and apply the veneer (direct or indirect type) to the entire existing facial surface without any tooth preparation. The perceived advantage of these "no prep" veneers is that little or no tooth structure is removed. Also, in the event of failure or if the patient does not like the veneer, it supposedly can be removed (being reversible), although in actuality, it is never easy to remove any bonded veneer without concomitant removal of some tooth structure (see also section No-Prep Veneers).

Several significant problems exist, however, with this approach. First, to achieve an esthetic result, if the tooth is otherwise of normal contour, the facial surface of such a restoration will be overcontoured, appearing and feeling unnatural. This observation is true for both direct and indirect veneers. An overcontoured veneer frequently results in gingival irritation with accompanying hyperemia and bleeding caused by bulbous and impinging gingival

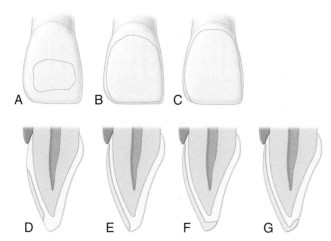

• **Fig. 9.32** Four types of veneers. A, Facial view of partial veneer that does not extend subgingivally or involve the incisal angle. B, Full veneer with window preparation design that extends to the gingival crest and terminates at the facioincisal angle. C, Full veneer with either a butt-joint incisal preparation design or an incisal-lapping preparation design extending subgingivally and including all of incisal surface. (Subgingival extension is indicated only for preparation of darkly stained teeth and is not considered routine.) D–G, Cross sections of the four types of veneers: partial veneer (D), full veneer with window preparation design (E), full veneer with butt-joint incisal preparation design (F), full veneer with incisal-lapping incisal preparation design (G).

contours. Second, with regard to direct veneers, the veneer is more likely to be dislodged when no tooth structure is removed before the etching and bonding procedures are done. If the veneer is lost, it can be replaced. The patient may live in constant fear, however, that it will happen again, possibly causing embarrassment.

The reversibility of no-prep veneers may seem desirable and appealing to patients from a psychologic standpoint; however, few patients who elect to have veneers wish to return to the original condition. In addition, removing full veneers with no damage to the underlying unprepared tooth, as noted earlier, is exceedingly difficult if not impossible. To achieve esthetically pleasing and physiologically sound results consistently, an intraenamel preparation is usually indicated. The only exception is in cases in which the facial aspect of the tooth is significantly undercontoured because of severe abrasion or erosion. In these cases, mere roughening of the involved enamel and defining of the peripheral margins are indicated.

Intraenamel preparation (or the roughening of the surface in undercontoured areas) before placing a veneer is strongly recommended for the following reasons:
1. To provide space for bonding and veneering materials for maximal esthetics without overcontouring
2. To remove the outer, fluoride-rich layer of enamel that may be more resistant to acid etching
3. To create a rough surface for improved bonding
4. To establish a definite finish line

Establishing an intraenamel preparation with a definite finish line is particularly important when placing indirectly fabricated veneers. Accurate positioning and seating of an indirectly made veneer are enhanced significantly if an intraenamel preparation is present.

Another controversy involves the location of the gingival margin of the veneer (see Fig. 9.32). Should it terminate short of the free gingival crest at the level of the gingival crest or apical of the gingival crest? The answer depends on the individual situation. If the defect or discoloration does not extend subgingivally, the margin of the veneer should not extend subgingivally. The position of the gingival margin of any veneer is dictated by the extent of the

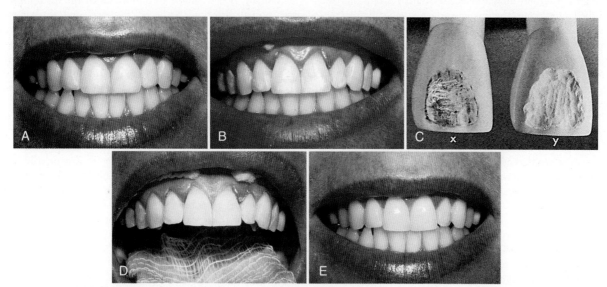

• **Fig. 9.33** Direct partial veneers. A, Patient with overcontoured direct full veneers. B, After removal of old veneer, localized white spots are evident. C, Models illustrate fault (x) and cavity preparation (y). The chamfered margins are irregular in outline. D, Intraenamel preparations for partial veneer restorations. E, Conservative esthetic result of completed partial veneers.

defects or discoloration and the amount of tooth structure that is visible with maximum smiling. If a patient exhibits a high smile line that exposes the entire facial surface of the tooth and if defects like fluorosis stains are generalized, then the margin of the veneer must be positioned at the level of the crest of tissue to optimize esthetics. However, the only logical reason for extending the margin subgingivally is if the gingival area is carious or defective, warranting restoration, or if it involves significantly dark discoloration that presents a difficult esthetic problem. No restorative material is as good as normal tooth structure, and the gingival tissue is never as healthy when it is in contact with an artificial material.

Three basic preparation designs exist for full veneers: (1) a window preparation, (2) a butt-joint incisal preparation, and (3) an incisal-lapping preparation (see Fig. 9.32). A window preparation is recommended for most direct composite veneers. It is also frequently used in cases of indirectly fabricated veneers where the outline form of the canine is intact and the patient is canine guided. This intraenamel preparation design preserves the functional lingual and incisal surfaces of maxillary anterior teeth, protecting the veneers from significant occlusal stress. This quality is of particular importance with direct composite veneers.

A window preparation design also is recommended for indirectly fabricated porcelain veneers in patients who exhibit a canine-guided pattern of lateral guidance and in whom the maxillary canines are of normal contour with little incisal wear or notching. By using a window preparation, the functional surfaces are better preserved in enamel (see Fig. 9.32E and, later, Fig. 9.41I). This design reduces the potential for accelerated wear of the opposing tooth that could result if the functional path involved porcelain on the lingual and incisal surfaces, as with incisal butt-joint or incisal-lapping designs.

For most indirectly fabricated porcelain veneers, either a butt-joint incisal design or an incisal-lapping approach is used. A butt-joint incisal design is used routinely in cases where no defects exist along the lingual aspect of the incisal edge. It is the simplest design and is used to easily provide adequate reduction of the tooth to accommodate the needed strength of the porcelain veneer in this area of the preparation (see Fig. 9.32F). An incisal-lapping preparation is indicated when the tooth being veneered needs lengthening or when an incisal defect warrants restoration. The extent of the lapping onto the lingual surface is generally dictated by the extent of the lingual incisal defect or by the amount of faciolingual resistance form desired for reinforcement of the incisal edge (see Fig. 9.32G and, later, Fig. 9.40).

The preparation and restoration of a tooth with a veneer should be carried out in a manner that provides optimal function, esthetics, retention, physiologic contours, and longevity. All of these objectives should be accomplished without compromising the strength of the remaining tooth structure. If the veneer becomes chipped, discolored, or worn, it usually can be repaired or replaced.

Darkly stained teeth, especially teeth discolored by tetracycline, are much more difficult to veneer with full veneers compared with teeth with generalized defects but that have normal underlying coloration (see Fig. 9.44). The difficulty is compounded further when the cervical areas are badly discolored. Usually, only the six maxillary anterior teeth require correction because they are the most noticeable when a person smiles or talks. The maxillary first premolars (and to a lesser extent the second premolars) also are included, however, if they too are noticeable on smiling.

Discolored mandibular anterior teeth are rarely indicated for veneers because the facioincisal portions are thin and usually subject to biting forces and attrition. Veneering mandibular teeth is discouraged if the teeth are in normal occlusal contact because it is exceedingly difficult to achieve adequate reduction of the enamel to compensate for the thickness of the veneering material. Also, if porcelain veneers are placed on mandibular teeth, the veneers may accelerate the wear of opposing maxillary teeth because of the abrasive nature of the porcelain. In most cases, the lower lip hides these teeth so esthetics is not a significant problem. Most patients are satisfied with the conservative approach of veneering only maxillary anterior teeth.

Direct Veneer Technique

Direct Partial Veneers

Small localized intrinsic discolorations or defects that are surrounded by healthy enamel are ideally treated with direct partial veneers (see Fig. 9.1B and C). Often practitioners place full veneers when only partial veneers are indicated. The four anterior teeth in Fig. 9.33A illustrate the clinical technique for placing partial veneers. These defects can be restored in one appointment with a light-cured composite. Preliminary steps include cleaning, shade selection, and isolation with cotton rolls or rubber dam. Anesthesia usually is not required unless the defect is deep, extending into dentin.

Fig. 9.33A shows four anterior teeth that had previously received direct composite veneers with no enamel preparation for the restoration of developmental white spot lesions. However, even after veneering, the white spots still show through the veneers. On removal of the defective veneers, the localized white spots are evident (see Fig. 9.33B). Models illustrating proper preparation are shown in Fig. 9.33C. The outline form is dictated solely by the extent of the defect and should include all discolored areas. The clinician should use a coarse, elliptical or round diamond instrument with air-water coolant to remove the defect. The use of water-air spray is also imperative so that the tooth can be maintained in a hydrated state. If dehydration is allowed to occur, it can cause the appearance of other white spots, which are artifacts and which will make defect assessment much more difficult (see Fig. 9.33D). After preparation, etching, and restoration of the defective areas (as described in the following paragraph), the finished partial veneers are seen (see Fig. 9.33E).

Usually, it is desirable to remove all of the discolored enamel in a pulpal direction. If the entire defect or stain is removed, a microfilled composite is recommended for restoring the preparation. Microfills are excellent "enamel replacement" materials because of their optical properties. If the tooth has been maintained in a hydrated state, the microfilled composite can be positioned on a trial basis to assess the accuracy of the shade prior to final restoration. Nanofilled composites also are excellent material choices for this technique. If a residual lightly stained area or white spot remains in enamel, however, an intrinsically less translucent composite can be used rather than extending the preparation into dentin to eliminate the defect. Most composites filled primarily with radiopaque fillers (e.g., barium glass) are more optically opaque with intrinsic masking qualities (in addition to being radiopaque). Use of these types of composites for the restoration of preparations with light, residual stains is most effective and conserves the tooth structure. In this example, all restorations are of a light-cured microfilled composite.

Direct Full Veneers

Extensive enamel hypoplasia involving all maxillary anterior teeth was treated by placing direct full veneers in this case (Fig. 9.34A). A diastema also was present between the central incisors. The patient desired to have the hypoplasia and the diastema corrected;

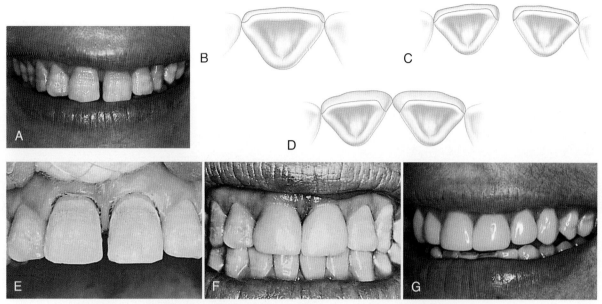

• **Fig. 9.34** Direct full veneers using light-cured composite. A, Enamel hypoplasia of maxillary anterior teeth. B, Typical preparation of facial surface for full veneer. C, The preparation is extended onto the mesial surface to allow closure of diastema. D, Full veneers restore proximal contact. E, Etched preparations of central incisors. F, Veneers completed on maxillary central incisors. G, Treatment completed with placement of full veneers on remaining maxillary anterior teeth.

examination indicated a good prognosis. A direct technique was used with a light-cured microfilled composite. Placing direct full composite veneers is very time consuming. Although all six teeth can be restored at the same appointment, it may be less traumatic for the patient and the dentist if the veneers are placed in two appointments. In this example, the central incisors were completed during the first appointment, and the lateral incisors and canines were completed during the second appointment.

After the teeth to receive the veneers are cleaned and a shade is selected, the area is isolated with cotton rolls and retraction cords. Both central incisors are prepared with a coarse, rounded-end diamond instrument. The window preparation typically is made to a depth roughly equivalent to half the thickness of the facial enamel, ranging from approximately 0.5 to 0.75 mm midfacially and tapering down to a depth of about 0.3 to 0.5 mm along the gingival margin, depending on the thickness of enamel (see Fig. 9.32). A well-defined chamfer at the level of the gingival crest provides a definite preparation margin for subsequent finishing procedures. The margins are not extended subgingivally because these areas are not defective. The preparation for all veneer types (both direct and indirect) normally is terminated just facial to the proximal contact except in the case of a diastema (see Fig. 9.34B). When interdental spaces exist, the preparations must be extended from the facial surfaces onto the mesial surfaces, terminating at the mesiolingual line angles (see Fig. 9.34C and D). This lingual extension of the preparation allows for proper reestablishment of the entire proximal contour of the tooth in the final restoration. The incisal edges were not included in the preparations in this example because no discoloration was present. In addition, preservation of the incisal edges better protects the veneers from heavy functional forces, as noted earlier for window preparations.

The teeth to be treated should be restored one at a time. After the etching, rinsing, and drying procedures (see Fig. 9.34E), the dentist applies and polymerizes the resin-bonding agent. The dentist places the composite on the tooth in increments, especially along

the gingival margin, to reduce the effects of polymerization shrinkage. The composite is placed in slight excess to allow some freedom in contouring. It is helpful to inspect the facial surface from an incisal view with a mirror to evaluate the contour before polymerization. After the first veneer is finished, the second tooth is restored in a similar manner (see Fig. 9.34F). In this case, the remaining four anterior teeth are restored with direct composite veneers (see Fig. 9.34G) at the second appointment. Chapter 8 describes the procedures used to insert and finish composite restorations. Another excellent example of direct composite veneers is seen in Fig. 9.35.

Indirect Veneer Techniques

Many dentists find that the preparation, placement, and finishing of several direct veneers at one time is too difficult, fatiguing, and time consuming. Some patients become uncomfortable and restless during long appointments. In addition, veneer shades and contours can be better controlled when made outside of the mouth on a cast. For these reasons, indirect veneer techniques are usually preferable. Indirect veneers are primarily made of (1) processed composite, (2) feldspathic porcelain, and (3) cast or pressed ceramic. Because of superior strength, durability, and conservation of the tooth structure, feldspathic porcelain bonded to intraenamel preparations has historically been the preferred approach for indirect veneering techniques used by dentists. Some pressed ceramic veneering materials offer comparable esthetic qualities but may require a deeper tooth preparation that is often located in dentin. Studies show that bond strengths to dentin decline over time and that porcelain veneers placed in intraenamel preparations offer the best long-term results.[35-38] However, newer, currently available pressed or castable ceramics are capable of being fabricated to much thinner dimensions, making them viable options for indirect fabrication as well.

Although two appointments are required for indirect veneers, chair time is reduced because much of the work has been done in

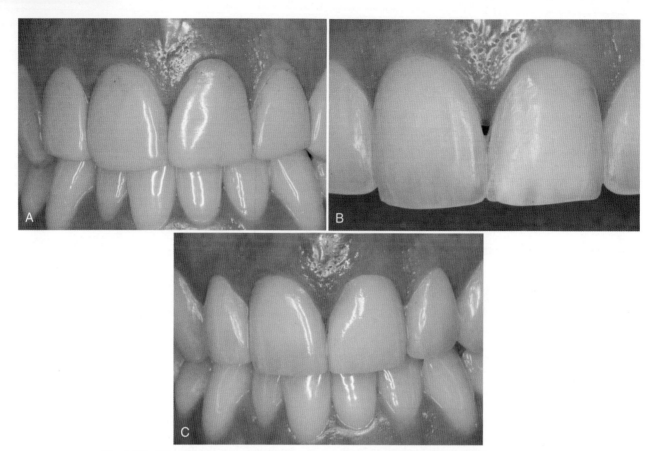

• **Fig. 9.35** Direct full veneers using light-cured composite for defective veneers. A, Defective composite veneers with marginal staining. B, Conservative intraenamel preparation. C, New direct composite veneers on maxillary anterior teeth. (Courtesy Dr. Robert Margeas.)

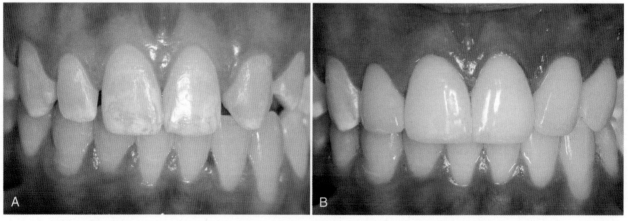

• **Fig. 9.36** No-prep veneers placed on maxillary anterior teeth. A, Before treatment. B, Immediately after placement of the no-prep veneers. (Courtesy Dr. Patricia Pereira.)

the laboratory. Excellent results can be obtained when proper clinical evaluation and careful operating procedures are followed. Indirect veneers are attached to the enamel by acid etching and bonding with light-cured resin cement.

No-Prep Veneers

As noted earlier (see section Veneers), one approach being used for indirect veneers is to place them on teeth with no tooth preparation. Although this "no prep" approach may at first appear desirable,

it can later cause problems if proper case selection is not done. No-prep veneers are best used when teeth are inherently undercontoured, when interdental spaces or open incisal embrasures are present, or when both conditions exist. Examples of successful no-prep veneers following these guidelines are seen in Figs. 9.36 and 9.37.

However, no-prep veneers can be problematic. First, no-prep veneers are inherently made thinner and consequently are more prone to fracture, especially during the try-in phase. Second, for

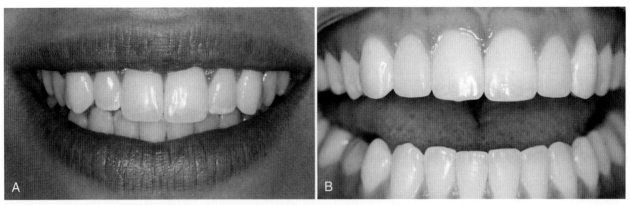

• **Fig. 9.37** No-prep veneers placed to restore undersized maxillary lateral incisors. A, Before treatment. B, After placement of the no-prep veneers. (Courtesy Dr. Gary Radz.)

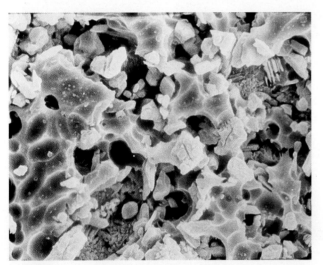

• **Fig. 9.38** Scanning electron micrograph (×31,000) of feldspathic porcelain etched with hydrofluoric acid. (Courtesy Dr. Steven Bayne.)

indirect no-prep veneers, interproximal areas are difficult to access for proper finishing. And third, as noted earlier, if case selection is not done properly and the teeth are already of normal contour, the resulting veneers inevitably will be overcontoured. Veneers that are overcontoured are not generally esthetic and often can result in impingement of gingival tissue, as noted earlier (see Fig. 9.31D). For these reasons, it is advisable in most cases to use a conservative, intraenamel preparation for the use of indirect veneers, as noted in the next section.

Etched Porcelain Veneers

The preferred type of indirect veneer is the etched porcelain (i.e., feldspathic) veneer. Porcelain veneers etched with hydrofluoric acid are capable of achieving high bond strengths to the etched enamel via a resin-bonding medium.[39-41] This porcelain etching pattern is shown in Fig. 9.38. In addition to the high bond strengths, etched porcelain veneers are highly esthetic, stain resistant, and periodontally compatible. The incidence of cohesive fracture for etched porcelain veneers is also very low.[36] However, as noted earlier, the key to the long-term success with etched porcelain veneers is the use of a *conservative intraenamel preparation*. Preparations into dentin should be avoided because virtually all problems associated with etched porcelain veneers (debonding, accelerated marginal staining, tooth sensitivity, etc.) occur when excessive amounts of dentin are exposed in the veneer preparation.

Tooth Preparation

Because the most important consideration in determining the success of etched porcelain veneers is tooth preparation, a systematic approach will be presented first, using a dentiform series, prior to reviewing the associated clinical procedures (Fig. 9.39). A veneer design using a butt-joint incisal edge will be illustrated first. The tooth used to illustrate the preparation sequence has intentionally been colored blue to allow better visualization of the involved steps. However, it is not recommended that this tooth marking be done clinically.

The veneer preparation is made with a tapered, rounded-end diamond instrument. It is critical that the tip diameter of the diamond be measured because the diamond will serve as the measuring tool in gauging proper reduction depth. A diamond with a tip diameter of 1 to 1.2 mm is recommended. The tip diameter of the diamond used in this series is 1.2 mm.

The first step in the veneer preparation is establishing the peripheral outline form. Position the diamond to half its depth (approximately 0.6 mm in this example) just facial to the proximal contact on either proximal surface, and then extend the bur, while maintaining its occlusogingival orientation, around the gingival area and then back up the opposite proximal area, again keeping the diamond positioned just facial to the proximal contact area (see Fig. 9.39A and B). In this example, a supragingival marginal position was maintained. Recall that clinically, the position of the gingival margin is determined by lip position (and the resulting display of teeth) and the gingival extent of the facial discoloration or defect being treated, as noted previously. If possible, a supragingival margin position is always considered desirable because it minimizes the potential for an adverse gingival response.

Facial reduction is achieved by first identifying and then reducing three separate facial zones: the incisal third, the middle third, and the gingival third (see Fig. 9.39C), in that order. To prepare the incisal zone of facial reduction, the diamond first is aligned parallel with the facial surface of the incisal third of the tooth. The diamond is then moved mesiodistally from line angle to line angle until the desired depth of approximately 0.6 mm is attained. Again, the tip of the diamond is used to gauge this reduction. Reduction depth can be verified by viewing the tip of the diamond in proximity to the unprepared tooth structure gingival to this reduced area when viewed from the proximal, facial, and incisal aspects (see Fig. 9.39D and E). Care also must be taken to round the mesial and distal facial line angles during this reduction sequence to ensure uniform facial reduction.

The middle third is reduced in a similar manner. By carefully watching the striations being created by the diamond mesiodistally during the reduction of the middle third, it is easy to see when the level of the previous incisal third reduction is reached (see Fig. 9.39F). When a similar reduction level has been reached, the striations in the middle one third will then extend into the area previously reduced in the incisal third. Stop immediately. *Do not go deeper.* Again, a reduction depth of approximately 0.6 mm is

desirable. Moreover, the reduction depth again can be verified by viewing the tip of the diamond in proximity to the unprepared tooth structure gingival to this reduced area when viewed from the proximal, facial, and incisal aspects. Care also must be taken to round the mesial and distal facial line angles during this reduction sequence to ensure uniform facial reduction.

Reduction of the gingival one third is straightforward and simply involves removal of the remaining "island" of unprepared tooth structure to a level consistent with the surrounding previously prepared tooth structure (see Fig. 9.39G and H).

Incisal reduction is made by orienting the diamond perpendicular to the incisal edge and then reducing the incisal edge to attain a

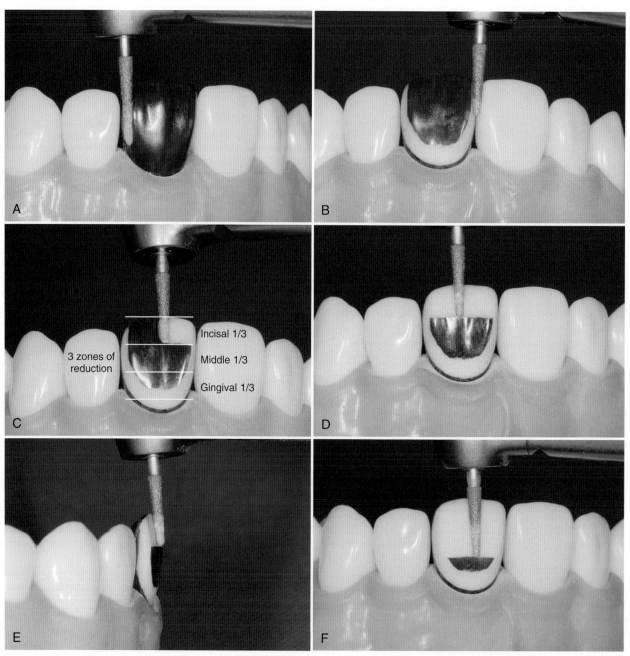

• **Fig. 9.39** Intraenamel preparation for an etched porcelain veneer with a butt-joint incisal edge design. A and B, The peripheral outline form is first established using a rounded-end diamond instrument. C–H, Facial reduction is achieved by first identifying and then reducing three separate facial zones: the incisal third, the middle third, and the gingival third (C), in that order.

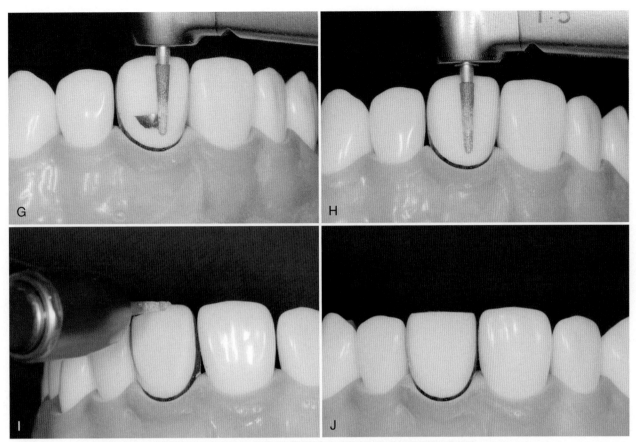

• **Fig. 9.39, cont'd** I, Incisal reduction is attained. J, The completed intraenamel preparation for an etched porcelain veneer with a butt-joint incisal edge.

minimum reduction of 1 mm or, more desirably, 1.5 mm (see Fig. 9.39I). Clinically, this reduction in depth will be gauged using an incisal reduction index. In this dentiform example, a minimum 1-mm incisal reduction depth was generated. Finally, round the facioincisal line angle with the side of the diamond to reduce internal stresses in the porcelain veneer. The final intraenamel preparation for an etched porcelain veneer using a butt-joint incisal edge design is seen in Fig. 9.39J.

Frequently, an incisal-lapping preparation is indicated if the patient has worn or defective areas on the lingual aspect of the incisal edge. Some operators also prefer this design because of enhanced adaptation of the veneer to the lingual preparation margin attributable to a "lap sliding" fit.

The preparation steps for the incisal-lapping preparation are identical to those for the butt-joint design, including the steps for incisal reduction; however, additional steps are required to attain the incisal-lapping feature. The first step in achieving this preparation design is to notch the mesial and distal incisal angles. The tip of the same diamond instrument used for the earlier steps of the veneer preparation is used to establish these notches. Using the diamond, extend the notches completely through the incisal angles faciolingually to a depth incisogingivally consistent with the desired amount of lapping of the lingual surface (Fig. 9.40A). For example, if a 0.5-mm lap of the lingual surface is desired, as in this example, the notches are prepared to a depth of 0.5 mm each accordingly (see Fig. 9.40B).

Once the incisal notches have been generated incisogingivally to a depth consistent with the desired amount of lingual lapping, the preparation of the lingual lap is made. Position the diamond into the tooth to a depth of approximately 0.6 mm (less if remaining faciolingual thickness of the incisal edge enamel is compromised) and extend the preparation across the lingual surface from notch to notch (see Fig. 9.40C). The resulting sharp incisal angles must then be rounded to finish the incisal-lapping portion of the preparation. Care must be taken to include any desired lingual defect. The gingival extent of the incisal lap is determined by the extent of any lingual defect. The final lapping portion of the preparation is seen in Fig. 9.40D. The facial view of the completed incisal-lapping preparation with a lingual lap of 0.5 mm is seen in Fig. 9.40E.

Clinical Procedures

The case of a patient with generalized fluorosis is used to illustrate the clinical procedures involved (Fig. 9.41A). A consult appointment is always recommended prior to initiating the veneer procedures. At this appointment, the actual procedures are discussed in detail, appropriate consents are obtained, and any needed records are generated, including shade selection, intraoral photographs, and impressions for diagnostic models and occlusal records. Laboratory communications are greatly enhanced through the inclusion of digital photographs. An excellent series of baseline photographs, including some with shade tabs positioned in the photographic field to document the preoperative shapes and shades of the involved teeth, should be made.

Although intraenamel preparations will be used, it is always recommended that patients be anesthetized during the appointment

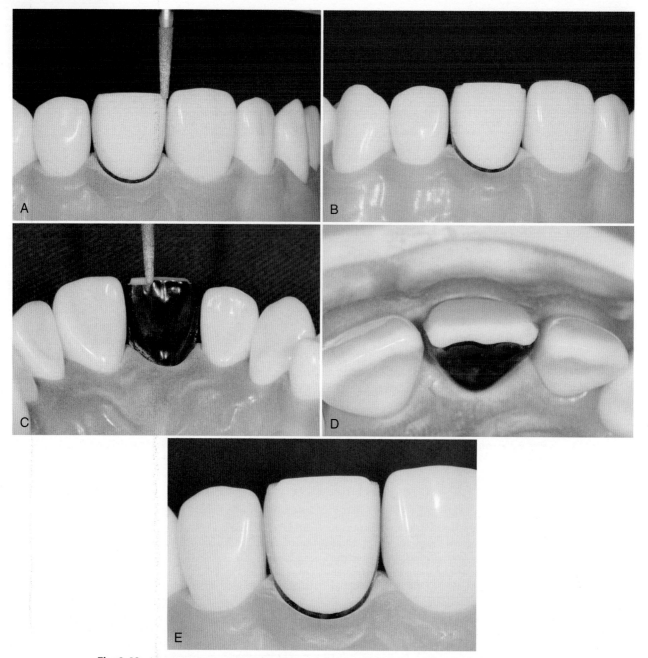

• **Fig. 9.40** Intraenamel preparation steps for an etched porcelain veneer with an incisal-lapping design. A and B, Incisal notches. C, Preparing the lingual-lapping portion of the prep. D and E, The completed intraenamel preparation viewed from the lingual and facial aspects for an etched porcelain veneer with an incisal-lapping design.

for tooth preparation to ensure maximum comfort for the patient and the dentist. Once the anesthetic is administered, preoperative records such as an incisal reduction index and those needed to facilitate temporization are made. An incisal reduction index is always recommended to accurately gauge the amount of incisal reduction during the preparation of teeth for etched porcelain veneers (Fig. 9.42; see also Fig. 9.41B–H). An incisal reduction index is made by recording the lingual and incisal contours of the anterior teeth to be prepared or the contours generated in a diagnostic wax-up. Typically a fast-setting silicone or polyvinyl siloxane elastomeric material is used to generate this record. If a diagnostic model has been made in which the incisal edge positions

of the final veneers will be different from the current teeth, the incisal reduction index should be made using the diagnostic model (see Fig. 9.42A and B). As in this case, if no change in the incisal edge positions of the involved teeth is desired, the reduction index can be made directly in the patient's mouth by recording the existing contours of the involved teeth. Once the facial excess has been trimmed away with a No. 12 surgical blade in a Bard-Parker handle, the incisal reduction index should be tried in the mouth to verify the accuracy of the index (see Fig. 9.41B).

The patient in this case has a high smile line and generalized defects that involve the entire facial surfaces of anterior teeth. Therefore a small diameter gingival retraction cord is placed in

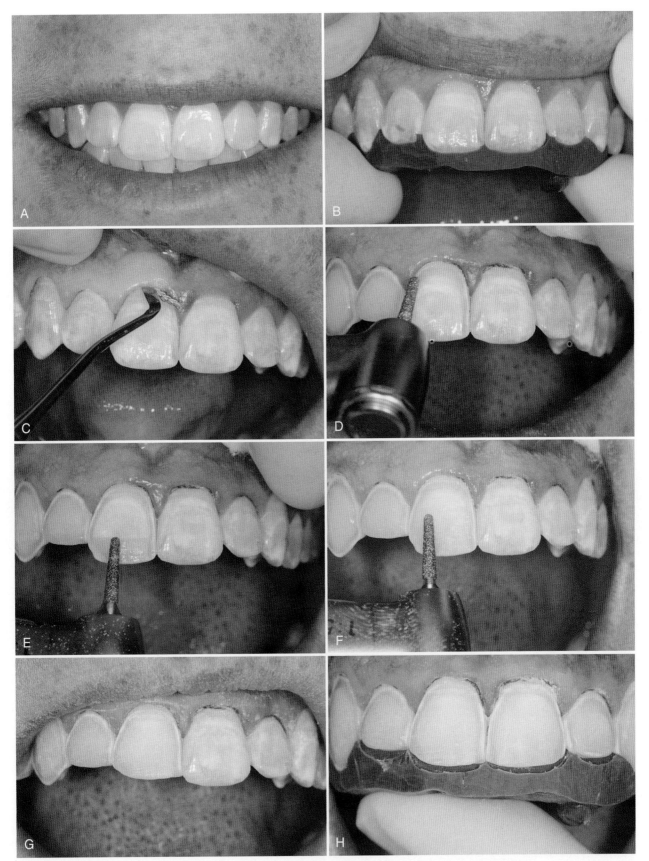

• **Fig. 9.41** Etched porcelain veneers using an intraenamel preparation. A, A patient with severe dental fluorosis. B, An incisal reduction index is made intraorally, since no significant change in incisal edge position is desired. C, Retraction cord is placed. D, The outline form is first established. E–G, Facial reduction is attained by using three zones of facial reduction. H, Incisal reduction is verified using the incisal reduction index.

Continued

• **Fig. 9.41, cont'd** I, Finished preparations for intraenamel preparations. Note the window preparations on canines and premolars. J, Retraction cord is placed for isolation. K, The fit of the veneer is assessed. L and M, Etching of the prepared maxillary central incisors. N and O, Adhesive is applied to the etched enamel and the tooth side of the porcelain veneer. P, The veneer is loaded with resin cement and seated on the tooth.

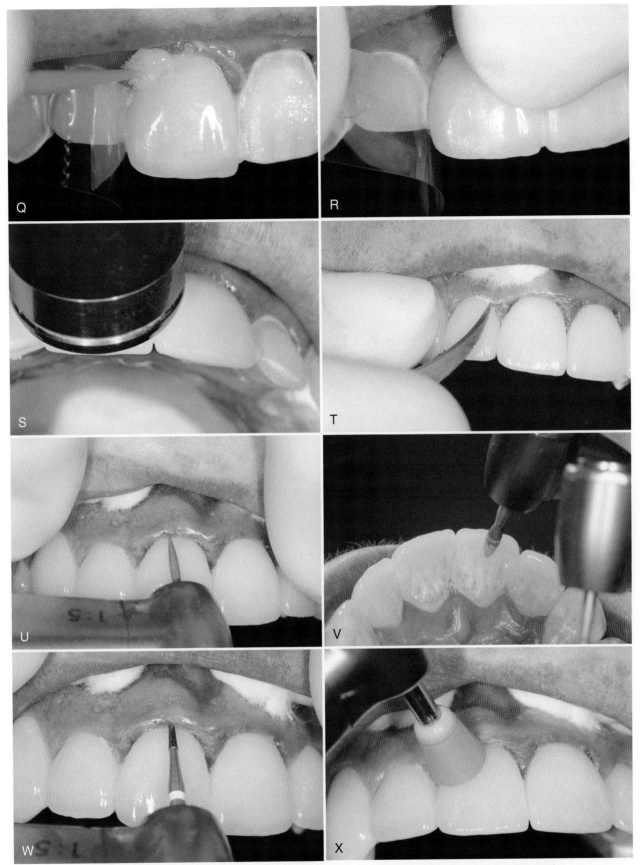

• **Fig. 9.41, cont'd**   Q, Excess cement is removed with a microbrush. R, Excess cement is removed interproximally through removal of polyester strip. S, Resin cement cured with intense curing light. T, No. 12 surgical blade in a Bard-Parker handle is used for removing excess cured resin cement. U and V, Diamond instruments used to "dress" marginal areas. W and X, 30-fluted carbide burs and diamond impregnated polishing instruments used to finish and polish veneer margins.   *Continued*

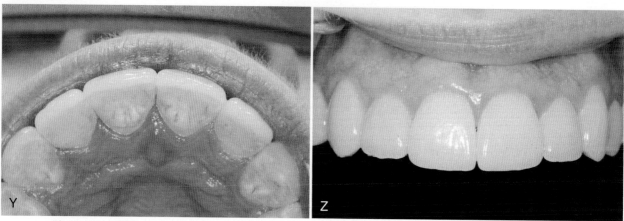

• **Fig. 9.41, cont'd** Y and Z, Finished etched porcelain veneers as viewed from the lingual and facial aspects.

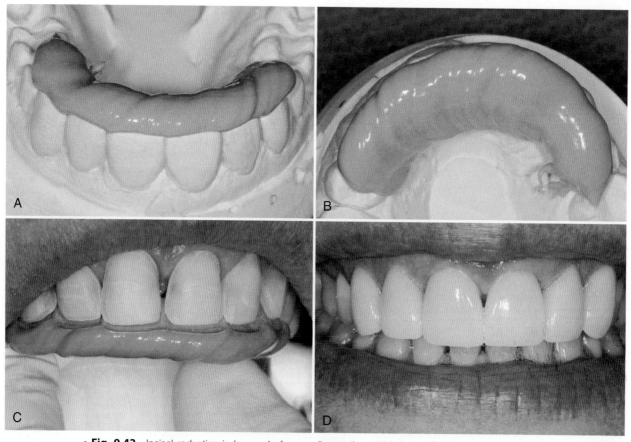

• **Fig. 9.42** Incisal reduction index made from a diagnostic model. A and B, A fast-set elastomeric material is used to record the lingual and incisal contours of the diagnostic model. C, Incisal reduction index is used to verify proper incisal preparation of teeth. D, Finished etched porcelain veneers.

anticipation of veneer margins that will be placed at the level of the free gingival margins (see Fig. 9.41C).

Incisal-lapping preparations for porcelain veneers are made on the maxillary central and lateral incisors consistent with the systematic step-by-step preparation procedures described earlier. The intraenamel preparations are made with a tapered, rounded-end diamond instrument to a depth of approximately 0.5 to 0.75 mm midfacially, diminishing to a depth of 0.3 to 0.5 mm along the gingival margins, depending on enamel thickness. The outline form is first established as noted earlier (see Fig. 9.41D). Facial

reduction is attained by using three zones of facial reduction as previously described (see Fig. 9.41E–G). Veneer interproximal margins should extend into the facial and gingival embrasures, without engaging an undercut, and yet should be located just facial to the proximal contacts.

Since this patient is young with beautifully shaped canines and also exhibits a canine-guided occlusion, a window type of preparation design was employed when preparing the maxillary canines. By restricting the window prep veneers to the facial surface entirely, functional contact will be maintained solely on tooth structure, thereby preventing accelerated wear of opposing teeth. Adequate incisal reduction is verified using the incisal reduction index as noted earlier (see Fig. 9.41H). The finished preparations are shown in Fig. 9.41I.

After the preparations are completed, an elastomeric impression is made and appropriate occlusal records generated. Digital photos of the prepared teeth (with and without appropriate shade tabs in the photographic field) also are recommended. In most cases, provisionals are fabricated for the prepared teeth, as described in the subsequent section on temporization (see Veneer Provisionalization). If a diagnostic wax-up was generated, veneer provisionals are necessary to assess the tooth contours generated in the wax-up intraorally. If no diagnostic wax-up was needed, occasionally temporary restorations are not required if the patient consents, because the preparations are shallow and involve only enamel. In these cases, the patient should be instructed to avoid biting hard foods and objects, to keep the areas clean with a soft bristled brush, and to expect the possibility of some mild sensitivity to hot and cold. It should be noted that the vast majority of veneer cases will warrant temporization.

After they have been fabricated in the laboratory, the porcelain veneers are returned to the dentist for cementation at the second appointment. The completed veneers must be inspected for cracks, overextended margins, and adequate internal etching (as evidenced by a frosted appearance). Marginal areas in particular should be inspected for proper etching so that an adequate seal occurs in these areas. Overextended marginal areas interproximally may preclude full seating of adjacent veneers. These areas can be trimmed carefully with a micron-finishing diamond instrument or flexible abrasive disk. Unless severe or inaccessible, most minor overextensions should be trimmed only after bonding the veneer to the tooth because of the risk of fracturing the porcelain.

After the prepared teeth are cleaned with a pumice slurry, rinsed, and dried, isolation is accomplished with a lip retractor (optional) and cotton rolls. A 5-cm by 5-cm (2-inch by 2-inch) cotton gauze is placed across the back of the patient's mouth to protect against aspiration or swallowing of an inadvertently dropped veneer. If the veneer margins closely approximate the gingiva, a small diameter retraction cord should be placed in the gingival crevice during try-in and cementation to prevent inadvertent contamination of the bonds from crevicular fluids (see Fig. 9.41J).

The fit of each veneer is evaluated on the respective individual tooth and adjusted if necessary. A No. 2 explorer should be used to assess marginal fit (see Fig. 9.41K). All of the veneers should be tried in place not only individually but also in adjacent pairs to ensure the fit of adjacent seated veneers. Veneers should be tried in place only on clean, dry teeth to eliminate any potential for contamination. If accidental contamination occurs, the veneer should be cleaned thoroughly with alcohol or acid etchant, rinsed, and dried before bonding.

Prior to cementation, a silane agent can optionally be applied to the internal surfaces of the veneers. The silane acts as a coupling agent, forming a chemical bond between the porcelain and the resin that increases bond strength of the resin to the porcelain.[42] It also improves the wettability of the porcelain. The primary source of retention with porcelain veneers still remains the etched porcelain surface itself. Only a modest increase in bond strength results from silanation of the porcelain; however, it is recommended because it also may reduce marginal leakage and discoloration.

A light-cured resin cement is recommended for bonding the veneer to the tooth because light-cured resins are more color stable and provide additional working time over the self-cured or dual-cured versions. Shade selection of the bonding medium is determined after the fit of the individual veneers has been evaluated and confirmed. Water can be used as an optical medium for try-in to assess the appearance of the veneers. With this technique, water is placed in a single central incisor veneer (or both central incisor veneers); placed on clean, dry teeth; and the appearance assessed. If the veneers are deemed acceptable in appearance, an untinted shade of the bonding resin is indicated. For the vast majority of etched porcelain veneers, an untinted shade of the bonding resin is recommended. Because etched porcelain veneers can be fabricated with inherent color gradients, characterizations, and even additional opaques when further masking of stains is needed, it is unusual that alternative shades or opaque resin bonding media are needed. Nonetheless, alternative shades or opaque versions of resin bonding cements are sometimes preferred by some dentists.

If alternative shades of resin cements are needed, shade selection is made by first placing a uniform layer of a selected shade of resin cement, approximately 0.5 mm in thickness, on the tooth side of a single veneer. Typically, a central incisor veneer is used to facilitate shade determination of the cement. The operatory light is turned away during shade assessment to prevent premature and inadvertent curing of the resin cement. The veneer is seated on a clean, dry, unetched tooth; the excess resin cement is removed with a brush; and the overall shade of the veneer is evaluated. After try-in, the veneer is removed quickly and stored in a container that is impervious to light to prevent curing of the cement. If the shade of the cement is determined to be appropriate, more of the same shade is added to the veneer just before bonding. If a different shade is deemed necessary, the existing shade is wiped from the inner aspect of the veneer with a disposable microbrush, and a new shade of resin cement is placed in the veneer. In the meantime, the assistant can remove residual cement of the previous shade from the tooth with a cotton pellet or brush. The veneer loaded with the new shade of cement is reseated and evaluated, as previously described.

Water-soluble try-in pastes that correspond to the same shades of resin cements also are available with many veneer bonding kits. These try-in pastes allow shade assessment without the risk of inadvertent premature curing of the cement because the try-in pastes are not capable of setting. However, after the try-in process with these try-in pastes, the veneers must be thoroughly cleaned, according to the manufacturer's instructions, to ensure that optimal bonding occurs. A light-cured resin cement of the same shade is used for final cementation.

The inherent shade of the veneer, characterization, and internal opaquing must be accomplished primarily during the fabrication of the veneer itself in the laboratory. Some additional masking can be accomplished chairside using an opaque resin-bonding medium at the time of bonding. However, excess use of opaque bonding resins also can reduce the "esthetic vitality" of the veneer, resulting in a poor esthetic outcome. Also, the overall shade of the veneer can be modified only slightly by the shade of cement selected. Significant changes in shading or masking ability cannot be accomplished chairside.

Prior to cementation of the veneers, the retraction cords are evaluated to ensure that they are tucked adequately into the gingival crevice. The tooth used for try-in to assess the shade of the resin-bonding medium should be cleaned again with a slurry of pumice to remove any residual resin or try-in paste that may preclude proper acid etching of the enamel.

A technique recommended for applying the veneers one at a time is presented here. Polyester strips are placed interproximally to prevent inadvertent bonding to the adjacent tooth, followed by etching, rinsing, and drying procedures. It is recommended that the two central incisors be etched and their veneers bonded first because of their critical importance esthetically. Etch the teeth to be bonded with a 35% to 37% phosphoric acid gel (see Fig. 9.41L). Following etching, rinsing, and drying, the preparations should exhibit a frosted appearance as evidence of an appropriately etched enamel surface (see Fig. 9.41M). An adhesive is applied to the etched enamel and the tooth side of the silane-primed porcelain veneer (see Fig. 9.41N and O). Next, a thin layer (0.5 mm) of the selected shade of light-cured resin cement is placed on the tooth side of the veneer, taking care not to entrap air. The first veneer is placed on the tooth and vibrated (carefully and lightly) into position with a blunt instrument or light finger pressure (see Fig. 9.41P). The margins of the veneer are examined with a No. 2 explorer to verify accurate seating. Next, the excess resin cement is removed with a disposable microbrush, always directing the microbrush in a gingival direction to prevent displacement of the veneer (see Fig. 9.41Q). The second veneer is placed and cleaned of excess cement in like manner. If a veneer cement with thick viscosity is used, the polyester strips can be carefully removed to facilitate removal of interproximal resin prior to curing (see Fig. 9.41R). However, the resin cement should be cured only after visual inspection reveals no excess resin remains in these critical interproximal areas.

Veneer margins are evaluated again before the veneer is exposed to the curing light. To ensure complete polymerization, the veneer should be cured for a minimum of 20 to 40 seconds each from the facial and lingual directions with a high-intensity, blue light-emitting diode (LED) light (see Fig. 9.41S). A light stream of air can be directed on the tooth during the curing sequence to prevent overheating from the curing light. After positioning and bonding of the first two veneers on the central incisors, the remaining veneers can be positioned carefully and bonded in like manner. Following proper positioning and bonding of all the veneers, any residual resin cement can be removed. A No. 12 surgical blade in a Bard-Parker handle is ideal for removing excess cured resin cement remaining around the margins (see Fig. 9.41T). Care must be exercised to ensure that the surgical blade is used only with a secure finger rest and using short shaving strokes, always directed parallel to the veneer margins. Removal of the retraction cord at this time facilitates access and visibility to the subgingival areas. If the marginal fit of the porcelain veneers is deemed acceptable and a favorable emergence profile exists, only removal of the excess cement is required.

If the porcelain margins are overextended beyond the cavosurface angles, an overhang is present, or the marginal areas are too bulbous, recontouring of these areas is required (especially along the gingival margins) to ensure proper physiologic contours and gingival health. A flame-shaped fine diamond instrument is used to carefully recontour and "dress" these areas (see Fig. 9.41U). Marginal areas should be confluent with the surrounding unprepared tooth surfaces when assessed with a No. 2 explorer. The lingual areas are always finished with an oval-shaped fine diamond instrument (see Fig. 9.41V). Because the use of a diamond instrument breaks the glazed surface, a series of appropriate instruments is used to restore a smooth surface texture. First, a rounded-end or bullet-shaped (or oval for lingual surfaces), 30-fluted carbide finishing bur (Midwest No. 9803 or Brasseler No. 7801) is used to plane the porcelain surface and to remove the striations created by the diamond instruments (see Fig. 9.41W). Studies show that the best results occur if the diamond instruments are used with air and water coolant, whereas the 30-fluted bur should be used dry.[43] Second, the porcelain is smoothed and polished with a series of abrasive rubber, porcelain polishing cups, and points (Dialite Porcelain Polishing Kit; Brasseler USA, Savannah, GA) (see Fig. 9.41X). Final surface luster is imparted by using a porcelain-polishing paste, applied with either a rubber Prophy cup or a felt wheel. This step is optional if a suitable polish has been attained with the polishing points and cups. The completed veneers are shown from incisal and facial views in Fig. 9.41Y and Z.

Etched porcelain veneers also can be used effectively to restore malformed anterior teeth conservatively. Malformed lateral incisors are shown in Fig. 9.43A. Incisal-lapping preparations that are extended well onto the lingual surface are used (see Fig. 9.43B). The resulting restorations are virtually comparable with "three-quarter crowns" in porcelain. The final esthetic results are shown in Fig. 9.43C.

Darkly discolored teeth are more difficult to treat with porcelain veneers. Several modifications in the veneering technique can be used to enhance the final esthetic result. First, opaque porcelain can be incorporated during the fabrication of the veneers to achieve more inherent masking. If the veneers are not inherently opaque, little chance exists for adequate masking of a darkly stained tooth. Typically, 5% to 15% opaque porcelain is required to achieve optimal masking. Exceeding 15% opaque porcelain dramatically reduces light penetration and results in a significant loss of esthetic vitality; the esthetic vitality or the realistic appearance of teeth depends on light penetration (see section Translucency, under Artistic Elements, earlier in the chapter). Second, a slightly deeper tooth preparation can be used to allow greater veneer thickness. The preparation should always be restricted to enamel, however, to ensure optimal bonding of the veneer to the tooth. Even with improved dentin-bonding agents, the bonds to dentin are less predictable or durable than the bonds to enamel because of the high variability and dynamic nature of dentin. Bonds to etched enamel are highly predictable and very durable.

Third, the laboratory can be instructed to use several coats of a die-spacing medium on the laboratory model to allow a slightly

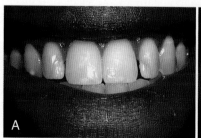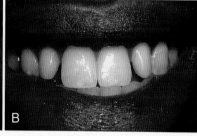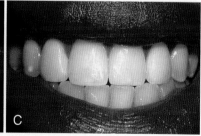

• **Fig. 9.43** Treatment of malformed teeth with porcelain veneers. A, Malformed lateral incisors. B, An incisal-lapping preparation similar to a three quarter crown in enamel is used. C, Final esthetic results.

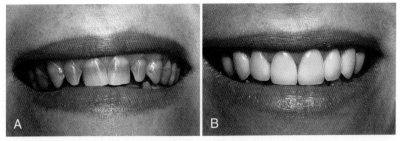

• **Fig. 9.44**   Darkly stained teeth treated with porcelain veneers. A, Tetracycline-stained teeth seen after preparation for porcelain veneers. B, After view of completed veneers.

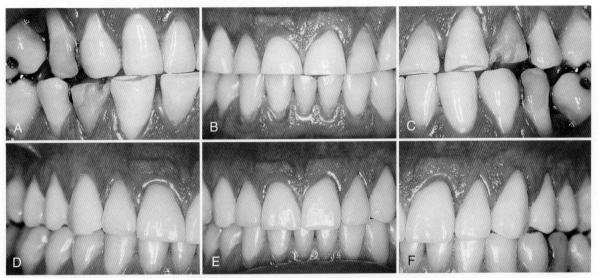

• **Fig. 9.45**   Pressed ceramic veneers (IPS Empress). A–C, Before treatment, facial views. D–F, Esthetic result after completed veneers. (Courtesy Dr. Luiz N. Baratieri.)

greater thickness of the resin-bonding medium. The die-spacing medium must not be extended closer than 1 mm to the margins to ensure adequate positioning of the veneer to the preparation during try-in and bonding and to provide for a slight internal space. A typical case of darkly discolored teeth showing prepared teeth and postoperative result is shown in Fig. 9.44.

Patients who have darkly stained teeth always should be informed that although porcelain (or composite) veneers can result in improved esthetics, they may not entirely eliminate or mask extremely dark stains. Because of the limited thickness of the veneers and the absolute necessity of incorporating intrinsic opacity, the realistic translucency or esthetic vitality of veneered teeth may never be comparable with that of natural, unaffected teeth (see Fig. 9.9). Full porcelain coverage with all-ceramic crowns may be indicated in some patients with severe discoloration because of the crown's greater capacity to restore esthetic vitality. Nonetheless, porcelain veneers are a viable option in most cases for patients who desire esthetic improvement without significant tooth reduction.

Pressed Ceramic Veneers

Another esthetic alternative for veneering teeth is the use of pressed ceramics (e.g., IPS Empress or e.max [Ivoclar Vivadent]). In contrast to etched porcelain veneers that are fabricated by stacking and firing feldspathic porcelain, pressed ceramic veneers are literally cast using a lost wax technique. Excellent esthetics is possible using pressed ceramic materials for most cases involving mild to moderate

discoloration. Because of the more translucent nature of pressed ceramic veneers, however, dark discolorations are best treated with etched porcelain veneers. The clinical technique for placing pressed ceramic veneers (e.g., IPS Empress) is not markedly different from that for feldspathic porcelain veneers, other than the need for a slightly greater tooth reduction depth.

The procedures for tooth preparation, try-in, and bonding of pressed veneers are the same as for etched porcelain veneers except that the marginal fit is superior. For that reason, often little marginal finishing is necessary. Only the excess bonding medium needs to be removed. A typical case involving pressed ceramic veneers, with before and after treatment views, is shown in Fig. 9.45.

Veneer Provisionalization

Because intraenamel preparations for etched porcelain veneers are by design very conservative, the resulting provisionals are inherently thin. Furthermore, they cannot be bonded in a similar manner to conventional provisionals for crowns, for example, because of the lack of inherent retention form. Moreover, since they are very thin, they cannot be made in the mouth and removed for trimming and subsequent cementing because of the high probability of fracture. Therefore veneer provisionals must be made and placed simultaneously intraorally.

Fig. 9.46 illustrates a typical case involving the fabrication of provisionals for etched porcelain veneers for maxillary anterior teeth. A clear polyvinyl siloxane material is used to make the preoperative impression from which the provisionals will be made. If no diagnostic model is needed and the existing contours of the teeth are to be replicated, the impression for the provisionals is made directly in the mouth. However, as in this case, if a diagnostic wax-up was generated (see Fig. 9.46A and B), the clear polyvinyl siloxane impression is made from this diagnostic model. Making the temporary from the diagnostic wax-up enables the clinician to see the contours of the wax-up manifested intraorally in the resulting provisionals. As seen in Fig. 9.46C, the impression itself is removed from the outer tray (no tray adhesive is used) and set aside for future use.

Following the preparation and impression of the teeth for porcelain veneers, the teeth to be temporized are "spot etched"

with 35% to 37% phosphoric acid. Only a 2-mm circle of enamel should be etched on the facial surface of each tooth to be veneered (see Fig. 9.46D and E). Because of the low viscosity of the bis-acryl temporary material, no bonding agent is required for bonding. The bis-acryl material will infiltrate the etched areas for microme-chanical bonding. These spot-etched areas will be the only areas to which the veneer provisionals will be bonded. If the entire tooth were etched, the veneer provisionals could not be readily removed. After spot etching, only small etched circles evidenced by a frosted appearance should be present on the surface of each prepared tooth (see Fig. 9.46F).

The etched teeth must be kept clean and dry at this point. The clear polyvinyl siloxane impression is quickly loaded with a

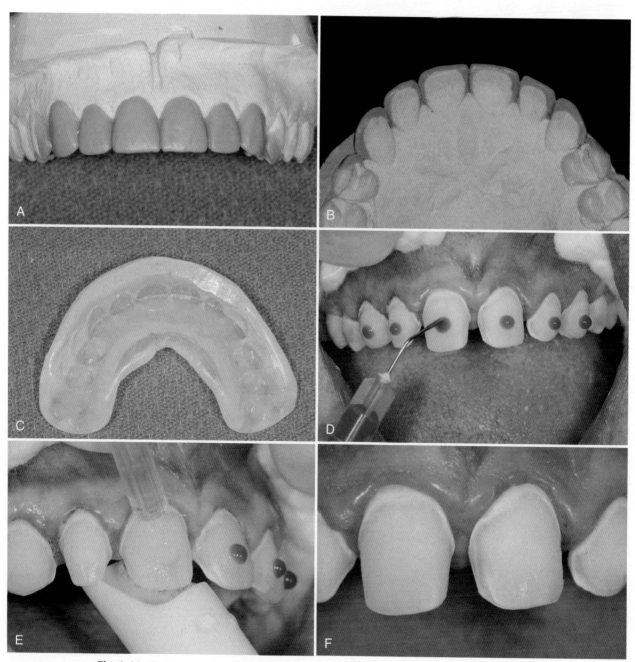

• **Fig. 9.46** Temporization for etched porcelain veneers. A and B, Diagnostic models in anticipation of etched porcelain veneers. C, Clear polyvinyl siloxane (PVS) impression made from diagnostic model. D–F, Spot-etched areas for retention of temporary veneers.

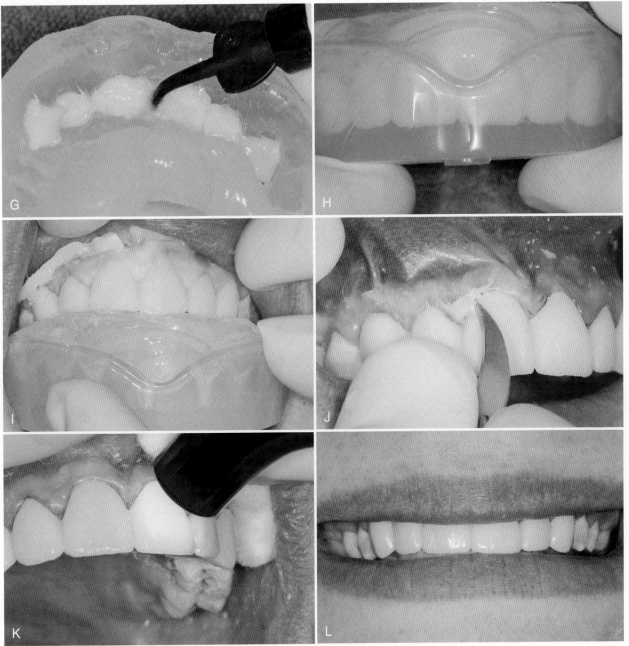

• **Fig. 9.46, cont'd**   G and H, Clear PVS impression is quickly loaded with bis-acryl temporary material, and positioned in the mouth. I and J, Impression is removed, and No. 12 blade in a Bard-Parker surgical handle is used to remove excess material. K, Glazing agent placed and cured. L and M, Final facial and lingual views of veneer provisionals.   *Continued*

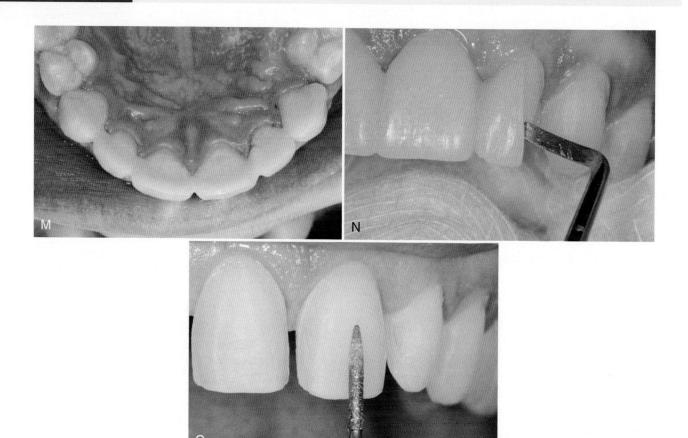

• **Fig. 9.46, cont'd** N and O, At delivery appointment, temporary veneers are removed with Black's spoon, and the spot-etched and bonded areas are relieved with a diamond.

self-curing bis-acryl temporary material and thereafter is immediately positioned in the mouth (see Fig. 9.46G and H). Once seated, finger pressure is applied to the peripheral areas of the flexible impression (since no outer hard tray is present) to express the excess material and "thin out" the resulting resin "flash."

When the bis-acryl temporary material has set, the clear impression is removed (see Fig. 9.46I). The gross excess "flash" material facially and lingually is removed with cotton pliers. Thereafter, a No. 12 blade held in a Bard-Parker surgical handle is used to *carefully* trim the excess temporary material around the margins of each tooth (see Fig. 9.46J). The same No. 12 blade is used to carefully trim excess material in the gingival embrasure areas as well.

A sharp large discoid applied parallel to the lingual margins is used to remove resin "flash" in the lingual concave areas. The temporary veneers are all joined together interproximally, increasing their collective strength and enhancing retention. A light-cured resin glazing agent is applied and cured to generate a smooth surface texture (see Fig. 9.46K). Final views of the finished provisionals are seen in Fig. 9.46L and M.

Appropriate adjustments can then be made intraorally in the provisionals to optimize occlusion and esthetics. A digital photograph of the final provisionals should be shared with the laboratory as a template for the final veneers. Patients must be instructed that they should not bite anything of any substance because of the weak nature of these veneers. These provisional veneers literally are more to accommodate esthetics and not function during the interim time until delivery of the final veneers.

As demonstrated in a different case, once the patient returns for the final try-in and cementation of the veneers, the provisionals are carefully removed by prying them from each tooth using a Black's spoon (see Fig. 9.46N). The provisionals can readily be removed since the only area where they actually are bonded to the tooth is the very small spot-etched, 2-mm circle on the facial surface of each prepared tooth. Once the veneer provisionals are removed, the areas that had been spot etched and bonded need to be lightly resurfaced with a flame-shaped diamond to ensure no residual resin-bonding agent is present that could preclude proper seating and bonding of the final veneers (see Fig. 9.46O).

Veneers for Metal Restorations

Esthetic inserts (i.e., partial or full veneers) of a tooth-colored material can be placed on the facial surface of a tooth previously restored with a metal restoration. For new castings, plans are made at the time of tooth preparation and during laboratory development of the wax pattern to incorporate a veneer into the cast restoration. After such a casting has been cemented, the veneer can be inserted, as described in the next section, except that the portion of mechanical retention of the veneer into the casting has been provided in the wax pattern stage.

Veneers for Existing Metal Restorations

Occasionally, the facial portion of an existing metal restoration (amalgam or gold) is judged to be distracting (Fig. 9.47A). A careful examination, including a radiograph, is required to determine

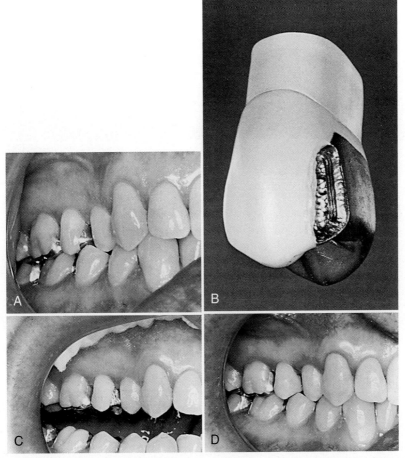

• **Fig. 9.47** Veneer for existing cast restoration. A, Mesiofacial portion of onlay is distracting to patient. B, Model of tooth and preparation. Note 90-degree cavosurface angle and retention prepared in gold and the cavosurface bevel in enamel. C, Clinical preparation ready for composite resin. D, Completed restoration.

that the existing restoration is sound before an esthetic correction is made. The size of the unesthetic area determines the extent of the preparation. Anesthesia is not usually required because the preparation is in metal and enamel. Preliminary procedures consist of cleaning the area with pumice, selecting the shade, and isolating the site with a cotton roll. When the unesthetic metal extends subgingivally, the level of the gingival tissue is marked on the restoration with a sharp explorer and a retraction cord is placed in the gingival crevice. Rubber dam isolation may be required in some instances.

A No. 2 carbide bur rotating at high speed with an air-water spray is used to remove the metal, starting at a point midway between the gingival and occlusal margins. The preparation is made perpendicular to the surface (a minimum of approximately 1 mm in depth), leaving a butt joint at the cavosurface margins. The 1-mm depth and butt joint should be maintained as the preparation is extended occlusally. All of the metal along the facial enamel is removed, and the preparation is extended into the facial and occlusal embrasures just enough for the veneer to hide the metal. The contact areas on the proximal or occlusal surfaces must not be included in the preparation. To complete the outline form, the preparation is extended gingivally approximately 1 mm past the mark indicating the clinical level of the gingival tissue.

The final preparation should have the same features as those described for veneers in new cast restorations. Mechanical retention is placed in the gingival area with a No. 1/4 carbide bur (using air coolant to enhance vision) 0.25 mm deep along the gingivoaxial and linguoaxial angles. Retention and esthetics are enhanced by beveling the enamel cavosurface margin (approximately 0.5 mm wide) with a coarse, flame-shaped diamond instrument oriented at 45 degrees to the external tooth surface (see Fig. 9.47B). After it is etched, rinsed, and dried, the preparation is complete (see Fig. 9.47C). Adhesive resin liners containing 4-methyloxy ethyl trimellitic anhydride (4-META), capable of bonding composite to metal, also may be used but are quite technique sensitive.[44] Manufacturers' instructions should be followed strictly to ensure optimal results with these materials. The composite material is inserted and finished in the usual manner (see Fig. 9.47D).

Repairs of Veneers

Failures of esthetic veneers occur because of breakage, discoloration, or wear. Consideration should be given to conservative repairs of veneers if the examination reveals that the remaining tooth and restoration are sound. It is not always necessary to remove all of the old restoration. The material most commonly used for making repairs is light-cured composite.

Small chipped areas on veneers often can be corrected by recontouring and polishing. When a sizable area is broken, it

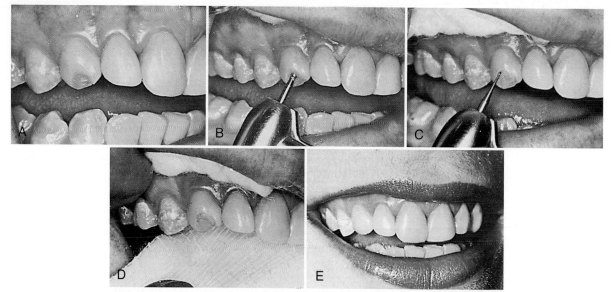

• **Fig. 9.48** Repairing a direct composite veneer. A, Fractured veneer on the maxillary canine. B, Preparation with rounded-end diamond instrument. C, Undercuts placed in existing veneer with a No. 1/4 bur. D, Completed preparation is shown isolated and etched. E, Veneer restored to original color and contour.

usually can be repaired if the remaining portion is sound (Fig. 9.48A). For direct composite veneers, repairs ideally should be made with the same material that was used originally. After cleaning the area and selecting the shade, the operator should roughen the damaged surface of the veneer or tooth (or both) with a coarse, tapered, rounded-end diamond instrument to form a chamfered cavosurface margin (see Fig. 9.48B). Roughening with microetching (i.e., sandblasting) also is effective. For more positive retention, mechanical locks may be placed in the remaining composite material with a small, round bur (see Fig. 9.48C). Acid etchant is applied to clean the prepared area and to etch any exposed enamel, which is then rinsed and dried (see Fig. 9.48D). Next, an adhesive is applied to the preparation (i.e., existing composite and enamel) and polymerized. Composite is added, cured, and finished in the usual manner (see Fig. 9.48E).

To repair porcelain veneers, a hydrofluoric acid gel, suitable for intraoral use (but only with a rubber dam in place), must be used to etch the fractured porcelain. Hydrofluoric acid gels are available in approximately 10% buffered concentrations that can be used for intraoral porcelain repairs if proper isolation with a rubber dam is used. Although caution still must be taken when using hydrofluoric acid gels intraorally, the lower acid concentration allows for relatively safe intraoral use. Full-strength hydrofluoric acid should *never* be used intraorally for etching porcelain. Isolation of the porcelain veneer to be repaired should always be accomplished with a rubber dam to protect gingival tissue from the irritating effects of the hydrofluoric acid. The manufacturer's instructions must be followed regarding application time for the hydrofluoric acid gel to ensure optimal porcelain etching. A lightly frosted appearance, similar to that of etched enamel, should be seen if the porcelain has been properly etched. A silane coupling agent may be applied to the etched porcelain surface before the adhesive is applied. Composite material is added, cured, and finished in the usual manner. Large fractures are best treated by replacing the entire porcelain veneer.

Acknowledgments

Portions of the section on artistic elements were reprinted with permission from Heymann HO: The artistry of conservative esthetic dentistry, *J Am Dent Assoc* 115(12E; special issue):14, 1987.

References

1. Goldstein RE: *Esthetics in dentistry*, Philadelphia, 1976, JB Lippincott.
2. Levin EI: Dental esthetics and the golden proportion. *J Prosthet Dent* 40:244, 1978.
3. Borissavlievitch M: *The golden number*, London, 1964, Alec Tiranti.
4. Preston JD: The golden proportion revisited. *J Esthet Dent* 5:247–251, 1993.
5. Ward DH: A study of dentists' preferred maxillary anterior tooth width proportions: comparing recurring esthetic dental proportions to other mathematical and naturally occurring proportions. *J Esthet Restor Dent* 19(6):324–339, 2007.
6. Sterrett JD, Oliver T, Robinson F, et al: Width/length ratios of normal clinical crowns of maxillary anterior teeth. *J Clin Periodontol* 26:153–157, 1999.
7. Magne P, Gallucci GO, Belser UC: Anatomic crown width/length ratios of unworn and worn maxillary teeth in white subjects. *J Prosthet Dent* 89:453–461, 2003.
8. Chiche GJ, Pinault A: *Esthetics of anterior fixed prosthodontics*, Chicago, 1994, Quintessence.
9. Sproull RC: Understanding color. In Goldstein RE, editor: *Esthetics in dentistry*, Philadelphia, 1976, JB Lippincott.
10. Dawson PE: *Evaluation, diagnosis, and treatment of occlusal problems*, ed 2, St. Louis, 1989, Mosby.
11. Graber TM, Vanarsdall RL: *Orthodontics: Current principles and techniques*, ed 3, St. Louis, 2000, Mosby.
12. Hattab FN, Qudeimat MA, al-Rimawi HS: Dental discolorations: an overview. *J Esthet Dent* 11:291, 1999.
13. Flynn M: Black teeth: a primitive method of caries prevention in Southeast Asia. *J Am Dent Assoc* 95:96, 1977.

14. Carver CC, Heymann HO: Dental and oral discolorations associated with minocycline and other tetracycline analogs. *J Esthet Dent* 11:43, 1999.

15. Haywood VB: History, safety, and effectiveness of current bleaching techniques and applications of the nightguard vital bleaching technique. *Quintessence Int* 23:471, 1992.

16. Haywood VB: Nightguard vital bleaching: A history and products update: Part 1. *Esthetic Dent Update* 2:63, 1991.

17. Titley KC, Torneck CD, Ruse ND: The effect of carbamide-peroxide gel on the shear bond strength of a microfill resin to bovine enamel. *J Dent Res* 71:20, 1992.

18. Sorensen JA, Martinoff JT: Intracoronal reinforcement and coronal coverage: a study of endodontically treated teeth. *J Prosthet Dent* 51:780, 1984.

19. Harrington GW, Natkin E: External resorption associated with bleaching of pulpless teeth. *J Endod* 5:344, 1979.

20. Madison S, Walton R: Cervical root resorption following bleaching of endodontically treated teeth. *J Endod* 16:570, 1990.

21. Lado EA: Bleaching of endodontically treated teeth: an update on cervical resorption. *Gen Dent* 36:500, 1988.

22. Haywood VB, Heymann HO: Nightguard vital bleaching: how safe is it? *Quintessence Int* 22:515, 1991.

23. Lado EA, Stanley HR, Weisman MI: Cervical resorption in bleached teeth. *Oral Surg Oral Med Oral Pathol* 55:78, 1983.

24. Holmstrup G, Palm AM, Lambjerg-Hansen H: Bleaching of discolored root-filled teeth. *Endod Dent Traumatol* 4:197, 1988.

25. Feinman RA, Goldstein RL, Garber DA: *Bleaching teeth*, Chicago, 1987, Quintessence.

26. Haywood VB, Heymann HO: Nightguard vital bleaching. *Quintessence Int* 20:173, 1989.

27. Sagel PA, Odioso LL, McMillan DA, et al: Vital tooth whitening with a novel hydrogen peroxide strip system: design, kinetics, and clinical response. *Compend Contin Educ Dent Suppl* (29):S10–S15, 2000.

28. Hall DA: Should etching be performed as a part of a vital bleaching technique? *Quintessence Int* 22:679, 1991.

29. Papathanasiou A, Kastali S, Perry RD, et al: Clinical evaluation of a 35% hydrogen peroxide in-office whitening system. *Compend Contin Educ Dent Suppl* 23:335–346, 2002.

30. American Dental Association Council on Scientific Affairs: Report on laser bleaching. *J Am Dent Assoc* 129:1484, 1998.

31. Shethri SA, Matis BA, Cochran MA, et al: A clinical evaluation of two in-office bleaching products. *Oper Dent* 28:488–495, 2003.

32. McCloskey RJ: A technique for removal of fluorosis stains. *J Am Dent Assoc* 109:63, 1984.

33. Croll TP, Cavanaugh RR: Enamel color modification by controlled hydrochloric acid-pumice abrasion: Part 1. Technique and examples. *Quintessence Int* 17:81, 1986.

34. Croll TP: Enamel microabrasion for removal of superficial dysmineralization and decalcification defects. *J Am Dent Assoc* 120:411, 1990.

35. Dumfahrt H, Schaffer H: Porcelain laminate veneers: A retrospective evaluation after 1-10 years of service. *Int J Prosthodont* 13:9–18, 2000.

36. Friedman MJ: A 15-year review of porcelain veneer failure: A clinician's observation. *Compend Contin Educ Dent Suppl* 19:625–636, 1998.

37. Hashimoto M, Ohno H, Kaga M, et al: Resin-tooth interfaces after long-term function. *Am J Dent* 14:211–215, 2001.

38. Meiers JC, Young D: Two-year composite/dentin durability. *Am J Dent* 14:141–144, 2001.

39. Calamia JR: Etched porcelain facial veneers: a new treatment modality based on scientific and clinical evidence. *N Y J Dent* 53:255, 1983.

40. Friedman MJ: The enamel ceramic alternative: porcelain veneers vs. metal ceramic crowns. *CDA J* 20:27, 1992.

41. Stangel I, Nathanson D, Hsu CS: Shear strength of the composite bond to etched porcelain. *J Dent Res* 66:1460, 1987.

42. Bayne SC, Taylor DF, Zardiackas LD: *Biomaterials science*, Chapel Hill, NC, 1991, Brightstar.

43. Haywood VB, Heymann HO, Kusy RP, et al: Polishing porcelain veneers: an SEM and specular reflectance analysis. *Dent Mater* 4:116, 1988.

44. Cooley RL, Burger KM, Chain MC: Evaluation of a 4-META adhesive cement. *J Esthet Dent* 3:7, 1991.

10

Clinical Technique for Amalgam Restorations

LEE W. BOUSHELL, ALDRIDGE D. WILDER, JR., SUMITHA N. AHMED

Dental amalgam (*silver amalgam* or simply *amalgam*) is a metallic, polycrystalline restorative material originally composed of a mixture of silver–tin alloy and mercury. Current alloys that are amalgamated with mercury are silver–tin–copper. The unset silver-colored mixture is pressed (condensed) into a tooth defect (cavitation) that has been specifically prepared to retain the amalgam. The material is then contoured to restore the tooth's form so that, when the material hardens, the tooth is returned to normal function (Fig. 10.1). Amalgam has been the primary direct restorative material in the United States for more than 150 years. It has been the subject of intense research and has been found to be safe and beneficial as a direct restorative material (see Chapter 13).[1-3] The cost-effective nature of amalgam restorations has benefited many people. According to the U.S. Public Health Service, "hundreds of millions of teeth have been retained that otherwise would have been sacrificed because restorative alternatives would have been too expensive for many people."[4]

In addition to being cost effective, amalgam has the unique property of being "self-sealing." Self-sealing occurs when percolation of oral fluids (i.e., microleakage) between the amalgam restoration and the prepared cavity walls results in corrosion of the amalgam and a subsequent accumulation of corrosion products in the microscopic space. Microleakage between the restoration and the adjacent tooth structure is reduced as corrosion products fill the space. The self-sealing process is self-limiting and requires several months. Amalgam is the only restorative material with an interfacial seal that improves over time.[5-7]

Amalgam was introduced to the United States in the 1830s. Initially, amalgam restorations were made by dentists filing silver coins and mixing the filings with mercury, creating a puttylike mass that was placed into the defective tooth. As knowledge increased and research intensified, major advancements in the formulation and use of amalgam occurred. Concerns about mercury toxicity in the use of amalgam were, however, expressed in many countries; concerns reached major proportions in the early 1990s.

Today, the popularity of amalgam as a direct restorative material has decreased.[8,9] The decline is attributed in part to increased interest in tooth-colored composite resin restorations and the minimally invasive nature of their preparation steps. Concerns have been raised that the preparation used when planning for amalgam may result in unnecessary weakening of teeth because of the demand for additional removal of tooth structure so as to accommodate amalgam's strength and retention requirements. While it is true that preparations for composite resin restorations may allow smaller, more conservative preparations for very early caries lesions, treatment of more advanced lesions may result in essentially the same amount of tooth structure loss regardless of the type of restorative material being used. The choice of a composite resin material over amalgam may be based on the assumption that both materials will perform equally well over time for all patients. However, a growing body of evidence suggests that the risk of developing secondary caries adjacent to amalgam restorations is at least two times less likely than that of composite resin restorations in high caries risk patients, and therefore the reduction/phase-out of dental amalgam may have been premature.[10,11] The decline of amalgam use is also due to perceived concerns over individual and environmental safety relative to the presence of elemental mercury in amalgam restorations. Safe, professional handling of mercury in mixing the amalgam mass, removal of old amalgam restorations, and amalgam scrap disposal is certainly appropriate and absolutely essential. Following best management practices for amalgam waste, as presented by the American Dental Association, results in appropriate amalgam use.[12]

Types of Amalgam Restorative Materials

Low-Copper Amalgam

Low-copper amalgams were primarily used before the early 1960s. When the setting reaction occurred, the material was subject to corrosion because of the formation of a tin–mercury phase (gamma-2). The corrosion led to the rapid breakdown of amalgam restorations. Subsequent research led to the development of high-copper amalgam materials. Currently low-copper amalgams are rarely used in the United States.

High-Copper Amalgam

High-copper amalgams are predominantly used today in the United States. In this book, unless otherwise specified, the term *amalgam*

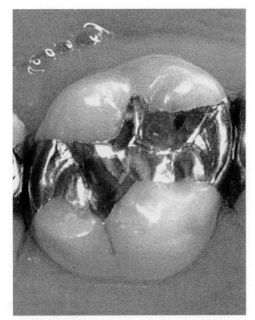

• **Fig. 10.1** Clinical example of an amalgam restoration. (From Hatrick CD, Eakle WS, Bird WF: *Dental materials: Clinical applications for dental assistants and dental hygienists,* ed 2, St. Louis, Saunders, 2011.)

refers to high-copper dental amalgam. The increase in copper content to 12% or greater designates an amalgam as a high-copper type. The advantage of the added copper is that it preferentially reacts with the tin and reduces the formation of the more corrosive phase (gamma-2) within the amalgam mass. This change in composition reduces the deleterious corrosion effects on the restoration. However, enough corrosion occurs at the amalgam–tooth interface to result in the sealing of the restoration, which reduces microleakage.[13,14] These materials may provide satisfactory clinical performance for more than 12 years.[15,16] High-copper amalgams are available with admixed or spherical alloy structure.

Admixed Amalgam

Admixed amalgam contains irregularly shaped and sized alloy particles, sometimes combined with spherical shapes, which are mixed to form a mass that is placed into the tooth preparation. The irregular shape of many of the particles results in a mass that requires greater condensation pressure (which many dentists prefer) and permits the dentist to displace matrix bands to generate proximal contacts more easily.

Spherical Amalgam

A spherical amalgam contains small, round alloy particles that are mixed with mercury to form the mass that is placed into the tooth preparation. Because of the shape of the particles, the material is condensed into the tooth preparation with little condensation pressure. This advantage is combined with its high early strength to provide a material that is well suited for very large amalgam restorations such as complex amalgams or foundations.[17]

New Amalgam Alloys

Because of the concern about mercury toxicity, new compositions of amalgam have been promoted as mercury-free or low-mercury amalgam restorative materials. Alloys with gallium or indium or alloys using cold-welding techniques have been presented as alternatives to mercury-containing amalgams. None of these new alloys have shown sufficient promise to become a universal replacement for current amalgam materials.[18-21]

Important Amalgam Properties

The linear coefficient of the thermal expansion of amalgam is 2.5 times greater than that of tooth structure, but it is closer to that of tooth structure than the linear coefficient of thermal expansion of composite.[22-24] Although the compressive strength of high-copper amalgam is similar to tooth structure, the tensile strength is lower, making amalgam restorations prone to fracture during flexure.[9,25,26] Usually, high-copper amalgam fracture is a bulk fracture, not a marginal fracture. All amalgams are brittle and have low edge strength. As such, the amalgam restoration must have sufficient bulk (usually 1.5–2 mm in any occlusally loaded area, depending on the position within the tooth) and a 90-degree marginal configuration.

Creep and flow relate to the deformation of a material under load over time. High-copper amalgams exhibit no clinically relevant creep or flow.[27,28] Because amalgam is metallic in structure, it also is a good thermal conductor. At minimum, a dentin desensitizer should be used immediately prior to amalgam placement to limit sensitivity secondary to rapid fluid movement in the dentinal tubules caused by thermal changes. A liner or base should be placed in areas of deep caries removal prior to amalgam placement to limit thermal sensitivity.

General Considerations for Amalgam Restorations

Restoration With Amalgam

Amalgam is effective as a direct restorative material because of its easy insertion into a tooth preparation and, when hardened, its ability to restore the tooth to proper form and function. The tooth preparation not only must remove the fault in the tooth and remove weakened tooth structure, but its form must also allow the amalgam material to function properly. The required tooth preparation form must allow the amalgam to (1) possess a uniform specified minimum thickness for strength (so that it will not flex and fracture under load), (2) produce a 90-degree amalgam angle (butt-joint form for maximum edge thickness) at the margin, and (3) be mechanically retained in the tooth (Fig. 10.2A and B). Amalgam restorations initially leak and therefore require steps to protect from pulpal sensitivity until self-sealing is able to occur (Fig. 10.3A).[13] After desensitizing the prepared tooth structure, mixing, inserting, carving, and finishing the amalgam are relatively fast and easy. The placing and contouring of amalgam restorations are generally easier than those for composite restorations.[29] For these reasons, it is considered a user-friendly material that is less technique (i.e., operator) sensitive as compared with composite.

Some practitioners have continued to use bonded amalgam restorations in their practice (see Fig. 10.3B). As noted in Chapter 4, this book does not promote the use of bonded amalgams.[30-33] The bonding of amalgam requires use of a dual-cure adhesive system to form a hybrid layer with the dentin followed by condensation of amalgam so that amalgam particles become intermingled with the curing adhesive resin. A bonded amalgam restoration, done properly, may seal the prepared tooth structure and may temporarily

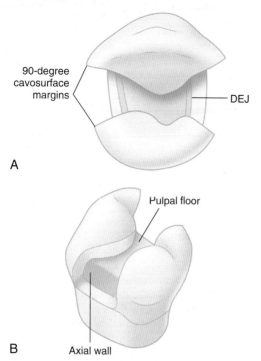

A

B

• **Fig. 10.2** A and B, Diagrams of Class II amalgam tooth preparations illustrating uniform pulpal and axial wall depths, 90-degree cavosurface margins, and occlusal convergence of walls.

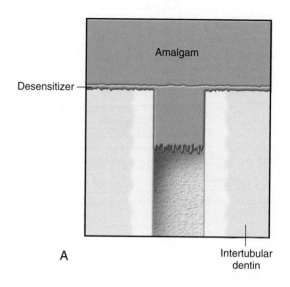

A

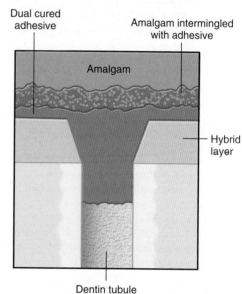

B

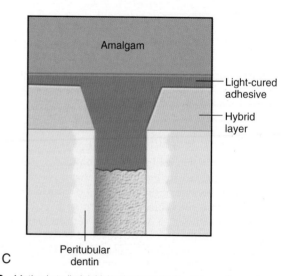

C

• **Fig. 10.3** Methods to limit initial pulpal sensitivity after amalgam placement. A, Dentin desensitization. B, Amalgam bonding (amalgam intermingled with adhesive resin). C, Dentin sealing (adhesive resin placed and cured before amalgam placement).

strengthen adjacent tooth structure. The strengthening and retention gained by bonding, however, is minimal and short term. Consequently, bonded amalgam restorations still require the same tooth preparation retention and resistance form as do nonbonded amalgam restorations.[34-35] Isolation requirements for a bonded amalgam restoration are the same as for a composite restoration.

Another amalgam technique uses light-cured adhesive to seal the dentin under the amalgam material (see Fig. 10.3C). This procedure, as is true of all procedures that use adhesive technology, requires proper isolation. The prepared tooth structure is etched (i.e., demineralized), primed, and sealed with adhesive. The adhesive is polymerized before insertion of the amalgam. This technique seals the dentinal tubules effectively.[36,37]

Uses of Amalgam

Amalgam is used for the restoration of many carious or fractured posterior teeth and in the replacement of failed restorations. Understanding the physical properties of amalgam and the principles of tooth preparation is necessary to produce amalgam restorations that provide optimal service. When properly placed, an amalgam restoration is able to provide many years of service.[38-43] Although improved techniques and materials are available, amalgam failures do occur. Much clinical time is spent replacing restorations that fail as a result of recurrent caries lesions, marginal deterioration (i.e., ditching), fractures, or poor contours.[44,45] Attention to detail throughout the procedure may significantly decrease the incidence of failures, however, and extend the life of the restoration.[46-48] Careful evaluation of existing amalgam restorations is important because they have the potential to provide long-term clinical service and should not be removed and replaced unless accurately identified to be defective or undermined by a secondary caries lesion.[49]

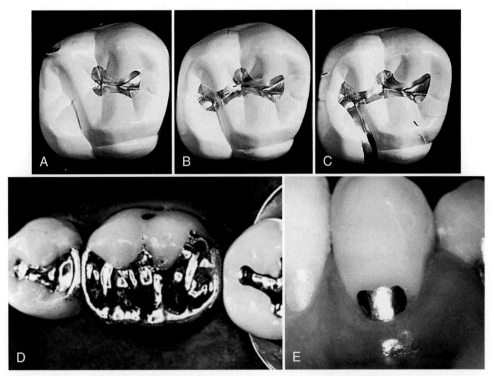

• **Fig. 10.4**   Amalgam restorations. A–C, Class I. D, Complex. E, Class V. (Most practitioners would restore all of these teeth with composite, except tooth No. 30.)

Because of its strength and ease of use, amalgam provides an excellent means for restoring large defects in nonesthetic areas.[50] A review of almost 3500 four-surface and five-surface amalgams revealed successful outcomes at 5 years for 72% of the four-surface and 65% of the five-surface amalgams. When considering complex amalgam restorations and discussing treatment options with patients, this result should be compared with the 5-year success rates for gold and porcelain crowns, which were 84% and 85%, respectively.[51]

Indications

Amalgam may be used for Class I, II, V, and VI restorations; for foundations; and for caries-control restorations (Figs. 10.4 and 10.5; see also Chapter 2). Occasionally amalgam may be utilized for Class III areas if isolation problems exist. Likewise, Class V amalgam restorations may be indicated in anterior areas where esthetics is not an important consideration and the patient has high caries risk.

Contraindications

Amalgams are contraindicated in patients who are allergic to alloy components. The use of amalgam in more prominent esthetic areas of the mouth may represent a relative contraindication. These areas include anterior teeth and, in some patients, premolars and molars. Amalgam should not be used when composite resin would offer more conservation of tooth structure and equal clinical performance.

Occlusal Factors

Amalgam generally has greater wear resistance than does composite in patients that have heavy occlusal function.[2,52,53] Amalgam also may be more appropriate than composite resin when there is little to no natural occlusal tooth structure remaining that requires the restoration to restore most or all of the occlusal contacts.[53]

Isolation Factors

Isolation of the operating field is important for moisture control, access, and visibility, to protect the patient from aspirating or ingesting foreign objects, protecting the pulp in the event of pulpal exposure, and protecting the operator medicolegally. However, minor moisture contamination of amalgam during the insertion procedure may not have as adverse an effect on the final restoration as the same contamination would for a composite restoration.

Operator Ability and Commitment Factors

The tooth preparation for an amalgam restoration is very exacting. It requires a specific design with depths that allow appropriate amalgam thickness and a precise marginal form. The failure of amalgam restorations is often related to inappropriate tooth preparation. However, the insertion and finishing procedures for amalgam are much easier than for composite.[29]

Advantages

Some of the advantages of amalgam restorations already have been stated, but the following list presents the primary reasons for the successful use of amalgam restorations over many years.
1. Ease of use
2. High compressive strength
3. Excellent wear resistance
4. Favorable long-term clinical research results
5. Lower cost than for composite restorations

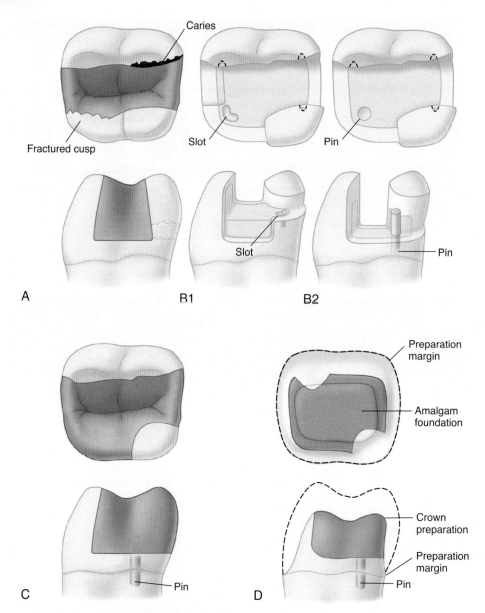

• **Fig. 10.5** Amalgam foundation. A, Defective restoration (defective amalgam, mesiolingual fractured cusp, distofaciocclusal caries). B, Tooth preparation with secondary retention, using slot (B1) and pin (B2). C, Amalgam foundation placed. D, Tooth with amalgam foundation prepared for crown. Note that dashed lines on the occlusal surface in B1 and B2 only indicate the position of the retention grooves on the facial and lingual walls of the proximal preparation. The grooves do not extend onto the occlusal surface.

Disadvantages

The primary disadvantages of amalgam restorations relate to esthetics and increased tooth structure removal during tooth preparation. The following is a list of these and other disadvantages of amalgam restorations.
1. Noninsulating
2. Nonesthetic
3. Less conservative tooth preparation than for composite restorations (more removal of tooth structure during tooth preparation)
4. More difficult tooth preparation than for composite restorations
5. Initial marginal leakage

The following sections begin with the introduction of general clinical techniques and associated concepts to be considered when restoring caries lesions or defects with dental amalgam. The general technique is then followed by specific discussion addressing the creation of Class I, II, III, V, VI, and Complex Amalgam restorations.

General Clinical Technique for Amalgam Restorations

Initial Clinical Procedures

Complete examination, diagnosis, and treatment planning must be completed before a patient is scheduled for operative appointments (except in emergencies). A brief review of patient's dental record (including medical factors), treatment plan, and radiographs should precede each restorative procedure. At the beginning of each appointment, the dentist should also carefully examine the operating site to confirm the diagnosis of the tooth or teeth scheduled for treatment.

Local Anesthesia

Local anesthesia is recommended for most operative procedures. Profound anesthesia contributes to comfortable and uninterrupted operation and usually results in a marked reduction in salivation.

Isolation of the Operating Site

Complete instructions for the control of moisture are given in Online Chapter 15. Isolation for amalgam restorations may be accomplished with a rubber dam, cotton rolls, with or without a retraction cord.

Other Preoperative Considerations

Preoperative assessment of the occlusion should be made. This step should occur before rubber dam placement. The dentist should identify not only the occlusal contacts of the tooth to be restored but also the contacts on the opposing and adjacent teeth. Knowing the preoperative location of occlusal contacts is important in planning the restoration outline form and in establishing the proper occlusal contacts on the restoration. Remembering the location of the contacts on adjacent teeth provides guidance in determining when the restoration contacts have been correctly positioned and adjusted.

A wedge placed preoperatively in the gingival embrasure is useful when restoring a proximal surface. This step causes slight separation of the operated tooth from the adjacent tooth and may help protect the adjacent proximal surface, the rubber dam, and the interdental papilla.

It is important to preoperatively visualize the anticipated extension of the tooth preparation. Because the tooth preparation requires specific depths, extensions, and marginal forms, the connection of the various parts of the tooth preparation should result in minimal tooth structure removal (i.e., as little as is necessary), while maintaining the strength of the cuspal and marginal ridge areas of the tooth as much as possible (Fig. 10.6). The projected facial and lingual extensions of a proximal box should be visualized before preparing the occlusal outline form through the marginal ridge of the tooth, reducing the chance of overextension while maintaining a butt-joint form of the facial or lingual proximal margins.

General Concepts Guiding Preparation for Amalgam Restorations

A solid comprehension of concepts presented in Chapter 4 is essential prior to the learning of information presented in the following sections. For an amalgam restoration to be successful, numerous steps must be accomplished correctly. After an accurate diagnosis is made, the dentist must create a tooth preparation that not only removes the defect (e.g., caries lesion, old restorative material, malformed structure) but also leaves remaining tooth structure as strong as possible by leaving as much dentin support

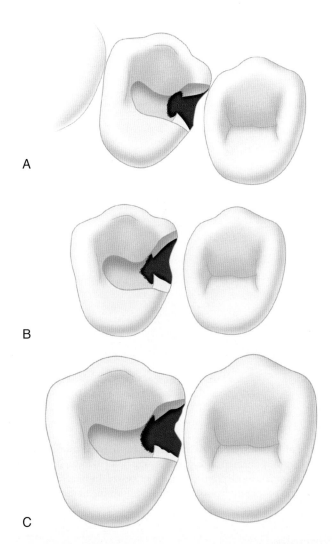

• **Fig. 10.6** Preoperative visualization of tooth preparation extensions when a cavitated caries lesion is present gingival to the proximal contact and in the central groove area. A, Rotated tooth (lingual extension owing to faulty central groove). B, Open proximal contact (preparation extended wider faciolingually to develop a proximal contact with appropriate physiologic proximal contours). C, Normal relationship.

as possible. Tooth preparation that conserves tooth structure is strongly recommended because it limits pulpal irritation and preserves the integrity of both the tooth and the subsequent restoration.[54-60]

Discussion in this chapter will include principles, techniques, and procedures using classic examples of amalgam preparations. However, clinically, the outline form of the preparation should always conform to the level of disease in the tooth and not necessarily to the examples presented here. Making the tooth preparation form appropriate for the use of amalgam as the restorative material is equally important. The physical properties of amalgam require that it be placed into a tooth preparation that provides for an approximately 90-degree or slightly greater occlusal cavosurface margin and 90-degree axial cavosurface margin (because of the amalgam's limited edge strength). The preparation must allow a minimum thickness of 1.5 to 2 mm so that the amalgam will not flex and fracture when under occlusal load (most amalgams fail by bulk fracture). The amalgam

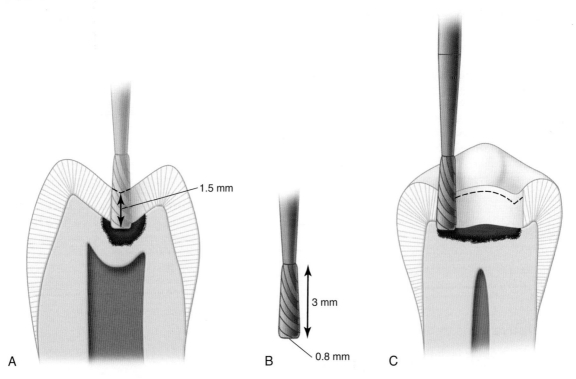

• **Fig. 10.7** Pulpal floor depth. A, Pulpal depth measured from central groove. B, No. 245 bur dimensions. C, Guides to proper pulpal floor depth: (1) one half the length of the No. 245 bur, (2) 1.5 mm, or (3) 0.2 mm inside (internal to) the dentinoenamel junction (DEJ).

must be placed into a prepared undercut form in the tooth so as to be mechanically retained (amalgam does not bond to tooth structure). After appropriate tooth preparation, the success of the final restoration depends on proper insertion, carving, and finishing of the amalgam material.

Principles

The basic principles of tooth preparation must be followed for amalgam tooth preparations to ensure clinical success. As presented in Chapter 4, the preparation for amalgam is discussed in two stages, for academic purposes, to facilitate student understanding of proper extension, form, and caries lesion removal. The initial stage (1) places the tooth preparation extension into sound tooth structure at the marginal areas (not pulpally or axially); (2) extends the depth (pulpally, axially, or both) at the periphery of the preparation to a prescribed, uniform dimension; (3) provides an initial form consistent with amalgam retention in the tooth; and (4) establishes the preparation external walls in a form that will result in a 90-degree amalgam margin upon restoration. The final stage of tooth preparation removes any remaining defect (caries lesion or old restorative material) and incorporates any additional preparation features (grooves, coves, slots, or pins) as needed to achieve the appropriate retention and resistance forms.

In academic institutions, assessing the tooth preparation after the initial preparation stage provides an opportunity to evaluate a student's knowledge and ability to extend the external walls properly and establish proper initial depth. If the student were to remove an extensive caries lesion in its entirety before any evaluation, the attending faculty would not know whether the prepared depths were obtained because of appropriate caries lesion removal or inappropriate overcutting of the tooth.

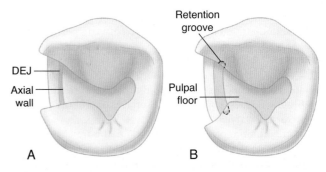

• **Fig. 10.8** Axial wall depth. A, If no retention grooves needed, axial depth 0.2 mm inside (internal to) the dentinoenamel junction (DEJ). B, If retention grooves needed (i.e., proximal divergence secondary to wide faciolingual caries lesion extension), axial depth 0.5 mm inside (internal to) the DEJ. Note that dashed lines on the occlusal surface only indicate the position of the retention grooves associated with the facial and lingual walls of the proximal preparation. The grooves do not extend onto the occlusal surface.

Initial Tooth Preparation

All initial depths of a tooth preparation for amalgam relate to the dentinoenamel junction (DEJ) except in the following two instances: (1) when the occlusal enamel has become significantly thinner and (2) when the preparation extends onto the root surface. The initial depth pulpally is 0.2 mm inside (internal to) the DEJ or 1.5 mm as measured from the depth of the central groove (Fig. 10.7), whichever results in the greater thickness of amalgam. The initial depth of the axial wall is 0.2 mm inside the DEJ when retention grooves are not used and 0.5 mm inside the DEJ when retention grooves are used (Fig. 10.8). The deeper extension allows placement of the retention groove without undermining marginal enamel. Axial depths on the root surface should be 0.75 to 1 mm deep so as to provide room for placement of retention grooves or coves.

Outline Form

The initial extension of the tooth preparation should be visualized preoperatively by estimating the extent of the defect, the preparation form requirements of the amalgam, and the need for adequate access and visibility to place the amalgam into the tooth. Enamel cavosurface margins must be left at 90 degrees or greater to limit the potential for enamel fracture. For enamel strength, the marginal enamel rods should be supported by sound dentin. These requirements for enamel strength must be combined with marginal requirements for amalgam (90-degree butt joint) when establishing the periphery of the tooth preparation (Fig. 10.9).

The preparation extension is dictated primarily by the existing caries lesion, old restorative material, or defect. Adequate extension to provide access for tooth preparation, caries lesion removal, matrix placement, and amalgam insertion also must be considered. When making the preparation extensions, every effort should be made to preserve the dentinal support (i.e., the strength) of cusps and marginal ridges.

When viewed from the occlusal, the facial and lingual proximal cavosurface margins of a Class II preparation should be 90 degrees (i.e., perpendicular to a tangent drawn through the point of extension facially and lingually) (see Fig. 10.9). In most instances, proximal caries lesions severe enough to require surgical intervention result in facial and lingual proximal walls that must be extended into the facial or lingual embrasure. This extension provides adequate access for performing the preparation (with decreased risk of damaging the adjacent tooth), easier placement of the matrix band, and easier condensation and carving of the amalgam. Such extension provides "clearance" between the cavosurface margin and the adjacent tooth (Fig. 10.10). Clearance also allows the operator to confirm that no voids exist at the proximal margins of the finished restoration. Occasionally the level of disease may not require extension of the proximal margins beyond the proximal contact. This is especially helpful in areas that are more esthetically demanding.

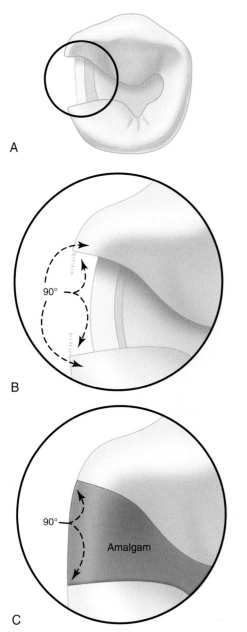

• **Fig. 10.9** Proximal cavosurface margins. A, Facial and lingual proximal cavosurface margins prepared at 90-degree angles to a tangent drawn through the point on the external tooth surface. B, A 90-degree proximal cavosurface margin produces a 90-degree amalgam margin; C, 90-degree amalgam margins.

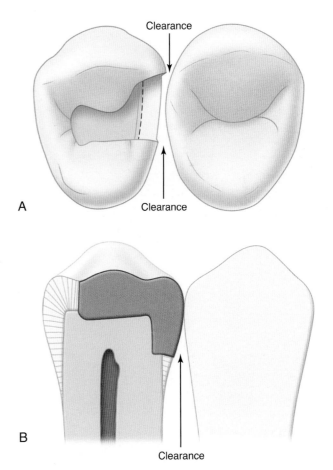

• **Fig. 10.10** Proximal box preparation clearance of adjacent tooth. A, Occlusal view. B, Lingual view of a cross section through the central groove.

Factors dictating the outline form are presented in greater detail in Chapter 4. They include caries lesion, old restorative material, inclusion of all of the defect, proximal or occlusal contact relationship, and the need for convenience form.

Cavosurface Margin

Enamel must have a marginal configuration of approximately 90 degrees or greater, and amalgam must have a marginal configuration of approximately 90 degrees. Marginal wall configurations with angles less than 90 degrees in enamel or amalgam are subject to fracture, as both of these materials are brittle. Preparation walls on the occlusal surface usually have obtuse enamel margins (representing the strongest enamel margin) and result in amalgam margins that are slightly less than 90 degrees (Figs. 10.11 and 10.12). Rounding of the central groove area when carving the occlusal amalgam enables the marginal configuration to be closer to 90 degrees (see Fig. 10.12). Preparation walls on vertical aspect (in the occlusogingival axis) of the tooth (facial, lingual, mesial, or distal) should result in

90-degree enamel walls (representing a strong enamel margin) (see Fig. 10.9) that meet the inserted amalgam at a butt joint (enamel and amalgam both having 90-degree margins).

Resistance Form

Resistance form preparation features help the tooth and the restoration resist fractures caused by occlusal forces. Resistance features that assist in preventing the tooth from fracturing include (1) maintaining as much tooth structure as possible (preserving the dentin supporting cusps and marginal ridges); (2) having pulpal and gingival walls prepared perpendicular to occlusal forces, when possible; (3) having rounded internal preparation angles; (4) removing unsupported or weakened tooth structure; and (5) placing slots and pins into the tooth as part of the final stage of tooth preparation, when indicated. The placement of slots and pins is considered a secondary resistance form feature and is discussed in the section Clinical Technique for Complex Amalgam Restorations. Resistance form features that assist in preventing the amalgam from fracturing include (1) adequate thickness of amalgam (at least 1.5–2 mm in areas of occlusal contact and 0.75 mm in axial areas); (2) amalgam margin of 90 degrees; (3) boxlike preparation form, which provides uniform amalgam thickness; and (4) rounded axiopulpal line angles in Class II tooth preparations. Many of these resistance form features may be achieved using the No. 330 or No. 245 bur.

Retention Form

Retention form preparation features retain (i.e., "lock") the restorative material in the tooth. For composite restorations, adhesion (bonding) provides most of the needed retention. Amalgam restorations must be mechanically retained in the tooth. Amalgam retention form (Fig. 10.13) is provided by (1) preparation of the

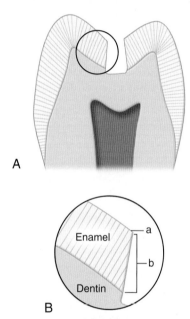

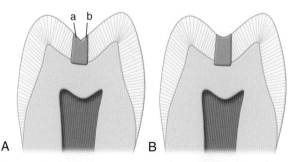

• **Fig. 10.11** Occlusal cavosurface margins. A, Tooth preparation. B, Occlusal margin representing the strongest enamel margin. Full-length enamel rods *(a)* and shorter enamel rods *(b)*.

• **Fig. 10.12** Amalgam form at occlusal cavosurface margins. A, Amalgam carved too deep resulting in acute angles *a* and *b* and stress concentrations within the amalgam, increasing the potential for fracture. B, Amalgam carved with appropriate anatomy, resulting in an amalgam margin close to 90 degrees, although the enamel cavosurface margin is obtuse.

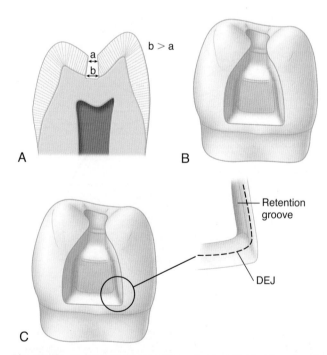

• **Fig. 10.13** Typical amalgam tooth preparation retention form features. A and B, Occlusal convergence of prepared walls (primary retention form). C, Retention grooves in proximal box (secondary retention form) if the proximal preparation is wide faciolingually.

vertical walls (especially facial and lingual walls) that converge occlusally (i.e., *primary retention*); (2) retention features such as grooves, coves, slots, and pins that are placed during the final stage of tooth preparation (i.e., *secondary retention*), and (3) engagement of the inserted amalgam into any surface irregularities in the preparation that may exist. Primary retention form features are achieved by the orientation and type of the preparation instrument such as the No. 330 or No. 245 pear-shaped carbide bur or diamond (see Fig. 10.7B). Secondary retention form features are discussed in subsequent sections.

Convenience Form

Convenience form includes features that allow adequate access and visibility of the operating site to facilitate tooth preparation and restoration. Convenience form includes extension of the outline form so that (1) the caries lesion may be accessed for removal, (2) the matrix may be placed, and (3) amalgam may be inserted, carved, and finished—all while maintaining resistance form.

Final Tooth Preparation

Removal of Defective Restorative Material and/or Soft Dentin

Any old restorative material or soft dentin remaining after the initial preparation will be located in the axial or pulpal walls (the extension of the peripheral preparation margins should have already been to sound tooth structure). Chapters 2 and 4 discuss (1) when to leave or remove old restorative material, (2) how to remove remaining soft dentin, and (3) what should be done to protect the pulp.

The removal of remaining soft dentin should be accomplished using the largest instrument that fits the carious area because it is least likely to penetrate the tooth in an uncontrolled manner. A hand instrument is more reliable than a rotating bur for judging the adequacy of removal of soft dentin. The removal of carious dentin should be stopped when the tooth structure feels firm unless exposure of the pulp becomes likely (see Chapter 2). This situation often occurs before all lightly stained or discolored dentin is removed.[61]

Pulp Protection

If the tooth preparation is of ideal or shallow depth, no liner or base is indicated. In deeper caries removal (where the remaining dentin thickness is judged to be 1–1.5 mm), a layer (i.e., 0.5–0.75 mm) of a resin-modified glass ionomer (RMGI) material should be placed (Fig. 10.14).[62,63] The RMGI insulates the pulp from thermal changes, bonds to dentin, releases fluoride, is strong enough to resist the forces of condensation, and reduces microleakage.[63-65] The RMGI is applied only over the deepest portion of the caries removal. It should be placed in small increments and should flow when it is touched to the dentin surface. The entire dentin surface should not be covered. Dentin peripheral to the liner should be available for support of the restoration.[66]

For pulpal protection in very deep caries removal (where the remaining dentin thickness is judged to be <0.5 mm and suspicion of potential microscopic pulpal exposure is increased), a thin layer (i.e., 0.5–0.75 mm) of a calcium hydroxide liner may be placed (Fig. 10.15). The calcium hydroxide liner may elicit tertiary dentin formation if the original odontoblasts are no longer vital. If the calcium hydroxide liner is used, it is placed by using the same

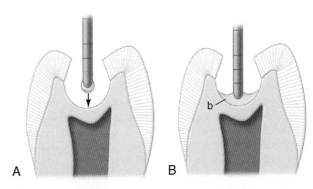

• **Fig. 10.14** Liner/Base application. A, Inserting resin-modified glass ionomer (RMGI) with periodontal probe. B, In moderately deep caries removal, a base *(b)* thickness of 0.5 to 0.75 mm is indicated.

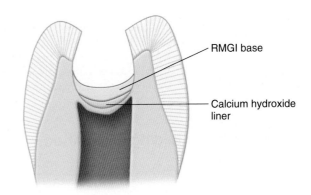

RMGI base

Calcium hydroxide liner

• **Fig. 10.15** Placement of calcium hydroxide liner and RMGI base.

instrument and the same technique as described for the RMGI liner. The calcium hydroxide liner should be placed only over the deepest portion of the caries removal (nearest the pulp). A layer of RMGI liner should be used to cover the calcium hydroxide.[67] The entire dentin surface should not be covered (see Figs. 10.14 and 10.15). The RMGI liner is recommended to cover the calcium hydroxide to resist the forces of condensation and to prevent dissolution over time by sealing the deeply excavated area.[64] Pulp exposure will require a direct pulp cap with calcium hydroxide or mineral trioxide aggregate (MTA), or endodontic treatment.[68]

Secondary Resistance and Retention Forms

Adequate resistance and retention form may no longer be present in the tooth preparation after caries lesion removal has resulted in excessive loss of vertical wall height. Therefore strategic features (such as the placement of grooves, coves, slots, pins) that enhance the resistance and retention form are added. Usually, the larger the tooth preparation, the greater the need for secondary resistance and retention forms.

Final Procedures: Debridement and Inspection

After the previous steps are performed, the completed tooth preparation should be cleaned of all debris (debridement) so that a careful inspection may be accomplished. The usual procedure in cleaning is to free the preparation of visible debris using short bursts of water spray from the air-water syringe followed by short bursts with the air syringe. If debris still clings to the preparation, it may be necessary to dislodge this material with an explorer, a small damp cotton pellet, or a commercially available applicator tip (i.e., a "microbrush") moistened with water. Excess water should be removed so as to allow a clear field for inspection. However, it is important not to desiccate the tooth by overuse of air as this may damage the odontoblasts associated with the desiccated tubules. The preparation should be viewed from all angles. Careful assessment should be made to ensure that the depths are proper, the external walls provide for enamel support and correct orientation for amalgam (i.e., that the preparation is retentive and the resultant restoration margins will not be prone to fracture), and the caries lesion has been removed as indicated. Preparation walls should be smooth and transitions should be gently rounded.[69] The cavosurface margin should be precise and clearly visualized.

Preparation Designs

Typical tooth preparation for amalgam has generally been referred to as *conventional tooth preparation*. A "box-only" tooth preparation is indicated if no occlusal caries lesion is present (i.e., only a proximal caries lesion is present). Fig. 10.16 illustrates various preparation designs. Appropriate details of specific tooth preparations are presented subsequently.

General Concepts Guiding Restoration With Amalgam

After tooth preparation, the tooth must be readied for the insertion of amalgam. Disinfectants may be used, but are not considered essential.[70,71] However, it is highly recommended that a dentin desensitizer (current commercial formulations contain 5% glutaraldehyde and 35% 2-hydroxyethyl methacrylate [HEMA] and water) be placed on the prepared dentin per manufacturer's instructions (see Fig. 10.3). This type of dentin desensitizer

cross-links tubular fluid proteins and, in the presence of HEMA, forms lamellar plugs in the dentinal tubules.[72] These plugs are thought to be responsible for reducing the potential for rapid tubular fluid movement and, thereby, the sensitivity of dentin. This step may occur before or after the matrix application.

Matrix Placement

A matrix primarily is used when a proximal surface is to be restored. The objectives of a matrix are to provide proper contact, provide proper contour, confine the restorative material, and reduce the amount of excess material. For a matrix to be effective, it should be easy to apply and remove, extend below the gingival margin enough that it can be engaged by a wedge, extend above the adjacent marginal ridge height so as to allow for proper condensation, and resist deformation during material insertion.

In some clinical circumstances, a matrix may be necessary for Class I or V amalgam restorations. Matrix application, along with wedging to increase interproximal space, may help protect the adjacent tooth from being damaged during preparation.

Mixing (Triturating) the Amalgam

Because of its superior clinical performance, high-copper amalgam is recommended. Preproportioned, disposable capsules are available in sizes ranging from 400 to 800 mg. Some precapsulated brands require activation of the capsules before trituration. The speed and time of trituration are factors that impact the setting reaction of the material. Alterations in either may cause changes in the properties of the inserted amalgam. Amalgam should be triturated (i.e., mixed) according to the manufacturer's directions. Correctly mixed amalgam should not be dry and crumbly; rather, it should retain sufficient "wetness" so as to aid in achieving a homogeneous and well-adapted restoration.[73] It is often necessary to make several mixes to complete the restoration, particularly for large preparations.

Insertion of the Amalgam

An amalgam carrier is used to transfer amalgam to the tooth preparation. Increments extruded from the carrier should be smaller (often only 50% or less of a full-carrier tip) for a small preparation, particularly during the initial insertion. A flat-faced, circular or elliptic condenser may be used to condense amalgam in the deeper areas of the preparation. The principal objectives during the insertion of amalgam are to condense the amalgam mass and to adapt it to the preparation walls and the matrix (when used). Thorough condensation is essential to produce a restoration free of voids, and helps to reduce marginal leakage.[74,75] Optimal condensation is necessary to minimize the mercury content in the restoration, which decreases corrosion and enhances restoration strength and marginal integrity.[75] Spherical amalgam is more easily condensed than admixed (lathe-cut) amalgam, but some practitioners prefer the handling properties of the admixed type. Condensation of amalgam that contains spherical particles requires larger condensers than are commonly used for admixed amalgam. Smaller condensers tend to penetrate a mass of spherical amalgam, resulting in less effective force to compact or adapt the amalgam within the preparation. In contrast, smaller condensers are indicated for the initial increments of admixed amalgam because it is more resistant to condensation pressure. This is because the area of a circular condenser face (nib) increases by the square of the diameter; doubling

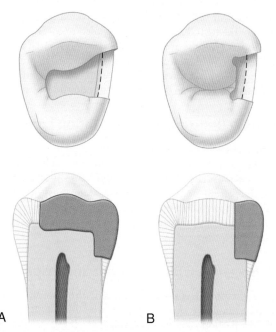

• **Fig. 10.16** Types of amalgam tooth preparations. A, Conventional. B, Box only.

the diameter requires four times more force for the same pressure per unit area. Each portion must be thoroughly condensed prior to placement of the next increment. Each condensed increment should fill only one third to one half the preparation depth. Each condensing stroke should overlap the previous condensing stroke to ensure that the entire mass is well condensed.

Lateral condensation (facially, lingually, and proximally directed condensation) is important in the proximal box portions of preparations to ensure confluence of the amalgam with the margins, the elimination of voids, and an adequate proximal contact. Generally, smaller amalgam condensers are used first, which allows the amalgam to be properly condensed into the internal line angles and secondary retention features. Subsequently, larger condensers are used. Amalgam preparations should be somewhat overfilled to ensure adequate condensation on the occlusal surface. The condensation of a mix should be completed within the time specified by the manufacturer (usually 2.5 to 3.5 minutes). Otherwise crystallization of the unused portion will be too advanced to react properly with the condensed portion. The mix should be discarded if it becomes dry, and another mix quickly made to continue the insertion.

Precarve Burnishing

To ensure that the marginal amalgam is well condensed before carving, the overpacked amalgam should be burnished immediately with a large burnisher, using heavy strokes mesiodistally and faciolingually, a procedure referred to as *precarve burnishing*. Precarve burnishing is useful to finalize the condensation, remove excess mercury-rich amalgam, and initiate the carving process. To maximize its effectiveness, the burnisher head should be large enough that in the final strokes it contacts the cusp slopes but not the preparation margins. Precarve burnishing produces denser amalgam at the margins of the occlusal preparations restored with high-copper amalgam alloys and initiates contouring of the restoration.[76,77]

Carving the Amalgam

The following discussion of carving (and shaping) of amalgam assumes the use of *sharp carving instruments*. All carving instruments dull with repeated use and sterilization cycles and, as a result, lose their efficiency. Carving a freshly condensed amalgam, which is setting and steadily getting harder, with a dull instrument requires the use of ever-increasing pressure on the instrument and increases the likelihood of losing control (slipping) and/or increasing the amount of time required to complete the carving. Always use sharp carving instruments!

The amalgam material selected for the restoration has a specific setting time. After precarve burnishing has been accomplished, the remainder of the accessible restoration must be contoured to achieve proper form and, as a result, function. The insertion (condensation) and carving of the material must occur before the material has hardened so much that it becomes uncarvable.

Occlusal Areas

A discoid–cleoid instrument may be used to carve the occlusal surface of an amalgam restoration. The rounded end (discoid) is positioned on the unprepared enamel adjacent to the amalgam margin and pulled parallel to the margin (Fig. 10.17). This removes any excess at the margin while not allowing the marginal amalgam to be carved below the preparation margins (i.e., "submarginated"). The pointed end (cleoid) of the instrument may be used to define

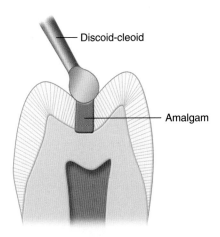

• **Fig. 10.17**   Carving the occlusal margins.

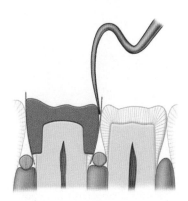

• **Fig. 10.18**   Defining the marginal ridge and the occlusal embrasure with an explorer.

the primary grooves, fossae, and cuspal inclines. The Hollenback carver is also useful for carving these areas.

The reproduction of grooves and fossae is necessary to provide appropriate mastication and sluiceways for the escape of food from the occlusal table. The mesial and distal fossae are carved to be inferior to the marginal ridge height, helping limit the potential for food to be wedged into the occlusal embrasure. Having rounded and relatively shallow occlusal anatomy also helps achieve a 90-degree amalgam margin on the occlusal surface and to ensure adequate occlusogingival dimension of the final amalgam restoration for strength (see Fig. 10.12B).

For multiple surface restorations (which require use of a matrix), the initial carving of the occlusal surface should be rapid, concentrating primarily on the marginal ridge height and occlusal embrasure areas. Occlusal embrasure areas are developed with a thin explorer tip or carving instrument by mirroring the contours of the adjacent tooth. The explorer tip is pulled along the inside of the matrix band, creating the occlusal embrasure form. When viewed from the facial or lingual direction, the embrasure form created should be identical to that of the adjacent tooth, assuming that the adjacent tooth has appropriate contour. Likewise, the height of the amalgam marginal ridge should generally be the same as that of the adjacent tooth (Figs. 10.18 and 10.19). If both these areas are developed properly, the potential for fracture of the marginal ridge area of the restoration while checking the occlusion is significantly reduced. Placing the initial carving emphasis on the occlusal areas for a

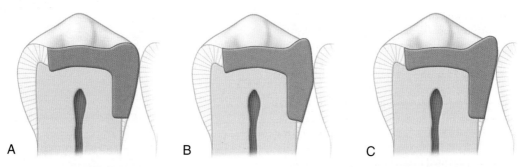

• **Fig. 10.19**   Proximal contour. A, Correct proximal contour. B, Incorrect marginal ridge height and occlusal embrasure form. C, The occlusogingival proximal contour is too straight, the contact is too high, and the occlusal embrasure form is incorrect.

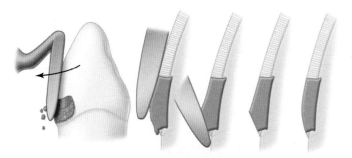

• **Fig. 10.20**   Positioning of the carving instrument to prevent overcarving amalgam and to develop the desired gingival contours.

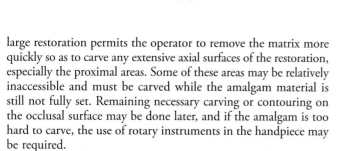

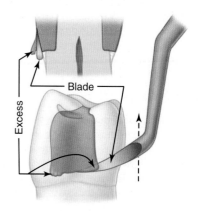

• **Fig. 10.21**   Gingival excess may be removed with amalgam knives.

large restoration permits the operator to remove the matrix more quickly so as to carve any extensive axial surfaces of the restoration, especially the proximal areas. Some of these areas may be relatively inaccessible and must be carved while the amalgam material is still not fully set. Remaining necessary carving or contouring on the occlusal surface may be done later, and if the amalgam is too hard to carve, the use of rotary instruments in the handpiece may be required.

Facial and Lingual Areas

Most facial and lingual areas are accessible and may be carved directly. The side of an explorer tine may be very effective in creating correct contours when the amalgam is early in its setting reaction. A Hollenbeck carver or base of the amalgam knife (scaler 34/35) is also useful for carving these areas. With regard to the cervical areas, it is important to remove any excess and develop the proper contour of the restoration, which is usually convex. The convexity is developed by using the occlusal and gingival unprepared tooth structure as guides for initiating the carving (Fig. 10.20). The marginal areas are blended together, resulting in the desired convexity and providing a physiologic contour that promotes the health of adjacent gingival tissue.

Proximal Embrasure Areas

The initial development of the occlusal embrasure of the proximal surface while the matrix is still in place has already been described. After removal of the matrix, the amalgam knife (or scaler 34/35) is an excellent instrument for removing proximal excess and developing proximal contours and embrasures (Figs. 10.21 and

10.22). The knife is positioned below the gingival margin and drawn occlusally to carefully shave off excess, to refine the proximal contour (below the contact) and the gingival embrasure form. The sharp tip of the knife also is beneficial in developing the facial and lingual embrasure forms. Care must be exercised in not carving away any of the contour necessary to create the desired proximal contact.

Development of proper proximal contour and contact is important for the physiologic health of interproximal soft tissue. Likewise, ensuring a smooth junction between the tooth and the amalgam is important. An amalgam overhang (excess of amalgam) may result in compromised gingival health. Voids at the cavosurface margins may result in recurrent caries lesion formation.

The proximal portion of the carved amalgam is evaluated by visual assessment (reflecting light into the contact area from the lingual and occlusal perspectives to confirm the dimensions and location of the proximal contact) and placement of very thin dental floss through the contact area. If dental floss is used, it must be used judiciously, ensuring that amalgam in the contact area is not inadvertently removed. A piece of floss may be inserted through the contact and into the gingival embrasure area by initially wrapping the floss around the adjacent tooth and exerting pressure on that tooth rather than the restored tooth while moving the floss through the contact area. When the floss is into the gingival embrasure area, it is wrapped around the restored tooth and moved occlusally and gingivally to determine whether excess exists and to smooth the proximal amalgam material. If excess material is detected along the gingival margin, the amalgam knife should again be used until a smooth margin is created.

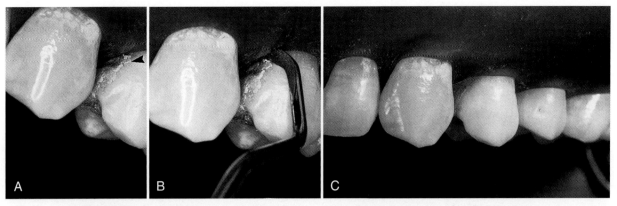

• **Fig. 10.22**   Removal of gingival excess of amalgam. A, Excess of amalgam *(arrowhead)* at the gingival corner of the restoration. B, Use of the amalgam knife for removal of gingival excess. C, Gingival corner of restoration with excess removed.

Postcarve Burnishing

Some operators prefer to *postcarve* burnish the amalgam surface by using a small burnisher. Postcarve burnishing is done by lightly rubbing the carved surface with a burnisher of suitable size and shape to improve smoothness and produce a satin (not shiny) appearance. The surface should not be rubbed hard enough to produce grooves in the amalgam. Postcarve burnishing may improve the marginal integrity of low- and high-copper amalgams and may improve the smoothness of the restoration.[78-80] Postcarve burnishing in conjunction with precarve burnishing may serve as a substitute for conventional polishing.[80]

Evaluation of Occlusal Contact Areas on the Restoration

After completion of the carving and the removal of the rubber dam, the occlusal contacts on the restoration must be evaluated. Even if the carving has been carefully accomplished, the restoration occasionally is "high," indicating premature occlusal contact. A piece of articulating paper is placed over the restoration and adjacent teeth, and the patient is instructed to close gently into occlusion. *It is essential that the teeth be completely dry for proper marking with articulating paper.* The patient is advised not to bite firmly because of the danger of fracturing the restoration, which is weak at this stage. The operator should visually assess the contact potential of the restored tooth and the extent of closure. If local anesthesia is still present, it may be difficult for the patient to tell when the teeth are in contact. After the patient has reopened the mouth and the articulating paper is removed, the following two features of the occlusal relationship suggest that the restoration is high: (1) Cusp tips of adjacent teeth are not in occlusal contact when it is known from the preoperative occlusal assessment that they should be touching, and (2) an opposing cusp prematurely occludes with the new restoration.

Contact areas on the amalgam should be assessed by the color imparted by the articulating paper. Deeply colored areas (heavy contacts) and those with light-colored centers (even heavier contacts) are reduced until all markings are uniformly of a light hue, and contacts are noted on adjacent teeth (Fig. 10.23). Heavy occlusal contacts are commonly referred to as "prematurities" or "high spots." Observing the bite opening between nearby teeth when the restoration is in contact indicates how much occlusal adjustment is indicated. For example, if the adjacent teeth are 0.5 mm apart

(by visual estimation), the high spot(s) should be reduced by approximately that amount. This observation may expedite the occlusal adjustment compared with making an insufficient adjustment and having to repeat closure-and-carving numerous times. The sequence of closure, observation, and carving is repeated until the appropriate surfaces of opposing teeth are touching.

Occlusal contacts on a cuspal incline or ridge slope are undesirable because they cause a deflective lateral force on the tooth. These should be adjusted until the resulting contact is stable (i.e., the occlusal contact should be perpendicular to the occlusal load where possible in maximum intercuspation, or, in other words, the occlusal force should be parallel to the long axis of the tooth).

To this point in the procedure, the patient has been instructed to close vertically into maximum intercuspation (i.e., "bite together on your back teeth"). After replacing the articulating paper over the tooth, the patient is asked to occlude lightly and to slide the teeth lightly from "side to side" to identify excursive interferences and "front to back" to identify protrusive interferences (see Chapter 1). Any additional occlusal marks are evaluated, and undesirable contact areas (interferences) are eliminated. Note that amalgam restorations carved completely out of occlusion (i.e., that are "over-carved") may allow supraeruptive tooth movement resulting in undesirable tooth contacts and this, too, should be avoided. Finally, the patient should be cautioned to protect the newly condensed restoration by not using it to chew firm food for 24 hours.

Finishing and Polishing of the Amalgam

Most amalgams do not require further finishing and polishing. These procedures are occasionally necessary, however, to (1) refine the anatomy, contours, and marginal integrity; and (2) refine the surface texture of the restoration. Additional finishing and polishing procedures for amalgam restorations are not attempted within 24 hours of insertion because crystallization of the restoration is incomplete.[73] If used, these procedures are often delayed until all of the patient's amalgam restorations have been placed, rather than finishing and polishing periodically during the course of treatment. An amalgam restoration is less prone to tarnish and corrosion if a smooth, homogeneous surface is achieved.[81-83] Polishing of high-copper amalgams is less important than it is for low-copper amalgams because high-copper amalgams are less susceptible to tarnishing and marginal breakdown.[56,82-87]

The finishing procedure may be initiated by use of a green carborundum or white alumina stone. (Fig. 10.24A). The green

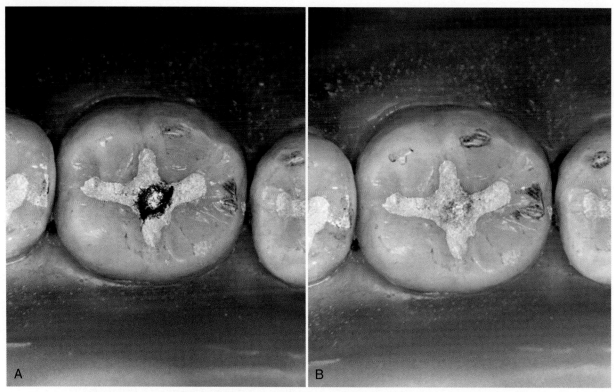

• **Fig. 10.23** Occluding the restoration. A, Heavy occlusal contacts on new amalgam should be adjusted. Articulating paper marks heavy contacts as dark areas, and it marks very heavy contacts as dark areas with light-colored, potentially shiny, centers. B, Amalgam should not be carved out of occlusion. Rather, it should have light occlusal contact or contacts, as indicated by faint markings.

stone is more abrasive than the white stone; the tip of either stone may be blunted on a diamond wheel before use. This helps prevent marring the center of the restoration while the margins are being adjusted. During the surfacing of amalgam, the stone's long axis is held at a 90-degree angle to the margins. Reduction of any occlusal contact should be avoided. After the stone is used, the margins should be reevaluated with the tine of an explorer and any additional discrepancies removed. The surface may be smoothed further using light pressure with an appropriate finishing bur (see Fig. 10.24B). A large, round finishing bur is generally used for this finishing step. If the groove and fossa features are not sufficiently defined, a small round finishing bur also may accentuate them without eliminating the occlusal contact areas. The long axis of the bur or stone should be at a ~45-degree angle to the margin to allow the unprepared tooth structure to guide the bur and prevent unnecessary removal of amalgam (see Fig. 10.24C). A smooth surface should be achieved before the polishing procedure is initiated. The finishing bur should remove the minor scratches that resulted from use of the green or white stone. Often, however, these scratches can be removed only with the use of rubber abrasive points.

The polishing procedure is initiated by using a coarse, rubber abrasive point at low speed and air-water spray to produce an amalgam surface with a smooth, satin appearance (see Fig. 10.24D and E). If the amalgam surface does not exhibit this appearance after only a few seconds of polishing, the surface was too rough at the start. In this instance, resurfacing with a finishing bur is necessary, followed by the coarse, rubber abrasive point to develop the satiny appearance. It is important that the rubber points be used at low speed (≤6000 revolutions per minute [rpm]) or just above "stall out" speed so as to limit the danger of point

disintegration (which may occur at high rotational speeds) and the danger of frictional temperature elevation of the restoration and the tooth. Temperature above 140°F [>60°C] is able to cause irreparable damage to the pulp, the restoration, or both. When overheated, the amalgam surface appears cloudy, even though it may have a high polish. This cloudy appearance indicates that mercury has been brought to the surface, which results in increased corrosion of the amalgam and loss of strength.[73]

Polishing with the coarse abrasive rubber point will result in a moderately polished surface. No deep scratches should remain on the amalgam surface. After the area is washed free of abrasive particles and dried, a high polish may be imparted to the restoration with a series of medium grit and fine-grit abrasive points (see Fig. 10.24F). As with the more abrasive points, the finer abrasive points must be used at a low speed. If a high luster does not appear within a few seconds, the restoration requires additional polishing with the more abrasive points. The system illustrated in Fig. 10.24 includes coarse-grit, medium-grit, and fine-grit rubber abrasive points. Using these points in sequence, from coarse to fine, produces an amalgam surface with a brilliant luster (see Fig. 10.24G). As an alternative to rubber abrasive points, final polishing may be accomplished using a rubber cup with flour of pumice followed by a high-luster agent such as precipitated chalk. Finishing and polishing of older, existing restorations may be performed to improve their contour, margins, surface, or anatomy, when indicated (Fig. 10.25).

These procedures should not leave the restoration undercontoured and should not alter the carefully designed occlusal contacts. The tip of an explorer should pass from the tooth surface to the restoration surface (and vice versa), without jumping or catching, thus

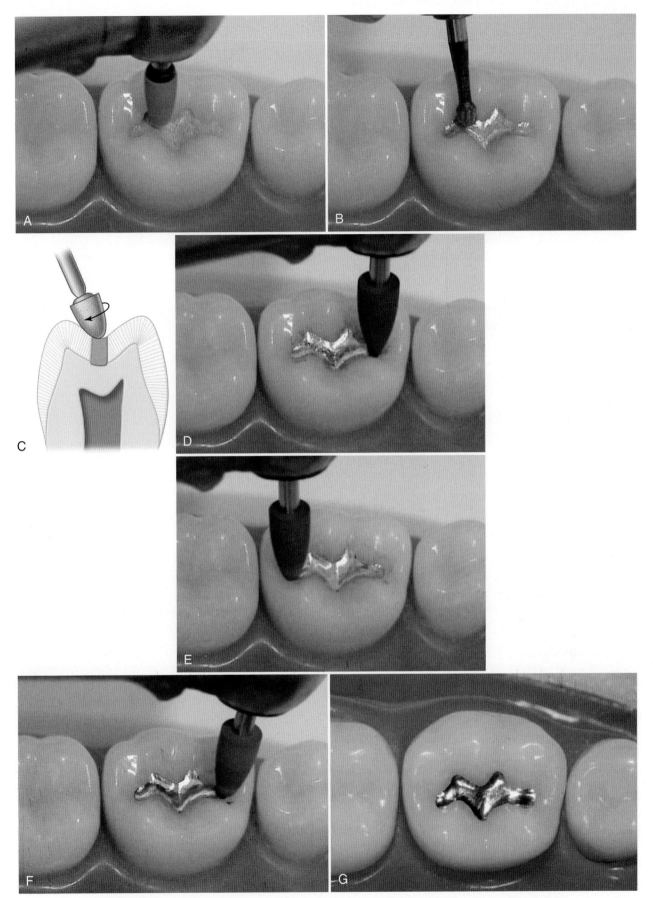

• **Fig. 10.24** Polishing the amalgam. A, When necessary, a carborundum or fine-grit alumina stone is used to develop continuity of surface from the tooth to the restoration. B, The restoration is surfaced with a round finishing bur. C, The stone's long axis or the bur's long axis is held at a right angle to the margin. D, Polishing is initiated with a coarse rubber abrasive point at low speed. E, The point should produce a smooth, satin appearance. F, A high polish is obtained with medium-grit and fine-grit abrasive points. G, Polished restoration. (Courtesy Aldridge D. Wilder, DDS.)

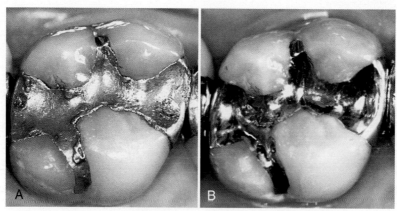

• **Fig. 10.25** A, Existing amalgam restoration exhibiting marginal deterioration and surface roughness. B, Same restoration after finishing and polishing.

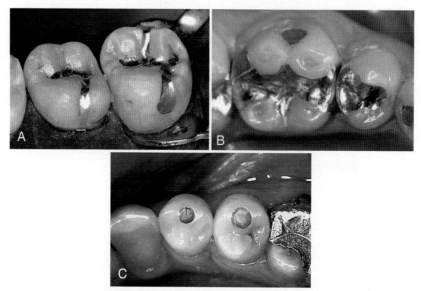

• **Fig. 10.26** Clinical examples of Class I, II, and VI amalgam restorations. A, Class I amalgam in the occlusal surface of the first molar. B, Class II amalgams in a premolar and molar. C, Class VI amalgams in premolars.

verifying continuity of contour across the margin. Every effort to avoid removal of adjacent tooth structure should be made.

Repairing an Amalgam Restoration

If an amalgam restoration fractures during insertion, generally all of the inserted amalgam must be removed and new amalgam condensed. If a small portion of amalgam fractures during insertion and the amalgam is still carvable, it may be possible to apply and condense newly triturated amalgam to repair the affected area. If a small void in the amalgam is discovered after the matrix is removed, for example, and if the amalgam is still carvable and the area is accessible, any poorly condensed amalgam in the void should be removed with an explorer or other instrument, and the void repaired with newly triturated amalgam. In cases where a new mix of amalgam is added to carvable existing amalgam, the "new" amalgam will adhere to the "old."

If a repair needs to be made to set, uncarvable amalgam, the defective area may be re-prepared as if it were a small restoration. Appropriate depth and retention form must be generated, sometimes

entirely within the existing amalgam restoration. If necessary, another matrix must be placed. A new mix of amalgam may be condensed directly into the defect.

Clinical Technique for Class I Amalgam Restorations

This section describes the use of amalgam for Class I restorations. Class I restorations restore defects on the occlusal surfaces of posterior teeth, the occlusal thirds of the facial and lingual surfaces of molars, and the lingual surfaces of maxillary anterior teeth (Fig. 10.26).

The procedural description for a small (i.e., "conservative") Class I amalgam restoration simply and clearly presents the basic information relating to the entire amalgam restoration technique, including tooth preparation and placement and contouring of the restoration. This basic procedural information may be expanded to describe Class I amalgam restoration of lesions/defects of all sizes. The maxillary first premolar is used for illustration in this section.

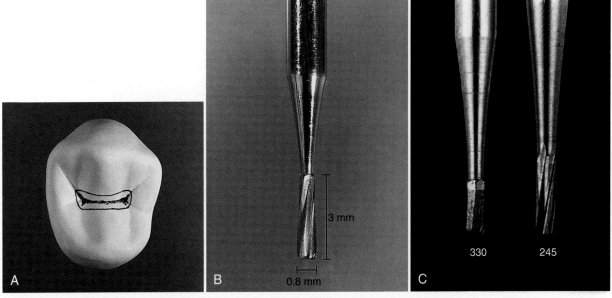

• **Fig. 10.27**   Class I preparation outline. A, Ideal outline includes all carious occlusal pits and fissures. B, Dimensions of head of a No. 245 bur. C, No. 330 and No. 245 burs compared.

Initial Clinical Procedures

A preoperative assessment of the occlusal relationship of the involved and adjacent teeth is necessary. After administration of local anesthetic, isolation of the operating field with the rubber dam is recommended.[73,88] The rubber dam may be applied in the few minutes necessary for onset of profound anesthesia before initiating the tooth preparation. Rubber dam isolation is especially indicated when removing deep caries (judged to be <1 mm from the pulp), during amalgam condensation, and for mercury hygiene. The rubber dam should be used for isolation of the operating site when a caries lesion is extensive. If caries removal exposes the pulp, pulp capping may be more successful if the site is isolated with a properly applied rubber dam. In addition, the dam prevents moisture contamination of the amalgam mix during insertion.[60] For a single maxillary tooth, where caries is not extensive, adequate control of the operating field may also be achieved with cotton rolls and high-volume evacuation.

Tooth Preparation for Class I Amalgam Restorations

This section describes the specific technique for preparing the tooth for a Class I amalgam restoration. It is divided into initial and final stages.

Initial Tooth Preparation

Initial tooth preparation is defined as establishing the outline form by extension of the external walls to sound tooth structure while maintaining a specified, limited depth (usually just inside the DEJ) and providing resistance and retention forms. The outline form for the Class I occlusal amalgam tooth preparation should include only the defective occlusal pits and fissures (in a way that sharp, angular, abrupt transitions in the marginal outline are avoided). Commonly, but not always, the marginal outline for maxillary premolars is butterfly shaped because of extension to include the developmental fissures facially and lingually. The ideal outline form for an amalgam restoration incorporates the following resistance

form principles that are basic to all amalgam tooth preparations of occlusal surfaces (Fig. 10.27A). These principles allow margins to be positioned in areas that are sound and subject to minimal occlusal loading while maintaining the strength and health of the tooth by conserving uncompromised tooth structure. The resistance principles are as follows:

1. Extending around the cusps to conserve tooth structure and prevent the internal line angles from approaching the pulp horns
2. Keeping the facial and lingual margin extensions as minimal as possible between the central carious fissure and the cusp tips
3. Extending the outline to include fissures, placing the margins on relatively smooth, sound tooth structure
4. Minimally extending into the marginal ridges (only enough to include the defect) without removing dentinal support
5. Eliminating a weak wall of enamel by joining two outlines that come close together (i.e., <0.5 mm apart)
6. Extending the outline form to include enamel undermined by the caries lesion
7. Using enameloplasty on the terminal ends of shallow fissures to conserve tooth structure
8. Establishing an optimal, conservative depth of the pulpal wall

A No. 245 bur, with a head length of 3 mm and a tip diameter of 0.8 mm, or a smaller No. 330 bur is recommended to prepare the Class I tooth preparation (see Fig. 10.27B and C). The silhouette of the No. 245 bur reveals sides slightly convergent toward the shank. This produces an occlusal convergence of the facial and lingual preparation walls, providing adequate retention form for the tooth preparation. The slightly rounded corners of the end of the No. 245 bur produce slightly rounded internal line angles that render the tooth more resistant to fracture from occlusal force.[89] The No. 330 bur is a smaller and pear-shaped version of the No. 245 bur and is also indicated for amalgam preparations (see Fig. 10.27C).

Class I occlusal tooth preparation is begun by entering the deepest or most carious pit with a "punch cut" using the No. 245 carbide bur at high speed with air-water spray. A punch cut is performed by orienting the bur such that its long axis parallels

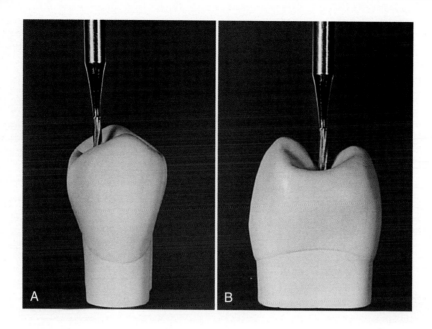

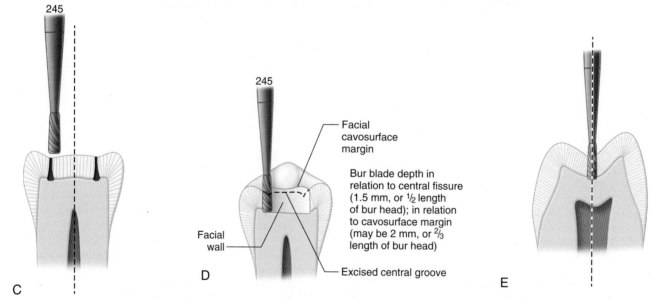

• **Fig. 10.28** A, No. 245 bur oriented parallel to long axis of tooth crown for entry as viewed from lingual aspect. B, The bur positioned for entry as viewed from the distal aspect. C, The bur is positioned over the most carious pit (distal) for entry. The distal aspect of the bur is positioned over the distal pit. D, Mesiodistal longitudinal section. Relationship of head of No. 245 bur to excised central fissure and cavosurface margin at ideal pulpal floor depth, which is just inside the DEJ. E, Faciolingual longitudinal section. Dotted line indicates the long axis of tooth crown and the direction of the bur.

the long axis of the tooth crown (Fig. 10.28A and B). The bur is inserted directly into the defective pit. When the pits are equally defective, the distal pit should be entered as illustrated. Entering the distal pit first provides increased visibility for the mesial extension. The bur should be positioned such that its distal aspect is directly over the distal pit, minimizing extension into the marginal ridge (see Fig. 10.28C). The bur should be rotating when it is applied to the tooth and should not stop rotating until it is removed from the tooth. On posterior teeth, the approximate depth of the DEJ is located at 1.5 to 2 mm from the occlusal surface. As the bur enters the pit, an initial target depth of 1.5 mm should be established. This is one half the length of the cutting portion of the No. 245 bur. The 1.5-mm pulpal depth is measured at the

central fissure (see Fig. 10.28D and E). The depth of the preparation is modified as needed so that the pulpal wall is established 0.1 to 0.2 mm into dentin. In other words, the depth of the prepared external walls should be 1.5 to 2 mm ("just inside the DEJ") (see Fig. 10.28D and E), depending on the cuspal incline. The length of the blades of an unfamiliar bur should be measured before it is used as a depth gauge.

Distal extension into the distal marginal ridge to include a fissure or caries occasionally requires a slight tilting of the bur distally (≤10 degrees). This creates a slight occlusal divergence to the distal wall to prevent undermining the marginal ridge of its dentin support (Fig. 10.29A–C). Because the facial and lingual prepared walls converge, this slight divergence does not compromise

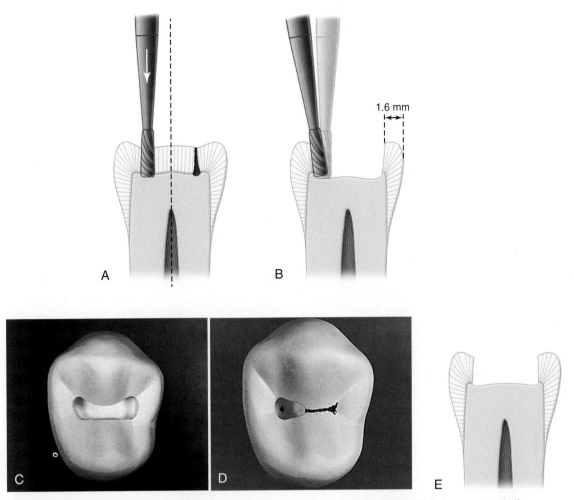

• **Fig. 10.29** A, Enter the pit with a punch cut to just inside the DEJ (depth of 1.5–2 mm or one half to two thirds the head length of the No. 245 bur). The 1.5-mm depth is measured at central fissure; the measurement of same entry cut at the prepared external wall is 2 mm. B, Incline the bur distally to establish proper occlusal divergence to distal wall to prevent removal of the dentin supporting the marginal ridge enamel when the pulpal floor is in dentin, and distal extension is necessary to include a fissure or caries lesion. For such an extension on premolars, the distance from the margin to the proximal surface (i.e., imaginary projection) must not be less than 1.6 mm (i.e., two diameters of bur end). C, Occlusal view of the initial tooth preparation that has mesial and distal walls that diverge occlusally. D, Distofacial and distolingual fissures that radiate from the pit are included before extending along the central fissure. E, Mesiodistal longitudinal section. The pulpal floors are generally flat but may follow the rise and fall of the occlusal surface.

the overall retention form. For premolars, the distance from the margin of such an extension to the proximal surface usually should not be less than ~1.6 mm, or two diameters of the end of the No. 245 bur (see Fig. 10.29B) measured from a tangent to the proximal surface (i.e., the proximal surface height of contour). For molars, this minimal distance is ~2 mm.

Minimal distal (or mesial) extension often does not require changing the orientation of the bur's axis from being parallel to the long axis of the tooth crown. In this case, the mesial and distal walls are parallel to the long axis of the tooth crown (or slightly convergent occlusally) (see Fig. 10.29D and E).

While maintaining the bur's orientation and depth, the preparation is extended distofacially or distolingually to include any fissures that radiate from the pit (see Fig. 10.29D). When these fissures require extensions of more than a few tenths of a millimeter,

however, consideration should be given to changing to a bur of smaller diameter or to using enameloplasty. Both of these approaches conserve the tooth structure and therefore minimize weakening of the tooth.

The bur's orientation and depth are maintained while extending along the central fissure toward the mesial pit, following the DEJ (see Fig. 10.29D and E). When the central fissure has minimal caries, one pass through the fissure at the prescribed depth provides the desired minimal width to the isthmus. Ideally the width of the isthmus should be just wider than the diameter of the bur. It is well established that a tooth preparation with a narrow occlusal isthmus is less prone to fracture.[90,91] As previously described for the distal margin, the orientation of the bur should not change as it approaches the mesial pit if the mesial extension is minimal. If the fissure extends farther onto the marginal ridge, the long axis

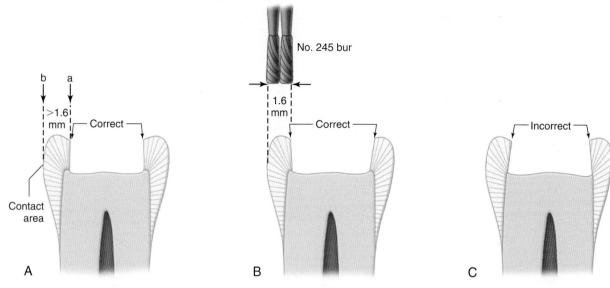

• **Fig. 10.30** The direction of the mesial and distal walls is influenced by the remaining thickness of the marginal ridge as measured from the mesial or distal margin *(a)* to the proximal surface (i.e., imaginary projection of proximal surface) *(b)*. A, Mesial and distal walls should converge occlusally when the distance from *a* to *b* is greater than 1.6 mm. B, When the operator judges that the extension will leave only 1.6-mm thickness (two diameters of No. 245 bur) of marginal ridge (i.e., premolars), the mesial and distal walls must diverge occlusally to conserve ridge-supporting dentin. C, Extending the mesial or distal walls to a two-diameter limit without diverging the wall occlusally undermines the marginal ridge enamel.

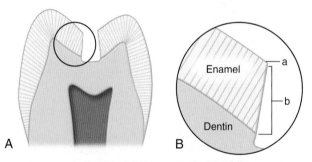

• **Fig. 10.31** A and B, The ideal and strongest enamel margin is formed by full-length enamel rods *(a)* resting on sound dentin supported on the preparation side by shorter rods, also resting on sound dentin *(b)*.

of the bur should be changed to establish a slight occlusal divergence to the mesial wall if the marginal ridge would be otherwise undermined of its dentinal support. Fig. 10.30 illustrates the correct and incorrect preparation of the mesial and distal walls. The remainder of any occlusal enamel defects is included in the outline, and the facial and lingual walls are extended, if necessary, to remove enamel undermined by the caries lesion.[92] The strongest and ideal enamel margin should be composed of full-length enamel rods attached to sound dentin, supported on the preparation side by shorter rods that are also attached to sound dentin (Fig. 10.31).

The Class I tooth preparation should have an outline form with gently flowing curves and distinct cavosurface margins. A faciolingual width of no more than 1 to 1.5 mm and a depth of 1.5 to 2 mm are considered ideal, but this goal is subject to the extension of the caries lesion. The pulpal floor, depending on the enamel thickness, is almost always in dentin (see Fig. 10.29C and E). Although conservation of the tooth structure is important, the convenience form requires that the extent of the preparation be adjusted to provide adequate access and visibility.

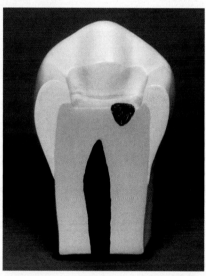

• **Fig. 10.32** Mesiodistal longitudinal section showing example of the pulpal floor in dentin and the caries lesion that is exposed after the initial tooth preparation. The caries lesion is surrounded by sound dentin on the pulpal floor for the resistance form.

This completes the initial amalgam preparation for a Class I caries lesion. The initial preparation should ensure that all the caries lesion is removed from the DEJ, resulting in a very narrow peripheral seat of healthy dentin on the pulpal wall surrounding any remaining caries located in the center of the pulpal wall. For the initial tooth preparation, the pulpal wall should remain at the initial ideal depth, even if any restorative material or soft caries lesion remains in the pulpal wall (Fig. 10.32). Remaining caries (and, if present, old restorative material) is removed during the final tooth preparation.

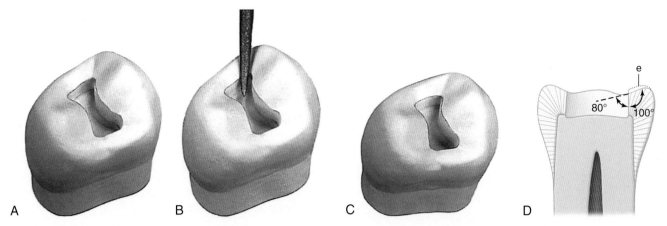

A   B   C   D

• **Fig. 10.33** Enameloplasty. A, Developmental defect at terminal end of fissure. B, Fine-grit diamond finishing instrument in position to remove the defect. C, Smooth surface after enameloplasty. D, The cavosurface angle should not exceed 100 degrees, and the margin–amalgam angle should not be less than 80 degrees. Enamel external surface *(e)* before enameloplasty.

Primary resistance form is provided by the following:

1. Sufficient area of relatively flat pulpal floor in sound tooth structure (i.e., the "peripheral seat") to resist forces directed in the long axis of the tooth and to provide a horizontal area for the restoration
2. Minimal extension of external walls (to conserve tooth strength)
3. Strong, ideal enamel margins
4. Sufficient depth (i.e., 1.5 mm) for adequate thickness of the restoration, providing resistance to fracture

The slight occlusal convergence of two or more opposing, external walls provides the primary retention form.

Usually, the No. 245 bur is used for extensions into the mesial and distal fissures. During such extensions, the remaining depth of the fissure may be viewed in cross section by looking at the wall being extended. When the remaining fissure is no deeper than one quarter to one third the thickness of enamel, enameloplasty is indicated. Enameloplasty refers to eliminating the developmental fault by removing it with the side of an appropriately shaped rotary finishing instrument, leaving a smooth surface (Fig. 10.33A–C). This procedure frequently reduces the need for further extension. The extent to which enameloplasty should be used cannot be determined exactly until the process of extending into the fissured area occurs, at which time the depth of the fissure into enamel may be observed. The surface left by enameloplasty should meet the tooth preparation wall, preferably with a cavosurface angle no greater than approximately 100 degrees; this would produce a distinct margin for amalgam of no less than 80 degrees (see Fig. 10.33D). If enameloplasty is unsuccessful in eliminating a mesial (or distal) fissure that extends to the crest of a marginal ridge or beyond, three alternatives exist:

1. Make no further change in the outline form.
2. Extend through the marginal ridge when margins would be lingual to the contact (Fig. 10.34).
3. Include the fissure in a conservative Class II tooth preparation.

The first alternative usually should be strongly considered except in patients at high risk for caries. Enameloplasty is not indicated if an area of occlusal contact is involved. In this case, the choices are either to consider the preparation completed (an option for patients at low risk for caries) or to extend the preparation to include the fissure as previously described.

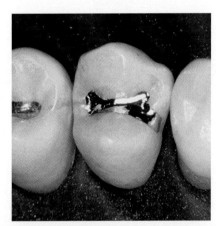

• **Fig. 10.34** Mesial fissure that cannot be eliminated by enameloplasty may be included in the preparation if the margins are able to be lingual of the occlusal contact.

A tooth may be found to have a large or "extensive" Class I caries lesion. A lesion is considered extensive if the distance between soft dentin and the pulp is judged to be less than 1 mm or when the faciolingual extent of the defect has involved much of the cuspal inclines. In this case, selective removal of soft dentin and insertion of a liner, if needed, may precede the establishment of outline, resistance, and retention forms. This approach protects the pulp as early as possible from any additional insult that may occur during tooth preparation. Normally, however, the outline, primary resistance, and primary retention forms are established through proper orientation of the No. 245 bur and appropriate extension of the preparation. As is the case for smaller caries lesions, an initial depth to reach the DEJ (measured approximately 1.5 mm at any pit or fissure and 2 mm on the prepared external walls) should still be established and maintained. The preparation is extended laterally at the DEJ to remove all enamel undermined by the caries lesion by alternately cutting and examining the lateral extension of the lesion. For a caries lesion extending up the cuspal inclines, it may be necessary to alter the bur's long axis to prepare a 90- to 100-degree cavosurface angle while maintaining the initial depth (Fig. 10.35). If not, an obtuse cavosurface angle may remain (resulting in an acute, or weak, amalgam margin), or the pulpal floor (over the pulp horns) may be prepared too deeply. Primary resistance form is obtained by extending the outline of the tooth preparation to include only undermined and defective tooth structure while preparing strong enamel walls and allowing strong cuspal areas to remain. Primary retention form is obtained by the occlusal convergence of the enamel walls. Secondary

retention form may result from undercut areas that are occasionally left in dentin (and that are not filled in by a liner or base) after peripheral removal of soft dentin. When extending the outline form, enameloplasty should be used in any indicated area (as described previously and in detail in Chapter 4).

When the defect extends to more than one half the distance between the primary groove and a cusp tip, reducing the cuspal tooth structure and restoring it with amalgam (also referred to as "capping the cusp") may be indicated as discussed in Clinical Technique for Complex Amalgam Restorations. When the distance is two thirds, cusp reduction and coverage is usually required because of the risk of cusp fracture during subsequent functional occlusal loading. Fig. 10.36 illustrates examples of large (extensive) Class I amalgam preparation outlines.

Final Tooth Preparation

The final tooth preparation includes (1) removal of remaining defective enamel and soft dentin on the pulpal floor as indicated; (2) pulp protection, where indicated; (3) procedures for finishing the external walls; and (4) final procedures of debridement (cleaning) and inspecting the preparation.

If several enamel pit-and-fissure remnants remain in the floor, or if a central fissure remnant extends over most of the floor, the floor should be deepened with the No. 245 bur to eliminate the defect or to uncover the caries lesion to a maximum preparation depth of 2 mm (Fig. 10.37). If these remnants are few and small, they may be removed with an appropriate carbide bur (Fig. 10.38). Removal of the remaining lesion (i.e., caries lesion that extends pulpally from the established pulpal floor) is best accomplished

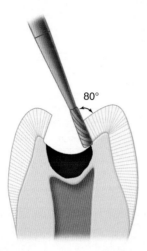

• **Fig. 10.35** Initial tooth preparation with an extensive caries lesion. When extending laterally to remove enamel undermined by the caries lesion, the bur's long axis is altered to prepare a 90- to 100-degree cavosurface angle. A 100-degree cavosurface angle on the cuspal incline results in an 80-degree marginal amalgam angle.

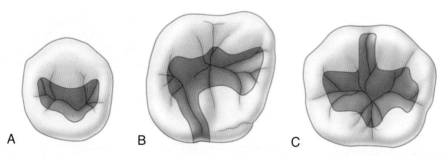

• **Fig. 10.36** Examples of more extensive Class I amalgam tooth preparation outline forms. A, Occlusal outline form in the mandibular second premolar. B, Occlusolingual outline form in the maxillary first molar. C, Occlusofacial outline form in the mandibular first molar.

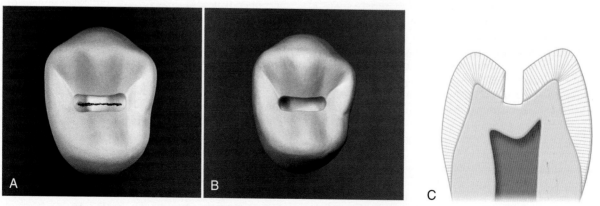

• **Fig. 10.37** Removal of enamel fissure extending over most of the pulpal floor. A, Full-length occlusal fissure remnant remaining on the pulpal floor after the initial tooth preparation. B and C, The pulpal floor is deepened to a maximum depth of 2 mm to eliminate the fissure or uncover dentin caries lesion.

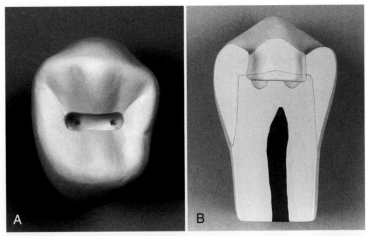

• **Fig. 10.38** Removal of enamel pit and fissure and dentin caries lesion that is limited to a few small pit-and-fissure remnants. A, Two pit remnants remain on the pulpal floor after the initial tooth preparation. B, Carious enamel and dentin caries lesion have been removed.

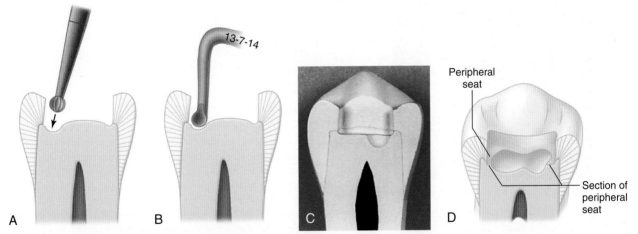

Peripheral seat

Section of peripheral seat

• **Fig. 10.39** A and B, Removal of dentin caries lesion is accomplished with round burs (A) or spoon excavators (B). C and D, The resistance form may be improved with a flat floor peripheral to the excavated area(s).

using a discoid-type spoon excavator or a slowly revolving round carbide bur of appropriate size (Fig. 10.39A and B).

The removal of carious dentin will not affect the resistance form of the tooth because the periphery would not need further extension. In addition, it will not affect the resistance form of the restoration as it will rest on the pulpal wall peripheral to the excavated area or areas. The peripheral pulpal floor should be at the previously described initial pulpal floor depth just inside the DEJ (see Fig. 10.39C and D). Usually, no secondary resistance or retention form features are necessary Class I amalgam preparations.

External walls may already have been finished during initial preparation steps; however, operator assessment of the external walls of the preparation is accomplished at this point, and any additional finish is accomplished as described previously and in Chapter 4. An occlusal cavosurface bevel is contraindicated in the tooth preparation for an amalgam restoration.[92] It is important to provide an approximate 90- to 100-degree cavosurface angle, which should result in 80- to 90-degree amalgam at the margins.[92] This butt-joint marginal area (which approximates 90-degree cavosurface marginal angles for both enamel and amalgam) allows strength

for both. Amalgam is a brittle material with low edge strength and tends to chip under occlusal stress if its angle at the margins is less than 80 degrees. The transition between the external and internal walls should be gently rounded.[93] The preparation should then be cleaned, carefully inspected as indicated previously in General Concepts Guiding Preparation for Amalgam Restorations, and any final modifications completed.

Other Class I Amalgam Preparations

Class I preparations, especially those in esthetically important areas, may be restored with composite because of their small size and the maximal thickness of enamel available for bonding. However, the following preparations may also be restored with amalgam:

1. Facial pit of the mandibular molar.
2. Lingual pit of the maxillary lateral incisor.
3. Occlusal pits of the mandibular first premolar.
4. Occlusal pits and fissures of the maxillary first molar.
5. Occlusal pits and fissures of the mandibular second premolar.

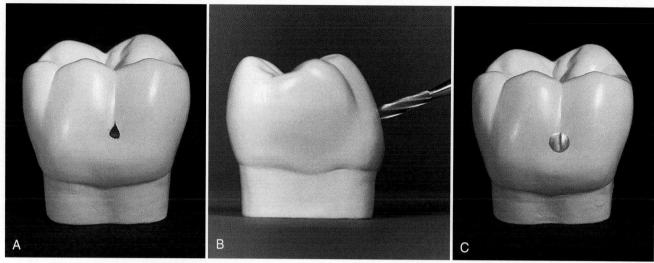

• **Fig. 10.40** Mandibular molar. A, Facial pit with a caries lesion. B, The bur positioned perpendicular to the tooth surface for entry. C, Outline of restoration.

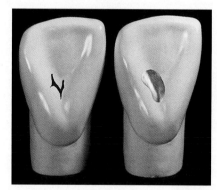

• **Fig. 10.41** Carious lingual pit and fissure and restoration on the maxillary lateral incisor.

Examples of some of these types of preparations and restorations are provided in Figs. 10.40, 10.41, 10.42, 10.43, 10.44, and 10.45.

Restorative Technique for Class I Amalgam Preparations

Desensitizer Placement

A dentin desensitizer is placed in the preparation according to manufacturer recommendations before amalgam condensation (Fig. 10.46).[72]

Matrix Placement

Generally matrices are unnecessary for a conservative Class I amalgam restoration except as specified in later sections.

Insertion and Carving of the Amalgam

The triturated amalgam (Fig. 10.47A) is placed into an amalgam well. The outline of the tooth preparation should be reviewed before inserting amalgam to establish a mental image that will later aid in carving amalgam to the cavosurface margin. Preoperative occlusal contact locations should be recalled (see Fig. 10.47B). Amalgam should be carefully condensed into the pulpal line angles (see Fig. 10.47C). The preparation should be overpacked 1 mm or more using heavy pressure (see Fig. 10.47D). This ensures that the cavosurface margins are completely covered with well-condensed amalgam. Final condensation over cavosurface margins should be done perpendicular to the external enamel surface adjacent to the margins. The overpacked amalgam should then be precarve burnished.

Finishing and Polishing of the Amalgam

With care, carving may begin immediately after condensation. Sharp discoid-cleoid carvers of suitable sizes are useful for this. The larger end of the discoid-cleoid instrument (No. 3/6) is used first, followed by the smaller instrument (No. 4/5) in regions not accessible to the larger instrument. Alternatively, the Hollenback carver may be used, with care not to overcarve the groove or fossa areas. All carving should be done with the edge of the blade perpendicular to the margins as the instrument is moved parallel to the margins. Part of the edge of the carving blade should rest on the unprepared tooth surface adjacent to the preparation margin (see Fig. 10.47F). Using this surface as a guide helps prevent overcarving amalgam at the margins and produces a continuity of surface contour across the preparation margins. During carving, thin amalgam should be removed from areas of enameloplasty. Thin amalgam left in these areas may fracture because of its low edge strength. Deep occlusal anatomy should not be carved into the restoration because these may thin the amalgam at the margins and weaken the restoration (see Fig. 10.47G). Undercarving leaves thin portions of amalgam (subject to fracture) on the unprepared tooth surface. The thin portion of amalgam extending beyond the margin is referred to as *flash*. The mesial and distal fossae should be carved slightly deeper than the proximal marginal ridges (see Fig. 10.47H).

After carving is completed, the outline of the amalgam margin should reflect the contour and location of the prepared cavosurface margin, revealing a regular (i.e., not ragged) outline with gentle curves. An amalgam outline that is larger or irregular is undercarved and requires further carving or finishing (Fig. 10.48). An amalgam restoration that is more than minimally overcarved (i.e., a submarginal defect >0.2 mm) should be replaced.[94] If the total carving time is short enough, the smoothness of the carved surface may be improved by wiping with a small, damp ball of cotton held with the cotton pliers. Alternatively, postcarve burnishing may be

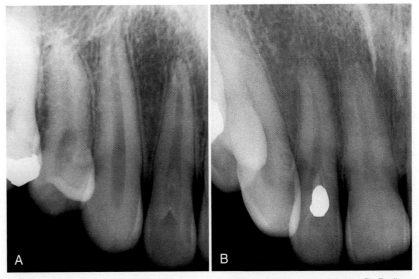

• **Fig. 10.42**   Maxillary lateral incisor. A, Preoperative radiograph of dens in dente. B, Radiograph of restoration after 13 years. (Courtesy Dr. Ludwig Scott.)

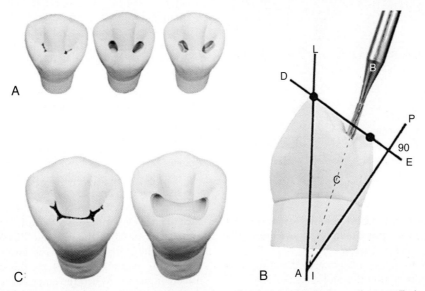

• **Fig. 10.43**   A, Preparation design and restoration of carious occlusal pits on the mandibular first premolar. B, Bur tilt for entry. The cutting instrument is held such that its long axis *(broken line, CI)* is parallel with the bisector *(B)* of the angle formed by the long axis of the tooth *(LA)* and the line *(P)* that is perpendicular to the plane *(DE)* drawn through the facial and lingual cusp points. This dotted line *(CI)* is the bur position for entry. C, Conventional outline, including occlusal pits and central fissure.

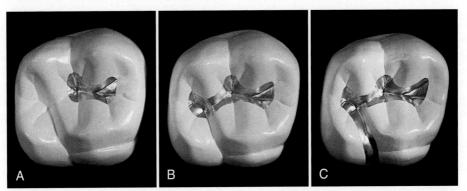

• **Fig. 10.44**   Maxillary first molar. A, Outline necessary to include the carious mesial and central pits connected by the fissure. B, Preparation outline extended from outline in *A* to include distal pit and connecting deep fissure in oblique ridge. C, Preparation outline extended from outline in *B* to include distal oblique and lingual fissures.

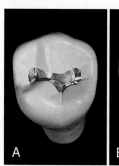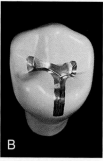

• **Fig. 10.45** Mandibular second premolar. A, Typical occlusal outline. B, Extension through the lingual ridge enamel is necessary when enameloplasty does not eliminate the lingual fissure.

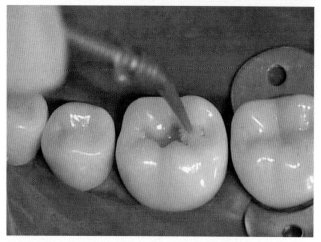

• **Fig. 10.46** Use of microbrush to apply the dentin desensitizer in the tooth preparation. (Courtesy Aldridge D. Wilder, DDS.)

utilized to refine the anatomy and leave a smooth, satin finish. All shavings from the carving procedure should be removed from the mouth with the aid of the oral evacuator.

The occlusion on the restoration is then evaluated and adjusted so that all markings on the restoration and adjacent teeth are uniform (see Fig. 10.23).

Extensive caries lesions require a more extensive restoration (which is a clear indication for amalgam as compared with composite resin). Use of amalgam in large Class I restorations provides good wear resistance and stable occlusal contact relationships. For very large Class I restorations, a bonding system may be used, although this book does not promote such use. The perceived benefits of bonded amalgams have not been substantiated.[85,95-99] Bonded amalgams have no advantage as compared with the conventional technique described above. Carving the extensive Class I restoration is often more complex because more cuspal inclines are included in the preparation. Appropriate contours, occlusal contacts, and groove/fossa anatomy must be provided. Finishing and polishing indications and techniques are as described previously.

Tooth Preparation for Class I Occlusolingual and Occlusofacial Amalgam Restorations

Occlusolingual amalgam restorations may be used on maxillary molars when a lingual fissure connects with the distal oblique fissure and distal pit on the occlusal surface (Fig. 10.49). Composite may also be used as the restorative material in smaller lesions.

After local anesthesia and evaluation of the occlusal contacts, the use of a rubber dam is generally recommended for isolation of the operating field. Alternatively, typical Class I preparations may be adequately isolated with cotton rolls.

Tooth Preparation

The initial tooth preparation involves the establishment of the outline, primary resistance, and primary retention forms, as well as initial preparation depth. The accepted principles of the outline form (previously presented) should be observed with special attention to the following:

1. The tooth preparation should be no wider than necessary; ideally, the mesiodistal width of the lingual extension should not exceed 1 mm except for extension necessary to remove carious or undermined enamel or to include unusual fissuring.
2. When indicated, the tooth preparation should be more at the expense of the oblique ridge, rather than centering over the fissure (weakening the small distolingual cusp).
3. Especially on smaller teeth, the occlusal portion may have a slight distal tilt to conserve the dentin support of the distal marginal ridge (Fig. 10.50).
4. The margins should extend as little as possible onto the oblique ridge, distolingual cusp, and distal marginal ridge.

These objectives help conserve the dentinal support (i.e., strength of the tooth) and aid in establishing an enamel cavosurface angle as close to 90 degrees as possible (Fig. 10.51). They also help to minimize deterioration of the restoration margins by locating the margins away from enamel eminences where occlusal forces may be concentrated.

The distal pit is identified with indirect vision and entered with the end of the No. 245 bur (Fig. 10.52A). The long axis of the bur usually should be parallel to the long axis of the tooth crown. The dentinal support and strength of the distal marginal ridge and the distolingual cusp should be conserved by positioning the bur such that it cuts more of the tooth structure mesial to the pit rather than distal to the pit (e.g., 70:30 rather than 50:50), if needed. The initial cut is to the level of the DEJ (a depth of 1.5–2 mm) (see Fig. 10.52B). At this depth, the pulpal floor is usually in dentin. When the entry cut is made (see Fig. 10.52C), the bur (maintaining the initial established depth) is moved to include any remaining fissures facial to the point of entry (see Fig. 10.52D). The bur is then moved along the fissure toward the lingual surface (see Fig. 10.52E). As with Class I occlusal preparations, a slight distal inclination of the bur is indicated occasionally (particularly in smaller teeth) to conserve the dentinal support and strength of the marginal ridge and the distolingual cusp. To ensure adequate strength for the marginal ridge, the distopulpal line angle should not approach the distal surface of the tooth closer than 2 mm. On large molars, the bur position should remain parallel to the long axis of the tooth, particularly if the bur is offset slightly mesial to the center of the fissure. Keeping the bur parallel to the long axis of the tooth creates a distal wall with slight occlusal convergence, providing favorable enamel and amalgam angles. The bur is moved lingually along the fissure, maintaining a uniform depth until the preparation is extended onto the lingual surface (see Fig. 10.52F). The pulpal floor should follow the contour of the occlusal surface and the DEJ, which usually rises occlusally as the bur moves lingually.

The mesial and distal walls of the occlusal portion of the preparation should converge occlusally because of the shape of the

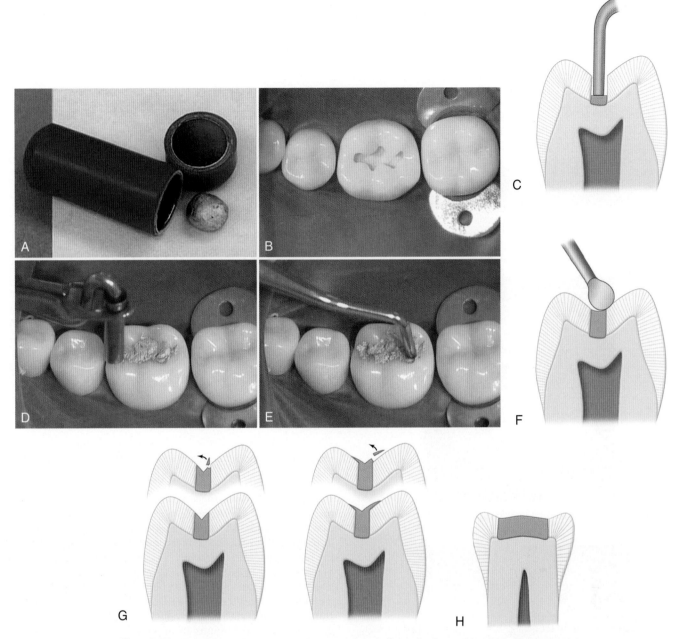

• **Fig. 10.47** *Restoration of occlusal tooth preparation. A, Properly triturated amalgam is a homoge-neous mass with slightly reflective surface. A properly mixed mass will flatten slightly if dropped on a tabletop. B, The operator should have a mental image of the outline form of the preparation before condensing amalgam to aid in locating the cavosurface margins during the carving procedure. C, Amalgam should be inserted incrementally and condensed with overlapping strokes. D and E, The tooth preparation should be overpacked to ensure well-condensed marginal amalgam that is not mercury rich. F, The carver should rest partially on the external tooth surface adjacent to the margins to prevent overcarving. G, Deep occlusal grooves invite chipping of amalgam at the margins. Thin portions of amalgam left on the external surfaces soon break away, giving the appearance that amalgam has grown out of the preparation. H, Carve fossae slightly deeper than the proximal marginal ridges. (A, From Darby ML, Walsh MM:* Dental hygiene: theory and practice, *ed 3, St. Louis, Saunders, 2010. B, D, and E, Courtesy Aldridge D. Wilder, DDS.)*

bur. If the slight distal bur tilt was required, the mesial and distal walls still should converge relative to each other (although the distal wall may be divergent occlusally, relative to the tooth's long axis). Convergence of the mesial and distal walls ensures occlusal retention form is adequate.

The lingual portion is prepared at this point by using one of two techniques. In one technique, the lingual surface is prepared with the bur's long axis parallel with the lingual surface (Fig. 10.53A and B). The tip of the bur should be located at the gingival extent of the lingual fissure. The bur should be controlled so that it does

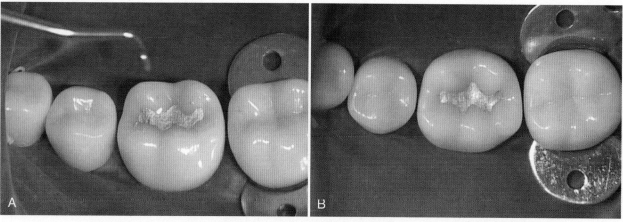

• **Fig. 10.48** A, Undercarved amalgam with flash beyond the margins. The restoration outline is irregular and larger than the preparation outline in Fig. 10.36B. B, Correctly carved amalgam restoration. (Courtesy Aldridge D. Wilder, DDS.)

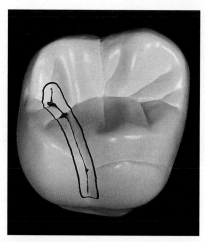

• **Fig. 10.49** Outline of margins for occlusolingual tooth preparation.

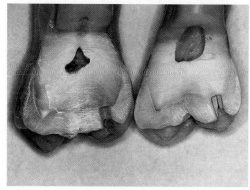

• **Fig. 10.50** Small distal inclination of the bur on smaller teeth may be indicated to conserve the dentinal support and the strength of the marginal ridge.

not "roll out" onto the lingual surface, which may "round over" or damage the cavosurface margin. The facial inclination of the bur must be altered as the cutting progresses to establish the axial wall of the lingual portion at a uniform depth of 0.5 mm inside the DEJ (see Fig. 10.53C). The axial wall should follow the contour of the lingual surface of the tooth with an axial depth of 0.2 mm inside the DEJ at the preparation periphery. When the caries lesion

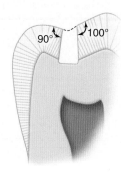

• **Fig. 10.51** Enamel cavosurface angles of 90 to 100 degrees are ideal.

affecting the lingual surface is wide mesiodistally, the resultant mesial and distal external walls may diverge to the lingual. In this case the amalgam will require retention grooves to prevent lingual displacement. An axial depth of 0.5 mm inside the DEJ is indicated if retentive grooves are required. A second, alternate approach to preparing the lingual aspect of the preparation may also be considered. In this case, the No. 245 bur is held perpendicular to the cusp ridge and then the lingual surface, as it extends the preparation from the occlusal surface gingivally (to include the entire defect). This technique also results in opposing preparation walls that converge lingually.

The No. 245 bur may be used with its long axis perpendicular to the axial wall to accentuate (i.e., refine) the mesioaxial and distoaxial line angles; this also results in the mesial and distal walls converging lingually because of the shape of the bur (see Fig. 10.53D and E). During this step, the axial wall depth is not altered (see Fig. 10.53F). The occlusal and lingual convergences usually provide a sufficient preparation retention form, and retention grooves are not needed.

The axiopulpal line angle must be rounded to limit the areas of stress concentration and ensure adequate preparation depth and amalgam thickness (Fig. 10.54). Initial tooth preparation of the occlusolingual preparation is now complete. As mentioned previously, enameloplasty may be performed to conserve the tooth structure and limit extension.

Additional retention in the lingual extension may be required if the extension is wide mesiodistally or if it was prepared without a lingual convergence. If additional retention is required, the No.

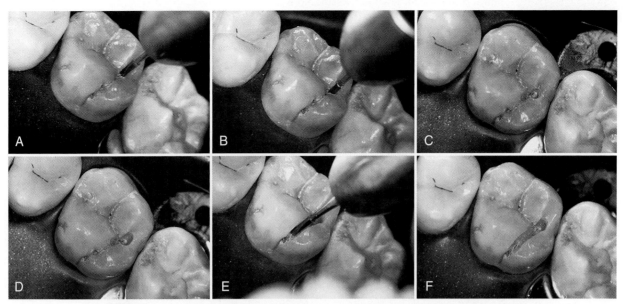

• **Fig. 10.52** Occlusolingual tooth preparation. A, No. 245 bur positioned for entry. B, Penetration to a minimal depth of 1.5 to 2 mm. C, Entry cut. D, The remaining fissures facial to the point of entry are removed with the same bur. E and F, A cut lingually along the fissure until the bur has extended the preparation onto the lingual surface.

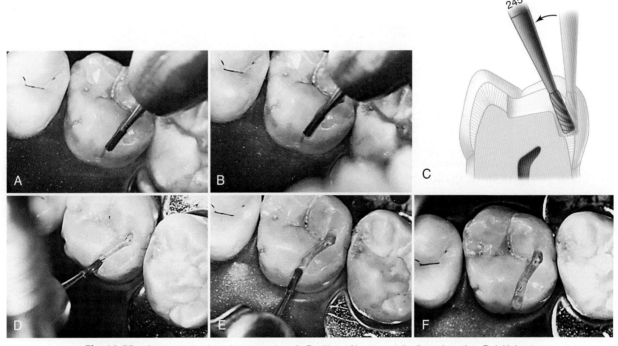

• **Fig. 10.53** Occlusolingual tooth preparation. A, Position of bur to cut the lingual portion. B, Initial entry of the bur for cutting the lingual portion. C, The inclination of the bur is altered to establish the correct axial wall depth. D and E, The bur is directed perpendicular to the axial wall to accentuate the mesioaxial and distoaxial line angles. F, The axial wall depth should be 0.2 to 0.5 mm inside the DEJ.

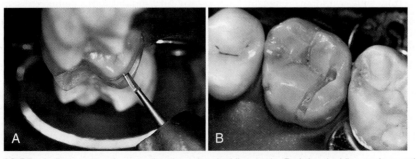

• **Fig. 10.54** A, Bur position for rounding the axiopulpal line angle. B, Axiopulpal line angle rounded.

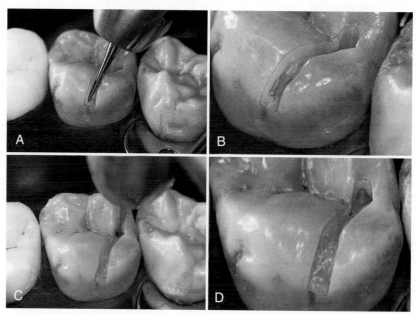

• **Fig. 10.55** Secondary retention form. A, Bur position for preparing groove in mesioaxial line angle. B, Completed groove is internal to the DEJ. C, Bur position for the retention cove in the faciopulpal line angle. D, Completed cove is internal to the DEJ.

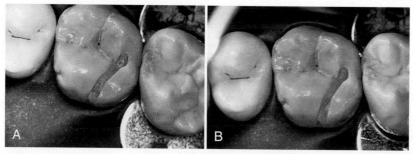

• **Fig. 10.56** A, Any remaining pit and fissure in enamel and soft dentin on established pulpal and axial walls are removed. B, Completed tooth preparation.

¼ or No. 169 bur may be used to prepare grooves into the mesioaxial and distoaxial line angles (Fig. 10.55A). If these angles are in enamel, the axial wall must be deepened to 0.5 mm axially of the DEJ to allow the grooves to be prepared in dentin and to not undermine enamel. The depth of the grooves at the gingival floor is one half the diameter of the No. ¼ bur. The cutting direction for each groove is the bisector of the respective line angle. The grooves are prepared in the mesioaxial and distoaxial line angles of the ideally positioned axial wall and 0.2 mm axial to the DEJ. The grooves should diminish in depth toward the occlusal surface, terminating midway along the axial wall (see Fig. 10.55B). The adequacy of the groove should be tested by inserting the tine of an explorer into the groove and detecting resistance to lingual movement. The depth of the groove should prevent the explorer from being withdrawn lingually. (See Secondary Resistance and Retention Forms for a description of placing retentive grooves in the proximal boxes of Class II amalgam preparations; the techniques are similar.)

Extension of a facial occlusal fissure may have required a slight divergence occlusally to the facial wall to conserve support of the facial ridge. If so, and if deemed necessary, the No. ¼ round bur may be used to prepare a retention cove in the faciopulpal line angle (see Fig. 10.55C and D). The tip of the No. 245 bur held parallel to the long axis of the tooth crown also might be used to prepare this cove. Care should be taken so as not to undermine the occlusal enamel. This retentive cove is recommended only if occlusal convergence of the mesial and distal walls of the occlusal portion is absent or inadequate.

The final tooth preparation is accomplished by removal of the remaining caries lesion on the pulpal and axial walls (Fig. 10.56) with an appropriate round bur, a discoid-type spoon excavator, or both. A RMGI is placed in areas of deep caries removal for pulpal protection. The external walls are finished. Any irregularities at the margins may indicate weak enamel that may be removed by the side of the No. 245 bur rotating at low speed. The preparation should then be cleaned, carefully inspected as indicated in General Concepts Guiding Preparation for Amalgam Restorations, and any final modifications completed.

Restorative Technique for Class I Occlusolingual or Occlusofacial Amalgam Preparations

Desensitizer Placement

A dentin desensitizer is placed over the prepared tooth structure and rinsed per manufacturer instructions. Excess moisture is removed using air stream without desiccating the dentin.

Matrix Placement (If Necessary)

Using a matrix to support the lingual portion of the restoration during condensation is occasionally necessary. A matrix is helpful to prevent "land sliding" during condensation and to ensure marginal adaptation and strength of the restoration. The Tofflemire matrix retainer is used to secure a matrix band to the tooth (as described later). Because this type of matrix band does not intimately adapt to the lingual groove area of the tooth (Fig. 10.57A), an additional step may be necessary to provide a matrix that is rigid on the lingual portion of the tooth preparation. If so, a piece of stainless steel matrix material (0.05 mm thick and 8 mm wide) is cut to fit between the lingual surface of the tooth and the band already in place (see Fig. 10.57B). The gingival edge of this segment of matrix material is placed slightly gingival to the gingival edge of the band to help secure the band segment. A quick-setting, rigid polyvinyl siloxane (PVS)–based material may be used between the sectional matrix and the Tofflemire matrix band, to prevent lingual displacement of the sectional matrix during condensation of the amalgam. Alternatively, green stick compound may be used. In

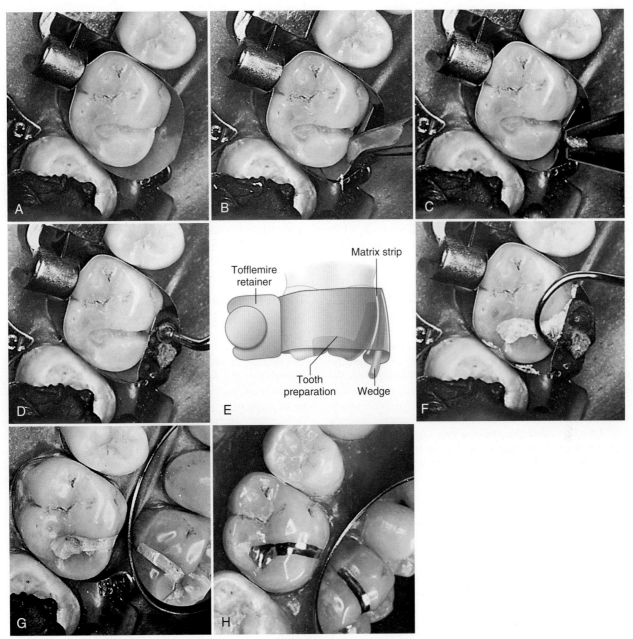

• **Fig. 10.57** Matrix for occlusolingual tooth preparation. A, Matrix band secured to the tooth with Tofflemire retainer. B, Positioning a small strip of stainless steel matrix material between the tooth and the band already in place. C, Inserting the wedge and the rigid supporting material. D, Compressing the rigid supporting material gingivally (or holding the steel strip in correct position while the material sets), which adapts the steel strip to the lingual surface. E, Cross section of the tooth preparation and the matrix construction. F, Using the explorer to remove excess amalgam adjacent to the lingual matrix. G, Carving completed. H, Polished restoration.

this case, the end of a toothpick wedge is covered with softened (heated) compound. The compound-coated wedge is then immediately inserted between the Tofflemire band and the cut piece of matrix material (see Fig. 10.57C). While the compound is still soft, a suitable burnisher is used to press the compound gingivally, securing the matrix tightly against the gingival cavosurface margin and the lingual surface of the tooth to provide a rigid, lingual matrix (see Fig. 10.57D and E). This matrix for the occlusolingual amalgam restoration is referred to as the *Barton matrix*. Occasionally the piece of strip matrix may be positioned appropriately by using only the wedge (without the rigid PVS or compound support).

Insertion of the Amalgam

Insertion of amalgam is accomplished as previously described in General Concepts Guiding Restoration with Amalgam and for the Class I occlusal tooth preparation. Condensation is begun at the gingival wall at the lingual component of the preparation. If a matrix is not used, care must be taken to ensure that "land sliding" of the amalgam does not occur because two adjoining surfaces of the tooth are being restored. For this technique, the last increments of amalgam may be condensed on the lingual surface with the side of a large condenser. Its long, broadly rounded contour approximates the rectangular shape of the lingual groove preparation. Appropriate care should be taken (when condensing the occlusal surface) to prevent fracturing the lingual amalgam. Another technique is to have the assistant secure the condensed lingual surface with a broad condenser nib, while the operator completes the condensation of the occlusal surface. Regardless of the technique used, the amalgam must be well condensed.

Contouring and Finishing of the Amalgam Restoration

When the preparation is sufficiently overfilled, carving of the occlusal surface may begin immediately with a sharp discoid-cleoid instrument or a Hollenback carver. All carving should be done with the edge of the blade perpendicular to the margin and the blade moving parallel to the margin. To prevent overcarving, the blade edge should be guided by the unprepared tooth surface adjacent to the margin. An explorer is used to remove excess amalgam adjacent to the lingual matrix before matrix removal (see Fig. 10.57F). After the occlusal carving is complete, the Tofflemire retainer is loosened from the band, and the band is removed with No. 110 pliers. The free ends of the band are pushed one at a time, lingually and occlusally, through the proximal contacts. After the lingual carving is complete (see Fig. 10.57G), the rubber dam is removed and the restoration is adjusted to ensure proper occlusion. Most amalgams do not require finishing and polishing. Fig. 10.57H illustrates a polished occlusolingual restoration.

Class I Occlusofacial Amalgam Restorations

Occasionally, mandibular molars exhibit fissures that extend from the occlusal surface through the facial cusp ridge and onto the facial surface. The preparation and restoration of these defects are very similar to those described for Class I occlusolingual amalgam restorations. Although these may be restored with composite, an illustration of preparation and restoration with amalgam is provided in Fig. 10.58. The amalgam restoration may be polished after it is completely set. The shape of abrasive points may need to be modified to allow optimal polishing (see Fig. 10.58I and J).

Clinical Technique for Class II Amalgam Restorations

Class II restorations restore defects that affect one or both of the proximal surfaces of posterior teeth (see Fig. 10.26B). Amalgam restorations that restore one or both of the proximal surfaces of the tooth may provide years of service to the patient when (1) the operating field is isolated, (2) the tooth preparation is correct, (3) the matrix is suitable, and (4) the restorative material is manipulated properly. Application of the principles discussed here will result in high-quality, durable Class II amalgam restorations.

Initial Clinical Procedures

Occlusal contacts should be marked with articulating paper before tooth preparation. A mental image of these contacts will serve as a guide in tooth preparation and restoration. Any opposing "plunging cusp" (that is not aligned well with the occlusal plane) or other sharply pointed cusp may need to be recontoured to reduce the risk of fracture of the new restoration. Before tooth preparation for amalgam, the placement of a rubber dam is generally recommended. It is especially beneficial when the caries lesion is extensive. If an existing defective restoration has rough proximal contacts, the restoration may be removed before rubber dam application. Soft dentin should be removed with the rubber dam in place, especially if pulpal exposure is a possibility. Insertion of an interproximal wedge or wedges is useful to depress and protect the rubber dam and underlying soft tissue, separate teeth slightly, and may serve as a guide to prevent gingival overextension of the proximal boxes.

Tooth Preparation for Class II Amalgam Restorations That Involve Only One Proximal Surface

This section introduces the principles and techniques of a Class II tooth preparation for an amalgam restoration involving a caries lesion on one proximal surface. A small, conservative mesiocclusal tooth preparation on the mandibular second premolar is presented to illustrate basic concepts. Composite may also be an acceptable restorative material for this preparation. Preoperative placement of a wedge ("pre-wedging") in the space adjacent to the proximal surface with the caries lesion will create space between the teeth. This lowers the risk of iatrogenic damage to the adjacent tooth during preparation.

Initial Tooth Preparation

Occlusal Outline Form (Occlusal Step)

The occlusal outline form of a Class II tooth preparation for amalgam is similar to that for a Class I tooth preparation. Using high speed with air-water spray, the operator enters the pit nearest the involved proximal surface with a punch cut using a No. 245 bur oriented as illustrated in Fig. 10.59A and B. The bur should be rotating when it is applied to the tooth and should not stop rotating until removed. Viewed from the proximal and lingual (facial) aspects, the long axis of the bur and the long axis of the tooth crown should remain parallel during the cutting procedures. The dentin caries lesion initially spreads at the DEJ; therefore the goal of the initial cut is to reach the DEJ. The DEJ location in posterior teeth is approximately 1.5 to 2.0 mm from the occlusal

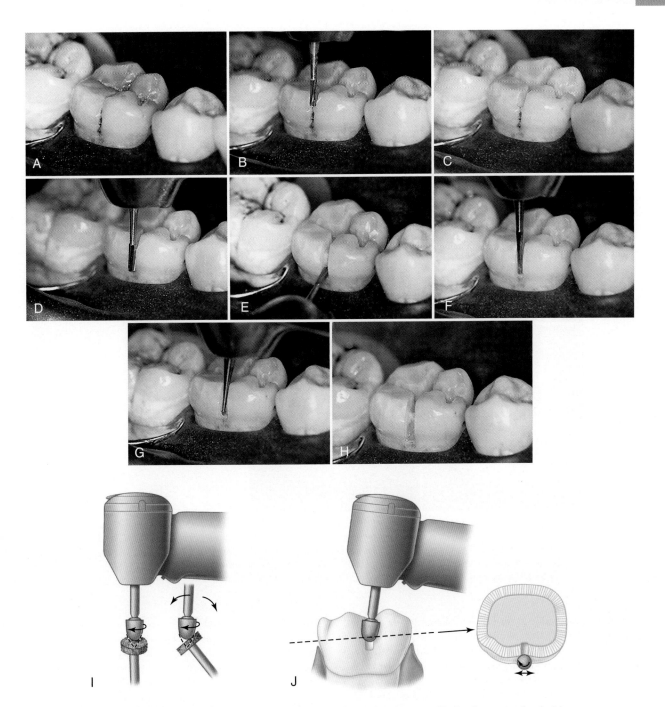

• **Fig. 10.58** Fissure extension. A, Facial occlusal fissure continuous with the fissure on the facial surface. B, Extension through the facial ridge onto the facial surface. C, Appearance of the tooth preparation after extension through the ridge. D, The facial surface portion of the extension is cut with the side of the bur. E, The line angles are sharpened by directing the bur from the facial aspect. F, Sharpening the line angles from the occlusal direction with a No. 169 L bur. G, Ensuring the retention form by preparing retention grooves with a No. ¼ round bur. H, Completed tooth preparation. I, The rubber polishing point may be reshaped (blunted as indicated) on a coarse diamond wheel. J, Proper orientation of the rubber point when polishing the facial surface groove area.

surface. As the bur enters the pit, a target depth of 0.1 to 0.2 mm into dentin (i.e., just into dentin) should be established. This depth is one half to two thirds the length of the cutting portion of a No. 245 bur, or approximately 1.5 mm as measured from the central fissure and 2 mm from the preparation external wall. While maintaining the same depth and bur orientation, the bur is moved to extend the outline to include the carious central fissure and the

opposite carious pit (see Fig. 10.59C and D). The isthmus width should be as narrow as possible, preferably no wider than one quarter the intercuspal distance.[54,55,100,101] Ideally the preparation should be the width of the No. 245 bur. Narrow restorations provide a greater length of clinical service.[57,60] Generally the amount of remaining tooth structure is more important to restoration longevity than is the restorative material used.[102] Ultimately, the

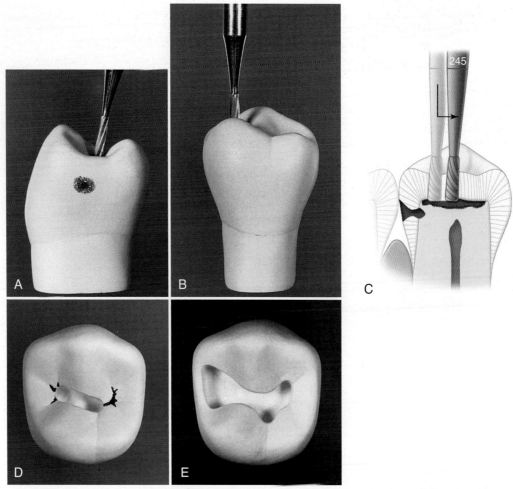

• **Fig. 10.59** Entry and occlusal step. A, Bur position for entry, as viewed proximally. Note the slight lingual tilt of the bur. B, Bur position as viewed lingually. C, The tooth is entered with a punch cut, and extension is done distally along central fissure at a uniform depth of 1.5 to 2 mm (1.5 mm at fissure; because of the inclination of the unprepared tooth surface, the corresponding measurement on the prepared wall is greater). D, Occlusal view of C. E, Completed occlusal step.

extension of the caries lesion at the DEJ will determine the amount of preparation extension and resultant width. The pulpal floor of the preparation should follow the slight rise and fall of the DEJ along the central fissure in teeth with prominent triangular ridges.

Maintaining the bur parallel to the long axis of the tooth crown creates facial, lingual, and distal walls with a slight occlusal convergence as well as external wall orientation favorable for amalgam use. The facial, lingual, and distal walls should be extended until a sound DEJ is reached. Proper extension will result in the formation of the peripheral seat, which aids in the primary resistance form. It may be necessary to tilt the bur to diverge occlusally at the distal wall if further distal extension would undermine the marginal ridge of its dentinal support. During development of the distal pit area of the preparation, extension to include any distofacial and distolingual developmental fissures radiating from the pit may be indicated. The distal pit area (in this example) provides a dovetail retention form, which will prevent mesial displacement of the completed Class II restoration. However, the dovetail feature is not required in the occlusal step of a single proximal surface preparation unless a fissure emanating from an occlusal pit indicates it. This type of retention form (i.e., form that provides resistance to mesial displacement of the restoration) also is provided by any

extension of the central fissure preparation that is not in a straight direction from pit to pit (see Fig. 10.59E). A dovetail outline form in the distal pit is not required if radiating fissures are not present.[103,104] Enameloplasty should be performed, where indicated, to conserve the tooth structure.

Before extending into the involved proximal marginal ridge (the mesial ridge, in this example), the final locations of the facial and lingual walls of the proximal box are estimated visually. Visual assessment prevents overextension of the occlusal outline form (i.e., occlusal step) where it joins the proximal outline form (i.e., proximal box). Fig. 10.60 illustrates visualization of the final location of the proximoocclusal margins before preparing the proximal box. Showing the view from the occlusal aspect, Fig. 10.61 illustrates a reverse curve in the occlusal outline of a Class II preparation, which often results when developing the mesiofacial wall perpendicular to the enamel rod direction while, at the same time, conserving as much of the facial cusp structure as possible.[101] The extension into the mesiofacial cusp is limited to that amount required to permit a 90-degree mesiofacial margin. Lingually, the reverse curve usually is minimal (if necessary at all) because of the relationship of the central fissure relative to the faciolingual position of the proximal contact.

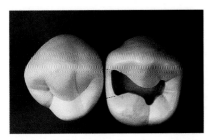

• **Fig. 10.60** Visualize final location of proximoocclusal margins *(dotted lines)* before preparing the proximal box.

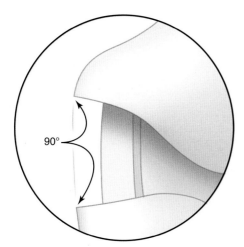

• **Fig. 10.61** The reverse curve in the occlusal outline usually is created when the mesiofacial enamel wall is parallel to the enamel rod direction. Lingually, the reverse curve is very slight, often unnecessary.

While maintaining the established pulpal depth and with the bur parallel to the long axis of the tooth crown, the preparation is extended mesially, stopping approximately 0.8 mm short of cutting through the marginal ridge into the contact area. The occlusal step in this region is made slightly wider faciolingually than in the Class I preparation because additional width is necessary for the proximal box. The proper depth of the occlusal portion of the preparation increases the strength of the restoration however, more than does faciolingual width (see Fig. 10.59C and E). Although this extension includes part of the mesial marginal ridge, it also exposes the marginal ridge DEJ. The location of the DEJ is an important guide in the development of the proximal preparation.

Proximal Outline Form (the Proximal "Box")

Before initiating the proximal outline form (i.e., the proximal "box"), the operator should visualize the desired final location of the facial and lingual walls relative to the contact. The objectives for the extension of the proximal margins are to (1) include all caries lesion, defects, or existing restorative material; (2) create approximately 90-degree cavosurface margins (i.e., butt-joint margins); and (3) establish (ideally) not more than 0.5-mm clearance with the adjacent proximal surface facially, lingually, and gingivally.

The initial procedure in preparing the outline form of the proximal box is the isolation of the proximal (i.e., in this case, mesial) enamel by the proximal ditch cut. While maintaining the same orientation of the bur, it is positioned over the DEJ in the pulpal floor next to the remaining mesial marginal ridge (Fig.

10.62A). The end of the bur is allowed to cut a ditch gingivally along the exposed proximal DEJ, two thirds at the expense of enamel and one third at the expense of dentin. The 0.8-mm-diameter bur end cuts approximately 0.5 to 0.6 mm into enamel and 0.2 to 0.3 mm into dentin. Pressure is directed gingivally and lightly toward the mesial surface to keep the bur against the proximal enamel, while the bur is moved facially and lingually along the DEJ. The ditch is extended gingivally just beyond the caries lesion or the proximal contact, whichever is greater (see Fig. 10.62B). Axial wall dentinal depths will vary based on the gingival extension of the preparation (see Fig. 10.62C). The axial wall follows the faciolingual contour of the proximal surface and the DEJ (see Fig. 10.62D).

It is necessary to visualize the completed mesiofacial and mesiolingual margins as right-angle projections of the facial and lingual limits of the ditch to establish the proper faciolingual ditch extension (see Fig. 10.62E). When preparing a tooth with a small lesion, these margins may clear the adjacent tooth by only 0.2 to 0.3 mm.[101] A guide for the gingival extension is the visualization that the finished gingival margin will be only slightly gingival to the gingival limit of the ditch. This gingival margin will likely clear the adjacent tooth by only 0.5 mm when treating an early cavitated proximal lesion (see Fig. 10.62F).[103] Recall that the caries lesion develops immediately gingival to the proximal contact and therefore the preparation will always result in gingival clearance, and that the amount of clearance will depend on the size of the caries lesion. Clearance of the proximal margins (i.e., mesiofacial, mesiolingual, gingival) greater than 0.5 mm is excessive, unless indicated to include the caries lesion, undermined enamel, or existing restorative material. The location of the final proximal margins (i.e., facial, lingual, gingival) should be established with hand instruments (i.e., chisels, hatchets, trimmers) and not the No. 245 bur, so as to prevent unnecessary overextension (see Fig. 10.62E). Extending gingival margins into the gingival sulcus should be avoided, where possible, because subgingival margins are more difficult to restore and may be a contributing factor to periodontal disease.[105-107]

The depth of the axial dentinal wall should be adjusted to approximately 0.5 mm if retention grooves are deemed necessary (i.e., if caries lesion removal requires placement/orientation of facial and lingual walls that are very divergent). This will allow the grooves to be prepared into the axiolingual and axiofacial line angles without undermining the proximal wall enamel. If the proximal ditch cut is entirely in dentin, the initial axial wall is too deep. Because the proximal enamel becomes thinner from the occlusal to the gingival aspect, the end of the bur comes closer to the external tooth surface as the cutting progresses gingivally (see Fig. 10.62B, C, and I). Premolars may have proximal boxes that are shallower pulpally than are molars because premolars typically have thinner enamel. In the tooth crown, the ideal dentinal depth of the axial wall of the proximal boxes of premolars and molars should be the same (two thirds to three fourths the diameter of the No. 245 bur [or 0.5–0.6 mm]).[101] When the extension places the gingival margin in cementum, the initial pulpal depth of the axiogingival line angle should be 0.7 to 0.8 mm (the diameter of the tip end of the No. 245 bur is 0.8 mm). The bur may shave the side of the wedge that is protecting the rubber dam and the underlying gingiva (see Fig. 10.62C).

The gingival extension of the proximal ditch may be measured by first noting the depth of the nonrotating bur in the ditch. The dentist removes the bur from the preparation and holds it in the facial embrasure at the same level to observe the relationship of

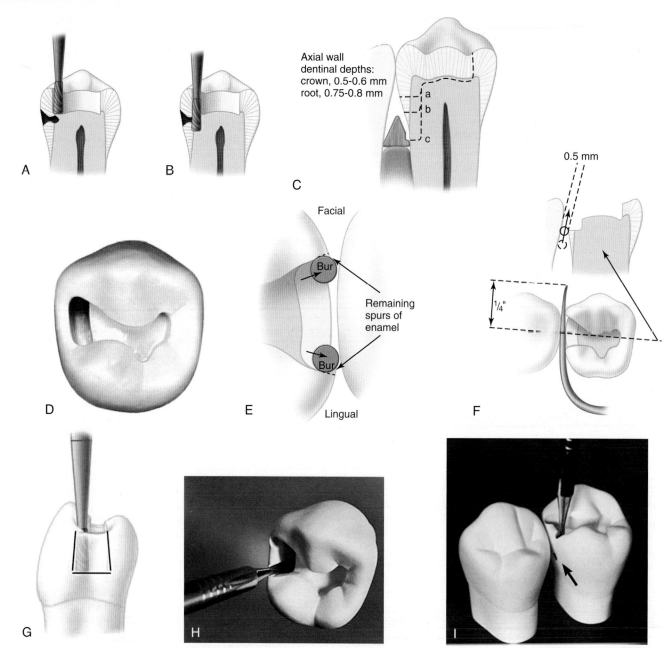

Axial wall dentinal depths: crown, 0.5-0.6 mm root, 0.75-0.8 mm

0.5 mm

Facial

Bur

Remaining spurs of enamel

Bur

Lingual

¼"

• **Fig. 10.62** Isolation of proximal enamel. A, Bur position to begin the proximal ditch cut. B, The proximal ditch is extended gingivally to the desired level of the gingival wall (i.e., floor). C, Variance in the pulpal depth of the axiogingival line angle as the extension of the gingival wall varies: *(a)* at minimal gingival extension; *(b)* at moderate extension; *(c)* at extension that places gingival margin in cementum, whereupon the pulpal depth is 0.75 to 0.8 mm and the bur may shave the side of wedge. D, The proximal ditch cut results in the axial wall that follows the outside contour of the proximal surface. E, The position of the proximal walls (i.e., facial, lingual, gingival) should not be overextended with the No. 245 bur, considering additional extension will occur when the remaining spurs of enamel are removed. F, When a small lesion is prepared, the gingival margin should clear the adjacent tooth by only 0.5 mm. This clearance may be measured with the side of the explorer. The diameter of the tine of a No. 23 explorer is ~0.5 mm at 6 mm from its tip. G, The faciolingual dimension of the proximal ditch is greater at the gingival level than at the occlusal level to provide occlusal convergence of the facial and lingual proximal box walls. H, To isolate and weaken the proximal enamel further, the bur is moved toward and perpendicular to the proximal surface. I, The side of the bur may emerge slightly through the proximal surface at the level of the gingival floor *(arrow)*.

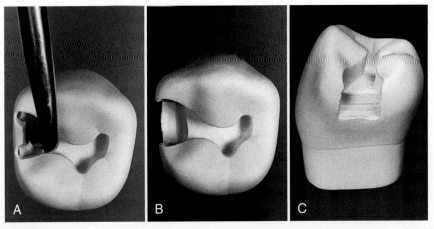

• **Fig. 10.63**   Removing isolated enamel. A, Using a spoon excavator to fracture the weakened proximal enamel. B, Occlusal view with the proximal enamel removed. C, Proximal view with the proximal enamel removed.

the end of the bur to the proximal contact. A periodontal probe also may be used.

The proximal ditch cut may diverge gingivally (i.e., converge occlusally) to ensure that the faciolingual dimension at the gingival aspect is greater than at the occlusal aspect (see Fig. 10.62G). The shape of the No. 245 bur will provide this divergence. The gingival divergence contributes to the retention form and provides for the desirable extension of the facial and lingual proximal margins to include defective tooth structure or old restorative material at the gingival level, while conserving the marginal ridge and providing for 90-degree amalgam at the margins on this ridge.[55]

Occasionally it is permissible not to extend the outline of the proximal box facially or lingually beyond the proximal contact to conserve the tooth structure.[103] An example of this modification is a narrow proximal lesion where broad proximal contact is present in a patient with low risk for caries. If it is necessary to extend 1 mm or more just to arbitrarily create clearance (i.e., to "break the contact"), the proximal margin is left in contact with the adjacent proximal surface. It is usually the facial margins that remain in contact as proximal caries lesions tend to develop slightly more toward the lingual.

The proximal extensions are completed when two cuts, one starting at the facial limit of the proximal ditch and the other starting at the lingual limit, extending toward and perpendicular to the proximal surface (until the bur is nearly through enamel at the contact level), are made (see Fig. 10.62H). The side of the bur may emerge slightly through the surface at the level of the gingival floor (see Fig. 10.62I); this weakens the remaining enamel by which the isolated portion is held. If this level is judged to be insufficiently gingival, additional gingival extension should be accomplished using the isolated proximal enamel, that is still in place, as a mental barrier to help the operator guide the bur. Ensuring the presence of the proximal enamel surface helps to limit the likelihood of iatrogenically damaging the proximal surface of the adjacent tooth. At this stage, however, the remaining wall of enamel often breaks away during cutting, especially when high speed is used. At such times, if additional use of the bur is indicated, a matrix band may be used around the adjacent tooth to limit potential marring of its proximal surface; however, the relative amount of protection afforded by the metal matrix material is very limited and serves more as a visual guide than an actual physical barrier. A No. 245 bur, rotating between 200,000 and 400,000 rpm,

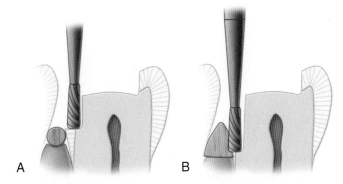

• **Fig. 10.64**   Wedging. A, A round toothpick wedge placed in the gingival embrasure protects the gingiva and the rubber dam during preparation of the proximal box. B, A triangular wedge is indicated when a deep gingival extension of the proximal box is anticipated because the wedge's greatest cross-sectional dimension is at its base. Consequently it more readily engages the remaining clinical tooth surface. Wedging increases the interproximal space and limits the potential for iatrogenic damage of adjacent tooth (or restoration) surfaces.

will rapidly cut through any matrix material and damage the adjacent proximal surface. The isolated enamel, if still in place, may be fractured with a spoon excavator (Fig. 10.63) or by mesial movement with the side of the nonrotating bur.

To protect the gingiva and the rubber dam when extending the gingival wall apically, a wooden wedge should already be in place in the gingival embrasure to depress soft tissue and the rubber dam.[55] A round toothpick wedge is preferred unless a deep gingival extension is anticipated (Fig. 10.64A). A triangular (i.e., anatomic) wedge is more appropriate for deep gingival extensions because the greatest cross-sectional dimension of the wedge is at its base; as the gingival wall is cut, the bur's end corner may shave the wedge slightly (see Fig. 10.64B). With a sharp enamel hatchet (10-7-14), bin-angle chisel (12-7-8), or both, the dentist cleaves away any remaining undermined proximal enamel (Fig. 10.65), establishing the proper orientation of the mesiolingual and mesiofacial walls. Proximal walls that result in cavosurface angles of 90 degrees are desired.[55] Cavosurface angles of 90 degrees ensure that no undermined enamel rods remain on the proximal margins and

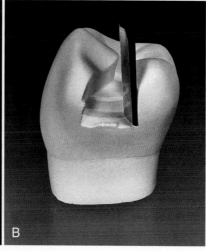
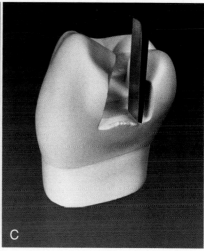

• **Fig. 10.65** Removing the remaining undermined proximal enamel with an enamel hatchet on the facial proximal wall (A), the lingual proximal wall (B), and the gingival wall (C).

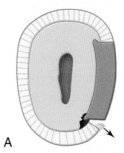
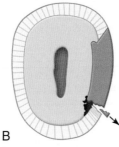
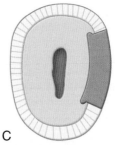

• **Fig. 10.66** Direction of mesiofacial and mesiolingual walls. A, Failure caused by a weak enamel margin. B, Failure caused by a weak amalgam margin. C, Proper direction to the proximal walls results in full-length enamel rods and 90-degree amalgam at the preparation margin. Retention grooves have been cut 0.2 mm inside the DEJ, and their direction of depth is parallel to the DEJ.

that the maximal edge strength of amalgam is maintained. The cutting edge of the instrument should not be aggressively forced against the gingival wall because this may cause a craze line (i.e., fracture) that extends gingivally in enamel, perhaps to the cervical line. Fig. 10.66 shows the importance of the correct direction of the mesiofacial and mesiolingual walls, dictated by enamel rod direction and the physical properties of amalgam. If hand instruments were not used to remove the remaining spurs of enamel, the proximal margins would have undermined enamel. To create 90-degree facial and lingual proximal margins with the No. 245 bur, the proximal margins would have to be significantly overextended for an otherwise conservative preparation. The weakened enamel along the gingival wall is removed by using the enamel hatchet in a scraping motion (see Fig. 10.65C).

When the isolation of the proximal enamel has been executed properly, the proximal box may be completed easily with hand-cutting instruments. Otherwise more cutting with rotary instruments is indicated. When a rotary instrument is used in a proximal box after the proximal enamel is removed, there is increased risk that the instrument may either mar the adjacent proximal surface or "crawl out" of the box into the gingiva or across the proximal margins. The latter mishap produces a rounded cavosurface angle, which results in a weak amalgam margin of less than 90 degrees if not corrected. The risk of this occurring is markedly reduced when high-speed operation is used. When finishing enamel margins

by using a rotary instrument, intermittent application of the bur along with air coolant alone (i.e., no water spray) is used to improve visualization and precision.

The primary resistance form is provided by (1) the pulpal and gingival walls being relatively level (i.e., perpendicular to forces directed along the long axis of the tooth); (2) restricting the extension of the walls to allow sufficient dentin support to remain (and therefore strong cusps and ridge areas) while at the same time establishing the peripheral seat; (3) restricting the occlusal outline form (where possible) to areas receiving minimal occlusal contact;[57] (4) use of a reverse curve to optimize the strength of the amalgam and tooth structure at the junction of the occlusal step and proximal box; (5) slight rounding of the internal line angles to reduce stress concentration in the tooth structure (automatically created by bur design except for the axiopulpal line angle); and (6) providing enough thickness of the restorative material to prevent its flexure and resultant fracture from the forces of mastication. The primary retention form is provided by the occlusal convergence of the facial and lingual walls and by the dovetail design of the occlusal step, if present.

After completing the initial tooth preparation, the adjacent proximal surface should be evaluated. An adjacent proximal restoration may require recontouring to reestablish the normal anatomic convex shape; this may be done with abrasive finishing strips, disks, finishing burs, or a combination of these. Any iatrogenic damage that compromises the convex adjacent proximal surface should be corrected by recontouring or restoration.

Final Tooth Preparation

Removing enamel pit-and-fissure remnants and soft dentin on the pulpal wall in Class II preparations is accomplished in the same manner as in the Class I preparation. Soft dentin is removed with a slowly revolving round bur of appropriate size, a discoid-type spoon excavator, or both. In general, the caries lesion removal should stop when a hard or firm feel, with an explorer or small spoon excavator, is achieved; this often occurs before all of the stained or discolored dentin is removed. The exception to this is when using the selective caries removal protocol (see Chapter 2). Removing enamel pit-and-fissure remnants and carious dentin should not affect the resistance form. To achieve an enhanced resistance form, the occlusal step should have pulpal seats at the initial preparation depth, perpendicular to the long axis of the tooth in sound tooth structure and peripheral to the excavated area (Fig. 10.67). Carious dentin in the axial wall is removed with appropriate round burs, spoon excavators, or both so as to conserve as much tooth structure as possible (Fig. 10.68).

Any remaining old restorative material (including base and liner) may be left if no evidence of a recurrent caries lesion exists, if its periphery is intact, and if the tooth has been asymptomatic (assuming the pulp is vital). This concept is particularly important if removal of all remaining restorative material may increase the risk of pulpal exposure. Appropriate steps to protect the pulp

should be taken as indicated in General Concepts Guiding Preparation for Amalgam Restorations.

After completion of the minimal gingival extension (i.e., the gingivoaxial line angle is in sound dentin), a remnant of the enamel portion of a caries lesion may remain on the gingival floor (wall), seen in the form of a decalcified (i.e., white, chalky) or faulty area bordering the margin (Fig. 10.69). This situation dictates further extension of a part or all of the gingival floor to place it in sound tooth structure. Extension of the entire gingival wall to include a large caries lesion may place the gingival margin so deep that proper matrix application and wedging become extremely difficult. Fig. 10.70A illustrates an outline form that extends gingivally in the central portion of the gingival wall to include a caries lesion that is deep gingivally, although leaving the facial and lingual gingival corners at a more occlusal position. This partial extension of the gingival wall permits wedging of the matrix band where otherwise it may be difficult and damaging to soft tissue. In this instance, the gingival wedge may not tightly support a small portion of the band. Special care must be exercised by placing small amounts of amalgam in this area first and thoroughly condensing with light pressure. In addition, care is exercised in carving the restoration in this area to remove any excess that may have extruded gingivally during condensation.

Fig. 10.70B illustrates removal of a caries lesion facially and gingivally beyond the conventional margin position. Such minor variations from the ideal preparation form permit conservation of healthy tooth structure. A partial extension of a facial or lingual wall is permissible if (1) the entire wall is not weakened, (2) the

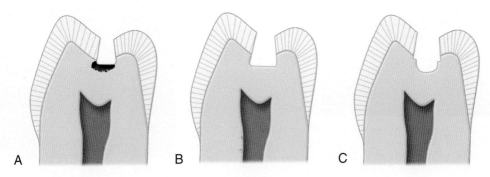

• **Fig. 10.67** Management of small- to moderate-sized caries lesion on the pulpal wall. A, Soft dentin extending beyond the ideal pulpal wall position. B, Incorrect lowering of the pulpal wall to include soft dentin. C, Correct extension facially and lingually beyond the soft dentin. Note the caries removal below the ideal pulpal wall level and the facial and lingual seats at the ideal pulpal wall level.

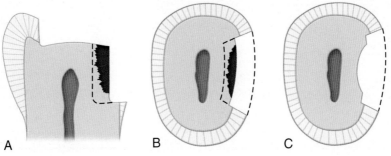

• **Fig. 10.68** Management of a moderate to extensive caries lesion. A and B, Soft dentin on the axial wall does not call for the preparation of the whole axial wall toward the pulp (dotted lines). C, Soft dentin extending pulpally from the ideal axial wall position is conservatively removed with a round bur.

extension remains accessible and visible, (3) sufficient gingival seats remain to support the restoration, and (4) a butt-joint fit at the amalgam–enamel margin (90-degree amalgam angle and 90-degree cavosurface angle) is possible.

Conserving as much tooth structure as possible by limiting the extensions of external walls helps to provide secondary resistance by limiting the risk of future tooth fracture from oblique forces. Ensuring that all internal line angles are rounded is necessary to limit areas of stress concentration in the remaining tooth structure and in the new restoration and improves secondary resistance of both. Use of the gingival margin trimmer or a bur to round the axiopulpal line angle (Fig. 10.71) helps to increase the bulk of restorative material and decrease the stress concentration within the restorative material.

The secondary retention forms for the occlusal and proximal portions of the preparation should be independent of each other. The occlusal convergence of the facial and lingual walls provide a sufficient retention form to the occlusal portion of the tooth preparation.

Proximal Retention Grooves

To enhance the retention form of the proximal portion, proximal grooves may be indicated to counter proximal displacement of the amalgam restoration.[55,108-110] The use of retention grooves in proximal boxes is controversial. It has been reported that proximal retention grooves in the axiofacial and axiolingual line angles may increase the fracture resistance and significantly strengthen the isthmus of a Class II amalgam restoration and that these grooves are significantly superior to the axiogingival grooves in increasing the restoration's fracture strength.[111-114] Other investigators have suggested, however, that retention grooves located occlusal to the axiopulpal line angle provide more resistance than do conventional grooves.[108] It also has been reported that proximal retention grooves are unnecessary in preparations that include dovetails, as part of the occlusal preparation, when high-copper amalgam is used.[109,115] Evidence suggests that retentive grooves may not be needed in conservative, narrow proximal boxes.[110] The use of retention grooves is recommended in tooth preparations with extensive proximal boxes. Generally the depth of the grooves should be approximately half of the diameter of the tip of the No. 169 or No. $\frac{1}{4}$ round bur (i.e., ~0.25–0.5 mm). The depth of retention grooves in extensively wide proximal boxes may need to be 0.5 mm or greater at the gingival aspect.

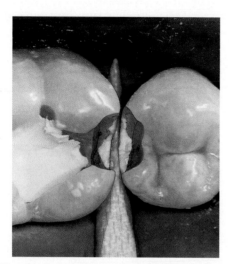

• **Fig. 10.69** Remnant of caries lesion bordering the enamel margin after insufficient gingival extension. Such a lesion indicates extending part or all of the gingival floor to place it in sound tooth structure. (Courtesy Dr. C. L. Sockwell.)

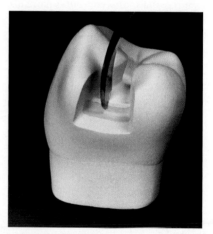

• **Fig. 10.71** Rounding the axiopulpal line angle.

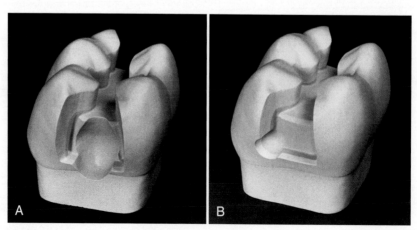

• **Fig. 10.70** A, Outline form that permits extension of the center portion of the gingival wall to facilitate proper matrix construction and wedging in situations where the caries lesion extends deep gingivally. B, Outline form that permits partial wall extension facially and gingivally to conserve the tooth structure.

Retention grooves are prepared with a No. 169 L or No. ¼ round bur with air coolant only (to improve visualization) and reduced speed (to improve tactile "feel" and control). The bur is placed in the properly positioned axiolingual line angle and directed (i.e., translated) to bisect the angle (Fig. 10.72) approximately parallel to the DEJ (Fig. 10.73). This positions the retention groove 0.2 mm inside the DEJ, maintaining the enamel support. The bur is tilted to allow cutting to the depth of the diameter of the end of the bur (which is initially positioned at the axiolinguogingival point angle) and to permit the groove to diminish in depth occlusally. The facial groove in the axiofacial line angle is prepared in a similar manner. When the axiofacial and axiolingual line angles are less than 2 mm in length, the tilt of the bur is reduced slightly so that the proximal grooves are extended occlusally to disappear midway between the DEJ and the enamel margin (see Fig. 10.72B and C).

The four characteristics or determinants of proximal grooves are (1) position, (2) translation, (3) depth, and (4) occlusogingival orientation (see Fig. 10.73). *Position* refers to the axiofacial and axiolingual line angles of initial tooth preparation (0.5 mm axial to the DEJ). *Translation* refers to the direction of movement of the axis of the bur. *Depth* refers to the extent of translation (i.e., depth of the retention groove). *Occlusogingival orientation* is considered when using the No. 169 L bur and refers to the tilt of

the bur. The tilt dictates the occlusal height of the groove, given a constant depth. When using the No. ¼ bur to prepare the proximal groove, the rotating bur is carried into the axiolinguogingival (or axiofaciogingival) point angle, then moved parallel to the DEJ to the depth of ~0.25 to 0.5 mm. It is then drawn occlusally along the axiolingual (or axiofacial) line angle, allowing the groove to become shallower and to terminate at the axiolinguopulpal (or axiofaciopulpal) point angle (or more occlusally if the line angles are <2 mm in length) (see Fig. 10.72D and E).

Regardless of the method used in placing the grooves, extreme care is necessary to prevent the removal of dentin that immediately supports the proximal enamel. In addition, it is essential that the grooves are not prepared entirely in the axial wall (i.e., incorrect translation [moving the bur only in an axial direction]) because groove placement in this area will not affect any resistance to proximal displacement of the amalgam (i.e., will not increase retention) and will increase the risk of iatrogenic pulpal involvement.

An improperly positioned axiofacial or axiolingual line angle must not be used as a positional guide for the proximal groove. If the axial line angle is too shallow, the groove may remove the necessary dentinal support of enamel. If the line angle is too deep, preparation of the groove may result in exposure of the pulp. *Retention grooves, when used, always should be placed 0.2 mm inside*

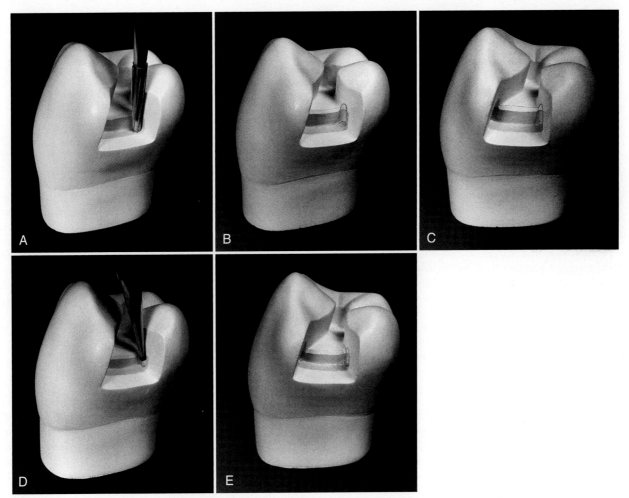

• **Fig. 10.72** Proximal retention grooves. A, Position of the No. 169 L bur to prepare the retention groove as the bur is moved lingually and pulpally. B, Lingual groove. Note the dentin support of the proximal enamel. C, Completed grooves. D, Grooves prepared with a No. ¼ round bur. E, Completed grooves.

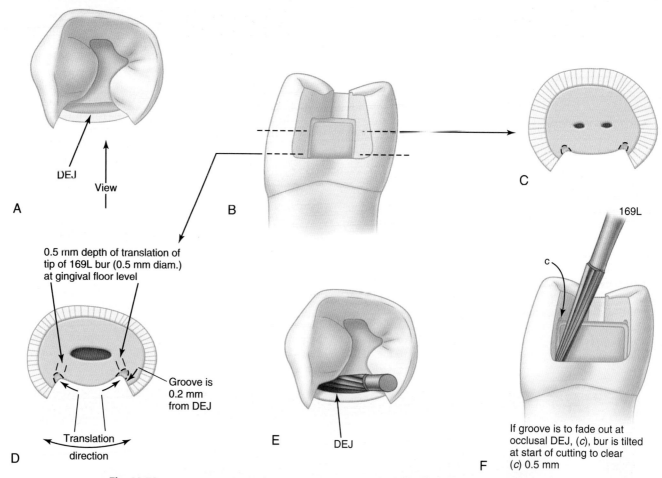

• **Fig. 10.73** Four characteristics of retentive grooves. A, Occlusal view of the mesioocclusal preparation before placement of the retention grooves. B, Proximal view of the mesioocclusal preparation. C and D, Position, translation, and depth. E and F, Occlusogingival orientation.

the DEJ of the facial and lingual proximal walls regardless of the depth of the axial wall and associated line angles.

Proximal Walls

The preparation walls and margins should not have unsupported enamel and marginal irregularities.[116] No occlusal cavosurface bevel is indicated in the tooth preparation for amalgam. Ideally, a 90-degree cavosurface angle (maximum of 100 degrees) should be present at the proximal margin. The occlusal line angle may be 90 to 100 degrees. This angle aids in obtaining a marginal amalgam angle of 90 degrees (≥80 degrees). Clinical experience has established that this "butt-joint" relationship of enamel and amalgam creates the strongest margin.[55] Amalgam is a brittle material and may fracture under occlusal load if its angle at the margin is less than 80 degrees.

A sharp mesial gingival margin trimmer (13-85-10-14, R and L) is used to remove unsupported gingival enamel by the establishment of a 90-degree gingival cavosurface angle at the gingival margin (Fig. 10.74). The resulting enamel gingival margin has a 6-centigrade (20-degree) gingival declination. The marginal configuration is angled no more than necessary to ensure that full-length enamel rods form the gingival margin and is no wider than the enamel (see Fig. 10.74). When the gingival margin is positioned gingival to the cementoenamel junction (CEJ) (i.e., on the tooth

root), the gingival cavosurface configuration is 90 degrees to the external surface of the root.[55] A sharp distal gingival margin trimmer (13-95-10-14, R and L) is similarly used for distal proximal preparations. Alternatively, the side of an explorer tine may be used to remove any friable enamel at the gingival margin. The tine is placed in the gingival embrasure apical to the gingival margin. With some pressure against the prepared tooth, the tine is moved occlusally across the gingival margin to "trim" the margin of friable, unsupported enamel.

Variations of Proximal Surface Tooth Preparations

This section describes variations in tooth preparation for some small Class II amalgam restorations. In most clinical situations, the restoration of these preparations would likely be with composite unless the patient has high caries risk. If amalgam is used, the features presented should be considered in the tooth preparation portion of the procedure.

Mandibular First Premolar

The technique of the Class II tooth preparation for amalgam for the mandibular first premolar must be modified because the

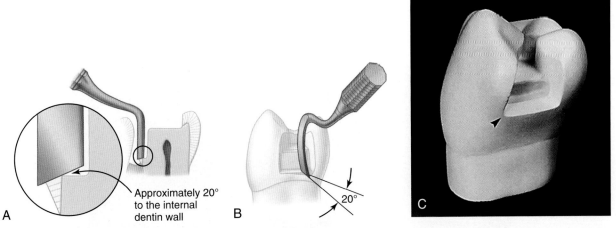

• **Fig. 10.74**   A, The marginal configuration of the enamel portion of the gingival wall is established with a gingival margin trimmer to ensure full-length enamel rods forming the gingival margin. B and C, The sharp angles at the linguogingival and faciogingival corners are rounded by rotational sweeping with a gingival margin trimmer.

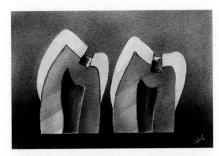

• **Fig. 10.75**   The mandibular first and second premolars are compared. Note differences in the sizes of the pulp chambers, lingual cusps, and direction of pulpal walls.

morphologic structure of this tooth is different from other posterior teeth. The relationship of the pulp chamber to the DEJ and the relatively small size of the lingual cusp are illustrated in Fig. 10.75. (This figure also illustrates the correct position of the pulpal wall and how it differs in position and orientation compared with the second premolar.) Incorrect preparation of the central groove area may weaken the lingual cusp, and excessive extension in a facial direction may approach or expose the facial pulp horn. When preparing the occlusal portion, the bur is tilted slightly lingually to establish the correct pulpal wall direction (see Fig. 10.43B).

The mandibular first premolar presents with unique occlusal morphology, most notably the presence of a large transverse ridge of enamel. Most often the coalescence of the enamel lobes is complete and no caries-prone central fissure results. Therefore a caries lesion in the mesial pit or distal pit may be included as part of the Class II preparation, but with an outline form that does not extend to or across the transverse ridge (Fig. 10.76A). The level of divergence of the facial and lingual proximal walls (see Fig. 10.76B) is such that secondary retention grooves are indicated (see Fig. 10.76C). If the opposite pit or proximal surface is faulty, it is restored with a separate restoration so as to not compromise the resistance form of the tooth.

For a preparation that does not cross the transverse ridge, the proximal box is prepared before the occlusal portion to prevent removing the tooth structure that will form the isthmus between the occlusal dovetail and the proximal box. The pit adjacent to the involved proximal surface is entered with the No. 245 bur. Immediately after the entry, the bur is directed into the proximal marginal ridge and then gingivally until the proximal DEJ is visible. The bur axis for the proximal ditch cut should be parallel to the tooth crown, which is tilted slightly lingually for mandibular posterior teeth (see Fig. 10.76C). The proximal enamel is isolated and the proximal box completed as previously described for the mandibular second premolar. The bur is then returned to the area of entry, and the occlusal step is prepared with a dovetail, if needed. When preparing the occlusal portion, the bur is tilted slightly lingual to establish the correct pulpal wall direction (which maintains the dentin support for the small lingual cusp and prevents encroachment on the facial pulp horn). The primary difference in tooth preparation on this tooth, compared with the preparation on other posterior teeth, is the facial inclination of the pulpal wall. The isthmus is broadened as necessary, but maintains the dovetail retention form. Fig. 10.76B illustrates the correct occlusal outline form. Removing any remaining caries lesion (if present) and inserting necessary liners, bases, or both precede the placement of proximal grooves and the finishing of the enamel margins (see Fig. 10.76C).

Maxillary First Molar

When mesial and distal proximal surface amalgam restorations are indicated on the maxillary first molar that has an unaffected oblique ridge, separate two-surface tooth preparations are indicated (rather than a mesioocclusodistal preparation). The use of two preparations is preferred because the strength of the tooth crown is significantly greater when the oblique ridge is intact.[55] The mesioocclusal tooth preparation is generally uncomplicated (Fig. 10.77A). Occasionally, extension through the oblique ridge and into the distal pit is necessary because of the extent of the caries lesion. The outline of the occlusolingual pit-and-fissure portion is similar to that of the Class I occlusolingual preparation. Fig. 10.77B and C illustrates a mesioocclusal preparation extended to include the distal pit and the outline form that includes the distal oblique and lingual fissures.

When the occlusal fissure extends into the facial cusp ridge and cannot be removed by enameloplasty, the defect should be eliminated by extension of the tooth preparation. Occasionally this may be accomplished by tilting the bur to create an occlusal divergence

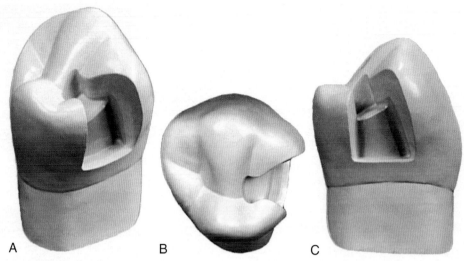

• **Fig. 10.76** The mandibular first premolar with a sound transverse ridge. A, A two-surface tooth preparation that does not include the opposite pit. B, Occlusal outline form. C, Proximal view of the completed preparation.

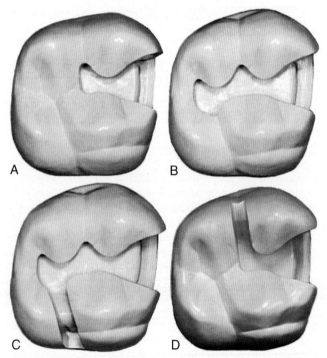

• **Fig. 10.77** Maxillary first molar. A, Conventional mesioocclusal preparation. B, Mesioocclusal preparation extended to include the distal pit. C, Mesioocclusolingual preparation, including the distal pit and the distal oblique and lingual fissures. D, Mesioocclusal preparation with facial fissure extension.

of the facial wall while maintaining the dentin support of the ridge. If it is not possible to eliminate this fault without extending the margin to the height of the cusp ridge or undermining the enamel margin, the preparation should be extended facially through the ridge (see Fig. 10.77D). The pulpal wall of this facial extension may have remaining enamel, but a depth of 1.5 to 2 mm is necessary to provide sufficient bulk of amalgam material for adequate strength (adequate resistance to flexure under load). For the best esthetic results, minimal extension of the proximal mesiofacial margin is indicated.

The distoocclusal tooth preparation may take one of several outlines, depending on the occlusal anatomy. The occlusal outline is determined by the pit-and-fissure pattern and by the amount and extension of the caries lesion. An extension onto the lingual surface to include a lingual fissure should be prepared only after the distolingual proximal margin is established. This approach may allow conservation of more tooth structure between the distolingual wall and the lingual fissure extension, resulting in more strength of the distolingual cusp. It is accomplished by preparing the lingual fissure extension more at the expense of the mesiolingual cusp than the distolingual cusp. Nevertheless, the distolingual cusp on many maxillary molars may be weakened during the distoocclusolingual tooth preparation because of the small cuspal portion remaining between the lingual fissure preparation and the distolingual proximal wall. In addition, removal of the caries lesion may reveal a weakened distolingual cusp. Reduction of the distolingual cusp and coverage with amalgam is often necessary to provide the proper resistance form (see the mesioocclusodistolingual [MODL] example in Clinical Technique for Complex Amalgam Restorations).

Maxillary First Premolar

A Class II amalgam tooth preparation involving the mesial surface of a maxillary first premolar requires special attention because the mesiofacial embrasure is esthetically prominent. The occlusogingival preparation of the facial wall of the mesial box should be parallel to the long axis of the tooth instead of converging occlusally to minimize an unesthetic display of amalgam in the faciogingival corner of the restoration. In addition, the facial extension of the mesiofacial proximal wall should be minimal so that the mesiofacial proximal margin of the preparation only minimally clears the contact as the margin is finished with an appropriate enamel hatchet or chisel (Fig. 10.78).

If the mesial proximal involvement (1) is limited to a fissure in the marginal ridge that is at risk for caries, (2) is not treatable by enameloplasty, and (3) does not involve the proximal contact, then the proximal portion of the tooth preparation is prepared by extending through the fault with the No. 245 bur so that the margins are lingual to the contact. Often this means that the proximal box is the faciolingual width of the bur, and the gingival

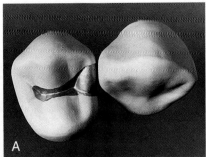
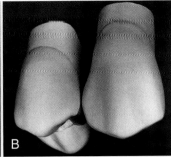

• **Fig. 10.78** To produce an inconspicuous margin on the maxillary first premolar, the mesiofacial wall does not diverge gingivally, and facial extension with a No. 245 bur should be minimal so that the mesiofacial proximal margin of the preparation minimally clears the contact as the margin is finished. A, Occlusal view. B, Facial view.

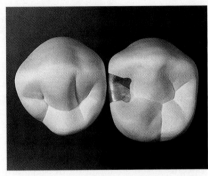

• **Fig. 10.79** A simple box restoration without the occlusal step is permissible when restoring a small proximal lesion in the tooth without either occlusal fissures or previously inserted occlusal restoration and when the involved marginal ridge does not support occlusal contact. The proximal grooves extend to the occlusal surface.

floor may be at the same depth as the pulpal floor. The retention form for this extension is provided by the slight occlusal convergence of the facial and lingual walls (see Fig. 10.34).

If the proximal caries lesion is limited to the mesiolingual embrasure, the mesial proximal contact should not be included in the tooth preparation. If only the lingual aspect of the mesial proximal contact is carious, the mesiofacial wall may be left in contact with the adjacent tooth (reducing the display of amalgam). A Class II tooth preparation involving the distal surface of the maxillary first premolar is similar to the preparation of the mandibular second premolar described earlier.

Box-Only Preparation

When restoring a small, cavitated proximal lesion in a tooth with neither occlusal fissures nor a previously inserted occlusal restoration, a proximal box preparation without an occlusal step has been recommended.[54,55] This preparation should be limited to a proximal surface with a narrow proximal contact (allowing minimal facial and lingual extensions) and a marginal ridge with no occlusal contact. To maximize retention, preparations with facial and lingual walls that almost oppose each other are recommended. As in the typical preparation, the facial and lingual proximal walls converge occlusally. Retention grooves are mandatory in box-only preparations.[117] The proximal retention grooves should have a 0.5-mm depth at the gingival point angle and extend occlusally to be visible in the occlusal outline form (Fig. 10.79).

Tooth Preparation for Class II Amalgam Restorations Involving Both Proximal Surfaces

Perhaps the best indications for the use of amalgam restorations are moderate and large Class II defects that include both proximal surfaces and much of the occlusal surface. This section describes factors to consider when amalgam is used for moderate and large Class II restorations. The tooth preparation techniques presented for a two-surface Class II restoration apply to larger Class II restorations as well. When the defect is large, however, certain modifications in tooth preparation may be necessary.

Occlusal Extensions

Larger Class II defects may require greater extension of the occlusal surface outline form. This may require extending into grooves that are fissured, extending the outline form up the cuspal inclines, or reducing and covering the cusps that have inadequate dentin support. These alterations may be accomplished easily by following the principles presented previously. The depth and extension of the initial preparation of fissures occur at the same initial pulpal floor depth (i.e., at the level of the DEJ) and follow the DEJ as the preparation is extended in a facial or lingual direction.

If an occlusal outline form extends up a cuspal incline, the extension also should maintain the pulpal floor at the level of the DEJ. This extension usually requires some alteration in the orientation of the No. 245 bur—a slight lingual tilt when extending in a facial direction and a slight facial tilt when extending in a lingual direction (see Fig. 10.35). Maintaining the correct pulpal floor depth preserves tooth structure and reduces the potential for pulpal encroachment. The prepared facial (or lingual) cavosurface margin still should result in a 90-degree amalgam margin. If it is necessary to extend through the cusp ridge onto the facial or lingual surface, the preparation is accomplished as described for the occlusolingual Class I restoration.

When the occlusal outline form extends from a primary fissure to within two thirds of the distance to a cusp tip, that cusp is usually sufficiently weakened so as to require reduction and coverage with the restoration. Leaving the cusp in a weakened state may be acceptable if the cusp is very large. Routine preparations in some teeth may predispose some cusps for reduction and coverage with amalgam. The small distal cusp of the mandibular first molars, the distolingual cusp of maxillary molars, and the lingual cusp of some mandibular premolars (especially first premolars) may be weakened when normal preparations of surrounding areas of the tooth are included. See the section Clinical Technique for Complex

Amalgam Restorations for information on when and how to reduce and cover cusps with amalgam.

Proximal Extensions

Larger Class II caries lesions often require larger proximal box preparations. These may include not only increased faciolingual or gingival extensions but also extension around a facial or lingual line angle. Large proximal box preparations may also need secondary retention features (i.e., retention grooves) for adequate retention form because the proximal external walls are excessively divergent. Extensive proximal boxes are usually prepared in the same fashion as more conservative proximal boxes but may require modifications. For increased faciolingual extensions, it may be necessary to tilt the No. 245 bur to include extensive proximal faults that are gingival to the contact area. Tilting the bur lingually when extending a facial proximal wall, or facially when extending a lingual proximal wall, conserves more of the marginal ridge and cuspal tooth structure. Although this action enhances preservation of some tooth structure strength, it results in a more occlusally convergent wall, which increases the difficulty of amalgam condensation in the gingival corners of the preparation.

When proximal extension around a line angle is necessary, it usually is associated with a reduction of the involved cusp (see Clinical Technique for Complex Amalgam Restorations). Such proximal extension is necessary because of a severely defective (or fractured) cusp or a cervical lesion that extends from the facial (or lingual) surface into the proximal area. Often these areas are included in the preparation by extending the gingival floor of the proximal box around the line angle, using the same criteria for preparation as the typical proximal box: (1) Facial (or lingual) extension results in an occlusogingival wall that has a 90-degree cavosurface margin, and (2) the axial depth is 0.5 mm inside the DEJ.

When the proximal defect is extensive gingivally, isolation of the area, tooth preparation, matrix placement, and condensation and carving of amalgam are more difficult. If the proximal box is extended onto the root surface, the axial wall depth is no longer dictated by the DEJ. Any root-surface preparation for amalgam should result in an initial axial wall depth of approximately 0.8 mm. This axial depth provides appropriate strength for amalgam, limits any potential pulp compromise, and creates enough dimension for the placement of ~0.25 to 0.5 mm deep retention grooves while preserving the strength of the adjacent, remaining marginal dentin and cementum. The extent of the preparation onto the root surface, the contour of the tooth, or both may require that the bur be tilted toward the adjacent tooth when preparing the gingival floor of the proximal box. This tilting may result in an axial wall that has two planes, the more gingival plane angled slightly internally. It also may cause more difficulty in retention groove placement. The more occlusal part of the axial wall may be overreduced if the bur is not tilted.

Examples of Moderate Class II Amalgam Tooth Preparations That Involve Both Proximal Surfaces

Mandibular Second Premolar

A moderate mesioocclusodistal tooth preparation in a mandibular second premolar is illustrated in Fig. 10.80. Note the similarity with the two-surface mesioocclusal preparation.

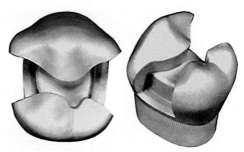

• **Fig. 10.80** Mesioocclusodistal (MOD) preparation on the mandibular second premolar that had a moderately sized MOD caries lesion.

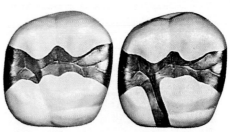

• **Fig. 10.81** Typical three- and four-surface restorations for the maxillary first molar. (See Fig. 10.167 for preparation of the distolingual cusp for coverage with amalgam.)

Mandibular First Premolar

When a mesioocclusodistal amalgam tooth preparation is needed for the mandibular first premolar, the support of the small lingual cusp may be conserved by preparing the occlusal step more at the expense of tooth structure facial to the central groove than lingual. In addition, the bur is tilted slightly lingually to establish the correct pulpal wall direction. Despite these precautions, the lingual cusp may need to be reduced for coverage with amalgam if the lingual margin of the occlusal step extends more than two thirds the distance from the central fissure to the cuspal eminence (see Clinical Technique for Complex Amalgam Restorations).

Maxillary First Molar

The mesioocclusodistal tooth preparation of the maxillary first molar may require extending through the oblique ridge to unite the proximal preparations with the occlusal step. Extending the preparation through the oblique ridge is indicated only if (1) the ridge is undermined by a caries lesion, (2) it is crossed by a deep fissure, or (3) occlusal portions of the separate mesioocclusal and distoocclusal outline forms leave less than 0.5 mm of the tooth structure between them. The remainder of the outline form is similar to the two-surface outline forms described previously in this chapter. Fig. 10.81 illustrates typical three-surface and four-surface restorations for this tooth.

Maxillary Second Molar With a Caries Lesion on the Distal Portion of the Facial Surface

Close examination of the distal portion of the facial surface of the maxillary second molar may reveal decalcification, cavitation, or both. When enamel is only slightly demineralized (i.e., softened and rough), polishing with sandpaper disks may eliminate the superficial fault. Careful brushing technique, daily use of fluoride (i.e., rinses, toothpaste), and periodic applications of a fluoride varnish may prevent further mineral loss. When decalcification is as deep as the DEJ and a distal proximal caries lesion is also present, however, the entire distofacial cusp may need to be reduced and included in a mesioocclusodistofacial tooth preparation. The facial lesion may be restored separately if it is judged that the distofacial cusp would not be significantly weakened if left unrestored by amalgam. In that case the mesioocclusodistal preparation would be restored first, followed by preparation and restoration of the facial lesion. When such sequential preparations are contraindicated, the preparation outline is extended gingivally to include the distofacial cusp (just beyond the caries lesion) and mesially to include the facial groove (Fig. 10.82). The No. 245 bur should be used to create a gingival floor (i.e., shoulder) perpendicular to the occlusal force when extending the distal gingival floor to include the affected facial surface. Inclusion of distofacial caries often indicates a gingival margin that follows the gingival tissue level. The width of the shoulder should be approximately 1 mm (or 0.5 mm inside the DEJ), whichever is greater. Some resistance form is provided by the shoulder. A retention groove should be placed in the axiofacial line angle of this distofacial extension, similar to the grooves placed in the proximal boxes. For additional retention a slot may be placed, as discussed in the section on Clinical Technique for Complex Amalgam Restorations.

Mandibular First Molar

The distal cusp on the mandibular first molar may be weakened when positioning the distofacial wall and margin. Facial extension of the distofacial margin to clear the distal contact often places the occlusal outline in the center of the cusp; this dictates relocation of the margin to provide a sound enamel wall and 90-degree amalgam that is not on a cuspal eminence. When the distal cusp is small or weakened or both, extension of the distal gingival floor and distofacial wall to include the distal cusp places the margin just mesial to the

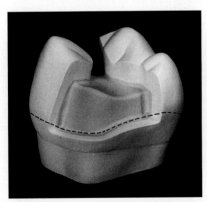

• **Fig. 10.82** Mesioocclusodistofacial preparation of the maxillary second molar showing extension to include moderate to extensive caries lesion in the distal half of the facial surface. The outline includes the distofacial cusp and the facial groove. The dotted line represents the soft tissue level.

distofacial groove. Fig. 10.83 illustrates the ideal distofacial extension and a preparation design that includes the distal cusp.

Modifications in Tooth Preparation for Proximal Surfaces

Slot Preparation for Root Caries

Older patients who have gingival recession that exposes cementum (or dentin) may experience caries lesion development on the proximal root surface that is appreciably gingival to the proximal contact (Fig. 10.84A). Assuming that the contact does not need restoring, the tooth preparation usually is approached from the facial direction and has the form of a slot (see Fig. 10.84B and E). A lingual approach is used when the caries is limited to the linguoproximal surface. Amalgam is particularly indicated for slot preparations if isolation is difficult.[5]

The initial outline form is prepared from a facial approach with a No. 2 or No. 4 bur using high speed and air-water spray. Outline form extension to sound tooth structure is at a limited depth axially (i.e., 0.75–1 mm at the gingival aspect [if no enamel is present], increasing to 1–1.25 mm at the occlusal wall [if the margin is in enamel]) (see Fig. 10.84B). If the occlusal margin is in enamel, the axial depth should be 0.5 mm inside the DEJ. During this extension, the bur should not remove any soft dentin from the axial wall deeper than the outline form initial depth. The remaining soft dentin (if any) is removed during final tooth preparation (see Fig. 10.84C). The external walls should form a 90-degree cavosurface angle. With a facial approach, the lingual wall should face facially as much as possible; this aids condensation of amalgam during insertion. The facial wall must be extended to provide access and visibility (convenience form) (see Fig. 10.84D). In the final tooth preparation, the No. 2 or No. 4 bur should be used to remove any remaining soft dentin on the axial wall. A liner or base (or both) is applied, as indicated.

A No. ¼ bur is used to create retention grooves in the occlusoaxial and gingivoaxial line angles, 0.2 mm inside the DEJ or 0.3 to 0.5 mm inside the cemental cavosurface margin (see Fig. 10.84D and E). The depth of these grooves is ~0.25 to 0.5 mm and the bur is directed to bisect the angle formed by the junction of the occlusal (or gingival) and axial walls. Ideally, the direction of the occlusal groove is slightly more occlusal than axial, and the direction of the gingival groove would be slightly more gingival than axial. A dentin desensitizer may be placed before or after application of the matrix. The matrix for the slot preparation is illustrated in Fig. 10.84F.

Rotated Teeth

Tooth preparation for rotated teeth follows the same principles as for normally aligned teeth. The outline form for a mesioocclusal tooth preparation on the rotated mandibular second premolar

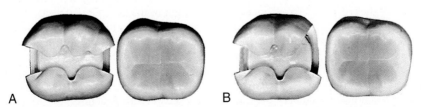

A   B

• **Fig. 10.83** Mandibular first molar. A, Ideal distofacial extension. B, Entire distal cusp included in preparation outline form.

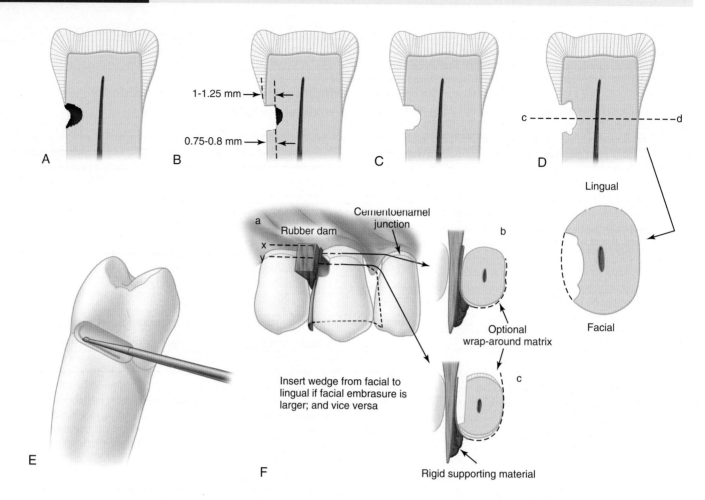

• **Fig. 10.84** Slot preparation. A, Mesiodistal longitudinal section illustrating a caries lesion. The proximal contact is not involved. B, Initial tooth preparation. C, Tooth preparation with soft carious dentin removed. D, The retention grooves are shown in longitudinal section, and the transverse section through plane *cd* illustrates the contour of the axial wall and the direction of the facial and lingual walls. E, Preparing the retention form to complete the tooth preparation. F, Matrix for slot preparation: *(a)* facial view of wedged matrix; *(b)* wedged matrix as viewed in transverse cross section *(x)*, gingival to gingival floor; *(c)* wedged matrix as viewed in transverse cross section *(y)*, occlusal to gingival floor.

(Fig. 10.85A) differs from normal in that its proximal box is displaced facially because the proximal caries lesion involves the mesiofacial line angle of the tooth crown. When the tooth is rotated 90 degrees and the "proximal" lesion is on the facial or lingual surface, and orthodontic correction is declined or ruled out, the preparation may require an isthmus that includes the cuspal eminence (see Fig. 10.85B). If the lesion is small, consideration should be given to slot preparation. In this instance, the occlusal margin may be in the contact area or slightly occlusal to it (see Fig. 10.85C).

Unusual Outline Forms

Outline forms should conform to the restoration requirements of the tooth and not to the classic example of a Class II tooth preparation. As mentioned earlier, a dovetail feature is not required in the occlusal step of a single proximal surface preparation unless a fissure emanating from the occlusal step is involved in the preparation. Another example is an occlusal fissure that is segmented by coalesced enamel (as illustrated previously for mandibular premolars and the maxillary first molars). This condition should be treated with individual amalgam restorations if the preparations are

separated by approximately 0.5 mm or more of sound tooth structure (Fig. 10.86).[54,104]

Adjoining Restorations

It is permissible to repair or replace a defective portion of an existing amalgam restoration if the remaining portion of the original restoration has adequate resistance and retention forms. Adjoining restorations on the occlusal surface occur more often in molars because the dovetail of the new restoration usually may be prepared without eliminating the dovetail of the existing restoration. Where the two restorations adjoin, care should be taken to ensure that the outline of the second restoration does not weaken the amalgam margin of the first (Fig. 10.87A). The intersecting margins of the two restorations should be at a 90-degree angle as much as possible. The decision to join two restorations is based on the assumption that the first restoration, or a part of it, does not need to be replaced and that the procedure for the single proximal restoration (compared with a mesioocclusodistal restoration) is less complicated and conserves tooth structure.

Occasionally, preparing an amalgam restoration in two or more phases is indicated, such as for a Class II lesion that is contiguous

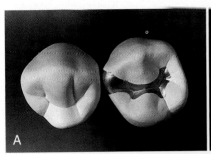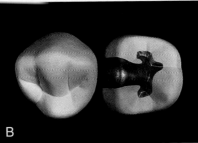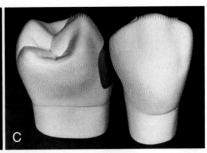

• **Fig. 10.85**   Restoration outlines for rotated teeth. A, Mesioocclusal outline for the mandibular premolar with 45-degree rotation. B, Mesioocclusal outline for the mandibular premolar with 90-degree rotation. C, Slot preparation outline for the restoration of a small mesial lesion involving the proximal contact of the mandibular premolar with 90-degree rotation.

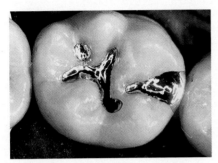

• **Fig. 10.86**   Restoration of the mesioocclusal tooth preparation, with the central fissure segmented by coalesced enamel.

with a Class V lesion. Preparing both lesions before placing amalgam introduces condensation problems that may be eliminated by preparing and restoring the Class II lesion before preparing and restoring the Class V lesion (see Fig. 10.87B). It is better to condense amalgam against a carious wall of the first preparation than to attempt condensation where no wall exists.

Abutment Teeth for a Removable Partial Denture

When the tooth is an abutment for a removable partial denture (RPD), the occlusoproximal outline form adjacent to the edentulous region may need additional extension if a rest seat is planned. Additional extension must be sufficient facially, lingually, and axially to allow for the rest seat to be in the proximoocclusal restoration without jeopardizing its strength. The facial and lingual proximal walls and the respective occlusal margins must be extended so that the entire rest seat may be prepared in the amalgam without encroaching on the restoration margins. If the rest seat is to be within the amalgam, it is recommended that a minimum of 0.5 mm of amalgam be present between the rest seat and the margins (Fig. 10.88A). The portion of the pulpal wall apical to the planned rest seat is deepened 0.5 mm so that the total depth of the axiopulpal line angle measured on the faciolingual wall is 2.5 mm (see Fig. 10.88B). A rest seat used for a tissue-borne (i.e., distal extension) partial denture may involve amalgam and enamel (see Fig. 10.88C). In this case, no modification of the outline form of the tooth preparation is indicated (see Fig. 10.88C). Note Fig. 10.88D illustrates the relationship of the tissue-borne RPD with the abutment tooth (see Fig. 10.88C).

All aspects of the Class II preparation, regardless of various levels of complexity, should be accomplished with precision. The preparation should then be cleaned, carefully inspected as indicated

in General Concepts Guiding Preparation for Amalgam Restorations, and any final modifications completed.

Restorative Technique for Class II Amalgam Preparations

Desensitizer Placement

A dentin desensitizer is placed on the prepared tooth structure per manufacturer instructions. Excess moisture is removed without desiccating the dentin.

Matrix Placement

The primary function of the matrix is to enable proper restoration of anatomic contours and contact areas. The qualities of a good matrix include (1) rigidity, (2) establishment of proper anatomic contour, (3) restoration of correct proximal contact relationships, (4) prevention of gingival excess, (5) convenient application, and (6) ease of removal. The following information presents the technique of placement for the universal (Tofflemire) and precontoured matrix systems.

Universal Matrix

The universal matrix system (designed by B.R. Tofflemire) is ideally indicated when three surfaces (i.e., mesial, occlusal, distal) of a posterior tooth have been prepared (Fig. 10.89). This system is also commonly used for the two-surface Class II restoration. A definite advantage of the Tofflemire matrix retainer is that it may be positioned on the facial or lingual aspect of the tooth. However, lingual positioning requires the contra-angled design of the retainer (which may be used on the facial aspect as well) (Fig. 10.90; also see Fig. 10.89). The retainer and the band are generally stable when in place. The retainer is separated easily from the band to expedite removal of the matrix system from the tooth. Matrix bands of various occlusogingival widths are available (see Fig. 10.89). A small Tofflemire retainer is available for use with the primary dentition.

The universal matrix band itself does not meet all the requirements of an ideal matrix band. The conventional, flat universal matrix band must be shaped (i.e., burnished) to reproduce natural anatomic contour and resultant proximal contact. Uncontoured bands are available in two thicknesses, 0.05 mm and 0.038 mm. Burnishing the thinner band to create contour is more difficult, and the band is less likely to retain its contour when tightened around the tooth. The uncontoured band must be burnished before assembling the matrix band and the retainer. Burnishing must

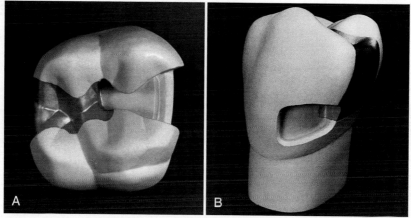

• **Fig. 10.87** Adjoining restorations. A, Adjoining mesioocclusal tooth preparation with distoocclusal restoration so that the new preparation does not weaken the amalgam margin of the existing restoration. B, Preparing and restoring a Class II lesion before preparing and restoring a Class V lesion contiguous with it eliminates condensation problems that occur when both lesions are prepared before either is restored.

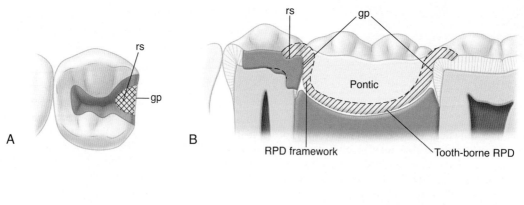

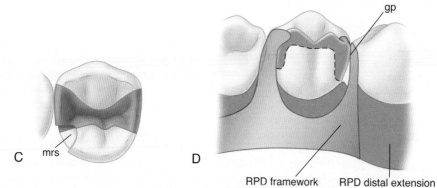

• **Fig. 10.88** Abutment teeth with Class II restorations designed for a removable partial denture (RPD). A, Occlusal view showing the location of the rest seat *(rs)* and the guide plane *(gp)* for a tooth-borne RPD. B, Cross-sectional view illustrating deepened pulpal wall in the area of the rest seat *(rs)* to provide adequate thickness of amalgam. Note the relationship of the guide planes *(gp)* to the tooth-borne RPD. C, Occlusal view showing the mesial rest seat *(mrs)* for the tissue-borne (i.e., distal extension) RPD prepared partly in a previous MOD amalgam restoration and partly in natural tooth structure. D, Lingual view of a distal extension RPD showing the relationship of the RPD to the Class II restoration and the guide plan *(gp)*. Note that the figure shows a M-D cross section through the MOD amalgam and the occlusal portion of the facial aspect of the distal marginal ridge is visible.

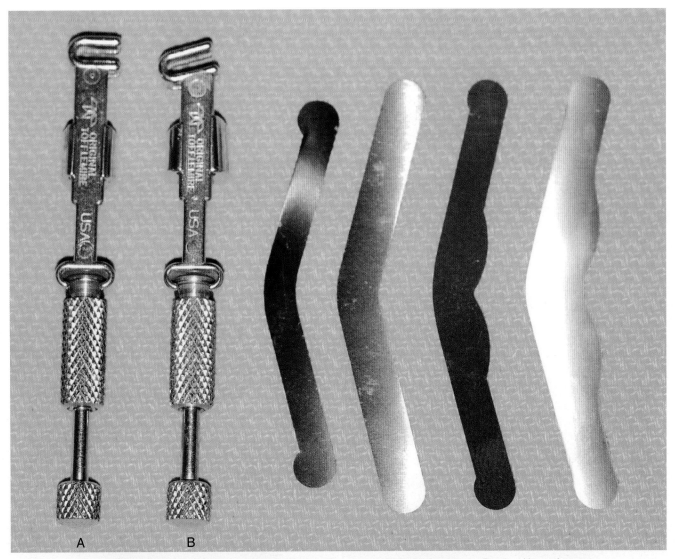

• **Fig. 10.89** Straight (A) and contra-angled (B) universal (Tofflemire) retainers. Bands with varying occlusogingival widths are available.

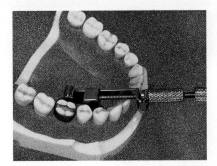

• **Fig. 10.90** Lingual positioning requires a contra-angled universal retainer.

occur in the areas corresponding to the proximal surface to be restored after the band is positioned around the tooth.

Precontoured bands for the universal retainer are commercially available and need little or no adjustment before being placed in the retainer or after being positioned around the tooth (Fig. 10.91). Although precontoured bands are more expensive, they generally are preferred over the uncontoured bands. The difference in cost

may be justified as less chair time is required during the restorative phase. When cotton roll isolation is used, the Tofflemire retainer helps hold the cotton roll in place (Fig. 10.92).

"Burnishing the matrix band" means that the metal band is intentionally deformed occlusogingivally with a suitable hand instrument to produce a rounded or convex surface that (when in place around the tooth) produces a restoration that is symmetric in contour with the adjacent proximal surface (Fig. 10.93). The No. 26-28 burnisher is generally recommended for burnishing the band. The band should be placed on a resilient paper pad because distortion of the metal matrix will not occur on a hard, nonresilient surface. The smaller round burnisher tip should first be used with firm pressure in back-and-forth, overlapping strokes along the length of the band until the band is deformed occlusogingivally in the appropriate areas. When the band is deformed, the larger egg-shaped end may be used to smooth the distorted band. If a convex surface is not obvious in the burnished areas when the band is removed from the pad, it has not been adequately burnished. The band may be burnished with the larger egg-shaped burnisher only, but more work is required to do so. It is not necessary to burnish the entire length of the band; focus effort only on distorting

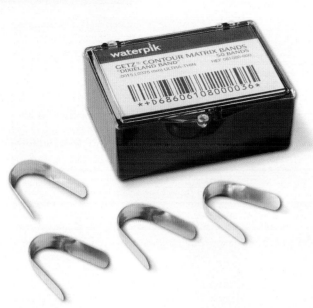

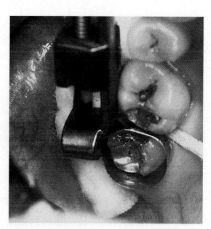

• **Fig. 10.92** Tofflemire retainer maintaining a cotton roll in the maxillary vestibule during condensation.

• **Fig. 10.91** Precontoured bands for a universal retainer. Pictured: Waterpik Getz Contour Matrix Bands. (Courtesy Water Pik Inc., Fort Collins, CO.)

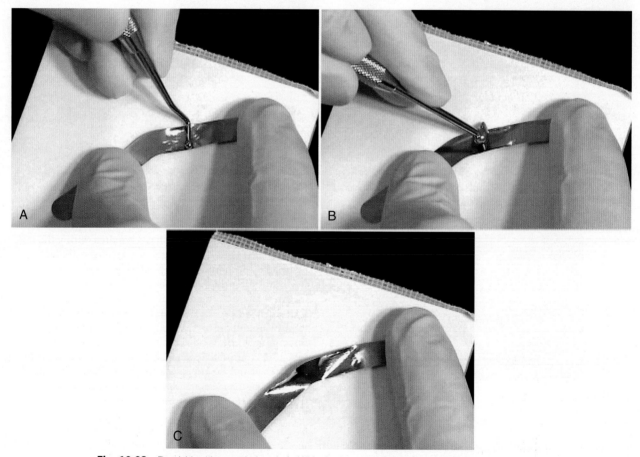

• **Fig. 10.93** Burnishing the matrix band. A, With the band on the pad, a small burnisher is used to deform the band. B, A large burnisher used to smooth the band contour. C, Burnished matrix band for mesioocclusodistal tooth preparation. (Courtesy Aldridge D. Wilder, DDS.)

the matrix where the proximal contact areas are planned to occur.

To prepare the retainer to receive the band, the larger of the knurled nuts is turned counterclockwise until the locking vise is positioned adjacent to the guide channel on the end of the retainer (Fig. 10.94A). Next, while holding the large nut, the dentist turns the smaller knurled nut counterclockwise until the pointed spindle is free of the slot in the locking vise (see Fig. 10.94B). The matrix band is folded end to end, forming a loop (see Fig. 10.94C). When the band is folded, the gingival edge has a smaller circumference as compared with the occlusal edge so as to accommodate the difference in tooth circumferences at the gingival and, the more occlusal, contact levels. The band is positioned in the retainer so that the slotted side of the retainer is directed gingivally to permit easy subsequent separation (in an occlusal direction) of the retainer from the band after the restoration has been inserted. This is accomplished by placing the occlusal edge of the band in the correct guide channel (i.e., right, left, or parallel to the long axis of the retainer), depending on the location of the tooth. The two ends of the band are placed in the slot of the locking vise so that the ends are aligned with the edge of the vise, and the smaller of the knurled nuts is turned clockwise to tighten the pointed spindle against the band within the locking vise (see Fig. 10.94D). If proximal wedges were used during tooth preparation, the wedges are removed at this point and the matrix band is fitted around the tooth (allowing the gingival edge of the band to be positioned at least 1 mm apical to the gingival margin). Damaging the gingival attachment with the sharp edge of the matrix band should be avoided. Care should be taken not to trap the rubber dam between the band and the gingival margin. If the dam material is trapped between the band and the tooth, the septum of the dam should be stretched and depressed gingivally to reposition the dam material. Once the matrix band is in place, the larger knurled nut is rotated clockwise to tighten the band slightly. The explorer should be used along the gingival margin to determine that the gingival edge of the band extends beyond the preparation margins. When the band is correctly positioned, the band is securely tightened around the tooth.

When one of the proximal margins is deeper gingivally, the Tofflemire mesioocclusodistal band may be modified to prevent damage to the gingival tissue or attachment on the more shallow side. The band may be trimmed for the shallow gingival margin, permitting the matrix to extend farther gingivally for the deeper gingival margin (Fig. 10.95).

The mouth mirror is positioned lingually to observe the proximal contours of the matrix through the interproximal space (Fig. 10.96). The occlusogingival contour should be convex, with the height of contour at proper contact level such that the metal band is touching the adjacent proximal surface in the precise location where the contact should occur. The matrix is also observed from an occlusal aspect allowing evaluation of the position of the contact area in a faciolingual direction. If proper proximal contour and contact is not observed, it may be necessary to remove the retainer and reburnish the band. Minor alterations in contour and contact may be accomplished without removal from the tooth. The backside of the blade of the 15-8-14 spoon excavator (i.e., Black spoon) is

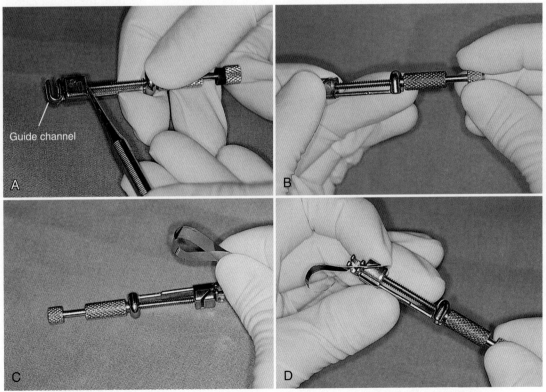

• **Fig. 10.94** Positioning the band in a universal retainer. A, Explorer pointing to the locking vise located immediately adjacent to the guide channel. B, The pointed spindle is released from the locking vise when the small knurled nut is turned counterclockwise. C, The band is folded to form a loop and to be positioned in the retainer (occlusal edge of band first). The gingival aspect of the vise is shown in this view. D, The spindle is tightened against the band in the locking vise. (From Daniel SJ, Harfst SA, Wilder RS: *Mosby's dental hygiene: Concepts, cases, and competencies,* ed 2, St. Louis, Mosby, 2008.)

excellent for improving contour in the area where the proximal contact is to occur. If a smaller burnishing instrument is used, the dentist should use care not to create a grooved or bumpy surface that would result in a restoration with an irregular proximal surface. Ideally the band should be positioned 1 mm apical to the gingival margin or deep enough to be engaged by the wedge (whichever is less) and 1 to 2 mm above the adjacent marginal ridge(s) to allow for adequate condensation of the amalgam in the marginal ridge areas. A minor modification of the matrix may be indicated for restoring the proximal surface that is planned for a guide plane for a RPD.

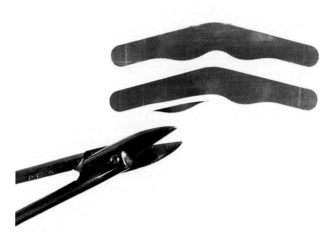

• **Fig. 10.95** The band may be trimmed for the shallower gingival margin, permitting the matrix to extend farther gingivally for the deeper gingival margin on the other proximal surface.

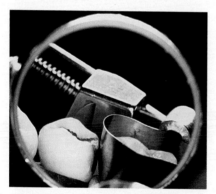

• **Fig. 10.96** Using a mirror from the facial or lingual position to evaluate the proximal contour of the matrix band.

After the matrix contour and extension are evaluated, a wedge is placed in the gingival embrasure(s) using the following technique: (1) Break off approximately 1.2 cm of a round toothpick; (2) grasp the broken end of the wedge with the No. 110 pliers; (3) insert the pointed tip from the lingual or facial embrasure (whichever is larger), slightly gingival to the gingival margin; and (4) wedge the band tightly against the tooth and margin (Fig. 10.97A). The wedge may be lightly moistened with water or a water-soluble lubricant to facilitate its placement. If the wedge is placed occlusal to the gingival margin, the band is pressed into the preparation, which will result in an abnormal concavity in the proximal surface of the restoration (see Fig. 10.97B). The wedge should not be so far apical to the gingival margin that the band will not be held tightly against the gingival margin. This improper wedge placement results in gingival excess of amalgam (i.e., amalgam "overhang") caused by the band moving slightly away from the margin during condensation of the amalgam. Such an overhang often goes undetected and may result in irritation of the gingiva or an area of plaque accumulation, which may increase the risk of secondary caries. If the wedge is significantly apical of the gingival margin, a second (usually smaller) wedge may be placed on top of the first to wedge adequately the matrix against the margin (Fig. 10.98). This type of wedging is particularly useful for patients whose interproximal tissue level has receded.

The gingival wedge should be tight enough to prevent any possibility of an overhang of amalgam in at least the middle two thirds of the gingival margin (see Fig. 10.98A and B). Occasionally, double wedging is permitted (if access allows), securing the matrix when the proximal box is wide faciolingually. *Double wedging* refers to using two wedges: one from the lingual embrasure and one from the facial embrasure (see Fig. 10.98E and F). Two wedges help ensure that the gingival corners of a wide proximal box may be properly condensed; they also help minimize gingival excess. Double wedging should be used only if the middle two thirds of the proximal margins are not able to be adequately wedged. Any amalgam excess that forms in the facial and lingual corners is accessible to carving, and therefore proper wedging to prevent gingival excess of amalgam in the middle two thirds of the proximal box (see Fig. 10.98B) is the primary objective.

Occasionally a concavity may be present on the proximal surface that is adjacent to the gingival margin. This may occur on a surface with a fluted root, such as the mesial surface of the maxillary first premolar (see Fig. 10.98G1). A gingival margin located in this area may be concave (see Fig. 10.98G2). To wedge a matrix band tightly against such a margin, a second pointed wedge may be inserted between the first wedge and the band (see Fig. 10.98G3 and G4).

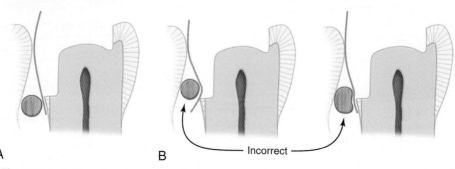

A   B   ── Incorrect ──

• **Fig. 10.97** A, Correct wedge position. B, Incorrect wedge positions.

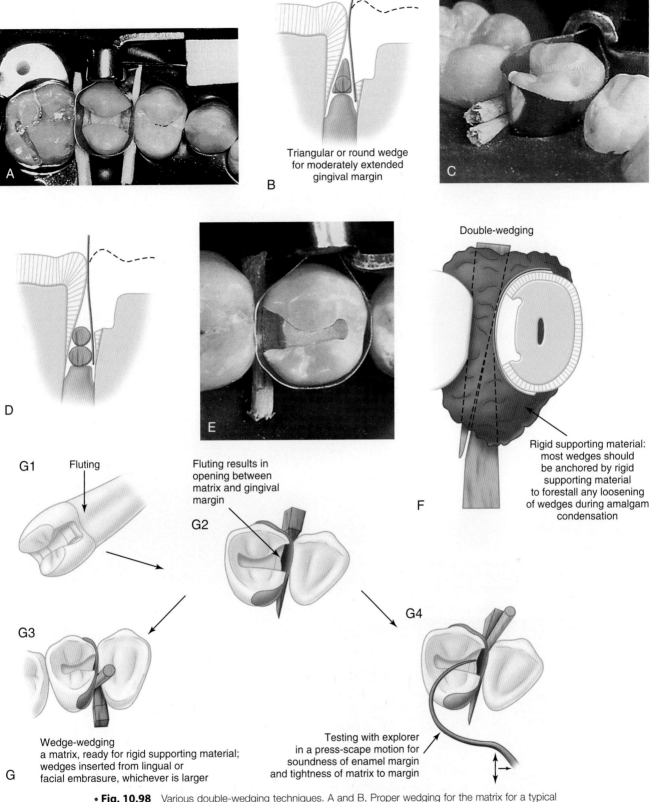

Triangular or round wedge
for moderately extended
gingival margin

Double-wedging

Rigid supporting material:
most wedges should
be anchored by rigid
supporting material
to forestall any loosening
of wedges during amalgam
condensation

Fluting

Fluting results in
opening between
matrix and gingival
margin

Wedge-wedging
a matrix, ready for rigid supporting material;
wedges inserted from lingual or
facial embrasure, whichever is larger

Testing with explorer
in a press-scape motion for
soundness of enamel margin
and tightness of matrix to margin

• **Fig. 10.98**   Various double-wedging techniques. A and B, Proper wedging for the matrix for a typical mesioocclusodistal preparation. C and D, Technique to allow wedging near the gingival margin of the preparation when the proximal box is shallow gingivally, the interproximal tissue level has receded, or both. E and F, Double wedging may be used with faciolingually wide proximal boxes to provide maximal closure of the band along the gingival margin. G, Another technique may be used on the mesial aspect of the maxillary first premolars to adapt the matrix to the fluted (i.e., concave) area of the gingival margin (G1, G2); a second wedge inserted from the lingual embrasure (G3); testing the adaptation of the band after insertion of the wedges from the facial aspect (G4).

The wedging action between teeth should provide enough separation of adjacent teeth to compensate for the thickness of the matrix band. This ensures a positive contact relationship after the matrix is removed (after the condensation and initial carving of amalgam). If a Tofflemire retainer is used to restore a two-surface Class II preparation, the single wedge must provide enough separation to compensate for two thicknesses of band material. The tightness of the wedge is tested by pressing the tip of an explorer firmly at several points along the middle two thirds of the gingival margin (against the matrix band) to verify that it cannot be moved away from the gingival margin (Fig. 10.99). As an additional test, the dentist

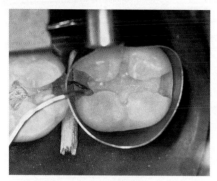

• **Fig. 10.99** Use of the explorer tip (with pressure) to ensure proper adaptation of the band to the gingival margin.

attempts to remove the wedge (using the explorer with moderate pressure) after first having set the explorer tip into the wood near the broken end. Moderate pulling should not cause dislodgment. Often the rubber dam has a tendency to loosen the wedge through rebounding of the dam stretched during wedge placement. Lubrication of the wedge and stretching the interproximal dam septa, in the direction opposite to the direction of wedge placement, before and during wedge placement may prevent rebound dislodgment. The stretched dam is released after the wedge is inserted.

Some situations may require a triangular wedge that is modified (by knife or scalpel blade) to conform to the approximating tooth contours (Fig. 10.100). The round toothpick wedge is usually the wedge of choice with conservative proximal boxes, however, because its wedging action is more occlusal (i.e., nearer the gingival margin) than with the triangular wedge (Fig. 10.101A and B).

The triangular (i.e., anatomic) wedge is recommended for a preparation with a deep gingival margin. The triangular wedge is positioned similarly to the round wedge, and the goal is the same. When the gingival margin is deep (cervically), the base of the triangular wedge more readily engages the tooth gingival to the margin without causing excessive soft tissue displacement. The anatomic wedge is preferred for deeply extended gingival margins because its greatest cross-sectional dimension is at its base (see Fig. 10.101C and D).

To maintain gingival isolation attained by an anatomic wedge placed before the preparation of a deeply extended gingival margin,

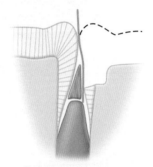

A Tall triangular wedge incorrect for minimally extended gingival margin

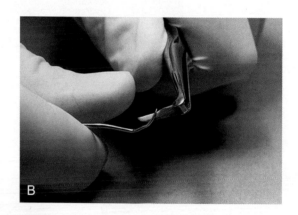

B

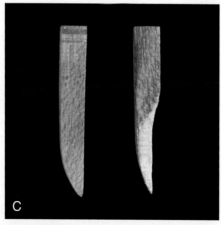

C

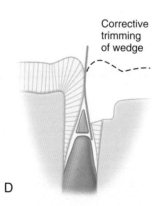

Corrective trimming of wedge

D

• **Fig. 10.100** Modified triangular (i.e., anatomic) wedge. A, Depending on the proximal convexity, a triangular wedge may distort the matrix contour. B, A sharp-bladed instrument may be used to modify the triangular steepness of the wedge. C, Modified and unmodified wedges are compared. D, Properly modified triangular wedge prevents distortion of the matrix contour.

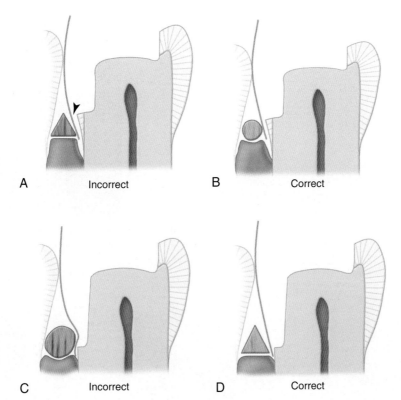

• **Fig. 10.101** Indications for the use of a round toothpick wedge versus a triangular (i.e., anatomic) wedge. A, As a rule, the triangular wedge does not firmly support the matrix band against the gingival margin in conservative Class II preparations *(arrowhead)*. B, The round toothpick wedge is preferred for these preparations because its wedging action is nearer the gingival margin. C, In Class II preparations with deep gingival margins, the round toothpick wedge crimps the matrix band contour if it is placed occlusal to the gingival margin. D, The triangular wedge is preferred with these preparations because its greatest width is at its base.

it may be appropriate to withdraw the wedge a small distance to allow passage of the band between the loosened wedge and the gingival margin. Tilting (i.e., canting) the matrix into place helps the gingival edge of the band slide between the loosened wedge and the gingival margin. The band is tightened, and the same wedge is firmly reinserted.

Supporting the matrix material with the blade of a Hollenback carver during the insertion of the wedge for the difficult deep gingival restoration may be helpful.[55] The tip of the blade is placed between the matrix and the gingival margin, and then the "heel" of the blade is leaned against the matrix and adjacent tooth (Fig. 10.102). In this position, the blade supports the matrix to help in positioning the wedge sufficiently gingivally and preventing the wedge from pushing the matrix into the preparation. After the wedge is properly inserted, the blade is gently removed.

All aspects of the band and wedge are assessed, and any desired final corrections are made. The matrix band and wedge must provide appropriate proximal contact and contour (see Fig. 10.96). After wedging, relaxing the tension of the band by turning the larger knurled nut of the Tofflemire retainer a quarter turn counterclockwise will help to ensure proximal contact. If loosening the Tofflemire band still does not allow for contact with an adjacent tooth, a custom-made band with a smaller angle may be used. Reducing the angle of the band increases the difference in length (i.e., circumferences) of the gingival and occlusal edges. To reduce the angle of the band, the operator folds it as shown in Fig. 10.103,

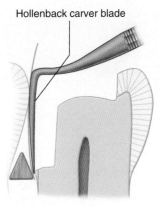

Hollenback carver blade

• **Fig. 10.102** Supporting the matrix with the blade of a Hollenback carver during wedge insertion.

burnishes for appropriate occlusogingival contour (in the contact areas), and inserts the band into the Tofflemire retainer.

Occasionally the interdental spacing is so large that a suitably trimmed tongue blade is required to wedge the matrix (Fig. 10.104). Occasionally it is impossible to use a wedge to secure the matrix band. In this case the band must be sufficiently tight to minimize the gingival amalgam excess. Because the band is not wedged, special care must be exercised to place small amounts of amalgam

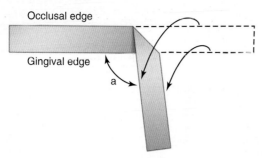

• **Fig. 10.103** The custom-made matrix strip is folded, as indicated by arrows. The smaller angle (a) compared with the angle of the commercial strip increases the difference between the lengths of the gingival and occlusal edges.

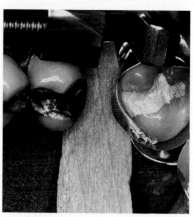

• **Fig. 10.104** A custom-made tongue blade wedge may be used when excessive space exists between adjacent teeth.

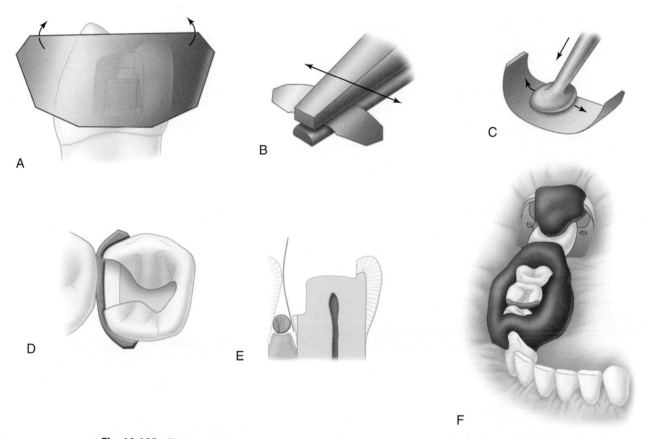

• **Fig. 10.105** Rigid material–supported sectional matrix. A, The shape of the stainless steel strip after trimming. B, The strip contoured to the circumferential contour of the tooth (fingers can be used). C, Burnishing the strip to produce occlusogingival contact contour (left and right arrows indicate the short, back-and-forth motion of the burnisher). D, Contoured strip in position. E, Matrix strip properly wedged. F, Completed rigid material–supported sectional matrix.

in the gingival floor and condense the first 1 mm of amalgam lightly but thoroughly in a gingival and lateral direction. The condensation of additional increments is then carefully continued in a gingival direction using a larger condenser with firm pressure. Condensation against an unwedged matrix may cause a gross extrusion of amalgam beyond the gingival margin. The excess amalgam must be removed with a suitable carver immediately after matrix removal.

Rigid-Material Supported Sectional Matrix

An alternative to the universal matrix band is the use of a properly contoured sectional matrix that is wedged and supported by a material that is rigid enough to resist condensation pressure. The supporting material selected must be easy to place and to remove. Examples include light-cured, thermoplastic, and quick-setting rigid polyvinyl siloxane (PVS) materials (Fig. 10.105). The gingival wedge is positioned interproximally to secure the band tightly at the gingival margin to prevent any excess of amalgam (i.e., over-hang). The wedge also separates teeth slightly to compensate for the thickness of the section of matrix material. The wedge is placed before the application of rigid supporting material.

The proximal surface contour of the matrix should allow the normal slight convexity between the occlusal and middle thirds of the proximal surface when viewed from the lingual (and facial) aspect. Proximal surface restorations often display an occlusogingival proximal contour that is too straight, thereby causing the contact relationship to be located too far occlusally (with little or no occlusal embrasure). This condition allows food impaction between teeth, with resultant injury to the interproximal gingiva and supporting tissues, and invites conditions leading to demineralization of the adjacent proximal surfaces. The proximal surface contour of the matrix should also provide the correct form to the proximal line angles, both facially and lingually. If these contours are not present, the facial and lingual embrasures of the restoration are too open, inviting food impaction and injury to underlying supporting tissues. Correct and incorrect contours and matrix correction steps are illustrated in Figs. 10.106 and 10.107.

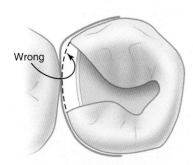

• **Fig. 10.106** Alteration of the sectional matrix contour to provide the correct form to the proximofacial line angle region.

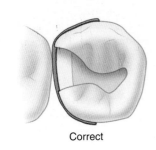

Correct

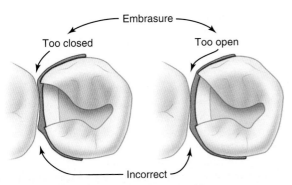

• **Fig. 10.107** Correct or incorrect facial and lingual embrasure form is determined by the shape of the sectional matrix strip.

The matrix should be tight against the facial and lingual margins on the proximal surface so that the amalgam may be well condensed at the preparation margins. In addition, when the matrix is tight against the tooth, minimal carving is necessary on the proximal margins after the matrix is removed.

Precontoured Sectional Matrix Strips

Commercially available sectional metal strips (e.g., Palodent System; DENTSPLY Caulk, Milford, DE) are precontoured and ready for application to the tooth (Fig. 10.108). These strips have limited application when used for amalgam because of their rounded contour. They usually are most suitable for mandibular first premolars and the distal surface of maxillary canines. The contact area of the adjacent tooth occasionally is too close to allow placement of the contoured Palodent strip without causing a dent in the strip's contact area, making it unusable.

Condensation and Carving of the Amalgam

Proper condensation of amalgam results in close material adaptation to the preparation walls (limiting marginal voids) and minimal inclusion of internal voids. In addition, careful overstepping condensation technique eliminates excess mercury and results in a stronger restoration that is less prone to corrosion. Care should be taken to choose condensers that are best suited for use in each part of the tooth preparation and that may be used without binding in the preparation or between the preparation and the matrix band.

Condensation should occur in the proximal box(es) first by transfer of enough amalgam with the amalgam carrier to fill the gingival portion by about 1 mm. This first increment is condensed in a gingival and lateral direction with sufficient force to adapt the amalgam to the gingival floor. Additional amalgam is carefully condensed against the proximal margins of the preparation and into the proximal retention grooves (if present). Firm, facially and lingually directed condensation (i.e., lateral condensation) with the side of the condenser should be accomplished along with the application of gingivally directed force (Fig. 10.109).[118] Condensation strokes in a gingival and lateral direction help to ensure that no voids occur internally or at the faciogingival or linguogingival line angles. Mesial (or distal) condensation of the amalgam in the proximal box is accomplished to ensure proper contour and proximal contact with the adjacent tooth.

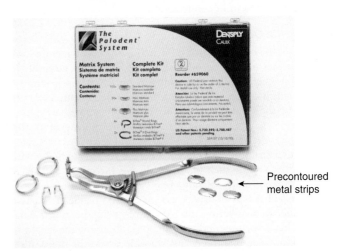

Precontoured metal strips

• **Fig. 10.108** Precontoured metal strips. (The Palodent System; courtesy of DENTSPLY Caulk, Milford, DE.)

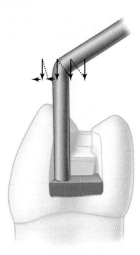

• **Fig. 10.109** Lateral and occlusogingival force is necessary to condense amalgam properly into the proximal grooves and into the angles at the junction of the matrix band and the margins of the preparation.

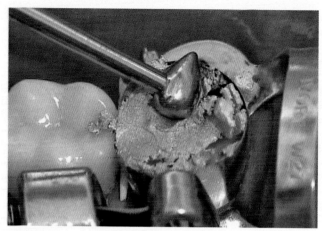

• **Fig. 10.110** Precarve burnishing with a large burnisher. (Courtesy Aldridge D. Wilder, DDS.)

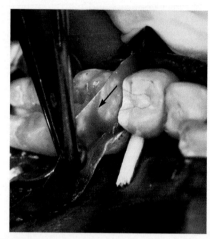

• **Fig. 10.111** Using No. 110 pliers, the matrix band should be removed in a linguoocclusal *(arrow)* or faciooocclusal direction (not just in an occlusal direction).

The procedure of adding and condensing continues until amalgam reaches the level of the pulpal wall. The size of the condenser is changed (usually to a larger one), if indicated, and amalgam is condensed in the remaining proximal portion of the preparation concurrently with the occlusal portion. It may be necessary to return to a smaller condenser when condensing in a narrow extension of the preparation or near the proximal margins. A smaller condenser face is more effective at condensing, provided it does not significantly penetrate the amalgam already in place. The occlusal margins are covered and overpacked by at least 1 mm using a large condenser, ensuring that the margins are well condensed, especially in the area of the marginal ridge.[119] Proper condensation of the amalgam in the marginal ridge area(s) reduces the risk of marginal ridge fracture during matrix removal. The plasticity and wetness of the amalgam mass should be monitored during condensation. Proper condensation requires that the mix should be neither wet (i.e., mercury rich) nor dry and crumbly (i.e., mercury poor). Amalgam that is beginning to set should be discarded and a new mix obtained to complete the condensation. Before carving procedures are initiated, precarve burnishing of the occlusal portion with a large egg-shaped or ball burnisher should be accomplished (Fig. 10.110).[79] As mentioned previously, precarve burnishing is a form of condensation.

Carving the Occlusal Portion

Carving of the occlusal portion (including the occlusal embrasure or embrasures) may be accomplished with the matrix assembly in place while the amalgam is reaching its initial set. Early removal of the band increases the risk of marginal ridge fracture. Careful carving of the occlusal portion should begin immediately after condensation and burnishing. Sharp discoid instruments of suitable size as well as the Hollenback carver may be effective at reestablishing the occlusal anatomy. The marginal ridge is carved confluent with the tooth's anatomy such that it duplicates the height and shape of the adjacent marginal ridge (see Fig. 10.18). An explorer or small Hollenback carver may be used to carefully define the occlusal embrasure. Remembering the pattern of occlusal contacts (that were evaluated before tooth preparation), observing the height of the adjacent marginal ridge, and knowing where the preparation cavosurface margins are located all aid in completing the carving of the occlusal surface, including the marginal ridge and occlusal

embrasure. If the restoration has extensive proximal involvement of the tooth, the occlusal carving should be accomplished quickly.

Removal of the Matrix Band and Completion of Carving

At the appropriate time, the matrix retainer first is removed from the band by turning the small knurled nut counterclockwise to retract the pointed spindle from the vice. The end of an index finger may be placed on the occlusal surface of the tooth and matrix band to provide stabilization while the retainer is removed. Next, any rigid supporting material, if used, is removed. The matrix band is removed next. The No. 110 pliers are used to tease the band free, from one contact area at a time, by pushing or pulling the band in a linguoocclusal (or faciooocclusal) direction and, if possible, in the direction of wedge insertion (Fig. 10.111). The wedge may be left in place to provide separation of teeth while the matrix band is removed, and then subsequently removed. By maintaining slight interdental separation, the wedge reduces the risk of fracturing the newly condensed marginal ridge(s). Band removal in a straight occlusal direction should be avoided so as to limit the risk of marginal ridge fracture.

Matrix band removal allows access to carve the proximal portions of the restoration. Efficient use of time is required so as to gain access to the proximal areas while the amalgam remains carvable.

Proper matrix form should result in a proximal surface that is nearly completed, with proper contact evident and minimal carving required except to remove a possible small amount of excess amalgam at the proximal facial and lingual margins, at the faciogingival and linguogingival corners, and along the gingival margin. Amalgam knives (scalers, No. 34 and No. 35) are ideal for removing gingival amalgam excess (see Figs. 10.21 and 10.22). They also are ideal for refining the embrasure form around the proximal contacts (see Fig. 10.19). The secondary (or "back") edges on the blades of amalgam knives are occasionally helpful, using a push stroke. The Hollenback carver No. 3 and (occasionally) the side of the explorer may also be suitable instruments for carving these areas. However, the explorer may not refine the margins and contour as effectively as the amalgam knife if the set of the amalgam is close to completion. When the proximal carving is completed, the occlusal surface contouring is completed. Occasionally, occlusal contouring may require the use of an abrasive stone or finishing bur if the setting of the amalgam is nearing completion.

When carving the margins of the restoration, the cutting surface of the carving instrument is held in a perpendicular orientation. Carving should be parallel to the margins, however, with the adjacent tooth surface being used to guide the carver. The existence of the proximal contact is verified visually by using the mouth mirror. When carving is completed, the rubber dam is removed and the occlusion is assessed and adjusted, as needed.

Abutment teeth for a tooth-supported RPD must provide amalgam contour to allow defining (by carving or [later] disking) a guide plane extending from the marginal ridge 2.5 mm gingivally. Normal proximal contour, rather than leaving an overcontour, is usually sufficient, however, and best for the development of a guide plane. Guide plane development results in a gingival embrasure between the natural tooth and RPD framework that is less open and less likely to trap food (see Fig. 10.88B and D).

An amalgam restoration of a proximal abutment tooth for a tissue-supported (i.e., distal extension) RPD is carved to provide a guide plan and adequate gingival embrasure space (see Fig. 10.88D). This allows for protection of the distogingival tissue, associated with the distal abutment, when occlusal loading of the RPD distal extension causes compression of the alveolar ridge soft tissue.

Before the patient is dismissed, thin unwaxed dental floss may be passed through the proximal contact(s) once to remove any amalgam shavings on the proximal surface of the restoration and to assess the gingival margin. Passing the floss multiple times through the contact area of an amalgam that is still early in its set may result in removal of some surface amalgam and loss of contact with the adjacent tooth. When positioned in the gingival embrasure, the floss is wrapped around the restored tooth and positioned apical to the gingival margin of the restoration. The floss is moved in an occlusogingival direction. The floss not only removes amalgam shavings but also smooths the proximal amalgam and detects any gingival overhang of amalgam. If an overhang is detected, further use of an amalgam knife is necessary.[120] Alternatively, a finishing strip may be used to remove the amalgam excess and finish the proximal surface gingival to the contact area. Floss also may be used to verify that the intensity of the contact is similar to that of neighboring teeth. Final rinsing and evacuation of the oral cavity is then accomplished. The patient is advised to avoid chewing with the restored tooth for 24 hours.

Finishing and Polishing of the Amalgam

Finishing and polishing of the occlusal surface of the Class II amalgam should follow the approach presented in General Concepts Guiding Restoration with Amalgam. Finishing and polishing of the proximal surface may be indicated where the proximal amalgam is accessible. This area usually includes the facial and lingual margins and areas occlusal to the contact. The remainder of the proximal surface is often inaccessible; however, the matrix band should have imparted sufficient smoothness to it.

If amalgam along the facial and lingual proximal margins was slightly overcarved, the enamel margin may be felt as the explorer tip passes from amalgam across the margin onto the external enamel surface. Finishing burs or sandpaper disks, rotating at slow speed, may be used to smooth the enamel–amalgam margin. Sandpaper disks also may be used to smooth and contour the marginal ridge. Inappropriate use of sandpaper disks may "ledge" the restoration around the contact, however, resulting in inappropriate proximal contours.

In small preparations, the facial and lingual proximal margins are generally inaccessible for finishing and polishing. Fine abrasive disks or the tip of a sharpened rubber polishing point or edge of a sharped abrasive rubber polishing cup may be used to polish the proximal portion that is accessible. When proximal margins are inaccessible to finishing and polishing with disks or rubber polishing points, and some excess amalgam remains (e.g., at the gingival corners and margins), amalgam knives occasionally may be used to trim amalgam back to the margin and to improve the contour, though a flame-shaped finishing bur may ultimately be required. Fig. 10.112 provides an example of a finished and polished Class II amalgam restoration.

Quadrant Dentistry

When several teeth in a quadrant have caries lesions, the experienced dentist usually treats them all at the same appointment rather than individually. Quadrant dentistry increases efficiency and reduces chair time for the patient. The use of the rubber dam is particularly important in quadrant dentistry. For maximal efficiency, when a quadrant of amalgam tooth preparations is planned, each rotary or hand instrument should be used on every tooth where it is needed before being exchanged.

When restoring a quadrant of Class II amalgam tooth preparations, it is permissible to apply matrix bands on alternate preparations in the quadrant and restore teeth two at a time. Banding adjacent preparations requires excessive wedging to compensate for a double thickness of band material and makes the control of proximal contours and interproximal contacts difficult. Extensive tooth preparations may need to be restored one at a time. If proximal boxes differ in size, teeth with smaller boxes should be restored first because often the proximal margins are inaccessible to carving if the larger adjacent box is restored first. In addition, smaller boxes may be restored more quickly and accurately because more tooth structure remains to guide the carver. If the larger proximal box is restored first, the gingival contour of the restoration may be damaged when the wedge is inserted to secure the matrix band for the second, smaller restoration. If the adjacent proximal boxes are similar in size, the banding of alternate preparations should be started with the most posterior preparation because this allows the patient to close slightly as subsequent restorations are inserted (Fig. 10.113).

Before restoring the second of two adjacent teeth, the proximal contour of the first restoration should be carefully established. Its anatomy serves as the guide to establish proper proximal contours leading to correct embrasure forms and contact position/size. If necessary, a finishing strip may be used to refine the contour of the first proximal amalgam (Fig. 10.114). The finishing strip is

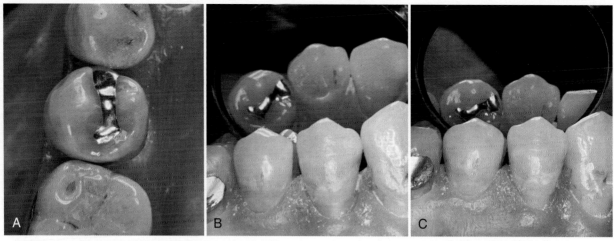

• **Fig. 10.112** Polished mesioocclusal amalgam restoration. Note the conservative extension. A, Occlusal view. B, Mesiofacial and occlusal views of the mesiofacial margin. C, Facial and occlusal views of the proximal surface contour and the location of the proximal contact.

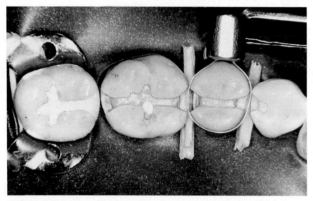

• **Fig. 10.113** Quadrant dentistry. Unless otherwise indicated, a quadrant of Class II preparations with similarly sized proximal boxes may be restored using two bands simultaneously if they are placed on every other prepared tooth. It is recommended that the most distal tooth be restored first.

indicated, however, only where the proximal clearance is present. Using a finishing strip between contacting amalgam restorations may compromise or eliminate the proximal contact. Properly placed amalgam restorations have the potential to last for decades (Fig. 10.115).

Clinical Technique for Class III Amalgam Restorations

Class III restorations are indicated for defects located on the proximal surface of anterior teeth that do not affect the incisal edge. Part of the facial or lingual surfaces also may be involved. The Class III amalgam restoration is rarely used and has been supplanted by tooth-colored restorations (primarily composite), which have become increasingly wear resistant and color stable. For esthetic reasons, use of amalgam is best suited for caries lesions that may be accessed from the lingual rather than from the facial. The Class III amalgam restoration is generally reserved for the distal surface of maxillary and mandibular canines if (1) the preparation is extensive with only minimal facial involvement, (2)

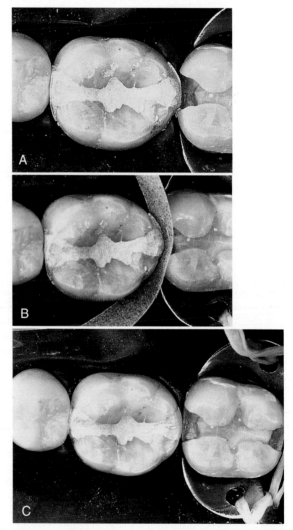

• **Fig. 10.114** When the first of two adjacent Class II preparations is restored, proper contour may be established by using a finishing strip before the second is restored. A, Before using the strip. B, Removing the over-contour. C, Verification of proper contour may be accomplished by viewing the restoration with a mirror from the occlusal, facial, and lingual positions. The proximal contour also may be evaluated after matrix placement by noting the symmetry between the restored surface and the burnished matrix band.

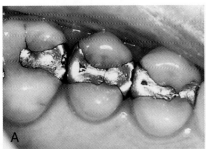 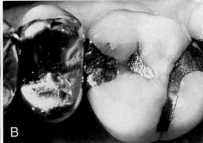 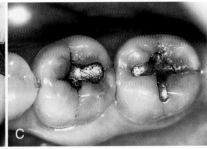

• **Fig. 10.115** Clinical examples of long-term amalgam restorations: A, 44-year-old amalgams; B, 58-year-old amalgams in the first molar; C, 65-year-old amalgams in molars. (A and B, Courtesy Drs. John Osborne and James Summitt.)

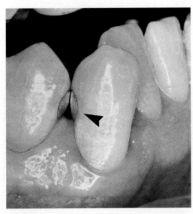

• **Fig. 10.116** Restoration for Class III tooth preparation using facial approach on mandibular canine. The restoration is 5 years old. (Courtesy Dr. C.L. Sockwell.)

the gingival margin primarily involves cementum, and/or (3) moisture control is difficult.

Initial Procedures

Appropriate review of the patient record (including medical history), treatment plan, and radiographs should be accomplished. Anesthesia is usually necessary when a vital tooth is to be restored. The gingival extension of the preparation should be anticipated. Prewedging in the gingival embrasure of the proximal site to be restored provides (1) better protection of soft tissue and the rubber dam, (2) better access because of the slight separation of teeth, and (3) better reestablishment of the proximal contact. The use of a rubber dam is generally recommended; however, cotton roll isolation is also acceptable.

Tooth Preparation for Class III Amalgam Restorations

A lingual access preparation on the distal surface of the maxillary canine is described here because the use of amalgam in that location is more likely. A facial approach for a mandibular canine may be indicated, however, if the lesion is more facial than lingual. The mandibular restoration is often not visible at conversational distance (Fig. 10.116). The outline form of the Class III amalgam preparation may include only the proximal surface. A lingual dovetail may be indicated if one existed previously or if additional retention is needed for a larger restoration.

Initial Tooth Preparation

Bur size selection depends on the size of the lesion. Bur options may include a No. 2 (or smaller) round bur or a No. 330 bur. The bur is positioned so that the entry cut penetrates into the caries lesion, which is usually slightly gingival to the contact area. Ideally the bur is positioned so that its long axis is perpendicular to the lingual surface of the tooth, but directed at a mesial angle as close to the adjacent tooth as possible. (The bur position may be described as perpendicular to the distolingual line angle of the tooth.) This position conserves the marginal ridge enamel (Fig. 10.117A–C). Penetration through enamel positions the bur so that additional cutting isolates the proximal enamel affected by the caries lesion and removes some or all of the soft dentin. In addition, penetration should be at a limited initial axial depth (i.e., 0.5–0.6 mm) inside the DEJ (see Fig. 10.117C and D) or at a 0.75- to 0.8-mm axial depth when the gingival margin is on the root surface (in cementum/dentin) (Fig. 10.118). This 0.75-mm axial depth on the root surface allows a 0.25-mm distance (the diameter of the No. ¼ bur is 0.5 mm) between the retention groove (which is placed later) and the gingival cavosurface margin. Soft dentin that is deeper than this limited initial axial depth is removed later during final tooth preparation.

For a small lesion, the facial margin is extended 0.2 to 0.3 mm into the facial embrasure (if necessary), with a curved outline from the incisal to the gingival margin (resulting in a less visible margin). The lingual outline blends with the incisal and gingival margins in a smooth curve, creating a preparation with little or no lingual wall. The cavosurface angle should be 90 degrees at all margins. The facial, incisal, and gingival walls should meet the axial wall at approximately right angles (although the lingual wall meets the axial wall at an obtuse angle or may be continuous with the axial wall) (Figs. 10.119 and 10.120). If a large round bur is used, the internal angles are more rounded. The axial wall should be uniformly deep into dentin and follow the faciolingual contour of the external tooth surface (see Fig. 10.120). The initial axial wall depth may be in firm dentin (i.e., shallow lesion), in soft dentin (i.e., moderate to deep lesion), or in existing restorative material, if a restoration is being replaced.

Incisal extension to remove carious tooth structure may eliminate the proximal contact (Fig. 10.121). It is important to conserve as much of the distoincisal tooth structure (i.e., sometimes referred to as the "incisal canopy") as possible to reduce the risk for subsequent fracture. When possible (i.e., when the incisal enamel has dentin support), it is best to leave the incisal margin in contact with the adjacent tooth.

When preparing a gingival wall that is near the level of the rubber dam or apical to it, it is beneficial to initially place a wedge

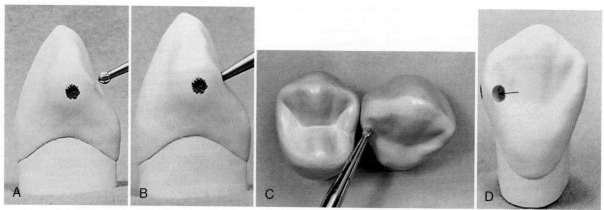

• **Fig. 10.117** Entry for Class III tooth preparation on maxillary canine. A, Bur position is perpendicular to the enamel surface at the point of entry. B, Initial penetration through enamel is directed toward cavitated, caries lesion. C, Initial entry should isolate the proximal enamel, while preserving as much of the marginal ridge as possible. D, Initial cutting reveals the DEJ *(arrow)*.

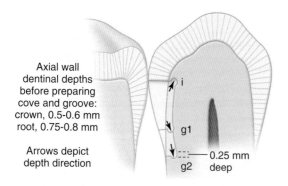

Axial wall dentinal depths before preparing cove and groove:
crown, 0.5-0.6 mm
root, 0.75-0.8 mm

Arrows depict depth direction

• **Fig. 10.118** Mesiodistal vertical section showing location, depth direction *(arrows)*, and direction depth of the retention form in Class III tooth preparations of different gingival depths. Incisal cove *(i)*; gingival groove *(g1)*, enamel margin; gingival groove *(g2)*, root-surface margin. Distance from outer aspect of g2 groove to margin is approximately 0.3 mm; bur head diameter is 0.5 mm; direction depth of groove is half this diameter (or approximately 0.3 mm [0.25 mm]).

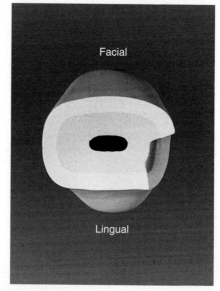

• **Fig. 10.120** Transverse section of mandibular lateral incisor illustrating that the lingual wall of a Class III tooth preparation may meet the axial wall at an obtuse angle and that the axial wall is a uniform depth into dentin and follows the faciolingual contour of the external tooth surface.

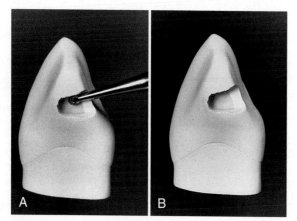

• **Fig. 10.119** Class III tooth preparation on maxillary canine. A, Round bur shaping the incisal area. The incisal angle remains. B, Initial shape of the preparation accomplished with a round bur.

in the gingival embrasure to depress and protect soft tissue and the rubber dam. As the bur is preparing the gingival wall, it may lightly shave the wedge. A triangular (i.e., anatomic) wedge, rather than a round wedge, is used for a deep gingival margin.

The initial tooth preparation is completed by using a No. ½ round bur to accentuate the axial line angles (Fig. 10.122A and B), particularly the axiogingival angle. This facilitates the subsequent placement of retention grooves and leaves the internal line angles slightly rounded. Rounded internal preparation angles permit more complete condensation of the amalgam. The No. ½ round bur also may be used to smooth any roughened, undermined enamel produced at the gingival and facial cavosurface margins (see Fig. 10.122C). The incisal margin of the minimally extended preparation is often not accessible to the larger round bur without damaging

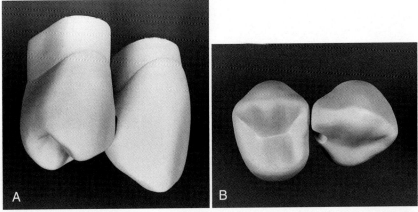

• **Fig. 10.121**   Distofacial (A) and incisal (B) views of the canine to show the curved proximal outline necessary to preserve the distoincisal corner of the tooth. The incisal margin of this preparation example is located slightly incisally of the proximal contact (but whenever possible, the margin may be in the contact area).

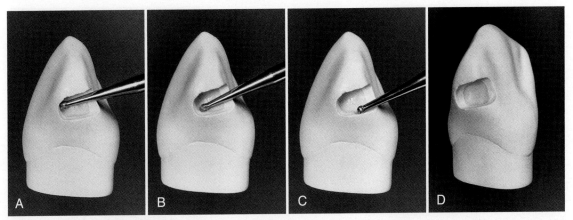

• **Fig. 10.122**   Refining proximal portion. A–C, A small, round bur is used to shape the preparation walls, define line angles, and initiate removal of any undermined enamel along the gingival and facial margins. D, Tooth preparation completed, except for the final finishing of the enamel margins and placement of secondary retention.

("marring") the adjacent tooth (see Fig. 10.122D). Further finishing of the incisal margin is presented later. At this point the initial tooth preparation is completed.

Final Tooth Preparation

Final tooth preparation involves removing any remaining soft dentin, protecting the pulp, developing secondary resistance and retention forms, finishing external walls, and debridement (cleaning)/inspecting. Any remaining soft dentin on the axial wall is removed by using a slowly revolving round bur (No. 2 or No. 4), appropriate spoon excavators, or both. (See Chapter 2 for the management of soft dentin.)

For the Class III amalgam restoration, resistance form against postrestorative fracture is provided by (1) cavosurface and amalgam margins of 90 degrees, (2) enamel walls supported by sound dentin, (3) sufficient bulk of amalgam, and (4) rounded preparation internal angles. The boxlike preparation form provides primary retention form. Secondary retention form is provided by a gingival groove, an incisal cove, and sometimes a lingual dovetail.

The gingival retention groove is prepared by placing a No. ¼ round bur (rotating at low speed) in the axiofaciogingival point angle. It is positioned in the dentin to maintain 0.2 mm of dentin between the groove and the DEJ. The rotating bur is moved lingually along the axiogingival line angle, with the angle of cutting generally bisecting the angle between the gingival and axial walls. Ideally the direction of the gingival groove is slightly more gingival than axial (and the direction of an incisal [i.e., occlusal] groove would be slightly more incisal [i.e., occlusal] than axial) (Fig. 10.123; see also Fig. 10.118).

Alternatively if less retention form is needed, two gingival coves may be used as opposed to a continuous groove. One each may be placed in the axiofaciogingival and axiogingivolingual point angles. The diameter of the ¼ round bur is 0.5 mm, and the depth of the groove should be ~0.25 to 0.5 mm. Note the location and depthwise direction of the groove, where the gingival wall remains in enamel (Fig. 10.124). When preparing a retention groove on the root surface (gingival wall in cementum or dentin), the angle of cutting is more gingival, resulting in the distance from the gingival cavosurface margin to the groove being approximately 0.3 mm (see Fig. 10.118). Careful technique is necessary in preparing the gingival retention groove. If the dentin that supports gingival enamel is removed, enamel is subject to fracture. In addition, if the groove is placed only in the axial wall, no effective retention form is developed and the risk of pulpal involvement is increased.

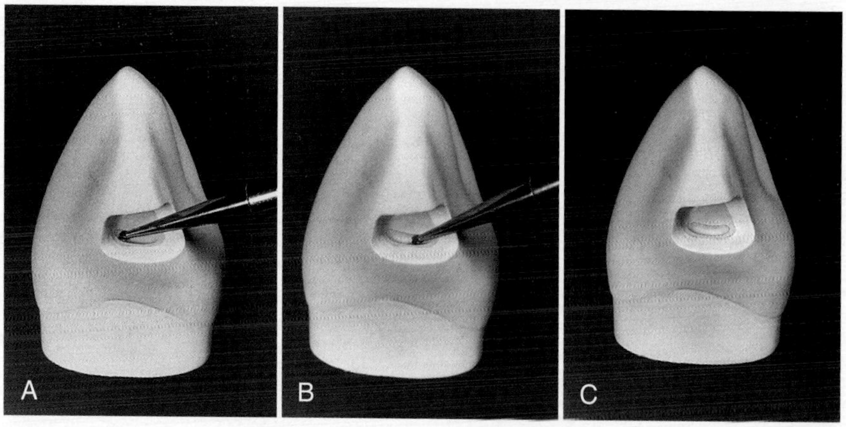

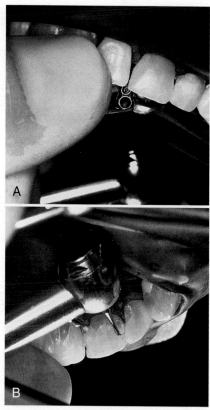

• **Fig. 10.123** Preparing the gingival retention form. A, Position of No. ¼ round bur in axiofaciogingival point angle. B, Advancing the bur lingually to prepare the groove along the axiogingival line angle. (See Fig. 10.118 regarding location, depth direction, and direction depth of groove.) C, Completed gingival retention groove.

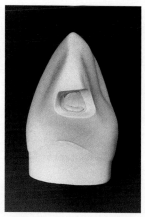

• **Fig. 10.124** Completed Class III tooth preparation for amalgam restoration.

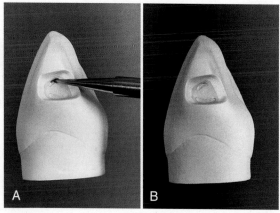

• **Fig. 10.125** Preparing the incisal retention cove. A, Position of No. ¼ round bur in the axioincisal point angle. B, Completed incisal cove.

• **Fig. 10.126** Use of the palm-and-thumb grasp to place the incisal retention cove. A, Hand position showing thumb rest. B, Handpiece position for preparing the incisal retention.

An incisal retention cove is prepared at the axiofacioincisal point angle with a No. ¼ round bur in dentin, being careful not to undermine enamel. It is directed similarly into the incisal point angle and prepared to half the diameter of the bur (Fig. 10.125). Undermining the incisal enamel should be avoided. For the maxillary canine, the palm-and-thumb grasp may be used to direct the bur incisally (Fig. 10.126). This completes the typical Class III amalgam tooth preparation (see Fig. 10.124).

A lingual dovetail is not required in small or moderately sized Class III amalgam restorations. It may be used in large preparations, especially preparations with excessive incisal extension in which additional retention form is needed. The dovetail may not be necessary (even in large preparations), however, if an incisal secondary retention form is possible (Fig. 10.127).

If a lingual dovetail is needed, it is prepared only after initial preparation of the proximal portion has been completed. Otherwise

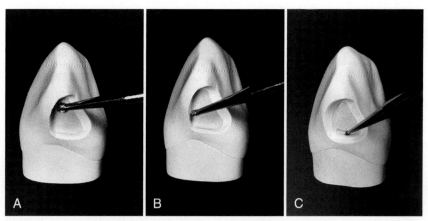

• **Fig. 10.127** Extensive Class III tooth preparation. A, Initial tooth preparation with No. 2 round bur. B, Defining line angles and removing undermined enamel with No. $\frac{1}{2}$ round bur. C, Placing the retention groove using No. $\frac{1}{4}$ round bur. Note the completed incisal cove.

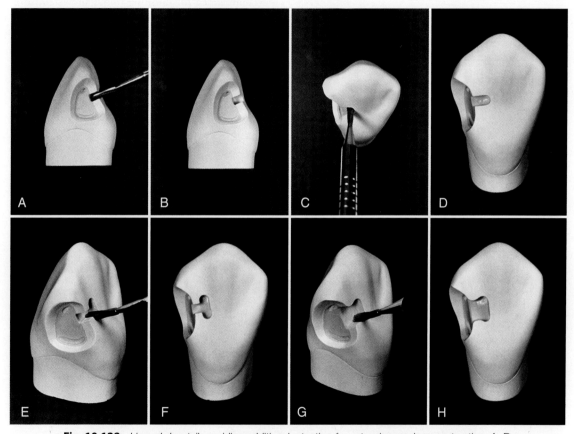

• **Fig. 10.128** Lingual dovetail providing additional retention for extensive amalgam restoration. A, Bur position at correct depth and angulation to begin cutting. B, Initial cut in beginning dovetail. C, Bur moved to most mesial extent of dovetail. D, If possible, cutting should not extend beyond the midlingual position. E, Bur cutting gingival extension of the dovetail. F, Incisal and gingival extensions of the dovetail. G, Completing the isthmus. The proximal and lingual portions are connected by the incisal and gingival walls in smooth curves. H, Completed lingual dovetail.

the tooth structure needed for the isthmus between the proximal portion and the dovetail may be removed when the proximal outline form is prepared. The lingual dovetail should be conservative, generally not extending beyond the mesiodistal midpoint of the lingual surface; this varies according to the extent of the proximal caries lesion. The depth of the axial wall of the dovetail should be just inside the DEJ and should be parallel to the lingual surface

of the tooth. The No. 245 bur is positioned in the proximal portion at the correct depth and angulation and moved in a mesial direction (Fig. 10.128A and B). The correct angulation places the long axis of the bur perpendicular to the lingual surface. The bur is moved to the point that corresponds to the most mesial extent of the dovetail (see Fig. 10.128C and D). The bur is then moved incisally and gingivally to create sufficient incisogingival dimension to the

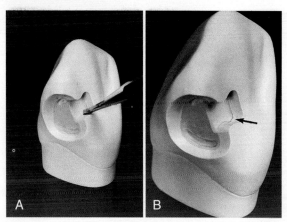

• **Fig. 10.129** Ensuring retention in lingual dovetail (often optional). A, Position of No. 33½ bur for cutting the retention cove. B, Preparation of the cove should not remove the dentinal support of the lingual enamel (arrow).

dovetail (approximately 2.5 mm) (see Fig. 10.128E and F). The incisal and gingival walls of the isthmus are prepared in smooth curves connecting the dovetail to the proximal outline form (see Fig. 10.128G and H).

The gingival margin trimmer may be used to round the axiopulpal line angle (i.e., the junction of the proximal and dovetail preparation). This increases the strength of the restoration at the junction of the proximal and lingual portions by providing bulk and limiting stress concentration. The slight lingual convergence of the dovetail's external walls (prepared with the No. 245 bur) usually provides a sufficient retention form. Retention coves, one in the incisal corner and one in the gingival corner (Fig. 10.129), may be placed in the dovetail to enhance retention. The coves are prepared with the No. ¼ round bur or the No. 33½ bur without compromising the dentinal support of the lingual enamel. This preparation may require deepening of the axial wall. Unsupported enamel is removed, the walls or margins are smoothed, and the cavosurface angles are refined, where indicated. The 8-3-22 hoe is recommended for finishing minimally extended margins (Fig. 10.130). If the gingival margin is in enamel, correct marginal configuration (approximately 20 degrees gingival declination) is

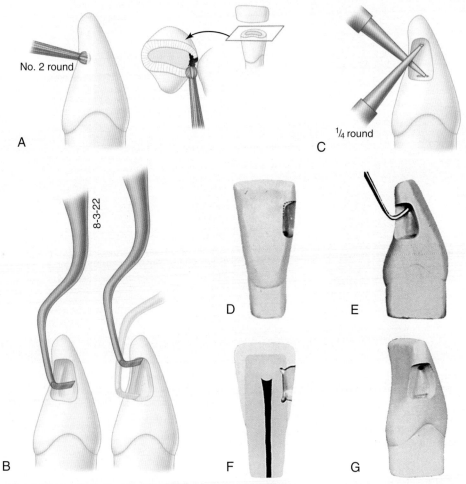

• **Fig. 10.130** Class III tooth preparation for amalgam restoration on the mandibular incisor. A, Entering the tooth from the lingual approach. B, Finishing the facial, incisal, and lingual enamel margins with an 8-3-22 triple angle hoe. Note how the secondary cutting edge of the blade is used on the lingual enamel. C, Placing incisal and gingival retention forms with No. ¼ round bur. D, Dotted line indicates the outline of the additional extension that is sometimes necessary for access in placing the incisal retention cove. E, Position of a bi-beveled hatchet to place the incisal retention cove. F, The axial wall forms a convex surface over the pulp. G, Completed tooth preparation. Note the gingival retention groove.

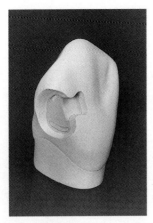

• Fig. 10.131 Completed distolingual Class III tooth preparation for amalgam.

necessary to ensure full-length enamel rods forming the cavosurface margin. All the walls of the preparation should meet the external tooth surface to form a right angle (i.e., butt joint) (Fig. 10.131; see also Fig. 10.124). The various steps involved in the preparation of the dovetail are shown in Fig. 10.132.

The completed tooth preparation should be cleaned of any residual debris and inspected. Careful assessment should be made to see that all of the caries lesion has been removed (as indicated), that the depth and retention are appropriate, and that cavosurface margins provide for sufficient amalgam bulk.

Restorative Technique for Class III Amalgam Preparations

Desensitizer Placement

A dentin desensitizer is placed on the prepared tooth structure per manufacturer instructions. Excess moisture is removed without desiccating the dentin.

Matrix Placement

The wedged, rigid material–supported sectional matrix may be used for the Class III amalgam restoration. It is essential to trim the lingual portion of the sectional matrix material correctly to avoid covering the preparation and blocking access for insertion of the amalgam. Stainless steel matrix material is obtained, 8 mm wide and 0.05 mm thick, which covers one third of the facial surface and extends through the proximal to the lingual surface. The lingual portion is trimmed at an angle that corresponds approximately to the slope of the lingual surface of the tooth (Fig. 10.133). The section of matrix is burnished on a resilient paper pad to create the desired proximal surface form. The sectional matrix is placed in position and wedged from the facial or lingual embrasure, whichever is greater. The facial and lingual portions of the matrix are stabilized with a rigid material (see Fig. 10.132G). Precontoured metallic matrices may be used (instead of custom-made matrices) if the contour of the precontoured matrix coincides with that of the proximal surface being restored. If the preparation is small and the matrix is sufficiently rigid, additional rigid material to support the matrix may not be required.

Condensation and Carving

Insertion of the amalgam, initial carving, matrix removal, wedge removal, and final carving are similar to the techniques for Class

II preparations. When properly placed, conservative restorations in incisors and canines are relatively inconspicuous (Fig. 10.134). Fig. 10.135 illustrates a Class III amalgam restoration in a mandibular incisor.

Finishing and Polishing

Finishing and polishing of the Class III amalgam should follow the approach presented in General Concepts Guiding Restoration with Amalgam.

Clinical Technique for Class V Amalgam Restorations

Class V restorations are indicated to restore defects on the facial or lingual cervical one third of any tooth. Class V amalgam restorations may be especially technique sensitive because of location, extent of the caries lesion, and limited access and visibility. Cervical caries lesions usually develop because of the chronic presence of an acidogenic biofilm located in the non–self-cleansing area just gingival to the height of contour. Patients with gingival recession are predisposed to Class V *root caries lesions* because dentin is more susceptible to demineralization than enamel. Patients with a reduced salivary flow caused by certain medical conditions (e.g., Sjögren's syndrome), medications, or head and neck radiation therapy are also predisposed to cervical and root caries lesions. These patients usually have less saliva to buffer the acids produced by oral bacteria. Class V restorations may be used to treat both cervical and root caries lesions. Incipient, smooth-surface enamel demineralization appears as a chalky white line just occlusal or incisal to the crest of the marginal gingiva (usually on the facial surface) (Fig. 10.136). These areas often are overlooked in the oral examination unless teeth are isolated with cotton rolls, free of debris, and dried gently with the air syringe. When the incipient cervical caries has not decalcified the enamel sufficiently to result in cavitation (i.e., a break in the continuity of the surface), the lesion may be remineralized by appropriate techniques, including patient motivation toward proper diet and hygiene. Occasionally an enamel surface that is only slightly cavitated may be treated successfully by smoothing with sandpaper disks, polishing, and treating with a fluoride varnish or infiltrated with a low viscosity resin in an attempt to prevent further demineralization, cavitation, and surgical management. Prophylactic, preventive treatment alone will be inadequate if the caries lesion has progressed to decalcify and soften enamel to an appreciable depth. In this instance, a Class V tooth preparation and restoration is indicated, particularly if the caries lesion has penetrated to the DEJ (Fig. 10.137A). When numerous cervical lesions are present (see Fig. 10.137B), high caries activity is obvious. In addition to the restorative treatment, the patient should be instructed and encouraged to implement an aggressive prevention program to avoid subsequent development of additional caries lesions. Class V amalgam restorations may be used anywhere in the mouth. As with Class III amalgam restorations, they generally are reserved for nonesthetic areas, for areas where access and visibility are limited and where moisture control is difficult, such as areas that are significantly deep gingivally. Because of limited access and visibility, many Class V restorations are difficult and present special problems during the preparation and restorative procedures.

Occasionally amalgam is preferred when the caries lesion extends gingivally enough that a mucoperiosteal flap must be reflected for adequate access and visibility (Fig. 10.138). Proper surgical technique must be followed, with special attention to complete debridement

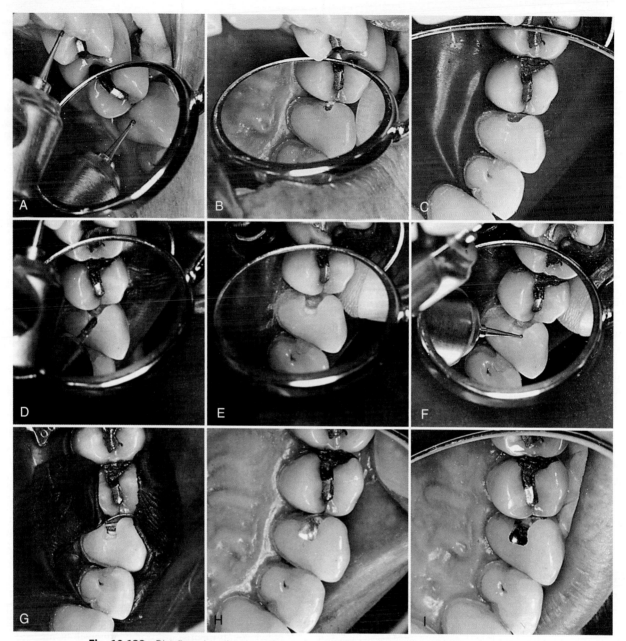

• **Fig. 10.132** Distolingual tooth preparation and restoration. A, Bur position for entry. B, Penetration made through the lingual enamel to the caries lesion. C, Proximal portion completed, except for the retention form. D, Preparing the dovetail. E, Completed preparation, except for the retention groove and the coves. F, Bur position for the incisal cove in the dovetail. G, Rigid material–supported sectional matrix ready for the insertion of amalgam. H, Carving completed and rubber dam removed. I, Polished restoration.

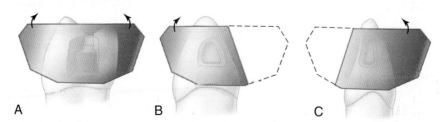

• **Fig. 10.133** Matrix strip design. A, Design required for rigid material–supported matrix for Class II tooth preparations. B, Alteration necessary for Class III preparation on the maxillary canine. C, Alteration necessary for the mandibular incisor. The strip material is cut to approximate the slope of the lingual surface.

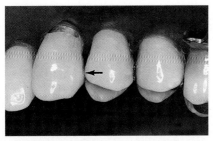

• **Fig. 10.134** Inconspicuous facial margin *(arrow)* of Class III amalgam restoration on the maxillary canine.

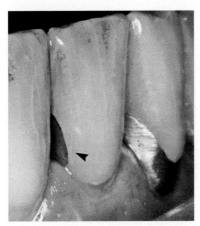

• **Fig. 10.135** Class III amalgam restoration on the mandibular incisor *(arrowhead)*.

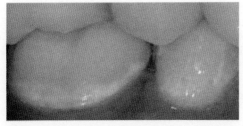

• **Fig. 10.136** Incipient caries lesions of enamel appear as white spots. The affected surface may be smooth (i.e., noncavitated). White spots are more visible when dried. (From Cobourne MT, DiBiase AT: *Handbook of orthodontics*, Edinburgh, 2010, Mosby.)

of amalgam particles before closure of the surgical site. Class V amalgam restorations usually are contraindicated in esthetically important areas because many patients object to metal restorations that are visible (Fig. 10.139). Generally Class V amalgams placed on the facial surface of mandibular canines, premolars, and molars are not readily visible. Amalgams placed on maxillary premolars and first molars may be visible.

Amalgam may be used in the cervical areas of partial denture abutment teeth because amalgam resists wear as clasps move over the restoration. Contours prepared in the restoration for clasp retentive areas may be achieved relatively easily and maintained when an amalgam restoration is used.

Initial Procedures

Proper isolation prevents moisture contamination of the operating site, enhances asepsis, and facilitates access and visibility. Moisture in the form of saliva, gingival sulcular fluid, or gingival hemorrhage must be excluded during caries lesion removal, liner application, and insertion and carving of amalgam. Moisture impairs visual assessment, may contaminate the pulp during caries lesion removal (especially with a pulpal exposure), and may negatively affect the physical properties of the amalgam. The gingival margin of Class V tooth preparations is often apical to the gingival crest. Such a gingival margin necessitates use of appropriate rubber dam and retainer, or displacement of the free gingiva with a retraction cord, to protect it and to provide access. Isolation helps eliminate seepage of sulcular fluid into the tooth preparation or restorative materials.

Isolation objectives are met through local anesthesia and use of (1) a cotton roll and a retraction cord or (2) a rubber dam and a suitable cervical retainer (Fig. 10.140). Isolation with a cotton roll and a retraction cord is satisfactory when properly performed (Fig. 10.141). This type of isolation is practical and probably the approach most often used. The retraction cord should be placed in the sulcus before initial tooth preparation to reduce the possibility of cutting instruments damaging the free gingiva. The cord should produce a temporary, adequate, atraumatic lateral displacement of the free gingiva. The cord may be treated with hemostatic preparations containing aluminum chloride or ferrous sulfate. Alternatively the cord may be treated with epinephrine; however, caution must be used as epinephrine on abraded gingiva is absorbed rapidly into the circulatory system and may cause an increase in blood pressure, elevated heart rate, and possible dysrhythmia. The retraction cord may be braided, twisted, or woven. The diameter of the cord should be easily accommodated in the gingival sulcus.

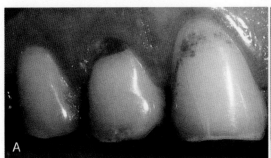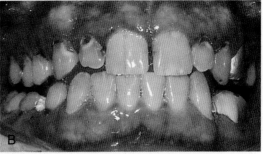

• **Fig. 10.137** Cervical caries lesions. A, Cavitation involving enamel and dentin in several teeth. B, Relatively high caries index is obvious when numerous cervical lesions are present. (From Perry DA, Beemsterboer PL: *Periodontology for the dental hygienist*, ed 3, St. Louis, 2007, Saunders.)

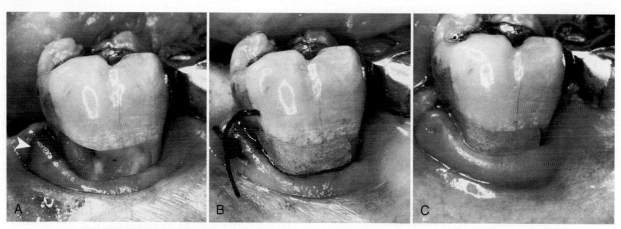

• **Fig. 10.138** Surgical access. A, Class V preparation requiring mucoperiosteal flap reflection with a releasing incision *(arrowhead)*. B, Completed restoration with suture in place. C, Suture removed 1 week after the procedure.

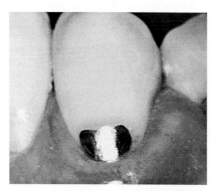

• **Fig. 10.139** Patients may object to metal restorations that are visible during conversation.

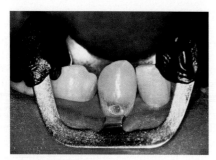

• **Fig. 10.140** A rubber dam and a No. 212 retainer may be required to isolate the caries lesion properly.

If significant blanching of the free gingiva is observed (or if too much pressure has to be applied to place the cord), an oversized cord may have been selected. If so, it should be exchanged for a cord of smaller diameter. An appropriate amount is cut to a length 6 mm longer than the gingival margin. Some operators prefer to place the cord in a dappen dish, wet it with a drop of hemostatic solution, and blot it with gauze (5 × 5 cm) to remove excess liquid. A braided or woven cord is usually easier to use because it does not unravel during placement. A larger cord may be inserted over the first cord if the sulcus is large enough to accommodate two cords. A thin, blunt-edged instrument blade or the side of an explorer tine may be used to gently insert the cord progressively into place. A slight backward direction of the instrument as it

steps along the cord helps prevent dislodgment of previously inserted cord (see Fig. 10.141). In addition, using a second instrument stepping along behind the first instrument may help prevent dislodgment of cord. Additionally using the air syringe or cotton pellets to reduce or absorb the sulcular fluid in the cord already placed is helpful during cord placement. The cord results in adequate retraction (displacement) in a short time. The cord may be moistened with the hemostatic solution before, during, or after placement if slight hemorrhage is anticipated or observed. Alternatively the cord may be used dry.

The cord usually remains in place during tooth preparation as well as insertion and initial carving of amalgam. While carving amalgam at the gingival margin, the presence of the cord may cause difficulty in detection of the unprepared tooth surface apical to the margin. This may limit proper carving, result in an over-contour and marginal excess. In this instance, after carving gross excess, the cord may be teased from the sulcus before the carving is completed.

Tooth Preparation for Class V Amalgam Restorations

Proper outline form for Class V amalgam tooth preparations results in extending the cavosurface margins to sound tooth structure while maintaining a limited axial depth of 0.5 mm inside the DEJ and 0.75 mm inside cementum (when on the root surface). The outline form for the Class V amalgam tooth preparation is determined primarily by the location and size of the caries lesion or old restorative material. Clinical judgment determines final preparation outline, especially when the cavosurface margins approach or extend into areas of enamel decalcification. The operator must observe the prepared enamel wall to evaluate the depth of the decalcified enamel and to determine if cavitation exists peripheral to the wall. When no cavitation has occurred and when the decalcification does not extend appreciably into the enamel, extension of the outline form often should cease. In some cases, if all decalcification were included in the outline form, the preparation would extend into the proximal cervical areas (if not circumferentially around the tooth). Such a preparation would be difficult and perhaps unrestorable. A full-coverage indirect restoration should be considered for teeth with extensive circumferential cervical decalcification (but only after caries risk has been reduced).

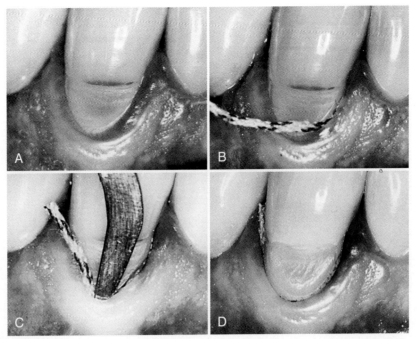

• **Fig. 10.141** Use of the retraction cord for isolation of a Class V lesion. A, Preoperative view. B, Cord placement initiated. C, Cord placement using a thin, flat-bladed instrument. D, Cord placement completed.

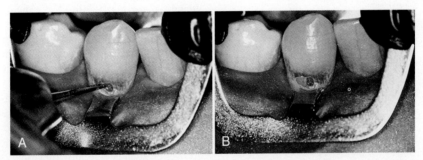

• **Fig. 10.142** Starting the Class V tooth preparation. A, Bur positioned for entry into caries lesion. B, The entry cut is the beginning of the outline form having a limited axial depth.

Initial Tooth Preparation

A Class V amalgam restoration is not used often in a mandibular canine, but it is presented here for illustration. The same general principles for tooth preparation apply for all other tooth locations. A tapered fissure bur of suitable size (e.g., No. 271) is used to enter the caries lesion (or existing restoration) to a limited initial axial depth of 0.5 mm inside the DEJ (Fig. 10.142). This depth is usually 1 to 1.25 mm total axial depth, depending on the incisogingival (i.e., occlusogingival) location. The enamel of the incisal (occlusal) external wall of the preparation is considerably thicker than the cervical. If the preparation is on the root surface, however, the initial axial depth is approximately 0.75 mm. The end of the bur at the initial depth may be in sound dentin, in soft dentin, or in old restorative material. The edge of the bur end may be used to penetrate the area; this is more efficient than using the flat end of the bur, reducing the possibility of the bur's tendency to "crawl" (i.e., move laterally instead of cut axially) on the external surface. When the entry is made, the bur orientation is adjusted to ensure that all external walls are perpendicular to the external tooth surface (i.e., parallel to the enamel rods) (Fig. 10.143). This requires frequent

changing of the bur orientation so as to accommodate the cervical mesiodistal and incisogingival (or occlusogingival) convexity of the tooth. The preparation is extended incisally, gingivally, mesially, and distally until the cavosurface margins are positioned in sound tooth structure such that an initial axial depth of 0.5 mm inside the DEJ (or 0.75 mm if on the root surface) is established. When extending mesially and distally, it may be necessary to protect the rubber dam from the bur by placing a flat-bladed instrument over the dam (Fig. 10.144). Because the axial wall follows the mesiodistal and incisogingival (or occlusogingival) contours of the facial surface of the tooth, it usually is convex in both directions (Fig. 10.145). In addition, the axial wall usually is slightly deeper at the incisal wall, where more enamel (i.e., approximately 1–1.25 mm in depth) is present than at the gingival wall, where little or no enamel (i.e., approximately 0.75–1 mm in depth) may be present. A depth of 0.5 mm inside the DEJ permits placement of necessary retention grooves without undermining enamel. This subtle difference in depth serves also to increase the thickness of the remaining dentin (between the axial wall and the pulp) in the gingival aspect of the preparation to aid in protecting the pulp.

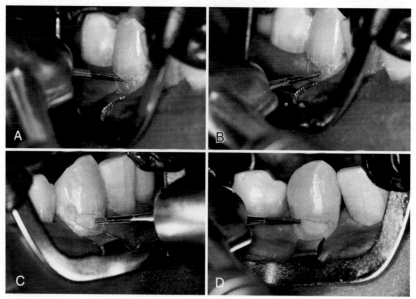

• **Fig. 10.143** When extending incisally (A), gingivally (B), mesially (C), and distally (D), the bur is positioned to prepare these walls perpendicular to the external tooth surface.

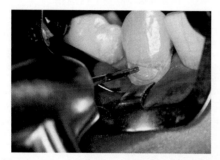

• **Fig. 10.144** The flat-bladed instrument protects the rubber dam from the bur.

Alternatively, an appropriate carbide bur (usually No. 2 or No. 4) may be used for the initial tooth preparation. Round burs are indicated in areas inaccessible to a fissure bur, which must be oriented perpendicular to the tooth surface. If needed, smaller round burs may also be used to define the internal angles in these preparations, enhancing proper placement of the retention grooves.

Final Tooth Preparation

Final tooth preparation involves the removal of any remaining soft dentin, pulp protection, retention form, the finishing of external walls, and cleaning/inspecting. Specifically any remaining soft axial wall dentin is removed (as indicated) with a No. 2 or No. 4 round bur. Any old restorative material remaining (including base and liner) may be left if (1) no evidence of recurrent caries exists, (2) the periphery of the base and liner is intact, and (3) the tooth is asymptomatic. With proper outline form, the axial line angles are already in sound dentin. If needed, an appropriate liner or base is applied.

Because the mesial, distal, gingival, and incisal walls of the tooth preparation are perpendicular to the external tooth surface, they usually diverge. Consequently this form provides no inherent retention, and retention form must be provided to retain the amalgam. A No. $\frac{1}{4}$ round bur is used to prepare two retention grooves, one along the incisoaxial line angle and the other along the gingivoaxial line angle (see Fig. 10.145). The handpiece is positioned so that the No. $\frac{1}{4}$ round bur is directed generally to bisect the angle formed at the junction of the axial wall and the incisal (i.e., occlusal) wall. Ideally the direction of the incisal (i.e., occlusal) groove is slightly more incisal (i.e., occlusal) than axial, and the direction of the gingival groove is slightly more gingival than axial. Alternatively, four retention coves may be prepared, one in each of the four axial point angles of the preparation (Fig. 10.146).

Using four coves instead of two full-length grooves conserves the dentin near the pulp, reducing the possibility of a mechanical pulp exposure. The depth of the grooves (or coves) should be approximately 0.25 to 0.5 mm. It is important that the retention grooves be adequate because they provide the only retention form to the preparation. Regardless, the grooves should not remove dentin immediately supporting enamel. In a large Class V amalgam preparation, extending the retention groove circumferentially around all the internal line angles of the tooth preparation may enhance the retention form.

If access is inadequate for use of the No. $\frac{1}{4}$ round bur, an angle-former chisel may be used to prepare the retention form. Additionally, a No. $33\frac{1}{2}$ bur may be used. Both methods result in retention grooves that are angular, but positioned in the same location and approximately to the same depth as when the No. $\frac{1}{4}$ round bur is used. The rounded retention form created with the No. $\frac{1}{4}$ round bur is generally preferred, however, because amalgam is able to be condensed into rounded areas more readily than into sharp areas, resulting in better adaptation of amalgam into the retention grooves. If necessary, suitable hand instruments (e.g., chisels, margin trimmers) are used to plane the enamel margins, verifying soundness and 90-degree cavosurface angles. Finally the preparation is cleaned of debris and inspected for completeness.

Large Preparations That Include Line Angles

A caries lesion on the facial (or lingual) surface may extend beyond the line angles of the tooth. Maxillary molars, particularly the second molars, are most commonly affected by these extensive defects (Fig. 10.147A). In this example, if the remainder of the

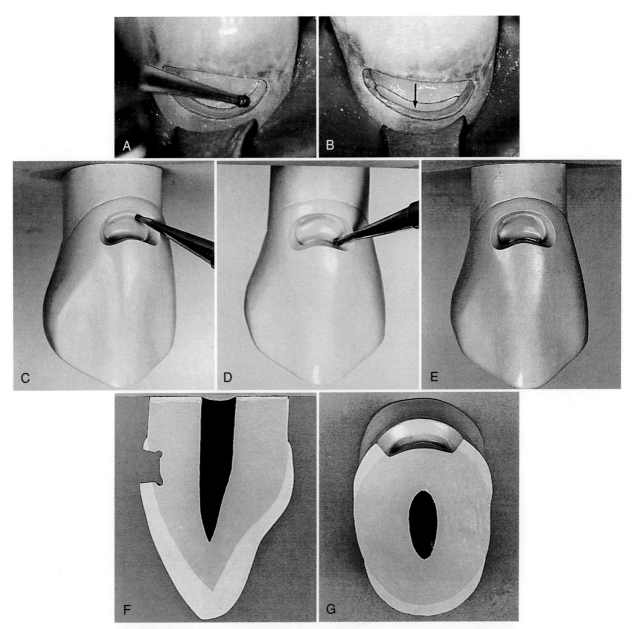

• **Fig. 10.145**   Retention form. A, A No. ¼ round bur positioned to prepare the gingival retention groove. B, Gingival retention groove *(arrow)* prepared along the gingivoaxial line angle generally to bisect the angle formed by the gingival and axial walls. Ideally the direction of preparation is slightly more gingival than pulpal. An incisal retention groove is prepared along the incisoaxial line angle and directed similarly. C and D, A groove is placed with a No. ¼ round bur along the gingivoaxial and incisoaxial line angles 0.2 mm inside the DEJ and ~0.25 – 0.5 mm deep. Note the slight pulpal inclination of the shank of the No. ¼ round bur. E, Facial view. F, Incisogingival section. Grooves depthwise are directed mostly incisally (gingivally) and slightly pulpally. G, Mesiodistal section.

distal surface is sound and the distal caries lesion is accessible facially, the facial restoration should extend around the line angle. This prevents the need for a Class II proximal restoration to restore the distal surface. However, the operator should strive not to overextend the occlusal wall of the distal surface preserving as much sound tooth structure as possible to support the distal marginal ridge. As much of the preparation as possible should be completed with a fissure bur. A round bur approximately the same diameter as the fissure bur is then used to initiate the distal portion of the preparation (see Fig. 10.147B and C). Smaller round burs should be used to accentuate the internal line angles of the distal portion.

Preparing the facial portion first provides better access and visibility to the distal portion. Occasionally hand instruments may be useful for completing the distal half of the preparation when space for the handpiece is limited (see Fig. 10.147D–F).

Grooves placed along the entire length of the occlusoaxial and gingivoaxial line angles help ensure retention of the restoration. The No. ¼ round bur is used as previously described to prepare the retention grooves. A gingival margin trimmer or a 7-85-2½ -6 angle-former chisel may be used in the distal half of the preparation to provide retention form when access for the handpiece is limited (see Fig. 10.147G and H).

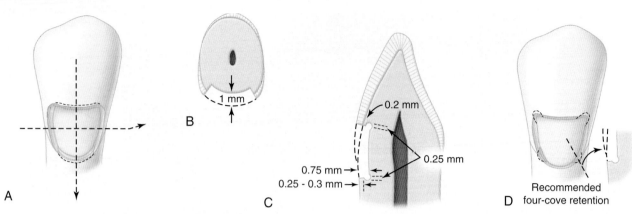

• **Fig. 10.146** A–C, Extended Class V tooth preparation (*A*) with the axial wall contoured parallel to the DEJ mesiodistally (*B*) and incisogingivally (*C*). The axial wall pulpal depth is 1 mm in the crown and 0.75 mm in the root. In addition, note location and direction depth (~0.25 – 0.5 mm) of the retention grooves and the dimension of the gingival wall (0.25 mm) from the root surface to the retention groove. D, Large Class V preparation with retention coves prepared in the four axial point angles.

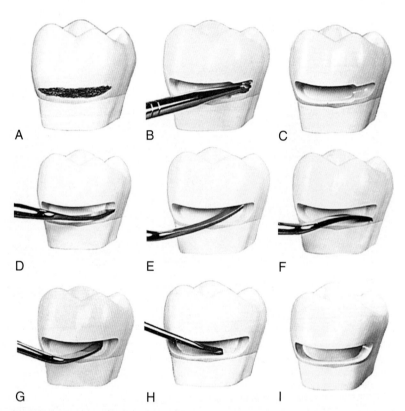

• **Fig. 10.147** Tooth preparation on a maxillary molar. A, Caries lesion extending around distofacial corner of the tooth. B and C, Distal extension is accomplished with round bur. D–F, A gingival margin trimmer may be useful in completing the distal half of the preparation when handpiece access is limited. G, A gingival margin trimmer may be used to provide the retention grooves. H, An angle-former chisel may be used to prepare the retention grooves in the distal portion of the preparation. I, Completed tooth preparation.

Because of the proximity of the coronoid process, access to the facial surfaces of maxillary molars, particularly the second molars, is often limited. Having the patient partially close and shift the mandible toward the tooth being restored improves access and visibility (Fig. 10.148).

If the Class V outline form approaches an existing proximal restoration, it is better to extend slightly into the bulk of the proximal restoration rather than to leave a thin section of the tooth structure between the two restorations (Fig. 10.149). In this illustration the previously placed amalgam serves as the distal wall of the preparation. When proper treatment requires Class II and V amalgam restorations on the same tooth, the Class II preparation and restoration is completed before initiating the Class V restoration. If the Class V restoration was accomplished first, it might be damaged by the matrix band and wedge needed for the Class II restoration.

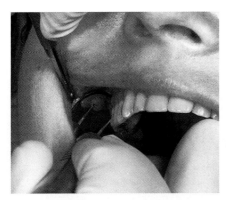

• **Fig. 10.148** The mandible shifted laterally for improved access and visibility.

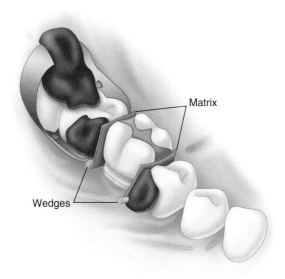

Matrix

Wedges

• **Fig. 10.150** Application of the matrix to confine amalgam in the mesial and distal extensions of the preparation.

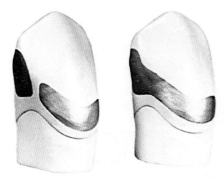

• **Fig. 10.149** When a Class V outline form closely approaches an existing restoration, the preparation should be extended to remove the remaining thin enamel wall to achieve adjoining restorations.

The preparation should then be cleaned, carefully inspected as indicated in General Concepts Guiding Preparation for Amalgam Restorations, and any final modifications completed.

Restorative Technique for Class V Amalgam Preparations

Desensitizer Placement

A dentin desensitizer is placed over the prepared tooth structure per manufacturer instructions. Excess moisture is removed without desiccating the dentin.

Matrix Placement

Most Class V amalgam restorations are accomplished without the use of any type of matrix. The most difficult condensation occurs in a tooth preparation with an axial wall that is convex mesiodistally. Two alternative methods for insertion may be used. The preferred method is the application of a matrix that confines amalgam in the mesial and distal portions of the preparation (Fig. 10.150). Short lengths of stainless steel matrix material, one each for the mesial and distal surfaces, are passed through the proximal contacts, carefully guided into the gingival sulcus, and wedged. The strips must be wide enough to extend occlusally through the respective proximal contacts and long enough to extend slightly past the facial line angles. The strip usually requires rigid material support for stability. The strips offer resistance against condensing the mesial and distal portions, which provides support for condensing the center of the restoration. The gingival edge of the steel strip often

must be trimmed to conform to the circumferential contour (level) of the base of the gingival sulcus to prevent soft tissue damage. Rather than using two short pieces, the operator may use a longer length that is passed through one proximal contact, extended around the lingual surface, and passed through the other contact, forming a U-shaped matrix. Trimming the gingival edge to conform to the interproximal soft tissue anatomy usually is more difficult with one matrix strip than when two strips are used.

A conventional Tofflemire band and retainer may be used with a window cut into the band, with a high-speed handpiece bur, to allow access to the preparation for condensation (Fig. 10.151). Alternatively, the tooth may be prepared and restored in sections without using a matrix. Each successive section of the preparation should be extended slightly into the previously condensed portion to ensure caries lesion removal.

Insertion and Carving of the Amalgam

The amalgam carrier is used to insert the mixed amalgam into the preparation in small increments (Fig. 10.152A). Amalgam is condensed into the retention areas first by using an appropriate condenser (see Fig. 10.152B). Amalgam is then condensed against the mesial and distal walls of the preparation (see Fig. 10.152C). Finally a sufficient bulk of amalgam is placed in the central portion to allow for carving the correct contour (see Fig. 10.152D). As the surface of the restoration becomes more convex, condensation becomes increasingly difficult. It is important to guard against the "land sliding" of amalgam during overpacking. A large condenser or flat-bladed instrument held against amalgam may help resist pressure applied elsewhere on the restoration (Fig. 10.153).

Carving may begin immediately after the insertion of amalgam (Fig. 10.154). All carving should be done using the side of the explorer tine or a Hollenback No. 3 carver held parallel to the margins. The side of the carving instrument always should rest on the unprepared tooth surface adjacent to the prepared cavosurface margin; this prevents overcarving or submargination of the restoration. The carving procedure is begun by removing excess amalgam to expose the incisal (or occlusal) margin. Removal of excess material

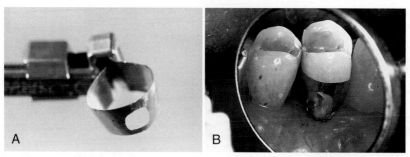

• **Fig. 10.151** Customized matrix band used to restore an area of proximal root caries. A, Conventional Tofflemire matrix with window cut into the band using a high-speed bur to allow access for condensation. B, Matrix in place around the tooth, allowing lingual access to preparation.

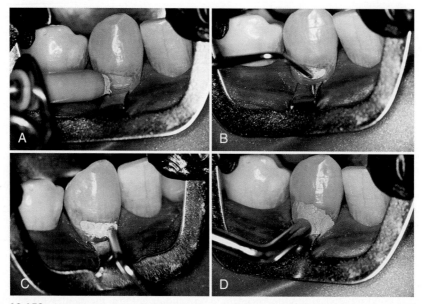

• **Fig. 10.152** Inserting amalgam. A, Place amalgam into the preparation in small increments. B, Condense first into the retention grooves with a small condenser. C, Condense against the mesial and distal walls. D, Overfill and provide sufficient bulk to allow for carving.

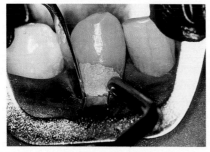

• **Fig. 10.153** Use a large condenser or a flat-bladed instrument to offer resistance to condensation pressure applied elsewhere on the restoration.

continues until the mesial and distal margins are exposed. Finally, material excess at the gingival margin is carved away. Carving the marginal areas should result in developing the desired convex contours in the completed restoration. Improper use of the carving instruments results in a poorly contoured restoration. Note in Fig. 10.20 how carving instruments are positioned to provide the desired contours. No amalgam excess should remain at the margins because amalgam may break away, creating a defect at the margin, or cause

gingival inflammation and increased risk of secondary caries from biofilm accumulation.

In some instances it is appropriate to change facial contours because of altered soft tissue levels (e.g., cervical lesions in periodontally treated patients). Facial contours may be increased (or relocated) only enough to prevent food impaction into the gingival sulcus and to provide access for the patient to clean the area. Overcontouring must be avoided as it results in reduced stimulation and cleansing of the gingiva during mastication.

When a rubber dam and the No. 212 cervical retainer have been used for isolation, the retainer is removed using care to open the jaws of the retainer wide enough to prevent damage to the surface of the restoration. The rubber dam is removed and the area is examined carefully to ensure that no amalgam particles remain in the sulcus.

When a retraction cord is used for isolation, it may interfere with carving any excess amalgam at the gingival margin. If so, removal of the gross excess of amalgam is followed by careful removal of the cord, followed by completion of the carving along the margin.

Finishing and Polishing of the Amalgam

If carving procedures were performed correctly, no finishing of the restoration should be required. A slightly moistened cotton

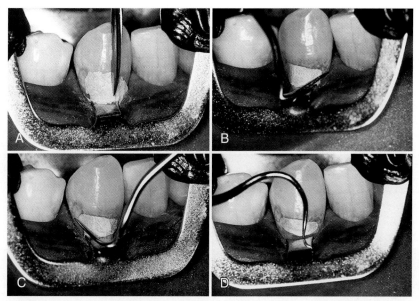

• **Fig. 10.154**   Carving and contouring the restoration. A, Begin the carving procedure by removing any excess and locating the incisal margin. B and C, An explorer may be used to remove the excess and locate the mesial and distal margins. D, Remove the excess and locate the gingival margin.

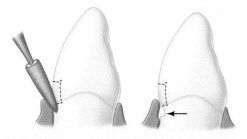

• **Fig. 10.155**   Incorrect use of a pointed stone at the gingival margin results in the removal of cementum, notching of the tooth structure gingival to the margin, or both.

pellet held in cotton pliers may be used to further smooth the carved restoration. Additional finishing and polishing of amalgam restorations may be necessary, however, to correct a marginal discrepancy or to improve contour. Care is required when using stones or any rotating cutting instruments on margins positioned below the CEJ because of the possibility of removing cementum, notching the tooth structure gingival to the margin, or both (Fig. 10.155). Fig. 10.156 illustrates reshaping a rubber abrasive point to allow optimal access to the gingival portion of a Class V amalgam restoration. A rubber abrasive cup may be preferred for finishing convex surfaces, like Class V restorations, if used carefully.

One measure of clinical success of cervical amalgam restorations is the length of time the restoration serves without failing (Fig. 10.157). Properly placed Class V amalgams have the potential to be clinically acceptable for many years. Some cervical amalgam restorations show evidence of failure, however, even after a short period. Inattention to tooth preparation principles, improper manipulation of the restorative material, and moisture contamination contribute to early failure. Extended service life of the restoration depends on the operator's care in following accepted treatment techniques and proper care by the patient. Any additional finishing and polishing of the Class V amalgam should follow the approach presented in General Concepts Guiding Restoration with Amalgam.

Clinical Technique for Class VI Amalgam Restorations

The Class VI tooth preparation is used to restore the incisal edge of anterior teeth or the cusp tip regions of posterior teeth (see Fig. 10.26C). Such tooth preparations are frequently indicated where attrition (loss of tooth substance from the occluding of food, abrasives, and opposing teeth) has removed enamel to expose the underlying dentin on those areas (Fig. 10.158). When the softer dentin is exposed, it wears faster than the surrounding enamel, resulting in "cupped-out" areas of the cusp tips. Intrinsic or extrinsic erosion also may be contributing to the excessive loss of tooth structure. Diagnostic steps, to identify the etiology of the tooth structure loss, are indicated and may involve referral for evaluation of potential gastroesophageal reflux disease. As the dentin support is lost, enamel begins to fracture away and more dentin is exposed, which often causes sensitivity. Sensitivity to hot and cold is a frequent complaint with Class VI lesions, and some patients are bothered by food impaction in deeper depressions. Enamel edges may become jagged and sharp to the tongue, lips, or cheek. Lip, tongue, or cheek biting is occasionally a complaint. Rounding and smoothing such incisoaxial (or occlusoaxial) edges is an excellent service to the patient. Early recognition and restoration of these lesions is recommended to limit the loss of dentin and the subsequent loss of enamel supported by this dentin.

The Class VI tooth preparation may be indicated to restore the hypoplastic pit occasionally found on cusp tips (Fig. 10.159). Such developmental faults are vulnerable to caries lesion formation, especially in high-risk patients, and should be restored as soon as they are detected.

Amalgam may be selected for posterior Class VI preparations because of its wear resistance and longevity. Moisture control for Class VI restorations is usually achieved with cotton roll isolation. Class VI amalgam preparations may be accomplished with a small tapered fissure bur (e.g., No. 169 L or 271) and involves extension to place the cavosurface margin on enamel that has sound dentin support (see Fig. 10.158B). The preparation walls may need to

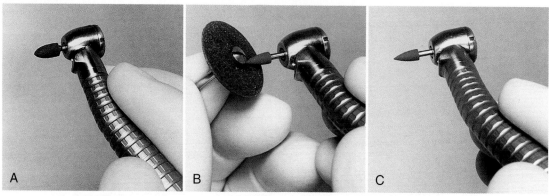

• **Fig. 10.156** Reshaping a rubber abrasive point against a mounted carborundum disk.

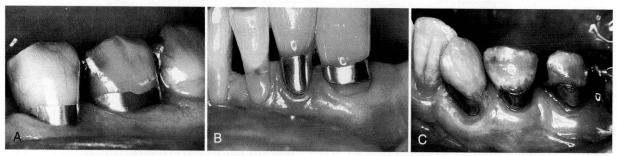

• **Fig. 10.157** A, Six-year-old cervical amalgam restorations. B, After 16 years, some abrasion and erosion are evident at the gingival margin of the lateral incisor and canine restorations. C, Twenty-year-old cervical amalgam restorations.

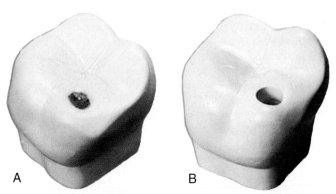

• **Fig. 10.158** Class VI preparation. A, Exposed dentin on the mesiofacial cusp. B, Tooth preparation necessary to restore the involved area.

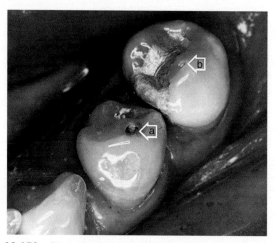

• **Fig. 10.159** Class VI lesions. Carious cusp tip fault on the first premolar (a). Noncarious fault on the second premolar (b).

diverge occlusally to ensure a 90-degree cavosurface margin. A depth of 1.5 mm is sufficient to provide bulk of material for strength. Retention of the restoration is ensured by the creation of small undercuts along the internal line angles similar to other areas where secondary retention is indicated. Conservative tooth preparation is particularly important with Class VI preparations because it is easy to undermine the enamel on incisal edges and cusp tips. The preparation should be cleaned, carefully inspected as indicated in General Concepts Guiding Preparation for Amalgam Restorations, and any final modifications completed. Insertion, carving, finishing, and polishing are similar to procedures described in General Concepts Guiding Restoration with Amalgam.

Some older patients have excessive occlusal wear of most of their teeth in the form of large concave areas with much exposed dentin. Teeth with excessive wear may require indirect restorations or, at least, efforts to limit further loss of tooth structure.

Clinical Technique for Complex Amalgam Restorations

Indications

Complex posterior restorations are indicated when tooth structure is missing due to cusp fracture, severe caries lesion development, or when replacement of existing restorative material is necessary. Complex amalgam preparations should be considered when large amounts of tooth structure are missing, when one or more cusps need to be covered, and when increased resistance and retention forms are needed (Fig. 10.160).[121] Complex amalgams may be used as (1) definitive (final) restorations, (2) foundations, (3) control restorations in teeth that have a questionable pulpal or periodontal prognosis, or (4) control restorations in teeth with acute or severe caries lesions. When determining the appropriateness of a complex amalgam restoration, the factors discussed in the following sections must be considered.

Resistance and Retention Forms

In a tooth with a severe caries lesion or existing restorative material, any undermined enamel or weak tooth structure subject to fracture must be removed and replaced. Usually a weakened tooth is best restored with a properly designed indirect (usually cast) restoration that prevents tooth fracture caused by mastication forces (see Online Chapter 18). In selected cases, amalgam preparations that improve the resistance form of a tooth may be designed (Fig. 10.161).

When conventional retention features are not adequate because of insufficient remaining tooth structure, the retention form may be enhanced by using auxiliary features such as slots and pins. The type of retention features needed depend on the amount of tooth structure remaining and the tooth being restored. As more tooth structure is lost, more auxiliary retention is required. Slots and pins provide additional resistance and retention form to the tooth when remaining vertical walls are inadequate.

Status and Prognosis of the Tooth

A tooth with a severe caries lesion that may require endodontic therapy or crown lengthening or that has an uncertain periodontal prognosis often is treated initially with a control restoration. A control restoration helps (1) protect the pulp from the oral cavity (i.e., fluids, thermal stresses, pH changes, bacteria), (2) provide an anatomic contour that is consistent with gingival health, (3) facilitate control of acidogenic biofilm and resultant caries risk, and (4) provide some resistance against tooth fracture (or propagation of an existing fracture). (See Chapter 2 for caries-control rationale and techniques.)

The status and prognosis of the tooth determine the size, number, and placement of retention features. Larger restorations generally require more retention. The size, number, and location of retention features demand greater care in smaller teeth. Carelessness may increase the risk of pulpal irritation or exposure.

Role of the Tooth in Overall Treatment Plan

The restorative treatment choice for a tooth is influenced by its role in the overall treatment plan. Although complex amalgam restorations are used occasionally as an alternative to indirect restorations, particularly due to cost savings, they often are used as foundations for full-coverage restorations. Abutment teeth for fixed prostheses may use a complex restoration as a foundation (Fig. 10.162). Extensive caries or previous restorations on abutment

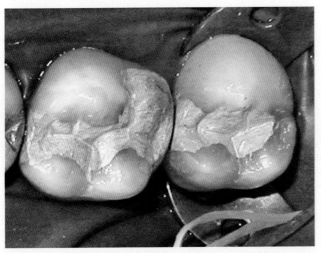

• **Fig. 10.160** Mesioocclusodistolingual (MODL) complex amalgam tooth No. 3.

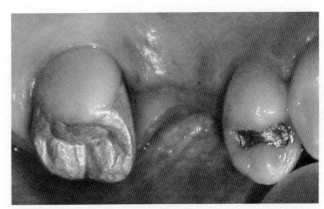

• **Fig. 10.162** Mesioocclusodistofacial (MODF) amalgam foundation for abutment tooth No. 15 in preparation for a 3 unit fixed partial denture.

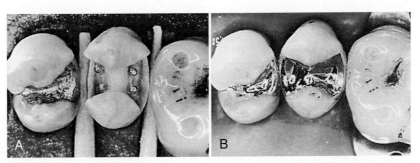

• **Fig. 10.161** Maxillary second premolar weakened by an extensive caries lesion and by the small fracture line extending mesiodistally on the center of the excavated dentinal wall. A, Minikin pins placed in the gingival floor improve resistance form after amalgam has been placed. B, Restorations polished.

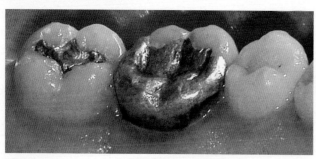

• **Fig. 10.163** Mesioocclusodistolingual (MODL) complex amalgam tooth #19.

teeth for removable prostheses generally indicate an indirect restoration for the resistance and retention forms and for development of external surface contours for retention of the prosthesis. A tooth may be treated with a complex direct restoration if adequate resistance and retention forms are provided. For patients with periodontal and orthodontic problems, the complex restoration may be the restoration of choice until the final phase of treatment, when indirect restorations may be preferred.

Occlusion and Economics

Complex amalgam restorations are sometimes indicated as interim restorations for teeth that require elaborate occlusal alterations, ranging from vertical dimension changes to correcting occlusal plane discrepancies. When cost of indirect restorations is a major factor for the patient, the complex direct amalgam restoration may be an appropriate treatment option, provided that adequate resistance and retention forms are included (Fig. 10.163).[122,123]

Age and Health of Patient

For some older patients and/or those who are debilitated, complex amalgam restoration may be the treatment preferred over the more expensive and time-consuming indirect restoration.

Contraindications

The complex amalgam restoration may be contraindicated if the tooth cannot be restored properly with direct restoration because of anatomic or functional considerations (or both). The complex amalgam restoration also may be contraindicated if the area to be restored has esthetic importance for the patient.

Advantages

Conservation of Tooth Structure

The preparation for a complex amalgam restoration is usually more conservative than the preparation for an indirect restoration.

Appointment Time

The complex restoration may be completed in one appointment. An indirect restoration generally requires at least two appointments unless it is done using a chairside computer-assisted design/computer-assisted machining (CAD/CAM) system.

Resistance and Retention Forms

Amalgam restorations with cusp coverage significantly increase the fracture resistance of weakened teeth compared with amalgam restorations without cusp coverage.[124] Resistance and retention forms may be significantly increased by the use of slots and pins (discussed in subsequent sections).

Reduced Cost

The complex amalgam restoration may be utilized to reinforce and stabilize compromised posterior teeth at a much reduced cost to the patient. It may serve as a definitive final restoration or an intermediate-term restoration with a long-term goal of indirect, more costly restoration and protection of the tooth.

Disadvantages

Tooth Anatomy

Proper contours and occlusal contacts and anatomy are sometimes difficult to achieve with large, complex restorations.

Resistance Form

Resistance form is more difficult to develop with a complex amalgam as compared to the preparation of a tooth for a cusp-covering onlay (skirting axial line angles of the tooth [see Online Chapter 18]) or a full crown. The complex amalgam restoration does not protect the tooth from fracture as effectively as a full-coverage indirect restoration.

Tooth Preparation for Complex Amalgam Restorations

In this section various types of Complex Amalgam preparation procedures are discussed before the restoration technique is presented. Also the word "vertical" is used to describe tooth preparation walls and other preparation aspects that are approximately parallel to the long axis of the tooth. The word "horizontal" is used to describe the walls and other aspects that are approximately perpendicular to the long axis of the tooth. Every effort should be made to protect the pulp as early as possible when accomplishing the procedures associated with complex amalgam restorations.

Preparation for Cusp Coverage Complex Amalgams

General concepts of initial tooth preparation presented in earlier sections apply to the complex amalgam preparations described here. When a caries lesion is extensive with resultant loss of dentin necessary to support occlusally loaded areas of the tooth, reduction of one or more of the cusps followed by coverage with amalgam may be indicated. When the facial or lingual extension exceeds two thirds the distance from a primary fissure toward the cusp tip (or when the faciolingual extension of the occlusal preparation exceeds two thirds the distance between the facial and lingual cusp tips), reduction of the cusp for coverage with amalgam usually is required for the development of adequate resistance form (Fig. 10.164A; see also Fig. 4.13). For cusps prone to fracture, coverage reduces the risk of fracture and extends the life of the restoration.[125,126] Complex amalgam restorations that cover one or more cusps have documented longevity of 72% after 15 years.[123,127]

The operator uses the bur to reduce the cusp, following the mesiodistal inclines of the cusp; this results in a uniform reduction (see Fig. 10.164B–E). If only one of two facial (or lingual) cusps is to be covered, the cusp reduction should extend slightly beyond the facial (or lingual) groove area, provide the correct amount of tooth structure removal, and meet the adjacent, unreduced cusp to create a 90-degree cavosurface margin. This approach results in adequate thickness and edge strength of the amalgam (see Fig. 10.164F and G). Cusp reduction and coverage reduce the amount of vertical preparation wall height and increase the need for the use of secondary retention features (Fig. 10.165). An increased retention form may be provided by proximal box retention grooves

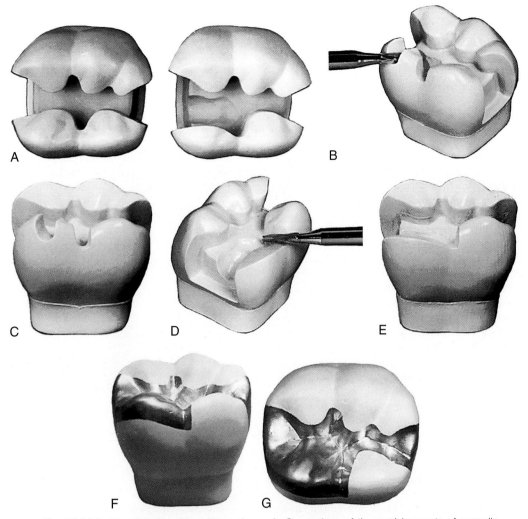

• **Fig. 10.164**   Covering the cusp with amalgam. A, Comparison of the mesial aspects of normally extended *(left)* and extensive *(right)* mesioocclusodistal tooth preparation. The resistance form of the mesiolingual cusp with extensive preparation is compromised and cusp coverage with amalgam is indicated. B, Preparing depth cuts. C, Depth cuts prepared. D, Reducing the cusp. E, Cusp reduced. F and G, Final restoration.

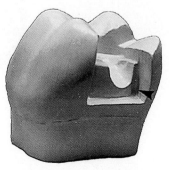

• **Fig. 10.165**   A retention groove is associated with the remaining vertical wall of a cusp requiring reduction.

but may require the use of slots and/or pins (as described in subsequent sections). If indicated, cusp reduction and coverage increase the resistance form of the tooth.[123,128]

Reduction of the unsupported cusp should be accomplished during the initial tooth preparation because it improves access and

visibility for subsequent steps. If the cusp to be reduced is located at the correct occlusal height before preparation, depth cuts should be made on the remaining occlusal surface of each cusp to be covered, using the side of a carbide fissure bur or a suitable diamond instrument (see Fig. 10.164B). The depth cuts should be a minimum of 2 mm for functional cusps and 1.5 mm for nonfunctional cusps.[126] These dimensions provide adequate strength for amalgam by preventing flexure of the restoration during loading. To reduce the cusp, the dentist orients the bur parallel to the cuspal incline (lingual incline for facial cusp reductions and facial inclines for lingual cusp reduction) and makes several depth cuts in the cusp (to a depth of 1.5 or 2 mm as indicated). The depth cuts provide guides for the correct amount of cusp reduction. Without depth cuts, after the beginning reduction of the cusp, the operator may no longer know how much more reduction is necessary. When using the restoration to correct an occlusal relationship, if the unreduced cusp height is located at less than the correct occlusal height, the depth cuts may be less. Likewise, if the unreduced cusp height is located higher than the correct occlusal height, the depth cuts may be deeper. The goal is to ensure that the final restoration has restored cusps with a minimal thickness of 2 mm of amalgam for functional cusps and 1.5 mm of amalgam for nonfunctional cusps (see Fig. 10.164C), while developing an appropriate occlusal relationship. Using the depth cuts as a guide, the reduction is completed to provide for a uniform reduction of tooth structure (see Fig. 10.164D). The occlusal contour of the reduced cusp should be similar to the normal contour of the unreduced cusp. Any sharp internal corners of the tooth preparation formed at the junction of prepared surfaces should be rounded to reduce stress concentration in the amalgam and improve its resistance to fracture from occlusal forces (see Fig. 10.164E). When reducing only one of two facial or lingual cusps, the cusp reduction should be extended just past the facial or lingual groove, creating a vertical wall against the adjacent unreduced cusp. Fig. 10.164F and G illustrate a final restoration.

Mandibular First Premolar

The lingual cusp of the mandibular first premolar may need to be reduced for coverage with amalgam if the lingual margin of the occlusal step extends more than two thirds the distance from the central fissure to the cuspal eminence (Fig. 10.166). Special attention is given to such cusp reduction because retention is severely diminished when the cusp is overreduced resulting in elimination of the lingual wall of the occlusal portion. Depth cuts of 1.5 mm aid the operator in establishing the correct amount of cusp reduction and in conserving a small portion of the lingual wall in the occlusal step. It is acceptable when restoring diminutive nonfunctional cusps, such as the lingual cusp of a mandibular first premolar, to reduce the cusp only 0.5 to 1 mm and restore the cusp to achieve an amalgam thickness of 1.5 mm. This procedure conserves more of the lingual wall of the isthmus for added retention form.

Maxillary First Molar

The procedure for reducing the distolingual cusp of a maxillary first molar for coverage is illustrated in Fig. 10.167. Extending the facial or lingual wall of a proximal box to include the entire

cusp is accomplished (if necessary) to include weak or carious tooth structure or existing restorative material. The lingual groove may be extended arbitrarily to increase the retention form (see Fig. 10.167B and C). When possible, opposing vertical walls should be formed to converge occlusally, to enhance the primary retention form (see Fig. 10.167C and D). The pulpal and gingival walls should be relatively flat and perpendicular to the long axis of the tooth. Secondary retention features may be indicated when the divergence of proximal walls results in limited primary retention form (see Fig. 10.167D). Mesial extension of the preparation into the mesiolingual cusp should be enough to allow placement of the distooblique and lingual groove within the amalgam restoration (see Fig. 10.167E).

Mandibular First Molar

Reducing the distal cusp is an alternative to extending the entire distofacial wall when the occlusal margin crosses the cuspal eminence (Fig. 10.168A; compare with Fig. 10.83). A minimal reduction

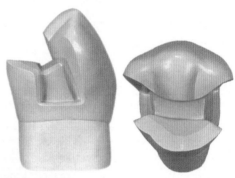

• **Fig. 10.166** Mandibular first premolar with the lingual cusp reduced for coverage with amalgam.

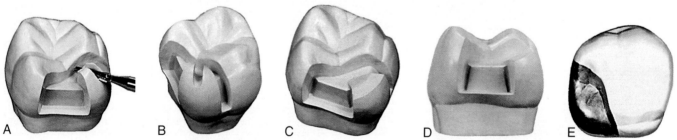

• **Fig. 10.167** Reduction of the distolingual cusp of the maxillary molar. A, Cutting a depth gauge groove with the side of the bur. B, Completed depth gauge groove. C and D, Completed cusp reduction. E, Distoocclusolingual complex amalgam.

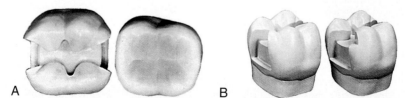

• **Fig. 10.168** Mandibular first molar. A, Reduction of the distal cusp is indicated when the occlusal margin crosses the cuspal eminence. B, Distofacial view of the distal cusp shown in A before reduction for coverage (left); the distal cusp after reduction (right). A reduction of 2 mm is necessary to provide for minimal 2-mm thickness of amalgam.

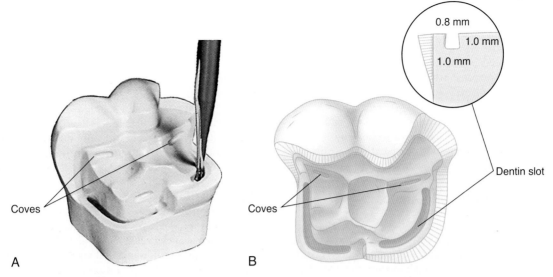

• **Fig. 10.169** Slots. A and B, With a No. 330 bur, dentinal slots are prepared approximately 1 mm deep and 0.5 to 1 mm inside the DEJ.

of 2 mm will allow a 2-mm thickness of amalgam over the reduced cusp (see Fig. 10.168B). The cusp reduction should result in a butt joint between the tooth structure and amalgam. When possible, reducing and covering the distal cusp is more desirable than extending the distofacial proximal margin because this conserves tooth structure of the functional cusp, and the remaining portion of the cusp helps in applying the matrix for the development of proper distofacial embrasure form. The plane of the reduced cusp should parallel the facial (or lingual) outline of the unreduced cusp mesiodistally and the cuspal incline emanating from the central groove faciolingually.

Tooth Preparation for Slot-Retained Amalgam Restorations

When loss of vertical coronal height is approximately 2 to 4 mm, then use of slots, in horizontal areas where no vertical walls remain, may be indicated to gain secondary retention form for the complex amalgam restoration (Figs. 10.169, 10.170, and 10.171). A slot is a horizontal retention groove in dentin (see Fig. 10.169). Slots are placed in the gingival floor of a preparation with a No. 330 bur (see Fig. 10.169B, inset). In general, slots should be about 1 mm wide and 1 mm deep, should be placed in the line-angle areas of the tooth, should be 2 to 4 mm in length (depending on the distance between remaining vertical walls), and be positioned 0.5 to 1 mm inside the DEJ. In general, one slot per missing axial line angle should be used. Increasing the width and depth of the slot does not increase the retentive strength of the amalgam restoration.[129] Slot length depends on the extent of the tooth preparation. A slot may be continuous or segmented, depending on the amount of missing tooth structure and whether pin retention is being planned (see subsequent sections). Shorter slots provide as much resistance to horizontal force as do longer slots.[130] Preparations with shorter slots fail less frequently than do preparations with longer slots.[130] Slot design should be such that it is independently retentive as a singular feature (the internal walls of the slot should be convergent) (see Fig. 10.169B, inset). In addition, the walls of the slot should work together with other vertical walls to create

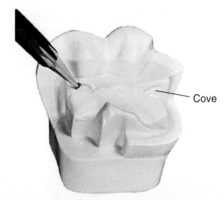

• **Fig. 10.170** Coves prepared in dentin with No. ¼ bur, where appropriate.

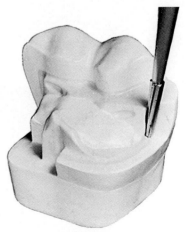

• **Fig. 10.171** Vertical grooves prepared in dentin with a No. ¼ round or No. 169L bur, where appropriate.

an overall convergence of the preparation so as to enhance retention of the restoration.

In addition to any slot placement, retention grooves and coves may be utilized in association with remaining vertical walls (Figs. 10.172 and 10.173). Coves and retention grooves should be prepared when possible. Coves are prepared in a horizontal plane, and grooves are prepared in a vertical plane.

Coves also may be used in preparations using slots (see Fig. 10.169). Proximal retention grooves, as described for wide Class II preparations, also are placed in the proximal box and in other locations where sufficient vertical tooth preparation permits (see Figs. 10.165 and 10.171).

Tooth Preparation for Pin-Retained Amalgam Restorations

When severe carious destruction or cusp fracture has resulted in the loss of 4 mm or more of vertical coronal height, consideration should be given to the use of a parapulpal retention pin to regain some of the lost vertical height. A *pin-retained amalgam* (also referred to as a "pin-amalgam") is defined as any restoration requiring the placement of one or more pins in dentin to provide adequate resistance and retention forms. Pins are used whenever adequate resistance and retention forms are not able to be established with slots, grooves, or undercuts only.[131] Pins placed into prepared pinholes (also referred to as *pin channels*) are used to provide auxiliary resistance and retention forms. The pin-retained amalgam

is an important adjunct in the restoration of teeth with extensive caries lesions or fractures.[132] Amalgam restorations including pins have significantly greater retention compared with restorations using boxes only or restorations relying solely on bonding systems.[133] However, caution is indicated when using pins. Preparing pinholes and placing pins may create craze lines or fractures and internal stresses in dentin.[134-136] Such craze lines and internal stress areas may have little or no clinical significance, but they may be important when minimal dentin is present. Preparation steps for pin retention have increased risk of penetrating into the pulp or perforating the external tooth surface. The use of pins decreases the tensile and horizontal strength of associated amalgam restorations.[137,138]

Types of Parapulpal Retention Pins

The most frequently used type of parapulpal pin is the self-threading pin. The pin-retained amalgam restoration using self-threading pins originally was described by Going in 1966.[139] Friction-locked and cemented pins, although still available, are rarely used (Fig. 10.174). The diameter of the prepared pinhole is 0.0381 to 0.1016 mm smaller than the diameter of the pin (Table 10.1). The threads engage dentin as the pin is inserted, thus retaining the pin. The elasticity (resiliency) of dentin permits insertion of a threaded pin into a hole of smaller diameter.[140] Although the threads of self-threading pins do not engage dentin for their entire width, self-threading pins are the most retentive of the three types of pins (Fig. 10.175), being three to six times more retentive than cemented pins.[141-143]

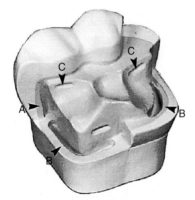

• **Fig. 10.172** Groove (A), slots (B), and coves (C).

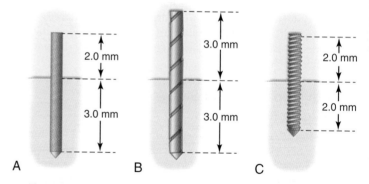

• **Fig. 10.174** Three types of pins. A, Cemented. B, Friction locked. C, Self-threading.

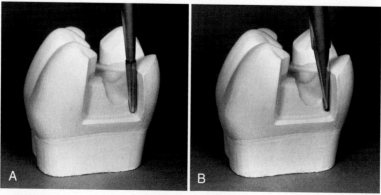

• **Fig. 10.173** Placement of retention grooves. A, Position of No. 169L bur to prepare the retention groove. B, Groove prepared with No. ¼ bur.

Vertical and horizontal stresses, potentially resulting in craze lines (cracks), are generated in dentin when a self-threading pin is inserted. Craze lines in dentin are related to the size of the pin. The insertion of 0.787-mm self-threading pins produces more dentinal craze lines than does the insertion of 0.533-mm self-threading pins.[144] Some evidence suggests, however, that self-threading pins may not cause dentinal crazing.[140] Pulpal stress is maximal when the self-threading pin is inserted perpendicular to the pulp.[145] The depth of the pinhole varies from 1.3 to 2 mm, depending on the diameter of the pin used.[146] Recommended pinhole depth is generally accepted to be 2 mm.

Several styles of self-threading pins are available. The Thread Mate System (TMS) (Coltène/Whaledent Inc., Cuyahoga, Ohio) is the most widely used self-threading pin system because of its (1) versatility, (2) wide range of pin sizes, (3) color-coding system, and (4) greater retentiveness.[147,148] TMS pins are available in gold-plated stainless steel or in titanium. Titanium alloy pins (Max Restorative Pins, Coltène/Whaledent Inc.) are also available.

Factors Affecting Retention of the Pin in Dentin and Amalgam

Type
With regard to the retentiveness of the pin in dentin, the self-threading pin is the most retentive, the friction-locked pin is intermediate, and the cemented pin is the least retentive.[141]

Surface Characteristics
The number and depth of the elevations (serrations or threads) on the pin influence the retention of the pin in the amalgam

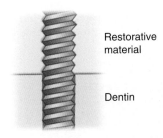

Restorative material

Dentin

• **Fig. 10.175** The complete width of the threads of self-threading pins does not engage dentin.

restoration. The shape of the self-threading pin results in the greatest retention of amalgam.

Orientation, Number, and Diameter
Placing pins in a nonparallel manner increases their ability to retain the restoration; however, bending pins to improve their retention in amalgam is not advised as the bends may interfere with adequate condensation of amalgam around the pin and decrease amalgam retention. In addition, bending also may weaken the pin and risk fracture of the adjacent dentin. Pins should be bent only to provide for an adequate amount of amalgam (approximately 1 mm) between the pin and the external surface of the finished restoration (on its lateral surface). Only the manufacturer's specific bending tool should be used to bend a pin, not other hand instruments (see subsequent section, Pin Insertion).

In general, increasing the number of pins increases their retention in dentin and amalgam. However, the potential benefit of increasing the number of pins must be compared with the potential problems. As the number of pins increases, (1) the crazing of dentin and the potential for fracture increase, (2) the amount of available dentin between the pins decreases, and (3) the strength of the amalgam restoration decreases.[149,150] Also, as the diameter of the pin increases, retention in dentin and amalgam generally increases. As the number, depth, and diameter of pins increase, the danger of perforating into the pulp or the external tooth surface increases. Numerous long pins also may severely compromise the condensation of amalgam and its adaptation to the pins. A pin technique (i.e., a balance between pin orientation, size, and number) that permits optimal retention with minimal danger to the remaining tooth structure should be used.[151]

Extension Into Dentin and Amalgam
Self-threading pin extension into dentin and amalgam should be approximately 1.5 to 2 mm to preserve the strength of dentin and amalgam.[141] Extension greater than this is unnecessary for pin retention and is contraindicated.

Pin Placement Factors and Techniques

Pin Size
Four sizes of TMS pins are available (Fig. 10.176), each with a corresponding color-coded drill (see Table 10.1). Familiarity with drill sizes and their corresponding colors is necessary to ensure that a proper-sized pinhole is prepared for the desired pin. It is

TABLE 10.1	The Thread Mate System (TMS) Pins					
Name	Illustration (Not to Scale)	Color Code	Pin Diameter (inches/mm)*	Drill Diameter (inches/mm)*	Total Pin Length (mm)	Pin Length Extending From Dentin (mm)
Regular (standard)		Gold	0.031/0.78	0.027/0.68	7.1	5.1
Regular (self-shearing)		Gold	0.031/0.78	0.027/0.68	8.2	3.2
Regular (two-in-one)		Gold	0.031/0.78	0.027/0.68	9.5	2.8
Minim (standard)		Silver	0.024/0.61	0.021/0.53	6.7	4.7
Minim (two-in-one)		Silver	0.024/0.61	0.021/0.53	9.5	2.8
Minikin (self-shearing)		Red	0.019/0.48	0.017/0.43	7.1	1.5
Minuta (self-shearing)		Pink	0.015/0.38	0.0135/0.34	6.2	1

*1 mm = 0.03937 inch.

difficult to specify a particular size of pin that is always appropriate for a particular tooth. Two determining factors for selecting the appropriate-sized pin are 1) the amount of dentin available to safely receive the pin and 2) the amount of retention desired. In the TMS system, the pins of choice for severely involved posterior teeth are the Minikin (0.48 mm) and, occasionally, the Minim (0.61 mm). The Minikin pins usually are selected to reduce the risk of dentin crazing, pulpal penetration, and root-surface perforation. The Minim pins usually are used as a backup in case the pinhole for the Minikin is overprepared or the pin threads strip dentin during placement resulting in a lack of Minikin pin retention in the dentin.

Larger diameter pins have the greatest retention.[152] For example, the Minuta (0.38 mm) pin is approximately half as retentive as the Minikin and one third as retentive as the Minim pin.[147,148] The Minuta is usually too small to provide adequate retention in posterior teeth. The Regular (0.78 mm) or largest diameter pin is rarely used because a significant amount of crazing in the tooth (dentin and enamel) may be created during its insertion.[144,153] Of the four types of pins, the Regular pin is associated with the highest incidence of dentinal crack communication with the pulp chamber.[136]

Number of Pins

Factors to be considered when deciding how many pins are required include (1) the amount of missing tooth structure, (2) the amount of dentin available to safely receive the pins, (3) the amount of retention required, and (4) the size of the pins. As a general rule, one pin per missing axial line angle should be used. The fewest pins possible should be used to achieve the desired retention for a given restoration. Although the retention of the restoration increases as the number of pins increases, an excessive number of pins may fracture the tooth and significantly weaken the amalgam restoration.

Pinhole Location

Factors that aid in determining the pinhole locations include (1) knowledge of normal pulp anatomy and external tooth contours, (2) a current radiograph of the tooth, (3) a periodontal probe, and (4) the patient's age. Although the radiograph is only a two-dimensional image of the tooth, it may give an indication of the position of the pulp chamber and the contour of the mesial and distal surfaces of the tooth. Consideration also must be given to the placement of pins in areas where the greatest bulk of amalgam will occur so as to compensate (through the reinforcing tendency of the amalgam restoration) for the weakening effect of the pins on the tooth structure.[154] Areas of occlusal contacts on the restoration must be anticipated because a pin oriented vertically and positioned directly below an occlusal contact point weakens amalgam significantly.[155] Occlusal clearance should be sufficient to provide 2 mm of amalgam over the pin.[156,157]

Several attempts have been made to identify the ideal location of the pinhole.[135,144,158,159] The following principles of pin placement are recommended. In the cervical third of molars and premolars (where most pins are located), pinholes should be located near the line angles of the tooth except as described later.[151,160] The pinhole should be positioned no closer than 0.5 to 1 mm to the DEJ or no closer than 1 to 1.5 mm to the external surface of the tooth, whichever distance is greater (Fig. 10.177). Before the final decision is made about the location of the pinhole, the operator should probe the gingival crevice carefully to determine if any abnormal contours exist that would predispose the tooth to an external perforation. The pinhole should be parallel to the adjacent external surface of the tooth.

The position of a pinhole must not result in the pin being so close to a vertical wall of tooth structure that condensation of amalgam against the pin or wall is jeopardized (Fig. 10.178A). It may be necessary to first prepare a recess in the vertical wall with the No. 245 bur to permit proper pinhole preparation and to

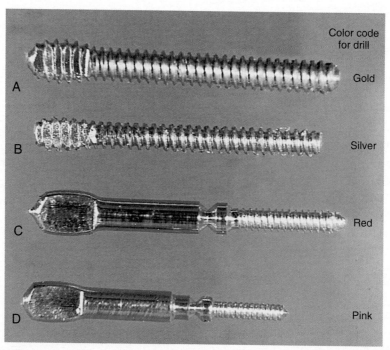

• **Fig. 10.176** Four sizes of the Thread Mate System (TMS) pins. A, Regular (0.78 mm). B, Minim (0.61 mm). C, Minikin (0.48 mm). D, Minuta (0.38 mm).

provide a minimum 0.5-mm clearance around the circumference of the pin for adequate condensation of amalgam (see Fig. 10.178B and C).[161] If necessary, after a pin is inappropriately placed, the operator should provide clearance around the pin to provide sufficient space for the smallest condenser nib to ensure that amalgam is condensed adequately around the pin. A No. 169L bur may be used, taking care not to damage or weaken the pin. Pinholes should be prepared on a flat surface that is perpendicular to the proposed direction of the pinhole. This will help prevent the drill tip from slipping or "crawling" and will allow a depth-limiting drill (discussed later) to prepare the pinhole as deeply as intended (Fig. 10.179).

Whenever three or more pinholes are placed, they should be located at different vertical levels on the tooth, if possible; this reduces stresses resulting from pin placement in the same horizontal plane of the tooth. Spacing between pins, or the interpin distance, must be considered when two or more pinholes are prepared. The optimal interpin distance depends on the size of pin to be used. The minimal interpin distance is 3 mm for the Minikin pin and 5 mm for the Minim pin.[160] Maximal interpin distance results in lower levels of stress in dentin.[162]

Several posterior teeth have anatomic features that may preclude safe pinhole placement. Fluted and furcal areas should be avoided.[160] External perforation may result from pinhole placement (1) over the prominent mesial concavity of the maxillary first premolar; (2) at the midlingual and midfacial bifurcations of the mandibular first and second molars; and (3) at the midfacial, midmesial, and middistal furcations of the maxillary first and second molars. Pulpal penetration may result from pin placement at the mesiofacial corner of the maxillary first molar and the mandibular first molar. Mandibular posterior teeth (with their lingual crown tilt), teeth that are rotated in the arch, and teeth that are abnormally tilted in the arch warrant careful attention before and during pinhole placement. When possible, the location of pinholes on the distal surface of mandibular molars and lingual surface of maxillary molars should be avoided. Obtaining the proper direction for preparing a pinhole in these locations is difficult because of the abrupt flaring of the roots just apical to the CEJ (Fig. 10.180). If the pinhole is placed parallel to the external surface of the tooth crown in these

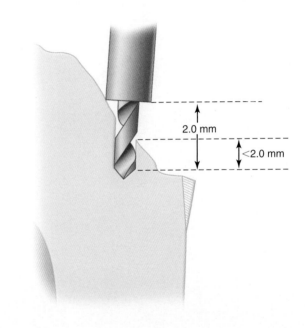

• **Fig. 10.179** Use of a depth-limiting drill to prepare a pinhole in the surface that is not perpendicular to the direction of the pinhole results in a pinhole of inadequate depth.

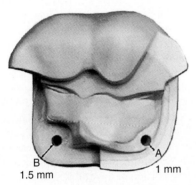

• **Fig. 10.177** Pinhole position. A, Position relative to the DEJ. B, Position relative to external tooth surface.

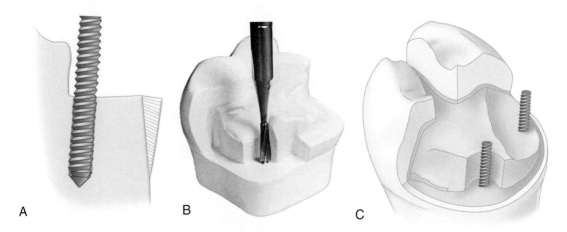

• **Fig. 10.178** A, Pin placed too close to the vertical wall such that adequate condensation of amalgam is jeopardized. B and C, Recessed area prepared in the vertical wall of the mandibular molar with a No. 245 bur to provide adequate space for amalgam condensation around the pin.

areas, penetration into the pulp is likely.[160] For mandibular second molars that are severely tilted mesially, care must be exercised to orient the drill properly to prevent external perforation on the mesial surface and pulpal penetration on the distal surface (Fig. 10.181). Because of limited interarch space, it is sometimes difficult to orient the twist drill (see subsequent section, Pinhole Preparation) correctly when placing pinholes at the distofacial or distolingual line angles of the mandibular second and third molars (Fig. 10.182).

When the pinhole locations have been determined, a No. ¼ round bur is first used to prepare a pilot hole (dimple) approximately one half the diameter of the bur at each location (Fig. 10.183). The purpose of this pilot hole is to permit more accurate placement of the twist drill and to prevent the twist drill from moving laterally (i.e., "crawling") when it has begun to rotate.

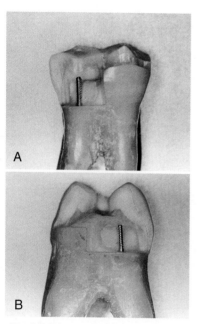

• **Fig. 10.180** Distal flaring of the mandibular molar (A) and palatal root flaring of the maxillary molar (B). Root angulation should be considered before pinhole placement.

Pinhole Preparation

The KODEX drill (a twist drill provided in the TMS system) should be used for preparing pinholes (Fig. 10.184). The aluminum shank of this drill, which acts as a heat absorber, is color coded to allow ready matching with the appropriate pin size (Table 10.2; see also Table 10.1). The drill shanks for the Minuta and Minikin pins are tapered to provide a built-in "wobble" when placed in a latch-type contra-angle handpiece. This wobble allows the drill to be "free floating" and to align itself as the pinhole is prepared. This feature minimizes the potential for dentinal crazing or the breakage of small drills.

Because the optimal depth of the pinhole into the dentin is 2 mm (only 1.5 mm for the Minikin pin), a depth-limiting drill should be used to prepare the hole (see Fig. 10.184). This type of drill is able to prepare the pinhole to the correct depth only when used on a flat surface that is perpendicular to the drill (see Fig. 10.178C; contrast with Fig. 10.179). When the location for starting a pinhole is not perpendicular to the desired pinhole direction, the location area should be flattened or the standard twist drill should be used (see Fig. 10.184). The standard twist drill has blades that are 4 to 5 mm in length, which would allow preparation of a pinhole with an effective depth. Creation of a flat area and use of the depth-limiting drill provide for a more predictable outcome and are recommended.

The technique of creating a properly aligned pinhole is as follows: (1) A pilot hole (dimple) is placed in the horizontal dentin surface to receive the pin; (2) the correct size twist drill (based on the pin size) is placed in a latch-type contra-angle handpiece; (3) the twist drill is placed in the gingival crevice beside the location for the pinhole and positioned such that it lies flat against the external surface of the tooth; (4) without changing the angulation obtained from the gingival crevice position, the handpiece is moved occlusally and the drill placed in the previously prepared pilot hole (Fig. 10.185A); (5) the drill is then viewed from a 90-degree angle to the previous viewing position to ascertain that the drill also is angled correctly in this plane (see Fig. 10.185B); (6) with the drill tip in its proper position and with the handpiece rotating at very low speed (300–500 rpm), pressure is applied to the drill until the depth-limiting portion of the drill is reached (see Fig. 10.185C and D); (7) the pinhole is prepared in one or two movements *without allowing the drill to stop rotating*. While still rotating, the drill is immediately removed from the pinhole.

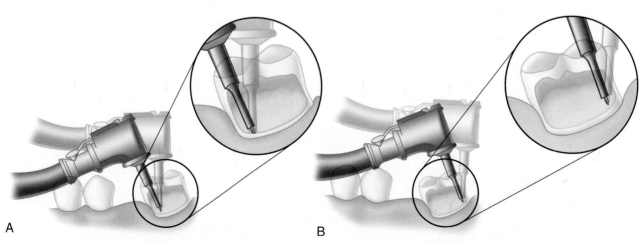

• **Fig. 10.181** Care must be exercised when preparing pinholes in mesially tilted molars to prevent external perforation on mesial surface (A) and pulpal penetration on the distal surface (B).

TABLE 10.2	The Thread Mate System (TMS) Link Series and Link Plus Pins					
Name	Illustration (Not to Scale)	Color Code	Pin Diameter (Inches/mm)*	Drill Diameter (Inches/mm)*	Pin Length Extending from Sleeve (mm)	Pin Length Extending From Dentin (mm)
Link Series						
Regular		Gold	0.031/0.78	0.027/0.68	5.5	3.2 (single shear)
Regular		Gold	0.031/0.78	0.027/0.68	7.8	2.6 (double shear)
Minim		Silver	0.024/0.61	0.021/0.53	5.4	3.2 (single shear)
Minim		Silver	0.024/0.61	0.021/0.53	7.6	2.6 (double shear)
Minikin		Red	0.019/0.48	0.017/0.43	6.9	1.5 (single shear)
Minuta		Pink	0.015/0.38	0.0135/0.34	6.3	1 (single shear)
Link Plus						
Minim		Silver	0.024/0.61	0.021/0.53	10.8	2.7 (double shear)

*1 mm = 0.03937 inch.

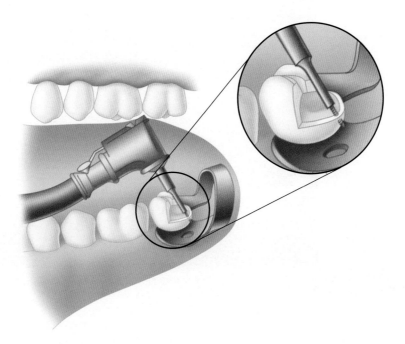

• **Fig. 10.182** When placing pinholes in molars and interarch space is limited, care must be exercised to prevent external perforation on distal surface.

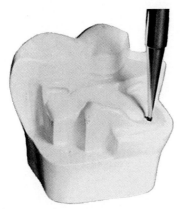

• **Fig. 10.183** Pilot hole (dimple) prepared with a No. ¼ bur.

Incorrect angulation of the drill may result in pulpal exposure or external perforation. If the proximity of an adjacent tooth interferes with placement of the drill into the gingival crevice, a flat, thin-bladed hand instrument is placed into the crevice and against the external surface of the tooth to indicate the proper angulation for the drill.[163] Using more than one or two movements, tilting the handpiece during the drilling procedure, or allowing the drill to rotate more than briefly at the bottom of the pinhole will result in a pinhole that is too large. The twist drill should never stop rotating (from insertion to removal from the pinhole) so as to limit the potential for binding and/or breakage while creating the pinhole.

Dull twist drills used to prepare pinholes may cause increased frictional heat and cracks in the dentin. Standlee et al. showed that a twist drill becomes too dull for use after cutting 20 pinholes

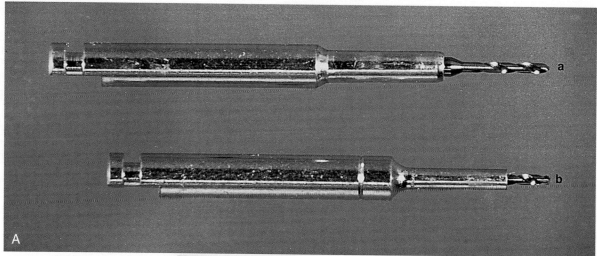

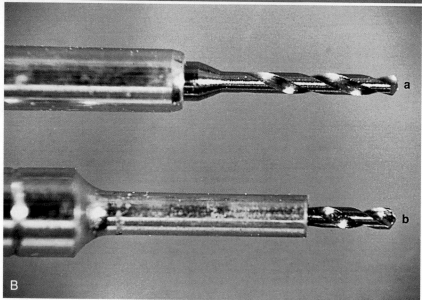

• **Fig. 10.184** A, Two types of KODEX twist drills: standard *(a)* and depth limiting *(b)*. B, Drills enlarged: standard *(a)* and depth limiting *(b)*.

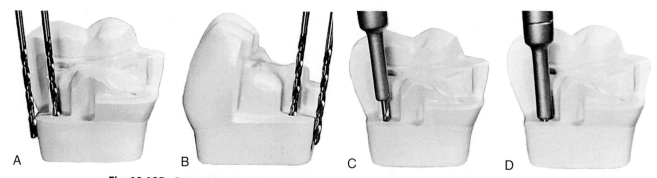

• **Fig. 10.185** Determining the angulation for the twist drill. A, Drill placed in the gingival crevice, positioned flat against the tooth, and moved occlusally into position without changing the angulation obtained. B, *A* repeated while viewing the drill from position 90 degrees left or right of that viewed in *A*. C and D, With twist drill at correct angulation, the pinhole is prepared in one or two thrusts until the depth-limiting portion of drill is reached and then removed while still rotating.

or less, and the signal for discarding the drill is the need for increased pressure on the handpiece.[164] Using a drill when its self-limiting shank shoulder has become rounded is contraindicated (Fig. 10.186). A worn and rounded shoulder may not properly limit pinhole depth and may permit pins to be placed too deeply.

Pin Design

Several designs are available for each of the four sizes of TMS self-threading pins: standard, self-shearing, two-in-one, Link Series, and Link Plus (Fig. 10.187). The Link Series pin is free floating in a plastic sleeve, which allows self-alignment as it is threaded into the pinhole (Fig. 10.188). When the pin reaches the bottom of the hole, the pin shears off at a machined narrow area, leaving a length of pin extending from dentin. The plastic sleeve is then discarded. The Minuta, Minikin, Minim, and Regular pins are available in the Link Series. Link Series pins are recommended because of their versatility, self-aligning ability, and retentiveness.[147]

Link Plus self-threading pins are also self-shearing and are available as single and two-in-one pins contained in color-coded plastic sleeves (Fig. 10.189). This design has a sharper thread, a shoulder stop at 2 mm, and a tapered tip to fit the bottom of the pinhole more readily as prepared by the twist drill. It also provides a 2.7-mm length of pin to extend out of dentin, which usually needs to be shortened with the use of a handpiece bur. Theoretically, and as suggested by Standlee et al., these innovations should reduce the stress created in the surrounding dentin as the pin is inserted and reduce the apical stress at the bottom of the pinhole.[164] Kelsey et al. reported that the two-in-one Link Plus first and second pins seat completely into the pinhole before shearing.[165]

The self-shearing pin has a total length that varies according to the diameter of the pin (see Table 10.1). It also consists of a flattened head to engage the hand wrench or the appropriate handpiece chuck for threading into the pinhole. When the pin approaches the bottom of the pinhole and begins to bind, the head of the pin shears off leaving a length of pin extending from dentin.

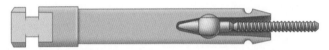

• **Fig. 10.188**   Cross-sectional view of Link Series pin.

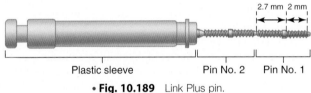

• **Fig. 10.189**   Link Plus pin.

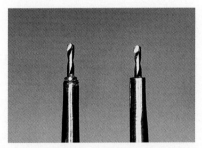

• **Fig. 10.186**   Minikin self-limiting drill with worn shank shoulder *(left)* compared with a new drill with an unworn shoulder *(right)*.

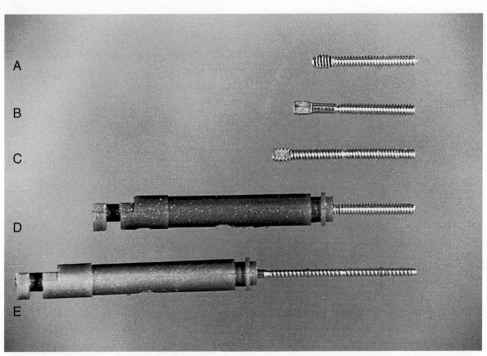

• **Fig. 10.187**   Five designs of the Thread Mate System (TMS) pins. A, Standard. B, Self-shearing. C, Two-in-one. D, Link Series. E, Link Plus.

The two-in-one pin is actually two pins in one, with each one being shorter than the standard pin. The two-in-one pin is approximately 9.5 mm in length and has a flattened head to aid in its insertion. When the pin reaches the bottom of the pinhole, it shears approximately in half, leaving a length of pin extending from dentin with the other half remaining in the hand wrench or the handpiece chuck. This second pin may be positioned in another pinhole and threaded to place in the same manner as the standard pin. The designs available with each size of pin are shown in Tables 10.1 and 10.2.

Selection of a particular pin design is influenced by the size of the pin being used, the amount of interarch space available, and operator preference. With minimal interarch space, the two-in-one design may be undesirable because of its length. It has been reported that 93% of Link Series and Link Plus two-in-one pins extended to the optimal depth of 2 mm.[166-169] Even so, both the two-in-one pin and the self-shearing pin may occasionally fail to reach the bottom of the pinhole.

Pin Insertion

The TMS utilizes hand wrenches to place the self-threading pins (Figs. 10.190A–C and 10.191A). Link Series and Link Plus pins are contained in color-coded plastic sleeves that fit a latch-type contra-angle handpiece or a specially designed plastic hand wrench (see Fig. 10.190D). In addition, handpiece chucks are available (Fig. 10.192). The results of studies are conflicting as to which method of pin insertion produces the best results. The latch-type handpiece is recommended for the insertion of the Link Series and the Link Plus pins. The hand wrench is recommended for the insertion of standard pins.

When using the latch-type handpiece, a Link Series or a Link Plus pin is inserted into the handpiece and positioned over the pinhole. The handpiece is activated at low speed until the plastic sleeve shears from the pin. The pin sleeve is then discarded. For low-speed handpieces with a low gear, the low gear should be used. Using the low gear increases the torque and increases the tactile sense of the operator. It also reduces the risk of stripping the threads in dentin during pin insertion.

A standard pin is placed in the appropriate hand wrench (see Fig. 10.191A) and slowly threaded clockwise into the pinhole until a definite resistance (indicating the pin has reached the bottom of the pin hole) is felt (see Fig. 10.191B). The pin should then be rotated one quarter to one half turn counterclockwise to reduce the dentinal stress created by the end of the pin that is pressing on dentin at the bottom of the pinhole.[170] The hand wrench should be removed from the pin carefully. If the hand wrench is used without rubber dam isolation, a gauze throat shield must be in place, and a strand of dental floss, approximately 30 to 38 cm in length, should be tied securely to the end of the wrench (Fig. 10.193) to prevent accidental swallowing or aspiration by the patient.

The lengths of the pins are evaluated after placement (see Fig. 10.191C). Any length of pin greater than 2 mm should be removed. A sharp No. ¼, No. ½, or No. 169L or 245 bur, at high speed and oriented perpendicular to the pin, may be used to remove the excess length (Fig. 10.194A). If oriented otherwise, the rotation

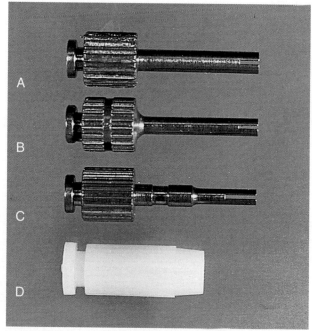

• **Fig. 10.190** Hand wrenches for the Thread Mate System (TMS) pins. A, Regular and Minikin. B, Minim. C, Minuta. D, Link Series and Link Plus.

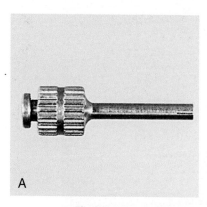 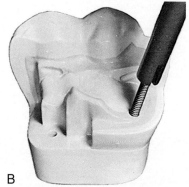 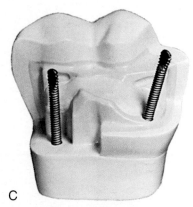

• **Fig. 10.191** A, Use of a hand wrench to place a pin. B, Threading the pin to the bottom of the pinhole and reversing the wrench one quarter to one half turn. C, Evaluating the length of the pin extending from dentin.

of the bur may loosen the pin by rotating it counterclockwise and unthreading it out of the pinhole. During removal of excess pin length, the assistant may apply a steady stream of air to the pin and have the high-volume evacuator tip positioned to remove the pin segment. Also, during removal of excess pin length, the pin may be stabilized with a small hemostat or cotton pliers. After placement, the pin should be tight, immobile, and not easily withdrawn. Every pin must be assessed with cotton pliers for stability immediately after placement.

The preparation is viewed from all directions with a mirror (particularly from the occlusal direction) to determine if any pins need to be bent so as to be positioned within the anticipated

contour of the final restoration such that there will be adequate bulk of amalgam between the pin and the external surface of the final restoration (see Fig. 10.194B and C). When pins require bending, the TMS bending tool (Fig. 10.195A) must be used. The bending tool should be placed on the pin where the pin is to be bent, and with firm controlled pressure, the bending tool should be rotated until the desired amount of bend is achieved (see Fig. 10.195B–D). Use of the bending tool allows placement of the fulcrum at some point along the length of the exposed pin. Other instruments should not be used to bend a pin because the location of the fulcrum would be at the orifice of the pinhole (i.e., the surface of the dentin). Force placed at this area may cause crazing or fracture of dentin, and the abrupt or sharp bend that usually results increases the chances of breaking the pin (Fig. 10.196). Also the operator has less control when pressure is applied with a hand instrument, and the risk of slipping is increased. Pins should only be bent if absolutely necessary, never simply to make them parallel or based on a notion that bending them will increase their relative retentiveness.

Possible Problems With Pins

Failure of Pin-Retained Restorations

The failure of pin-retained restorations might occur at any of five different locations (Fig. 10.197). Failure may occur (1) within the restoration (restoration fracture), (2) at the interface between the pin and the restorative material (pin–restoration separation), (3) within the pin (pin fracture), (4) at the interface between the pin

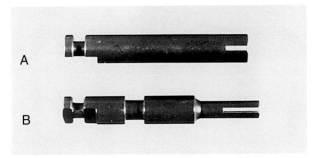

• **Fig. 10.192** Handpiece chucks for the Thread Mate System (TMS) regular self-shearing and Minikin pins (A) and TMS Minuta pins (B).

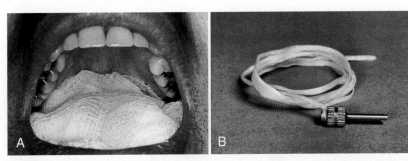

• **Fig. 10.193** Precautions to be taken if a rubber dam is not used. A, Gauze throat shield. B, Hand wrench with 30 to 38 cm of dental tape attached.

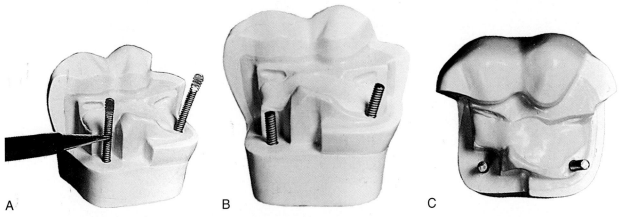

• **Fig. 10.194** A, Use of sharp No. ¼ bur held perpendicular to the pin to shorten the pin. B and C, Evaluating the preparation to determine the need for bending the pins.

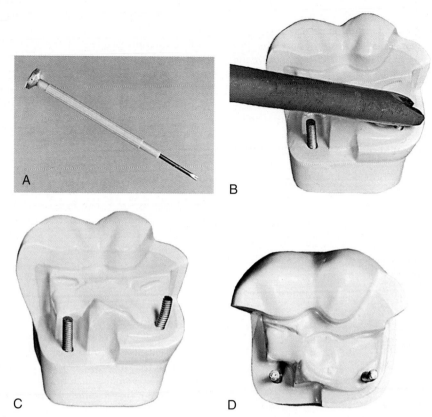

• **Fig. 10.195** A, The Thread Mate System (TMS) bending tool. B, Use of the bending tool to bend the pin. C and D, The pin is bent to a position that provides adequate bulk of amalgam between the pin and the external surface of the final restoration.

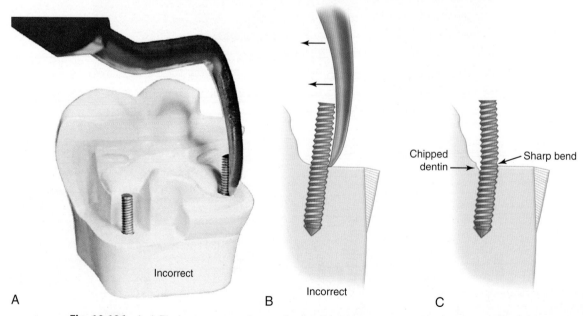

• **Fig. 10.196** A, A Black spoon excavator or other hand instrument should not be used to bend the pin. B and C, Use of hand instruments may create a sharp bend in the pin and fracture dentin.

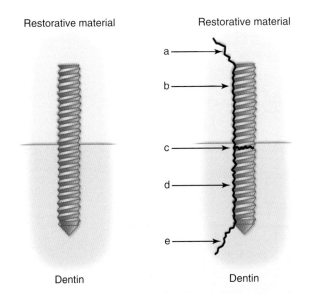

Restorative material   Restorative material

Dentin   Dentin

• **Fig. 10.197** Five possible locations of failure of pin-retained restorations: fracture of restorative material (a), separation of pin from restorative material (b), fracture of pin (c), separation of pin from dentin (d), fracture of dentin (e).

and dentin, and (5) within dentin (dentin fracture). Failure is more likely to occur at the pin–dentin interface than at the pin–restoration interface. The operator must keep these areas of potential failure in mind at all times and apply necessary principles to reduce failure risk.

Broken Drills and Broken Pins

Occasionally, a twist drill breaks if it is stressed laterally or allowed to stop rotating before it is removed from the pinhole. Use of a sharp twist drill helps to limit the possibility of drill breakage. Pins also may break during bending if care is not exercised. The treatment for broken drills and broken pins is to choose an alternative location, at least 1.5 mm remote from the broken item, and prepare another pinhole and place another pin. Removal of a broken pin or drill is difficult, if not impossible, and usually should not be attempted.

Loose Pins

Self-threading pins sometimes do not engage dentin properly because the pinhole was inadvertently prepared too large or a self-shearing pin failed to shear, resulting in stripped-out dentin. The pin should be removed from the tooth and the pinhole re-prepared with the next largest size drill, and the appropriate pin should be inserted. Preparing another pinhole of the same size as the original, 1.5 mm from the original pinhole, also is acceptable.

As described earlier, a properly placed pin may be loosened while being shortened with a bur, if the bur is not held perpendicularly to the pin and the pin stabilized. A loose pin may be removed from the pinhole by holding a rotating bur parallel to the pin and lightly contacting the surface of the pin; this causes the pin to rotate counterclockwise out of the pinhole. A second attempt should be made with the same-size pin. If the second pin fails to firmly engage the dentin, a larger hole is prepared, and the appropriate pin is inserted. Preparing another pinhole of the same size 1.5 mm from the original pinhole also is acceptable.

Penetration Into the Pulp and Perforation of the External Tooth Surface

Penetration into the pulp or perforation of the external surface of the tooth is obvious if hemorrhage occurs in the pinhole after removal of the drill. Usually the operator is able to perceive when pulp penetration or root perforation has occurred by an abrupt loss of resistance of the drill to hand pressure. Also if a standard or Link Series pin continues to thread into the tooth beyond the 2-mm depth of the pinhole, this is an indication of a penetration or perforation. A pulpal penetration might be suspected if the patient is anesthetized and has sudden sensitivity when the pinhole is being completed or the pin is being placed. However, if the patient still has profound pulpal anesthesia, pulpal penetration of the pinhole or pin may not be perceived.

Pulpal penetration is treated as any other small mechanical exposure if the tooth has been asymptomatic. When preparation of the pinhole causes a pulp exposure, any hemorrhage is controlled. A calcium hydroxide liner is placed over the opening of the pinhole, and another hole is prepared 1.5 mm away. If the exposure is discovered as the pin is being placed, the pin is removed and the area of pulp penetration treated as described. Although certain studies have shown that the pulp tolerates pin penetration when the pin is placed in a relatively sterile environment, it is not recommended that pins be left in place when a pulpal penetration has occurred.[157,171] If the pin were left in the pulp, (1) the depth of the pin into pulpal tissue would be difficult to determine, (2) considerable postoperative sensitivity might ensue, and (3) the pin location might complicate subsequent endodontic therapy. Regardless of the method of treatment rendered, the patient must be informed of the pulpal penetration or root perforation at the completion of the appointment. The affected tooth should be evaluated periodically using appropriate diagnostic tests including radiographs. The patient should be instructed to inform the dentist if any discomfort develops.

Because most teeth receiving pins have had extensive caries, restorations, or both, the health of the pulp is likely compromised. The ideal treatment of a pulpal penetration for such a compromised tooth generally is endodontic therapy. Furthermore, endodontic treatment should be strongly considered when such a tooth is to receive an indirect restoration.

An external perforation might be suspected if an unanesthetized patient senses pain when a pinhole is being prepared or a pin is being placed in a tooth that has had endodontic therapy. Observation of the angulation of the twist drill or the pin may help in the determination of whether a pulpal penetration or external perforation has occurred. Perforation of the external surface of the tooth may occur occlusal or apical to the gingival attachment. Careful probing and radiographic examination must be used to accurately diagnose the location of a perforation. The method of treatment for a perforation often depends on the experience of the operator and the particular circumstances of the tooth being treated.

Three options are available for perforations that occur occlusal to the gingival attachment: (1) The pin may be cut off flush with the tooth surface and no further treatment rendered; (2) the pin may be cut off flush with the tooth surface and the preparation for an indirect restoration extended gingivally beyond the perforation; or (3) the pin may be removed, if still present, and the external aspect of the pinhole enlarged slightly and restored with amalgam. Surgical reflection of gingival tissue may be necessary to render adequate treatment. The location of perforations occlusal to the attachment often determines the option to be pursued.

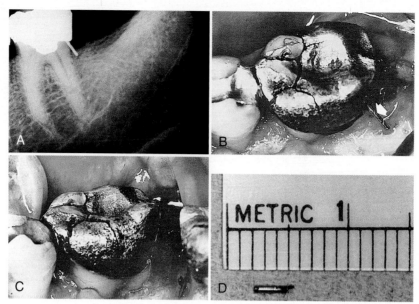

• **Fig. 10.198** External perforation of a pin. A, Radiograph showing the external perforation of a pin. B, Surgical access to extruding pin *(arrow)*. C, Pin cut flush with the tooth structure and crown-lengthening procedure performed. D, Length of pin removed.

Two options are available for perforations that occur apical to the gingival attachment: (1) Reflect the tissue surgically, perform any necessary ostectomy, enlarge the pinhole slightly, and restore with amalgam; or (2) perform a crown-lengthening procedure and place the margin of a cast restoration gingival to the perforation (Fig. 10.198). As with perforations located occlusal to the gingival attachment, the location of the perforation and the design of the present or planned restoration help determine which option to pursue. As with pulpal penetration, the patient must be informed of the perforation and the proposed treatment. The prognosis of external perforations is favorable when they are recognized early and treated properly.

Considerations for the Use of Slots or Pins

Slot retention may be used in conjunction with pin retention or as an alternative to it.[172] Some operators use slot retention and pin retention interchangeably. Others more frequently use slot retention in preparations with vertical walls that allow retention grooves to oppose one another. Pin retention is used more frequently in preparations with few or no vertical walls. Slots are particularly indicated in short clinical crowns and when cusp reduction has been limited to 2 or 3 mm.[172] More tooth structure is removed in slot preparation as compared with pin placement; however, slots are less likely to (1) create microfractures in dentin, (2) perforate the tooth surface, or (3) penetrate into the pulp. Slot placement does not elicit an inflammatory response, whereas medium-sized self-threading pins may elicit an inflammatory response if placed within 0.5 mm of the pulp.[158] The retention potential of slots and pins is similar.[173-176]

Tooth Preparation for Amalgam Foundations

An amalgam foundation may be used as part of the initial restoration of a severely involved tooth. The tooth is restored so that the restorative material (amalgam, composite, or other) serves to replace lost tooth structure necessary to provide retention and resistance forms for the final indirect restoration (e.g., crown or bridge retainer). The retention of the foundation material should not be compromised by tooth reduction during the final preparation for the indirect restoration. The foundation also should provide the resistance form against forces that otherwise might fracture the remaining tooth structure.

In contrast to a conventional complex amalgam restoration, an amalgam foundation may not depend primarily on the remaining coronal tooth structure for support. Instead it may rely mainly on secondary preparation retention features (proximal retention grooves, coves, slots, pins). A temporary or caries-control restoration may serve as a foundation, but only if the retention and resistance forms of the restoration are appropriate.

A temporary or caries-control restoration is used to restore a tooth when definitive treatment is uncertain or when several teeth require immediate attention for control of caries lesions. It also may be used when a tooth's prognosis is questionable. A temporary or control restoration might depend only on the remaining coronal tooth structure for support, however, using few auxiliary retention features. When preparing a tooth for either a foundation or a temporary restoration, remaining unsupported enamel may be left (except at the gingival aspect) to aid in forming a matrix for amalgam condensation. In this case the remaining unsupported enamel will subsequently be removed when the preparation for the indirect restoration is accomplished. Occasionally, when providing a temporary or control restoration, sufficient retention and resistance forms are included in the preparation to meet the requirements of a foundation.

As a rule, foundations are placed in anticipation of full-coverage indirect restorations. Not all teeth with foundations, however, need to be immediately restored with full-coverage crowns. For example, amalgam may be used as a definitive partial-coverage restoration of endodontically treated teeth if only minimal coronal damage has occurred.[177] The greatest influence on fracture resistance is the amount of remaining tooth structure; therefore restorations that conserve natural tooth structure are preferred.[178]

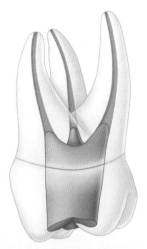

• **Fig. 10.199** Pulp chamber retention with 2- to 4-mm extension of the foundation into the canal spaces.

Amalgam and composite resin are the direct restorative materials used for foundations. RMGIs may be used to block out minor undercut areas of the preparation for an indirect restoration that do not draw. Amalgam may be preferred by some clinicians because it is easy to use and it is strong. While slots and threaded pins may be used for secondary retention in vital teeth, prefabricated posts and cast post/cores are used to provide additional retention for the foundation material in endodontically treated teeth receiving foundations. Prefabricated posts and cast post/cores are generally used on anterior teeth or single-canal premolars that have little or no remaining coronal tooth structure. Note, however, that there must be adequate remaining natural tooth structure to allow creation of a ferrule so as to achieve long-term clinical success. The pulp chamber and entrance to the root canals of endodontically treated molar teeth typically provide retention for foundations, and it is not necessary to use any form of intraradicular retention (i.e., post material extended further into the root canal space) (Fig. 10.199).

Slot and/or Pin Retention of Foundations

The technique of tooth preparation for a foundation depends on the type of retention that is selected—slot retention, pin retention, or both. The techniques have in common the axial location of the retention. Slots and pins for the retention of amalgam foundations are placed slightly more axial (farther inside the DEJ) than indicated for definitive complex amalgam restorations. The actual pulpal positioning depends on the type of indirect restoration that has been planned. The preparation for an indirect restoration should not eliminate or cut into the foundation's retentive features.

Severely broken teeth with few or no vertical walls, in which an indirect restoration is indicated, may require a pin-retained foundation. The main difference between the use of pins for foundations and the use of pins in definitive complex restorations is the distance of the pinholes from the external surface of the tooth.[179] For foundations, the pinholes must be located farther from the external surface of the tooth (farther internally from the DEJ), and more bending of the pins may be necessary to allow for adequate axial reduction of the foundation without exposing the pins during the cast-metal tooth preparation. Any removal of the restorative material from the circumference of the pin would compromise its retentive effect. If the material is removed from

more than half the diameter of the pin, any retentive effect of the pin probably has been eliminated.

The location of the pinhole from the external surface of the tooth for foundations depends on (1) the occlusogingival location of the pin (external morphology of the tooth), (2) the type of restoration to be placed (e.g., a porcelain-fused-to-metal [PFM] requires more reduction than a full gold crown), and (3) the type of margin to be prepared. Preparations with heavily chamfered margins at a normal occlusogingival location require slot and pin placement at a greater axial depth. The length of the pins also must be adjusted to permit adequate occlusal reduction without exposing the pins. Proximal retention grooves still should be used, wherever possible.

Completion of all final preparation steps is accomplished as described previously. An RMGI liner/base may be applied as indicated. A liner or base should not extend closer than 1 mm to a slot or a pin.

Pulp Chamber Retention of Foundations

The pulp chamber may be effectively used to retain an amalgam foundation in multirooted, endodontically treated teeth. This alternative to the use of slots/pins is recommended when (1) dimension of the pulp chamber is adequate to provide retention and bulk of amalgam, and (2) dentin thickness in the region of the pulp chamber is adequate to provide rigidity and strength to the tooth.[180] Additional extension of 2 to 4 mm into the root canal space is recommended when the pulp chamber height is 2 mm or less (see Fig. 10.199).[181] When the pulp chamber height is 4 to 6 mm in depth, no advantage is gained from additional extension into the root canal space. After matrix application, amalgam is thoroughly condensed into the pulp chamber (and radicular space if indicated) and the coronal portion of the tooth. Natural undercuts in the pulp chamber and the divergent root canals provide the necessary retention form. The resistance form against forces that otherwise may cause tooth fracture is improved by gingival extension of the crown preparation approximately 2 mm beyond the foundation onto sound tooth structure to establish the necessary ferrule once the indirect restoration is in place. This extension should have a total taper of opposing walls of less than 10 degrees.[182] If the pulp chamber height is less than 2 mm, the use of a prefabricated post, cast post and core, pins, or slots should be considered for additional retention of the foundation material.

The preparation should then be cleaned, carefully inspected as indicated in General Concepts Guiding Preparation for Amalgam Restorations, and any final modifications completed.

Restorative Technique for Complex Amalgam Preparations

Desensitizer Placement

A dentin desensitizer is placed over the prepared tooth structure per manufacturer instructions. Excess moisture is removed without desiccating the dentin.

Matrix Placement

One of the most difficult steps in restoring a severely compromised posterior tooth is development of a satisfactory matrix to assist in formation of the anatomic shape of the restoration. Fulfilling the objectives of a matrix is complicated by possible gingival extensions, missing line angles, and restoration of reduced cusps typical of complex tooth preparations.

Universal Matrix

The Tofflemire retainer and band may be used successfully for most amalgam restorations (Fig. 10.200). Use of the Tofflemire retainer requires sufficient tooth structure to retain the band after it is applied. Even when the Tofflemire retainer is placed appropriately an opening may remain next to an area of the preparation tooth structure. In this case a closed system may be developed as illustrated in Fig. 10.201. A strip of matrix material that is long enough to extend from the mesial to the distal corners of the tooth is prepared. The strip must extend into these corners sufficiently that the band, when tight, holds the strip in position. Also it must not extend into the proximal areas, or a ledge would result in the restoration contour (see Fig. 10.201F).

The Tofflemire retainer is loosened one half turn, and the strip of matrix material is inserted next to the opening between the matrix band and the tooth. The retainer is then tightened and the matrix is completed. Sometimes it is helpful to place a small amount of rigid material (hard-setting polyvinyl siloxane [PVS] or compound or light-cured flowable resin) between the strip and the open aspect of the band retainer to stabilize and support the strip (see Fig. 10.201G and H).

When little tooth structure remains and deep gingival margins are present, the Tofflemire matrix may not function successfully, and the AutoMatrix system (DENTSPLY Caulk, Milford, DE) may be an alternative method (Fig. 10.202).

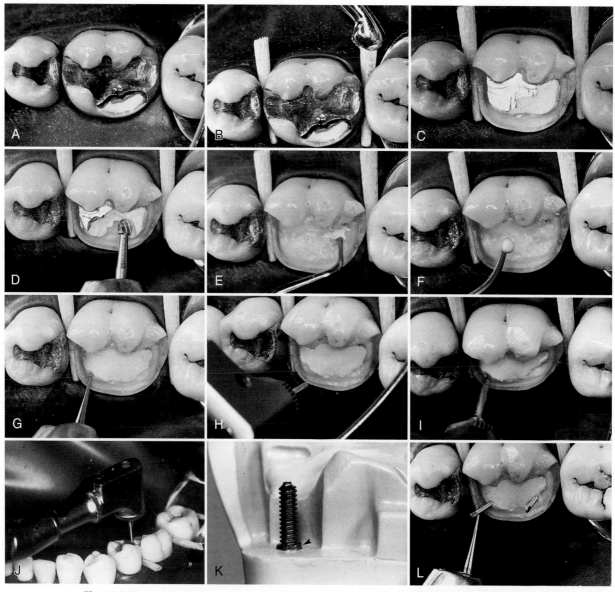

• **Fig. 10.200** A, Mandibular first molar with fractured distolingual cusp. B, Insertion of wedges. C, Initial tooth preparation. D and E, Removal of any soft dentin and/or any remaining old restorative material as indicated. F, Application of a liner and a base (if necessary). G, Preparation of pilot holes. H, Alignment of the twist drill with the external surface of the tooth. I, Preparation of pinholes. J, Insertion of Link pins with a slow-speed handpiece. K, Depth-limiting shoulder *(arrowhead)* of inserted Link Plus pin. L, Use of a No. ¼ bur to shorten pins.

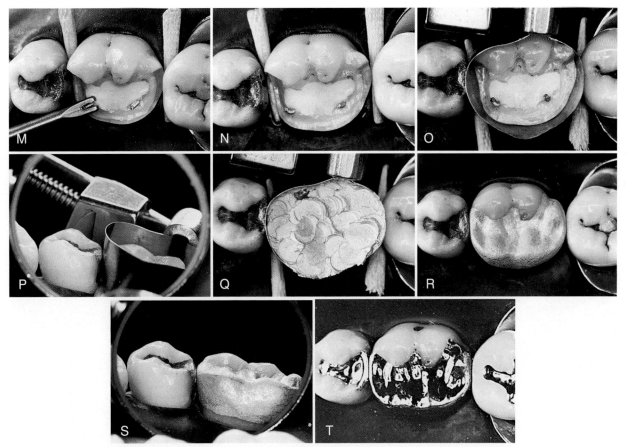

• **Fig. 10.200, cont'd** M, Bending pins (if necessary) with a bending tool. N, Final tooth preparation. O, Tofflemire retainer and matrix band applied to the prepared tooth. P, Reflecting light to evaluate the proximal area of the matrix band. Q, Preparation overfilled. R, Restoration carved. S, Reflecting light to evaluate the adequacy of the proximal contact and contour. T, Restoration polished.

AutoMatrix

The AutoMatrix is a retainerless matrix system designed for any tooth regardless of its circumference and height. AutoMatrix bands are supplied in three widths: (1) 4.76 mm, (2) 6.35 mm, and (3) 7.94 mm. The medium band is available in two thicknesses (0.038 mm and 0.05 mm). The 4.76, 6.35, and 7.94 mm band widths are available in the 0.05 mm thickness only. Advantages of this system include (1) convenience, (2) improved visibility because of absence of a retainer, and (3) ability to place the autolock loop on the facial or lingual surface of the tooth. Disadvantages of this system are that (1) the band is flat and difficult to burnish and is sometimes unstable even when wedges are in place, and (2) development of proper proximal contours and contacts may be difficult. Use of the AutoMatrix system is illustrated in Fig. 10.203.

Regardless of the type of matrix system used, the matrix must be stable during condensation of the amalgam. The matrix should extend beyond the gingival margins of the preparation enough to provide support for the matrix and to permit appropriate wedge stabilization. The matrix should extend occlusally beyond the marginal ridge of the adjacent tooth by 1 to 2 mm. If the matrix for a complex amalgam restoration is not stable during condensation, a homogeneous restoration will not be developed. An improperly condensed amalgam may disintegrate when the matrix is removed, or eventually fail because of lack of sufficient strength secondary to internal voids or fractures. Matrix stability during condensation is especially important for slot-retained amalgam restorations. If the matrix is not secure during condensation, it may slip out of position causing separation of the main bulk of the amalgam from its retentive slots or pins.

Insertion, Contouring, and Finishing of Amalgam

A high-copper alloy is strongly recommended for the complex amalgam restoration because of excellent clinical performance and high early compressive strengths.[183-185] Spherical alloys have a higher early strength than admixed alloys, and spherical alloys may be condensed more quickly and with less pressure so as to ensure good adaptation in slots and around the pins. However, proximal contacts may be easier to achieve with admixed alloys because of their condensability. Alloys that provide extended working time are necessary to allow adequate time for condensation, removal of the matrix band, and final carving. Because complex amalgam restorations usually are quite large, a slow-set or medium-set amalgam may be selected to provide more time for the carving and adjustment of the restoration.

Regardless of the type of alloy chosen, care must be taken to condense the amalgam thoroughly in and around the retentive features of the preparation. If a mix of amalgam becomes dry or crumbly, a new

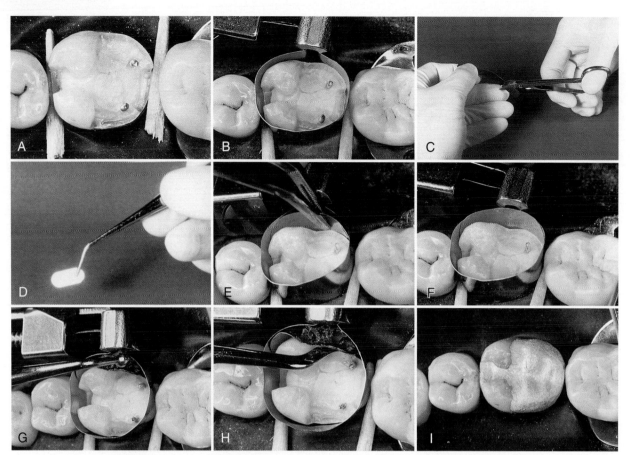

• **Fig. 10.201** Technique for closing the open space of the Tofflemire matrix system. A, Tooth preparation with wedges in place. B, Open aspect of the matrix band next to the prepared tooth structure. C and D, Cutting an appropriate length of the matrix material. E, Insertion of a strip of the matrix material. F, Closed matrix system. G and H, Placement of the rigid supporting material between the strip and the matrix band, and contouring, if necessary. I, Restoration carved.

mix is triturated immediately. Placement of a whole freshly mixed mass of amalgam (instead of using the amalgam carrier to place increments of amalgam) increases the rate of completely filling the defect. Special care must be taken when this technique is used to ensure the amalgam is well adapted in and around all retentive areas and at all margins.

With a complex (or any large) amalgam, carving time must be properly allocated. The time spent on carving occlusal anatomy (while the matrix is still in place) must be shortened to allow adequate time for carving the more inaccessible gingival margins and the proximal and axial contours (after the matrix is removed). The bulk of excess amalgam on the occlusal surface is removed and the initial anatomic contours are rapidly developed, especially the marginal ridge heights and cuspal inclines, with a discoid carver and/or Hollenback carver. The occlusal embrasures are defined by running the tine of an explorer against the internal aspect of the matrix band. Appropriate marginal ridge heights and embrasures reduce the potential of fracturing the marginal ridge when the matrix is removed.

Matrix removal is crucial when completing complex amalgam restorations, especially slot-retained restorations.[172] If the matrix is removed prematurely, the newly placed restoration may fracture immediately adjacent to the areas where amalgam has been condensed into the slot(s). Any rigid material supporting the matrix

is removed with an explorer or a Black spoon. Tofflemire matrices are removed first by loosening and removing the retainer while the wedges are still in place. Leaving the wedges in place may help prevent fracturing the freshly condensed amalgam. It may be beneficial to place a fingertip on the occlusal surface of the restored tooth to stabilize the matrix while loosening and removing the retainer from the band. This is to reduce the risk of fracturing the freshly inserted amalgam while applying the force necessary to loosen the retainer. The matrix is removed by sliding each end of the band in an oblique direction (i.e., moving the band facially or lingually while simultaneously moving it in an occlusal direction). Moving the band obliquely toward the occlusal surface minimizes the possibility of fracturing the marginal ridge. Preferably the matrix band should be removed in the same direction as the wedge placement to prevent dislodging the wedges. AutoMatrix bands are removed by using the system's instruments and, after the band is open, by the same technique described for Tofflemire-retained matrices. Carving of the restoration is then continued (see Figs. 10.200R and 10.203N).

Wedges are then removed, and the gingival excess on the proximal surface is removed with an amalgam knife or explorer. Facial and lingual contours are developed with a Hollenback carver, amalgam knife, or explorer to complete the carving (see Figs. 10.200R and S and 10.201I). Appropriately shaped rotary instruments are used

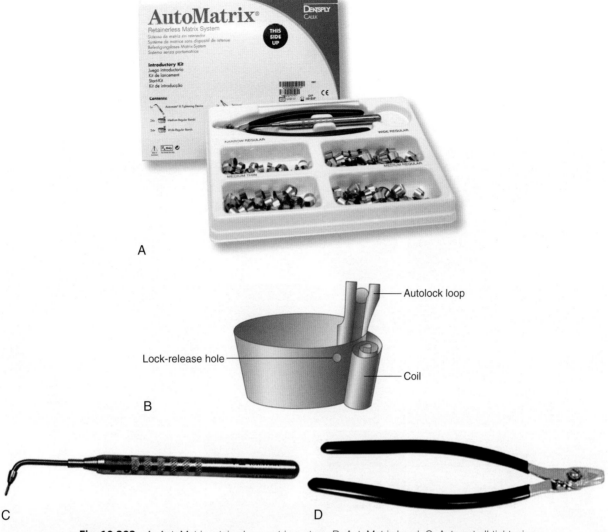

• **Fig. 10.202**   A, AutoMatrix retainerless matrix system. B, AutoMatrix band. C, Automate II tightening device. D, Shielded snippers. (A, Courtesy Dentsply Caulk, Milford, DE.)

to complete the occlusal contouring if amalgam has become so hard that the force needed to carve with hand instruments might fracture portions of the restoration.

Each proximal contact is evaluated by using a mirror occlusally and lingually to ensure that no light can be reflected between the restoration and the adjacent tooth at the level of the proximal contact (see Fig. 10.200S). When the proper proximal contour or contact is not achieved in a large, complex restoration, it may be possible to prepare a conservative "ideal" two-surface tooth preparation within the initial amalgam to restore the proper proximal surface contours. Amalgam forming the walls of this "ideal" preparation must have sufficient bulk to prevent future fracture.

The rubber dam is removed and the occlusal surface of the amalgam is adjusted to obtain appropriate occlusal contacts. Thin, unwaxed dental floss may be carefully passed through the proximal contacts one time to remove amalgam shavings and to smooth the proximal surface of amalgam. Amalgam excess and loose particles are removed from the gingival sulcus by moving the floss occlusogingivally and faciolingually. The patient should be cautioned not to chew with the restoration for 24 hours. Fast-setting high-copper amalgam may be prepared for an indirect restoration within 30 to 45 minutes after insertion of the foundation. Further finishing and polishing of the complex amalgam may be accomplished, if desired, as early as 24 hours after placement (see Fig. 10.200T).

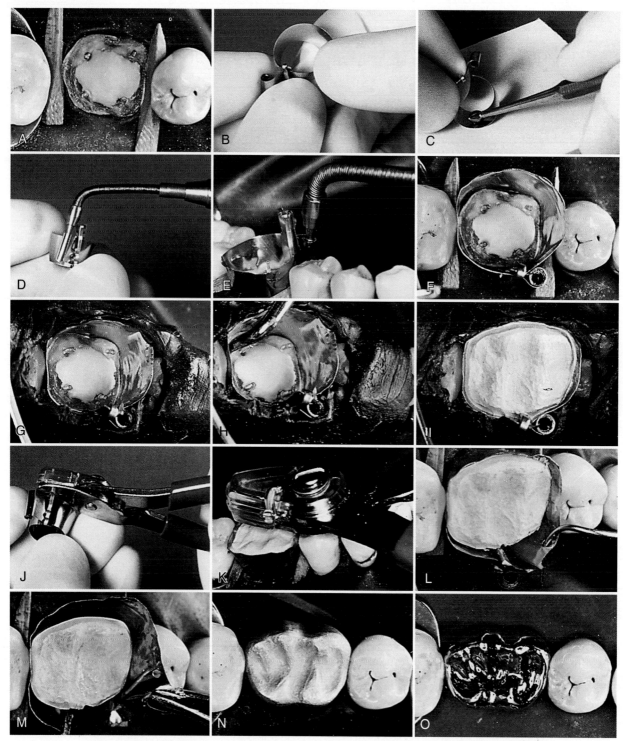

• **Fig. 10.203** Application of AutoMatrix for developing a pin-retained amalgam crown on the mandibular first molar. A, Tooth preparation with wedges in place. B, Enlargement of the circumference of the band, if necessary. C, Burnishing the band with an egg-shaped burnisher. D–F, Placement of the band around the tooth, tightening with an Automate II tightening device, and setting wedges firmly in place. G, Application of the green compound. H, Contouring of the band with the back of a warm Black spoon excavator so the softened compound will allow matrix deformation. I, Overfilling the preparation and carving the occlusal aspect. J and K, Use of shielded snippers to cut an autolock loop. L, Separating the band with an explorer. M, Removing the band in an oblique direction (facially with some occlusal vector). N, Restoration carved. O, Restoration polished.

Summary

Dental amalgam remains a predictable, cost-effective, and safe means for the restoration of posterior (and some anterior) teeth that are missing various amounts of tooth structure. The design of a successful tooth preparation must be based on the material properties of dental amalgam and the successful use of primary and secondary means of restoration retention. Complex preparations use retention grooves/coves in remaining vertical walls as well as slots, pins, and customized matrix designs to effect successful restorations. Restoration of normal anatomic contours and therefore normal clinical function may be readily accomplished with dental amalgam.

References

1. American Dental Association Council on Scientific Affairs: Dental amalgam: update on safety concerns. *J Am Dent Assoc* 129:494–503, 1998.
2. Collins CJ, Bryant RW, Hodge KL: A clinical evaluation of posterior composite resin restorations: 8-year findings. *J Dent* 26:311–317, 1998.
3. Lauterbach M, Martins IP, Castro-Caldas A, et al: Neurological outcomes in children with and without amalgam-related mercury exposure: seven years of longitudinal observations in a randomized trial. *J Am Dent Assoc* 139:138–145, 2008.
4. Corbin SB, Kohn WG: The benefits and risks of dental amalgam: current findings reviewed. *J Am Dent Assoc* 125:381–388, 1994.
5. Burgess JO: Dental materials for the restorations of root surface caries. *Am J Dent* 8:342, 1995.
6. Gottlieb EW, Retief DH, Bradley EL: Microleakage of conventional and high-copper amalgam restorations. *J Prosthet Dent* 53:355, 1985.
7. Hilton TJ: Can modern restorative procedures and materials reliably seal cavities? In vitro investigations: part 2. *Am J Dent* 15:279, 2002.
8. Berry TG, Summitt JB, Chung AK, et al: Amalgam at the new millennium. *J Am Dent Assoc* 129:1547–1556, 1998.
9. Dunne SM, Gainsford ID, Wilson NH: Current materials and techniques for direct restorations in posterior teeth: silver amalgam: part 1. *Int Dent J* 47:123–136, 1997.
10. Bernando M, Luis H, Martin MD, et al: Survival and reasons for failure of amalgam versus composite restorations placed in a randomized clinical trial. *J Am Dent Assoc* 138:775–783, 2007.
11. Opdam NJM, Bronkhorst EM, Loomans BA, et al: 12-year survival of composite vs. amalgam restorations. *J Dent Res* 89:1063–1067, 2010.
12. American Dental Association: Amalgam waste: ADA's best management practices. *ADA News* 35:1, 2004.
13. Ben-Amar A, Cardash HS, Judes H: The sealing of the tooth/amalgam interface by corrosion products. *J Oral Rehabil* 22:101–104, 1995.
14. Liberman R, Ben-Amar A, Nordenberg D, et al: Long-term sealing properties of amalgam restorations: an in vitro study. *Dent Mater* 5:168–170, 1989.
15. Letzel H, van 't Hof MA, Marshall GW, et al: The influence of the amalgam alloy on the survival of amalgam restorations: a secondary analysis of multiple controlled clinical trials. *J Dent Res* 76:1787–1798, 1997.
16. Mahler DB: The high-copper dental amalgam alloys. *J Dent Res* 76:537–541, 1997.
17. Suchatlampong C, Goto S, Ogura H: Early compressive strength and phase-formation of dental amalgam. *Dent Mater* 14:143–151, 1995.
18. Osborne JW: Photoelastic assessment of the expansion of direct-placement gallium restorative alloys. *Quintessence Int* 30:185–191, 1999.
19. Osborne JW, Summitt JB: Direct-placement gallium restorative alloy: a 3-year clinical evaluation. *Quintessence Int* 30:49–53, 1999.
20. Venugopalan R, Broome JC, Lucas LC: The effect of water contamination on dimensional change and corrosion properties of a gallium alloy. *Dent Mater* 14:173–178, 1998.
21. Kiremitci A, Bolay S: A 3-year clinical evaluation of a gallium restoration alloy. *J Oral Rehabil* 30(6):664–667, 2003.
22. Bullard RH, Leinfelder KF, Russell CM: Effect of coefficient of thermal expansion on microleakage. *J Am Dent Assoc* 116:871–874, 1988.
23. Williams PT, Hedge GL: Creep-fatigue as a possible cause of dental amalgam margin failure. *J Dent Res* 64:470–475, 1985.
24. Combe EC, Burke FJT, Douglas WH: Thermal properties. In Combe EC, Burke FJT, Douglas WH, editors: *Dental biomaterials*, Boston, 1999, Kluwer Academic Publishers.
25. Bryant RW: The strength of fifteen amalgam alloys. *Aust Dent J* 24:244–252, 1979.
26. Murray GA, Yates JL: Early compressive and diametral tensile strengths of seventeen amalgam alloy systems. *J Pedod* 5:40–50, 1980.
27. Mahler DB, Adey JD: Factors influencing the creep of dental amalgam. *J Dent Res* 70:1394–1400, 1991.
28. Vrijhoef MM, Letzel H: Creep versus marginal fracture of amalgam restorations. *J Oral Rehabil* 13:299–303, 1986.
29. Dilley DC, Vann WF, Jr, Oldenburg TR, et al: Time required for placement of composite versus amalgam restorations. *J Dent Child* 57:177, 1990.
30. Dias de Souza GM, Pereira GD, Dias CT, et al: Fracture resistance of teeth restored with the bonded amalgam technique. *Oper Dent* 26:511, 2001.
31. Mahler DB, Engle JH: Clinical evaluation of amalgam bonding in class I and II restorations. *J Am Dent Assoc* 131:43, 2000.
32. Smales RJ, Wetherell JD: Review of bonded amalgam restorations and assessment in a general practice over five years. *Oper Dent* 25:374, 2000.
33. Summitt JB, Burgess JO, Berry TG, et al: Six-year clinical evaluation of bonded and pin-retained complex amalgam restorations. *Oper Dent* 29:261, 2004.
34. Gorucu J, Tiritoglu M, Ozgünaltay G: Effects of preparation designs and adhesive systems on retention of class II amalgam restorations. *J Prosthet Dent* 78:250–254, 1997.
35. Winkler MM, Moore BK, Allen J, et al: Comparison of retentiveness of amalgam bonding agent types. *Oper Dent* 22:200–208, 1997.
36. Ben-Amar A, Liberman R, Rothkoff Z, et al: Long term sealing properties of Amalgam bond under amalgam restorations. *Am J Dent* 7:141–143, 1994.
37. Olmez A, Ulusu T: Bond strength and clinical evaluation of a new dentinal bonding agent to amalgam and resin composite. *Quintessence Int* 26:785–793, 1995.
38. Bjertness E, Sonju T: Survival analysis of amalgam restorations in long-term recall patients. *Acta Odontol Scand* 48:93, 1990.
39. Downer MC, Azli NA, Bedi R, et al: How long do routine restorations last? A systematic review. *Br Dent J* 187:432, 1999.
40. Letzel H, van 't Hof MA, Marshall GW, et al: The influence of the amalgam alloy on the survival of amalgam restorations: a secondary analysis of multiple controlled clinical trials. *J Dent Res* 76:1787, 1997.
41. Mjör IA, Jokstad A, Qvist V: Longevity of posterior restorations. *Int Dent J* 40:11, 1990.

42. Osborne JW, Norman RD: 13-year clinical assessment of 10 amalgam alloys. *Dent Mater* 6:189, 1990.

43. Osborne JW, Norman RD, Gale EN: A 14-year clinical assessment of 12 amalgam alloys. *Quintessence Int* 22:857, 1991.

44. Maryniuk GA: In search of treatment longevity—a 30-year perspective. *J Am Dent Assoc* 109:739, 1984.

45. Maryniuk GA, Kaplan SH: Longevity of restorations: survey results of dentists' estimates and attitudes. *J Am Dent Assoc* 112:39, 1986.

46. Jokstad A, Mjor IA: The quality of routine class II cavity preparations for amalgam. *Acta Odontol Scand* 47:53, 1989.

47. Kreulen CM, Tobi H, Gruythuysen RJ, et al: Replacement risk of amalgam treatment modalities: 15-year results. *J Dent* 26:627, 1998.

48. Smales RJ: Longevity of low- and high-copper amalgams analyzed by preparation class, tooth site, patient age, and operator. *Oper Dent* 16:162, 1991.

49. Bader JD, Shugars DA: Variations in dentists' clinical decisions. *J Public Health Dent* 55:181, 1995.

50. Plasmans P, Creugers NH, Mulder J: Long-term survival of extensive amalgam restorations. *J Dent Res* 77:453–460, 1998.

51. Martin JA, Bader JD: Five-year treatment outcomes for teeth with large amalgams and crowns. *Oper Dent* 22:72–78, 1997.

52. Mair LH: Ten-year clinical assessment of three posterior resin composites and two amalgams. *Quintessence Int* 29:483–490, 1998.

53. Ferracane JL: Resin-based composite performance: Are there some things we can't predict? *Dent Mater* 29(1):51–58, 2013.

54. Almquist TC, Cowan RD, Lambert RL: Conservative amalgam restorations. *J Prosthet Dent* 29:524, 1973.

55. Markley MR: Restorations of silver amalgam. *J Am Dent Assoc* 43:133, 1951.

56. Berry TG, Laswell HR, Osborne JW, et al: Width of isthmus and marginal failure of restorations of amalgam. *Oper Dent* 6:55, 1981.

57. Osborne JW, Gale EN: Relationship of restoration width, tooth position and alloy to fracture at the margins of 13- to 14-year-old amalgams. *J Dent Res* 69:1599, 1990.

58. Goel VK, Khera SC, Gurusami S, et al: Effect of cavity depth on stresses in a restored tooth. *J Prosthet Dent* 67:174, 1992.

59. Lagouvardos P, Sourai P, Douvitsas G: Coronal fractures in posterior teeth. *Oper Dent* 14:28, 1989.

60. Osborne JW, Gale EN: Failure at the margin of amalgams as affected by cavity width, tooth position, and alloy selection. *J Dent Res* 60:681, 1981.

61. Fusayama T: Two layers of carious dentin: diagnosis and treatment. *Oper Dent* 4:63, 1979.

62. Hebling J, Giro EM, Costa CA: Human pulp response after an adhesive system application in deep cavities. *J Dent* 27:557, 1999.

63. Hilton TJ: Cavity sealers, liners, and bases: current philosophies and indications for use. *Oper Dent* 21:134, 1996.

64. Eliades G, Palaghias G: In-vitro characterization of visible-light-cured glass-ionomer liners. *Dent Mater* 9:198, 1993.

65. Wieczkowski G, Jr, Yu XY, Joynt RB, et al: Microleakage evaluation in amalgam restorations used with bases. *J Esthet Dent* 4:37, 1992.

66. Robbins JW: The placement of bases beneath amalgam restorations: review of literature and recommendations for use. *J Am Dent Assoc* 113:910, 1986.

67. Hilton TJ: Sealers, liners, and bases. *J Esthet Restor Dent* 15:141, 2003.

68. Rasaratnam L: Review suggests direct pulp capping with MTA more effective than calcium hydroxide. *Evid Based Dent* 17(3):94–95, 2016, doi:10.1038/sj.ebd.6401194.

69. Terkla LG, Mahler DB, Van Eysden J: Analysis of amalgam cavity design. *J Prosthet Dent* 29(21):204–209, 1973.

70. Goho C, Aaron GR: Enhancement of anti-microbial properties of cavity varnish: a preliminary report. *J Prosthet Dent* 68:623, 1992.

71. Vlietstra JR, Sidaway DA, Plant CG: Cavity cleansers, *Br Dent J* 149:293, 1980.

72. Schüpbach P, Lutz F, Finger WJ: Closing of dentinal tubules by Gluma desensitizer. *Eur J Oral Sci* 105:414, 1997.

73. Anusavice KJ, editor: *Phillips' science of dental materials*, ed 11, St. Louis, 2003, Mosby.

74. Mahler DB: The amalgam-tooth interface. *Oper Dent* 21:230, 1996.

75. Symons AL, Wing G, Hewitt GH: Adaptation of eight modern dental amalgams to walls of Class I cavity preparations. *J Oral Rehabil* 14:55, 1987.

76. Bauer JG: A study of procedures for burnishing amalgam restorations. *J Prosthet Dent* 57:669, 1987.

77. Lovadino JR, Ruhnke LA, Consani S: Influence of burnishing on amalgam adaptation to cavity walls. *J Prosthet Dent* 58:284, 1987.

78. Kanai S: Structure studies of amalgam II: effect of burnishing on the margins of occlusal amalgam fillings. *Acta Odontol Scand* 24:47, 1966.

79. May KN, Wilder AD, Leinfelder KF: Clinical evaluation of various burnishing techniques on high-copper amalgam [abstract]. *J Prosthet Dent* 61:213, 1982.

80. May KN, Jr, Wilder AD, Jr, Leinfelder KF: Burnished amalgam restorations: a two-year evaluation. *J Prosthet Dent* 49:193, 1983.

81. Straffon LH, Corpron RE, Dennison JB, et al: A clinical evaluation of polished and unpolished amalgams: 36-month results. *Pediatr Dent* 6:220, 1984.

82. Collins CJ, Bryant RW: Finishing of amalgam restorations: a three-year clinical study. *J Dent* 20:202, 1992.

83. Drummond JL, Jung H, Savers EE, et al: Surface roughness of polished amalgams. *Oper Dent* 17:129, 1992.

84. Moffa JP: The longevity and reasons for replacement of amalgam alloys [abstract]. *J Dent Res* 68:188, 1989.

85. Summitt JB, Burgess JO, Berry TG, et al: Six-year clinical evaluation of bonded and pin-retained complex amalgam restorations. *Oper Dent* 29:261, 2004.

86. Mayhew RB, Schmeltzer LD, Pierson WP: Effect of polishing on the marginal integrity of high-copper amalgams. *Oper Dent* 11:8, 1986.

87. Osborne JW, Leinfelder KF, Gale EN, et al: Two independent evaluations of ten amalgam alloys. *J Prosthet Dent* 43:622, 1980.

88. Council on Dental Materials, Instruments, and Equipment: Dental mercury hygiene: summary of recommendations in 1990. *J Am Dent Assoc* 122:112, 1991.

89. Sockwell CL: Dental handpieces and rotary cutting instruments. *Dent Clin North Am* 15:219, 1971.

90. Blaser PK, Lund MR, Cochran MA, et al: Effect of designs of Class 2 preparations on resistance of teeth to fracture. *Oper Dent* 8:6, 1983.

91. Vale WA: Tooth preparation and further thoughts on high speed. *Br Dent J* 107:333, 1959.

92. Gilmore HW: Restorative materials and tooth preparation design. *Dent Clin North Am* 15:99, 1971.

93. Mahler DB, Terkla LG: Analysis of stress in dental structures. *Dent Clin North Am* 2:789, 1958.

94. Restoration of tooth preparations with amalgam and tooth-colored materials: Project ACCORDE student syllabus, Washington, D.C., 1974, US Department of Health, Education, and Welfare.

95. Dias de Souza GM, Pereira GD, Dias CT, et al: Fracture resistance of teeth restored with the bonded amalgam technique. *Oper Dent* 26:511, 2001.

96. Mahler DB, Engle JH: Clinical evaluation of amalgam bonding in class I and II restorations. *J Am Dent Assoc* 131:43, 2000.

97. Smales RJ, Wetherell JD: Review of bonded amalgam restorations and assessment in a general practice over five years. *Oper Dent* 25:374, 2000.

98. Ziskind D, Venezia E, Kreisman I, et al: Amalgam type, adhesive system, and storage period as influencing factors on microleakage of amalgam restorations. *J Prosthet Dent* 90:255, 2003.

99. Lindemuth JS, Hagge MS, Broome JS: Effect of restoration size on fracture resistance of bonded amalgam restorations. *Oper Dent* 25:177, 2000.

100. Larson TD, Douglas WH, Geistfeld RE: Effect of prepared cavities on the strength of teeth. *Oper Dent* 6:2, 1981.

101. Rudda JC. Modern class II amalgam tooth preparations. *N Z Dent J* 68:132, 1972.

102. Joynt RB, Davis EL, Wieczkowski G, Jr, et al: Fracture resistance of posterior teeth with glass ionomer-composite resin systems. *J Prosthet Dent* 62:28, 1989.

103. Osborne JW, Summitt JB: Extension for prevention: Is it relevant today? *Am J Dent* 11:189, 1998.

104. Summitt JB, Osborne JW: Initial preparations for amalgam restorations: extending the longevity of the tooth-restoration unit. *J Am Dent Assoc* 123:67, 1992.

105. Leon AR: The periodontium and restorative procedures: a critical review. *J Oral Rehabil* 4:105, 1977.

106. Loe H: Reactions of marginal periodontal tissues to restorative procedures. *Int Dent J* 18:759, 1968.

107. Waerhaug J: Histologic considerations which govern where the margins of restorations should be located in relation to the gingivae. *Dent Clin North Am* 4:161, 1960.

108. Summitt JB, Howell ML, Burgess JO, et al: Effect of grooves on resistance form of conservative class 2 amalgams. *Oper Dent* 17:50, 1992.

109. Crockett WD, Shepard FE, Moon PC, et al: The influence of proximal retention grooves on the retention and resistance of class II preparations for amalgam. *J Am Dent Assoc* 91:1053, 1975.

110. Summitt JB, Osborne JW, Burgess JO, et al: Effect of grooves on resistance form of Class 2 amalgams with wide occlusal preparations. *Oper Dent* 18:42, 1993.

111. Della Bona A, Summitt JB: The effect of amalgam bonding on resistance form of class II amalgam restorations. *Quintessence Int* 29:95, 1998.

112. Görücü J, et al: Effects of preparation designs and adhesive systems on retention of class II amalgam restorations. *J Prosthet Dent* 78:250, 1997.

113. Mondelli J, Ishikiriama A, de Lima Navarro MF, et al: Fracture strength of amalgam restorations in modern Class II preparations with proximal retentive grooves. *J Prosthet Dent* 32:564, 1974.

114. Mondelli J, Francischone CE, Steagall L, et al: Influence of proximal retention on the fracture strength of Class II amalgam restorations. *J Prosthet Dent* 46:420, 1981.

115. Sturdevant JR, Taylor DF, Leonard RH, et al: Conservative preparation designs for Class II amalgam restorations. *Dent Mater* 3:144, 1987.

116. Khera SC, Chan KC: Microleakage and enamel finish. *J Prosthet Dent* 39:414, 1978.

117. Summitt JB, Osborne JW, Burgess JO: Effect of grooves on resistance/retention form of Class 2 approximal slot amalgam restorations. *Oper Dent* 18:209, 1993.

118. Duncalf WV, Wilson NHF: Adaptation and condensation of amalgam restorations in Class II preparations of conventional and conservative design. *Quintessence Int* 23:499, 1992.

119. Jokstad A, Mjor IA: Cavity design and marginal degradation of the occlusal part of Class II amalgam restorations. *Acta Odontol Scand* 48:389, 1990.

120. Pack AR: The amalgam overhang dilemma: a review of causes and effects, prevention, and removal. *N Z Dent J* 85:55, 1989.

121. Van Nieuwenhuysen JP, D'Hoore W, Carvalho J, et al: Long-term evaluation of extensive restorations in permanent teeth. *J Dent* 31:395–405, 2003.

122. Martin JA, Bader JD: Five-year treatment outcomes for teeth with large amalgams and crowns. *Oper Dent* 22:72–78, 1997.

123. Smales RJ: Longevity of cusp-covered amalgams: survivals after 15 years. *Oper Dent* 16:17–20, 1991.

124. Mondelli RF, Barbosa WF, Mondelli J, et al: Fracture strength of weakened human premolars restored with amalgam with and without cusp coverage. *Am J Dent* 11:181–184, 1998.

125. Davis R, Overton JD: Efficacy of bonded and nonbonded amalgam in the treatment of teeth with incomplete fractures, *J Am Dent Assoc* 131:469–478, 2000.

126. McDaniel RJ, Davis RD, Murchison DF, et al: Causes of failure among cuspal coverage amalgam restorations: a clinical survey *J Am Dent Assoc* 131:173–177, 2000.

127. Robbins JW, Summitt JB: Longevity of complex amalgam restorations. *Oper Dent* 13:54–57, 1988.

128. Mondelli RF, Barbosa WF, Mondelli J, et al: Fracture strength of weakened human premolars restored with amalgam with and without cusp coverage. *Am J Dent* 11:181, 1998.

129. Chan CC, Chan KC: The retentive strength of slots with different width and depth versus pins. *J Prosthet Dent* 58:552–557, 1987.

130. McMaster DR, House RC, Anderson MH, et al: The effect of slot preparation length on the transverse strength of slot-retained restorations. *J Prosthet Dent* 67:472–477, 1992.

131. Christensen GJ: Achieving optimum retention for restorations. *J Am Dent Assoc* 135:1143–1145, 2004.

132. Mozer JE, Watson RW: The pin-retained amalgam. *Oper Dent* 4:149–155, 1979.

133. Fischer GM, Stewart GP, Panelli J: Amalgam retention using pins, boxes, and Amalgambond. *Am J Dent* 6:173–175, 1993.

134. Boyde A, Lester KS: Scanning electron microscopy of self-threading pins in dentin. *Oper Dent* 4:56–62, 1979.

135. Standlee JP, Caputo AA, Collard EW, et al: Analysis of stress distribution by endodontic posts. *Oral Surg Oral Med Oral Pathol* 33:952–960, 1972.

136. Webb EL, Straka WF, Phillips CL: Tooth crazing associated with threaded pins: a three-dimensional model. *J Prosthet Dent* 61:624–628, 1989.

137. Going RE, Moffa JP, Nostrant GW, et al: The strength of dental amalgam as influenced by pins. *J Am Dent Assoc* 77:1331–1334, 1968.

138. Welk DA, Dilts WE: Influence of pins on the compressive and horizontal strength of dental amalgam and retention of pins in amalgam. *J Am Dent Assoc* 78:101–104, 1969.

139. Going RE: Pin-retained amalgam. *J Am Dent Assoc* 73:619–624, 1966.

140. Pameijer CH, Stallard RE: Effect of self-threading pins. *J Am Dent Assoc* 85:895–899, 1972.

141. Moffa JP, Razzano MR, Doyle MG: Pins—a comparison of their retentive properties. *J Am Dent Assoc* 78:529–535, 1969.

142. Perez E, Schoeneck G, Yanahara H: The adaptation of noncemented pins. *J Prosthet Dent* 26:631–639, 1971.

143. Vitsentzos SI: Study of the retention of pins. *J Prosthet Dent* 60:447–451, 1988.

144. Dilts WE, Welk DA, Laswell HR, et al: Crazing of tooth structure associated with placement of pins for amalgam restorations. *J Am Dent Assoc* 81:387–391, 1970.

145. Trabert KC, Caputo AA, Collard EW, et al: Stress transfer to the dental pulp by retentive pins. *J Prosthet Dent* 30:808–815, 1973.

146. Dilts WE, Welk DA, Stovall J: Retentive properties of pin materials in pin-retained silver amalgam restorations. *J Am Dent Assoc* 77:1085–1089, 1968.

147. Eames WB, Solly MJ: Five threaded pins compared for insertion and retention. *Oper Dent* 5:66–71, 1980.

148. Hembree JH: Dentinal retention of pin-retained devices. *Gen Dent* 29:420–422, 1981.

149. Khera SC, Chan KC, Rittman BR: Dentinal crazing and interpin distance. *J Prosthet Dent* 40:538–543, 1978.

150. Wing G: Pin retention amalgam restorations. *Aust Dent J* 10:6–10, 1965.

151. Courtade GL, Timmermans JJ, editors: *Pins in restorative dentistry*, St. Louis, 1971, Mosby.

152. Dilts WE, Duncanson MG, Jr, Collard EW, et al: Retention of self-threading pins. *J Can Dent Assoc* 47:119–120, 1981.

153. Durkowski JS, Harris RK, Pelleu GB, et al: Effect of diameters of self-threading pins and channel locations on enamel crazing. *Oper Dent* 7:86–91, 1982.

154. Mondelli J, Vieira DF: The strength of Class II amalgam restorations with and without pins. *J Prosthet Dent* 28:179–188, 1972.

155. Cecconi BT, Asgar K: Pins in amalgam: a study of reinforcement. *J Prosthet Dent* 26:159–169, 1971.

156. Dilts WE, Mullaney TP: Relationship of pinhole location and tooth morphology in pin-retained silver amalgam restorations. *J Am Dent Assoc* 76:1011–1015, 1968.

157. Dolph R: Intentional implanting of pins into the dental pulp. *Dent Clin North Am* 14:73–80, 1970.

158. Felton DA, Webb EL, Kanoy BE, et al: Pulpal response to threaded pin and retentive slot techniques: a pilot investigation. *J Prosthet Dent* 66:597–602, 1991.

159. Caputo AA, Standlee JP: Pins and posts—why, when, and how. *Dent Clin North Am* 20:299–311, 1976.

160. Gourley JV: Favorable locations for pins in molars. *Oper Dent* 5:2–6, 1980.

161. Caputo AA, Standlee JP, Collard EW: The mechanics of load transfer by retentive pins. *J Prosthet Dent* 29:442–449, 1973.

162. Dilts WE, Coury TL: Conservative approach to the placement of retentive pins. *Dent Clin North Am* 20:397–402, 1976.

163. Standlee JP, Collard EW, Caputo AA: Dentinal defects caused by some twist drills and retentive pins. *J Prosthet Dent* 24:185–192, 1970.

164. Standlee JP, Caputo AA, Collard EW: Retentive pin installation stresses. *Dent Pract Dent Rec* 21:417–422, 1971.

165. Kelsey WP, III, Blankenau RJ, Cavel WT: Depth of seating of pins of the Link Series and Link Plus Series. *Oper Dent* 8:18–22, 1983.

166. Barkmeier WW, Cooley RL: Self-shearing retentive pins: a laboratory evaluation of pin channel penetration before shearing. *J Am Dent Assoc* 99:476–479, 1979.

167. Barkmeier WW, Frost DE, Cooley RL: The two-in-one, self-threading, self-shearing pin: efficacy of insertion technique. *J Am Dent Assoc* 97:51–53, 1978.

168. Garman TA, Binon PP, Averette D, et al: Self-threading pin penetration into dentin. *J Prosthet Dent* 43:298–302, 1980.

169. May KN, Heymann HO: Depth of penetration of Link Series and Link Plus pins. *Gen Dent* 34:359–361, 1986.

170. Irvin AW, Webb EL, Holland GA, et al: Photoelastic analysis of stress induced from insertion of self-threading retentive pins. *J Prosthet Dent* 53:311–316, 1985.

171. Abraham G, Baum L: Intentional implantation of pins into the dental pulp. *J South Calif Dent Assoc* 40:914–920, 1972.

172. Robbins JW, Burgess JO, Summitt JB: Retention and resistance features for complex amalgam restorations. *J Am Dent Assoc* 118:437–442, 1989.

173. Bailey JH: Retention design for amalgam restorations: pins versus slots. *J Prosthet Dent* 65:71–74, 1991.

174. Garman TA, Outhwaite WC, Hawkins IK, et al: A clinical comparison of dentinal slot retention with metallic pin retention. *J Am Dent Assoc* 107:762–763, 1983.

175. Outhwaite WC, Garman TA, Pashley DH: Pin vs. slot retention in extensive amalgam restorations. *J Prosthet Dent* 41:396–400, 1979.

176. Outhwaite WC, Twiggs SW, Fairhurst CW, et al: Slots vs. pins: a comparison of retention under simulated chewing stresses. *J Dent Res* 61:400–402, 1982.

177. Smith CT, Schuman N: Restoration of endodontically treated teeth: a guide for the restorative dentist. *Quintessence Int* 28:457–462, 1997.

178. Oliveira Fde C, Denehy GE, et al: Fracture resistance of endodontically prepared teeth using various restorative materials. *J Am Dent Assoc* 115:57–60, 1987.

179. Lambert RL, Goldfogel MH: Pin amalgam restoration and pin amalgam foundation. *J Prosthet Dent* 54:10–12, 1985.

180. Nayyar A, Walton RE, Leonard LA: An amalgam coronal-radicular dowel and core technique for endodontically treated posterior teeth. *J Prosthet Dent* 43:511–515, 1980.

181. Kane JJ, Burgess JO, Summitt JB: Fracture resistance of amalgam coronal-radicular restorations. *J Prosthet Dent* 63:607–613, 1990.

182. Shillingburg HT, Jr, editor: *Fundamentals of fixed prosthodontics*, ed 3, Chicago, 1997, Quintessence.

183. Leinfelder KF: Clinical performance of amalgams with high content of copper. *Gen Dent* 29:52–55, 1981.

184. Osborne JW, Binon PP, Gale EN: Dental amalgam: clinical behavior up to eight years. *Oper Dent* 5:24–28, 1980.

185. Eames WB, MacNamara JF: Eight high copper amalgam alloys and six conventional alloys compared. *Oper Dent* 1:98–107, 1976.

11

Periodontology Applied to Operative Dentistry

PATRICIA A. MIGUEZ, THIAGO MORELLI

This chapter presents an overview of the periodontal structures and their importance in restorative dentistry. Following a review of the anatomy and physiology of the periodontal tissues, periodontal contributory factors affecting restorative dentistry are discussed. The impact of periodontal therapy as part of the restorative treatment and the effect of the restorative treatment on the periodontium will also be presented.

The proximity of many dental restorations to the periodontium makes their relationship inseparable. To maintain a healthy periodontium and avoid chronic periodontal inflammation, restorations should be designed and performed properly. Dental restorations that reestablish function and esthetics, when required, and are supported by a healthy periodontium should be the goal of any restorative procedure.

When necessary, periodontal therapy to eliminate or control the etiologic factors that contribute to periodontal disease should be performed prior to restorative procedures. Timely periodontal therapy can avoid unesthetic results such as undesired position of the gingival margins. Healthy gingival tissues that frame the dentition are crucial to maintain the oral health and to enhance esthetics.

Basic Concepts of the Periodontium Relevant for Restorative Dentistry

The Gingiva

From an anatomic point of view, the gingiva represents the masticatory mucosa that is bound to the teeth and covers the alveolar processes. The gingiva involves the alveolar crest, the interdental bony septa, and part of the alveolar process to the mucogingival junction in continuity to the lining alveolar mucosa.[1]

The gingiva is described as free, attached, and interdental gingiva, with the free gingival groove and mucogingival junction as main anatomical landmarks (Fig. 11.1). The *free gingiva* is unattached and often characterized by the sulcus depth. It can be distinguished from the attached gingiva by the free gingival groove. The free gingival groove is present in only about one third of the normal gingiva with similar occurrence between different genders and deciduous/permanent dentitions.[2]

The *attached gingiva* is firmly attached to the periosteum of the alveolar process. The attached gingiva is clinically characterized by a firm and pink gingiva surrounding the dentition and separated from the mucosa by the mucogingival junction. In a series of radiographic studies, Ainamo and colleagues demonstrated the relative stable position of the mucogingival junction over time and suggested that the zone of attached gingiva increases with age due to teeth and alveolar process eruption.[3-5] The widest band of attached gingiva is present on the buccal aspect of central and lateral incisors; the narrowest band is present at the buccal area of canines and first premolars.

The *interdental gingiva* consists of the gingival tissues that fill the embrasures below the interproximal contact points in anterior teeth. In posterior teeth where the interproximal contact points are broad, the interdental gingiva is formed from the buccal and lingual papillae bridged by the col.

The Cementum

The cementum is an avascular, multiunit, mineralized connective tissue with variable phenotypes (i.e., cellular, acellular, fibrillar, afibrillar) and functions. The principal function of the cementum is tooth anchorage (Fig. 11.2). Due to its dynamic restorative nature and adaptability, the cementum is important for the maintenance of the occlusal relationships and for the integrity of the root surface.[6]

The Alveolar Bone

The alveolar processes house the teeth and are composed of the outer cortical plates of compact bone, the trabecular bone, and the alveolar bone proper (the bundle bone around teeth)[7] (see Fig. 11.2). The cortical plates are built from bony lamellae and are thinner in the maxilla and thicker in the posterior mandible. The alveolar bone proper is located adjacent to the periodontal ligament.

The Periodontal Ligament

The periodontal ligament (PDL) occupies the space between the cementum and the alveolar bone (see Fig. 11.2). The PDL is a

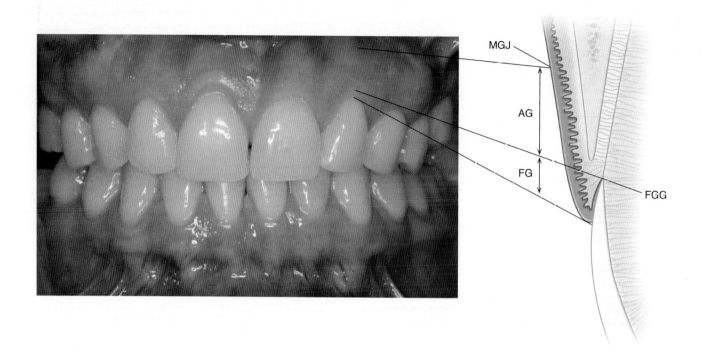

• **Fig. 11.1** Free gingiva *(FG)* and attached gingiva *(AG)* are parts of the gingiva and limited by the anatomical landmarks mucogingival junction *(MGJ)* and free gingival groove *(FGG)*.

multifunctional unit of connective tissue that contains numerous cells, fibers, rich vasculature, and cellular components—osteoblasts, osteoclasts, fibroblasts, epithelial rests of Malassez, odontoblasts, cementoblasts, macrophages, and undifferentiated mesenchymal cells. The extracellular matrix consists of collagen fibrils and other noncollagenous proteins[8] and pluripotent dynamic stem cells.[9]

From a functional point of view, the PDL participates in tooth anchorage, bone tissue development and homeostasis, nutrition-metabolic circulation, and innervation.[7] Its width varies from 0.15 to 0.4 mm and is adapted to functional demands within this narrow range.[8]

The Biologic Width

The term biologic width, a genetically driven structure, refers to the combined vertical dimension of the junctional epithelium and the supraalveolar connective tissue (Fig. 11.3). This dentogingival complex acts as a seal around the cervical portion of the tooth and has a self-restoration capacity. For instance, epithelial attachment mechanically separated from the tooth surface during periodontal probing or flossing reattaches to the original level in approximately 5 days.[10] In health, the epithelial attachment terminates at the apical end of the junctional epithelium. In diseased tissues, it terminates at the coronal aspect of the connective tissue, or apical to the junctional epithelium.[11,12]

Gargiulo and colleagues studied the dentogingival dimensions in healthy human specimens using autopsy material from 30 subjects, completing measurements in a total of 287 teeth. One of their observations was that the epithelial–connective tissue complex as a whole migrates apically during passive eruption. Moreover, they noted that during the different phases of development and passive eruption, the connective tissue zone had the

most consistent dimension. The junctional epithelium was the most variable area.[13] Years later, Vacek and colleagues focused on the implication of biologic width dimensions for restorative dentistry. They conducted another cadaveric study in pursuit of the minimum biologic dimensions that can be tolerated by the tissues. The authors confirmed the findings of the previous study in terms of the variability of the individual components. In addition, they recognized that the biologic width was greater in posterior teeth and the junctional epithelium was significantly longer in teeth with restorations.[14] The mean biologic width was found to be 1.91 mm, which consisted of junctional epithelium (1.14 mm) and connective tissue attachment (0.77 mm). The mean sulcus depth was found to be 1.32 mm (Table 11.1; see Fig. 11.3).

Violating the biologic width by placing restorative margins within or apical to the junctional epithelium will lead to disturbance of the biologic seal and penetration of bacteria and their by-products leading to gingival inflammation, attachment loss, and recession or pocket formation. In that event, the biologic width can only be restored by apical reestablishment of the supracrestal connective tissue.[15]

The Gingival Display

In a healthy smile, the lip rises to the level of or slightly apical to the gingival margins of the maxillary anterior teeth, revealing 1 to 2 mm of gingiva. When more than 2 mm of gingival tissue is shown upon smiling this is described as a "gummy smile" and considered unesthetic. Different etiologic factors have been described in the literature for this excessive gingival display (Fig. 11.4).[16]

Excessive gingival display has been associated with excessive maxillary bone growth. In this case individuals may have longer lower third facial height, shorter upper lips, and consequently

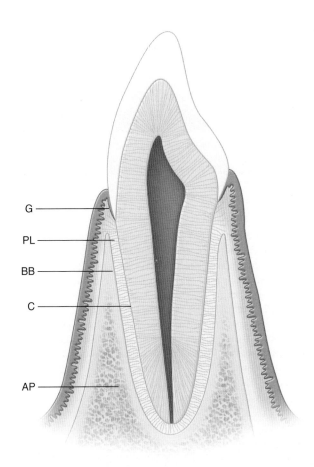

• **Fig. 11.2** The periodontium surrounds and supports the teeth and is composed of gingiva *(G)*, periodontal ligament *(PL)*, bundle bone *(BB)*, cementum *(C)*, and alveolar process *(AP)*.

TABLE 11.1	Biologic Width Components and Dimensions (mm and Range)	
	Gargiulo et al. 1961	Vacek & Gher 1994
Sulcus	0.69 (0.61–1.76)	1.32 (0.26–6.03)
Junctional epithelium	0.97 (0.71–1.35)	1.14 (0.32–3.27)
Connective tissue	1.07 (1.06–1.08)	0.77 (0.29–1.84)
Biologic width	2.04	1.91

more eruption of the maxillary teeth. A multidisciplinary approach including potentially combined orthodontic therapy and orthognathic surgery is indicated to move the maxillary complex apically and address this esthetic concern. Recently, surgical techniques for lip repositioning have been described as alternatives to orthognathic surgery.[17,18] A comprehensive evaluation is always indicated to avoid frustration with unexpected results.

Another etiologic factor for excessive gingival display is the delayed migration of the gingival margin commonly known as altered passive eruption. As teeth erupt, the gingival margin migrates apically to a level at or about 1 mm coronal to the cementoenamel junction (CEJ). The failure of gingival tissues to move apically

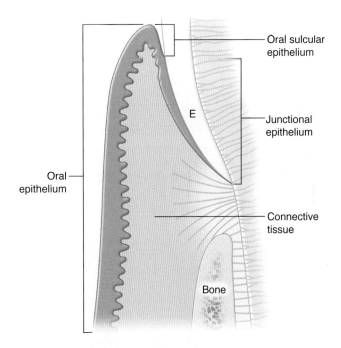

• **Fig. 11.3** The biologic width combines the vertical dimension of the junctional epithelium and the supraalveolar connective tissue. The oral sulcular epithelium lines the clinical gingival sulcus, which is occlusal to the biological width. *E,* enamel.

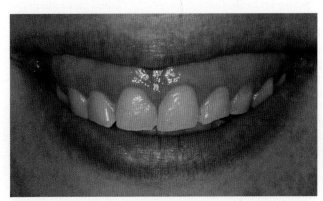

• **Fig. 11.4** "Gummy smile" showing more than 2 mm of gingival tissue during smile. (Courtesy Dr. Tony Crivello.)

results in excessive gingival display (Fig. 11.5). Surgical intervention is usually beneficial in individuals with thick, fibrotic, and noninflamed gingival tissue with a probing depth of 3 to 4 mm coronal to the CEJ. To ascertain the type of surgical intervention needed, the clinician is referred to the classification and treatment recommendations described by Coslet and colleagues.[19] Considerations in the decision between crown lengthening and gingivectomy are described later in this chapter.

Challenges in Periodontal Health Affecting Restorative Dentistry

Periodontal Disease

Periodontitis is an immune-inflammatory infection of the tooth-supporting structures and a major cause of tooth loss among adults.

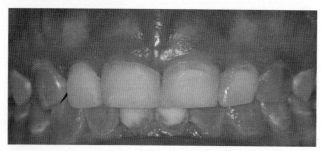

• **Fig. 11.5** Example of altered passive eruption where the gingival margin failed to move apically and closer to the cementoenamel junction, resulting in excessive gingival display. (Courtesy Dr. André Ritter.)

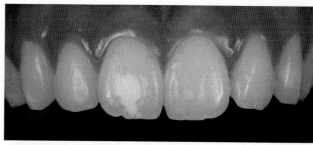

• **Fig. 11.6** Thin and scalloped biotype often shows transparency within the clinical gingival sulcus when a periodontal probe is inserted. It is often associated with tapered or triangular anatomic crown shapes with small interproximal contact areas.

It has been recognized as one of the current most prevalent infectious diseases, affecting nearly 50% of the American population.[20] Associations with overall systemic conditions and numerous risk factors or indicators such as diabetes, smoking, age, genetics, immunosuppression, and obesity have been identified as these may increase the severity and distribution of periodontal disease.[21]

A healthy periodontium is important to achieve long-term success with optimum comfort, function, and esthetics for any restorative procedure. In the presence of active periodontal diseases, such as gingivitis or periodontitis, periodontal therapy should be performed prior to most restorative procedures in order to eliminate and/or control the etiologic factors contributing to tissue damage.

Active periodontitis is diagnosed by clinical and radiographic evaluations. It is characterized clinically by deep probing depths, inflammation (bleeding on probing or visual bleeding), and subgingival calculus. Radiographically, active periodontitis is characterized by alveolar bone loss. Signs of successful periodontal therapy are the resolution of gingival inflammation, which can be achieved with efficient oral hygiene habits and nonsurgical and/or surgical periodontal therapy. Administration of antibiotics is indicated in some situations.[22]

Similar to periodontitis, gingivitis is also diagnosed by gingival inflammation characterized by edematous, spongy, and red gingiva. Bleeding on probing is usually present as well. However, there is no loss of the periodontal attachment often characterized by radiographic bone loss. Different than periodontitis, gingivitis may be controlled with adequate oral hygiene and adult prophylaxis only. Periodontitis requires scaling and root planing to remove subgingival plaque and calculus deposits. Severe cases may require concomitant antibiotic therapy and periodontal surgery to reestablish a healthy periodontium. A healthy periodontium is important to establish a controlled and clean field for restorative procedures and to maintain the integrity and esthetics of restorative treatments.

The Importance of Maintenance Therapy

The end of active periodontal treatment, nonsurgical or surgical, is not the end of periodontal therapy. Only maintenance therapy can secure the long-term success of periodontal treatment. The effect of maintenance therapy is evident when comparing tooth loss, amount of bone loss, changes in attachment level and probing depth, tooth mobility, and the progression of furcation involvement between patients with and without regular maintenance visits. It should be noted that tooth loss, while being the ultimate end point, may occur for reasons other than periodontal disease.

Furthermore, the decision to extract a tooth is subjective and may depend on the preference and philosophy of the practitioner. Nevertheless, studies have shown that patients in periodic maintenance therapy preserve more teeth than those who fail to comply.[23,24] Changes in attachment level and probing depth are surrogate end points and are objective; however, the cutoff point determines the sensitivity of the parameters used. Longitudinal studies indicate that patients in a periodic maintenance therapy schedule may have less mean annual attachment loss than non-compliant patients.[25,26]

Although maintenance therapy can be very effective in stabilizing the progression of periodontal disease in most patients, a subset of patients (2%–4%) and sites may suffer from progressive attachment loss regardless of regular maintenance schedule.[27,28] As mentioned earlier, several risk factors such as smoking, stress, and genetic background can influence disease progression.[29]

Gingival Biotypes

The gingival architecture depends on the type of gingival biotype. Generally the periodontium has been described as having two basic forms: a thick and flat biotype or a thin and scalloped biotype.[30,31] Each biotype has its own distinct characteristics and the clinician must be mindful of these to achieve a stable dento-gingival complex.

The thin and scalloped biotype frequently responds to gingival inflammation with gingival recession and is usually associated with tapered or triangular anatomic crown shapes with small interproximal contact areas (Fig. 11.6). Thin bone support with underlying dehiscences and/or fenestrations is a common finding in individuals with thin biotype. On the other hand, thick and flat biotype often responds to gingival insults with deep pocket depth formation, and it is usually associated with square anatomic crowns with broad interproximal contact areas (Fig. 11.7). The stability of the bone crest and position of the free gingival margin are positively correlated to the thickness of the alveolar bone and gingival tissue. This was confirmed by Stetler and Bissada who showed that there was less inflammation and shrinkage when subgingival restorations were placed in individuals with thick gingival biotype.[32]

Furcation Involvement

The furcation forms with the presence of two or more roots in a tooth and is therefore most common in molars. It is assumed that furcations increase the surface area of teeth for periodontium attachment and thus provide additional periodontal support.

However, this unique structure also renders neighboring periodontium more susceptible to destruction.

Exposure of the furcation with its involvement may occur as a result of bone loss during progression of periodontal disease or of surgical treatment as part of the restorative therapy. The diagnosis of furcation involvement is crucial because it is related to tooth prognosis. The degree of furcation involvement dictates the treatment for the tooth, as there is an association between the severity of furcation involvement and tooth longevity.[33] For proper diagnosis, thorough clinical and radiographic examinations must occur. Usually the furcation is examined with a specific probe such as the Nabers probe (Fig. 11.8), a 12-mm curved probe with 3-mm markings. Placing the tip of the Nabers probe against the tooth and moving it in an apical direction aids in detection of furcation involvement. The depression of the furca may also be examined in a similar manner.

Unfortunately, even though special care is taken during clinical examinations, furcation involvement, especially in maxillary molars, is difficult to detect. The assessment of furcation areas tends to be inaccurate because of great variations in root anatomy. It is further complicated by limited access due to adjacent teeth or soft tissue coverage. Radiographs provide an essential aid to clinical examinations; however, there are also limitations associated with the diagnosis of furcation involvement using radiographic images. The inherent two-dimensional presentation of conventional radiographic images limits the recognition of furcations.

Treatment options for furcation-involved teeth are generally based on the nature and extent of the furcation involvement. In general, treatment modalities are selected based on the classification of the furcation involvement. Several classification systems have been designed to determine the severity of furcation-involved teeth. The most commonly used is the Hamp classification. It classifies furcation involvement into three different grades:

- Grade I: horizontal penetration of the Nabers probe less than 3 mm
- Grade II: horizontal penetration of the Nabers probe more than 3 mm, but not through the furcation
- Grade III: through penetration of the Nabers probe from buccal to lingual[34] (Fig. 11.9).

Other factors, such as size and divergence of roots, root trunk length, crown-root ratio, and volume of remaining bone, are also important. Grade I furcation is generally treated with scaling and root planing. A clinical study evaluated the efficacy of scaling and root planing in Grade I furcation involvement and showed a 100% survival rate during a 5-year evaluation series.[34] Open flap debridement and furcation plasty may be indicated in some situations where prosthetic treatment is needed. Grades II and III furcations are also treated initially with scaling and root planing. However, the need for surgical treatment, such as open flap debridement or guided tissue regeneration, may be indicated to improve tooth prognosis. An investigation on the effects of nonsurgical treatment on periodontally involved teeth with furcation involvement showed a 90.7% survival rate during a 5- to 12-year period. Out of the failures, 60% were on teeth with Grade III furcation and 30% on teeth with Grade II furcation. That demonstrates the limitations of nonsurgical therapy to treat severe furcation involvement.[35] A retrospective study looking at the long-term survival of maxillary furcation-involved teeth in patients who had received treatment and were on maintenance showed decent prognosis with only 12% of involved molars being lost in 24 years.[33]

Open Proximal Contacts

Interestingly, open proximal contacts do not have a direct effect on periodontal disease progression despite its reported indirect impact on the periodontium. In 1980, Hancock and colleagues analyzed 40 males with open proximal contacts between their teeth and could not demonstrate a significant correlation between open contacts, gingival inflammation, and deep probing depths. On the other hand, open contacts were significantly related to food impaction, which demonstrated a significant correlation with higher gingival inflammation and deeper probing depths.[36] Jernberg and collaborators reported similar findings in regard to gingival inflammation and pocket depths. In their study, however, open proximal contacts demonstrated direct effect on the development

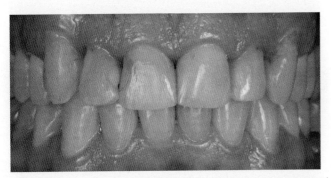

• **Fig. 11.7** Thick and flat biotype often shows more pronounced "orange peel" surface characteristics of the attached gingiva. It is often associated with square anatomic crowns with broad interproximal contact areas.

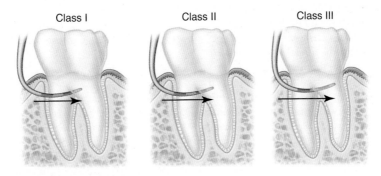

Class I   Class II   Class III

• **Fig. 11.8** Furcation involvement classified into three different grades or Classes by Hamp. Usually the furcation is examined with a specific probe such as the Nabers probe. The probe is placed against the tooth and moved in an apical direction as to try to find the entrance of the furcations.

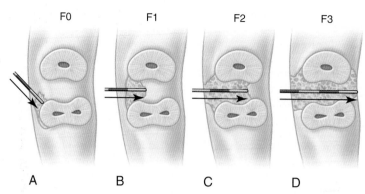

F0   F1   F2   F3

A   B   C   D

• **Fig. 11.9** A, F0 indicates no furcation penetration with the Nabers probe. B, F1 grade or Class I indicates horizontal penetration of the Nabers probe up to 3 mm. C, F2 grade or Class II indicates horizontal penetration of the Nabers probe more than 3 mm, but not through the furcation. D, F3 grade or Class III indicates through penetration of the Nabers probe from buccal to lingual.

of periodontal disease. A total of 104 adults were evaluated and open proximal contacts were found to be significantly correlated with deeper probing depths and higher clinical attachment loss.[37] To reduce the influence of open proximal contacts, it is appropriate to restore (close) them as long as overhangs are not created. Adequate oral hygiene instructions should always be part of the therapy.

Enamel Pearls

Enamel pearls are ectopic globules of enamel adherent to the tooth found most often in furcation regions of maxillary second and third molars.[38] They consist primarily of enamel, but dentin and even pulpal tissues can be found in some cases. The mean occurrence of enamel pearls in humans is 2.9% with a high occurrence of 9.7% among the Eskimo population.[38] Ectopic enamel such as enamel pearl is highly associated with attachment loss[39] and its removal is therefore indicated. Histologic observations demonstrate that enamel pearls have most of the structural features of enamel but with less orderly organization.[40] Its development is not well understood.

Cervical Enamel Projection

Cervical enamel projections (CEPs) are ectopic deposits of enamel apical to the CEJ with a tapering form and extending toward or entering the furcation. Since connective tissue does not attach to enamel, CEPs have been demonstrated to be an etiologic factor in furcation defects (Fig. 11.10). Bissada and Abdelmalek analyzed 1138 molars in Egyptian skulls and showed that CEPs were present in 8.6% of the cases. CEPs were present in approximately 50% of the cases where the furcation was involved.[41] The authors reported that CEPs were more frequently present in mandibular second molars followed by maxillary second molars. In another study CEPs were present in 67.9% of the studied population (45.2% molars). Molars with furcation involvement had CEPs in 82.5% of the cases, whereas molars without furcation involvement had CEPs in 17.5% of the cases. The most affected tooth was the mandibular first molar followed by the maxillary first molar.[42]

The impact of CEPs on periodontal health depends on the extent of the projection. In 1964 Masters and Hoskins introduced a classification system for CEPs, which is still in use[43]:

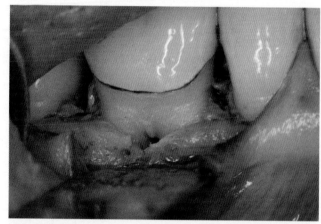

• **Fig. 11.10** Cervical enamel projection present on the furcation of a mandibular molar. Note the furcation defect caused by lack of connective tissue attachment to the apically located enamel leading to increased bacterial colonization and apical migration in the furcation. (Courtesy Dr. Tony Crivello.)

- Grade 1: Short but distinct change in the contour of CEJ extending toward the furcation
- Grade 2: CEP approaches the furcation, without making contact with it
- Grade 3: CEP extends into the furcation

Considering CEPs are a contributory factor to periodontal disease, especially in furcation areas, its removal or at least reduction is indicated. However, this should be done carefully to avoid irreversible damage to the tooth.

Cemental Tears

The cemental tear is a fragment of cementum that detaches from the tooth, usually after trauma, causing isolated bone loss (vertical bone defects) (Fig. 11.11). It should be taken into consideration as a differential diagnosis for root fracture. Due to its low incidence, most studies available are case reports. Treatment involves surgical debridement, removal of the cementum fragment, and periodontal regeneration, if indicated. Several case reports demonstrate that the area can be successfully maintained after surgical treatment.[44,45]

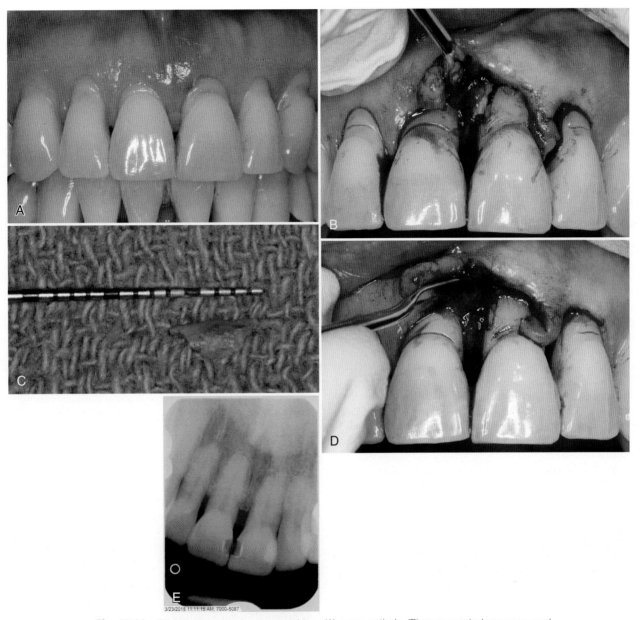

• **Fig. 11.11** Clinical case showing cemental tear (A) preoperatively, (B) upon surgical exposure, and (C) fractured cement. The mesiofacial root area on tooth No. 9 after removal of cemental tear is shown in D. Radiographic diagnosis may not always be possible (E). (Courtesy Dr. David Semeniuk.)

Palatoradicular Grooves

The radicular or palatal groove is a developmental anomaly in which an infolding of the inner enamel epithelium and Hertwig epithelial root sheath create a groove that passes from the cingulum of maxillary incisors apically onto the root.[46] Palatal grooves may act as funnels, which facilitate the accumulation of biofilm in the depth of the groove. The area is inaccessible to both patients and clinicians, and the prognosis for involved teeth, with diagnosed bone loss around the area, is poor. Hou and Tsai evaluated 404 maxillary incisors and reported that the palatal groove was present in 30.2% of lateral incisors, 5.9% of central incisors, and 4% of both maxillary incisors.[47] When indicated, treatment consists of odontoplasty to remove or reduce the groove. When odontoplasty is not possible, the groove may be restored with a biologically acceptable restorative material (see Materials, later in this chapter).

Tooth Position

Various parameters of tooth malposition have been correlated with periodontal disease.[48] The main influence of tooth malposition is the effect on plaque accumulation due to more difficult hygiene around malpositioned teeth. However, when oral hygiene is properly done, tooth malposition is not a significant factor causing plaque accumulation and consequent gingival inflammation.[49]

Occlusion

The role of traumatic occlusion in periodontal disease is extremely controversial. Consensus exists, however, that traumatic occlusion is not an initiating factor but can act as a contributory factor for periodontal disease. Nunn and Harrel evaluated the effects of traumatic occlusion on periodontal disease and concluded that occlusal discrepancy is an independent risk factor for periodontal disease.[50] Records from 24 years showed that teeth with initial occlusal discrepancies demonstrate significantly worse prognosis, and deeper probing depths and mobility. Trauma from occlusion has also been linked to higher risk for furcation involvement.[51]

Based on the evidence suggesting that traumatic occlusion may influence the course of periodontal disease, minor occlusal adjustments with the purpose of achieving better periodontal treatment outcomes are recommended.[52]

Periodontal Procedures Relevant to Restorative Dentistry

Crown Lengthening

A healthy periodontium is important to achieve long-term success and optimum comfort, function, and esthetics for any restorative procedure. As mentioned earlier, the relationship between restorations and periodontium must be respected for a successful treatment outcome. Even if gingivitis or periodontitis are not present, one should not proceed with restorative treatment without further consideration of the future relationship between restoration and supporting tissues. In this regard, biologic width preservation is critical.

When violation of the biologic width—namely placement of the restorative margin beyond the gingival sulcus and invading the junctional epithelium and connective tissue boundaries—is anticipated, crown lengthening of the tooth in question needs to be performed so the margin of the restoration is coronal to these biologic structures. As previously described, the mean depth of the sulcus is 1.32 mm; thus placing a restoration beyond 1 mm into the sulcus is potentially disruptive of the biologic width.

Crown lengthening is defined as the removal of bone tissue with concomitant removal or repositioning of the soft tissue around the tooth. The goal of this therapy is to increase the clinical crown and consequently preserve the biologic width. Typically, crown lengthening is needed to avoid impingement of the biologic width often occurring due to presence of subgingival caries or deep restorative margins. The procedure may also be recommended to correct esthetic unpleasant situations such as a "gummy smile." Failing to recognize the need for crown lengthening prior to restorative procedures often leads to invasion of biologic width leading to inflammation (gingivitis) and bone loss (periodontitis), pain associated with inflammatory remodeling of the periodontium, local soft and hard tissue defects, compromised esthetics, and problematic retention of restoration in some instances.

Padbury and colleagues suggested that the biologic width is preserved when the restoration is placed allowing for approximately 2 mm for the connective tissue and junctional epithelium and 1 mm for the sulcus. Further, ideally an additional 0.5 to 1 mm should be added coronally to create a safe distance from the alveolar bone crest to the restorative margin. A 3- to 4-mm distance from gingival margin to the alveolar crest ensures periodontium healing after tooth preparation with quick reestablishment of the junctional epithelium and connective tissue integrity, which avoids continuous inflammation around the tooth.[53,54]

Current research and clinical observations show that there is variation in biologic width measurements among individuals and teeth, and that the 3-mm distance is the minimum necessary to avoid periodontal breakdown around subgingival restorative margins.[55] Wagenberg and colleagues, in fact, have suggested to

aim for a 5-mm distance from bone to the restorative margin when possible.[56] The challenge is that periodontists have a tendency to remove less bone than needed due to the nature of their specialty (i.e., preservation of the periodontium).[57] Thus aiming for 5 mm will direct the surgeon to achieve the necessary removal of the minimum 3 mm. Other authors have also discussed that individual variations in biologic width dimensions will be accounted for if more than 3-mm distance is ensured after surgery.[58] Several studies have reported that subgingival margins of restorations, even without overhangs, have more plaque accumulation, gingival inflammation, and development of periodontal pockets than supragingival ones.[59,60] In a 26-year prospective cohort, Schatzle and colleagues showed a 0.5-mm increased mean loss of attachment in patients with restorations with subgingival margins after 10 years of function.[61]

It is important to remember that the periodontium biotype plays a key role in the periodontal response. Normally if the periodontium is thin and scalloped, recession will follow the inflammatory process caused by the restoration margin. If the periodontium is thick and flat and thus soft tissue stability is more likely, there is a higher likelihood of a moatlike lesion around the tooth to appear on the alveolar bone, leading to increased bleeding, sensitivity on probing, and pocket formation.[53,62] Timely recommendation of crown lengthening to avoid such issues is a crucial step toward tissue health, predictable esthetics, and patient satisfaction.

There are situations, however, where clinical crown lengthening may not be indicated and alternative treatment options should be explored. These include limitations caused by position of the furcation, reduced attachment levels, and esthetic issues. For instance, a tooth with a short trunk may limit the amount of crown lengthening that can be performed as the procedure could expose the furcation and compromise tooth prognosis (Fig. 11.12). In that event, avoiding violation of biologic width may not be possible and the surgical procedure may not be performed or may be only partially performed, leading to a compromised restorative treatment. In general, all subgingival margins compromise and impact the periodontium. Herrero and colleagues found that in areas of difficult access such as the lingual and distolingual surfaces of molars, surgeons removed an average of 0.4 mm of bone short of the 3-mm goal. A higher degree of inflammation leading to bone loss is expected in these areas since proper crown lengthening was not performed.[57]

Another common scenario where biologic width is violated and difficult to manage is crown fractures extending below the gingival margin. Crown lengthening is often necessary for proper restoration of fractured teeth (Fig. 11.13). In the case of fracture of anterior teeth, crown lengthening surgery will significantly impact the tooth clinical and consequently esthetic display (as well as of the adjacent teeth) due to the removal of bone and subsequent apical repositioning of the gingival margin (Fig. 11.14). There are situations where orthodontic extrusion is indicated to minimally affect the gingival margin levels in the anterior sextant or esthetic area. Crown lengthening may follow the orthodontic extrusion. Camargo in 2007 stated that forced tooth eruption via orthodontic extrusion is the technique of choice when clinical crown lengthening is necessary on isolated teeth in the esthetic zone.[63]

For optimal outcome, proper healing of the periodontal tissues after crown lengthening is necessary. The type of periodontium (thick and flat versus thin and scalloped) and the location (anterior versus posterior) generally dictate the extent of healing time. Direct restorations can be made as soon as there is initial tissue shrinkage

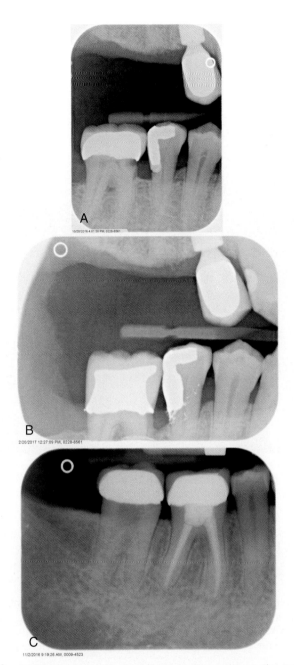

• **Fig. 11.12** A, Tooth No. 30 with secondary caries on the mesial surface leading to invasion of biologic width (beyond the clinical gingival sulcus). Note that tooth No. 29 has a restoration with deep and open margin violating the biologic width on the distal surface. B, After compromised crown lengthening surgery and crown replacement. To avoid furcation exposure (note the short trunk of tooth No. 30), the amount of crown lengthening was limited. C, Another clinical case showing an example of a long trunk on teeth No. 30 and No. 31, which would allow for a non-compromised crown lengthening surgery since furcation would likely not be at a risk of exposure.

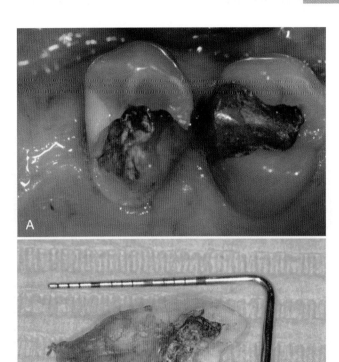

• **Fig. 11.13** A, Endodontically treated bicuspid presents with a large coronal subgingival fracture. B, Poor crown–root ratio can be appreciated indicating that crown lengthening would not be recommended on this tooth to expose the fractured surface for restoration. Extraction was recommended.

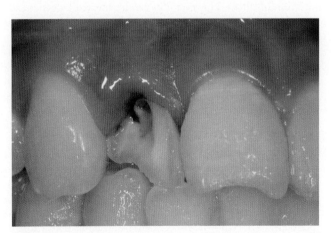

• **Fig. 11.14** Fractured anterior tooth No. 7. Esthetics must be carefully considered when treatment planning the restoration of anterior fractured teeth. Crown lengthening may compromise the esthetic outcome and be contraindicated. (Courtesy Dr. Eduard Epure.)

if the margin is supragingival and hemostasis/trauma to the tissue is not anticipated. For indirect full-coverage restorations, clinical studies indicate that the clinician should wait approximately 6 to 8 weeks before proceeding with final preparation and impression in posterior teeth.[64] In anterior esthetic cases, the periodontal biotype needs to be taken into consideration before proceeding with restorative treatment. In a thick and flat periodontium, the

gingiva tends to bulk postoperatively prior to moving coronally and flatten as maturation occurs in the first 6 to 8 weeks. Further flattening may continue to occur beyond the initial maturation phase. In a thin and scalloped periodontium, there is usually recession immediately after surgery and in some cases "creeping attachment" occurs in the months after initial maturation. One study demonstrated that probing depths stabilized at 6 weeks but recession ranging from 2 to 4 mm continued to develop between 6 and 24 weeks.[65] Thus, in areas of esthetic concern, postponing final margin placement and restoration for 6 to 8 months may be desirable to ensure gingival margin stability. To better predict results, an accurate diagnosis of thick versus thin biotype should be done.[66] Finally it is important to be knowledgeable of situations where crown lengthening is not indicated. Besides the previously mentioned risk of exposing furcation and causing esthetic issues in the anterior dentition, other limitations/contraindications are teeth with significantly reduced periodontal support; endodontically infected teeth that should not be treated prior to resolution of the periapical lesion; extensive need for osseous removal, which would compromise the stability of adjacent teeth; and inadequate crown-to-root ratio after surgery.

Gingivectomy

Unlike crown lengthening, gingivectomy does not involve hard tissue but rather just gingival excess removal to expose the clinical crown. For a successful gingivectomy procedure, careful treatment planning after detailed examination is crucial. Diagnosis and management of the etiology are critical for a positive outcome. In the case of gingival overgrowth, the soft tissue should not rebound provided the etiology for overgrowth is addressed (e.g., triggering medications, local trauma) and good oral hygiene is exercised. Plaque control is critical for overgrowth control in cases involving drugs that may stimulate tissue reaction and where medication replacement is not possible.[67] In the case of altered passive eruption, where there is excess of soft tissue due to altered apical migration of the gingiva, the tissue removed does not regrow provided absence of coronal positioning of the bone. When gingival tissue is removed to expose the clinical crown but the removal alters the dimension of the sulcus and junctional epithelium, the tissue regrows to establish at least approximately 1 mm of junctional epithelium and 1 mm of sulcus. However, this can be affected by genetically predetermined dimensions. Crown lengthening would be indicated to remove the bone and reposition the gingival margin apically.

Some of the clinical scenarios to consider gingivectomy versus crown lengthening are (1) subgingival caries/access for proper restoration, (2) tooth fracture, (3) inadequate retention, (4) altered passive eruption, and (5) other esthetic concerns such as gingival overgrowth or defects.

Subgingival Caries/Access for Proper Restoration

When subgingival caries present, at least 3 mm of sound tooth structure are needed from the margin of the final cavity preparation (not the caries lesion) to the alveolar bone crest (Fig. 11.15); otherwise crown lengthening is recommended. It is important to emphasize that open flap and bone contour correction is warranted if periodontal breakdown with evidence of osseous defect due to caries impinging the biologic width is present.

Tooth Fracture

Crown lengthening is almost always necessary for subgingival crown-root fractures, to avoid continuous periodontal breakdown in the site. Subgingival fractures are normally already affecting biologic width considering their presentation. In the unusual situations where the biologic width is adequate after a subgingival fracture, it is very likely that crown lengthening will be necessary after tooth preparation for a crown, for instance, because the crown preparation is often placed more apically to where the fracture happened. When the fracture is not treated for several weeks or

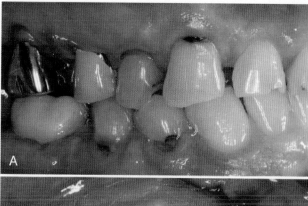
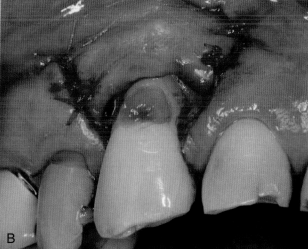

• **Fig. 11.15** A, Subgingival caries on teeth No. 6, No. 28, and No. 29. Ideally the cavitated areas need to be exposed surgically to allow for proper restoration. Further, a 3-mm distance for biologic width establishment is needed from the margin of the tooth preparation to the alveolar bone crest to promote best tissue health. B, Tooth No. 6 with caries excavated, immediately after crown lengthening procedure. (Courtesy Dr. Bruno Herrera.)

months, the periodontium and bone remodel on the site, moving away from the fracture margin, creating a bony ledge and a crater (moatlike defect) around the tooth. The area is likely to stay inflamed and become uncomfortable for the patient if not corrected.

Inadequate Retention

Extensively compromised teeth due to extensive fractures and/or caries lesions often need to be altered prior to final restoration. When there is a need to create a ferrule in a tooth that will receive a post-and-core restoration, crown lengthening may be needed to facilitate its placement without violation of the biologic width and adequate retention form. There is an overall consensus that 1.5 to 2 mm of ferrule is necessary for adequate retention of crowns and protection of the integrity of the remaining tooth structures. Crown lengthening may not be necessary if adequate ferrule can be achieved without violation of the biologic width. However, additional retention may be necessary; otherwise gingivectomy may be performed to temporarily remove gingival tissue.[68]

Gegauff highlighted that an attempt to gain adequate ferrule via crown lengthening procedure can negatively affect the tooth mechanical properties.[69] The apical relocation of the crown margin after crown lengthening procedures leads to a thinner cross section in the ferrule area. Further, there is a reduction in the crown-to-root

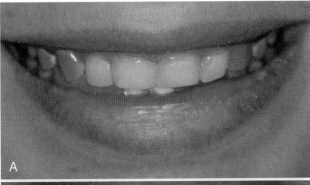

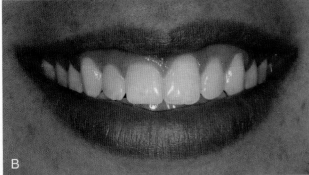

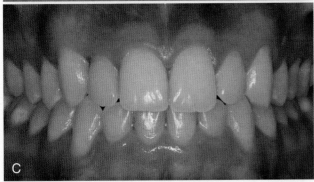

• **Fig. 11.16** Altered passive eruption often results in a flat gingival contour and squared-shaped anterior teeth (A) or uneven gingival contours such as the case in *B*, where discrepancies can be noted between teeth No. 7 and No. 10, and teeth No. 8 and No. 9. Case (B) with gingival discrepancy corrected by gingivectomy (C). (A, Courtesy Dr. André Ritter; B, C, Photo credit: Dr. Akshay Kumarswamy, Mumbai, India.)

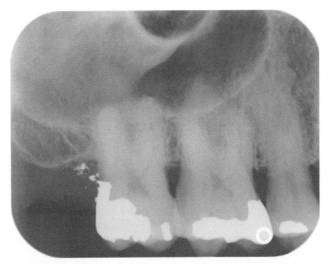

• **Fig. 11.17** Tooth No. 2 with ill-fitting amalgam restoration at the subgingival distal margin. Distal wedge should have been performed prior to restoration to facilitate access for proper restorative treatment.

CEJ to the alveolar crest, there is enough keratinized tissue, and there is no evidence of bone defect (see Fig. 11.16B and C). The location of the bone in relationship to the CEJ and the mucogingival junction are important parameters in treatment of altered passive eruption. They can be determined with bone sounding and clinical and radiograph examination. Gingivectomy is not advised when the band of keratinized tissue is insufficient (<3 mm).

Distal Wedge

Distal wedge is commonly performed on the distal surface of molars (tuberosity or the retromolar pad) to facilitate hygiene, access and help eliminate periodontal pockets, or facilitate access for proper restorative treatment (Fig. 11.17). The procedure is either complete removal of the tissue (if there is abundant amount of keratinized tissue even after removal) or partial ablation of tissue (to spare keratinized tissue). In any case, after tissue removal, soft tissue coverage of the bone and more coronal tooth exposure is achieved. A direct restoration can be performed immediately after the surgical procedure provided adequate operating field isolation is achieved.

Noncarious Cervical Lesions and Mucogingival Surgery

Noncarious cervical lesions (NCCLs) are characterized by the loss of tooth structure at the cervical area of a tooth due to abfraction, abrasion, and/or erosion (Fig. 11.18). These lesions are noncarious but may need to be managed provided one or more of these factors are present: (1) The patient is concerned with esthetics, (2) there is substantial tooth sensitivity that does not resolve with other treatment options (i.e., desensitizing agents), (3) the lesion is progressing and there is risk of pulpal exposure, or (4) the lesion is progressing and the tooth integrity is at risk.

To deliver the best possible treatment preserving the natural contour and integrity of the gingival tissues around the affected tooth or teeth, options other than restoration only are available and should be considered. In the event of gingival recession and/or lack of keratinized/attached gingiva with concomitant presence of a NCCL, careful evaluation of the site should be performed to

ratio that also may negatively affect the outcome of the treatment. Orthodontic extrusion may be another option to expose tooth structure in some clinical situations of inadequate retention. Yet crown-to-root ratio and apical location of the ferrule also will occur in orthodontic extrusion.

Altered Passive Eruption

Crown lengthening or gingivectomy can also be indicated for esthetic reasons only or before restoring a tooth that has altered passive eruption. Altered passive eruption is the diagnosis when a significant amount of anatomic crown is covered by gingiva due to failure of proper apical migration of the soft tissue that covers the crown of the tooth. Often the patient displays a gummy smile with squared-looking teeth (Fig. 11.16A).[70] This condition affects esthetics and also increases plaque accumulation as the sulcus depth promotes easy apical plaque migration.[71] Gingivectomy may be performed when there is a distance of more than 3 mm from the

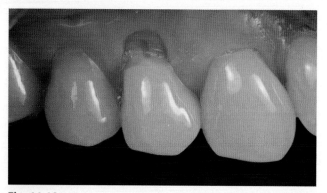

• **Fig. 11.18** Noncarious cervical lesions are characterized by the loss of tooth structure at the cervical area of a tooth and multifactorial etiology. Treatment may involve soft tissue grafting of the area depending on extent of lesion and periodontal condition with or without concomitant tooth restoration.

determine the appropriate treatment: restoration, soft tissue coverage (graft), or a combined approach.

Predictable soft tissue root coverage of recessions with subcutaneous connective tissue graft can be accomplished with recessions that fall under the Miller classification of Class I and Class II.[72] The Miller classification has been widely used to classify recessions based on the amount of tissue loss in relationship to the mucogingival junction, width of the tissue loss around the facial or lingual aspect of the tooth, and loss of soft and hard interproximal tissue[73] (Fig. 11.19):

- Class I: Marginal tissue recession that does not extend to the mucogingival junction. There is no periodontal loss (bone or soft tissue) in the interdental area, and 100% root coverage can be anticipated.
- Class II: Marginal tissue recession that extends to or beyond the mucogingival junction. There is no loss of interdental bone or soft tissue, and 100% of root coverage can be expected.

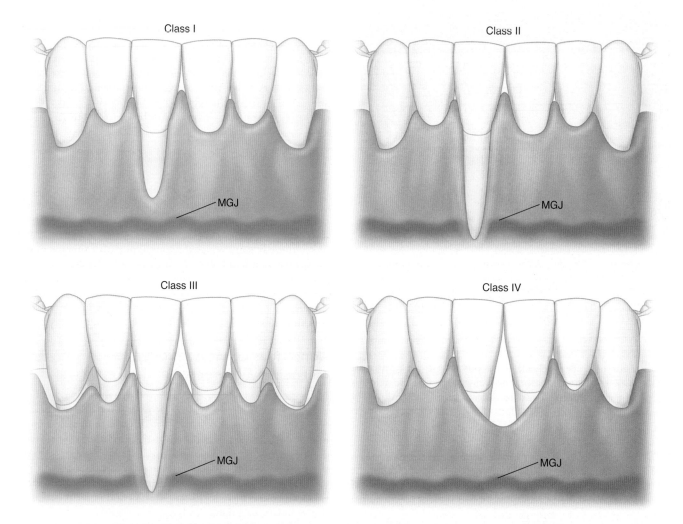

• **Fig. 11.19** Miller classification of gingival recessions. Class I: recession does not extend to the mucogingival junction *(MGJ)*. Class II: recession extends to or beyond the MGJ; 100% of root coverage can be expected for Class I and II. Class III: recession extends to or beyond the MGJ with loss of interdental tissue or there is malpositioning leading to inability to cover 100% of the root surface. Class IV: recession extends to or beyond the MGJ where there is advanced loss of interdental tissues and root coverage is not anticipated.

- Class III: Recession that extends to or beyond the mucogingival junction. There is loss of interdental bone and/or soft tissue or there is malpositioning of the teeth leading to inability to cover 100% of the root surface.
- Class IV: Marginal tissue recession that extends to or beyond the mucogingival junction where there is advanced loss of interdental tissues and root coverage is not anticipated.

After gingival grafting, full root coverage can usually be expected up to the level of the interdental bone. However, soft tissue coverage of a cervical lesion that is located mostly in enamel is not recommended.[74] Indeed, no true tissue–tooth attachment is expected to happen between the grafted soft tissue and the tooth enamel to help stabilize the graft. Further, such location is typically at a far distance from the bone, which restricts vascular supply to support the grafted tissue in that area. Clinical researchers have reported that NCCLs, just like interdental tissue loss, are a significant negative factor in the prognosis of gingival root coverage.[75] The authors did not elaborate on the possible reason. It is possible that occlusion and hygiene factors are involved in the lower success of grafting of NCCLs.

The following rationale is followed when treating a NCCL. Lesions that exceed approximately 2 mm in axial depth typically need restoration. This will depend on progression rate, symptomatology, and desire to restore. Aside from diagnosing and treating the etiology, fast-developing lesions should be restored. Restoration also may be indicated for NCCLs that continue symptomatic after attempts to reduce sensitivity with desensitizing products. Soft tissue grafting in addition to restoration may be recommended when there is lack of attached gingiva or a thin tissue biotype.[74]

Grafting only is indicated in cases of limited tooth loss (lesion depth <2 mm). That is based on the need for grafting due to recession or lack of keratinized/attached gingiva. While Miller Class I and Class II cases have good prognosis, the long-term stability has been questioned.[75] That said, the patient may opt for periodic application of desensitizing products in lieu of the surgical procedure. A randomized clinical trial evaluating the outcome of connective tissue graft and resin-modified glass ionomer restorations for the treatment of gingival recession and NCCLs concluded that graft alone or graft with restoration showed increased attachment level and soft tissue coverage for up to 2 years in patients with Miller Class I recessions.[76]

When considering mucogingival surgery, the keratinized tissue and attached gingiva levels must be evaluated. There is a difference between attached and keratinized gingiva. Keratinized gingiva involves the attached and the free gingival tissue. Since the attached gingiva is bound to the underlying periosteum, the clear presence of keratinized gingiva is seen as protective of the periodontium against inflammation and bone loss. Recommendations have been made to increase the band of keratinized/attached gingiva prior to subgingival restorations that will be in close proximity with the gingival margin (or subgingivally after grafting). The presence of a narrow keratinized tissue band (i.e., less than 2 mm) has been linked to an increased chance of gingivitis.[32] However, others have found that gingival health can be maintained with little or no keratinized tissue in the absence of plaque accumulation and inflammation.[77,78] Soft tissue grafting to increase the band of keratinized/attached gingiva may be recommended in patients with poor hygiene and restorations in close proximity to the gingival tissues.

Another indication for mucogingival surgery includes teeth that lack adequate band of keratinized/attached gingiva and that will undergo orthodontic therapy. Increasing the keratinized/attached gingiva band may be necessary to avoid gingival recession.[79] This is particularly significant for patients with thin periodontium. Despite this, teeth should always be moved inside of their alveolar housing to minimize chances of recession. Recessions cannot be predictably covered when the position of the tooth in the arch is far outside the alveolar plate. Soft tissue grafting may be of different types and have different indications such as free gingival graft, connective tissue graft, pedicle flap, among others.

Effect of Restorative Treatment on the Periodontium

In the previous section we reviewed the impact and indications of surgical procedures in restorative dentistry such as crown lengthening, gingivectomy, distal wedge, and mucogingival surgery. Often these procedures are crucial prior to proper restorative treatment. Conversely, it is also important to understand the impact of restorative procedures on periodontal health to prevent periodontal breakdown. It is critically important to understand the possible effects of restorative therapy (e.g., biologic width violation, materials, margins of restorations, provisional restorations, retraction cord trauma) on the periodontium.

Biologic Width Violation

Much has already been discussed in this chapter about the importance of biologic width preservation. Violation of the biologic width is often a result of caries removal and consequent preparation of the tooth for direct or indirect restorations leading to damage of the junctional epithelium and the connective tissue above the alveolar crest. The contact of the restoration margin with the junctional epithelium or the connective tissue below the gingival sulcus allows for bacterial colonization of the area. Recruitment of inflammatory cells and chronic inflammation of the site follow.[55] While polishing of the restoration may alleviate plaque accumulation and inflammation, there is extensive evidence of inflammation leading to bone resorption in sites with biologic width violation. The inflammatory process is usually aggravated with indirect restorations as the marginal gap of a well-fitted crown is normally larger than that of a direct restoration. Sorensen and colleagues reported on marginal fit in relation to percentage bone loss and gingival flow and found positive correlation between marginal discrepancy of restorations and periodontal defects.[80] In summary, proper placement of the margin of the restoration (direct or indirect) in respect of the biologic width is critical.

Materials

Besides careful placement of restorations to avoid marginal overhangs, voids, and rough restorations in close proximity to the periodontium, biocompatible materials should be favored.

Mineral trioxide aggregate (MTA) appears to have a significant improved tissue response and bone formation compared to composite resins, amalgams, and glass ionomers.[81] The common response from other materials is the formation of fibrous connective tissue that will connect them to the alveolar bone. Despite this, MTA is not the material of choice for situations where the material is close to the gingiva, as it does not have the mechanical properties required to sustain occlusal stresses.[82] Further, a coronal restoration in contact with soft tissues would not need to promote bone growth but rather a healthy soft tissue response.

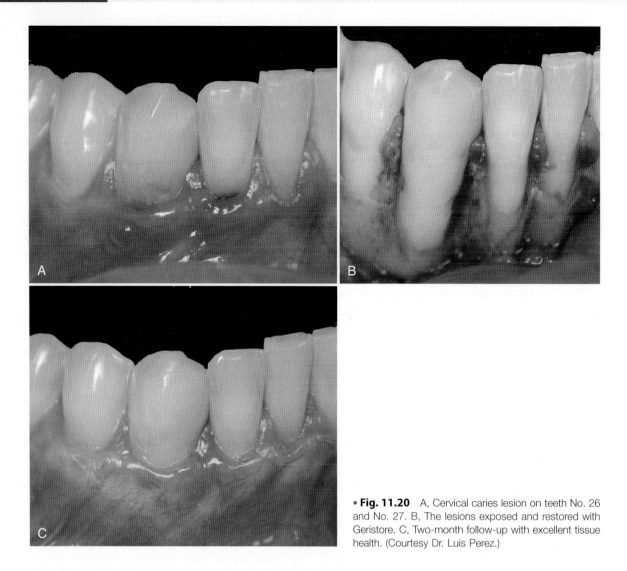

• **Fig. 11.20** A, Cervical caries lesion on teeth No. 26 and No. 27. B, The lesions exposed and restored with Geristore. C, Two-month follow-up with excellent tissue health. (Courtesy Dr. Luis Perez.)

Gomes and colleagues reported that the periodontal response to resin-modified glass ionomers was more favorable than the response to amalgam and composite resins in an animal study after 124 days.[83] In another more recent study, Sakallioglu and colleagues studied the release of inflammatory markers in gingival crevicular fluid in humans after restorations with metaloceramic, composite resin, and amalgam restorations. Results showed a significant increase in certain inflammatory peptides compared to controls (enamel surface) for all groups with amalgam showing the highest levels after 4 weeks.[84]

Known for its biocompatibility, Geristore (DenMat, Lompoc, CA) is a dual-cure, hydrophilic resin-modified glass ionomer often recommended when the periodontium is extensively involved. Its manufacturer recommends it as liner, in direct pulp capping, in Class V and conservative Class I and Class II restorations, in root caries lesions, in subgingival restorations for fractured roots and resorption lesions, in root perforations, and as retrograde filling material. Research has shown that Geristore has better or similar adhesion to tooth structures than some of the other glass ionomers and presents low microleakage.[85-88] Its biocompatibility has been extensively studied with mostly positive results being reported.[89-91] Geristore has shown to allow for better growth and cell morphology, and has improved toxicity profile of human gingival fibroblasts

compared to Ketac Fil (3M Oral Care, St. Paul, MN) and IRM (Dentsply Sirona, York, PA).[90]

Gupta and colleagues showed that Geristore had superior biocompatibility compared to MTA and glass ionomer when tested on human periodontal ligament cells.[89] A clinical study by Dragoo showed that Geristore was not different in terms of probing depth and gingival inflammation than other resin-based materials such as Dyract (Dentsply Sirona) and Photac Fil (3M Oral Care).[92] It was concluded that a material with biocompatibility, dual-cure capability, insolubility in oral fluids, low coefficient of thermal expansion, low polymerization shrinkage, and low microleakage is ideal for subgingival restorations. Such properties are found in Geristore, which appears to be the preferred material among clinicians for cases where teeth are in need of subgingival restorations[93] (Fig. 11.20).

Provisional Restorations and Restorative Margins

The margins of indirect restorations are often placed subgingivally for esthetic purposes, to provide preparation margin in tooth structure rather than in restorative material (restorative foundation), or for additional retention. However, even when placed at gingival

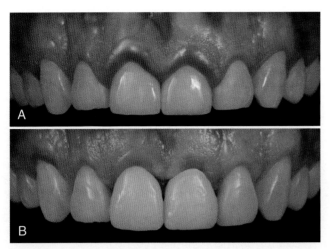

• **Fig. 11.21** A, Full-coverage restorations on teeth No. 8 and No. 9 with inadequate marginal preparation, crown adaptation, and invasion of biologic width causing gingival inflammation. B, Improved tissue health after crown lengthening to reestablish the biologic width and well-adapted temporary restoration.

level or slightly into the sulcus, some inflammatory tissue reaction will occur[94] (Fig. 11.21A). The presence of localized periodontal pathology has been found with indirect metaloceramic restorations independently of the supragingival or subgingival location of the margin. However, marginal adaptation is correlated with severity of inflammation.[94] To minimize the probability of tissue recession or chronic local inflammatory response, a well-adapted provisional restoration should always be placed and tissue reaction ideally observed for several weeks prior to final impression and placement of the final restoration. A tissue that is healthy after the provisional restoration is in place for several days or weeks is a good indication of no violation of the biologic width and that the periodontium will respond well to the final restoration margins (Fig. 11.21B). A well-adapted provisional restoration also will facilitate gingival retraction and final impression and ensure that the tissue will rebound atraumatically (after impression).

When a poorly contoured provisional restoration is placed, the inflammatory process starts and can be perpetuated after the final restoration is cemented as the area remains injured.[95] It is important to correct margins and roughness of any provisional as soon as detected to prevent and/or reverse damage leading to loss of periodontal attachment.

Further, placement of provisional restorations prior to proper initial healing after crown lengthening or gingivectomy can be problematic as it is not easy to determine the exact location where the alveolar crest and the biologic width will be reestablished. Despite the periodontal procedure performed, the result may still be violation of the biologic width with development of an inflammatory lesion after surgery. When there is need for immediate or early provisionalization after surgery, the restoration should rest

on supragingival margins. This early provisionalization can help with the soft tissue contouring and maintenance or papilla regrowth during the healing phase.[96] Further, some have advocated immediate provisionalization after crown lengthening surgery.[97] Such practice is only advised to extremely experienced periodontal-restorative teams and mostly indicated for patients with well-known positive tissue response to restorative procedures. Finally, to obtain a well-fitting provisional, it is important to understand that the tooth preparation/restoration margins need to be easily visualized and have enough intracoronal depth to allow for thickness of material without overhanging margins.

Besides provisional restorations, any final indirect or direct restoration (even well fitting) harbors more plaque and bacteria than enamel and challenges the supportive periodontium.[98] Thus in the case of a poorly contoured restoration, periodontal breakdown and recurrent caries at the restoration–tooth interface is probable in the long term.

Retraction Cord and Impressions

When the tooth is receiving an indirect restoration, gingival displacement is usually needed to adequately capture the preparation margins with either physical or digital impression methods.[99] This gingival displacement, or retraction, can be done mechanically, chemically, or surgically (electrosurgery or laser). Retraction cords have been shown to cause a reversible gingival displacement that is greater than other types of materials (i.e., paste or foam).[100] Others have found that all retraction techniques cause temporary gingival displacement with inflammation with Ultrapak (Ultradent Products, Inc., South Jordan, UT) cord without impregnation of hemostatic agent causing most bleeding but fastest recovery compared to Magic FoamCord (Coltène, Altstätten, Switzerland) and Expasyl (Kerr Corporation, Orange, CA).[101] In this study, all retraction techniques caused an acute injury after 1 day of retraction, which took 1 week to heal in the Ultrapak and the Magic FoamCord groups. The Expasyl group had the highest gingival index of inflammation and showed the slowest healing. Its use may also cause tooth sensitivity. In another study, the Magic FoamCord system was a less traumatic method of gingival retraction compared to cords in slightly subgingival preparations. However, the material was less effective than the single cord retraction technique in preparations with margins deeper than 2 mm.[102]

When evaluating gingival retraction cords versus electrosurgery, Wostmann and colleagues did not find any significant difference in the quality of the marginal fit of the crowns as long as the impression technique utilized two (light and heavy) impression materials.[103] To date there is no comparison between laser, electrosurgery, cord, and cordless materials in regard to gingival health and quality of impression. It is currently accepted that retraction systems cause some temporary damage to the integrity of the gingival tissues; however, the soft gingival tissue heals in a few days provided there is adequate marginal adaptation of the temporary restoration.

Summary

When planning restorations, thorough evaluation of periodontal health, impact of restorative treatment on periodontium, and patient perceptions of esthetics and understanding of oral health is warranted. Respecting the periodontium boundaries while restoring tooth structures is vital for the success of the restorative treatment and the overall oral homeostasis. Ill-fitting restorations and undiagnosed periodontal defects in teeth that will be restored can complicate treatment and lead to further disturbance of periodontal health. Although periodontal disease is primarily caused by dental plaque, there are modifying and significant alterations caused by restorative treatment that contribute to the establishment and progression of periodontal breakdown.

References

1. Schroeder HE, Listgarten MA: The gingival tissues: the architecture of periodontal protection. *Periodontol 2000* 13:91–120, 1997.
2. Ainamo J, Loe H: Anatomical characteristics of gingiva. A clinical and microscopic study of the free and attached gingiva. *J Periodontol* 37(1):5–13, 1966.
3. Ainamo A: Influence of age on the location of the maxillary mucogingival junction. *J Periodontal Res* 13(3):189–193, 1978.
4. Ainamo J, Talari A: The increase with age of the width of attached gingiva. *J Periodontal Res* 11(4):182–188, 1976.
5. Ainamo A, Ainamo J: The width of attached gingiva on supraerupted teeth. *J Periodontal Res* 13(3):194–198, 1978.
6. Bosshardt DD, Selvig KA: Dental cementum: the dynamic tissue covering of the root. *Periodontol 2000* 13:41–75, 1997.
7. Hassell TM: Tissues and cells of the periodontium. *Periodontol 2000* 3:9–38, 1993.
8. Nanci A, Bosshardt DD: Structure of periodontal tissues in health and disease. *Periodontol 2000* 40:11–28, 2006.
9. Seo BM, Miura M, Gronthos S, et al: Investigation of multipotent postnatal stem cells from human periodontal ligament. *Lancet* 364(9429):149–155, 2004.
10. Taylor AC, Campbell MM: Reattachment of gingival epithelium to the tooth. *J Periodontol* 43(5):281–293, 1972.
11. Magnusson I, Listgarten MA: Histological evaluation of probing depth following periodontal treatment. *J Clin Periodontol* 7(1):26–31, 1980.
12. Fowler C, Garrett S, Crigger M, et al: Histologic probe position in treated and untreated human periodontal tissues. *J Clin Periodontol* 9(5):373–385, 1982.
13. Gargiulo AW, Wentz FM, Orban B: Dimensions and relations of the dentogingival junction in humans. *J Periodontol* 32:261–267, 1961.
14. Vacek JS, Gher ME, Assad DA, et al: The dimensions of the human dentogingival junction. *Int J Periodontics Restorative Dent* 14(2):154–165, 1994.
15. Tal H, Soldinger M, Dreiangel A, et al: Periodontal response to long-term abuse of the gingival attachment by supracrestal amalgam restorations. *J Clin Periodontol* 16(10):654–659, 1989.
16. Kokich VG: Esthetics: the orthodontic-periodontic restorative connection. *Semin Orthod* 2(1):21–30, 1996.
17. Sanchez IM, Gaud-Quintana S, Stern JK: Modified lip repositioning with esthetic crown lengthening: A Combined approach to treating excessive gingival display. *Int J Periodontics Restorative Dent* 37(1):e130–e134, 2017.
18. Bhola M, Fairbairn PJ, Kolhatkar S, et al: LipStaT: The lip stabilization technique: Indications and guidelines for case selection and classification of excessive gingival display. *Int J Periodontics Restorative Dent* 35(4):549–559, 2015.
19. Coslet JG, Vanarsdall R, Weisgold A: Diagnosis and classification of delayed passive eruption of the dentogingival junction in the adult. *Alpha Omegan* 70(3):24–28, 1977.
20. Eke PI, Dye BA, Wei L, et al: Update on prevalence of periodontitis in adults in the United States: NHANES 2009 to 2012. *J Periodontol* 86(5):611–622, 2015.
21. Williams RC, Offenbacher S: Periodontal medicine: the emergence of a new branch of periodontology. *Periodontol 2000* 23:9–12, 2000.
22. Mombelli A: Antimicrobial advances in treating periodontal diseases. *Front Oral Biol* 15:133–148, 2012.
23. Becker W, Becker BE, Berg LE: Periodontal treatment without maintenance. A retrospective study in 44 patients. *J Periodontol* 55(9):505–509, 1984.
24. Axelsson P, Lindhe J: The significance of maintenance care in the treatment of periodontal disease. *J Clin Periodontol* 8(4):281–294, 1981.
25. Wennstrom JL, Serino G, Lindhe J, et al: Periodontal conditions of adult regular dental care attendants. A 12-year longitudinal study. *J Clin Periodontol* 20(10):714–722, 1993.
26. Rosling B, Serino G, Hellstrom MK, et al: Longitudinal periodontal tissue alterations during supportive therapy. Findings from subjects with normal and high susceptibility to periodontal disease. *J Clin Periodontol* 28(3):241–249, 2001.
27. Hirschfeld L, Wasserman B: A long-term survey of tooth loss in 600 treated periodontal patients. *J Periodontol* 49(5):225–237, 1978.
28. McFall WT, Jr: Tooth loss in 100 treated patients with periodontal disease. A long-term study. *J Periodontol* 53(9):539–549, 1982.
29. Fardal O, Linden GJ: Tooth loss and implant outcomes in patients refractory to treatment in a periodontal practice. *J Clin Periodontol* 35(8):733–738, 2008.
30. Ochsenbein C, Ross S: A reevaluation of osseous surgery. *Dent Clin North Am* 13(1):87–102, 1969.
31. Weisgold AS: Contours of the full crown restoration. *Alpha Omegan* 70(3):77–89, 1977.
32. Stetler KJ, Bissada NF: Significance of the width of keratinized gingiva on the periodontal status of teeth with submarginal restorations. *J Periodontol* 58(10):696–700, 1987.
33. Ross IF, Thompson RH, Jr: A long term study of root retention in the treatment of maxillary molars with furcation involvement. *J Periodontol* 49(5):238–244, 1978.
34. Hamp SE, Nyman S, Lindhe J: Periodontal treatment of multirooted teeth. Results after 5 years. *J Clin Periodontol* 2(3):126–135, 1975.
35. Dannewitz B, Krieger JK, Husing J, et al: Loss of molars in periodontally treated patients: a retrospective analysis five years or more after active periodontal treatment. *J Clin Periodontol* 33(1):53–61, 2006.
36. Hancock EB, Mayo CV, Schwab RR, et al: Influence of interdental contacts on periodontal status. *J Periodontol* 51(8):445–449, 1980.
37. Jernberg GR, Bakdash MB, Keenan KM: Relationship between proximal tooth open contacts and periodontal disease. *J Periodontol* 54(9):529–533, 1983.
38. Moskow BS, Canut PM: Studies on root enamel (2). Enamel pearls. A review of their morphology, localization, nomenclature, occurrence, classification, histogenesis and incidence. *J Clin Periodontol* 17(5):275–281, 1990.
39. Hou GL, Tsai CC: Cervical enamel projection and intermediate bifurcational ridge correlated with molar furcation involvements. *J Periodontol* 68(7):687–693, 1997.
40. Risnes S, Segura JJ, Casado A, et al: Enamel pearls and cervical enamel projections on 2 maxillary molars with localized periodontal disease: case report and histologic study. *Oral Surg Oral Med Oral Pathol Oral Radiol Endod* 89(4):493–497, 2000.
41. Bissada NF, Abdelmalek RG: Incidence of cervical enamel projections and its relationship to furcation involvement in Egyptian skulls. *J Periodontol* 44(9):583–585, 1973.
42. Hou GL, Tsai CC: Relationship between periodontal furcation involvement and molar cervical enamel projections. *J Periodontol* 58(10):715–721, 1987.
43. Masters DH, Hoskins SW: Projection of cervical enamel into molar furcations. *J Periodontol* 35:49–53, 1964.
44. Chou J, Rawal YB, O'Neil JR, et al: Cementodentinal tear: a case report with 7-year follow-up. *J Periodontol* 75(12):1708–1713, 2004.
45. Ishikawa I, Oda S, Hayashi J, et al: Cervical cemental tears in older patients with adult periodontitis. Case reports. *J Periodontol* 67(1):15–20, 1996.
46. Gound TG, Maze GI: Treatment options for the radicular lingual groove: a review and discussion. *Pract Periodontics Aesthet Dent* 10(3):369–375, quiz 76, 1998.
47. Hou GL, Tsai CC: Relationship between palato-radicular grooves and localized periodontitis. *J Clin Periodontol* 20(9):678–682, 1993.
48. Geiger AM, Wasserman BH, Turgeon LR: Relationship of occlusion and periodontal disease. 8. Relationship of crowding and spacing to periodontal destruction and gingival inflammation. *J Periodontol* 45(1):43–49, 1974.

49. Ingervall B, Jacobsson U, Nyman S: A clinical study of the relationship between crowding of teeth, plaque and gingival condition. *J Clin Periodontol* 4(3):214–222, 1977.

50. Nunn ME, Harrel SK: The effect of occlusal discrepancies on periodontitis. I. Relationship of initial occlusal discrepancies to initial clinical parameters. *J Periodontol* 72(4):485–494, 2001.

51. Wang HL, Burgett FG, Shyr Y: The relationship between restoration and furcation involvement on molar teeth. *J Periodontol* 64(4):302–305, 1993.

52. Burgett FG, Ramfjord SP, Nissle RR, et al: A randomized trial of occlusal adjustment in the treatment of periodontitis patients. *J Clin Periodontol* 19(6):381–387, 1992.

53. Padbury A, Jr, Eber R, Wang HL: Interactions between the gingiva and the margin of restorations. *J Clin Periodontol* 30(5):379–385, 2003.

54. Ingber JS, Rose LF, Coslet JG: The "biologic width"–a concept in periodontics and restorative dentistry. *Alpha Omegan* 70(3):62–65, 1977.

55. Matthews DC, Tabesh M: Detection of localized tooth-related factors that predispose to periodontal infections. *Periodontol 2000* 34:136–150, 2004.

56. Wagenberg BD, Eskow RN, Langer B: Exposing adequate tooth structure for restorative dentistry. *Int J Periodontics Restorative Dent* 9(5):322–331, 1989.

57. Herrero F, Scott JB, Maropis PS, et al: Clinical comparison of desired versus actual amount of surgical crown lengthening. *J Periodontol* 66(7):568–571, 1995.

58. Pontoriero R, Carnevale G: Surgical crown lengthening: a 12-month clinical wound healing study. *J Periodontol* 72(7):841–848, 2001.

59. Jansson L, Blomster S, Forsgardh A, et al: Interactory effect between marginal plaque and subgingival proximal restorations on periodontal pocket depth. *Swed Dent J* 21(3):77–83, 1997.

60. Orkin DA, Reddy J, Bradshaw D: The relationship of the position of crown margins to gingival health. *J Prosthet Dent* 57(4):421–424, 1987.

61. Schatzle M, Land NP, Anerud A, et al: The influence of margins of restorations of the periodontal tissues over 26 years. *J Clin Periodontol* 28(1):57–64, 2001.

62. Almeida AL, Esper LA, Sbrana MC, et al: Relationship between periodontics and restorative procedures: surgical treatment of the restorative alveolar interface (rai)–case series. *J Indian Prosthodont Soc* 13(4):607–611, 2013.

63. Camargo PM, Melnick PR, Camargo LM: Clinical crown lengthening in the esthetic zone. *J Calif Dent Assoc* 35(7):487–498, 2007.

64. Dowling EA, Maze GI, Kaldahl WB: Postsurgical timing of restorative therapy: a review. *J Prosthodont* 3(3):172–177, 1994.

65. Bragger U, Lauchenauer D, Lang NP: Surgical lengthening of the clinical crown. *J Clin Periodontol* 19(1):58–63, 1992.

66. De Rouck T, Eghbali R, Collys K, et al: The gingival biotype revisited: transparency of the periodontal probe through the gingival margin as a method to discriminate thin from thick gingiva. *J Clin Periodontol* 36(5):428–433, 2009.

67. Moffitt ML, Bencivenni D, Cohen RE: Drug-induced gingival enlargement: an overview. *Compend Contin Educ Dent (Jamesburg, NJ : 1995)* 34(5):330–336, 2013.

68. Hempton TJ, Dominici JT: Contemporary crown-lengthening therapy: a review. *J Am Dent Assoc* 141(6):647–655, 2010.

69. Gegauff AG: Effect of crown lengthening and ferrule placement on static load failure of cemented cast post-cores and crowns. *J Prosthet Dent* 84(2):169–179, 2000.

70. Alpiste-Illueca F: Altered passive eruption (APE): a little-known clinical situation. *Med Oral Patol Oral Cir Bucal* 16(1):e100–e104, 2011.

71. Dello Russo NM: Placement of crown margins in patients with altered passive eruption. *Int J Periodontics Restorative Dent* 4(1):58–65, 1984.

72. Tatakis DN, Chambrone L, Allen EP, et al: Periodontal soft tissue root coverage procedures: a consensus report from the AAP Regeneration Workshop. *J Periodontol* 86(2 Suppl):S52 S55, 2015.

73. Miller PD, Jr: A classification of marginal tissue recession. *Int J Periodontics Restorative Dent* 5(2):8–13, 1985.

74. Allen EP, Winter RR: Interdisciplinary treatment of cervical lesions. *Compend Contin Educ Dent (Jamesburg, NJ : 1995)* 32(Spec5):16–20, 2011.

75. Pini-Prato G, Magnani C, Zaheer F, et al: Influence of inter-dental tissues and root surface condition on complete root coverage following treatment of gingival recessions: a 1-year retrospective study. *J Clin Periodontol* 42(6):567–574, 2015.

76. Santamaria MP, da Silva Feitosa D, Casati MZ, et al: Randomized controlled clinical trial evaluating connective tissue graft plus resin-modified glass ionomer restoration for the treatment of gingival recession associated with non-carious cervical lesion: 2-year follow-up. *J Periodontol* 84(9):e1–e8, 2013.

77. Wennstrom J, Lindhe J, Nyman S: Role of keratinized gingiva for gingival health. Clinical and histologic study of normal and regenerated gingival tissue in dogs. *J Clin Periodontol* 8(4):311–328, 1981.

78. Wennstrom J, Lindhe J: Role of attached gingiva for maintenance of periodontal health. Healing following excisional and grafting procedures in dogs. *J Clin Periodontol* 10(2):206–221, 1983.

79. Geiger AM: Mucogingival problems and the movement of mandibular incisors: a clinical review. *Am J Orthod* 78(5):511–527, 1980.

80. Sorensen SE, Larsen IB, Jorgensen KD: Gingival and alveolar bone reaction to marginal fit of subgingival crown margins. *Scand J Dent Res* 94(2):109–114, 1986.

81. Schwartz RS, Mauger M, Clement DJ, et al: Mineral trioxide aggregate: a new material for endodontics. *J Am Dent Assoc* 130(7):967–975, 1999.

82. Nielsen MJ, Casey JA, VanderWeele RA, et al: Mechanical properties of new dental pulp-capping materials. *Gen Dent* 64(1):44–48, 2016.

83. Gomes SC, Miranda LA, Soares I, et al: Clinical and histologic evaluation of the periodontal response to restorative procedures in the dog. *Int J Periodontics Restorative Dent* 25(1):39–47, 2005.

84. Sakallioglu EE, Lutfioglu M, Sakallioglu U, et al: Gingival crevicular fluid levels of neuropeptides following dental restorations. *J Appl Biomater Funct Mater* 13(2):e186–e193, 2015.

85. Ashcraft DB, Staley RN, Jakobsen JR: Fluoride release and shear bond strengths of three light-cured glass ionomer cements. *Am J Orthod Dentofacial Orthop* 111(3):260–265, 1997.

86. Arora R, Deshpande SD: Shear bond strength of resin-modified restorative glass-ionomer cements to dentin–an in vitro study. *J Indian Soc Pedod Prev Dent* 16(4):130–133, 1998.

87. Nup C, Boylan R, Bhagat R, et al: An evaluation of resin-ionomers to prevent coronal microleakage in endodontically treated teeth. *J Clin Dent* 11(1):16–19, 2000.

88. Stockton LW, Tsang ST: Microleakage of Class II posterior composite restorations with gingival margins placed entirely within dentin. *J Can Dent Assoc* 73(3):255, 2007.

89. Gupta SK, Saxena P, Pant VA, et al: Adhesion and biologic behavior of human periodontal fibroblast cells to resin ionomer Geristore: a comparative analysis. *Dent Traumatol* 29(5):389–393, 2013.

90. Al-Sabek F, Shostad S, Kirkwood KL: Preferential attachment of human gingival fibroblasts to the resin ionomer Geristore. *J Endod* 31(3):205–208, 2005.

91. Al-Hiyasat AS, Al-Sa'Eed OR, Darmani H: Quality of cellular attachment to various root-end filling materials. *J Appl Oral Sci* 20(1):82–88, 2012.

92. Dragoo MR: Resin-ionomer and hybrid-ionomer cements: part II, human clinical and histologic wound healing responses in specific periodontal lesions. *Int J Periodontics Restorative Dent* 17(1):75–87, 1997.

93. Gultz JP, Scherer W: The use of resin-ionomer in restorative procedures. *N Y State Dent J* 64(6):36–39, 1998.

94. Passariello C, Puttini M, Virga A, et al: Microbiological and host factors are involved in promoting the periodontal failure of metalo-ceramic crowns. *Clin Oral Investig* 16(3):987–995, 2012.

95. Dragoo MR, Williams GB: Periodontal tissue reactions to restorative procedures. *Int J Periodontics Restorative Dent* 1(1):8–23, 1981.

96. Zucchelli G, Mazzotti C, Monaco C: A standardized approach for the early restorative phase after esthetic crown-lengthening surgery. *Int J Periodontics Restorative Dent* 35(5):601–611, 2015.

97. Tseng SC, Fu JH, Wang HL: Immediate temporization crown lengthening. *Compend Contin Educ Dent (Jamesburg, NJ : 1995)* 32(3):38–43, 2011.

98. Waerhaug J: Presence or absence of plaque on subgingival restorations. *Scand J Dent Res* 83(1):193–201, 1975.

99. Nemetz H, Donovan T, Landesman H: Exposing the gingival margin: a systematic approach for the control of hemorrhage. *J Prosthet Dent* 51(5):647–651, 1984.

100. Prasanna GS, Reddy K, Kumar RK, et al: Evaluation of efficacy of different gingival displacement materials on gingival sulcus width. *J Contemp Dent Pract* 14(2):217–221, 2013.

101. Al Hamad KQ, Azar WZ, Alwaeli HA, et al: A clinical study on the effects of cordless and conventional retraction techniques on the gingival and periodontal health. *J Clin Periodontol* 35(12):1053–1058, 2008.

102. Beier US, Kranewitter R, Dumfahrt H: Quality of impressions after use of the Magic FoamCord gingival retraction system–a clinical study of 269 abutment teeth. *Int J Prosthodont* 22(2):143–147, 2009.

103. Wostmann B, Rehmann P, Trost D, et al: Effect of different retraction and impression techniques on the marginal fit of crowns. *J Dent* 36(7):508–512, 2008.

12

Digital Dentistry in Operative Dentistry

DENNIS J. FASBINDER, GISELE F. NEIVA

Digital technology, computerized dentistry, and digital dentistry are general terms used to describe the clinical application of computer-assisted design, computer-assisted machining (CAD/CAM). The restorative dentistry application of CAD/CAM technology is the fabrication and delivery of permanent restorations for teeth and implants. For the past 30 years the incorporation of dental CAD/CAM into direct patient care has provided a way for dentists to deliver esthetic ceramic restorations in a single dental appointment.

There are three sequences involved in the CAD/CAM process.[1] An intraoral scanner or camera is used to accurately record the hard and soft tissue geometry of the patient's intraoral condition to a computer program in the first sequence. This is commonly referred to as a digital impression. A proprietary software design program is used to create a virtual restoration (the volume proposal) in the second sequence. The software programs have the capability of controlling and editing the various parameters of the restoration such as emergence profile, proximal contact, and occlusal relationships. Once the proposal of the restoration has been completed, a computer-controlled device is used to produce the restoration in the third sequence. The most common device uses a subtractive process to machine (i.e., grind or mill, depending on whether carbide burs or diamonds are used) the final restoration from a preformed block of a variety of restorative materials. Understanding these three sequences provides a basis for deciding how best to implement the technology in the dental office and also creates a simple way to categorize various systems in the marketplace.

Digital impression systems are designed to accurately record the intraoral geometry and then transmit the files to a dental laboratory for design and fabrication of the desired restoration. There is minimal if any opportunity for the dentist to design any aspect of the restoration on digital impression systems. They were developed to leverage the digital recording process to take advantage of the comfort and efficiency of not using conventional impression materials as well as the convenience and accuracy of digital transmission of the case to the dental laboratory.

Chairside CAD/CAM systems employ all three sequences of the CAD/CAM process in the dental office. They also record intraoral scans but provide, in addition, a software program for designing restorations as well as milling units to fabricate the restoration during a single dental appointment. They are designed to leverage the efficiency of a single appointment procedure for the delivery of ceramic restorations. Chairside CAD/CAM systems are the primary focus of the chapter because they allow the dentist complete control of the design, fabrication, and delivery of the restoration in the office during a single appointment.

Clinical Application

Treatment planning considerations for CAD/CAM restorations are not significantly different from ceramic restorations done with conventional impression materials and techniques. The CAD/CAM system represents an alternative means of restoration fabrication, not the restoration per se. The type of restoration (inlay, onlay, crown), the choice of material to be used, the desired occlusal relationships, and ability to isolate the tooth preparation for delivery of the restoration are several primary factors to consider rather than the restoration fabrication process itself. A case in point is that the predictable ability to isolate a subgingival margin for adhesive cementation is a much more important factor to consider than whether the ceramic restoration is fabricated with a conventional or digital impression technique. Nonetheless, there are a few specific considerations relative to the use of digital impressions. The relative size of the camera may be a concern for patients with a restricted ability to open wide. Generally, if there is sufficient vertical space to complete the tooth preparation with a dental handpiece, there is sufficient space for use of a digital camera. However, patients with a severe gag reflex may appreciate the use of a digital impression more than conventional impression since there is no physical contact with the intraoral tissues by a tray or impression material when recording a digital impression.

Chairside CAD/CAM Systems

Dr. Francois Duret conceptualized the first chairside CAD/CAM system in 1973. The first functioning chairside CAD/CAM prototype was introduced in the 1980s through the collaboration between a Swiss prosthodontist, Dr. Werner Mörmann, and an Italian electrical engineer, Marco Brandestini. Dr. Mörmann's vision was to use CAD/CAM technology to deliver esthetic ceramic restorations with improved longevity in a single appointment that avoided the deleterious consequences polymerization shrinkage caused in composite restorations.[2,3] The CEREC 1 unit marked the introduction of the CEREC system in 1985 with the first clinical trials reported in 1987.[4] The system has evolved through a series of hardware and software innovations and upgrades that culminated with the introduction of the first color-streaming powder-free intraoral camera in 2012, the CEREC Omnicam (Fig. 12.1).[5,6] The Omnicam is the imaging camera of the CEREC AC acquisition unit. The Omnicam is connected to a chairside computer with the three-dimensional design software and a liquid crystal display (LCD) monitor. The CEREC system is electronically connected to a milling unit. The newest version is a dry grinding

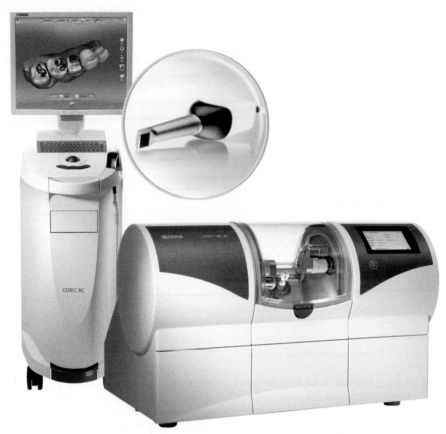

• **Fig. 12.1** CEREC OmniCam and MCX milling chamber. (Courtesy Dentsply Sirona.)

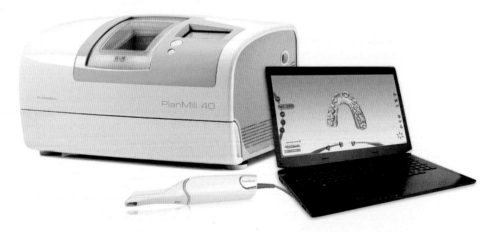

• **Fig. 12.2** PlanFit chairside CAD/CAM system. (Courtesy D4D Technologies.)

and wet milling unit that is the first in-office means by which to dry mill zirconia. Single-visit, full-contour, milled zirconia restorations are then further processed by sintering and glazing the restoration in the CEREC SpeedFire sintering furnace. This is the first in-office zirconia sintering furnace that can sinter preshaded CEREC zirconia material (CEREC Zirconia) in 10 to 15 minutes, as compared to the multiple hours that are generally necessary for sintering laboratory processed zirconia restorations.

An increasing number of chairside systems have been introduced since the late 2000s. The E4D Dentist System (D4D Technologies) was introduced in 2008 with its DentaLogic software offering a true three-dimensional virtual model.[7] The E4D Dentist System has an intraoral laser scanner, mobile Design Center with DentaLogic software, and a separate milling unit with a dedicated CAM server computer. The milling unit has two opposing electric motors that automatically change between three different diamonds depending on the specifics of the restoration dimensions. The milling unit has a dedicated computer server, which allows independent operation separate from the Design Center (after completion and transmission of the case design) (Fig. 12.2).

The CS 3500 is a powder-free intraoral scanner that was introduced in 2013. The Carestream system allows for in-office design using CS Solutions Restore software and in-office fabrication using the CS 3000 milling unit. The digital files may also be uploaded to a dental laboratory via CS Connect as they are compatible with a number of commercial laboratory design programs such as 3Shape (3Shape) and Exocad (Exocad Gmbh). Some of the unique features of the intraoral scanner include a disposable tip and a guiding light, which indicates a successful scan. The Carestream system has chairside capability for only a limited number of applications, including inlays, onlays, and crowns.

Chairside CAD/CAM systems are able to produce inlays, onlays, veneers, and crowns. Some systems also have the ability to fabricate short-span fixed partial dentures as well as temporary restorations in the dental office. Additional applications, such as implant abutments, fixed partial dentures, and orthodontic appliances, are unique to specific systems (Table 12.1).

Tooth Preparation Principles for CAD/CAM Restorations

Guidelines for tooth preparation for all-ceramic restorations are generally based on the specific geometries and thickness dimensions required to provide optimum strength for the selected ceramic material. For example, the occlusal reduction for a full-contour zirconia crown is less than that required for a leucite-reinforced or feldspathic porcelain crown, even if both materials are fabricated with a chairside CAD/CAM system. However, there are several preparation guidelines that enhance the accuracy of the CAD/CAM restoration due to their influence on the imaging and fabrication process, such as smooth contours, rounded transitions, and uniform pulpal floor.

A concept unique to CAD/CAM restorations has been termed "undermilling" or "overmilling." These terms have been applied to both grinding and milling processes. Any preparation geometry smaller than the dimension of the milling instruments presents a potential problem. Either the instrument must cut away more restorative material to ensure the restoration seats completely (overmilling) or it does not remove the smaller geometry (undermilling), leaving restorative material that will prevent complete seating of the restoration. Utilization of a preparation geometry with smooth contours, gently flowing curves, and rounded transition angles helps to limit the potential for overmilling and ensure an accurate internal adaptation of the restoration.

Crowns

Tooth preparation for CAD/CAM-fabricated crowns is essentially the same as for laboratory-fabricated ceramic crowns. The margin design for an all-ceramic crown requires a bulk of ceramic at the margin to avoid the risk of ceramic chipping or fracture. This is best accomplished with a shoulder, sloped shoulder, or heavy chamfer margin (Fig. 12.3). All of these margin geometries are equally useful for chairside CAD/CAM crowns as long as the internal angles are rounded (i.e., not sharp or angular) to facilitate internal adaptation of the crown. The occlusal and axial reduction requirements are determined based on the specific material properties of the ceramic material selected for the crown. Axial reduction for CAD/CAM ceramic crowns should be 1 to 1.2 mm for the monolithic ceramic materials as there is no opaque inner coping that needs to be covered (veneered). A greater variation in occlusal

TABLE 12.1	Clinical Applications for Chairside CAD/CAM Systems						
System	Inlays/Onlays	Crowns	Veneers	FPDs	Implant Abutment	Orthodontic Application	CBCT Compatible
CEREC (Dentsply Sirona)							
BlueCam	X	X	X	X	X	X	X
OmniCam	X	X	X	X	X	X	X
PlanFit (Planmeca)	X	X	X	X	–	–	X
CS Solutions (Carestream)	X	X	X	–	–	–	X

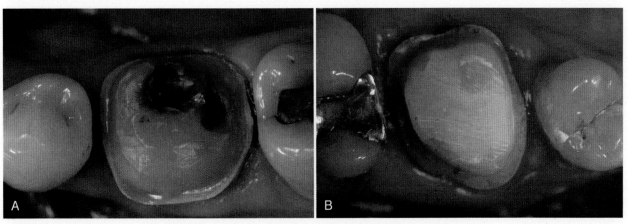

• **Fig. 12.3** A and B, Examples of chairside CAD/CAM crown preparations.

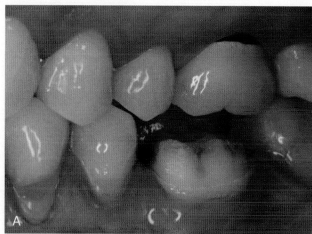

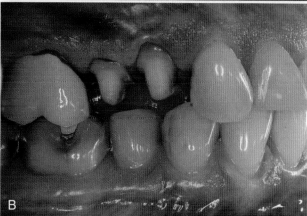

• **Fig. 12.4** A and B, Examples of the occlusal clearance for chairside CAD/CAM crown preparations.

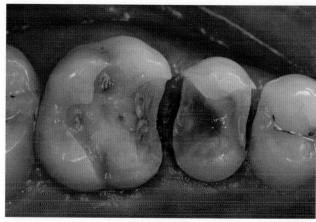

• **Fig. 12.5** Onlay preparations for teeth #3 and #4 relying primarily on the adhesive bond of the resin cement for retention of the restoration.

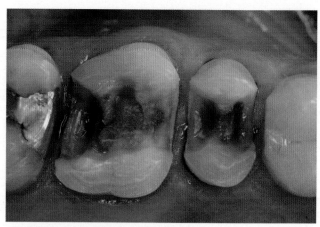

• **Fig. 12.6** Full cuspal onlay preparation for tooth #3 and MODL onlay for #4 with smooth and rounded internal angles.

reduction may be expected as a function of the material selected. Most glass ceramic materials require a minimum of 1.5 mm occlusal reduction in the central fissure area and over nonfunctional cusps and 2 mm over functional cusps (Fig. 12.4). Laboratory-based (*in vitro*) research studies suggest that full-contour zirconia crowns may be fabricated with an occlusal thickness of 1 mm without compromising the strength of the crown. Additionally, the manufacturer of lithium disilicate blocks has recently announced that e.maxCAD crowns now only require a 1-mm occlusal reduction; however, this claim still requires independent validation. All angles of the preparation should be rounded to facilitate accurate internal adaptation and needless overcutting of the internal surface of the crowns during milling.

It is not uncommon to identify significant undercuts in a crown preparation as a result of prior large restorations or caries excavation. Undercuts will be accurately recorded by the digital camera and be present in the calculated virtual model in the CAD software program. However, the milling process will not duplicate any internal undercuts in the preparation that might prevent seating of the restoration. These undercuts would subsequently be filled in with the resin cement. Alternatively, undercuts could be blocked out using the software program during design of the restoration. This process is not recommended, however, as it could ultimately result in an internal inaccuracy as the digital model is altered. Therefore, if blockout is necessary, it is best accomplished with an appropriate dentin substitute material, as indicated, prior to digital scanning.

Inlays and Onlays

CAD/CAM inlay and onlay preparations are primarily adhesive-style preparations that rely on the adhesion of the resin cement to dentin and enamel for retention of the restoration (Fig. 12.5). These preparations are divergent and relatively nonmechanically retentive in design as this provides a more conservative preparation than the requirement for mechanical resistance through grooves, slots, or boxes. The internal aspect of the preparation should avoid sharp divots or concavities, and all internal angles should be rounded (Fig. 12.6). Occlusal reduction should be uniform and of sufficient thickness to provide optimum strength of the selected ceramic material similar to crown preparations. Preparation should allow for a minimum of 1.5 mm of ceramic thickness in the central fossa and over nonfunctional cusps, and 2 mm over functional cusps. All cavosurface margins should be strategically placed away from the contact position of the opposing cusp(s) and be well defined (smooth) for easy identification in the design software. Beveled margins must be avoided, as thin areas of ceramic are prone to fracture.[8,9] Similarly, the preparation isthmus should be at least 2 mm in faciolingual width so as to avoid inlay/onlay fracture (Fig. 12.7).

CAD/CAM onlay preparations do not require the creation of a ferrule with the ceramic restoration as used with metal castings (Fig. 12.8). On the contrary, a ferrule may actually interfere with

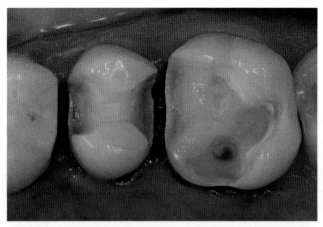

• **Fig. 12.7** Inlay preparation for tooth #13 and onlay preparation for tooth #14 with smooth flowing outline form and crisp cavosurface margins.

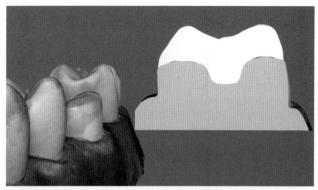

• **Fig. 12.10** Modified butt-joint margin with a football-shaped diamond for improved esthetic blending of the onlay margin.

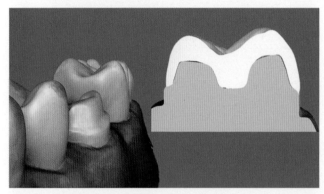

• **Fig. 12.8** Ferrule margin design with opposing walls for mechanical retention more appropriate for cast-metal restorations.

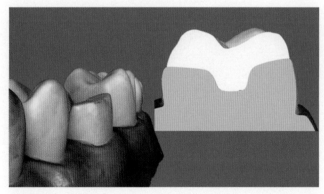

• **Fig. 12.9** Preferred butt-joint margin design for ceramic onlay preparation.

proper seating of the restoration due to undermilling of the relatively parallel walls and/or sharp transitions. Alternatively the system may significantly overmill the intaglio surface of the restoration, thinning the restoration further. Both undermilling and overmilling are detrimental to the final onlay restoration. Consequently, a butt-joint margin is preferred as it allows for proper thickness of the ceramic material at the margin, reducing the incidence of marginal fracture (Fig. 12.9). Unfortunately, this marginal design often causes a visible demarcation between the tooth and the restoration. Hence, when the blend of the restoration and the tooth is

of esthetic concern, a modification of the facial butt-joint margin is necessary. The cavosurface margin may be modified with a football-shaped diamond at a 45-degree angle, creating opportunity for a transition of ceramic thickness over the underlying enamel while maintaining a bulk of ceramic at the margin for physical strength of the ceramic (Fig. 12.10). An *in vitro* study on ceramic preparations for conservative restoration of endodontically treated teeth reported a significant improvement in the marginal and internal fit of the ceramic restoration with this modified-margin design relative to both a ferrule and 90-degree butt-joint margin.[10]

Chairside CAD/CAM Clinical Workflow

The clinical workflow to design and fabricate a chairside CAD/CAM restoration is relatively similar for all currently available systems, with noticeable differences in the unique cameras, software programs, and milling chambers of marketed systems (Fig. 12.11A–L workflow sequence). The tooth preparation, including the margins, must be visible by retraction of soft tissues and isolated from moisture contamination so that the camera may accurately capture a digital image of the preparation. The opposing arch is also recorded, as well as a scan of the dentition in maximum intercuspation from the facial aspect. The computer software virtually articulates the opposing models using the scan of the facial surfaces so the appropriate occlusal relationships for the restoration may be designed. The restoration design is initiated by identifying the margins of the planned restoration to identify the limits of the restoration design. The software utilizes data from adjacent and opposing teeth to generate a proposed (virtual) restoration, which may then be edited by a series of tools unique to each software program. The design software enables control of the emergence profile of the restoration, occlusal anatomy, planned occlusal contacts, and size and intensity of proximal contacts. Once the design of the restoration is complete, it is transmitted to the milling unit so the fabrication process may create the volumetric shape of the restoration out of an industrially produced block of ceramic material. Although a variety of chairside fabrication processes may be imagined, subtractive grinding or milling processes of ceramic blocks are accomplished based on the volumetric design created with the software design program. Most restorations may be designed and milled within 10 to 15 minutes to allow for delivery of the restoration at the same appointment. Extended machining times may be required for more complex geometries of fixed partial dentures or implant restorations. Slower machining may be preferred for thin margins, such as for porcelain veneers, in order to prevent chipping during fabrication. Certain systems allow for fine machining modes, which slow the advancement of the block at each pass of the diamonds/burs (or allow for a smoother second machining pass), so as to refine the surface contour. Final glaze firing and/or external surface polishing follows clinical confirmation of the anatomy and marginal adaptation of the resultant restoration. The final restoration is adhesively cemented with resin cement.

Chairside CAD/CAM software programs also offer various design techniques that provide the opportunity to copy a pretreatment or prototype tooth form onto the recorded tooth preparation. The copy function minimizes the need for restoration editing following the proposal of the restoration, which is especially useful in clinical situations requiring the restoration of fractured abutment teeth for removable partial dentures (RPD). Existing rest seat and proximal contours are copied from the pretreatment tooth and subsequently applied to the recorded tooth preparation. The new ceramic restoration will then have very good adaptation to the existing RPD. The copy-design process is also very useful for anterior restorations through use of a diagnostic wax-up containing strategically planned contours of the restorations. These contours may be virtually copied onto the recorded preparation, digitally perfected, and then transmitted for milling.

Chairside Restorative Materials

Dental material manufacturers produce monolithic materials for chairside CAD/CAM restorations generally referred to as "blocks." The blocks are dense, homogeneous materials that have been industrially produced under ideal conditions so as to limit the presence of internal flaws (porosity or voids). Limited inclusion of flaws enables maximization of the physical properties of the

Text continued on p. 443

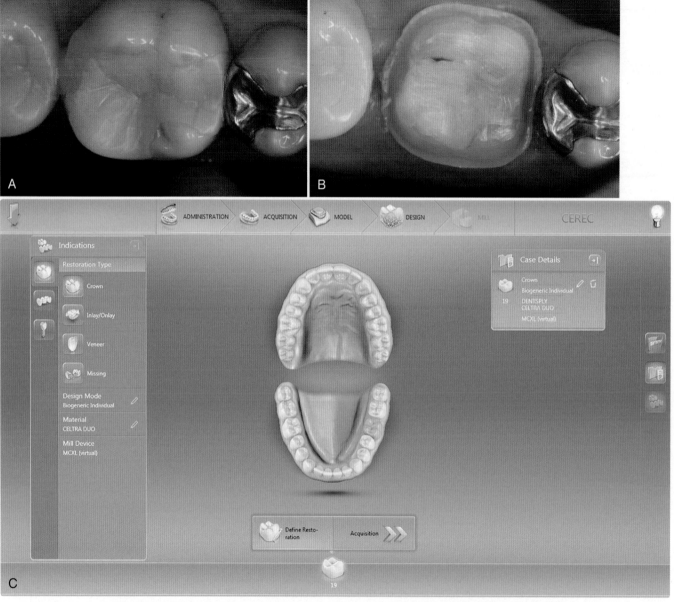

• **Fig. 12.11** Chairside CAD/CAM workflow using the CEREC system. A, Preoperative view of tooth #19. B, All-ceramic crown preparation for tooth #19. C, Case identification in the Administrative Phase.

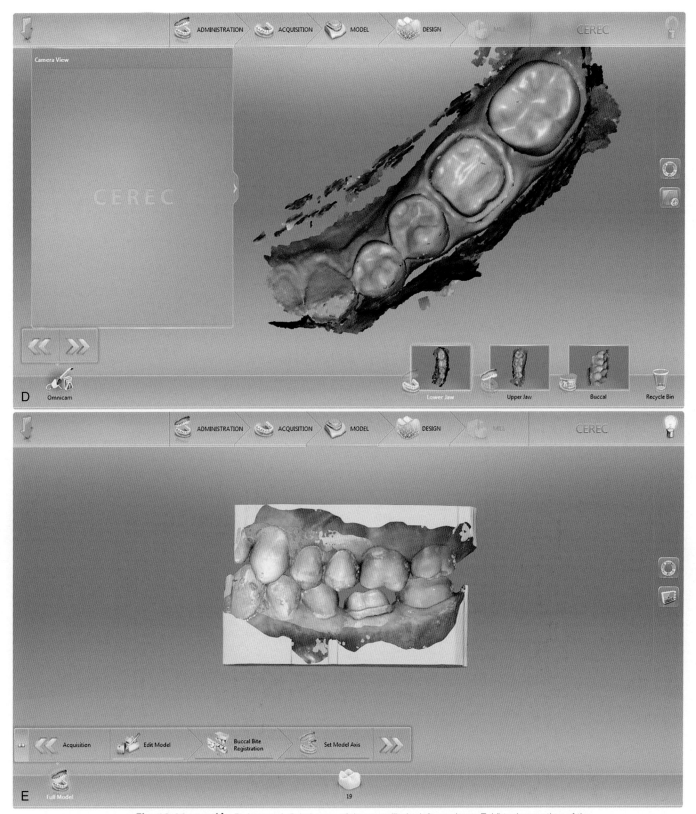

• **Fig. 12.11, cont'd**   D, Intraoral digital scan of the mandibular left quadrant. E, Virtual mounting of the opposing digital models.   *Continued*

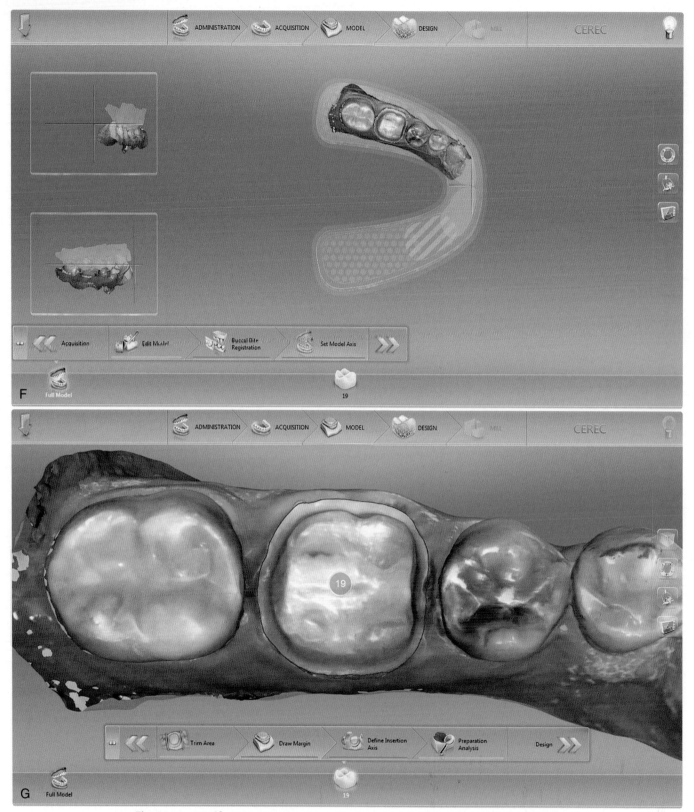

• **Fig. 12.11, cont'd** F, The Model Axis is set for the model. G, The crown margin is identified.

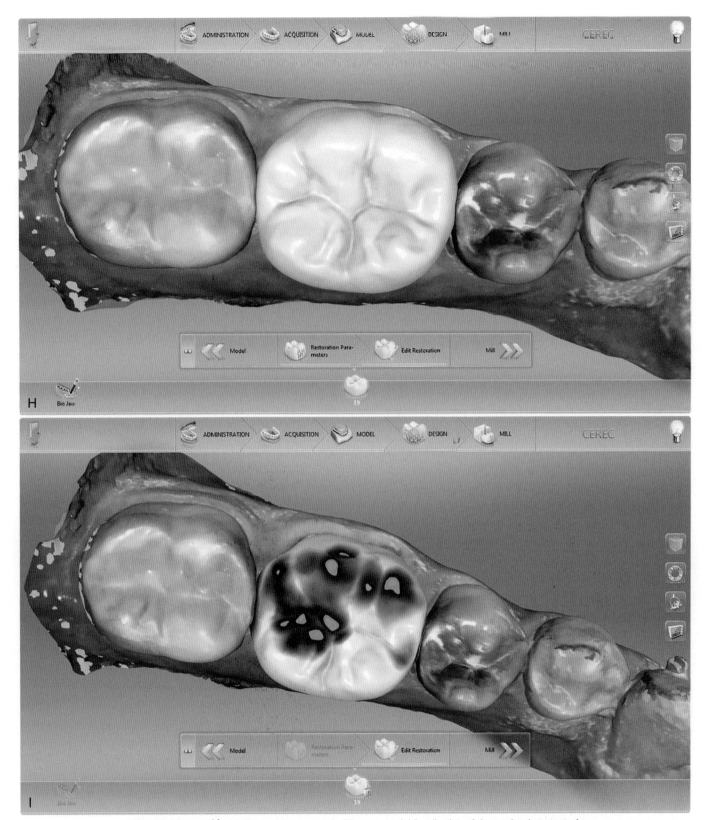

• **Fig. 12.11, cont'd** H, Biogeneric proposal of the crown. I, Visualization of the occlusal contacts for refinement.

Continued

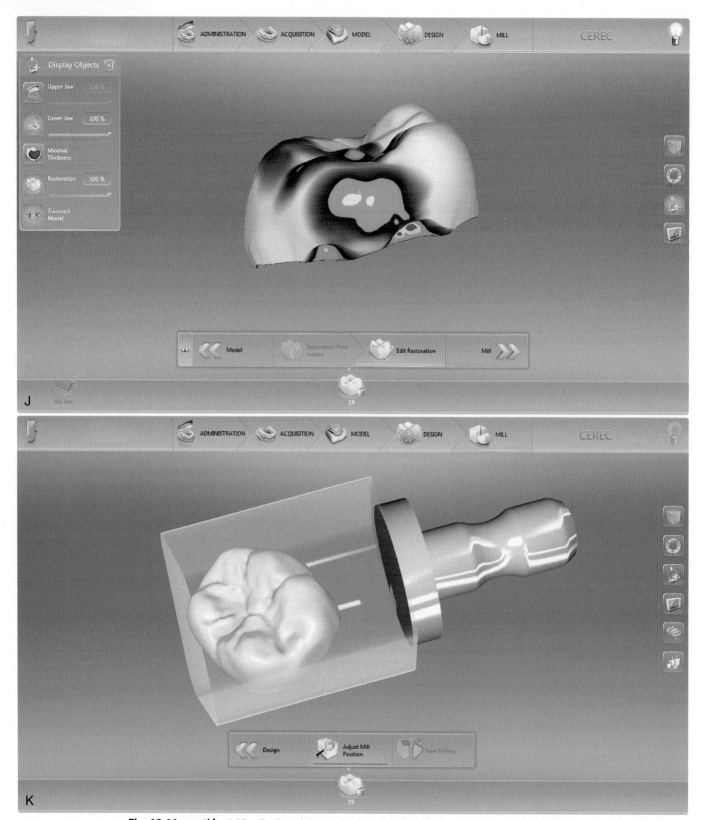

• **Fig. 12.11, cont'd** J, Visualization of the proximal contact for refinement. K, Crown proposal in the proposed mill block (Celtra Duo).

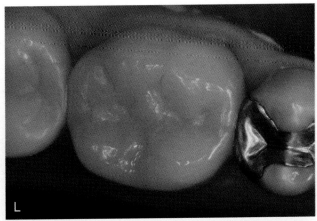

• **Fig. 12.11, cont'd** L, Delivered Celtra Duo ceramic crown for tooth #19. (C–K, Courtesy Dentsply Sirona.)

TABLE 12.2	**Restorative Material Options for Chairside CAD/CAM Systems**				
Material	**Brand**	**CEREC**	**PlanFit**	**CS Solution**	
Adhesive ceramic					
Leucite-reinforced	IPS EmpressCAD (Ivoclar)	X	X	–	
Feldspathic	Vita Mark II (Vita)	X	X	X	
	Sirona Blocs (Dentsply Sirona)	X	–	–	
High-strength ceramic					
Lithium disilicate	IPS emaxCAD (Ivoclar)	X	X	–	
Zirconia-reinforced lithium-silicate	Celtra Duo (Dentsply Sirona)	X	–	–	
Lithium-silicate	Obsidian (Glidewell)	–	X	–	
Resilient ceramic (resin nano ceramic)	Lava Ultimate (3M)	X	X	X	
	Enamic (Vita)	X	X	X	
	Cerasmart (GC America)	X	–	–	
Composite resin	Paradigm MZ100 (3M)	X	–	–	
	Brilliant Crios (Coltene)	X	–	–	
Zirconia (full contour)	CEREC Zirconia (Dentsply Sirona)	X	–	–	
Provisional acrylic materials	TelioCAD (Ivoclar)	X	X	–	
	Vita CAD-Temp (Vita)	X	–	–	

material. The blocks are attached to mandrels that are specific to the various brands of chairside CAD/CAM milling units.

The first CAD/CAM block was created as a result of the collaboration between Dr. Werner Mörmann and the Vita Corporation. The Vita Mark I blocks were originally created out of feldspathic porcelain and eventually evolved into the current generation of feldspathic blocks, Vita Mark II. Since then the CAD/CAM market has expanded to include multiple formulations of ceramic materials.

Chairside CAD/CAM materials may be divided among a number of categories based on material composition for ease in understanding their properties and clinical applications.[11,12] These categories include (Table 12.2):

1. Adhesive ceramics (feldspathic, leucite-reinforced) that must be etched and adhesively bonded to the tooth structure
2. High-strength ceramics (lithium disilicate, zirconia reinforced lithium silicate) with improved strength properties compared to the adhesive ceramic materials
3. Resilient ceramics that do not require a porcelain furnace and must be adhesively bonded to the tooth

4. Composite materials that have a resin matrix
5. Full-contour zirconia that may be cemented to the tooth
6. Provisional materials used for temporary restorations

The adhesive ceramic category includes both fine-grained feldspathic porcelain and leucite-reinforced porcelain. These materials contain a significant glass component resulting in increased translucency allowing them to have an improved "chameleon" effect. The chameleon effect may be described as the ability to reflect the color of the surrounding tooth structure and thus blend into the existing tooth shade (Fig. 12.12). These materials have a moderate flexural strength on the order of 100 to 175 megapascals (MPa). The glass component of these materials allows them to be etched with hydrofluoric acid for micromechanical adhesive bonding. Adhesive bonding is critical to their long-term success because the glass matrix makes them brittle. These materials do not have enough inherent physical strength to be cemented with resin-modified glass ionomer or traditional glass ionomer cements. The adhesive resin cement not only provides retention for the restoration but, by virtue of its adhesive properties, contributes to the physical strength of the ceramic to resist fracture by limiting flexure under

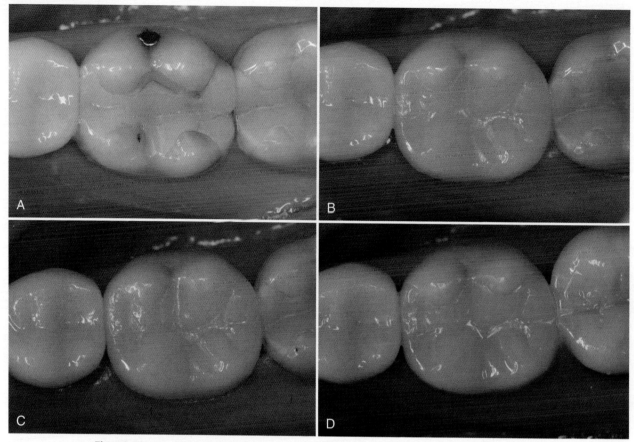

• **Fig. 12.12** Vita Mark II (Vita) onlay for tooth #30. A, Preoperative view of tooth #30. B, Vita Mark II onlay delivered. C, Vita mark II onlay at the 3-year recall. D, Vita mark II onlay at the 5-year recall.

occlusal load. Vita Mark II (Vita) and Sirona Blocks (Dentsply Sirona) are both feldspathic porcelain blocks with a fine-grained particle size that averages 4 microns and a flexural strength of 100 MPa.[13,14]

The leucite-reinforced glass ceramic was initially introduced as ProCAD (Ivoclar) and later evolved into IPS EmpressCAD (Ivoclar) with a similar crystal structure as IPS Empress 1 (Ivoclar). EmpressCAD has a finer particle size of 1 to 5 microns that is evenly dispersed 35% to 45% by volume using a proprietary manufacturing process. It comes in two levels of translucency as well as multishaded blocks.[13] The manufacturer-reported flexural strength is 160 MPa, which is within the range of what is reported independently in the literature. EmpressCAD also has a light scattering behavior that allows for a natural chameleon effect (Fig. 12.13).

There are several higher strength glass ceramic materials available for chairside CAD/CAM restorations. IPS e.maxCAD (Ivoclar) is composed of lithium disilicate and has a significantly greater flexural strength and fracture toughness than other adhesive glass ceramics.[15,16] The manufacturer provides the IPS e.maxCAD block in a partially crystallized state (160 MPa, 40% crystalized by volume) to allow for easier and more efficient grinding of the material. After the restoration has been fabricated, it must be subjected to a two-stage firing cycle in a ceramic furnace under vacuum to complete the crystallization process and achieve the maximum flexural strength potential of the material (500 MPa). The resulting glass ceramic restoration has a grain size of approximately 1.5 microns with a 70% crystal volume incorporated in a glass matrix. The crystallization

firing also creates optimum translucency for the material (Fig. 12.14). Celtra Duo (Dentsply Sirona) is a zirconia-reinforced lithium silicate (ZLS) material that is another example of ceramic with high strength. The ZLS microstructure has high content of ultrafine glass ceramic crystals (<1 μm) and 10% zirconia content. It is provided by the manufacturer in a fully crystallized state that may be either hand polished or glaze fired in a ceramic furnace prior to delivery. Hand polishing the restoration results in a material that has a flexural strength of 210 MPa, while glazing it in a porcelain oven results in a restoration with a flexural strength of 370 MPa. Celtra Duo is available in shades A1, A2, A3, A3.5, and B2 in both high and low translucencies (Fig. 12.15). NICE! (Straumann) is another fully crystallized zirconia-reinforced lithium silicate block that has recently been introduced for chairside CAD/CAM restorations.

The Resilient Ceramic category of chairside CAD/CAM blocks [Lava Ultimate (3M), Enamic (Vita), and Cerasmart (GC America)] includes materials that have a resin matrix (instead of a glass matrix) that, according to manufacturers, allows greater force absorption capability without fracture. The added feature of these materials is that no additional firing is required allowing for a very efficient delivery process following fabrication of the restoration. All three materials (Lava Ultimate, Cerasmart, and Enamic) exhibit flexural strength properties similar to human dentin, and are indicated for single-unit restorations. In contrast, the low stiffness properties of these materials may be considered disadvantageous from a bonding perspective, as marginal seal debonding due to material flexure might occur.[17] Therefore treating the intaglio surface of the

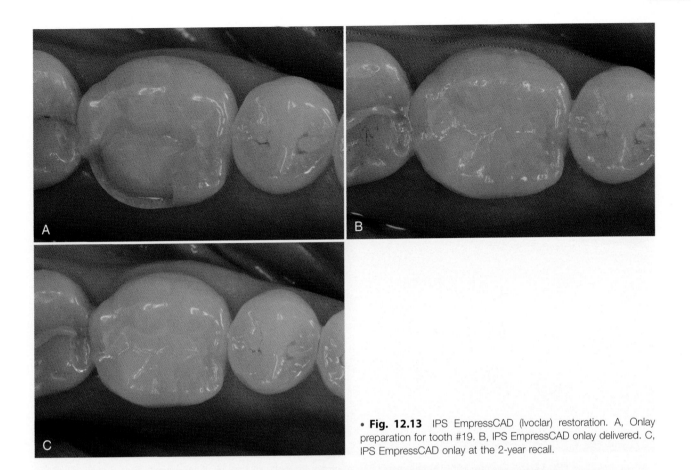

• **Fig. 12.13** IPS EmpressCAD (Ivoclar) restoration. A, Onlay preparation for tooth #19. B, IPS EmpressCAD onlay delivered. C, IPS EmpressCAD onlay at the 2-year recall.

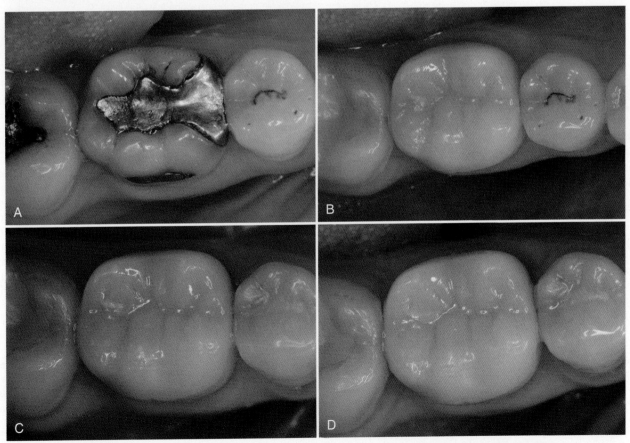

• **Fig. 12.14** IPS emaxCAD (Ivoclar) crown for tooth #30. A, Preoperative view of tooth #30. B, IPS emaxCAD crown delivered. C, IPS emaxCAD crown at 2-year recall. D, IPS emaxCAD crown at 4-year recall.

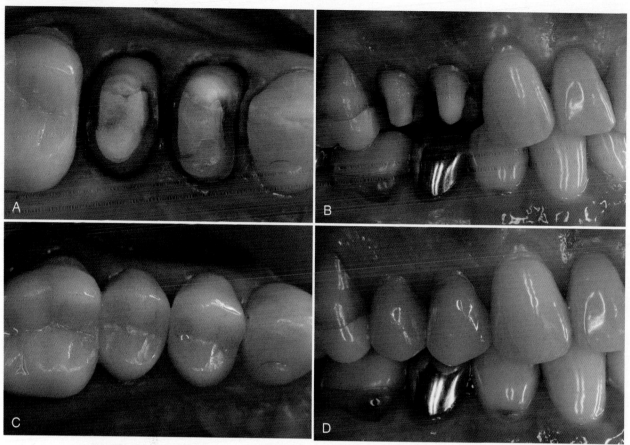

• **Fig. 12.15** Glazed Celtra Duo (Dentsply Sirona) crown for teeth #4 and #5. A, All-ceramic crown preparations for teeth #4 and #5. B, Facial view of all-ceramic crown preparations from the facial. C, Delivered glazed Celtra Duo crowns for teeth #4 and #5. D, Facial view of delivered Celtra Duo glazed crowns.

restoration with sandblasting technique as well as selecting a total-etch approach combined with adhesive cementation is considered to be imperative. Because resilient ceramics are less dense they mill faster, with a smaller incidence of margin chipping during milling compared to glass-containing materials.[17]

Lava Ultimate (3M) is a nanoceramic material that contains 20 nanometers (nm) size silica particles, 4 to 11 nm size zirconia particles, and agglomerated nanosize particles of silica and zirconia, all embedded in a highly cross-linked polymer matrix with an approximately 80% ceramic load. Lava Ultimate has a reported flexural strength of 170 MPa and it is indicated for inlays and onlays but not for crowns (Fig. 12.16).[17,18]

Cerasmart (GC America) is described by the manufacturer as a flexible nanoceramic with a resin matrix containing homogeneously distributed nanoceramic filler particles. The material is a high-density composite resin with 71% silica and barium glass nanoparticles filler by weight.[17] The reported flexural strength of Cerasmart is 230 MPa and it is indicated for inlays, onlays, and crowns.[17]

Enamic (Vita) is described by the manufacturer as a resin-based (14 wt%) hybrid ceramic comprised of a dual interpenetrating structure of a leucite-based and zirconia-reinforced ceramic network (86 wt%). The mechanical properties of the material are in between glass ceramics and highly filled composites.[19] The ceramic network provides wear resistance; however, it makes the material more brittle and susceptible to fracture. The polymer network is capable of improving the fracture resistance of the material due to its capability of undergoing plastic deformation.[20] The manufacturer recommends the material for inlays, onlays, and crowns and reports that flexural strength of Enamic is 150 MPa, which is significantly lower than Lava Ultimate or Cerasmart. This is in line with the results of an independent study (approximately 135 ± 25 MPa).[17]

Composite resin block materials are gaining in interest as the efficiency of chairside designing and milling a CAD/CAM restoration has improved. The chairside CAD/CAM workflow allows for easier control of proximal contours, contacts, and occlusal relationships for larger, more complex multisurface composite restorations compared to incremental hand placement of direct composite materials. Paradigm MZ100 (3M) is a composite block based on Z100 composite chemistry and relies on a proprietary processing technique to maximize the degree of cross-linking in the bis-GMA polymer-based composite material. It has zirconia-silica filler, which is radiopaque, and is 85% filled by weight with an average particle size of 0.6 micron.[21] The manufacturer reported flexural strength of Paradigm MZ100 is 150 MPa. An independent study reported slightly higher value 157 ± 30 MPa, which was not significantly different than the flexural strength reported for EmpressCAD.[17] Brilliant Crios (Coltene) is a recently introduced reinforced composite block containing amorphous silica and glass ceramic particles in a cross-linked methacrylate matrix.

The most recent material innovation for chairside CAD/CAM restorations was the introduction, in 2016, of CEREC Zirconia

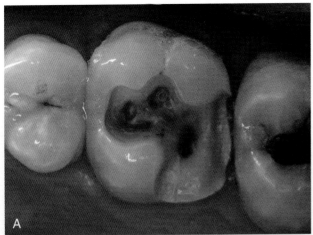

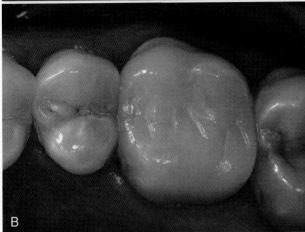

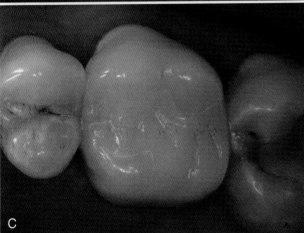

• **Fig. 12.16** Lava Ultimate (3M) onlay for tooth #14. A, Onlay preparation for tooth #14. B, Lava ultimate onlay delivered for tooth #14. C, Lava Ultimate onlay at the 3-year recall.

(Dentsply Sirona). This material is a precolored, full-contour zirconia that may be processed efficiently for a single-appointment delivery. The fast production time is a result of the simultaneous introduction of the SpeedFire (Dentsply Sirona) furnace that is able to sinter the zirconia restorations in under 20 minutes. Zirconia has a flexural strength and fracture toughness that is generally at least three times as great as glass ceramic materials.[22] CEREC zirconia has a manufacturer reported flexural strength of over 900 MPa; therefore it is suitable for crowns as well as short-span fixed partial dentures (FPDs) that may be cemented with traditional cements.

A unique property of zirconia is that it shrinks volumetrically approximately 22% to 24% when sintered. The CEREC software program automatically compensates for the degree of shrinkage in the milled restoration. When the restoration design is ready for milling, the bar code on the zirconia block is input into the software program. The bar code contains the precise amount of expected shrinkage of the particular zirconia block as determined by the manufacturer. The software virtually expands the designed restoration by this degree and an enlarged restoration is milled. The CEREC software automatically programs the SpeedFire furnace to sinter the milled zirconia restoration and firing shrinkage results in a final restoration that accurately fits the preparation. The sintering process takes 10 to 15 minutes for crowns and more than 25 minutes for FPDs. Subsequent glaze firing and surface color characterization is optional. Glazing of the zirconia restoration may be accomplished in the SpeedFire furnace or in a conventional porcelain furnace.

CAD/CAM blocks for provisional restorations are also available for chairside fabrication of long-term provisional crowns and FPDs. The chairside CAD/CAM process avoids the air-inhibited layer present on conventional self-cure or VLC acrylics as well as polymerization shrinkage. Vita CAD-Temp blocks (Vita) are made from a highly cross-linked, microfilled polymer and are available in extended block sizes, including 40 mm and 55 mm lengths, to accommodate multiple unit FPDs. Telio CAD (Ivoclar) is a millable cross-linked polymethyl methacrylate block that is part of the Telio System (a self-curing composite, desensitizer, and cement). The Telio CAD material is also available in 40 mm and 55 mm size blocks.

Accuracy of Digital Impressions

It is axiomatic that the accuracy of the final restoration depends on the accuracy of the recorded dimensions of the tooth preparation. This is true for both conventional and digital impressions. The accuracy of the margin fit and internal adaptation of any restoration is limited by the geometry of the tooth preparation and the limitations of the recording medium. The tooth preparation must be well isolated from moisture contamination and adjacent soft tissues if an accurate digital impression is to be made.

Current technology will not allow the digital capture of the tooth preparation through saliva, blood, or soft tissue. A simple way to think about digital impressions is that the camera can only accurately record what is clearly visible to the eye of the operator. Careful control of the scanning environment ensures an accurate surface reproduction with the digital impression.

Conventional impression materials require lateral and cervical retraction of the soft tissues for an accurate impression. Lateral space must be adequate to ensure sufficient impression material to resist tearing at the margin. Cervical space, generally 1 mm cervical to the margin, is required for accurate assessment of the recorded margin in the impression. Digital impressions have the advantage that soft tissues only need be retracted laterally in order to visualize the margin.

Digital impressions provide excellent immediate feedback relative to the recorded tooth preparation. Digital magnification of the image, in many cases up to 20 times lifesize, facilitates critical evaluation of the tooth preparation while the patient is still in the chair. Preparation corrections may be accomplished immediately. Additionally, inadequately captured areas may be immediately reimaged without the need to redo the entire impression, as is the case with conventional impression materials.

Research Relative to CAD/CAM Systems

Dentists have ongoing concern that restoration adaptation to tooth preparations allows for optimal clinical performance. The CEREC system was the initial chairside CAD/CAM system introduced to the dental marketplace and has over 30 years of both laboratory and clinical research documenting the relative accuracy of the fit of CEREC chairside CAD/CAM restorations. Digital camera technology has evolved from a single image capture process (RedCam) to the LED-based BlueCam to the present video version (OmniCam). The fit of CEREC restorations have consistently been considered accurate irrespective to the version of the image capturing device used. Cook and Fasbinder compared marginal fit and internal adaptation of crowns fabricated on virtual models made from the CEREC 3 infrared laser camera (RedCam) and CEREC BlueCam.[10] No significant difference was found in the margin fit and internal adaptation of CEREC crowns fabricated with either RedCam or BlueCam. The average marginal gap was 67 ± 18 μm for all groups evaluated.

Marginal adaptation (or margin fit) plays a critical role in long-term clinical performance of CAD/CAM restorations; when the adaptation of the restoration to the preparation is poor it leads to greater discrepancies at the margin. Restoration adaptation has been thoroughly investigated in the literature. Whereas some internal space is necessary to accommodate the resin cement, most authors are in agreement that margin openings under 100 μm would be desirable. A systematic review evaluated the fit and margin adaptation of CAD/CAM restorations.[23] Two electronic databases were searched for articles published between 2000 and 2012 and cross-matched against predetermined inclusion and exclusion criteria. A total of 230 studies were reviewed and 90 were selected for the meta-analysis, including data on 26 different CAD/CAM systems. The authors concluded that restorations fabricated using CAD/CAM systems have better internal fit than restorations fabricated using traditional methods. The marginal gap of crowns, made from a variety of primarily ceramic materials, ranged from 10 to 110 μm, often with gaps less than 80 μm. It was reported that the limitation of CAD/CAM systems is not achieving a precise margin fit, but the reliability of doing so over a large set of restorations.

Margin fit is also an indicator of accuracy of restorations. An in vitro study by Seelbach et al. compared the accuracy of ceramic crowns fabricated from scans using Lava COS, CEREC AC, and iTero digital impressions with two different conventional impression techniques.[24] A stainless steel master model was scanned 10 times each with the Lava COS and iTero (Cadent) systems, and zirconia crowns were made from each digital impression. The master model was scanned 10 times with the CEREC AC (BlueCam) system and 10 EmpressCAD crowns were fabricated. Ten putty-wash impressions using a single step and a two-step technique were made and zirconia crowns were made from each impression. There was no statistically significant difference in the marginal fit of the crowns fabricated using Lava COS (48 ± 25 μm), CEREC AC (30 ± 17 μm), iTero (41 ± 16 μm), and the single-step putty-wash technique (33 ± 19 μm), whereas the mean margin fit for the two-step putty-wash technique (60 ± 30 μm) was significantly

higher than that of the other methods ($P < 0.05$). The mean internal fit was 29 ± 7 μm for Lava COS, 88 ± 20 μm for CEREC AC, 50 ± 2 μm for iTero, 36 ± 5 μm for single-step putty-wash technique, and 35 ± 7 μm for two-step putty-wash technique. There was no significant difference in the mean internal fit for all groups ($P > 0.05$) except the CEREC AC ($P < 0.05$).

Another study compared the fit of Lava DVS zirconia crowns fabricated using Lava COS digital impressions to Vita Rapid Layering Technique crowns using digital impressions with the CEREC AC system.[25] Two posterior crowns were fabricated for each of 14 patients using each digital impression technique on the same tooth preparation. The replica technique was used with all crowns to measure the clinical adaptation and margin fit. The study reported that crowns made with the Lava COS system had a statistically significant better mean marginal fit (51 ± 38 μm) when compared to crowns fabricated using the CEREC system (83 ± 51 μm); however, this difference in fit was below the accepted clinical threshold of 100 μm and therefore it may not be clinically relevant.

Lee et al. investigated the margin fit of ceramic crowns from two different digital impression systems and the CEREC chairside CAD/CAM system.[26] Crowns were fabricated from digital impressions using the Lava COS and Cercon systems and from digital impressions using the CEREC BlueCam and compared to PFM crowns made with a conventional impression technique. The mean marginal gaps were 70.5 ± 34.4 μm for the PFM crowns, 87.2 ± 22.8 μm for Lava, 58.5 ± 17.6 μm for Cercon, and 72.3 ± 30.8 μm for CEREC BlueCam. There were no significant differences in the marginal fit among most of the groups except that Cercon crowns presented significantly smaller marginal gaps than Lava crowns ($P < 0.001$). However, once again this difference in fit was below the accepted clinical threshold of 100 μm and therefore may not be clinically relevant.

Another study investigated different chairside CAD/CAM systems relative to margin fit of ceramic crowns.[27] Three lithium disilicate crown fabrication techniques were included: CEREC 3D BlueCam, E4D laser scanner, and a lost-wax, heat-pressed technique (IPS Empress 1). Microcomputed tomography was used to measure margin discrepancies on the crowns. Heat-pressed crowns had a mean vertical misfit of 36.8 ± 13.9 μm and CEREC crowns had mean vertical misfit of 39.2 ± 8.7 μm, both of which were statistically significantly smaller than the mean vertical misfit recorded for the E4D crowns, 66.9 ± 31.9 μm ($P < 0.05$). In addition, the authors suggested that clinically acceptable fit should be equal or less than 75 μm. The percentage of crowns with a vertical misfit under the 75 μm reported was 83.8% for CEREC and heat-pressed technique, whereas only 65% of the E4D crowns had vertical misfit under that value, potentially indicating better fit accuracy for CEREC and heat-pressed technique.

Ender and Mehl evaluated the in vivo precision of impressions using conventional and digital methods.[28] The conventional methods used were metal full-arch tray or triple tray with PVS material. In addition, eight digital impression systems were also evaluated: Lava True Definition Scanner and Lava COS (3M ESPE), iTero (Cadent), Trios (3Shape), Trios Color (3Shape), as well as CEREC BlueCam (Software 4.0), CEREC BlueCam (Software 4.2), and CEREC Omnicam (Dentsply Sirona). Five subjects each received three quadrant impressions with each of the impression methods. The impressions were superimposed within each test impression group, for each patient, using CAD software (Geomagic Qualify 12, 3D Systems). A perfect match (misfit of zero) would indicate ideal precision, with increasing values from zero gradually indicating poorer precision. The precision for all methods ranged from 18.8 ± 7.1 μm for the metal full-arch tray to 58.5 ± 22.8 μm with the triple tray. The conventional metal full-arch tray had statistically best precision of all groups, followed by True Def (21.7 ± 7.4 μm), Trios (25.7 ± 4.9 μm), Trios Color (26.1 ± 3.8 μm), and group BlueCam 4.0 (34.2 ± 10.5 μm). No statistically significant difference was found between BlueCam 4.2 (43.3 ± 19.6 μm), OmniCam (37.4 ± 8.1 μm), Lava COS (47.7 ± 16.1 μm), iTero (49 ± 12.4 μm), and conventional triple tray impressions (58.5 ± 22.8 μm). The authors concluded that despite significant differences found, all of the digital impression systems were capable of producing quadrant impression with precision that was clinically acceptable.

Hack and Patzalt measured the ability of six intraoral scanners to accurately capture a single molar abutment tooth in vitro.[29] The scanners tested included iTero, True Def, PlanScan, CS 3500, Trios, and CEREC Omnicam. A master typodont model of a single crown preparation was scanned with a highly accurate industrial benchtop scanner, and the digital file from the benchtop scanner was compared to the digital scans of the intraoral scanners using a CAD software program (Geomagic Qualify). Precision was measured by superimposing the benchtop scanner digital file onto the digital files recorded by each scanner and evaluated for three-dimensional deviations. Similar to a previously mentioned study, a perfect match (misfit of zero) would indicate ideal precision, with increasing values from zero gradually indicating poorer precision. The authors reported most accurate precision values for the Trios (4.5 ± 0.9 μm), followed by True Def (6.1 ± 1 μm), iTero (7 ± 1.4 μm), CS3500 (7.2 ± 1.7 μm), CEREC OmniCam (16.2 ± 4 μm), and PlanScan (26.4 ± 5 μm). Statistically significant differences were reported between all scanners and CEREC Omnicam ($P < 0.05$) as well as between all scanners and PlanScan ($P < 0.05$). The authors concluded that, even though there were differences in levels of accuracy, all scanners investigated produced clinically acceptable accuracy.

A more recent systematic review also evaluated the marginal fit of single-unit all-ceramic crowns fabricated after conventional and digital impressions. The search included studies published from January 1989 through December 2014. From the original 63 articles that were identified, 12 were selected (both in vitro and in vivo) after applying the inclusion and exclusion criteria. For in vitro studies mean marginal fit of crowns fabricated after conventional impressions was 58.9 μm (95% CI: 41.1–76.7 μm), whereas for digital impressions it was 63.3 μm (95% CI: 50.5–76 μm). However, for in vivo studies the results were reversed with mean marginal fit of crowns fabricated after digital impressions 56.1 μm (95% CI: 46.3–65.8 μm), whereas for digital impressions it was 79.2 μm (95% CI: 59.6–98.9 μm). The authors reported low overall risk of bias of the included studies as well as moderate heterogeneity, mostly due to the variety of intraoral scanners and ceramic materials in the studies included. The result of the meta-analysis indicated no statistically significant difference in marginal gap of single-unit ceramic restorations fabricated after conventional or digital impressions. The authors suggested that the digital workflow exceeds clinically acceptable standards and performs equal to conventional impressions.[30]

The PlanFit and CS Solutions systems have been more recently introduced for chairside CAD/CAM restorations and have very limited published research on margin fit and internal adaptation. One study measured the marginal fit of E4D fabricated crowns on typodont preparations completed by 62 different clinicians.[31] Each of the crown preparations was judged as good, fair, or poor

by using both a replica technique and visual examination looking at common criteria for ceramic restorations. The quality of the preparation influenced the accuracy of the margin fit in ways that were statistically significant. Ideal preparations had a mean margin fit of 38.5 ± 9 μm, fair preparations had 58.3 ± 12 μm, and poor preparations had 90.1 ± 23 μm. A second in vitro study measured the margin fit and internal adaptation of E4D fabricated emaxCAD crowns.[32] Mean margin fits varied from 79.32 ± 63.18 μm for buccal margins to 50.39 ± 35.98 μm for lingual margins. Additional independent studies are warranted for a more precise assessment of margin fit and internal adaptation of PlanFit and CS Solutions restorations.

Clinical Longevity of CAD/CAM Restorations

The clinical performance of chairside CAD/CAM restorations has been studied so as to assess relative longevity in the oral environment. Long-term randomized clinical trials are considered the most robust study design for the purpose of proper assessment of clinical longevity. However, there is considerable amount of variation in the dental literature when searching for independent randomized studies on clinical longevity of chairside CAD/CAM restorations. The vast majority of the publications report on the long-term clinical performance of CEREC restorations primarily because the CEREC System has been available since the early 1990s whereas other systems have been more recently introduced. Systematic reviews represent invaluable tools to synthesize the results of these multiple and varied clinical studies; however, the conclusions of systematic reviews are only as valuable as the quality of the studies they seek to combine.

Wittneben and coworkers evaluated the clinical performance of CAD/CAM restorations in a systematic review.[33] The authors performed an electronic search of all publications on clinical performance of CAD/CAM restoration between 1985 and 2007. Studies were selected following specific inclusion criteria. The included publications comprised 14 prospective and 2 retrospective studies on the chairside CEREC System (CEREC 1 and 2) as well as the laboratory system Celay, providing follow-up data from 2 to 10 years. The search yielded data on a total of 1957 restorations with a mean exposure time of 7.9 years. The restorations included mostly posterior crowns, but some studies evaluated inlays, onlays, endocrowns, and anterior crowns. A total of 170 failures were reported, at a rate of 1.75% failure per year. The most common modes of failure described were fractures of the restoration or tooth. The estimated survival rate for CEREC single-tooth restorations was 91.6% (95% CI: 1.22%–2.52%). Restorations fabricated with feldspathic porcelain had the highest 5-year survival rate, which contrasted with the lowest 5-year survival rate for glass ceramic. At 5 years, ceramic onlays performed equally as successful as crowns; however, the authors identified a significant lack of randomized studies as well as a shortage of scientific evidence longer than 3 years.

Among the CEREC literature, several of the studies published data on CAD/CAM generated feldspathic porcelain restorations. Posselt and Kerschbaum conducted a retrospective study on the clinical performance of 2328 inlays and onlays for 794 patients in a private practice setting. A total of 35 failures were reported over 9 years. The Kaplan-Meier survival probability reported was 97.4% at 5 years and 95.5% at 9 years for CEREC inlays and onlays. According to the authors, failure rate was not significantly influenced by restoration size, tooth vitality, previous presence of deep caries, type of tooth treated, or whether the restoration was located in the maxilla or mandible. The most common type of failure reported was tooth extraction.[34] A 10-year prospective clinical trial on feldspathic CEREC 1 inlays and onlays reported a Kaplan-Meier survival probability of 90.4% after 10 years for 200 restorations placed in private practice. The restorations were placed in 108 patients (62 female, 46 male). The mean age of the patients was 37 years (range 17 to 75 years). All patients presented with good dental care and a low risk for caries. The restorations were fabricated chairside using Vita MK I feldspathic ceramic and were delivered with adhesive technique with luting composite resin instead of resin cement. A total of 15 restorations (8%) failed in 10 years, primarily due to either restoration or tooth fracture.[35] In a follow-up report of that study, the authors reported less than 3% drop in survival rate for the same restorations at 17 years, with reported Kaplan-Meier survival probability of 88.7%. Six restorations failed during the 7-year period between evaluations, once again primarily due to either restoration or tooth fracture.[36] Compared to clinical studies using early versions of the CEREC system, these more recent studies reported better survival probabilities.

The clinical survival of CAD/CAM restorations is influenced by the adhesive cementation, which in turn is maximized with the presence of enamel margins. This was well demonstrated by a longitudinal study on clinical performance of nonretentive feldspathic CAD/CAM overlays (occlusal veneers). A single operator placed 310 CEREC overlays paying particular attention to keeping preparation margins within enamel whenever possible. After 8 years of follow-up, 286 paired onlays were available for evaluation and the calculated survival rate was 99.3%. The only two fractures observed in this study were on maxillary premolars of one patient with occlusal parafunction.[37] The clinical success of these restorations was likely due to the predictable bonding that is often achieved whenever the all-ceramic preparation is within enamel. In addition, an experienced operator may have influenced such remarkable performance, as more inexperienced operators did not achieve similar results. For example, a short-term prospective randomized controlled clinical trial looked at the clinical performance of 68 paired feldspathic CEREC onlays (Vitablock Mark II) that were cemented with a self-adhesive cement (RelyX Unicem, 3M ESPE). The influence of selective enamel etching was evaluated so each patient had one onlay cemented with the self-etch technique and the other one after selective etching. Statistically significant changes were observed for marginal adaptation and marginal discoloration between baseline and 2 years but no statistically significant difference in clinical performance was recorded between the two different cementation groups. Two onlays debonded, one from each group; two onlays fractured from the self-etch group. The 2-year failure rate for CEREC feldspathic onlays was 5.1% for the self-etch technique and 1.7% for the selective etching group. The authors concluded that selective enamel etching did not statistically significantly influence the results.[38] However, the failure to find significance could be attributed to the short follow-up time. Long-term clinical trials indicate that failures tend to continue to increase over time.

A long-term randomized clinical trial was designed to access the longitudinal performance of 80 inlays machined from either a composite resin material (Paradigm MZ100) or feldspathic ceramic (Vitablocks Mark II), cemented with a dual-cured resin cement (RelyX ARC) using a total-etch bonding technique. At the 10-year recall 89% of the inlays were available for evaluation. No statistically significant difference in margin adaptation was evident between the two materials; however, a significant decrease in margin adaptation was noted when inlays of both materials were compared to baseline values due to margin wear of the adhesive luting cement over time. Composite inlays had fewer fractures in 10 years, with a calculated survival rate of 95% for Paradigm MZ100 inlays versus 87.5% for Vitablocks Mark II. The calculated annual failure rates were 0.5% for composite inlays and 1.25% for ceramic inlays.[39]

The vast majority of publications report on feldspathic CAD/CAM materials because they were the first blocks available for chairside milling. More recent studies have evaluated newer CAD/CAM materials. A randomized clinical study compared leucite-reinforced (Paradigm C, 3M ESPE) and feldspathic (Vita Mark II, Vita) CEREC onlays cemented with a self-etching, self-adhesive resin cement (RelyX Unicem, 3M ESPE). No statistically significant differences in the clinical performance were noted between the two materials at 3 years.[40] This trend continued to be observed at the 5-year follow-up as no statistically significant difference was noted in margin adaptation between the two materials either at 5 years or when results were compared to baseline values. However, an increased trend for localized crevice formation was noted over time and a statistically significant difference was found between baseline and 5-year data for both materials when more discriminative criteria were applied.[41]

Chairside CAD/CAM systems were initially limited to the fabrication of inlays and onlays since crowns were not possible with the milling instruments first introduced; therefore most of the initial studies focus on chairside all-ceramic inlays and onlays. With the advent of newer materials and evolution of the milling systems, an increased number of publications focus on chairside CAD/CAM crowns. Reich and coworkers reported a short-term clinical study on the performance of chairside CAD/CAM IPS e.maxCAD crowns fabricated with the CEREC system. Forty-one full-contour e.maxCAD crowns were placed in 34 patients and 39 were available for the 24-month recall. Kaplan-Meier analysis revealed a 2-year survival rate of 97.4%. However, the failures observed were not due to crown fracture; one crown exhibited secondary caries and two crowns received root canal treatment.[42] In contrast, a large longitudinal clinical study evaluated the clinical performance of 100 IPS e.maxCAD CEREC crowns at 2, 4, and 5 years.[43-45] All crowns were fabricated and delivered at a single appointment. The first 62 crowns were placed with either a self-etching bonding agent and resin cement or a self-adhesive resin cement. The last group consisted of 38 crowns that were delivered using an experimental self-etching, self-curing cement. No crown failures were reported during the first 24 months, therefore the 2-year survival rate was 100%. A total of five failures were recorded at 5 years, four crowns debonded (three of which had been delivered with the experimental cement that never made it to market), and one crown fractured, for a 95% survival rate at 5 years. This study is currently ongoing and the optimistic trends continue to be observed.

There is considerable published clinical research on chairside CAD/CAM technology that has revealed it to be a valuable tool for the delivery of high-quality restorations delivered during a single appointment. The ability to adhesively bond ceramic restorations at the time of restoration fabrication minimizes the occurrence of postoperative sensitivity while allowing for more conservative tooth preparation as no preparation retention is required to retain a temporary restoration. Research studies have assessed an extensive variety of resin-based, porcelain, glass ceramic, and high-strength ceramic materials that may be used to provide restorative solutions for inlays, onlays, veneers, and full crowns.

Conclusion

The clinical application of CAD/CAM technology has developed through a continuous evolution of the hardware and software. A variety of restorative materials are available to offer alternative solutions for a variety of clinical problems. Laboratory and clinical research has documented the accuracy, longevity, and effectiveness of CAD/CAM fabricated restorations. The efficient treatment workflow provides an opportunity for patient-centered treatment in one appointment. The evidence-based reliability, as well as the perceived value of same-day dentistry, has helped secure a permanent spot for CAD/CAM dentistry in operative dentistry practice.

References

1. Beuer F, Schweiger J, Edelhoff D: Digital dentistry: an overview of recent developments for CAD/CAM generated restorations. *Br Dent J* 204:505–511, 2008.
2. Mörmann WH, Brandestini M, Lutz F, et al: Chairside computer-aided direct ceramic inlays. *Quintessence Int* 20:329–339, 1989.
3. Mörmann WH: Chairside computer-generated ceramic restorations: the CEREC third generation improvements. *Pract Periodontics Aesthet Dent* 4(7):9–16, 1992.
4. Mörmann WH, Gotsch T, Krejci I, et al: Clinical status of 94 CEREC ceramic inlays after 3 years in situ. In Mörmann WH, editor: *International symposium on computer restorations*, Chicago, 1991, Quintessence, pp 355–363.
5. Mehl A, Hickel R: Current state of development and perspectives of machine-based production methods for dental restorations. *Int J Comput Dent* 2:9–35, 1999.
6. Mormann WH: The evolution of the CEREC system. *J Am Dent Assoc* 137(9 Suppl):7S–13S, 2006.
7. Severance G, Swann L: The Take Care approach to treatment planning, preparation and design for CAD/CAM restorations. *Oral Health* 99(3):47–52, 2009.
8. Qualtrough AJ, Cramer A, Wilson NH, et al: An in vitro evaluation of the marginal integrity of a porcelain inlay system. *Int J Prosthodont* 4:517–523, 1991.
9. Wilson NHF, Wilson MA, Wastell DG, et al: Performance of Occlusion in butt-joint and bevel-edged preparations: five-year results. *Dent Mater* 7:92–98, 1991.
10. Cook KT, Fasbinder DJ: Marginal and internal adaptation of CAD/CAM endocrown preparation designs [abstract 1022]. *J Dent Res* 91(specialA):2012.
11. Fasbinder DJ: Materials for chairside CAD/CAM restorations. *Compend Contin Educ Dent* 31(9):702–709, 2010.
12. Fasbinder DJ: Chairside CAD/CAM: an overview of restorative material options. *Compend Contin Educ Dent* 33(1):50–58, 2012.
13. Charlton DG, Roberts HW, Tiba A: Measurement of select physical and mechanical properties of 3 machinable ceramic materials. *Quintessence Int* 39:573–579, 2008.
14. Buso L, Oliveira-Júnior OB, Hiroshi Fujiy F, et al: Biaxial flexural strength of CAD/CAM ceramics. *Minerva Stomatol* 60(6):311–319, 2011.
15. Albakry M, Guazzato M, Swain MV: Biaxial flexural strength, elastic moduli, and x-ray diffraction characterization of three pressable all-ceramic materials. *J Prosthet Dent* 89(4):374–380, 2003.
16. Belli R, Geinzer E, Muschweck A, et al: Mechanical fatigue degradation of ceramics versus resin composites for dental restorations. *Dent Mater* 30(4):424–432, 2014.
17. Awada A, Nathanson D: Mechanical properties of resin-ceramic CAD/CAM restorative materials. *J Prosthet Dent* 114(4):587–593, 2015.
18. Albero A, Pascual A, Camps I, et al: Comparative characterization of a novel CAD/CAM polymer-infiltrated-ceramic network. *J Clin Exp Dent* 7(4):e495–e500, 2015.
19. Della Bona A, Corazza PH, Zhang Y: Characterization of a polymer-infiltrated ceramic-network material. *Dent Mater* 30(5):564–569, 2014.
20. El Zhawi H, Kaizer MR, Chughtai A, et al: Polymer infiltrated ceramic network structures for resistance to fatigue fracture and wear. *Dent Mater* 2016, pii: S0109-5641(16)30362-1. doi:10.1016/j.dental.2016.08.216. [Epub ahead of print].
21. Rusin RP: Properties and applications of a new composite block for CAD/CAM. *Compend Contin Educ Dent* 22(6 Suppl):35–41, 2001.
22. Guazzato M, Albakry M, Ringer SP, et al: Strength, fracture toughness and microstructure of a selection of all-ceramic materials. Part II. Zirconia-based dental ceramic. *Dent Mater* 20:449–456, 2004b.
23. Boitelle P, Mawussi B, Tapie L, et al: A systematic review of CAD/CAM fit restoration evaluations. *J Oral Rehabil* 41:853–874, 2014.
24. Seelbach P, Brueckel C, Wostmann B: Accuracy of digital and conventional impression techniques and workflow. *Clin Oral Investig* 17(7):1759–1764, 2013, doi:10.1007/s00784-012-0864-4. [Epub 2012 Oct 21].
25. Brawek PK, Wolfart S, Endres L, et al: The clinical accuracy of single crowns exclusively fabricated by digital workflow – comparison of two systems. *Clin Oral Investig* 17(9):2119–2125, 2013.
26. Lee KH, Yeo IS, Wu BM, et al: Effects of computer-aided manufacturing technology on precision of clinical metal-free restorations. *Biomed Res Int* 2015:619027, 2015, doi:10.1155/2015/619027. [Epub 2015 Oct 18].
27. Neves FD, Prado CJ, Prudente MS, et al: Micro-computed tomography evaluation of marginal fit of lithium disilicate crowns fabricated by using chairside CAD/CAM systems or the heat-pressing technique. *J Prosthet Dent* 112:1134–1140, 2014.
28. Ender A, Zimmermann M, Attin T, et al: *In vivo* precision of conventional and digital methods for obtaining quadrant dental impressions. *Clin Oral Investig* 20:1495–1504, 2016.
29. Hack GD, Patzalt SBM: Evaluation of the accuracy of six intraoral scanning devices: an in-vitro investigation. *ADA Professional Product Review* 10(4):1–5, 2015.
30. Tsirogiannis P, Reissmann DR, Heydecke G: Evaluation of the marginal fit of single-unit, complete-coverage ceramic restorations fabricated after digital and conventional impressions: a systematic review and meta-analysis. *J Prosthet Dent* 2016, pii: S0022-3913(16)00139-6. doi:10.1016/j.prosdent.2016.01.028. [Epub ahead of print].
31. Renne W, McGill ST, VanSickle Forshee K, et al: Predicting marginal fit of CAD/CAM crowns based on the presence of or absence of common preparation errors. *J Prosthet Dent* 108:310–315, 2012.
32. Plourde J, Harsono M, Fox L, et al: Marginal and internal fit of E4D CAD/CAM all-ceramic crowns. *J Dent Res* 90(SpecA):638, 2011.
33. Wittneben JG, Wright RF, Weber HP, et al: A systematic review of the clinical performance of CAD/CAM single-tooth restorations. *Int J Prosthodont* 22(5):466–471, 2009.
34. Posselt A, Kerschbaum T: Longevity of 2328 chairside Cerec inlays and onlays. *Int J Comput Dent* 6(3):231–248, 2003.
35. Otto T, De Nisco S: Computer-aided direct ceramic restorations: a 10-year prospective clinical study of Cerec CAD/CAM inlays and onlays. *Int J Prosthodont* 15(2):122–128, 2002.
36. Otto T, Schneider D: Long-term clinical results of chairside Cerec CAD/CAM inlays and onlays: a case series. *Int J Prosthodont* 21(1):53–59, 2008.
37. Arnetzl GV, Arnetzl G: Reliability of nonretentive all-ceramic CAD/CAM overlays. *Int J Comput Dent* 15(3):185–197, 2012.
38. Schenke F, Federlin M, Hiller KA, et al: Controlled, prospective, randomized, clinical evaluation of partial ceramic crowns inserted with RelyX Unicem with or without selective enamel etching. Results after 2 years. *Clin Oral Investig* 16(2):451–461, 2012, doi:10.1007/s00784-011-0516-0. [Epub 2011].
39. Fasbinder DJ, Neiva GF, Dennison JB, et al: Clinical performance of CAD/CAM generated Composite inlays after 10 years. *J Cosmetic Dentistry* 28(4):134–145, 2013.

40. Fasbinder DJ, Neiva GF, Dennison JB, et al: Clinical evaluation of CAD/CAM-generated ceramic onlays. *J Dent Res* 90(SpecA): Abstract #378. 2011.

41. Fasbinder DJ, Neiva GF, Dennison JB, et al: Clinical evaluation of CAD/CAM-generated onlays: 5-year report. *J Dent Res* 92(SpecA): abstract #177. 2013.

42. Reich S, Fischer S, Sobotta B, et al: A preliminary study on the short term efficacy of chairside computer-aided design/computer-aided manufacturing-generated posterior lithium disilicate crowns. *Int J Prosthodont* 23(3):214–216, 2010.

43. Fasbinder DJ, Dennison JB, Heys D, et al: A clinical evaluation of chairside lithium disilicate CAD/CAM crowns. A two-year report. *J Am Dent Assoc* 141:10S–14S, 2010.

44. Fasbinder DJ, Dennison JB, Heys D, et al: Clinical evaluation of lithium disilicate chairside CAD/CAM crowns at four years. *J Dent Res* 91(SpecA): abstract #645. 2012.

45. Fasbinder DJ, Dennison JB, Heys D, et al: Five-year clinical evaluation of lithium disilicate chairside CAD/CAM crowns. *J Dent Res* 94(SpecA): abstract #247. 2015.

13

Dental Biomaterials

TERENCE E. DONOVAN, TAISEER A. SULAIMAN, GUSTAVO MUSSI STEFAN OLIVEIRA, STEPHEN C. BAYNE[a], JEFFREY Y. THOMPSON[a]

This chapter discusses dental biomaterials with the practicing dentist and dental student in mind. As such, it is not meant to be an in-depth review of materials that would be of interest to material scientists. The chapter discusses dental biomaterials from the perspective of the clinician trying to make a decision about, for example, what composite resin material, dental adhesive system, or impression material is best for his or her practice in order to provide optimum care for patients.

These decisions are often important because, in addition to clinical time, materials themselves are very expensive and the cost of premature failure of a restoration and subsequent replacement is considerable. Most materials are brought to the marketplace with little or no clinical testing. Practicing dentists are basically doing the clinical testing for manufacturers. Understanding the basic nature and composition of dental materials can allow clinicians to make educated decisions related to new materials and avoid catastrophic outcomes (Fig. 13.1).

Contemporary dental practitioners are expected to practice "evidence-based" dentistry.[1-4] The evidence-based diagram (Fig. 13.2) shows the top of the hierarchy is filtered information from meta-analyses and systematic reviews of published randomized controlled trials (RCTs). However, the reality is that it takes at least 10 years from the introduction of a new material before 5-year RCTs are published. Most currently published (2017) systematic reviews are of limited value to the clinician, because the clinical trials included in the reviews are usually very weak and poorly designed.[5] Thus in the absence of good "evidence," it is essential that dentists understand the composition of commonly used dental materials and the functions of each component of those materials.

Dental materials have a number of important physical and mechanical properties that will be described in the next section. One of the most important properties is "technique sensitivity." A material is described as technique sensitive when different operators get different outcomes when using that material. Materials that are low in technique sensitivity are desirable, and manufacturers strive to develop materials that are not technique sensitive. A good example of this is seen with dental adhesives. Dental adhesives have evolved over many years and as many as seven generations have been described. For many years, the fourth generation of dental adhesives was identified as the best system, but dentists have had variable results with it, as it required three separate steps (etch, prime, bond) and involved the vague concept of "moist"

dentin. These materials were indeed "technique sensitive." Subsequent generations attempted to simplify the bonding procedure and make it less technique sensitive, but in fact made it less effective. Dentists who understood the fourth generation of bonding agents and who were meticulous in their technique achieved excellent clinical results. Those who did not understand these materials and/or were less meticulous in their technique got less successful outcomes.

One material that is very low in technique sensitivity is silver amalgam (Fig. 13.3). A short time after placement of a silver amalgam restoration, oral fluids penetrate the microscopic space between the amalgam and tooth structure.[6] This process, called percolation, results in the deposition of corrosion products and effectively seals the interface between the amalgam and the tooth. This process of "self-sealing" occurs irrespective of the skill and knowledge of the operator, which makes silver amalgam one of the least technique sensitive materials.

The discussion on technique sensitivity leads to the concept that there are two parts to the successful use of dental materials: material selection and material manipulation. Dentists must select the most appropriate restorative material based on knowledge of the disease process, knowledge of materials appropriate for dealing with the dental defect, and knowledge of expected outcomes of the proposed intervention. Appropriate material manipulation of the selected material requires knowledge about the material and meticulous attention to details such as isolation, bonding technique, incremental buildup, curing time, matrix selection, and many other variables. Thus, both material selection and proper manipulation of the selected material are critical to clinical success.

Dentists have variable approaches to their adoption of new materials and procedures. Some are very conservative and patiently wait for high quality of evidence prior to using a new material or technique. Others, described as "early adopters," eagerly utilize every new material or technique the instant it comes on market, and others are between the two extremes. There is room in the profession for all three groups, but it is clear that early adopters must have an excellent knowledge and understanding of both the selection and the manipulation of dental materials.

THE BOTTOM LINE

1. Understanding the composition and nature of dental materials is important to obtain optimum clinical outcomes.
2. Materials are brought to the market with almost no clinical testing.

---

[a]Drs. Bayne and Thompson were inactive authors in this edition.

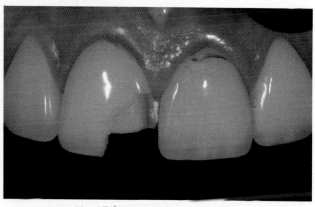

• **Fig. 13.1** Fractured porcelain veneer.

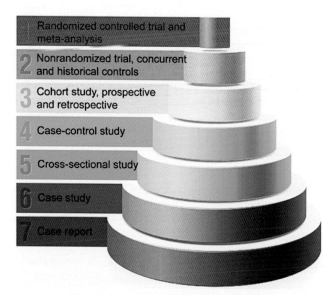

| Randomized controlled trial and meta-analysis |
| Nonrandomized trial, concurrent and historical controls |
| Cohort study, prospective and retrospective |
| Case-control study |
| Cross-sectional study |
| Case study |
| Case report |

• **Fig. 13.2** Evidence-based medicine pyramid.

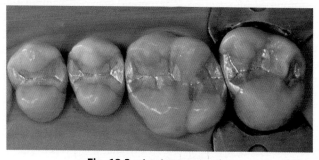

• **Fig. 13.3** Amalgam restorations.

3. Premature clinical failures of dental restorations are extremely costly to dental practices.
4. The evidence base for restorative materials is not robust.
5. The relative technique sensitivity of a material is an important attribute.
6. Both material selection and material manipulation are important.

Physical, Mechanical, and Optical Properties

A number of important physical and mechanical properties of dental materials can be identified. This section will discuss some of these properties and illustrate how they might be important to the long-term clinical success of a restoration. The discussion will also attempt to answer the question, "Does a comparison of physical properties of dental materials help predict clinical success or failure?"[2] This section is not meant to be an exhaustive description of all of the physical and mechanical properties that can be evaluated in dental materials. The reader is referred to any of the excellent contemporary textbooks on dental materials for that discussion. Rather, it is intended to be a brief description of several properties of dental materials that might be critical for clinical success.

One important point to be considered when evaluating studies on physical and mechanical properties is that materials should be tested in the mode in which they are used. Many in vitro studies fail to do this. One example is dental cements. Clinically cements are used in thin films between 15 and 100 microns. It is physically impossible to test a sample of this dimension, so tests on dental cements are done on samples that are not clinically relevant. Thus any in vitro data generated that is related to physical and mechanical properties of dental cements should not be used to infer significant clinical implications.

The following is an incomplete list and description of physical and mechanical properties of dental materials and some examples of why they are important.

Dimensional Change. Dimensional change is the percent shrinkage or expansion of a material, which usually occurs as a result of the setting reaction. One example is with composite resin. Basically composite resin materials consist of inert filler particles in a matrix of resin, usually mostly bisphenol A glycidyl methacrylate (Bis-GMA). The resin material undergoes a polymerization reaction as it sets, with individual monomers joining to become long-chain polymers that then cross-link to form the polymer matrix. During the process, the material undergoes polymerization shrinkage. With contemporary hybrid composite resin materials, the shrinkage is between 2.4% and 2.8%. If not accounted for in the placement technique, this amount of shrinkage can lead to clinically significant contraction gaps between the margin of the preparation and the composite resin restoration. This can result in microleakage, postoperative sensitivity, and recurrent caries.

Another example is with elastomeric impression materials. These also set with a polymerization reaction that results in shrinkage. This shrinkage can be controlled with use of custom impression trays that provide a 1- to 2-mm cross-sectional thickness of the material and proper use of tray adhesives, which ensures the direction of shrinkage is toward the tray.[7] Use of stock trays results in excessive thicknesses of impression material that may result in undesirable distortion of the impression.

Thermal Coefficient of Expansion (COE). The COE is defined as the amount a material expands per unit length if heated 1 degree higher. Waxes have the highest COE of all dental materials. When the lost wax process is used, wax patterns should be invested as soon as possible after margination to ensure that there is no distortion of the wax pattern due to normal fluctuations in room temperature (Table 13.1).

This property can be very important when dealing with materials that have cores with veneering materials. An example is metal-ceramic crowns. The feldspathic porcelain veneer, which provides excellent esthetic result with such restorations, is very brittle and must be supported with a rigid material (metal alloy).

TABLE 13.1	Linear Thermal Coefficient of Expansion of Dental Materials in the Temperature Range 20°C to 50°C
Material	Coefficient (× 10⁶/°C)
Human teeth	8–15
Ceramics	8–14
Glass ionomer base	10–11
Gold alloys	12–15
Dental amalgam	22–28
Composites	25–68
Unfilled acrylics and sealants	70–100
Inlay wax	300–1000

TABLE 13.2	Thermal Conductivity of Different Materials Used in Dentistry
Material	Thermal Conductivity (cal/sec/cm²[°C/cm])
Unfilled acrylics	0.0005
Zinc oxide–eugenol cement	0.0011
Human dentin	0.0015
Human enamel	0.0022
Composites	0.0025
Ceramic	0.0025
Zinc phosphate cement	0.0028
Dental amalgam	0.055
Gold alloys	0.710

When fabricating metal-ceramic restorations the crowns must be heated to a high temperature several times to sinter the veneering ceramic. Then the units must be cooled to bench temperature. If the COEs of the metal alloy and veneering porcelains are not closely matched, stresses can build up in the veneering porcelain that result in cracking or fracture of the ceramic. This can occur at the time of fabrication or later in clinical service. Generally the COE of the metal alloy is reduced with the addition of platinum, and the COE of the porcelain is increased with the addition of sodium. Whatever the mechanism used, it is clear the COEs of both the core and veneering material must be closely matched (Fig. 13.4).

It is often thought that the COEs of restorative materials must be matched with the COE of tooth structure. If they are not matched, the ingestion of hot beverages (e.g., coffee) and cold foods and beverages (e.g., ice cream and beer) could result in uneven expansion and contraction of the restoration and tooth, resulting in microleakage. The reality is foods and beverages do not surround the tooth/restoration complex for a long enough time frame to effect any significant change in the temperature of the tooth restoration.

Thermocycling of tooth restoration samples is frequently done during in vitro studies, and many incorrectly believe this is intended to mimic intraoral conditions. Samples are alternately placed in water at 5°C and 55°C for a specified dwell time. This is generally done to artificially age the samples and to stress the bond being tested. This thermocycling takes advantage of the differing COEs of the restorative material and tooth structure to stress the bond and accelerate the failure rate to shorten the necessary testing time.

Percolation. The process of fluids entering the microscopic space between a restorative material and the wall of the cavity preparation is called percolation. This is not a beneficial process with materials such as composite resins, but works wonderfully with materials such as silver amalgam. When percolation occurs with amalgam, corrosion products build up at the tooth-restoration interface and effectively seal it, usually 6 weeks after placement of the amalgam. With modern high copper amalgams with reduced gamma-2 phase, this phenomenon occurs but takes slightly longer to create an effective seal (Fig. 13.5; Table 13.2).

Thermal Conductivity. Thermal conductivity is the rate at which thermal changes are conducted through a material. Materials with

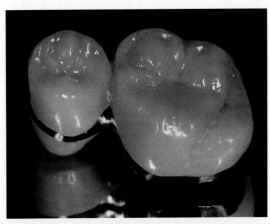

• **Fig. 13.4** Metal-ceramic restorations.

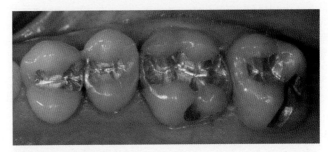

• **Fig. 13.5** Teeth numbers 12, 13, 14, 15 restored with amalgam restorations. Percolation = corrosion product = seal.

high thermal conductivity are good conductors of hot and cold, and could be a factor in postoperative sensitivity. This is the rationale for placing bases and/or liners with cavity preparations that are close to the pulp. Bases and liners have low thermal conductivity and thus are efficient insulators (see Table 13.2).

There is speculation by some that these bases and liners are not needed because dentin itself is a good insulator. However, often the thickness of dentin over the pulp may be minimal, so it is usually recommended that the thickness of remaining dentin plus the thickness of the base or liner should be at least 2 mm.

It is interesting to note that amalgam is an excellent thermal conductor whereas composite resin is an effective insulator; however, the incidence of postoperative sensitivity is significantly higher with composite resin restorations than with amalgam restorations. This demonstrates that the phenomenon of postoperative sensitivity is multifactorial and complex, and not due to thermal conductivity alone.

Layered zirconia restorations experience a rate of veneer chipping about eight times that of metal-ceramic restorations. The etiology of this chipping is multifactorial, but one of the potential causes is the thermal conductivity of the zirconia core. The thermal conductivity is extremely low, and zirconia can be considered an insulator. The consequence of this is that when a layered zirconia restoration is removed from the sintering oven, the core cools very slowly and the veneering ceramic cools past its glass transition temperature while the core continues to cool and shrink. The net result of this interaction is that stress is built up in the veneering ceramic, which is later released via clinical chipping of the veneering material. New firing cycles involving slower cooling rates seem to have reduced the incidence of chipping in recent years.[8]

Creep. Creep is defined as time dependent plastic deformation of a material under static load or constant stress. This property is important with silver amalgam. Conventional low copper amalgam materials have high creep values and exhibit poor marginal integrity over time as the amalgam creeps into a thin layer and then breaks off creating marginal ditching. Contemporary high copper amalgams have low creep values and maintain good marginal integrity as a function of time.

Creep is one of the few properties that has a demonstrated ability to predict clinical performance. Amalgam materials with low creep values perform well clinically when compared with amalgams with high creep values.

Electrical Properties. The three major electrical properties in dentistry are galvanism, tarnish, and corrosion. Galvanism occurs whenever different metals are in contact with one another in the presence of an electrolyte (saliva). Clinically, this can occur when a gold crown is placed adjacent to an existing amalgam restoration or vice versa. Gold crowns adjacent to metal-ceramic crowns can have a similar result as there are over 277 different commercially available porcelain bonding alloys. The clinical symptoms resemble an "electrical shock" or the presence of a metallic taste. These symptoms typically are self-limiting and are not considered serious problems (Fig. 13.6).

Tarnish is a surface phenomenon resulting in unesthetic discoloration of dental alloys, similar to tarnish of commonly used silverware (Fig. 13.7). It does not result in physical breakdown of the alloy. It is important to note that the term "noble metal" connotes that the metal is resistant to tarnish in the oral cavity. The major noble metals used in dentistry are gold, platinum, and palladium. Others are rhodium, ruthenium, iridium, and osmium. Alloys should contain a minimum 45% noble metal to prevent intraoral tarnishing. Chromium is a metal that prevents tarnish in base metal alloys. One metal that is precious but not noble is silver.

Corrosion is chemical or electrochemical dissolution of metals in oral fluids. The varying pHs in the oral environment create the possibility of corrosion, although in fact it is a rare occurrence. Corrosion of prefabricated metal endodontic dowels with flawed endodontically treated teeth has been seen occasionally. In these cases it is believed that fracture of the endodontically treated tooth occurred first, allowing contact of oral fluids with the post resulting in corrosion. The other possibility is that the corrosion occurred first followed by fracture due to the production of corrosion products (Fig. 13.8).

Solubility. Solubility is the relative tendency to dissolve in oral fluids. This was a major problem with the first direct esthetic restorative material, silicate cement. This cement was a powder

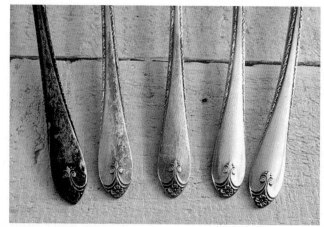

• **Fig. 13.7** Tarnish of silverware. Dental alloys may undergo the same discoloration in the oral environment.

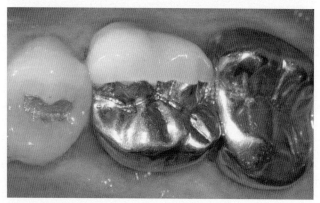

• **Fig. 13.6** The generation of electrical currents due to contact of dissimilar metals in an electrolyte is known as galvanism.

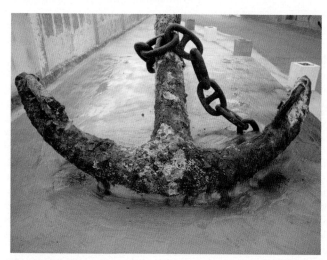

• **Fig. 13.8** Example of corrosion due to electrochemical dissolution in water.

liquid system, the powder being ground alumino-silicate glass and the liquid phosphoric acid. When mixed, it formed a paste that was inserted into the prepared cavity and when set and finished provided a restoration suitable for class III restorations that was expected to provide only 3 to 5 years of service. The reason for this short time of service was that silicate cements were soluble in oral fluids. An unexpected benefit of this problem was that as the alumino-silicate glass dissolved, it released high concentrations of fluoride. When the partially dissolved restoration was removed for replacement, recurrent caries was never found due to this high level of fluoride release (Fig. 13.9).

Conventional nonresin-based dental cements had variable levels of solubility; for example, zinc-oxide eugenol (ZOE) cements that are often used for provisional restorations are quite soluble in oral fluids. From a practical standpoint, this means that provisional restorations should not be cemented for more than 6 weeks if ZOE is used. At that time, the provisional restorations should be removed, cleaned, and recemented.

The relative solubility of conventional nonresin cements made it necessary to provide precisely fitting definitive restorations. Cast gold restorations provide an extremely long time of service cemented with zinc-phosphate cement, providing they have precision of fit. Poorly fitting cast gold restorations provide a short term of service as they are simply chunks of metal in a sea of cement.

Solubility of dental cements is typically measured with a 24-hour in vitro solubility test where a sample of cement is immersed in a solute for 24 hours and the amount of dissolved cement is calculated.[9] Long-term (6 months) in vivo solubility tests are preferred. These types of studies indicate that there are small differences between cements in long-term solubility, but importantly find there are significant differences among patients in regard to solubility. Some patients dissolve considerable amounts of cement, while other patients demonstrate minimal solubility. The causes of this phenomenon are not known.

Glass ionomer cements perform poorly in 24-hour in vitro solubility testing because they are quite soluble in the first 24 hours after mixing. However, they perform very well in 6-month in vivo testing, and in fact are the best of the conventional nonresin cements in that parameter. This means they must be protected from saliva immediately after cementation using excellent isolation and coating with petroleum jelly or varnish.

Optical Properties. Optical properties of bulk materials include interactions with visible light that involve reflection, refraction, absorption (and fluorescence), or transmission. The radiation typically involves different intensities for different wavelengths (or energies) over the range of interest (spectrum). Any of these interactive events can be measured using a relative scale or an absolute scale. When the electromagnetic radiation is visible light, the amount of reflection can be measured in relative terms as gloss or in absolute terms as percent reflection. Visible light absorption can be measured in absolute terms as percent absorption (or transmission) for every wavelength (in the visible spectrum). Color is a perception by an observer of the distribution of wavelengths. The same color sensation may be produced by different absorption spectra (metamerism). An individual's eye is capable of sensing dominant wavelength, luminous reflectance (intensity), and excitation purity. Variations among individuals' abilities to sense these characteristics give rise to varying perceptions of color.

The quality of color is measured by the Commission Internationale de l'Eclairage system as tristimulus values and reported as color differences (ΔL^*, Δa^*, and Δb^*) compared with standard conditions.

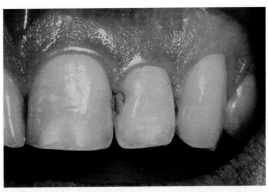

• **Fig. 13.9** Class III cavity restored with silicate cement after 3 years. Notice the poor resistance to solubility and color change. No evidence of recurrent carries.

Radiation of another wavelength may be preferentially absorbed (e.g., x-rays). Composites that contain lithium, barium, strontium, or other good x-ray absorbers may appear radiopaque (radiodense) in dental radiographs. Materials that are good absorbers (for whatever form of radiation) are described as opaque.

The appearance of a dental restoration is a combination of events of surface reflection, absorption, and internal scattering. The scattering simply may deflect the path of the radiation during transmission (refraction), or it may reflect the radiation internally from varying depths back out of a solid to the observer (translucency). Enamel naturally displays a high degree of translucency; translucency is a desirable characteristic for restorative materials attempting to mimic enamel. A tooth that is isolated and kept from any contact with oral moisture (saliva) soon develops a transient whiter appearance. Refractive index is the angle of changed path for a standard wavelength of light energy under standard conditions (Fig. 13.10).

Compressive Strength, Tensile Strength, Diametral Tensile Strength, Flexural Strength, and Fracture Toughness. All of these are mechanical properties of materials that are tested utilizing nonclinical samples and thus are only useful when comparing the tested material to a known standard. Compressive strength tests use cylindrical samples. Tensile tests can be done with certain materials such as wires but cannot be used with materials such as dental cements. Diametral tensile strength tests use discs and apply the force to an edge. Because these tests do not test the material in the mode in which it is used, data obtained from the tests are of little value in predicting clinical performance but may be useful in comparing a new product to a standard (Fig. 13.11).

Flexural strength testing has become popular for evaluating new ceramic materials. Many of the newer ceramics such as lithium disilicate and monolithic zirconia have vastly improved flexural strength compared to feldspathic porcelain or leucite reinforced ceramic. However, that data in itself does not automatically ensure improved clinical performance, because ceramic crowns do not fracture because of a lack of strength. They fracture because of inherent defects called Griffith flaws, which are incorporated into the restorations during fabrication. These defects propagate under occlusal stress and due to static fatigue, and eventually result in catastrophic failure. These newer materials may well provide improved clinical performance because the techniques used in fabrication (pressing and machining) result in fewer inherent defects, and the phase transformation capability of zirconia prevents defects from propagating after initiation.

Fracture toughness determination may be one of the most valuable in vitro tests because it evaluates failure initiating from a predetermined defect. It is possible that materials with improved fracture toughness may show improved clinical performance.

Elastic Modulus. Elastic modulus is a measure of the relative stiffness or rigidity of a material (Fig. 13.12). The elastic modulus is the ratio of stress over strain and is the slope of the straight-line portion of a stress-strain diagram. It is a measure of how the material will deform when placed under stress. A material with a high elastic modulus will be stiff; a material with a low elastic modulus will be flexible.

Ceramic materials have a very high elastic modulus and are very brittle. These materials are frequently bonded to a core material to support the ceramic veneer and prevent fracture. It is critical that the core material have an elastic modulus equal to or higher than that of the ceramic material, because if the core material flexes, the ceramic will fracture.

Another area where the modulus of elasticity of a material is important is in the restoration of noncarious cervical lesions (NCCLs). One potential etiology of NCCLs is tooth flexure leading to cervical breakdown. Traditionally, materials with a low elastic modulus such as microfilled composite resins and resin modified glass ionomers have been more successful in restoring NCCLs than stiff materials such as hybrid composite resins.[10] Contemporary adhesive systems are now highly filled and, because they have a low elastic modulus, can act as stress breakers during tooth flexure, permitting successful restoration with stiffer composite resins.

Load-to Failure Testing Versus Fatigue Testing. The traditional approach to testing the strength of dental restorations is load-to-failure testing. With load-to-failure testing, a restoration is fabricated and cemented/bonded to the prepared tooth or die and then loaded with a testing machine and the forces increased until the restoration fractures. If the load at which the restorations fail exceeds the maximum bite force in the area of the restoration, it is then deemed that materials will provide excellent clinical performance. Data generated from load-to-failure testing can be very misleading and do not provide predictive information on clinical performance.

Several problems with load-to-failure testing can be identified. Clinically, teeth and restorations generally fail by defect propagation. Load-to-failure testing does not take this into account. The loads at which failure occurs with load-to-failure testing are much higher than the loads at which clinical failure occurs.[11] The failures with

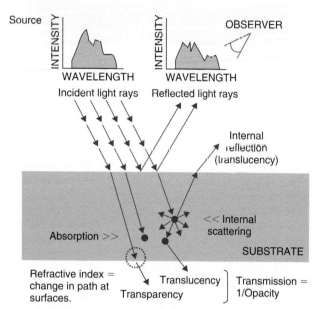

• **Fig. 13.10** Schematic summary of interactions of electromagnetic radiation with materials. The color perceived by the observer is the result of several interactions between substrate and incoming radiation producing reflection, internal scattering, absorption, fluorescence, and transmission.

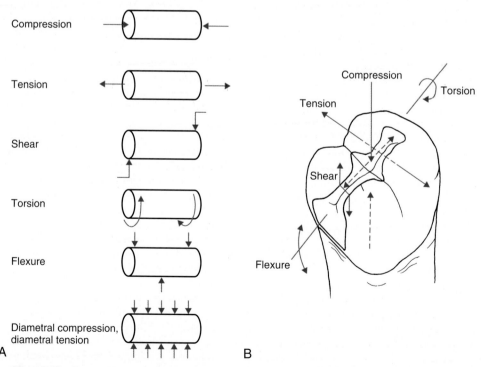

• **Fig. 13.11** Examples of directions of loading. A, Uniaxial loading of cylinder. B, Uniaxial loading of a mesioocclusal amalgam restoration.

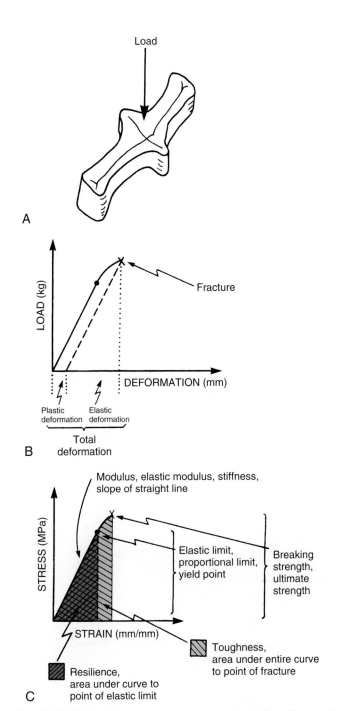

A

B

C

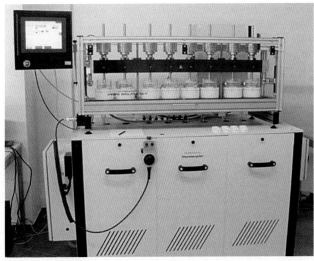

• **Fig. 13.13** Eight-chamber chewing simulator.

• **Fig. 13.12** Schematic summary of mechanical properties with respect to amalgam restoration in function. A, Occlusal loading of Class I amalgam restoration. B, Load/deformation curve describing behavior of amalgam. C, Normalization of load/deformation curve to stress-strain curve with important characteristics of curve indicated. (Mechanical responses depend on temperature and strain rate involved.)

load-to-failure testing initiate at the occlusal surface of the restoration being tested while clinically restorations fail by defect propagation from defects at the tooth cement surface. Finally, the fracture pattern of failed restorations with load-to-failure testing results in the restoration fracturing in multiple fragments. Clinically, failure usually occurs with the restoration breaking into two pieces.

One major argument against load-to-failure testing is that restorations do not fail because the patient bites down with incredible force on a restoration, but rather they fail by defect propagation due to low occlusal forces over a long period of time. In order to make in vitro testing more clinically related, fatigue testing using cyclic loading machines has become increasingly popular (Fig. 13.13).

Fatigue testing using cyclic loading is considerably more relevant than load-to-failure testing because it much more closely mimics the clinical situation. Fortunately, many major research organizations have made the considerable investment in cyclic loading machines and more and more fatigue studies are appearing in the peer reviewed literature. It is important to note that dental fatigue testing is in its infancy and many factors need to be considered when attempting to bring the study environment closer to the clinical situation.

Some of the variables that need to be considered include loading force, number of cycles, loading frequency, and antagonist material. Whether or not to include a simulated periodontal ligament is an important consideration. Whether to fatigue under water or dry is also a consideration. With ceramic materials, it is critical to fatigue under water as it has been proven that ceramic materials fail at half the load under water as in air. This is because of the presence of static fatigue with ceramic materials under water or saliva. The use of thermocycling, the type of abutment or die material, the use of vertical plus lateral movements, and the use of anatomic versus flat samples are all important considerations when designing a fatigue study.

The bottom line is that load-to-failure studies have no clinical relevance whatsoever and should not be published. While recognizing that designing appropriate fatigue studies is challenging, it is clear that these types of studies are going to play an increasingly important role in dental materials research.

Wettability. Wettability is a measure of the affinity of a liquid for a solid as indicated by the spreading of a sessile drop (Fig. 13.14).

This might be best explained by the state of a raindrop on a freshly waxed car. It will bead up, indicating a high contact angle and low wettability. Similarly, placing a drop on air abraded versus polished metal will result in a spreading drop (low contact angle; good wettability) on the former and a beaded drop (high contact angle; poor wettability) on the latter.

Early versions of addition reaction silicone impression material were extremely hydrophobic and difficult to pour. Modern elastomeric impression materials contain nonionic surfactants, which render them more hydrophilic and considerably easier to pour because the surface is more wettable and forms a lower contact angle with liquids.

Hardness Testing. The surface hardness of a material is often of interest and is determined by use of some form of indenter. Basically the indenting tool is dropped onto the surface of the material with a specified load, and the size of the defect created on the material is measured using a microscope. There are different hardness tests that are optimally used with specific materials. These include Knoop, Vickers, Barcol, Brinell, and Rockwell hardness testing (Fig. 13.15). The difference between these testers is the shape and material of the indenter and the force used.

One area where hardness testing is frequently used is in determining the degree of polymerization of composite resin materials. The harder the surface, the greater the degree of conversion. Studies generally compare the hardness of the top surface (closest to the light) and the hardness of the bottom surface. Some of the variables that have been tested include intensity of the light, thickness of

the composite resin increment, curing through ceramics, and distance of the light from the resin.

Bond Strength Testing. In the adhesive era there is a need to test the bond of one material to another, and the bond of materials to enamel and dentin. There have been hundreds of studies published on bond strength in recent years. These studies are useful for comparing the relative bond strength of product X to product Y but have relatively low ability to predict clinical performance.[12]

The most common bond strength test is the shear bond strength test. This test is used frequently because it is easy to perform, but the clinical relevance is minimal. Another approach is the microtensile bond strength test. This test became popular because it was initially thought that 8 to 10 samples could be obtained from a single tooth; however, subsequent evaluation determined that data from these samples needed to be combined and in reality only 1 sample was obtained from each tooth. This bond strength test is extremely technique sensitive and produces data with wide standard deviations. It is not clear that the predictive data from microtensile bond strength testing is more predictive of clinical performance than shear bond testing.

It is clear that many bonds are quite strong initially but deteriorate over time. Thus it is imperative that bond strength testing must include initial testing plus testing after storage in water, thermocycling, or fatigue.

Biologic Properties. Biologic properties of biomaterials are concerned with toxicity and sensitivity reactions that occur locally, within the associated tissue, and systemically. It is possible to evaluate local toxic effects on cells by clinical pulp studies or by tissue culture tests. Unset materials may release cytotoxic components; however, in clinical situations this problem is rarely evident. Two

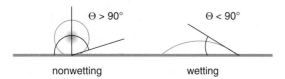

• **Fig. 13.14** Schematic drawing of the contact angle determining wettability. Contact angles less than 90 degrees are considered to be wetting and hydrophilic. Contact angles larger than 90 degrees are considered nonwetting and hydrophobic.

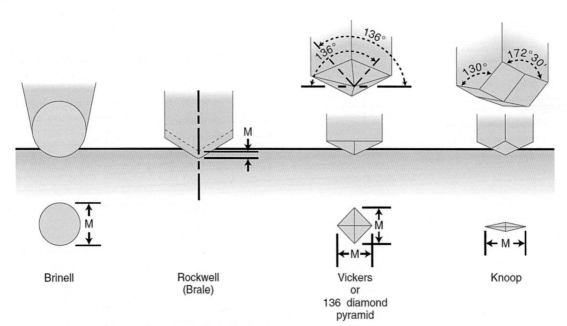

• **Fig. 13.15** Shapes of hardness indenter points *(upper row)* and the indentation depressions left in material surfaces *(lower row)*. The measured dimension *M* that is shown for each test is used to calculate hardness. The following tests are shown: Brinell test—a steel ball is used, and the diameter of the indentation is measured after removal of the indenter. Rockwell test—a conical indenter is impressed into the surface under a minor load *(dashed line)* and a major load *(solid line)*, and *M* is the difference between the two penetration depths. In the Vickers or 136-degree diamond pyramid test, a pyramidal point is used and the diagonal length of the indentation is measured. In the Knoop test, a rhombohedral pyramid diamond tip is used and the long axis of the indentation is measured. (From Anusavice KJ, Shen C, Rawls RH: *Phillips' science of dental materials,* ed 12, Elsevier, St. Louis, 2013.)

important clinical factors determining toxicity are the exposure time and the concentration of the potentially toxic substance.

Generally, restorative materials harden quickly or are not readily soluble in tissue fluids (or both). Potentially toxic products do not have time to diffuse into tissues. Even more importantly, the concentration makes the poison. Some authorities believe that if the amount of material involved is small, the pulp or other tissues can transport and excrete it without significant biochemical damage. Others believe there is no threshold. A threshold level for toxicity is one below which no effect can be detected.

This section is not meant to be an exhaustive description of all physical and mechanical properties of dental materials. It is intended to highlight some of the more important properties and to describe some clinical examples where these properties might be important. Even though these properties are important, it is imperative to understand that in vitro studies of physical and mechanical properties are poor indicators of clinical performance. As fatigue studies become more sophisticated and clinically relevant, in vitro studies may become more predictive.

THE BOTTOM LINE

1. A large number of physical and mechanical properties of dental materials can be evaluated with in vitro testing.
2. When testing materials, whenever possible they should be tested in the mode in which they are used.
3. Bond strength studies have little relevance to clinical performance.
4. Static in vitro studies of physical and mechanical properties yield minimal data that are predictive of clinical performance.
5. Ceramic materials should be fatigue tested under water.
6. Fatigue testing with cyclic loading is promising but complex.

Direct Restorative Materials

Silver Amalgam

Silver amalgam has been used for the restoration of teeth for well over a century.[6] It has been the most popular restorative material over that period of time, having been used in over 75% of single tooth restorations placed in the past 100 years (see Fig. 13.3).

The use of silver amalgam in North America has diminished somewhat in recent years due to a dramatic reduction in caries rate coupled with a high interest in esthetics and concern for the potential toxicity of mercury.

Nonetheless, silver amalgam will continue to be an important restorative material for many years to come. It will likely be especially valuable in many of the developing countries where dental caries continues to be a major problem and where resources required to deliver alternative (more sophisticated) restorative dentistry options are not available. Additionally, silver amalgam continues to be one of the best materials available for core buildups of extensively damaged teeth to support crowns and fixed partial dentures.

Silver amalgam has had a fascinating and controversial history ever since its introduction to North America by the Crawcour brothers in the 1830s. The actions of these charlatans resulted in the first amalgam war and the infamous "amalgam pledge" that was finally rescinded in 1850. A period of scientific investigation followed, championed by individuals such as Flagg and Hickock, and culminated in G.V. Black's publication of his formula for silver amalgam in 1896 (Fig. 13.16).

In the 1930s the writings of a German physician, Stock, stimulated research into the biocompatibility of silver amalgam, and specifically the effects of mercury. In what could be called the

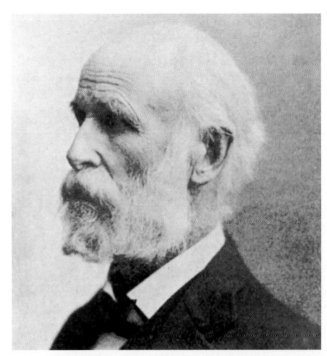

• **Fig. 13.16** G.V. Black. Father of operative dentistry. (From Kock CRD: *History of dental surgery,* vol 1, Chicago, 1909, National Art Publishing.)

second amalgam war, claims and counterclaims were made, and eventually organized dentistry accepted the belief that amalgam was safe. The first American Dental Association (ADA) Specification (#1) for a dental material was established for silver amalgam, and Stock later went on to repudiate his own writings.

The composition of silver amalgam did not change substantially from the publication of Black's formula until the 1960s when high copper amalgam was introduced to the profession by two Canadian researchers (Fig. 13.17).

As subsequent clinical research would clearly demonstrate, the high copper formulations that are almost exclusively used today are clinically superior to the conventional amalgam materials that had been used up to that time. As Greener has explained, the discovery of high copper amalgam was a case of "serendipity of the highest order," yet it remains as one of the most important advances in dental materials in the past 50 years.[6]

Advantages of Silver Amalgam

Silver amalgam has been and will continue to be such a popular restorative material because it possesses a number of well-defined advantages. It is one of the easiest of all restorative materials to manipulate, it can be placed into the prepared cavity in a plastic state, and then it can be carved and shaped to physiologic form before it hardens. Once hardened, it has excellent physical properties that allow it to perform well in the long term as a restorative material in posterior teeth. It is strong enough to provide very predictable long-term service in conservative restorations, and is also valuable as an interim restorative material in very large restorations.

The basic strength of silver amalgam, coupled with the fact that it can be placed relatively rapidly in a single appointment, make it a very cost-effective material. It is less expensive by a wide margin than any of the alternative restorative materials.

Silver amalgam has one additional important advantage: its ability to automatically seal the cavity preparation. This ability,

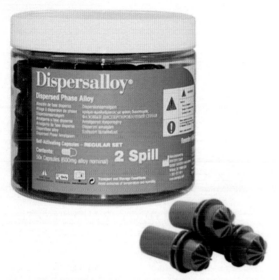

• Fig. 13.17 Dispersalloy (dispersed phase alloy) high copper amalgam. (Courtesy Dentsply.)

TABLE 13.3	Amalgam Alloy Composition	
Element	Alloy %	Principal Function
Ag	70%	Strength
Sn	16%	Expansion
Cu	13%	Strength
Zn	1%	Deoxidizer

which is a result of the buildup of corrosion products at the interface between the amalgam and the cavity margins, makes silver amalgam unique among restorative materials. A seal can be produced with excellent technique with some of the alternative materials, but none are as user friendly as amalgam, which creates a seal independent of the operator. Several months are required before the seal becomes complete, especially with high copper amalgam formulations; but once attained, it is a very effective barrier against recurrent caries.

Because it requires some time for the seal resulting from deposition of corrosion products to materialize, a method of obtaining a temporary seal at the time of placement is recommended. This used to be accomplished by placing two or three coats of copal varnish on the enamel and dentin surfaces of the prepared cavity. This copal varnish created an initial seal that would eventually be replaced by the percolation process as corrosion products gradually formed at the interface. In contemporary practice copal varnish is obsolete, and sealing the cavity with a desensitizing agent such as Gluma Desensitizer or G5 prior to amalgam placement is indicated.

Composition

Silver amalgam is supplied to the dentist as a powder or metallic pellets that are then mixed together with liquid mercury in a high-speed triturator to form a plastic mass that can be placed into a prepared cavity. The plastic material allows sufficient working time for successful placement and then sets to form a strong and durable restoration that can provide long-term clinical service.

Amalgam formulations differ from one another both chemically in terms of chemical composition and physically in terms of the size and shape of the alloy particles that are mixed with mercury. These physical and chemical variations result in differences in handling characteristics of the material and in the clinical results that are ultimately attained.

From a chemical standpoint, amalgam can be divided into two groups, *conventional amalgam*, which is similar to Black's formulation, and *high copper amalgam*, which represents the state of the art. Table 13.3 lists the components of both types of amalgam alloy prior to mixing with mercury and also indicates the function of each component.

It is useful to understand the chemical reactions that occur with both types of amalgam, as such an understanding will explain the differences in their clinical performance.

A set amalgam is a true eutectic, and micrographic evaluation reveals three distinct phases: gamma, gamma-1, and gamma-2. The reaction for conventional amalgam may be written as follows:

$$\underset{\text{(AgSn)}}{\text{gamma}} + \underset{\text{(Hg)}}{\text{mercury}} \rightarrow \underset{\text{(AgSn)}}{\text{gamma}} + \underset{\text{(AgHg)}}{\text{gamma-1}} + \underset{\text{(SnHg)}}{\text{gamma-2}}$$

The gamma phase, which consists of unreacted silver and tin, is the major component of the unreacted alloy and is also present in the set amalgam. It is suspended in a matrix of gamma-1, which is the reaction product of silver and mercury. The gamma phase is very strong and corrosion resistant, whereas the gamma-1 phase is less strong and is more corrosion susceptible. The gamma-2 phase, the reaction product of tin-mercury, is also suspended in the gamma-1 matrix. It is the weakest and most corrosion susceptible of the three phases. The major difference between conventional and high copper amalgams is the near elimination of the gamma-2 phase in the high copper amalgams. Elimination of this phase produces a much stronger and clinically superior restoration.

Laboratory studies show that high copper amalgams display less creep than conventional amalgams. The main clinical manifestation of this superiority is improved edge strength, which results in a lack of marginal ditching over the long term (Fig. 13.18).

The chemical reaction for high copper amalgams may be written as follows:

$$\underset{\text{(AgSn)}}{\text{gamma}} + \underset{\text{(AgCu)}}{\text{copper}} + \underset{\text{(Hg)}}{\text{mercury}} \rightarrow \underset{\text{(AgSn)}}{\text{gamma}} + \underset{\text{(AgHg)}}{\text{gamma-1}} + \underset{\text{(CuSn)}}{\text{CuSn}}$$

With such amalgam formulations, where the alloy contains 9% to 30% copper, the copper will preferentially react with the tin and thus prevent formation of the gamma-2 phase. Again, the elimination of this gamma-2 phase strengthens the resultant amalgam and is clinically manifest in improved marginal integrity and minimal marginal ditching over time.

The discovery of high copper amalgams was basically an accident. The metallurgists who developed the first commercial product added small metal spheres to the irregularly shaped alloy particles in an attempt to "dispersion strengthen" the set amalgam. The concept was that the spheres would fit into the interstices between the larger irregular particles and this would make the amalgam stronger. They happened to use copper spheres for this initial product, and it was the elimination of the gamma-2 phase as a result of the added copper that resulted in the improved clinical performance of the alloy, rather than the imagined dispersion strengthening. In fact, it has never been demonstrated that dispersion strengthening is a viable modality.

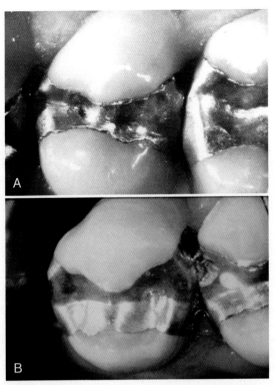

• **Fig. 13.18** A, Conventional amalgam restoration. B, High copper amalgam restoration.

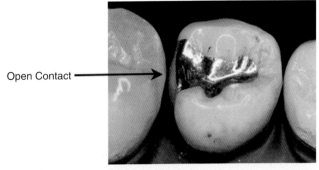

Open Contact

• **Fig. 13.19** Open proximal contact in a Class II amalgam restoration.

TABLE 13.4	Compressive Strength (MPa) of Different Brands of Amalgam Alloys After 1 Hour and 24 Hours	
Alloy	1 hr	24 hrs
Velvalloy	18,000	55,000
Dispersalloy	33,000	64,500
Phasealloy	12,900	65,700
Tytin	34,900	75,000
Valiant	47,800	76,500

Commercial amalgams can also differ from one another in the shape of the alloy particles. The two major types are *admixed* alloys and *spherical* alloys. Both types of alloys produce clinically successful restorations, but the handling characteristics of each are very different.

With traditional amalgam materials, the alloy particles are formed by cutting a block of alloy with a lathe. This method forms relatively large, irregular particles. With admixed alloys, small spheres formed by atomizing the liquid alloy are added to the mix in the hope that a denser final amalgam will result. Such an alloy is termed an admixed alloy, and is the most common material in use today.

Such alloys require considerable force during condensation of the amalgam to ensure optimum packing of the material and intimate adaptation of the amalgam to the cavity walls. Strength of these alloys is time dependent, and 24-hour compressive strength is considerably greater than 1-hour strength (Table 13.4). These alloys should be carved and burnished, and final polishing should be delayed for at least 24 hours.

Spherical alloys handle much differently than admixed alloys. Generally speaking they require slightly less mercury in the initial mix due to the small size of the spherical particles. The consistency of the mix is often described as "buttery," and the amalgam is easily placed into the cavity and adapted to the cavity walls with a minimum of pressure. However, because the fresh amalgam mix will not resist a moderate amount of condensation pressure, it is somewhat difficult to attain an adequate proximal contact in Class II restorations (Fig. 13.19). With experience, this deficiency can be overcome with excellent clinical technique.

Spherical amalgams attain much higher early (1 hour) strengths than do admixed amalgams, and the final (24 hours) compressive strengths are also generally higher. The gain in early strength may possibly reduce the incidence of isthmus fractures due to occlusal force exerted shortly after placement of the amalgam; however,

there is no clinical data that would support that. It may also allow preparation of the freshly placed amalgam 15 minutes after insertion in those situations where it is being used as a build-up prior to crown fabrication. The gains in final compressive strength are likely of minor importance.

Evaluation of Silver Amalgam Materials

Dental materials are generally initially evaluated in the laboratory and subsequently in patients in controlled clinical trials. Laboratory tests are of minimal value in differentiating clinical performance between different alloys. The only laboratory test that has proven to be of predictive value in the clinical setting is that of "creep." Alloys with low creep values typically demonstrate excellent marginal integrity over time in clinical trials.[13] Generally high copper amalgams display low creep values and are clinically successful alloys.

Thus an amalgam alloy should be selected on the basis of proven clinical performance. Other variables, such as quality control, and handling characteristics also may play a role in the decision to select a given alloy. Thus today it would be a reasonable choice to select a high copper formulation that has a consistency and rate of set that is desired by the individual practitioner. In fact, the intelligent practitioner may well choose to keep a couple of different formulations on inventory and choose the appropriate formulation to match the specific clinical situation.

For example, many prefer an admixed zinc containing alloy for the majority of conventional restorations where a dry field can be maintained and where achieving good interproximal contact is desirable. They would choose a spherical zinc containing alloy in those situations where a dry field can be maintained but using strong condensation force is difficult, for example when restoring a Class V lesion on the distobuccal of a maxillary second molar. Such a formulation is also desirable when building up an extensively broken down tooth prior to preparing that tooth for a cast crown. Here the high early strength is useful, as is the ease of condensation especially when small slots, potholes, and small undercut areas are utilized as the primary retentive features. Finally, a nonzinc spherical alloy is useful in those situations where adequate moisture control is not possible, such as certain Class V situations and surgical endodontics where amalgam is used to seal the small prepared cavity in the root apex.

Manipulation of Silver Amalgam

The quality of a given mix of silver amalgam is controlled by the quality of the product as supplied to the dentist, and can be modified by the manipulation of that product by the dentist. The manipulative variables include the mercury/alloy ratio, trituration, condensation, and carving and finishing of the restoration.

In general terms, the less mercury that remains in the final restoration, the better it will be both in terms of strength and corrosion resistance. Thus the initial mix should be made with only as much mercury as is required to make an adequate mix. With most admixed alloys this will be about 50% mercury, whereas with spherical alloys it will be slightly less. Proper condensation and carving technique will remove a significant amount of mercury from the material, thus enhancing final strength. In the past care had to be taken with mercury dispensers to maintain control of the mercury/alloy ratio, but today the majority of practitioners utilize precapsulated products. This is beneficial in that it allows precise control of the mercury/alloy ratio, minimizes handling of the mercury, and minimizes the mercury vapor aerosol created during trituration.

Mixing the amalgam is called trituration. Adequate trituration of the amalgam is essential to produce a workable mass and to ensure optimum physical properties. Each brand of amalgam has specific instructions regarding optimum time and speed of trituration. The instructions are specific for each brand of amalgamator. The longer and the faster an amalgam is mixed, the more rapidly it will set. The manufacturers' guidelines for mixing should be followed and can be modified slightly to obtain a faster or slower setting material.

Condensation of the amalgam is probably the most critical manipulative variable. Adequate condensation results in intimate adaptation of the amalgam to the cavity walls, as well as a denser material to maximize strength. The prepared cavity is always overfilled and carved back to proper anatomic contour. This is because condensation results in a mercury-rich superficial layer, which is removed during the carving procedure. The resultant amalgam surface has considerably less mercury and subsequently superior physical properties.

The most common error made by dentists is under condensation. This results in poor adaptation to the cavity walls, increased microleakage, and recurrent caries. The final amalgam is weaker and more fracture prone, and cannot be polished nearly as well as a properly condensed amalgam.

With the high copper formulations currently in use, both precarve and postcarve burnishing is recommended. This is generally accomplished with a large, egg-shaped burnisher. The amalgam is carved after achieving a firm set, with careful attention being paid to eliminating all marginal flash and carving the amalgam flush with the margins of the cavity preparation. Any marginal flash will eventually fracture, and it is rare that it fractures right at the margin. Inevitably, marginal ditching will occur.

After carving back to anatomic form, the restoration is lightly burnished to a smooth sheen. The restoration may be polished after 24 hours. There are no solid clinical data that support the routine polishing of amalgam restorations, but certainly highly polished restorations are more comfortable for the patient and will be less likely to retain bacterial plaque. Polishing amalgams also indicates a certain amount of pride in workmanship and is a source of great personal satisfaction.

Bonded Amalgams

With adhesive dentistry becoming so popular in recent years, many innovative techniques in all areas of restorative dentistry have been proposed. One of the most intriguing is the concept of *"bonded"* amalgams. This technique has the advantages of forming an instant seal of the prepared cavity, a more conservative preparation design, and the *potential* to strengthen the prepared tooth and reduce the long-term incidence of cuspal fracture.[14] The word *potential* is stressed because the concept of tooth strengthening has not been proven clinically at the time of writing.

Bonded amalgams utilize any one of the current generation of enamel/dentin bonding agents to seal the dentin and "bond" the amalgam to the prepared tooth. The amalgam is condensed into polymerizing dual cure resin that is placed on conditioned dentin and etched enamel. The amalgam or the oxide of amalgam will chemically bond to the resin, and the resin is bonded to the tooth structure primarily by micromechanical retention. Thus the resin will partially retain the amalgam in place, reducing the need to create retentive undercuts in the tooth. Elimination of these undercuts, which have been shown to weaken cusps, coupled with the potential strengthening effect may improve the long-term prognosis of these restorations. Clinical research thus far has shown that bonded and nonbonded amalgams perform equally well. There seems to be little advantage to bonding amalgams, and the technique is more complex and time consuming.

THE BOTTOM LINE

1. Silver amalgam has been an important restorative material for many years and will continue to be an important material for years to come.
2. Advantages of silver amalgam are excellent physical properties, cost, long-term service, and the ability to self-seal the cavity.
3. Amalgam is the most user-friendly material in restorative dentistry.
4. High copper amalgams are superior to conventional amalgams demonstrating excellent marginal integrity over time. This is due to elimination of the gamma-2 phase (tin-mercury).
5. It is easier to create a good proximal contact with admixed versus spherical alloys.
6. Spherical alloys can be prepared 15 minutes after insertion and are indicated for amalgam core buildups.
7. Proper condensation of the amalgam is the most important manipulative variable.
8. Bonding amalgam to tooth structure is possible, but there is minimal clinical benefit.

Mercury and Silver Amalgam

Silver amalgam contains between 43% and 52% mercury when it is freshly mixed, prior to condensation into the prepared cavity. The procedures of condensation, precarve burnishing, and carving remove a portion of this mercury. The remainder of the mercury remains in the finished restoration. Because high doses of mercury vapor can cause serious systemic illness, this mercury remaining in silver amalgam restorations has been a source of continued controversy for over a century.[6,15] This controversy continues unabated today in spite of a total lack of scientific evidence demonstrating a link between silver amalgam and systemic disease. In fact, quite to the contrary, ample scientific data support the continued use of silver amalgam and document its enviable record of safety.

Historical Review

Amalgam has been the source of controversy ever since it was first introduced to North America by the Crawcour brothers in 1836. These charlatans from France placed their version of amalgam, called "Royal Mineral Succedaneum," into the teeth of patients at carnivals and medicine shows. The material, which was derived from filings from silver coins mixed with large amounts of mercury, tended to expand significantly on setting. This resulted in an incredibly high incidence of postoperative pain, tooth fracture, and elevated occlusal contacts. These postoperative sequelae, coupled with the use of a potentially toxic material such as mercury, precipitated the first amalgam war.

The debate raged furiously for many years, dividing organized dentistry into two main camps. One group—naturally intrigued with the possibilities of a truly plastic material that could be placed into the mouth in a softened state, conformed to the cavity preparation in the tooth, and then hardened—sought to continue to use the material and to experiment with modified formulations. The other group—which comprised the main body of organized dentistry at the time—chose to outlaw amalgam and in fact drafted the now infamous "Amalgam Pledge." The essence of the pledge was that the signer agreed to never consider using silver amalgam. Anyone wishing to belong to the organization was required to sign this pledge.

In 1850 the Amalgam Pledge was rescinded and a period of scientific experiment began, led by individuals such as Hickock, Flagg, and others. This period culminated in 1897 when Black published his formula for amalgam alloy. This alloy, and minor variations thereof, was the type essentially used by all North American dentists until the serendipitous discovery of modern high copper alloy by Innes and Youdelis in 1963.[16] Because silver amalgam is relatively strong, inexpensive, and essentially user friendly, it became the most popular restorative material for posterior teeth in the latter half of the 20th century and continues to be used extensively today. In spite of this popularity and tremendous utility, silver amalgam has had to survive periodic attacks relative to its safety.

A second amalgam war resulted from the writings of a German medical doctor named Stock. His writings appeared in the European medical literature and consisted of anecdotal reports related to mercury toxicity in patients with silver amalgam restorations. No controlled scientific data was reported, and in fact Stock later repudiated that information in his own articles in the 1940s. However, at the time, his statements were sufficiently provocative that scientists initiated a number of studies that would eventually help to establish the safety of this fine material.

In the 1990s, renewed controversy surrounding amalgam resulted in what might be called the third amalgam war. This particular episode in the turbulent history of amalgam has been precipitated by a combination of renewed scientific investigation coupled with an unprecedented amount of charlatanism and media hype.[17] To the uninformed, the safety of silver amalgam is once again in question. This doubt concerning its safety, coupled with an ever-increasing demand by the public for tooth-colored posterior restorations and a concomitant decrease in the incidence of caries in developed countries, has resulted in a drastic reduction in the use of silver amalgam. The reduction in the caries rate is a remarkable achievement, and the desire for more esthetic restorative materials is understandable. However, the widespread practice of removing functional amalgam restorations in the name of patient safety is to be deplored. This results in unwarranted loss of tooth structure, unnecessary expense, and, especially if the replacement restoration is tooth colored, limited longevity.

Perhaps a brief review of the classical and contemporary literature on the topic of mercury in silver amalgam will clarify the issue. For those who would prefer to simply receive the bottom line on this issue, it is this: There is absolutely no scientific evidence to indicate that silver amalgam restorations pose a health risk of any kind to patients. There is a large body of well-conducted and controlled scientific literature to support this statement. Unwarranted removal of amalgam restorations in order to prevent or cure systemic health conditions is wrong and in fact is considered unethical in many jurisdictions.

Classical Research

There are a number of classic studies that had established the safety of silver amalgam to the satisfaction of the scientific community up until the findings of the 1980s. The broad body of this research has been the subject of an excellent review by Bauer and First in 1982, and only a few classic papers will be reported here.[18] The first of these was conducted primarily to repudiate the writings of Stock, published in 1931.[19] A selenium sulfide mercury detector was used to determine if mercury vapor was released from the surface of silver amalgam. The solubility of amalgam in a number of acidic solutions was also tested. No mercury vapor was detected, nor was there any tendency of the amalgam to dissolve in any of the solutes tested. The results of this study corroborated the commonly held belief that the mercury in silver amalgam is chemically reacted and tied up within the body of the amalgam restoration.

A second study that was part of a multifaceted evaluation of industrial mercury measured urinary mercury in patients with multiple amalgam restorations versus patients with no amalgam restorations.[20] No differences in urinary mercury were found, lending credence to the belief that mercury from silver amalgam did not contribute to the overall body burden of mercury.

As part of an in-depth study of mercury in amalgam, Frykholm radioactively labeled mercury and then placed multiple amalgam restorations in a number of patients.[21] He then monitored the amount of radioactivity in the urine over time. The level of radioactivity rose after the restorations were placed, and then dropped back to zero after 8 days. This indicated that there is a small but measurable exposure to mercury vapor when amalgams are placed, but the mercury is then excreted a few days after placement.

Thus, based on these studies, years of use of the material with few reported side effects, and numerous other studies, most authorities were confident of the safety of silver amalgam. However, new studies reported in the 1980s and 1990s have questioned that conclusion.

Research Questioning the Safety of Silver Amalgam

In 1981 researchers at the University of Iowa reported that small amounts of mercury vapor were released from the surface of amalgam restorations when patients chewed gum.[22] This finding has since been confirmed by other researchers.[23] Presumably, sufficient heat is generated during mastication that a miniscule amount of mercury vapor is released intraorally. A portion of this mercury vapor will undoubtedly be absorbed into the bloodstream. This fact has been accepted by the scientific community, but considerable debate has occurred concerning the actual amount of mercury that is released and whether or not it represents a risk for the patient. This will be discussed in some depth in the subsequent section.

Additional research has established that patients with multiple amalgam restorations have slightly higher blood mercury levels than do patients with no amalgam restorations.[24] Autopsy studies have also shown that patients with multiple amalgam restorations have slightly elevated levels of mercury in the kidneys and in certain areas of the brain.[25,26] Again, the debate hinges on the question of whether these relatively minor elevations of mercury have any demonstrable clinical consequence. At this time, the evidence supporting the safety of amalgam is overwhelming, and there is not a shred of scientific data to support the negative viewpoint.

Much of the emotional outcry against silver amalgam has resulted not from scientific data reported in peer reviewed journals, but from anecdotal stories and sensationalized media coverage of such anecdotal information. Such anecdotal data are simply not admissible in scientific circles. In these case histories, patients have experienced a vague series of symptoms, and an approximate diagnosis is made but not necessarily confirmed. Solid baseline data are never recorded, and some treatment, in this case usually removal of some or all of the existing amalgam restorations, is performed. Rarely is this done in a controlled manner; and often the treatment is carried out concomitantly with a number of additional therapies, including a regime of various medications, alteration in diet, etc. The patient may report some short-term amelioration in symptomatology, again in a very subjective manner. This improvement may or may not be real; if real, it could be a result of any one of the therapies that have been utilized or it could be the result of a placebo effect. No attempt seems to have been made to gather long-term data or to present that data in the scientific literature.

Critique of Anti–Amalgam Research

Most of the hysteria regarding mercury and amalgam has resulted from the anecdotal accounts mentioned previously. These reports have virtually no scientific validity. Medicine and dentistry have made tremendous strides in the past century, by insisting that all proscribed therapies be based on data from controlled scientific studies. Adhering to the scientific method has been essential in developing sound techniques of diagnosis and predictable therapeutic modalities. To be guided by anecdotal reports would be tantamount to returning to the days of witchcraft and medicine shows.

It is important to understand that what is of consequence in this discussion is mercury vapor. Liquid mercury and particulate amalgam are of no importance except to the extent that mercury vapor may be emitted from their surface. High levels of mercury vapor can produce definite neurologic symptoms and be toxic to certain target organs such as the kidney. These effects are essentially toxic in nature. True allergy or hypersensitivity to mercury is extremely rare. It is often claimed that certain individuals are "hypersensitive" to mercury; however, this is an inappropriate use of the term. The implication is that these individuals and perhaps their neurologic and/or immune systems are negatively affected by extremely low doses of mercury. There is virtually no scientific evidence to support this claim.

The critical factor in evaluating the scientific literature related to mercury in amalgam is to determine the actual amount of mercury exposure a patient might receive from his or her amalgam restorations. Mercury, like most elements or therapeutic agents, has a classic dose-response curve (Fig. 13.20). With these therapeutic agents at very low doses, no clinical manifestations are observed; at slightly higher doses a therapeutic effect may be seen, with untoward side effects increasing as the dose is increased. At even higher doses, toxic effects become apparent. In the worst-case scenario the mercury exposure to a patient with amalgams in all of their posterior teeth would represent a dose in the first category, and virtually no clinical manifestations would be evident.

This statement may be made with absolute assurance when comparing the exposure of mercury that would occur from silver amalgam to that allowed a worker who has occupational exposure to mercury vapor. As with other potentially toxic materials, a safe level of mercury vapor that can be tolerated without untoward effects has been established by industrial safety boards. That level is known as the *threshold limit value (TLV)*. This level has been adjusted downward over the years as more and more is known

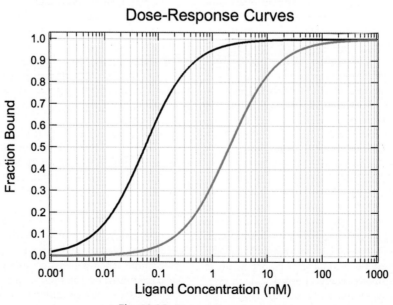

• **Fig. 13.20** Dose-response curves.

about mercury vapor and its effects. That level is currently either 50 μg/m³ (U.S. Occupational Safety and Health Administration [OSHA]) or 25 μg/m³ (World Health Organization [WHO]) and represents the amount of mercury vapor that can be safely allowed in the air for workers who spend 8 hours/day, 40 hours/week in that environment. The worst dose a patient could receive from 10 or 12 amalgam restorations would be about 1/100 of the current TLV.[27]

The actual dose that a patient might receive from amalgams has been the focus of a spirited debate in the literature. Vimy and colleagues calculated that the dose could be as high as 10 μg/day, but their results have been assaulted by other researchers; and it is generally accepted that this number is at least 10 times higher than reality.[28-30] It must be understood that the machines utilized to measure intraoral mercury are not designed to do that, but are used to measure mercury vapor in the air of a well-ventilated room. Thus certain calculations are required to convert the number retrieved from the mercury detector to the actual dose to the patient. Flow rates, respiration rates, and other factors must also be accounted for. When these factors are considered, Mackert concluded that the maximum potential dose to a patient would be in the area of 1.2 μg/day.[29] This number is in close agreement with the adjusted calculations of Berglund, an independent researcher who estimated the dose at 1.7 μg/day.[30]

Thus, the dose of mercury vapor to a patient from 10 or 12 amalgam restorations is extremely low and has virtually no clinical consequences. To put it into perspective, the amount of mercury vapor a patient could absorb per day from his or her amalgams would be 1/10 to 1/20 of that which they receive from a normal healthy diet.[31] Recently, calculations related to dose have estimated that for the most sensitive of patients to demonstrate even minor symptoms of mercury poisoning, patients would have to have 450 to 500 amalgam restorations in place.[32] Of course, this is patently impossible and illustrates that the doses of mercury vapor received by patients from their amalgam restorations are indeed miniscule.

A great deal has been made in the media of studies in sheep and in primates, which purport to demonstrate extremely high concentrations of mercury in the kidneys and other organs as a result of amalgam placement. Reduced organ function in these animals has also been reported. Rather than criticizing these extremely flawed studies, it is more pertinent to review existing human data on mercury concentration in these end organs and the function of these organs. From the autopsy studies mentioned previously, the concentration of mercury in the kidneys of humans with 10 to 12 amalgam restorations has been shown to be 0.38 μg/mg, which is 12 to 20 times less than that reported in the animal studies.[25] More importantly, an evaluation of enzyme function, a critical index of overall organ function, has demonstrated that patients with multiple amalgams have no diminution of normal kidney function.[33] In fact, this study demonstrated that there was no difference between patients with multiple amalgams and patients with no amalgam restorations in terms of kidney function.

Research Supporting the Continued Use of Silver Amalgam

It is clear that there is no scientific data to indicate that silver amalgam poses any significant health risk for patients. It is equally clear that there is an impressive body of research that demonstrates that amalgam is completely safe. The articles by Langan and Fan, as well as the more recent paper by Mackert, review the contemporary literature published subsequent to Bauer's initial review article.[27,34]

Brodsky published a classic epidemiologic article regarding the pregnancy outcome of dental personnel.[35] Using a large patient sample of women either employed in a dental office or married to a dentist, the outcome of pregnancy was compared to that of a nondental group. The underlying assumption of the study was that dental personnel are exposed to much higher concentrations of mercury vapor than are the general population. Thus, if mercury vapor exposure in the concentrations experienced in dental offices was a problem, a difference in pregnancy outcome between the two groups would be expected to emerge. The results of the study indicated that there was absolutely no difference between the two groups in any of the indices evaluated (spontaneous abortion, stillbirth, birth defects, etc.). It must be emphasized that the levels of mercury vapor to which dental personnel are routinely exposed, while usually within the established TLV, are far greater than those that any patient would ever be exposed to as a consequence of his or her amalgam restorations.

Directly related to this finding is the general health of American dentists. The American Dental Association has conducted surveys on the health of its member dentists for a number of years. The data are gathered at the annual meetings of the ADA. These surveys have unequivocally demonstrated that, in spite of their chronic exposure to higher than normal levels of mercury vapor, American dentists are slightly healthier than the general population. If indeed low levels of mercury vapor exposure were etiologic of various autoimmune and other disorders, one would expect an epidemic of such maladies to occur in the dental population. Such is clearly not the case.

Concern has been expressed regarding the potential for mercury in amalgam to suppress the level of circulating lymphocytes in the bloodstream. Most of this concern is based on a report that purported to demonstrate that patients with amalgams had suppressed numbers of T lymphocytes.[36] The scientific validity of this report has been questioned particularly in terms of sample size (three patients) and lack of controls. A recent study with ample numbers of patients has reported absolutely no difference in white blood cell populations (including T lymphocytes) in patients with and without amalgam restorations.[37] As mentioned, additional research has noted that the function of several organ systems is completely normal in patients with multiple amalgams and identical to that of patients with no amalgams.

Mercury is a neurotoxin that has been speculated to play a role in the pathogenesis of Alzheimer disease. An evaluation of 129 Roman Catholic nuns from 75 to 102 years of age indicated that existing amalgams are not associated with lower performance scores on eight different cognitive function tests.[38] Data-related amalgam status and dental history were correlated with mercury levels in the brain at autopsy of 68 patients with Alzheimer disease and a control group of 33 subjects without the disease.[39] There was no significant association with the number, surface area, or history of having amalgam restorations with differences in brain levels of mercury or Alzheimer disease.

It has also been speculated that long-term exposure to low levels of mercury vapor from amalgams can cause or exacerbate neurodegenerative diseases such as amyotrophic lateral sclerosis, multiple sclerosis, and Parkinson disease. An extensive review evaluated existing epidemiologic investigations and concluded that these studies had failed to provide evidence of a role of amalgam in these degenerative diseases and there is no clear evidence supporting the removal of amalgams.[40]

Several countries have suggested that women should not receive dental amalgams during pregnancy because it could possibly result in children with low birth weight. A population-based case control study of over 1000 women with low-birth-weight infants and over 4400 women who had normal-birth-weight infants found no evidence that silver amalgam fillings placed during pregnancy increased low-birth-weight risk.[41] A recent Norwegian study of over 108,000 pregnancies that occurred between 1999 and 2008 evaluated the number of amalgams in the mother's teeth and pregnancy outcome.[42] Investigators found no relation between the number of amalgam restorations and the incidence of preterm birth, low birth weight, malformation, or stillbirth.

A number of independent health agencies have extensively reviewed the issues of safety and efficacy of silver amalgam in recent years and have all concluded that available data do not justify either the discontinuance of use of amalgam or the removal of existing amalgam restorations. These agencies include the Food and Drug Administration (FDA) in 1991 and 2002, WHO along with the FDI World Dental Federation in 1997, the National Institutes of Health (NIH) and the National Institute of Dental Research in 1991, and the U.S. Public Health Service in 1993.[43,44] The National Council Against Health Fraud warns consumers about dentists recommending unnecessary removal of serviceable amalgam restorations and states, "Promoting a dental practice as mercury-free is unethical because it falsely implies that amalgam fillings are dangerous and that mercury-free methods are superior."[45]

The Life Sciences Research Office, a nonprofit scientific organization in Bethesda, Maryland, released results of its independent review of all articles published on this topic between 1996 and 2004. Among 950 published articles, 300 were accepted based on the scientific methodology. The report concluded that "there is little evidence to support a causal relationship between silver fillings and human health problems."[46]

Two very important randomized controlled clinical trials were published in the *Journal of the American Medical Association* in 2006.[47,48] One was called the New England Children's Amalgam Trial and the other, the Casa Pia Children's Trial. Both studies included over 500 children who received multiple restorations of either composite resin or amalgam. One of the trials was 5 years in duration, the other 7 years. They measured subtle neurobehavioral effects to determine if there were any negative effects due to amalgam. Both studies basically found that there were no neurobehavioral effects that could be attributed to amalgam. In fact the very scant data suggested that composite resin may have more effects than amalgam, but the data were of very low scientific validity.[49-51] The studies also showed that composite resin restorations needed to be repaired or replaced 7 times more than amalgam restorations and that composite resin restorations were 2.5 times more likely to have recurrent caries.

Environmental Impact

Concerns have been raised regarding the impact mercury in amalgam has on the environment. Major environmental sources of mercury include volcanoes (50%), coal combustion (33%), and gold production (6%). Amalgam's only contribution in this area is in waste disposal, largely through mercury resulting from crematories, and is less than 1% of the total. Many jurisdictions require dental offices to utilize sophisticated amalgam separators, and a 2016 FDA regulation requires all offices in the United States to install such separators within 3 years.

In January 2013, a number of nations signed the Minamata Convention in Geneva. This meeting was convened to discuss the influence of mercury on health and the environment. Discussions on amalgam were a small part of that meeting, and there were no curbs imposed on the use of silver amalgam. The group declared that the use of amalgam should be reduced in coming years through improved preventive measures and that research should be encouraged to develop materials that will work as good or better than amalgam.

An analysis of the data presented in this section leads to the conclusion that mercury in silver amalgam restorations poses absolutely no problem for dental patients. This conclusion has been reached by experts in the field, by consumer interest groups, and by thorough reviews by governmental agencies.

Impact of Unwarranted Amalgam Removal

A small minority of the profession currently recommends to their patients that their existing serviceable amalgam restorations should be removed as a health precaution. This is not only incorrect, but also unscrupulous, dishonest, and unethical. Removal of an amalgam restoration requires loss of additional tooth structure—sometimes considerable amounts of tooth structure if an indirect restoration that requires a certain amount of "draw" is to replace the amalgam. This additional loss of tooth structure, coupled with the inevitable inherent operative trauma, can result in compromise of the pulpal tissues and eventually in the necessity for endodontic therapy.

The restorative alternatives to silver amalgam all carry with them certain disadvantages. Cast gold, while undoubtedly the finest possible posterior restorative service, is rather expensive (currently 10 times the cost of amalgam) and time consuming.[52] The cost of well-done cast gold restorations is simply prohibitive for many patients. The tooth colored alternatives are also more expensive, with direct composite resin restorations costing about 3 times the cost of an amalgam, while indirect resin or porcelain inlays are closer to 10 times as expensive. None of these tooth colored alternatives has a clinical track record of success equal to that of amalgam, and some of the procedures must be considered to be essentially experimental at this time. Suffice it to record here that some of the problems with them are fracture, excessive wear, microleakage at the cervical margin, and extreme technique sensitivity.

One other tragic situation that has occurred frequently in recent times is the false hope given to patients suffering from incurable diseases such as multiple sclerosis and other autoimmune conditions that by removing their amalgam restorations they would be cured. Amalgam is not the cause of such ailments; nor is amalgam removal the cure. The authors have personally met many individuals inflicted with such dreaded diseases who have undergone great suffering and expense in having their amalgams removed only to have the symptoms continue.

THE BOTTOM LINE

1. Small amounts of mercury vapor are released from the surface of silver amalgam restorations during mastication.
2. The amount of mercury vapor released is very small and poses no risk to the integrity of the restoration or to the systemic health of the patient.
3. There are virtually no published scientific papers validating the belief that mercury in silver amalgam is potentially dangerous to patients.
4. There is an ample and growing body of research that demonstrates the safety of silver amalgam.
5. This research plus the over 100-year history of use of the material supports its continued use.

6. While mercury in silver amalgam poses no health risk to dental patients, even in dental offices where excellent mercury hygiene is practiced, dental personnel are occupationally exposed to higher levels of mercury vapor than the general population. This is due to vapor that is released when amalgams are placed and, even more importantly, when they are removed, or when teeth with amalgam core buildups are prepared for crowns. While the levels of mercury vapor to which dental personnel are routinely exposed are well above those of the general population, they are generally below the current TLV. This occupational exposure to mercury vapor poses no risk as long as proper procedures for mercury hygiene are utilized. All dental personnel should be familiar with the procedures essential for the proper practice of mercury hygiene.

Composite Resins

History

Prior to the introduction of composite resin materials, dentists had two types of tooth colored restorative materials that could be utilized to restore carious defects in anterior teeth: silicate cement and poly(methyl methacrylate) (PMMA).

Silicate cements were supplied as a powder and liquid, with the main constituent of the powder being ground alumino-silicate glass and the liquid phosphoric acid. These materials demonstrated decent initial esthetics but had poor physical properties and color stability and most importantly dissolved readily in oral fluids.

Silicate restorations were expected to serve 3 to 5 years, at which time they would have to be replaced. The main advantage of this material was that as it dissolved, it released substantial amounts of fluoride, with the result that recurrent caries almost never occurred with silicate restorations (see Fig. 13.9).

The second available tooth colored direct material was PMMA (Fig. 13.21). These materials were also supplied as a powder and liquid. The powder was essentially ground prepolymerized methyl methacrylate and initiator, and the liquid was monomeric methyl methacrylate. PMMA materials provided good initial esthetics but also had poor physical properties and lacked color stability; however, their main disadvantage was considerable polymerization shrinkage (three times the shrinkage of modern composites) resulting in large contraction gaps between the restoration and the cavity margins. These gaps permitted significant microleakage that resulted in a very high incidence of recurrent caries.

Thus, while PMMA materials were chronologically developed later than silicate materials, they were actually inferior in terms of clinical performance.

Glass ionomer restorative materials were developed in the 1970s and later evolved into resin-modified glass ionomer materials.[53] These materials are currently indicated for the restoration of root caries lesions.

Composite Resin Materials

These materials were introduced to the profession in 1955 by Dr. Raphael Bowen.[54] It is interesting to note that the discovery of the concept of acid-etching enamel by Dr. Michael Buonocore occurred almost at the same time.[55]

The initial composite resin materials were superior to their predecessors (silicate and PMMA) in terms of physical properties, color stability, solubility, and clinical performance. However, these initial materials were not suitable for use in posterior teeth and

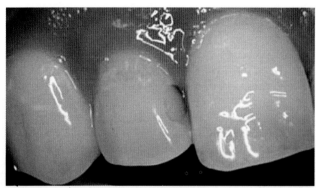

• **Fig. 13.21** Class III cavity restored with poly(methyl methacrylate) (PMMA).

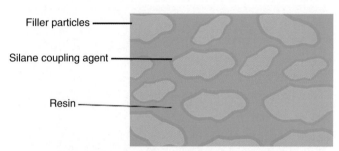

• **Fig. 13.22** Main components of composite resins.

had problems resulting from polymerization shrinkage even though the amount of that shrinkage was substantially less than the shrinkage of PMMA materials. Composite resin materials have evolved constantly over the past 50 years and contemporary composite resin materials are vastly superior to the original material in both clinical performance and esthetic potential.

Composition of Composite Resin Materials

There are three main components of all composite resin materials (Fig. 13.22). These are the resin matrix; filler particles, which vary in composition, size, and shape; and silane coupling agents, which chemically bind the filler particles to the matrix.

The resin matrix of most North American composite resin materials is Bis-GMA. Some composite resins utilize urethane dimethacrylate (UDM) as the matrix and both resins are substantially equivalent in terms of clinical performance. Bis-GMA was synthesized from a type of epoxy by Bowen. It sets by means of a polymerization reaction and its major advantage over methyl methacrylate is that the monomeric molecule is substantially larger than monomeric methyl methacrylate. This results clinically in significantly less polymerization shrinkage.

The filler particles in composite resin are composed of quartz or silica, and vary considerably in terms of size and shape (Fig. 13.23). The incorporation of fillers into the resin matrix increases the strength of the material and further reduces the amount of polymerization shrinkage.

There are two rules regarding filler particles in composite resins. The first is the more filler, the better. Increasing the relative amount of filler in a material increases the strength and reduces the amount of polymerization shrinkage. Most modern composites experience a 2.4% to 2.8% polymerization shrinkage. A contemporary composite resin material for restorations should contain at least 75% filler by weight. Most modern materials meet or exceed this specification.

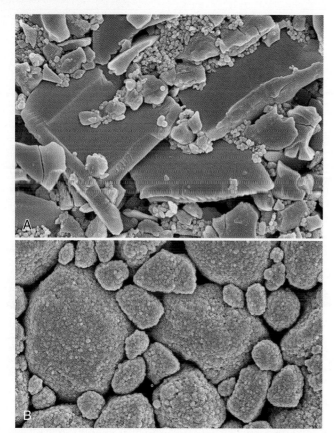

• **Fig. 13.23** A and B, SEM of composite resin displaying different sizes and shapes of filler particles. (Images courtesy Dr. Jorge Perdigao.)

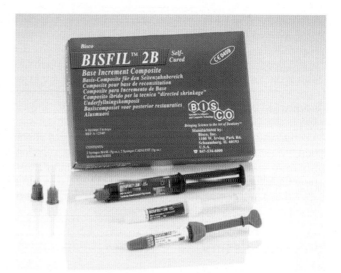

• **Fig. 13.24** Chemical cure composite resin. (Courtesy BISCO.)

According to Polymerization Reaction Initiation

The polymerization reaction for composite resin materials can be initiated chemically or with visible light.

Chemical Cure. Initial composite resin materials were chemically initiated and were called chemical-cure, auto-cure, or self-cure composite resins. These materials had a limited working time and suffered from poor long-term color stability as they contained tertiary amines that turned yellow or orange after several years of service. Chemical cure materials are used today primarily as core materials for the buildup of extensively damaged teeth (Fig. 13.24).

Light Cure. The original light-cure materials were cured using ultraviolet light, but contemporary composite materials all utilize visible light, which will activate the initiator (camphorquinone). Light-cure materials have the substantial advantage of being able to cure on command and thus provide essentially infinite working time so that the restoration can be sculpted and shaped into final form prior to polymerization. They are also color stable due to the elimination of the tertiary amines (Fig. 13.25).

Dual Cure. Dual-cure composite resin materials, which utilize both chemical cure and light cure technologies, are primarily used as cements or core materials. With these materials, the setting reaction is initiated by exposure to visible light but the reaction will slowly continue over time in the absence of light (Fig. 13.26).

According to Filler Particle Size

Early composite resin materials utilized rather large filler particles and are called "macrofilled" composite resins. As esthetic composite bonding became popular, manufacturers developed composite resin materials with very small fillers that are called "microfilled" composite resins. Modern composite resin materials contain a variety of sizes of filler and are called "hybrid" composite resins. The evolutionary trend has been to develop hybrid composite resin materials with smaller and smaller fillers. Thus, contemporary hybrid composite resin materials may be subdivided into subgroups of "microhybrid" and "nanohybrid" composite resin materials. Other categories of contemporary composite resin materials include "flowable" composite resins and "packable" composite resins.

Macrofilled Composite Resin Materials. The original composite resin materials were macrofilled composite resins. These materials had a relatively high level of loading (approximately 75% by weight), with particles that ranged in size between 4 and 40 microns.

The second rule regarding filler particles is the smaller the average filler particle size, the better. Materials with small filler particles are inherently more polishable, retain their polish for longer periods, and have improved wear resistance. One difficulty that manufacturers have faced is that it is difficult to maintain a high filler content with very small filler particles. This is because small filler particles possess a high ratio of surface area to weight, and this resulted in materials that were not usable with high filler content. Modern technology has resulted in a constant evolution of materials, the crux of which has been the ability to create useful materials with a high filler content using smaller and smaller particles.

The filler particles are chemically bound to the resin matrix by silane coupling agents. Silanes are complex, bifunctional molecules that have two different end groups, one of which bonds to the filler particle and the other bonds to the matrix. The use of silane allows for stronger bonding of the filler to the matrix, which improves wear resistance, and also permits the incorporation of more filler into a given amount of resin matrix. The silanization process is complex and involves coating the particles with silane and then utilizing acetone washes to thin the thickness of the silane to a monomolecular layer.

Composite resin materials also contain numerous other components including pigments, viscosity diluents, cross-linking agents, and initiators.

Classification of Composite Resin Materials

Several different classifications for composite resin restorative materials have been proposed over the years—for example, according to polymerization reaction initiation or according to size of filler particles.

Commercial examples of macrofilled composite resins include Adaptic (Johnson & Johnson, New Brunswick, NJ) and Concise (3M Oral Care, St. Paul, MN). Because of the relatively high loading these materials were quite strong, but the rather large size of the filler particles resulted in two significant disadvantages.

First, these materials were not polishable. The filler particles were harder than the abrasives used to polish them. As these materials were polished, the relatively soft matrix was worn away, thus

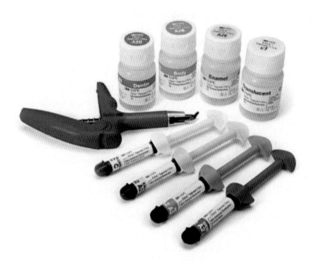

• **Fig. 13.25** Light cure composite resin. (Courtesy 3M.)

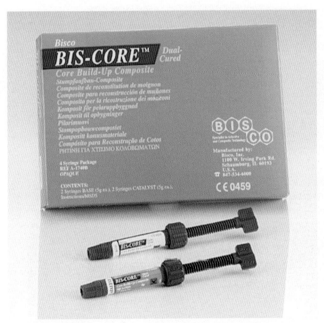

• **Fig. 13.26** Dual cure composite resin. (Courtesy BISCO.)

exposing the large, hard fillers; and the more these materials were polished, the rougher they got. This is obviously a problem for an "esthetic" restorative material (Fig. 13.27).

Second, these large particles could be "plucked" from the surface of a posterior restoration by opposing cusp tips and result instantly in a quantum loss of restorative material (40 microns). Thus the materials had very poor wear resistance, a major deficiency clearly demonstrated in early clinical trials (Fig. 13.28).

Microfilled Composite Resin Materials. The poor polishability of macrofilled composite resins directly led to the introduction of microfilled composite resin materials. These materials had a relatively low level of filler loading (45%–55% by weight), with a uniform filler particle size of 0.04 microns. This resulted in restorations that were very polishable and thus provided an excellent esthetic result. The low level of filler loading resulted in a material with a low modulus of elasticity (MOE), which made it unsuitable for stress bearing restorations. These materials were contraindicated for Class IV restorations and for the restoration of posterior teeth. This low modulus of elasticity made these materials the material of choice for the restoration of NCCLs, which many consider to have a flexural etiology.

The low MOE allows the material to flex along with the tooth. Commercial examples of microfilled composite resin materials include Silux Plus (3M Oral Care, St. Paul, MN), Renamel (Cosmedent, Chicago, IL), Durafil VS (Kulzer, South Bend, IN), and A110 (3M Oral Care, St. Paul, MN). Current evidence indicates that microfilled composite resins may not be needed because the filled bonding agents act as stress breakers.

Hybrid Composite Resin Materials. Hybrid composite resin materials have a combination of small and large filler particles, to combine high filler loading with a sufficient quantity of small particles to ensure improved wear resistance and also permit adequate polishability. These materials have been in use since the early 1980s and have proven to be excellent materials for both anterior and posterior restorations. Most contemporary hybrids have a filler content of 75% to 80% by weight, and the trend has been to produce materials with smaller and smaller average filler particle size. With most contemporary materials the largest filler particle would be in the range between 1 and 2 microns. These materials are quite strong, polishable, and have wear resistance equivalent to amalgam (6–15 microns/year). The esthetic potential of these materials is excellent and many products offer a wide range of shades and translucencies. Typical commercial products in the hybrid category include Herculite XRV (Kerr Corporation, Orange, CA), Z100 (3M Oral Care, St. Paul, MN), and TPH (DENTSPLY Sirona, York, PA).

The most contemporary hybrid composite resin materials have been described as microhybrids and nanohybrids. These materials contain a mixture of small and smaller particles and have excellent handling characteristics and esthetic potential. High filler loading is made possible with advanced technology that permits the formation of clusters of very small particles that reduce surface area yet function as individual nanoparticles to ensure adequate wear resistance.

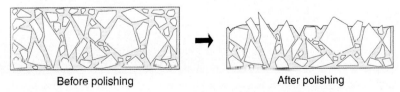

Before polishing → After polishing

• **Fig. 13.27** Schematic illustration of macrofilled composite resin before and after polishing.

Commercial products in this category include Esthet-X (DENTSPLY Sirona, York, PA), Point 4 (Kerr Corporation, Orange, CA), and Filtek Supreme (3M Oral Care, St. Paul, MN) (Fig. 13.29). The major advantage of nanocomposites is that they polish to a very high luster and they maintain that luster over time.

Packable (Condensable) Composite Resin Materials. Several products have been introduced to the market in recent years that have been described as "packable" or "condensable" composite resins. These materials have been designed by manufacturers to possess handling characteristics similar to amalgam.

These materials are basically hybrid composite resins to which large fillers have been added that can be condensed or packed in a manner similar to amalgam.

The addition of these large fillers has resulted in documented poor wear resistance of some of these materials. While some dentists prefer the handling characteristics of these materials, it is doubtful that the benefits of improved handling offset the reduction in clinical performance that has been demonstrated by some of these products.

Flowable Composite Resin Materials. In recent years manufacturers have introduced a group of materials designated as "flowable" composite resin materials. These materials represent a wide range of products, with filler content ranging between 35% and 65% by weight. These materials are very convenient to use because their viscosity allows them to be injected into the cavity preparation with a syringe. However, as would be expected, the reduction in filler content is accompanied by reduced physical properties and increased polymerization shrinkage. The use of these materials should be restricted to "niche" functions such as a 0.5-mm-thick liner under large posterior composite restorations.

Low Shrinkage Composite Resin Materials

Most modern hybrid composite resin materials exhibit linear polymerization shrinkage of between 2.2% and 2.4%. This amount of shrinkage, if not compensated for by clinical technique, can

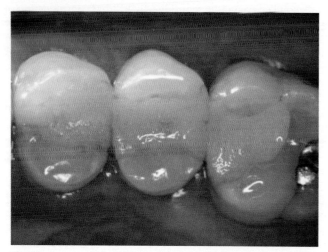

• **Fig. 13.28** Teeth numbers 12, 13, 14 restored with macrofilled composite resin.

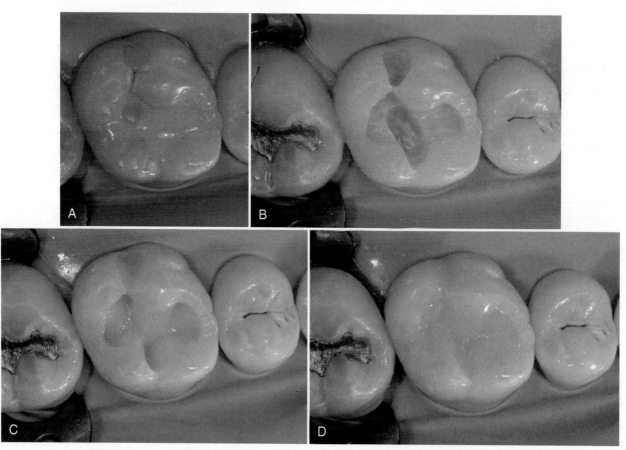

• **Fig. 13.29** A–D, Tooth number 15 restored with a hybrid composite resin. (Photos courtesy Dr. Phillip Timmins.)

result in contraction gap formation, microleakage, postoperative sensitivity, and a potential to develop recurrent caries.

Some manufacturers have introduced products to the market that are described as "low shrinkage" composite resin materials. The linear shrinkage of these materials ranges between 1.4% and 1.7%. The reduction in shrinkage has been accomplished by technology that permits higher filler loading. These materials have not undergone extensive clinical testing at the time of writing. More clinical evidence of their efficacy is essential before they can be recommended for routine use.

Recently, composite resin materials based on silorane technology have been introduced on an experimental basis. These materials use a resin polymer that exhibits very low shrinkage and thus does not depend on increased filler loading.

As with other low shrinkage materials, more clinical evidence is required before these materials can be considered for routine use.

Bulk-Fill Composite Resin Materials

Bulk-fill resin materials were recently introduced to allow clinicians to divert from using an incremental layering technique when placing composite restorations, thus simplifying the procedure and reducing chair time. This technique was developed to minimize negative effects of polymerization-induced shrinkage stress and curing light penetration. The undesired side effects—a time-consuming and complex clinical procedure—contribute significantly to make composite restorations technique sensitive.[56]

Different from traditional composites, which are typically restricted to increments of 2 mm or less, these materials are designed to be used in increments of 4 to 5 mm.[57,58] Common manufacturers' claims involve greater depth of cure and lower polymerization-induced shrinkage stress. Although these composites are usually referred to as if they were clearly identifiable as a class of materials—bulk-fill composites—scientific evidence contradicts the assumptions that they would behave similarly.[59,60] The variety in handling characteristics, as well as physical and mechanical properties, is a direct consequence of the wide range of different compositions used by manufacturers, largely related to their filler content.[61]

The different types of bulk-fill composites currently available can be categorized as *flowable base bulk-fill composites* and *full-body bulk-fill composites*. Flowable base bulk-fill composites require a conventional composite as the occlusal increment and therefore are used for dentin replacement only; full-body bulk-fill composites can replace dentin and enamel in a single increment.[60] Overall, bulk-fill composites are more translucent than other composite resin materials. To a certain extent, this is attained by decreasing the filler content and increasing the filler size. Increased translucency facilitates light penetration, which is closely associated with depth of cure and increased polymerization rates toward the deepest areas of the restoration.[62] Evidence appears to support light-curing times of at least 20 seconds.[60] Despite the large array of materials being marketed, bulk-fill composites appear to deliver an increased depth of cure and reduced polymerization-induced shrinkage stress.[63,64]

Manipulative Variables With Composite Resin Restorative Materials

The contemporary clinician has a wide variety of quality composite resin restorative materials from which to choose. *How* these chosen materials are manipulated in the clinical setting is more important to long-term results than *which* material is chosen. The following narrative will briefly discuss some of the important variables when using composite resin restorative materials.

I. Most contemporary composite resin materials are cured or set by means of exposure to visible light using a curing light. In general, most composite resin materials should not be cured in thick sections, and the recommended thickness of an increment of composite resin is about 2 mm. Curing sections greater than 2 mm may result in insufficient curing of the undersurface of the composite resin material. The depth of cure is determined by a number of variables:
   - The shade of the composite resin
   - The thickness of the material
   - The irradiance of the curing light, and the time of cure

II. Curing lights should be checked periodically with a radiometer (most curing lights have one built in) to ensure that the light emitted is of sufficient output irradiance to efficiently cure the material. The light should be held in close proximity to the material (the closer the light, the greater the irradiance) and the composite resin should be exposed to the light for a sufficient time frame. In this regard, the manufacturers' recommended curing times should be closely followed.

III. The major deficiency of composite resins is their inherent polymerization shrinkage (2.2%–2.4%). This can result in the formation of substantial contraction gaps between the restorative material and the cavity margin, which can result in postoperative sensitivity and recurrent caries. The shrinkage of composite resin materials cannot be avoided, but the stress created by the shrinkage can be reduced by the placement technique. Reducing polymerization shrinkage stress can result in intact restoration margins and the prevention of microleakage.

There are five primary strategies that can be used to reduce polymerization shrinkage stress:

- The first is to create a relatively thick primed layer with the chosen dentin bonding agent. OptiBond FL (Kerr Corporation, Orange, CA) has a relatively high amount of filler content and, when properly used, will result in a thick primed layer. This primed layer has a relatively low modulus of elasticity and can thus deform slightly when the composite resin is curing and shrinking and thus absorb some of the stress and maintain the integrity of the tooth/restoration bond.

- The second strategy is to use a thin liner (0.5 mm) of resin-modified glass ionomer (Vitrebond Plus, 3M Oral Care, St. Paul, MN) under the composite resin restoration. These materials bond predictably to tooth structure and also have a low modulus of elasticity to absorb the shrinkage stress.

- The third option is to place a thin layer (0.5 mm) of flowable composite resin as a liner. This again will theoretically effectively absorb the shrinkage stress.

- A fourth concept that may be used to reduce shrinkage stress is the use of "soft-start" polymerization.[65] This approach utilizes a number of procedures to prolong the gel phase of the setting reaction of the composite resin material. The theory is that the longer the setting composite can maintain a gel or flowable condition, the better it can distribute the stresses resulting from shrinking. Procedures to do this include the use of ramped lights, pulse curing, or simply holding the curing light some distance from the material for the initial exposure. Several clinical and laboratory studies have demonstrated the effectiveness of soft-start polymerization, while other studies have demonstrated limited benefit.

- The final approach to reduce stress is to place the composite resin in increments, always keeping in mind the concept of

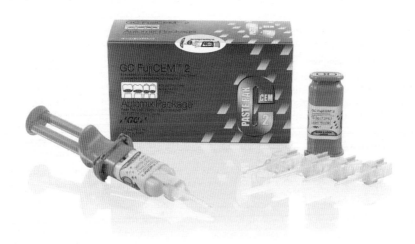

• **Fig. 13.30** Glass ionomer restorative material. (Courtesy GC.)

"C-factor."[66] The C-factor relates to the configuration of the cavity walls, and is the relative ratio between the bonded surface area of the composite resin to the unbonded surface area.

A class IV composite restoration has a wealth of unbonded surface area and a relatively small bonded area and thus has a low C-factor. The unbonded composite resin material will shrink toward the bond, thus reducing the shrinkage stress.

On the other hand, small Class I cavities have a high C-factor because they have a huge bonded area and relatively small unbonded area. When these restorations are cured, there is a high amount of competition for the bond, and the result is that the weakest bond (pulpal floor) gives away under the shrinkage stress creating a fluid-filled gap below the restoration and a high likelihood of postoperative sensitivity. These restorations should be placed in anatomical increments so that the material can shrink freely in one direction and thus eliminate or reduce the shrinkage stress.

Summary and Conclusions About Composite Resin Materials

Contemporary composite resin materials have improved significantly over the years. Today's materials have good wear resistance and a wide variety of shades and translucencies. They are quite polishable and provide excellent esthetics.

However, the major disadvantage of composite resin materials is the inherent polymerization shrinkage. This results in a significant level of technique sensitivity. Composite resin restorations must be placed with excellent isolation (rubber dam), in conjunction with meticulous bonding procedures. The placement technique itself is critical, as is meticulous finishing and polishing. Properly placed, composite resin materials can provide a very esthetic and durable restoration, and the results are gratifying to both patients and clinicians.

THE BOTTOM LINE

1. There is a significant interest by the public in tooth colored restorative materials.
2. Composite resin restorative materials have improved significantly over the years.

3. High filler content (75% weight) of small filler particles (0.04–1 micron) is the key to that improvement.
4. Polymerization shrinkage (2.4%–2.8%) is the main disadvantage of composite resin materials. This can be accounted for with proper technique.
5. Composite resins must be used in conjunction with contemporary bonding systems.
6. Excellent isolation is critical to success with composite resin materials.

Glass Ionomer Restorative Materials

Glass ionomers (GI) were introduced to the profession by Wilson and Kent in the early 1970s, and since then have evolved into a number of unique dental materials.[53] These materials tend to be misunderstood by many in the profession, and as a result many clinicians underutilize glass ionomer materials, whereas other clinicians tend to overutilize glass ionomers and use them in situations where they are clearly not indicated. This section describes available glass ionomer products and also provides specific indications and contraindications for the clinical use of glass ionomer materials (Fig. 13.30).

Glass ionomer materials are used as dental cements/luting agents, cavity liners, pit-and-fissure sealants, restorative materials (primarily Class V), bases, and core buildup materials. Based on clinical trials and physical properties testing, the efficacy of GI for pit-and-fissure sealants and for large core buildups is questionable.

All GI materials have a number of features in common. While some materials have multiple setting mechanisms, the basic GI setting reaction is an acid-base reaction with polyacrylic acid acting on and partially dissolving alumino-silicate glass. This results in a "burst" of fluoride release at a very high level, but this burst of fluoride release is completed in 24 hours. After that, there is a continual low-level release of fluoride that is likely well below the threshold necessary to protect against secondary caries. Most publications on GI materials state that GI is a fluoride releasing material, which implies protection from secondary caries. However, GI materials must be "recharged" with fluoride, which can then be re-released in order to provide protection. This ability for GI materials to act as "reservoirs" for fluoride will be discussed later.

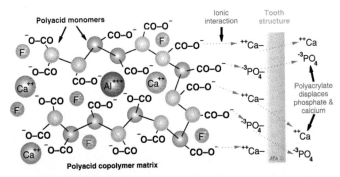

• **Fig. 13.31**   Schematic illustration of ionic interaction between glass ionomer ions and tooth structure. (From Albers HF: *Tooth-colored restoratives: principles and techniques*. 2002, PMPH-USA.)

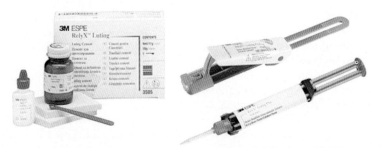

• **Fig. 13.32**   Three different dispensing methods for RMGI cements: powder liquid, clicker, and automix. (Courtesy 3M.)

Glass ionomer materials form very predictable bonds to both enamel and dentin. The bonds are weak chemical (chelation) bonds, but are predictable, effective, and durable (Fig. 13.31). In general, GI materials have inferior physical properties compared to amalgam and resin composite.

Types of Glass Ionomer Materials

Dental Cements/Luting Agents

Conventional Glass Ionomer Cements

Conventional glass ionomer cements are supplied as powder-liquid materials, with the primary component of the powder being ground aluminosilicate glass, and the liquid consisting of polyacrylic acid with small amounts of itaconic and tartaric acid. Examples include Fuji Type I and Ketac-Cem. The setting reaction is a chemical acid-base reaction.

These cements bond to tooth structure and have good physical properties compared to the "gold standard" cement, zinc phosphate. They release fluoride although it is doubtful that this is of any clinical significance.

The main disadvantage of these cements is that they have been associated anecdotally with an increased incidence of postoperative sensitivity. Clinical trials have demonstrated that this sensitivity is likely related to technique (e.g., overdrying the prepared tooth) or contamination of the setting cement by saliva. With proper technique, the level of postcementation sensitivity should be very low.

Conventional GI cements have decreased in popularity in recent years because of the development of resin-modified GI cements.

Resin-Modified Glass Ionomer Cements

Resin-modified glass ionomer (RMGI) cements are the most popular cements available today. Examples include Rely-X Luting and Rely-X Luting Plus cements, Fuji Plus and Fuji-Cem cements. Resin monomers have been incorporated into these materials, and thus these cements have two setting reactions: the classic acid-base reaction and a chemical-cure resin reaction.

Resin-modified GI cements bond to tooth structure and possess the same fluoride release characteristics as conventional GI cements. As a result of the addition of resin, they also possess superior physical properties, have improved handling characteristics, and are less technique sensitive.

Resin-modified GI cements have almost totally replaced zinc phosphate cement and are indicated for cementation of gold inlays, onlays, partial veneer and full veneer crowns and fixed partial dentures, metal-ceramic crowns and fixed partial dentures, and monolithic and layered zirconia crowns and fixed partial dentures. The manipulation of RMGI cements is relatively simple, making them relatively free of technique sensitivity. They are supplied with three different dispensing techniques (Fig. 13.32).

The original cement was supplied as a powder and liquid. It is important with powder/liquid cements to closely follow the manufacturer's directions regarding the ratio of powder to liquid. A later version of RMGI was the development of a "clicker" dispenser. With this product, it was simply a matter of dispensing the correct amount of cement and mixing. This simplified approach was partially responsible for RMGI cements gaining the lion's share of the cement market. The latest innovation has been the development of "automix" dispensers. With these devices the operator simply dispenses the mixed cement into the restoration and proceeds with cementation.

A short note on dispensing devices: It is clear from research conducted at the University of Washington and at the University of North Carolina that the same brand of cement manipulated by different dispensing systems has significantly different physical properties.[67] Whether or not this has clinical significance remains to be determined.

The prepared tooth should be cleaned with pumice or an intraoral air particle abrasion device if available. The use of a desensitizer such as Gluma Desensitizer or G5 is optional, but has been shown to not only *not* interfere with bonding, but actually slightly enhances it with RMGI cements. A small amount of cement should be placed in the restoration and the restoration should be seated with firm finger pressure and then completely seated with the "dynamic seating" technique. The cement should be protected from saliva contamination while setting and should be allowed to set completely before removing the excess cement.

Many manufacturers of RMGI cements and some brands of resin cements are suggesting the operator should "preset" the excess setting cement with 5 seconds exposure to a curing light to plasticize the excess cement. The excess cement can then be removed readily with one or two deft moves with an explorer. This is not recommended as it is likely that cement just under the margin will also be removed along with the excess cement.

Glass Ionomer Restorative Materials

Resin-Modified Glass Ionomers

Glass ionomer materials have been formulated for use as restorative materials, with their primary function being restoration of noncarious cervical lesions and root caries lesions. The original materials were chemically similar to GI cements with higher glass content and increased particle size. Examples of these materials would be Fuji II and Ketac Cem. These materials have essentially been replaced with RMGI restorative materials, which are less technique sensitive, have better physical properties, show improved esthetics, and display vastly improved handling characteristics. Examples of RMGI restorative materials are Fuji II LC, Fuji Filling LC, Vitremer Restorative Material, and Ketac Nano.

The setting reactions of these materials are complex. All undergo the classic GI acid-base reaction as well as a light-activated resin polymerization reaction. Some also have an additional chemical-cure reaction and can set in the absence of light.

Resin-modified glass ionomer restorative materials are indicated for root caries lesions due to their excellent adhesion to tooth structure and fluoride release. They are also recommended for repair of recurrent caries around existing indirect restorations. (Removal of the existing restoration is generally preferred in these situations, but is not always practical.) RMGI restorative materials are the materials of choice for the restoration of NCCLs where esthetics is NOT of primary importance. RMGI materials have an excellent clinical history of retention with NCCLs, due to excellent adhesion and low elastic modulus, but the long-term esthetic result is compromised. Resin-modified glass ionomer restorative materials are contraindicated in stress bearing situations.

When placing RMGI restorations, the following technique is suggested. First, obtain the appropriate shade match. Then obtain the appropriate isolation with a retraction cord/cotton roll or preferably rubber dam. Complete the cavity preparation and then clean the preparation with the dedicated conditioner. Conditioners are formulations of 10% to 20% polyacrylic acid, which clean the smeared layer of dentin without opening the dentinal tubules and removing the smear plug. Follow the manufacturer's directions carefully. Some conditioners are designed to be washed off prior to placing the restorative material, while others are not. Mix the material. Some materials are mixed in a triturator (automixed), some are powder/liquid, and some are dispensed with a clicker. With Ketc-Nano, do not attempt to place the material until 30 to 40 seconds after mixing as it is initially very sticky and difficult to handle. Place and shape the material and light-cure for the recommended time, typically 20 to 40 seconds. Finish and polish. Placement of a surface glaze material is optional.

Reinforced Glass Ionomers

A number of reinforced glass ionomer materials have been introduced over the years in an attempt to expand the indications for GI materials. The following is a partial listing of such materials:

- Miracle Mix (Fuji II plus amalgam alloy particles)
- Ketac Silver (a glass cermet where the silver particles are chemically attached to the glass)
- Ketac Molar and Fuji IX (self-cure GI with increased aluminosilicate glass concentrations, polyacrylic acid, and polycarboxylic acid)
- Fuji IX
- Equia and Equia Forte
- Chem-fil Rock

Manufacturers claim that these materials are indicated as core buildup materials for extensively damaged or endodontically treated teeth. The physical properties of these materials are inferior to silver amalgam and resin composite, and thus they should *not* be used for core buildups. They can be used as bases and blockout materials.

Fuji IX is one of the most popular of these materials. It is indicated as a base under large composite resin restorations, as the intermediary material in an indirect pulp cap procedure, and as a temporary restorative material to replace missing restorations, broken cusps, etc. Fuji IX is mixed in an automix device. A conditioner of 10% polyacrylic acid is placed on the tooth for 20 seconds and washed off prior to placing Fuji IX.

Cavity Liners

There are several GI materials that have been specifically formulated to serve as liners. Among the most popular are Vitrebond and Vitrebond Plus. Both of these materials are light cured, and the difference between them is that Vitrebond is a powder/liquid material and Vitrebond Plus is dispensed with a "clicker." Liners are materials that are used at a thickness of no more than 0.5 mm under either amalgam or composite restorative materials. Their function is to seal deep dentin exposed during caries removal with the goal of having about 2 mm of thickness of cavity liner and remaining dentin between the restorative material and the pulp.

Glass ionomer liners are recommended when excavation of caries results in a remaining thickness of dentin that is likely less than 2 mm. They are optional any time the depth of a cavity preparation exceeds the depth of a "minimal" preparation.

Manipulation of glass ionomer cavity liners is straightforward. Complete the cavity preparation and clean and dry the cavity. Do *not* desiccate. Mix the lining material and place into the preparation in a thin layer (no more than 0.5 mm) using a Dycal applicator or similar instrument. Light-cure for 20 seconds. Now regular bonding procedures are completed when placing composite resin restorations, or Gluma Desensitizer or G5 is applied if placing an amalgam restoration.

A Note on Fluoride Release and Secondary Caries Prevention. Dentists understand that fluoride is an effective caries reducing agent and manufacturers understand that dentists will buy any material that contains fluoride. Dentists would likely purchase fluoride releasing tires if someone would manufacture them. However, it is critical to understand that the effectiveness of fluoride as a caries preventive agent is dose related. Fluoride releasing amalgam or composite resin has no chance of reducing caries because the dose of released fluoride is so low.

Glass ionomer–based materials are unique in that the set material consists of an aqueous polygel that permits ion exchange in the oral cavity. This allows glass ionomer–based restorative materials to absorb topically applied fluoride from toothpastes, gels, etc., and slowly re-release that fluoride over 24 hours.

An almost universal misconception is that all GI materials release fluoride and that this released fluoride is effective in preventing secondary caries. As noted in the introduction, all GI materials do release fluoride. There are two phases to this fluoride release. The first occurs primarily in the first 24 hours after mixing and is described as a "burst" of fluoride release resulting from dissolution of the glass particles in the material by polyacrylic acid. After this 24-hour period, there is a sustained fluoride release over time, but this level of fluoride release is likely far below the therapeutic level essential to prevent secondary caries.

To reach a potentially therapeutic level, it is essential that GI materials are regularly (3×/day) exposed to sources of fluoride (e.g., toothpastes, gels, mouth rinses) that will allow the GI material to uptake fluoride and slowly re-release it into the surrounding environment.[68] Research has demonstrated that this does occur on a predictable long-term basis.

Repeated exposure is essential if the GI material is to act as a reservoir for fluoride. It is unlikely that a GI-based luting cement, in a 25-μm film thickness under a properly fabricated indirect restoration, would be able to absorb and re-release fluoride at a therapeutic level. A GI base or liner under a sealed restoration would not be exposed to fluoride to be absorbed and re-released. Similarly, under a leaking restoration, these materials would not be exposed to sufficient fluoride to be effective against recurrent caries. The reason these materials are preferred as bases and cavity liners is because of their predictable bond and seal of the underlying dentin, not because of their ability to prevent secondary caries.

Thus, the only GI materials that have legitimate potential for prevention of secondary caries are GI restorative materials such as Fuji II LC, Ketac Nano, and Fuji IX. It is important to understand that these materials will only be effective if they receive regular exposures to fluoride (multiple exposures/day).

Polyacid Modified Composites (Compomers)

Polyacid modified composites or compomers were released in the 1990s. They are modestly filled composite resin materials to which has been added some prereacted glass ionomer material. The important distinction between a glass ionomer product and a compomer is that there is *no acid-base glass ionomer reaction* with compomers. Examples of compomer products are Dyract, Compoglass, and F2000. Compomers are intended to be used in non–stress-bearing situations; and they have adequate esthetics, ease of handling, adhesion to tooth structure, but poor physical properties. They do release fluoride, but at a very low level, less than 10% of the release of glass ionomers. Thus it is unlikely that compomers have any meaningful effect on the incidence of secondary caries. There are likely no indications for use of compomers in contemporary dentistry.

THE BOTTOM LINE

1. Glass ionomer materials are useful for several clinical applications in restorative dentistry.
2. Glass ionomer materials provide predictable long-term bonds to enamel and dentin.
3. Resin-modified glass ionomer cement is the most popular cement in restorative dentistry and is indicated for cementation of metal castings and zirconia and porcelain-fused-to-metal based restorations.
4. Resin-modified glass ionomer liners have an excellent track record as lining materials used in films no thicker than 0.5 mm.
5. Resin-modified glass ionomer lining cements should be used to provide a liner/dentin thickness of 2 mm from the pulp.
6. Resin-modified glass ionomer restorative materials provide satisfactory service for the restoration of root caries and noncarious cervical lesions.
7. Reinforced glass ionomer materials should not be used for core buildups.
8. Glass ionomer materials do not provide protection from secondary caries with their inherent fluoride release.
9. Glass ionomer and RMGI materials may provide protection from secondary caries as a result of their ability to act as fluoride reservoirs. In order to accomplish this, they must be regularly exposed to topical fluoride from toothpastes, gels, mouthwashes, etc.

Adhesive Dentistry

Bonding to Enamel

Of the many important scientific advances in restorative dentistry in the past century, perhaps none is as important as the discovery by Buonocore in 1955 of acid etching enamel.[51] Buonocore was investigating the use of phosphoric acid to clean fissures in molar teeth and recognized the retention potential of the etched enamel surface when he examined it microscopically (Fig. 13.33).

The first practical application of his discovery was pit-and-fissure sealants, although routine use of sealants was not to become popular for many years. The concomitant introduction of the first composite resin material by Raphael Bowen in 1957 made possible current concepts of adhesive dentistry.[50] It is worth noting that the concept of bonding composite resin materials to tooth structure did not become popular until the mid-1970s. It is also worth noting that at the present time (2017) the resin bond to acid-etched enamel is the most important bond in adhesive dentistry.

The original acid etchant was the liquid from zinc-phosphate cement, which was basically phosphoric acid. This has been replaced by brightly colored gels (Fig. 13.34A), which aid in ensuring the phosphoric acid is completely washed off the tooth. Phosphoric acid concentrations vary from 30% to 40% with the most common one being 37%. While extended application times may be okay

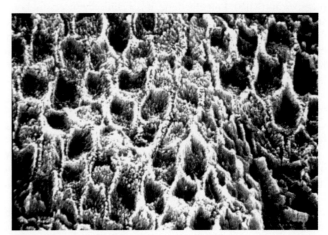

• **Fig. 13.33** SEM image of enamel surface etched with phosphoric acid.

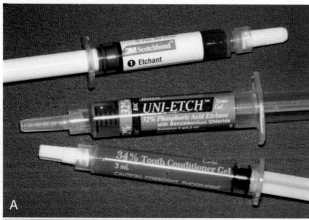

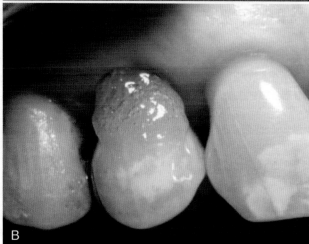

• **Fig. 13.34** A, Phosphoric acid gel. B, Etching of the enamel surface with phosphoric acid gel.

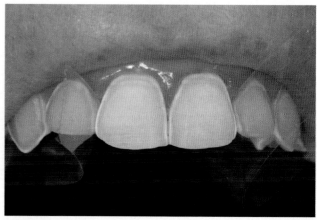

• **Fig. 13.35** Enamel surface appearance after applying the acid etchant. Notice the chalkiness of the enamel surface.

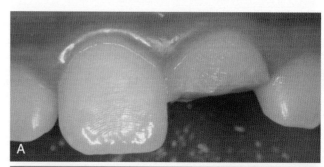

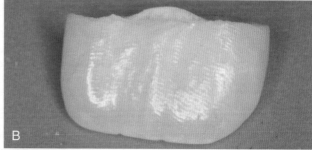

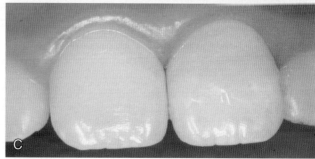

• **Fig. 13.36** A, Fractured tooth #9. B and C, Fragment piece was saved and bonded back in place.

on enamel, there is no benefit in applying the gel for more than 15 seconds (Fig. 13.34B). The operator should always verify that an etch pattern has been achieved before proceeding with bonding (Fig. 13.35).

The acid-etched enamel/resin bond has been studied extensively and is a very predictable long-term bond. This bond is a purely *mechanical bond*, with shear bond strength usually exceeding 20 megapascals (MPa). Properly done, it is a clinically successful bond and should result in sealed margins with composite resin restorations. This is important to reduce microleakage and prevent secondary caries, which is a common cause of failure with composite resin restorations. It's worth repeating that the acid-etched enamel/resin bond is the most important bond in restorative dentistry.

The acid-etched enamel/resin bond is useful for providing retention for Class IV restorations, and for sealing the margins of Class I, II, III, and V restorations. It is also useful for bonding fragments of teeth fractured due to trauma (Fig. 13.36).

The process of etching enamel with phosphoric acid is an example of a "differential acid attack," a process that has been used in industry for many years. A specific acid will preferentially attack one phase of a multiphasic substrate and leave behind a microscopically rough, retentive surface. Phosphoric acid is used to etch enamel, nitric acid is used to etch base metal, and hydrofluoric acid is used to etch feldspathic porcelain. The surfaces created on each of these substrates are similar in appearance and provide

mechanical bonds to resin that are equal to or greater than the bonds to etched enamel.

These concepts have resulted in the use of a number of very conservative resin-retained modalities for restoring teeth. One of these procedures is the Maryland bridge (Fig. 13.37), which is a conservative method of replacing missing teeth. Clinical trials have demonstrated that these resin-retained restorations have clinical longevity comparable to conventional fixed partial dentures. A

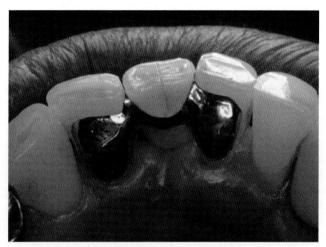

• **Fig. 13.37** Maryland bridge.

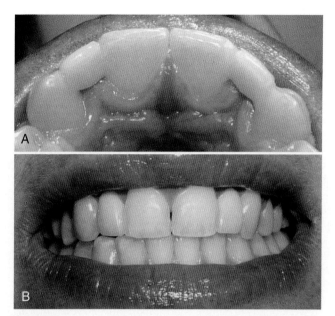

• **Fig. 13.38** A and B, Missing teeth 7 and 10 restored with a Carolina bridge.

similar concept is the use of bonded metal rests to provide support for removable partial dentures.

Perhaps the most popular of these modalities has been bonded porcelain laminate veneers. Simonsen and Calamia are credited with the first study on etching porcelain with hydrofluoric acid and Harold Horn wrote the first article describing porcelain veneers.[69,70] With conservative intraenamel preparations, these restorations can provide many years of successful service and have a survival rate of 95% at 15 years.[71]

The survival rate of all-ceramic crowns is improved if they are etched and bonded in place. Posterior bonded ceramic restorations in the form of inlays, onlays, and crowns are popular today and must be bonded in place. Etched porcelain pontics can be bonded to etched enamel of the abutment teeth to fabricate a "Carolina" bridge. These are primarily meant to be long-term provisionals for patients with congenitally missing lateral incisors during their teenage years prior to placing an implant (Fig. 13.38).

In summary, the acid-etched enamel/resin bond is a strong, reliable, mechanical bond that has proven to be useful with many different clinical procedures. It is the most important bond in adhesive restorative dentistry.

THE BOTTOM LINE
1. The acid-etched enamel/resin bond is the most important bond in adhesive restorative dentistry.
2. Enamel etchants are 30% to 40% phosphoric acid.
3. Normal etch time is 15 seconds.
4. If the etched surface is not achieved after 15 seconds, etch again until it is obvious.
5. Isolation is imperative. Any contamination of the etched surface prior to bonding will negatively affect the bond.
6. The etched-enamel/resin bond is a durable mechanical bond. It can provide adequate retention for restorations such as porcelain laminate veneers and can also result in sealed margins with direct composite resin restorations.

Bonding to Dentin

Bonding to acid-etched enamel is a rather straightforward procedure that has been used effectively for many years. Bonding to dentin, however, has proven to be a much more difficult process. Research into dentin bonding began in the late 1970s and it continues to be an active area of both clinical and laboratory research. Dentin bonding has grown through many generations, and the process has been one of evolution and simplification. The following narration will describe the evolution of dentin bonding agents in some detail and will identify preferred adhesives at the time of writing (2017).

The first three generations of dentin bonding agents (DBAs) were generally ineffective, and the fourth generation DBAs introduced in the 1990s were one of the most effective bonding agents ever available until recently. However, the number of steps in the fourth generation DBAs makes their use technique sensitive, and many dentists reported poor results when using them. Most of the later generations of DBAs were designed by the manufacturers to be simpler to use, but that simplification has generally resulted in diminished clinical performance.

There are three main groups of DBAs: initial bonding agents that were generally ineffective, etch-and-rinse bonding agents that include the fourth and fifth generations, and self-etching primers. Basically the contemporary dentist must decide on whether to use an etch-and-rinse product or a self-etch product. Recent products have been marketed that can be used either as a self-etch, selective etch, or etch-and-rinse materials.

There are a number of factors that have made bonding to dentin more difficult than bonding to enamel.

I. The compositions of enamel and dentin are different (Table 13.5). The major differences are that dentin is much less mineralized and has much more water content than enamel.

II. Dentin is a heterogeneous substrate. One of the major factors in this regard is the dentinal tubules. Superficial dentin, close to the dentinoenamel junction (DEJ), has a relatively small number of tubules and the orifices of the tubules are small. Thus there is a large amount of intertubular dentin to bond to and successful dentin bonding is relatively predictable and easy. With deep dentin, there are more tubules and the orifices of the tubules are wider, so there is little intertubular dentin to bond to (Fig. 13.39). Bonding to deep dentin is difficult and unpredictable.

III. Dentin is a dynamic substrate. It changes after bonding occurs. It also contains enzymes called matrix-metalloproteinases (MMPs), which can be activated by the bonding procedure.

These activated MMPs gradually break down the collagen matrix and hybrid layer. The result of this is that dentin bonds tend to decrease significantly with time.

Initial Bonding Agents

For practical purposes, the first three generations of DBAs can be clumped together and called "initial" bonding agents. These materials were ineffective because at the time they were formulated dental scientists believed resin-based materials were deleterious to the pulp. Thus these materials were designed to bond to minerals in the smeared layer of dentin, which scientists believed would protect the pulp from the resinous bonding agents.

The smeared layer of dentin is 3 to 5 microns thick and consists of ground dentin, fragments from the rotary instruments, denatured protein, and both live and dead bacteria (Fig. 13.40). It does have a significant protective function, but most importantly for dentin bonding, it is not firmly attached to the underlying dentin. Thus when shrinking polymers such as DBAs are bonded to it, the smeared layer becomes detached from the underlying dentin.

These initial DBAs formed excellent bonds to etched enamel, and weak bonds to dentin. Most importantly, however, they had significant microleakage that lead to both postoperative sensitivity and recurrent caries.

Etch-and-Rinse Bonding Agents (Previously Called "Total-Etch")

The ineffectiveness of the initial DBAs led to the development of total-etch systems in the late 1980s. Credit must be given to Fusayama and Nakabyashi from Japan for developing this concept and to Bertolotti for recognizing the value of their work and introducing it to North America. John Kanca also deserves credit

for creating the first effective total-etch product developed in North America. Kanca has suggested that total-etch DBAs be called "etch-and-rinse" DBAs to clearly differentiate them from the self-etch products developed later on.

These DBAs constitute the fourth and fifth generations of DBAs. The fourth-generation DBAs were multiple bottle systems that required three distinct procedures for bonding. These steps are as follows: (1) The tooth (enamel and dentin) is etched and then rinsed. (2) A primer is placed. (3) A bonding agent is placed and cured. The primer bonded to enamel and dentin, and sealed the dentin. The bonding agent bonded to the primer and to the restorative material. Inherent to this process was the necessity of bonding to "moist" dentin, and the difficulty of precisely defining exactly what "moist" meant led to many dentists having difficulty using these products successfully. Commercial products of fourth generation DBAs include All-Bond 2 (Bisco, Inc.), Scotchbond Multi-Purpose (3M Oral Care, St. Paul, MN), OptiBond FL (Kerr Corporation, Orange, CA), and Tenure Multi-Purpose (Den-Mat).

The technique sensitivity of the fourth-generation DBAs led directly to the development of the fifth-generation DBAs, which were basically single bottle systems and were easier to use. With these systems only two steps are required: (1) The tooth is etched and rinsed, and (2) priming and bonding are carried out as a single

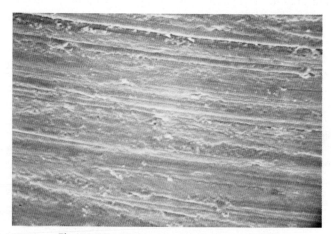

• **Fig. 13.40** SEM image of smear layer of dentin.

TABLE 13.5	Composition of Enamel and Dentin	
	Enamel	**Dentin**
Mineral	80%	45%
Organic	2%	30%
Water	12%	25%

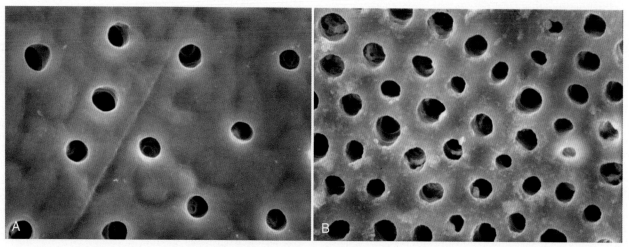

• **Fig. 13.39** A, Superficial intertubular dentin. B, Deep intertubular dentin. (Photos courtesy Dr. Ed Swift.)

step, because both the primer and the bonding agent are in the same bottle. While this procedure is a significant simplification, it still requires bonding to "moist" dentin, which remains a dilemma for many dentists. Commercial examples of fifth-generation DBAs include One-Step Plus (Bisco, Inc.), Adper Single Bond Plus (3M Oral Care, St. Paul, MN), OptiBond SOLO Plus (Kerr Corporation, Orange, CA), and Tenure Quick (Den-Mat).

Many of the initial fourth-generation products were not particularly successful because the manufacturers were still not convinced it was safe to use phosphoric acid on dentin. Thus they used two different etching agents, one for enamel and one for dentin. For example, an early version of Scotchbond Multi Purpose used only one acid to etch both enamel and dentin; however, it was a weak (10% maleic) acid. Maleic acid works well on dentin, but again does not adequately etch enamel. As stated several times in the section on acid-etching enamel, the most important bond in adhesive restorative dentistry is the resin bond to acid-etched enamel.

Today's fourth-generation DBAs all use 30% to 40% phosphoric acid to etch both enamel and dentin, as research has shown conclusively that it is both safe and effective. The components of the primers include a hydrophilic monomer such as HEMA, PENTA, BPDM, and now MDP in a volatile carrier such as acetone or ethyl alcohol and water. One of the keys to successfully using fourth-generation DBAs is to completely volatilize this carrier. This can be done by air thinning or by use of high volume vacuum. The components of bonding agents are Bis-GMA and a hydrophilic monomer such as HEMA.

The fifth-generation DBAs are similar in composition, but components of both the primer and bonding agent are in the same bottle.

Almost all contemporary fourth-generation and fifth-generation DBAs contain quartz filler particles to improve strength, reduce shrinkage, and provide a thicker primed layer. Research has shown that DBAs with a thicker primed layer are generally more efficacious than those with a thin primed layer.

Etch-and-rinse DBAs basically remove the smeared layer of dentin, and etch both enamel and dentin. Etching dentin is often called "conditioning." Etching dentin involves removing a small amount of mineral from the superficial layer of dentin. This exposes bundles of collagen, which the primer can infiltrate and form the "hybrid" layer, composed of infiltrated collagen, mineralized dentin, and the primer. The bond is primarily to etched intertubular dentin. Bonding to the peritubular dentin around the dentinal tubules is difficult and ineffective. Resin tags look spectacular in SEMs but provide no real benefit in dentin bonding (Fig. 13.41).

Superficial dentin has an abundance of intertubular dentin and allows predictable successful bonding. With deep dentin there is relatively little intertubular dentin available due to the presence of multiple large orifice tubules. Predictable bonding is difficult with deep dentin, and a resin-modified glass ionomer may be placed over deep dentin prior to etching and bonding.

Comparing the fourth and fifth generations of etch-and-rinse DBAs, it is clear the fourth generation has the best clinical performance. The fourth-generation DBAs have three separate steps: (1) The enamel and dentin are etched and rinsed, (2) the primer is applied, and (3) the bonding agent is applied and cured. With the fifth-generation DBAs, the enamel and dentin are etched and rinsed, and the priming and bonding steps are done simultaneously. Clinical research has shown clearly that the fourth-generation (three-step) DBAs provide superior clinical performance when compared to the fifth-generation (two-step) DBAs.

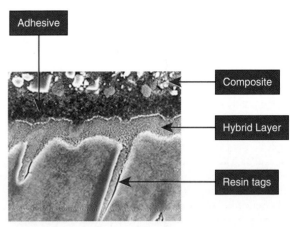

• **Fig. 13.41** SEM image of the hybrid layer and resin tags.

The sequencing of the bonding procedures and their rational will be given in "The Bottom Line" at the end of this chapter.

Self-Etching Primers

Self-etching primers are basically acidic monomers that etch through the smeared layer of dentin. The primers are simply applied and light cured. They are not rinsed off. Since the smeared layer is usually not completely removed, the dentinal tubules remain sealed and postoperative sensitivity is almost completely eliminated.

There are two types of self-etching primers. One type has two bottles. The first bottle is the self-etching primer that is placed on the prepared tooth and dried. The second bottle is the bonding agent that is placed over the primer and cured prior to placing the restorative material. Commercial products in this category are Clearfil SE Bond (Kuraray America, Inc., New York, NY), Simplicity (Apex Dental Materials, Inc., Lake Zurich, IL), Opti-Bond XTR (Kerr Corporation, Orange, CA), and All-Bond SE (Bisco, Inc.).

The second type of self-etching primer is the single bottle systems that have the primer and bonding agent in the same bottle. Current research has shown that the single bottle materials are not reliable and should be avoided at this time. Commercial products in this category include Xeno IV (DENTSPLY Sirona, York, PA) and Adper Prompt-L-Pop (3M Oral Care, St. Paul, MN).

Self-etching primers create very predictable bonds to dentin and eliminate postoperative sensitivity, but they have one major problem: They form weak bonds with uncut enamel. If the proposition that the acid-etch/resin bond to enamel is the most important bond in adhesive restorative dentistry is accepted, this is a significant deficiency. Clinical trials using self-etching primers frequently report marginal staining after 3 or 4 years indicating microleakage at the enamel/restoration margin. Clinicians using self-etching primers should consider using the selective etch procedure to obtain a better bond to enamel. That technique will be described in the "Bottom Line" section of this chapter.

In summary, the etch-and-rinse DBAs have two groups. One group has three distinct steps including etching, priming, and bonding. The other group has two steps, etching then priming and bonding simultaneously. The self-etch materials also have two groups. The best self-etch materials have two steps, etching and priming simultaneously and then bonding. The other group etches, primes, and bonds all at once.

New Developments

While today's DBAs are clearly superior to early generations of DBAs, research has demonstrated that the bonds to dentin deteriorate over time. This is partially due to hydrolysis of the DBAs and also to breakdown of the collagen matrix in the hybrid layer due to the action of MMPs activated during the bonding procedure. Part of the problem seems to be that many DBAs are too hydrophilic and act as semipermeable membranes allowing water-tree formation and osmotic blistering. Newer products are considerably less hydrophilic than their predecessors.

The use of 2% chlorhexidine (Consepsis, Ultradent Products; Cavity Cleanser, Bisco, Inc.) after etching seems to be somewhat effective in inhibiting the ability of MMPs to break down the hybrid layer, although this has not yet become a common practice. Kerr Corporation has introduced a product called OptiBond XTR, which is the first self-etch material to demonstrate enamel bonding equivalent to that of the fourth-generation DBAs. The long-term clinical efficacy of such bonds has yet to be determined, but laboratory testing has been promising.

A major development in dentin bonding has been the expiration of the patent held by Kuraray on the monomer MDP. This is the chief ingredient in Clearfil SE Bond, which has been shown in long-term clinical trials to be as effective as the fourth-generation etch-and-rinse materials. This is a mild two-step self-etching primer, which has proven to be a very effective DBA and also does not activate MMPs. Many of the major manufacturers have now incorporated MDP into their DBAs, and it is anticipated that they will be effective. For example, 3M Oral Care has introduced a new product called Scotchbond Universal that purportedly can be used in the self-etch, selective-etch, or etch-and-rinse modes. This adhesive utilizes the monomer MDP. Laboratory tests indicate that superior bond to enamel is achieved using the etch-and-rinse procedure. For the different bonding protocols, please refer to Chapter 5.

THE BOTTOM LINE

1. Dentin bonding agents have evolved rapidly over the past few decades.
2. Contemporary DBAs are considerably more effective than early generations.
3. Modern DBAs contain fillers, which result in a thicker primer layer and seemingly improved efficacy.
4. Contemporary DBAs are either etch-and-rinse materials or self-etching primers.
5. Etch-and-rinse DBAs are either three-step (fourth-generation) or two-step (fifth-generation) materials. Both groups are effective, but clinical trials have clearly demonstrated the superiority of the three-step systems.
6. Both etch-and-rinse materials involve bonding to "moist" dentin. An effective technique for bonding to "moist" dentin will be described later in this section.
7. Self-etching primers are supplied as either two-step or one-step products. The one-step products are not recommended at this time.
8. Most self-etching primers do not completely remove the smeared layer of dentin, and postoperative sensitivity is rarely reported with these products.
9. Enamel bonds are compromised with most self-etching primers. This deficiency may be overcome using the "selective etch" technique that will be described later on in this section.
10. Bonding to superficial dentin is more predictable than bonding to deep dentin. With deep cavities a thin resin-modified glass ionomer liner should be used.
11. Successful dentin bonding requires the formation of a hybrid layer resulting from resin penetration into a collagen matrix that is partially demineralized by etching with either phosphoric acid or acidic monomers.
12. Dentin bonds tend to deteriorate over time.

Bases and Cavity Liners in the Adhesive Era

Bases and cavity liners have been used for many years in restorative dentistry. With the development of more effective adhesives, the use of materials as bases and liners has diminished. The topic of bases and cavity liners is quite controversial today and there is a general lack of consensus among authorities, practitioners, and educational institutions as to indications for such materials.[72] The following is a brief description of materials used as bases, liners, varnishes, and sealing agents available today.

Base Materials

To begin, a base is any substance placed under a restoration that blocks out undercuts in the preparation, acts as a thermal or chemical barrier to the pulp, and/or controls the thickness of the overlying restoration (Fig. 13.42).

Any dental cement mixed to a very thick consistency can be used as a base. Zinc-phosphate, polycarboxylate, zinc oxide-eugenol (IRM), and glass ionomer cements have all been historically used as bases for direct and indirect restorations.

The primary contemporary function of a base is to block out undercuts for indirect restorations, to seal the dentin against leakage in deep cavities, and to act as replacement dentin with large composite resin restorations to reduce the volume of composite resin. The contemporary material most often utilized for these functions is Fuji IX (GC America, Alsip, IL), which is a reinforced, self-cure glass ionomer.

Liner Materials

A cavity liner is a fluid paste applied in a thin layer as a protective barrier between dentin and the restorative material. Liners should *not* be used in layers thicker than 0.5 mm.

A number of materials have been used historically, including calcium hydroxide, zinc oxide-eugenol, glass ionomer, and resin-modified glass ionomer. Calcium hydroxide (e.g., Dycal, DENTSPLY

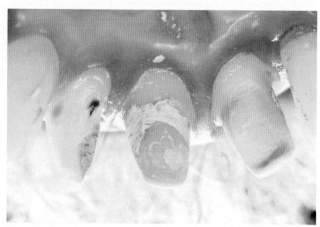

• **Fig. 13.42** Base material used to block out undercuts in the preparation of teeth 9 and 10.

Sirona, York, PA) and resin-modified glass ionomer (e.g., Vitrebond, 3M Oral Care, St. Paul, MN; Fuji Lining Cement, GC America, Alsip, IL) lining materials are the most commonly used. Resin-modified glass ionomers are used most frequently, as few clinical situations today call for the use of calcium hydroxide.

Resin-modified glass ionomer liners (Vitrebond and Vitrebond Plus) are supplied as powder/liquid or paste/paste systems, respectively. They are light activated and have improved handling characteristics and physical properties compared to regular glass ionomer lining materials. They bond very predictably to dentin, provide an excellent seal, and are very compatible with the pulp. Typically they are used as a thin liner (0.5 mm) over dentin in deep cavity preparations (Fig. 13.43).

Calcium-hydroxide materials have a very high pH (9–14), are antibacterial, and promote sclerosis, hence reducing permeability. They must not be used as a base because they have very poor physical properties and should only be placed as a very thin (0.5 mm) liner over the deepest portion of the cavity preparation. Calcium hydroxide materials have traditionally been used when performing a direct pulp cap, as the high pH irritates the pulp tissues and stimulates the production of secondary dentin. Calcium hydroxide has largely been replaced by bioactive cements such as mineral trioxide aggregate (MTA) and biosilicate cement (Biodentine, Lancaster, PA) for this function. Direct pulp capping should only be considered with teeth with no record of spontaneous pain and no radiographic evidence of periapical pathology.

Cavity varnish is a solution of a natural gum or synthetic resin in an organic solvent. Copal varnish (Copalite, Temrex, Freeport, NY) has been traditionally used under amalgam restorations to reduce initial levels of marginal leakage. Cavity varnishes are no longer popular and have been replaced by cavity sealers.

A cavity sealer is a liquid primerlike material that seals the dentin surface prior to placing definitive restorative materials. Current products used as cavity sealers under silver amalgam restorations are Gluma Desensitizer (Kulzer, South Bend, IN) and G5 desensitizer (Clinician's Choice, New Milford, CT). These sealers contain both HEMA and glutaraldehyde and are very effective sealing agents for dentin.

Clinical Recommendations

When using bases and liners, it should be remembered that the ultimate goal is to have a minimum of 2 mm of tooth structure or a combination of tooth structure base and liner between the restorative material and the pulp.[73]

Amalgam

It is no longer considered necessary to use bases to build up deep cavity preparations to "ideal" form. With deep preparations close to the pulp, a very small liner of calcium hydroxide may be placed, followed by a thin liner of resin-modified glass ionomer (Vitrebond Plus). As an alternative, the calcium hydroxide liner may be omitted. Deep preparations that are not close to the pulp should receive a thin RMGI liner. Gluma Desensitizer or G5 should be applied to all preparations, including those in which liners have been placed.

Composite Resin

For any preparation deeper than a minimal preparation, a thin resin-modified glass ionomer liner should be placed in the deepest portion of the preparation. In this situation (deep dentin), dentin adhesives tend to be less effective because there is less intertubular dentin to interact with and form an effective hybrid layer. With posterior composite resin preparations where the proximal box ends close to or beyond the CEJ, a resin-modified glass ionomer liner should be placed to reduce postoperative sensitivity. Adhesive bonding systems *must* be used with all composite resin restorations regardless of whether a lining material has been placed.

Cast-Metal Indirect Restorations

Deep restorations should receive a RMGI liner prior to impression making. With very deep lesions, vitality testing must be done before administration of local anesthetic to determine the need for endodontic therapy. Resin-modified glass ionomer, Fuji IX, or other base materials can be used to block out undercuts. Gluma Desensitizer or G5 should be applied immediately after tooth preparation prior to making the provisional restoration.

THE BOTTOM LINE

1. There is still a need for bases and liners in the adhesive era.
2. Bases are primarily used to block out undercuts.
3. Liners should be used in a thin film, no greater than 0.5 mm thick.
4. Resin-modified glass ionomers are used with deep caries prior to bonding because bonding to deep dentin with available dentin

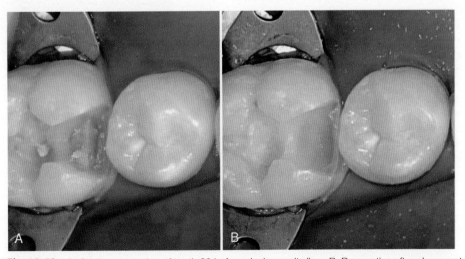

• **Fig. 13.43**   A, Cavity preparation of tooth 30 before placing cavity liner. B, Preparation after placement of cavity liner.

bonding agents is not predictable due to the lack of intertubular dentin.

5. Cavity sealers should be used routinely under amalgam restorations.

Indirect Restorative Materials

Impression Materials

When fabricating indirect tooth-supported or implant-supported restorations, accuracy of the impression is critical. It is clear that impression materials have improved steadily over the past 50 years, and the contemporary clinician has a great number of excellent impression materials to choose from. While it is clear that contemporary impression materials are vastly superior to their predecessors in the 1960s and 1970s, the quality of impressions sent to commercial dental laboratories has failed to show a concomitant improvement (Fig. 13.44).[74]

The major deficiency seen with these impressions is failure to record the entire prepared cervical margin in the impression. A second deficiency is failure to follow the fundamental principles in the manipulation of impression materials. Use of flexible plastic stock trays ignores the need to control bulk and risk the possibility of hydraulic distortion, especially with use of heavy body and/or putty materials.[75] Putty-wash materials are also used extensively, often in an inappropriate manner resulting in impressions with less than optimal accuracy.

The primary cause of these problems is a lack of appreciation of the principles of manipulation of impression materials and poor decisions related to margin placement and gingival displacement techniques. Many dentists are excited about the ability to make optical impressions, and the technology related to optical impressions is impressive; however, it is clear that dentists who cannot predictably make a traditional impression will not be able to predictably make an optical impression.

Classification of Impression Materials

There are two main types of impression materials: nonelastic impression materials, which are used primarily in removable prosthodontics, and elastic impression materials (Fig. 13.45). There are two types of elastic impression materials: water-based and elastomeric (rubberlike) impression materials. The two types of water-based impression materials are reversible and irreversible hydrocolloid (alginate). There are four types of elastomeric impression materials: polysulfide rubber (also known as rubber base, thiokol rubber, and mercaptan rubber); polyether; condensation silicone; and addition reaction silicone (also known as polyvinyl siloxane (PVS) impression material).

This section will outline the ideal properties of impression materials. Critical manipulative variables will be highlighted in the subsequent section. Properties to be discussed include accuracy, elastic recovery, dimensional stability, flow, flexibility, workability, hydrophilicity, shelf life, patient comfort, and economics.

Accuracy

There are three main factors related to accuracy of impression materials: fine detail reproduction, dimensional accuracy, and elastic recovery, which will be discussed separately. According to ADA #19, elastomeric impression materials used to fabricate precision castings must be able to reproduce fine detail 25 microns or less. All currently available impression materials meet this specification.

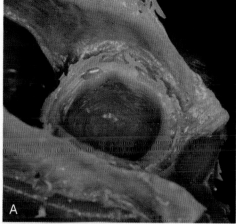
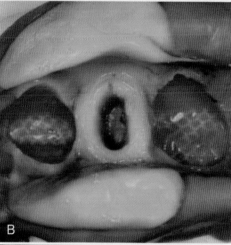
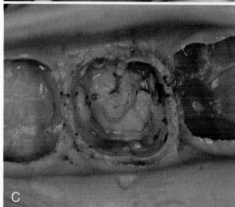

• **Fig. 13.44** A–C, Examples of poor intraoral impressions.

Classification of Impression Materials

1. Nonelastic Impression Materials
2. Elastic Impression Materials

A. Water-Based Impression Materials
1. Irreversible Hydrocolloid
2. Reversible Hydrocolloid

B. Elastomeric Impression Materials
1. Polysulfide Rubber
2. Polyether
3. Condensation Silicone
4. Addition Reaction Silicone (PVS)

• **Fig. 13.45** Classification of impression materials.

Polyvinyl siloxane is the best in this regard and reversible hydrocolloid is the worst. It is not likely that improved ability to record fine detail results in improved accuracy of the final restoration, because the limiting factor in this area is the ability of the gypsum die materials to record fine detail. The corresponding specification for gypsum die materials related to fine detail is 50 microns. Some die materials can provide better fine detail reproduction than the 50-micron specification but fall short of the impression materials in this regard.

There are differences in the ability of different viscosities of elastomeric impression materials to record fine detail. Typically the lower the viscosity, the better the ability to record fine detail. Putty viscosities in general are very poor in this regard and are only required to record fine detail of 75 microns.[76] Some putty-wash techniques result in putty recording some or the entire gingival margin, which has a deleterious effect on the accuracy of the gypsum die.

A second aspect is dimensional accuracy, which is evaluated by measuring tooth-to-tooth distances in the same quadrant and also cross-arch distances. There is some evidence that reversible hydrocolloid is slightly superior to the elastomers in this respect, but it is likely of limited clinical significance.[77]

All of the available contemporary impression materials provide superb accuracy if they are manipulated correctly. Although PVS materials are likely to be slightly more accurate than other impression materials, differences in accuracy are not likely to be clinically significant.

Elastic Recovery
Elastic recovery is the ability to flow into an undercut, set in that position, and then spring around the undercut on removal of the impression and rebound to its original shape. No impression material has 100% elastic recovery; and for all impression materials, the greater the depth of the undercut, the greater the permanent distortion of the impression material is.[78,79] Polyvinyl siloxane impression materials have the best elastic recovery at over 99% with a specific test undercut. This elastic recovery coupled with excellent dimensional stability make it the material of choice for clinicians who prefer to double pour impressions to obtain a backup die.

At one time, dentists were cautioned to wait 30 minutes prior to pouring impressions to allow maximum elastic recovery to occur. With contemporary impression materials, this delay is no longer necessary as elastic recovery occurs almost instantly. Keeping in mind the greater the depth of the undercut, the greater the distortion, an important procedure is to always block out undercuts in tooth preparations prior to impression making. This often occurs when preparing teeth with existing restorations. Many dentists fail to do this, assuming the laboratory can block out the undercuts on the die. While this is possible, blocking out the undercuts with resin-modified glass ionomer materials will reduce the overall distortion due to improved elastic recovery.

Dimensional Stability
One of the most important properties when selecting an impression material is dimensional stability. An ideal impression material would be dimensionally stable over time, allowing the impression to be poured at the convenience of the operator. This is extremely important in contemporary dentistry, as most dentists have opted to not pour up their own impressions and instead send them to dental laboratories to be poured. The time between removal of an impression from the mouth and the time when it is poured by the laboratory varies considerably, and if the impressions are mailed to the lab, it will be well over 24 hours.

Dimensional stability of an impression material is determined by the composition of the material, its susceptibility to imbibition and syneresis, and the volatility of the by-product of the setting reaction.[80] Impressions made from water-based impression materials, such as reversible and irreversible hydrocolloid (alginate), are approximately 80% water, which evaporates at room temperature. This evaporation can result in clinically significant distortion of the impression. Because of this evaporation (syneresis), water-based impression materials should be poured within 10 minutes after removal from the mouth. Water-based impression materials are also subject to imbibition or the absorption of water. The common practice of wrapping alginate impressions with wet paper towels should be avoided, as the impression material will absorb water from the towel (imbibition), which results in distortion of the impression. These impressions are properly stored in sealed plastic bags prior to pouring.

The by-product of the setting reaction of condensation silicone impression materials is ethyl-alcohol, which evaporates rapidly at room temperature. Impressions made with condensation silicone should be poured within 30 minutes of removal from the mouth.

The by-product of the setting reaction of polysulfide rubber (rubber base) impression materials is water (Fig. 13.46). This evaporates more slowly than it does from water-based impression materials, but is still significant. Thus impressions made with polysulfide rubber should be poured within 30 minutes.

Polyether impression materials have no volatile by-product of the setting reaction but are sufficiently hydrophilic to absorb water from the atmosphere. This absorption is dependent on relative humidity (RH); and if the RH is over 50%, absorption of water is sufficient to cause clinically significant distortion.[81] Polyether impressions should be poured within 1 hour and should never be mailed to a dental laboratory.

There is no by-product of the setting reaction for PVS impression materials, so PVS impressions possess almost unlimited dimensional stability. If impressions are to be mailed to the dental laboratory, the only reasonable material to use is PVS. Indeed, the case can

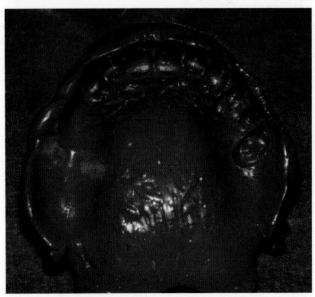

• **Fig. 13.46** Rubber base impression material.

be made that if the impression is going to be poured by a local laboratory, it is safer to use PVS because there is no way to be certain it will be poured at the appropriate time. This exceptional dimensional stability, coupled with the excellent elastic recovery of PVS impression materials, make it the best choice for clinicians who prefer to double pour impressions to obtain a backup die. Table 13.6 displays discussed impression materials and recommended pouring times.

Flow and Flexibility

Impression materials need to flow readily into the minute details of cavity preparations and accurately capture grooves, pinholes, and cervical margin detail. Most brands of impression material provide light body or syringe materials with low viscosity to accomplish this. These are used with heavy body materials in a tray to provide more rigidity to the impression and assist in forcing the low viscosity material into the gingival sulcus and accurately and completely capture the prepared cervical margin.

Many early versions of low viscosity PVS impression materials had excellent flow characteristics but tended to flow away from the prepared tooth after injection of the impression material. This created problems when attempting to make an impression of several prepared teeth at one time. The composition of most contemporary PVS and polyether materials has been modified to render them more thixotropic, and stay in place when they are syringed around the prepared teeth, but then flow readily when the heavy body tray materials are placed over top of them.

Set impression materials vary considerably from one another with regard to flexibility. Polyether impression materials tend to be more rigid than other materials. This can present a problem with long, thin preparations of mandibular incisors or periodontally involved teeth. Fracture of the delicate gypsum dies is a common occurrence due to the rigidity of polyether materials. Another problem related to this rigidity is tearing of the impression material in the gingival sulcus. While the tear strength of polyether impression materials is excellent, the amount of force required to remove the rigid impression may exceed the tear strength of the material. More recent formulations of polyether materials are less rigid than early versions but are still more rigid than PVS materials.

Set PVS materials are relatively rigid but seem to fall below the threshold where problems with fracture of dies are common. Although rarely used today, reversible hydrocolloid impression material is the least rigid of all impression materials and may be the material of choice when making impressions of multiple prepared periodontally involved teeth.

With dual-arch impressions, it is advantageous to use a relatively rigid material. Many of the commonly used trays for dual-arch impressions are somewhat flexible, and a rigid impression material can compensate for this flexibility. Polyether impression materials work well in this regard. Many PVS products have heavy body versions that also provide the essential rigidity.

Workability

Impression materials were originally supplied as two tubes for each viscosity. One tube was labeled as the base, the other the catalyst (Fig. 13.47). The base and the catalyst were different colors, and equal lengths of each were dispensed on a mixing pad. The materials were mixed until the material became a uniform color with no streaks. When making a clinical impression, one pad with heavy body material was used and one with light body material. The materials were mixed simultaneously, the light body material loaded into an impression syringe and the heavy body material loaded into a tray. This process required excellent coordination between the dentist and assistant(s); thus impression making was a stressful procedure.

Contemporary materials are supplied with "automix" handheld devices. This is a substantial improvement and results in a standardized mix with fewer inherent porosities, increased working time, and economic savings due to less waste of material. Even better are sophisticated electronic mixing devices such as the Pentamix (3M Oral Care, St. Paul, MN).

Working times of impression materials vary by the manufacturer, and most automix devices provide materials with standard-set and quick-set capabilities. When making a single crown impression with a quadrant or dual-arch tray, the operator may opt for a quick-set material with a shorter working time. When making a full-arch impression with multiple prepared teeth, it might be prudent to choose a material with a longer working time. When making an impression with several prepared teeth, another option to extend working time is to refrigerate the low viscosity material, which increases working time without sacrificing accuracy.[82]

Hydrophilicity

Reversible hydrocolloid impression materials are truly hydrophilic and can effectively make accurate impressions in the presence of moisture. *All elastomeric impression materials require a completely dry field to make a successful impression.*

Polyether impression materials are hydrophilic as witnessed by their tendency to absorb water from the atmosphere. However, polyether impression materials absolutely require a dry preparation surface to make an accurate impression.

TABLE 13.6	Multiple Impression Materials and Recommended Pouring Time	
Impression Material	**Pour Time**
Water based	10 minutes
Polysulfide rubber	30 minutes
Condensation silicone	30 minutes
Polyether rubber	60 minutes
Polyvinyl siloxane	At operator convenience

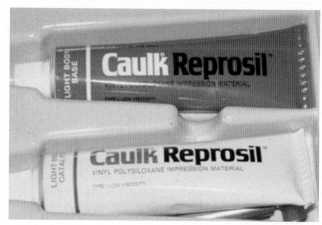

• **Fig. 13.47** Two-tube impression material: base and catalyst.

The manufacturers of many contemporary PVS impression materials claim their products are "hydrophilic," and incorrectly imply that their materials can effectively make impression in the presence of blood and/or saliva. The hydrophilicity of a material is measured by the contact angle a sessile drop makes with the material. If the contact angle is below a specific value, the material can be called hydrophilic. Many contemporary PVS impression materials meet that criterion, and therefore the manufacturers are technically correct. However, the implication that these materials can make impressions in a wet environment is totally incorrect.[83,84] These materials require a dry environment to make successful impression.

The advantage these "hydrophilic" PVS materials have is they are significantly easier to pour. Early versions of PVS were hydrophobic and very difficult to pour. They also released hydrogen for approximately 3 hours after setting, so delaying pouring for that period was recommended. Contemporary PVS materials have nonionic surfactants grafted onto the polymer chains, which makes them hydrophilic and thus easier to pour. They also contain small quantities of spongy palladium, which absorbs hydrogen and allows pouring of the impression immediately upon removal from the mouth.

Shelf Life

The exact shelf life of impression materials is not known, but it is inadvisable to use impression materials that have passed the expiration date established by the manufacturer. Dentists must become familiar with manufacturers' codes for the materials they are using and ensure that current materials are consistently utilized. It is arbitrarily suggested that no more than a 6-month supply of impression material should be kept on hand at any time.

Patient Comfort

Contemporary impression materials are far more patient friendly than the old polysulfide materials, which were messy, had a bad taste and odor, and permanently stained clothing. Reversible hydrocolloid materials were uncomfortable for patients because they required the use of bulky, water-cooled trays. Contemporary impression materials are essentially odorless and tasteless.

The rigidity of polyether impression materials can be a disadvantage, especially if the patient has existing fixed prostheses or multiple open gingival embrasures due to periodontal disease. In these situations, it is advisable to use a more flexible material, and to block out the undercuts with utility wax prior to impression making. The use of the dual-arch impression technique, where indicated, is also pleasant for patients in that it requires a minimum amount of material and avoids the necessity for opposing arch impressions.

When full-arch impressions are indicated, the use of a custom tray is advocated. Many studies indicate that custom trays are more accurate than stock trays and the level of patient comfort is substantially improved. In addition, significantly less material is used, which offsets the costs of fabricating the custom trays.

The ultimate in patient comfort with impression making is the use of optical impressions. Digital impressions are becoming more and more popular and are very patient friendly. Imaging systems are becoming more economical and it is anticipated that the majority of impressions made in the next decade will be made optically. It is important to point out that while optical impressions for single tooth preparation are as accurate as conventional impressions, the same factors that result in failed contemporary impressions will result in failed optical impressions.

Economic Factors

There can be significant differences between the costs of different impression materials. Reversible hydrocolloid impression material is considerably less expensive than elastomeric impression materials. However, there is a significant cost involved with using reversible hydrocolloid, considering conditioning and tempering baths need to be purchased along with an appropriate selection of water-cooled stock trays. Polyether and PVS materials are comparable in costs at about $12 per impression. Competing elastomeric materials are less expensive and are popular in underdeveloped countries.

It is likely true, however, that the cost of impression materials is of minimal consequence in most contemporary practices. Practitioners can reduce costs by using automix devices, by using the dual-arch technique where indicated, by using custom trays when full-arch impressions are indicated, and by reducing the need for remakes by making successful impressions on the first attempt.

THE BOTTOM LINE
1. Many excellent impression materials are available to the contemporary clinician.
2. The quality of impressions sent to commercial dental laboratories needs improvement.
3. All contemporary impression materials are sufficiently accurate if manipulated properly.
4. The only impression material that should be mailed to commercial laboratories is PVS.
5. Polyvinyl siloxane materials have the best fine detail reproduction, elastic recovery, and dimensional stability of all impression materials.

Principles of Impression Material Manipulation

Proper manipulation of impression materials is probably more important in determining the accuracy of an impression than which type of material is selected. This section will discuss the important manipulative variables that must be considered when making impressions for indirect restorations.

Control of Bulk

Impression materials shrink when setting. Irreversible hydrocolloid and elastomers shrink due to polymerization reactions, and reversible hydrocolloid undergoes thermoplastic shrinkage as it cools from the warm to cool state. The effect of this shrinkage can be controlled by paying close attention to the bulk of impression material used. Water-based impression materials are most accurate when used with a uniform cross-sectional thickness of 4 to 6 mm. This means that successful impressions can be made using stock trays that will provide approximately 4- to 6-mm thickness of material.

Elastomeric impression materials are most accurate when used with a cross-sectional thickness of 1 to 2 mm.[7] Use of a stock tray with elastomers results in excess thicknesses of impression material, which possibly could result in an inaccurate impression. Elastomeric full-arch impressions are best made using a custom tray that will provide the desired cross-sectional thickness of impression material (Fig. 13.48).

Numerous studies have evaluated the accuracy of elastomeric impressions made in stock trays versus impressions made in custom trays. Almost all conclude that impressions made in custom trays are more accurate, yet very few North American dentists routinely use custom trays.[85]

The difference in cross-sectional thickness of impression material in a stock tray versus a custom tray is only about 2 mm, but that difference does reduce the accuracy of the impression.[86] This mandates that custom trays be fabricated with precision. Custom trays should be fabricated on the diagnostic cast using one layer of base plate wax as a spacer. Trays can be fabricated with PMMA, photo-cure bisacryl (Triad, DENTSPLY Sirona, York, PA), or PVS. PMMA trays should be fabricated at least 24 hours in advance to ensure stability.

Occlusal stops are critical for proper orientation of the tray in the patient's mouth. Three occlusal stops are ideal, with at least one stop posterior to the prepared teeth. Stops should be placed on nonfunctioning cusp tips to minimize distortion in the area of the stops. The stops are prepared by removing the base plate wax from the nonfunctioning cusp tips with a hand instrument (Fig. 13.49). The wax spacer should be covered with tin foil before making the tray to facilitate removal of the wax from the tray and to prevent incorporation of a wax residue on the internal surface of the tray. This can happen due to the inherent exotherm reaction that occurs during the setting of the PMMA tray material. This residue can interfere with the proper functioning of tray adhesives.

Adhesion of the Impression Material to the Tray

It is imperative that the impression material adheres to the tray. With proper adherence, the impression material shrinks *toward* the tray as it polymerizes, creating a slightly larger die. Adhesion is achieved using specific chemical tray adhesives. Adhesives must be specifically matched with the impression material. They should be painted in a thin layer on the internal portion of the tray and the tray borders (Fig. 13.50). The tray should be painted 7 to 15 minutes prior to impression making to permit formation of an adequate bond strength of the impression material to the tray.[87]

Pouring of Impression Materials

One of the most important manipulative variables with impression materials is the time limit after removal from the mouth to when the impression is poured with the appropriate gypsum product.[88] The factors that determine when an impression should be poured are discussed in depth in the previous section (see Table 13.6).

Viscosity Control

Impression materials are supplied in a number of viscosities ranging from very low viscosity to very high viscosity putty materials. The main difference between these materials with different viscosities is in the amount of inert filler material in the impression material. With low viscosity materials, there is relatively little inert filler and thus more chemical reagent. Low viscosity materials are excellent at recording fine detail, but also undergo more polymerization shrinkage during the setting reaction. Thus the optimum method of impression making is to use only as much low viscosity material as is necessary to capture the fine detail of the prepared margin, grooves, and boxforms of the preparation; and the bulk of the impression should be made with high viscosity material. This high viscosity material has correspondingly more inert filler and less reagent and displays less polymerization shrinkage on setting. The heavy body material also assists in pushing the low viscosity, light body material into the gingival sulcus.

Monophase PVS and polyether materials are supplied by many manufacturers. In theory, such materials do not provide the same level of accuracy as provided by the proper use of a combination of low viscosity/high viscosity materials, but the actual differences in accuracy are likely not clinically significant. The convenience of having to use only one viscosity of material makes monophasic materials very practical.

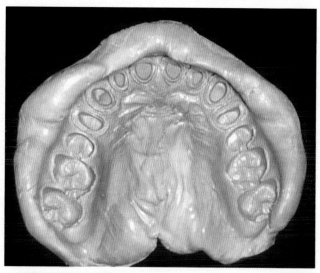

• **Fig. 13.48** Full-arch impression taken with a custom tray.

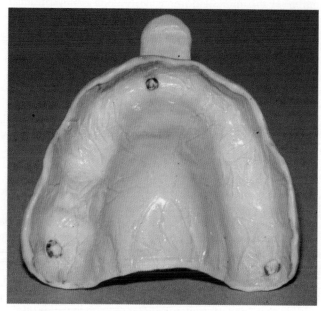

• **Fig. 13.49** Custom tray showing three occlusal stops.

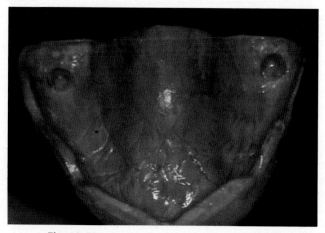

• **Fig. 13.50** Custom tray coated with tray adhesive.

Adequate Mixing

As discussed in the previous section, almost all impression materials today come with an automix system. This provides optimum mixing with fewer inherent voids, extends the essential working time of the materials, and reduces waste because the materials are loaded from the dispenser directly into the syringe or tray.

Disinfection

Microorganisms in the oral cavity can be transmitted from impressions to the dental laboratory. Dentists must disinfect impressions prior to pouring the cast or sending the impression to the laboratory.

The first step of any disinfection technique is to rinse the impression thoroughly in cold tap water. This step removes a significant portion of the microorganisms from the impression. Disinfection techniques involve spraying the impression with disinfection agents or immersion of the impression materials in chemical agents such as sodium hypochlorite. Polyvinyl siloxane materials are stable in this regard, but special care must be taken with water-based materials and polyethers to ensure that adequate immersion times are used to eliminate microorganisms but that extended immersion times are avoided to prevent excess imbibition of the disinfecting solution and distortion of the impression.

Polyvinyl Siloxane Impression Materials and Latex

Polyvinyl siloxane impression materials have been available since the mid-1970s and have continued to evolve and improve.[89] Polyvinyl siloxane impression materials are easily the best selling impression materials on the North American market, and they have the best fine detail reproduction and the best elastic recovery of all available impression materials. Polyvinyl siloxane materials have remarkable dimensional stability and are odorless and tasteless and pleasant for patients. They are provided in a wide variety of viscosities, rigidities, and working and setting times so they can be used in a variety of clinical situations.

Polyvinyl siloxane impression materials have one major disadvantage: They have a significant interaction with latex (rubber dam and latex gloves). Any contact of unpolymerized PVS material with latex results in inhibition of polymerization of the impression material. This can occur if the dentist or assistant mixes putty materials while wearing latex gloves or even if latex gloves were worn prior to mixing. Direct inhibition of polymerization also can occur if the impression material is in contact with a rubber dam.

Indirect inhibition of polymerization also can occur intraorally when latex gloves contact tooth preparations and the surrounding periodontal tissues during tooth preparation or gingival displacement procedures.[90-93] Such inhibition of polymerization is often subtle and limited to small isolated areas of the surface of the impression. It is often not detected with the initial inspection of the impression and may be noticed only after pouring and separation of the gypsum cast. The presenting signs of inhibited polymerization are a film of unset material in isolated areas or the presence of a sticky, slippery substance on the surface of the impression (Fig. 13.51). It is similar to the feel and appearance of the oxygen-inhibited layer that is seen with photo-cure composite resin restorative materials.

Although these isolated areas of inhibited polymerization are subtle and not easy to detect (Fig. 13.52), depending upon their location they can render an impression unusable. Clinicians must inspect impressions and recovered casts carefully to ensure contamination of critical areas has not occurred.

The mechanism of inhibition of polymerization is thought to be a result of contamination of the chloroplatinic acid catalyst of the PVS material with unreacted sulfur, which is present in natural latex gloves. Synthetic latex gloves, vinyl gloves, and the powder commonly found on gloves do not cause this inhibition of polymerization. Sulfur-containing gingival displacement chemicals do *not* cause inhibition of polymerization.[94]

Clinicians should avoid touching tooth preparations and adjacent gingival areas with latex gloves. When this is not avoidable, wearing vinyl gloves over the latex gloves is recommended. Once contamination of the preparations has occurred, cleaning with water and other agents is not effective in removing the contamination. Routine cleansing of tooth preparations with flour of pumice may be indicated prior to impression making.

Contemporary PVS impression materials may not be as sensitive to latex as the products that were used in the 1990s. It does appear that direct contact of contemporary PVS with latex or nitrile gloves will result in inhibited polymerization; however, these materials are not susceptible to indirect contamination.[95] It appears this reduced sensitivity is a result of changes to the impression materials rather than changes in gloves and rubber dam materials. Contemporary PVS materials have increased concentrations of platinum in the chloroplatinic acid catalyst, which makes it less sensitive to sulfur. Also nonionic surfactants have been grafted onto the polymer chains and these surfactants may act as a separating medium and prevent the sulfur from contacting the catalyst.

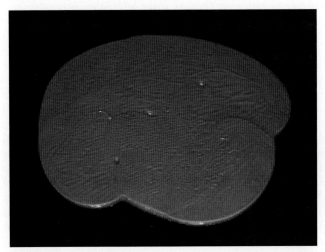

• **Fig. 13.51** Unpolymerized polyvinyl siloxane material due to handling of the material with latex gloves.

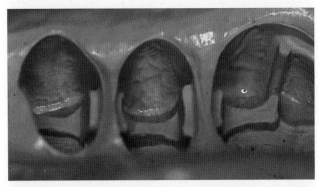

• **Fig. 13.52** Impression displaying areas of inhibited polymerization of the prepared teeth.

Putty-Wash Impression Techniques

While the recommended technique for full-arch impressions is use of heavy body/light body viscosities of impression material in a custom tray, many dentists prefer to make "putty-wash" impressions.[80] There are three approaches to putty-wash impressions. One approach is appropriate and acceptable, another can provide acceptable impressions but has some potential drawbacks, and a third approach is unacceptable.

An excellent technique for putty-wash impressions is to use the putty material to fabricate a custom tray. It is fabricated in the same manner as with PMMA materials or light cure materials. One layer of base plate wax is placed over the diagnostic cast as a spacer, and wax is removed from nonfunctioning cusp tips to provide occlusal stops. A putty impression is made in a stock tray, producing a PVS putty custom tray (Fig. 13.53).

A second approach is to use a relieved putty impression. In this technique, a preoperative putty impression is made intraorally prior to tooth preparation. Plastic sheets may be placed over the teeth to prevent putty material from entering gingival embrasures. In the area where the teeth are to be prepared, putty impression material is removed with a bur or scalpel to provide relief, and the impression is "washed" or relined with low viscosity PVS material.

This approach can be successful, but there are two potential problems. It is difficult to confine the wash materials to the area of the relieved impression, and some wash material enters the unrelieved impression. This results in an inaccurate occlusal pattern for the resultant cast. Thus the entire impression rather than just the relieved area should be "washed." This creates the problem of hydraulic distortion of the putty material as the impression is seated in the mouth. This is impossible to detect on a clinical level but may have a deleterious effect on the accuracy of the impression and resulting restoration.

The third approach to putty-wash impressions is the "simultaneous" technique. With this technique a stock tray is loaded with putty material, and the syringe material is injected around the prepared tooth or teeth. The tray containing the putty material is squashed over the syringe material, and the impression is made with the putty and syringe material setting simultaneously. This approach is unacceptable because it is impossible to control the thickness of the impression material, and excess bulk is used. It is impossible to control what material records the margin detail of the preparation(s). Usually portions of the prepared margin are captured in the putty, and putty materials are essentially deficient in their ability to record marginal detail (Fig. 13.54).

THE BOTTOM LINE

1. Water-based impression materials are most accurate with a uniform cross-sectional thickness of 4 to 6 mm. This allows impressions made with these materials to be made in a stock tray.
2. Elastomeric impression materials are most accurate when made with a uniform thickness of 1 to 2 mm. This implies the routine use of custom trays.
3. The rational for custom trays is to make impressions with a uniform cross-sectional thickness of 1 to 2 mm.
4. Custom trays can be made with PMMA, putty, and photo-cure bisacryl.
5. Occlusal stops should be placed on nonfunctioning cusp tips.
6. Low viscosity materials should be used only around the prepared teeth.
7. Specific impression adhesives should be used and applied to custom trays 7 to 15 minutes prior to making the impression.
8. Impressions should be poured at appropriate times for each type of material.
9. Impressions should be disinfected prior to pouring or sending to the laboratory.
10. Some putty-wash techniques are superior to others.

Gypsum Products

Gypsum products are widely used in a variety of applications in restorative dentistry. In many situations, obtaining maximum accuracy and strength with the selected gypsum product is critical to the long-term success of the restoration or prosthesis to be fabricated. To predictably attain such success, the clinician must first *select* the optimum product for the use intended and then must *manipulate* the gypsum product properly.[96,97]

Fortunately there are a relatively small number of gypsum products available, and the critical manipulative variables are rather simple. However, many dentists consistently select inappropriate materials for the task at hand. Additionally, even though proper

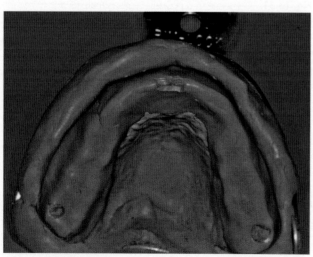

• **Fig. 13.53** Polyvinyl siloxane putty custom tray.

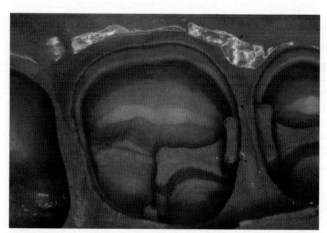

• **Fig. 13.54** Impression taken utilizing the "simultaneous technique." Notice portions of the margin captured with putty material, which may result in lack of details.

manipulation of gypsum is not complicated, it is frequently ignored, thus compromising both strength and accuracy.

The Nature of Gypsum Products

Mineral gypsum exists naturally as calcium-sulfate *dihydrate* and is treated by the manufacturer to remove water. It is then supplied to the dentist as a powder, which chemically is calcium-sulfate *hemihydrate*. The dentist then adds water, and a chemical reaction occurs converting the gypsum back to the *dihydrate* form. The chemical reaction for these processes may be written as follows:

$$Ca_2SO_4 \bullet 2\,H_2O + HEAT \rightarrow Ca_2SO_4 \bullet 0.5\,H_2O + 1.5\,H_2O$$

$$Ca_2SO_4 \bullet 0.5\,H_2O + 1.5\,H_2O \rightarrow Ca_2SO_4 \bullet 2\,H_2O + HEAT$$

Differences in the various types of gypsum exist due to the conditions under which the water is removed during the manufacturing process, the size and shape of the particles of the hemihydrate, and the effects of various chemical additives. From a practical standpoint, the properties of a given gypsum product can be predicted from the water/powder ratio suggested by the manufacturer, and an understanding of the concept of gaging water.

A finite quantity of water is required to chemically react with a given amount of gypsum powder supplied as calcium-sulfate hemihydrate. This amount of water is the same, whether the material to be mixed is Type I, Type II, Type III, Type IV, or Type V gypsum. However, depending upon the size and shape of the gypsum crystals, an additional amount of water is required to produce a workable mix of material. This extra water is known as gaging water. This gaging water does not react chemically and remains trapped within the matrix of the setting gypsum. With time (24 hours), most of this water evaporates, leaving air-filled voids in the set gypsum. As a general rule, the greater the porosity of a set gypsum material, the weaker it will be. It will also display diminished abrasion resistance and greater expansion, although this latter factor is somewhat variable depending upon whatever additives are present in the formulation.

For example, the recommended water/powder ratio for a Type II gypsum product is 45 cc/100 gm. For a Type III product it is 30 cc/100 gm, and for a Type IV stone it is 22 cc/100 gm. With 100 gm of each of these gypsum products, approximately 19 cc of water will be used up in the ensuing chemical reaction. The rest of the water will be unreacted and will eventually result in porosity in the set gypsum. The gaging water in the products would be 26 cc, 11 cc, and 3 cc for Types II, III, and IV, respectively. Thus, a cast from a Type II stone would be porous, weak, and have poor abrasion resistance. Casts from the Type IV materials would have the least porosity and the greatest strength and abrasion resistance. Casts from the Type III materials would be intermediate between the Type II and IV products.

Understanding the nature of the setting reaction for gypsum is essential to understanding the clinical behavior of the materials. When the calcium-sulfate hemihydrate is mixed with water, insoluble crystals of calcium-sulfate dihydrate form and begin to precipitate from the mass. These crystals, which can be visualized three dimensionally as resembling sea urchins, serve as precipitation centers or nuclei of crystallization (Fig. 13.55).

As the reaction proceeds, more and more nuclei precipitate out and all continue to grow in an outward direction. The branches of these growing crystals intermesh and intercept one another, creating a tendency for the crystals to be pushed apart. This results practically in a net volumetric expansion (Fig. 13.56). Continued

mixing while the reaction is underway can result in increased expansion because of the breakup of the gypsum crystals creating many more nuclei of crystallization.

Classification of Gypsum Products

Gypsum products are classified as Types I through V, and described by ADA Specification #25 (Table 13.7). Types I and II are plaster products. Type III is commonly known as dental stone or hydrocal. Types IV and V are high strength dental stones, also called improved dental stone or densite. The old terms *alpha* and *beta* calcium-sulfate dihydrate have been deemed obsolete because there is no actual chemical difference between the two types, and all differences are a result of the physical characteristics of the gypsum particles.

Type I dental stones are referred to as "impression plaster," and are typically weak, quick setting, and possess relatively low expansion values, as additives cause the materials to "set" before the normal setting expansion (due to crystalline growth) can occur. The primary use for Type I stones today is in mounting casts in an articulator. The minimum expansion displayed by these materials coupled with their quick setting capabilities make them ideal for this task. Because virtually zero expansion is desirable in a mounting stone and because expansion is bulk related, the two-stage mounting technique is recommended. With this technique, the cast is attached to the mounting ring with as small an increment of plaster as is deemed practical. After this material has set, a subsequent mix may be made and added to the initial mix for strength and cosmetic purposes. Impression plaster is also useful in certain indexing procedures, such as the soldering of fixed restorations, occlusal registrations, and in implant dentistry.

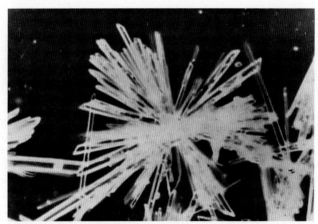

• **Fig. 13.55** Crystal of calcium-sulfate dihydrate.

TABLE 13.7	Classification of Gypsum Products
Type I	Impression plaster
Type II	Model plaster
Type III	Dental stone (hydrocal)
Type IV	Improved dental stone
Type V	Die stone high expansion

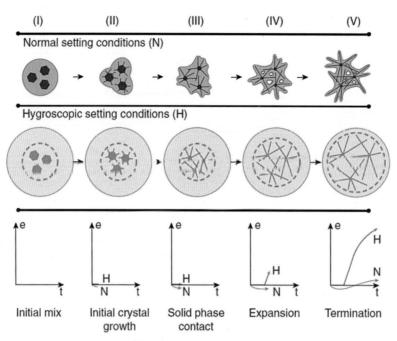

• **Fig. 13.56** Diagrammatic representation of the setting expansion of gypsum products. In the top row, the crystal growth is inhibited by the surface tension of water surrounding the growing crystals. In the middle row, the gypsum mixture *(the area surrounded by the dashed circle)* is immersed in water during setting *(represented by the larger solid circle)*; the immersion water provides more room for longer crystal growth. The bottom row shows the expansion *(e)* over time *(t)* for hygroscopic setting expansion *(H)* and normal setting expansion *(N)*. (From Anusavice KJ, Shen C, Rawls RH: *Phillips' science of dental materials,* ed 12, Elsevier, St. Louis, 2013; adapted from Mahler DB, Ady AB: An explanation for the hygroscopic setting expansion of dental gypsum products. *J Dent Res* 39:378-379, 1960.)

Type II dental stones are referred to as "model plaster" and have little use in restorative dentistry, although they are often utilized for the fabrication of diagnostic casts. These materials are weak and suffer from excessive expansion, which is desirable only in certain situations.

Type III gypsum is commonly referred to as "dental stone." Dental stone is considerably stronger and more resistant to abrasion than plaster. It also exhibits much less expansion. This product is used extensively in restorative dentistry for the fabrication of diagnostic casts, opposing arch casts, and in removable prosthodontics where a high strength stone may actually be a disadvantage when attempting to recover a processed prosthesis from a denture flask.

Type IV gypsum, often referred to as densite or improved dental stone, is commonly called "die stone." This stone is quite strong and abrasion resistant, and demonstrates low expansion values. It is used primarily for the fabrication of precision casts and dies in the lost wax process.

Type V gypsum is a high strength and high expansion stone, and is utilized today in the fabrication of casts and dies for metal-ceramic restorations, particularly when the casting shrinkage of the metal utilized is high and warrants extra expansion in the dies (Fig. 13.57).

Selection and Manipulation of Gypsum Products

The selection of gypsum products is relatively simple, with the main variables being the strength and expansion desired for any specific procedure. Once the appropriate product is selected, proper

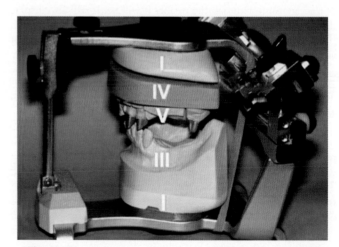

• **Fig. 13.57** Cast model showing four types of gypsum products.

manipulation is essential to ensure that the maximum physical properties of the material are attained.

The most important manipulative variable is paying attention to the proper water to powder ratios. Gypsum is best purchased in prepackaged envelopes. This ensures purity and prevents contamination that may occur when using bulk gypsum, and also provides a consistent volume of powder. Distilled water should be used and measured carefully with a pipette or glass cylinder. Often tap water contains minerals and other contaminants that can affect the setting reaction.

Controlling porosity in the set cast is critical to achieving maximum strength. This is accomplished in several ways. Adhering to the correct water/powder ratio helps this initially by minimizing the amount of gaging water. Next, the powder is always added to the water rather than the other way around. This minimizes air inclusions that occur when the water is added to the powder. Vacuum mixing should be utilized whenever dental stones or improved dental stones are mixed. The mixing times recommended by the manufacturer should be closely adhered to. Impressions should also be poured utilizing vibration devices to prevent air entrapment.

Separating the set cast from the impression must be done at the appropriate time. First the gypsum must have attained sufficient strength to avoid fracture during removal. Generally speaking, waiting 45 minutes to 1 hour will accomplish this. Additionally, especially when using water-based impression materials such as reversible or irreversible hydrocolloid, separation should occur within this time frame to avoid interaction between the impression material and the surface of the set gypsum. Such interaction would deleteriously affect the surface of the stone cast.

In most cases, handling of the casts should be avoided for 24 hours. There is a dramatic difference between the wet strength (1 hour) and dry strength (24 hours) of gypsum products. If casts are trimmed or margins on dies delineated before maximum strength is attained, it is likely that such casts and dies could be excessively abraded. Also gypsum casts are very susceptible to erosion by water during trimming. This can be minimized by soaking the aged (24 hours) cast in a solution of slurry water for 1 to 2 minutes prior to trimming. It will also prevent sludge from the trimming process from adhering to the surface of the cast. An alternative approach is to soften a sheet of base plate wax and adapt it to the surface of the cast prior to trimming. This will effectively prevent water contamination and sludge adherence.

Casting Investments

The lost wax process was introduced to the profession in 1907 by Taggart.[98] In order to fabricate a precise gold casting, it is necessary to balance a number of expansions and contractions related to dental materials (Fig. 13.58).

One of the major shrinkage factors in the process is the casting shrinkage of the metal alloys as they cool from the liquidus temperature to bench temperature. This shrinkage is roughly proportional to melting temperature: The higher the melting temperature the greater the shrinkage of the alloy. Type III gold alloys shrink approximately 1.2% while base metal alloys have double the casting shrinkage at 2.4%. This shrinkage must be compensated in the entire process. The major mechanism for accomplishing this is the use of casting investments.

There are three major types of casting investments. Gypsum bonded investments are primarily used with gold casting alloys. Phosphate bonded investments, also known as high-heat investments, are primarily used with porcelain bonding alloys because they can withstand the higher temperatures required to melt porcelain bonding alloys. Ethyl-silicate investments are primarily used with removable partial denture castings.

With gypsum bonded investments there are three major components. The refractory is composed of materials such as cristobalite, tridymite, and quartz. The refractory supplies most of the thermal expansion of the investment through the process of inversion. As the investment is heated in a burnout oven, the

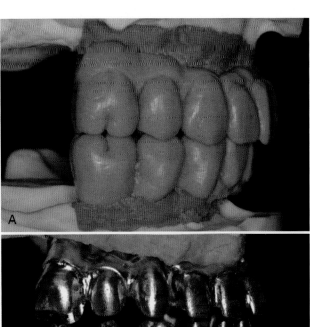
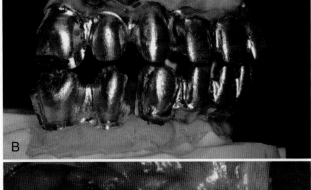
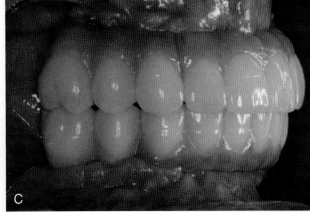

• **Fig. 13.58** A, Wax-up of maxillary and mandibular arches. B, Metal casting of maxillary and mandibular arches. C, Final restoration of maxillary and mandibular arches.

investment expands in proportion to the increase in temperature. Then a significant amount of expansion suddenly occurs when a specific temperature, called the inversion temperature, is reached. This expansion occurs as a result of a change in crystalline form of the refractory; it changes from the alpha crystalline form to the beta crystalline form. This form change is associated with specific expansion, called inversion (Fig. 13.59).

The second component of gypsum bonded investments is the binder. The binder is basically gypsum, starting out as calcium sulphate hemihydrate powder converting to calcium-sulphate dihydrate after being mixed with water. The setting reaction of gypsum is associated with expansion, which contributes along with the thermal expansion to compensate the casting shrinkage of the alloy.

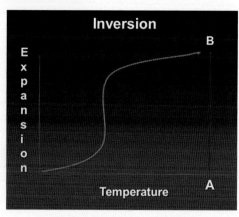

• **Fig. 13.59** Inversion diagram.

The third component of gypsum bonded investments is the modifier, which may take the form of oxidizing agent or reducing agent, depending on the commercial product.

There are three types of expansion associated with gypsum bonded investments. The first and most important is thermal expansion as a result of refractory expansion, as described previously. The second is setting expansion provided by the setting reaction of the gypsum binder. The third type is hygroscopic expansion provided by soaking the ceramic liner of the casting ring. At one time, asbestos was used for this function. The liner allows the investment and casting to be easily removed from the casting ring after casting is completed. By soaking it in water before placing it into the ring, the liner supplies a small amount of gaging water to the setting gypsum, which in turn allows a small amount of extra expansion. NOTE: There is a separate type of investment called a hygroscopic investment. These are very accurate investments that rely primarily on hygroscopic expansion and will not be described here because they are rarely used at this time.

Phosphate bonded investments were developed to provide the extra expansion required with metal alloys that melt at high temperatures and also had to be formulated to withstand those higher melting temperatures. Phosphate bonded investments come with a "special liquid" that is basically liquid silica. The liquid replaces some of the water used to mix the investment, and the basic rule is the more liquid silica, the greater the expansion of the investment.

Ethyl-silicate investments are used with removable partial denture framework castings. Basically the master cast is blocked out and duplicated with an ethyl-silicate investment. The wax-up is completed on the ethyl-silicate cast and the cast and framework are invested in ethyl-silicate investment; the wax pattern is burnt out and cast with chrome-cobalt alloy.

Manipulation of casting investments is relatively simple. First the appropriate investment materials must be selected. Then the most important variable is use of precise water to powder ratios. In the case of phosphate bonded investments, liquid to powder ratios are used, with the liquid being part water and part special liquid, depending on the amount of expansion required. Investments are vacuum mixed and poured into different sized molds, depending on the size of the casting.

After waiting a minimum of 1 hour, the casting ring is placed into a cold oven, subjected to a controlled burnout, and the restoration is cast.

THE BOTTOM LINE

1. Casting investments are an integral part of the lost wax process.
2. The three types of casting investments are gypsum bonded, phosphate bonded, and ethyl silicate investments.
3. Gypsum bonded investments are used with cast gold; phosphate bonded investments are used with porcelain bonding alloys, and ethyl-silicate investments with removable partial denture frameworks.
4. Casting investments compensate for casting shrinkage of the alloy.
5. Three types of expansion occur with casting investments: thermal, setting, and hygroscopic. The most important expansion is thermal.
6. Special liquid (liquid silica) is used with phosphate bonded investments to allow for the precise amount of expansion depending on the alloy used.

Gold Alloys

Cast gold restorations have been used in dentistry ever since Taggart introduced the lost wax process in 1907.[98] Properly done cast gold restorations provide the longest term survival of all types of restorations. A recent study of 1314 cast gold restorations in place from 1 to 55 years demonstrated that at 30 years, the failure rate was 4.5% (Fig. 13.60).[52] Pure (100%) gold is too soft for use in the oral cavity so it must be alloyed with other metals to produce the essential physical properties.

Gold foil is 98% pure gold and direct gold foil restorations have been placed for many years and provide long-term service with non–stress-bearing restorations (Fig. 13.61). Metals that are

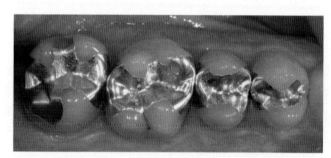

• **Fig. 13.60** Cast gold restorations after 37 years.

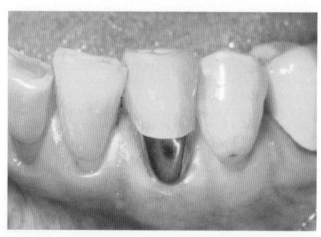

• **Fig. 13.61** Gold foil restoration (98% gold) restoring a noncarious cervical lesion.

alloyed with gold in dental casting alloys include platinum and/ or palladium for both strength and passivity, silver and copper for strength, and zinc and indium as deoxidizers. Gold is used because it is a noble metal and does not tarnish in the oral cavity. All noble metals share that property. The major noble metals used in dentistry are gold, platinum, and palladium. Nobility is determined by an element's position in the periodic table. Silver is a precious metal, but is not noble as it easily tarnishes in the oral cavity.

There are four types of gold alloy, Types I, II, III, and IV (Table 13.8). Type I gold alloy has the highest concentration of gold at 98%; it is considered a "soft" gold and is indicated in non–stress-bearing situations such as Class V inlays. Type II gold contains approximately 77% gold and is typically used with gold inlays and restorations with finishable margins, as these alloys can be burnished to attain maximum marginal integrity. Type III gold, with a concentration of 72% gold, is the most commonly used gold alloy in dentistry; it is used to fabricate crowns and fixed partial dentures. Type IV gold has the lowest concentration of gold (69%), and was used for the fabrication of removable partial denture frameworks at one time but rarely for that purpose now. It is still used for the fabrication of custom cast dowel and cores, as it is the strongest of the gold alloys and is less expensive due to the lower concentration of gold.

Type I gold is the softest, with the highest concentration of gold; Type IV is the hardest, with the lowest concentration of gold. Types I and IV gold are rarely used at this time, thus the most used alloys in contemporary dentistry are Types II and III.

One technique that can be used to improve marginal integrity of cast gold restorations is heat treatment. To heat treat a gold alloy, the alloy must have a copper content of 12%. Metal alloys can exist in one of three states. With a eutectic mixture, distinct phases can be identified in the microstructure. A good example of a eutectic would be amalgam where gamma, gamma-1, and gamma-2 phases can easily be identified in a micrograph. Eutectic mixtures are hard and brittle.

The second state seen with metal alloys is as an intermetallic compound. With intermetallic compounds there are no distinct phases, but there is molecular ordering, and these alloys are hard and strong. After heat hardening treatment, gold alloys exist as intermetallic compounds. When gold alloys are heat softened, they exist as a solid solution. With solid solutions there is a total lack of molecular order with randomization, and solid solutions are soft and burnishable.

The heat treatment procedure begins by heat softening. The alloy is melted and cast and immediately quenched in cold water. This transforms the alloy into a solid solution, which again is soft and burnishable. The restoration is then taken to the mouth and the finishable margins are burnished to achieve maximum marginal integrity. Then the alloy is heat hardened to render it hard and strong. To accomplish this, the restoration is heated in an oven and then slowly cooled to bench temperature. This transforms the alloy into an intermetallic compound, which will be hard and strong and provide optimum clinical service.

Cast gold restorations unquestionably provide the longest service of any restoration available in dentistry. The use of cast gold has declined significantly in recent years primarily due to the profession's obsession with esthetics and also due to the cost of gold. Most recent graduates of dental schools have not been taught how to fabricate gold restorations with a high level of precision. This is an unfortunate situation. Dentists are encouraged to contact any one of many study clubs that teach the concepts of cast gold restorations and add this wonderful modality to their armamentarium.

TABLE 13.8	Types of Gold Alloys Used in Dentistry		
Type	Au	Hardness	Indication
I	98%	Soft	Class V
II	77%	↑	Inlays
III	72%		Crowns
IV	69%	Hard	RPDs

Porcelain Bonding Alloys

Prior to the introduction of porcelain-fused-to-metal technology, the clinician had only two options for the esthetic restoration of extensively broken down anterior teeth. One was the classic feldspathic porcelain jacket crown, which generally displayed inferior marginal fidelity and had a high incidence of fracture. The second option was heat-processed acrylic resin bonded to metal. The acrylic resin was mechanically bonded to the metal using beads and other mechanical retentive features. Type III or IV gold alloys were generally used for these restorations. The major disadvantage of these crowns and fixed partial dentures was the poor wear resistance of the resin veneering materials. At time intervals ranging from 3 to 5 years, the resin veneer would typically begin to age, demonstrating clinically evident wear and staining.

In late 1962 metal-ceramic restorations were patented and introduced to the profession by Weinstein, Katz, and Weinstein.[99] Original research in this area began with typical gold casting alloys, simply because they had been used in dentistry ever since Taggert had introduced the lost wax process to the profession in 1907. Four major alterations needed to be made to these alloys before clinical success could be expected.

1. The melting temperature needed to be raised because the gold alloys melted at temperatures well below the fusing temperatures of porcelain. This was achieved by the addition of an appropriate amount of platinum to the gold alloy.
2. Strength of the alloy needed to be increased. Any flexure in the metal substructure would result in catastrophic fracture of the porcelain veneer. Conventional gold alloys are far too flexible. Again, the addition of platinum was a major factor in improving the strength of the alloy.
3. The thermal coefficients of expansion and contraction of the metal alloy and the veneering porcelain needed to be more closely matched. The COE of the alloy was reduced to a great extent again by the inclusion of platinum, and the COE of the veneering ceramic was raised with the addition of sodium.
4. Predictable bonding of the porcelain to the metal needed to be achieved. Mechanisms of porcelain to metal bonding will be dealt with in more depth later on in this chapter. With these early alloys, chemical bonding was achieved with the inclusion of trace elements such as indium, zinc, and tin. These elements produced a consistent oxide on the surface of the alloy that would provide a chemical bond with the tetravalent oxides in the opaque porcelains.

These early porcelain bonding alloys contained a high percentage of gold (85%) and were used extensively through the 1960s and early 1970s. Although the physical properties of these high gold alloys were less than ideal, the main impetus for research into alternative alloys was the sudden increase in the price of gold in the late 1970s that approached $1000/ounce. Since that time a number of alternative alloy systems have been introduced and have been extensively researched. The following analysis is given to assist the clinician in alloy selection for this important clinical modality. It is important to understand that the dentist should determine which alloy should be used for each restoration. This important choice should not be delegated to the laboratory technician.

Classification

Because the physical properties of an alloy can be predicted from their component elements, it is useful to classify porcelain bonding alloys according to their composition. Often alloys are casually referred to as "precious," "semiprecious," or "nonprecious" metals, usually based on the approximate gold content of the alloy. These terms lack precision, and several alloy groups with significantly different physical properties could be legitimately termed "semiprecious" (Fig. 13.62).

A more meaningful classification is to use the *nobility* of an alloy to designate the appropriate group to which a metal alloy should be assigned. The nobility of an element is determined by its position in the periodic table, and is a measure of its passivity in the oral environment. The noble metals most commonly used in restorative dentistry are gold, platinum, and palladium. Iridium, rhodium, ruthenium, and osmium are also designated as noble metals. Silver, which has a tendency to tarnish in oral fluids, is generally not considered as a noble metal. Silver is a precious metal, which signifies only that the metal has some intrinsic value. The word "precious" has nothing to do with tarnish potential.

Thus porcelain bonding alloys can be classified into two major groups: noble alloys and base metal alloys. There are three subgroups of noble alloys and three subgroups of base metal alloys (Table 13.9).

They can be differentiated from one another in terms of composition and in terms of certain attributes and physical properties such as strength, fit of castings, and bond potential with porcelain, biocompatibility, and economic considerations. Table 13.10 compares the alloy systems in terms of these variables.

Composition

High gold alloys typically contain a high percentage of gold, usually in the range of 80% to 85%. The alloy is strengthened with the addition of 7% to 10% platinum, and trace elements such as indium, zinc, and tin are added to provide an oxide layer for predictable porcelain bonding. These alloys predominated until the price of gold skyrocketed in the mid-1970s. Examples of commercial alloys in this category are Jelenko-O (J.F. Jelenko Co., Armonk, NY), Silhouette 850SL (Leach and Dillon, N. Attleboro, MA), and SMG-3 (J.M. Ney Co., Bloomfield, CT).

High noble alloys have a gold content typically in the range of 50% to 55% gold. Palladium is present in the range of 35% to 40%, along with the trace elements essential for bonding. These alloys may or may not contain silver. If more than 12% silver is present, it may cause a tendency for the porcelain to take on a greenish hue. Small amounts of silver may improve the wettability of the metal coping with the opaque porcelain, although this has not been scientifically established. Examples of this type of alloy include Olympia (J.F. Jelenko, Armonk, NY), USC Ceramic Alloy (Leach and Dillon, N. Attleboro, MA), and W2 and W3 (Williams Gold Co., Buffalo, NY).

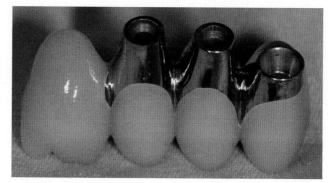

• **Fig. 13.62** Porcelain-fused-to-metal fixed dental prosthesis.

TABLE 13.9	Classification of Metal-Porcelain Alloys	
Noble Metal Alloys	**Base Metal Alloys**
High gold	Nickel-chrome-beryllium
Low gold	Chrome-cobalt
Palladium-silver	Titanium

TABLE 13.10	Comparison of Multiple Alloys According to Different Variables			
	High Au	**Low Au**	**Ag-Pd**	**Base**
Composition	85% Au, 7% Pt	58% Au, 38% Pd	60% Pd, 38% Ag	65% Ni, 20% Cr
Strength	0.5 mm	0.3 mm	0.3 mm	0.1 mm
Fit	-	++	+	–
Bond	++	++	+	–
Biocompatibility	++	++	+	–
Cost	$100	$52	$34	$6

Palladium-silver alloys are composed primarily of high concentrations of palladium (60%) and silver (30%). With such high concentrations of silver, discoloration of the porcelain is obviously a consideration unless special precautions are taken during firing. Use of the alloy W1 (Williams Gold Co., Buffalo, NY) along with the low sodium content porcelain specified by the same manufacturer can eliminate this problem. Another example of a palladium-silver alloy is Silhouette 150 (Leach and Dillon, N. Attleboro, MA).

There are three groups of *base metal alloys*. The first, *nickel-chromium alloy*, is the most common of the three and typically contains about 65% nickel for strength, 20% chromium for passivity, and 2% beryllium for castability and control of oxide formation. Commercial products representing this type of alloy include Rexillium III (Jeneric Pentron) and Lite-Cast B (Williams Gold Co., Buffalo, NY). Nonberyllium alloys are commercially available but should not be considered for clinical use. Note: Beryllium is critical to help control oxide formation with base metal alloys; however, it has been associated with the development of berylliosis, a serious occupational pulmonary condition, and laboratory technicians are at risk. The American Dental Association will no longer certify beryllium-containing alloys.

Chromium-cobalt alloys are commercially available and primarily marketed as "biocompatible" base metal alloys because they are nickel and beryllium free. Other than the exclusion of these elements, these alloys have little to recommend them and thus should not be used. Because they contain approximately twice as much cobalt as they do chromium, it has been suggested that these metals should be designated cobalt-chromium alloys. It is now possible to very accurately mill chrome-cobalt frameworks, which removes one of the major disadvantages (poor fit) of these alloys. There is little evidence at this time that the problems associated with excess oxide formation with these alloys have been solved.

Titanium alloys have become available recently, and copings are currently formed both by casting and by a combination of copy-milling and spark-gap erosion. Both of these systems must be considered experimental at this time and should be used only under strict protocol in an institutional setting. The other issue with titanium fused-to-metal is that veneering ceramics with very low COEs are required, and the esthetic results achieved with these ceramics are poor. Thus only the nickel-chrome-beryllium alloys should be considered for use by the practitioner.

Strength

Strength of a porcelain bonding alloy is of paramount importance to the long-term longevity of the restoration. Any flexure whatsoever in the metal substructure will result in catastrophic failure (fracture) of the porcelain veneer. The greater the number of units in any fixed partial denture framework, the greater is the potential for flexure. An alloy will ideally possess strength in relatively thin sections to allow for minimal tooth reduction and permit the fabrication of delicate frameworks. These substructures will then permit the creation of embrasure forms and connector designs that will allow for optimum cleansibility and the development of physiologic crown contours.

One of the major disadvantages of the high gold alloys is the relative lack of strength possessed by these metals. This lack of strength can be compensated by bulking up the framework and the occlusogingival dimension of the connector areas. This can compromise embrasure form and produce overcontoured restorations. A minimum cross-sectional thickness of 0.5 mm is suggested for use with these alloys. High gold alloys should only be used with single crown restorations on anterior teeth. In this situation, high gold alloys have an advantage because they do not produce a dark oxide, and intense opaque porcelains do not need to be used to block out the color of the oxide. Because of the reduced bite force with anterior teeth compared to posterior teeth, the strength of the gold framework is adequate.

The high noble and palladium-based alloys are considerably stronger than the high gold alloys, and a minimum cross-sectional thickness of only 0.3 mm is required. This reduction of thickness required is only 0.2 mm, but it is extremely significant clinically. The nickel-chrome-beryllium alloys are very strong and can survive with a minimal thickness of only 0.1 mm, although it is very difficult to work within such a tight tolerance without running the risk of perforation of the metal coping.

Fit of Castings

A most important factor in long-term success with cast restorations is achieving excellent marginal integrity. A number of factors totally independent of the alloy utilized are important in this regard.

However, there are also differences in the ability of the various alloy systems to predictably produce excellent margins.

Several studies have evaluated the castability of these alloy systems.[100] Variations were found due to the different specific gravities of the alloys and due to variations in melting temperatures. However, current research has established that there is a "metal-mold equilibrium" for each alloy and investment combination that will produce an optimum casting in terms of completeness and the quality of the surface of the casting. This equilibrium is defined as the difference between the melting temperature of the alloy and the temperature of the mold into which the alloy is cast. Once this optimum temperature differential is established, excellent castings can be achieved with all of the systems under discussion. This finding, plus the development of induction casting machines, has determined castability is no longer a concern with any of the alloy systems.

When metal alloys are cast they solidify from the liquid to the solid state and then subsequently cool to room temperature. Casting shrinkage occurs during this time. This shrinkage occurs in three stages: (1) when the liquid metal cools from the melting temperature to the solidification temperature; (2) when it undergoes the transformation from the liquid to the solid state; and (3) when the solidified metal cools to room temperature. It is likely that this latter stage is where the most significant shrinkage occurs.

There are major differences in the amount of casting shrinkage that occurs with the various alloy systems. Casting shrinkage is a function of the melting temperature: The higher the melting temperature of the alloy, the greater will be the casting shrinkage. This shrinkage of course must be compensated by equivalent expansion of the investment. There is some question that this can be accomplished with adequate precision with the alloys possessing the highest melting temperatures. This is especially a problem with large multiunit castings.

Type III gold alloys shrink approximately 1.2%. Gypsum bonded investments can compensate very accurately for this amount of shrinkage. High gold porcelain bonding alloys shrink slightly more at about 1.3%. The casting shrinkage of the high noble and palladium based alloy systems is slightly higher than that of the high gold alloys. Compensation for this shrinkage is accomplished with high heat phosphate bonded investments, using specific amounts of liquid silica to control the expansion. The more silica used, the greater is the expansion.

The nickel-chrome-beryllium alloys shrink 2.4%, which is double the shrinkage of a Type III gold alloy. Early studies with these alloy systems indicated that the castings were too tight and failed to seat adequately. This was simply a result of lack of adequate expansion provided by the investment materials utilized in the investigation. Today it is possible to provide adequate expansion with modern investments. However, the difficulty of producing an accurate casting increases as the expansions and contractions of the materials involved increase. This is particularly true when dealing with castings with nonuniform amounts of bulk, and large multiunit castings. It is difficult to solder base metal alloy units, and as a result, fixed partial dentures fabricated with this alloy are often cast in one piece. A diminution in the quality in the fit of the castings is likely to occur when this is done.

A third factor related to fit of castings is distortion of the metal coping during firing of the porcelain veneer. Clinicians have long noted subjectively that metal copings that fit very well prior to firing the porcelain do not fit nearly as well after firing. The distortion that occurs is a function of both the composition of the alloy and the margin geometry utilized. Additionally, research has shown that not only do individual copings distort, but so do entire frameworks for larger fixed partial dentures. Because the majority of the distortion seems to occur during the degassing process, the major factor in this latter type of distortion seems to be release of stresses induced in the casting process.

As noted previously, distortion varies with the composition of the alloy. The higher the melting temperature of an alloy, the less distortion will likely occur. Thus the high gold alloys, which have melting temperatures closest to the sintering temperatures of the porcelain, tend to distort the most. High noble and the palladium-based alloys distort somewhat less, while base metal alloys tend to distort very little. However, this latter fact should not be taken to construe that there is no change in fit of base metal castings during porcelain application. In fact the quality of the fit is diminished considerably with base metal castings as a result of inevitable *oxide* formation on the internal of the castings. This oxide layer, which is substantial with base metal alloys, can interfere with seating of the casting and result in marginal opening.

Of course distortion can be minimized with the intelligent use of cervical marginal geometry. Shoulder and shoulder-bevel margins distort relatively little, even with high gold alloys, and should be utilized routinely in nonesthetic situations. Framework distortion can be minimized by proper alloy selection, use of custom sager trays, and use of the postsoldering procedure where indicated.

When all factors are taken into account, it would appear that the high noble/palladium-silver/high palladium alloys would have an advantage over the other systems in terms of the ability to achieve consistently excellent marginal integrity.

Bonding to Porcelain

Clearly the formation of a predictable bond to porcelain is an essential property of an alloy intended for crown and bridge prosthodontics. There are three main mechanisms of porcelain bonding: mechanical, chemical, and compression bonding. The most important of these by far is chemical bonding. However, it is prudent to take advantage of all three methods.

Mechanical bonding occurs due to the inherent microscopically rough metal surface that exists after the degassing procedure. Van der Waal forces play a role here, as does the improved wetting that occurs when the surface of the alloy is air-abraded with 50-micron aluminum-oxide particles prior to applying the opaque porcelain. It has been estimated that such mechanical bonding should constitute only about 10% of the total bond of the porcelain to the metal.

Compression bonding occurs as a result of the slight thermal coefficient of expansion mismatch that exists between the porcelain and a compatible alloy. When a metal-ceramic restoration is taken from the muffle of a porcelain oven and allowed to cool, the metal coping will cool first and begin to shrink slightly. This will pull the overlying porcelain under compression. This compression stress contributes to the overall bond strength. We take advantage of this by attempting to get a "wrap around" effect with our cutback design, both buccolingually and interproximally.

Chemical bonding is the most important means of bonding porcelain to metal. The opaque porcelains are specially formulated with tetravalent oxides that will bond to oxides formed on the surface of the metal. The metallic oxides either form naturally or are induced from trace elements during the degas cycle, and ideally will form a monomolecular layer on the surface of the alloy (Fig. 13.63).

Chemical bonding with the noble metal alloys has been extensively studied and is very predictable. Trace elements such as indium,

zinc, and tin are added to the alloy to provide the oxide required as well as refine the grain structure. The metal coping is run through a degas or oxidation cycle to induce the oxide onto the surface. At least 50% new metal is used each time a coping is cast to prevent depletion of the trace elements from the mix. Light air abrading with aluminum-oxide is recommended with many alloys to prevent excess oxide formation.

Chemical bonding is much less predictable with the base metal alloys. The problem with these alloys is with the oxide layer. There is simply too much of an oxide layer, and while the bond failure may occur at either the interface between the metal and the oxide or between the oxide and the opaque, it most frequently occurs within the thick oxide layer itself.

Most porcelain bond tests are flawed in that they all allow for a considerable amount of compression bonding. Thus base metal alloys can appear to possess good ability to bond to porcelain as measured by these tests. However, a majority of the reported bond will be compression bonding, which can fail catastrophically at any time. As stated previously, the major problem is the thickness of the oxide layer, which propagates each time the porcelain is fired. The main function of beryllium in a base metal alloy is to help control the oxide layer in addition to improving the castability of the alloy. In the former function, the beryllium is only partially successful. Nonberyllium base metal alloys have no control of the oxide layer and hence should be avoided.

The tendency of base metal alloys to form thick oxide layers is also problematic when attempting to solder fixed partial dentures. The problem here is that the alloys form the oxide layer before

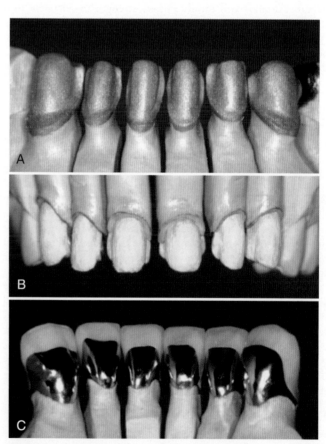

• **Fig. 13.63**   A, Noble metal alloy copings. B, Opaque porcelain applied to noble metal alloy copings. C, Finalized porcelain-fused-to-metal crowns.

the solder can melt and join with the parent metal. This interposed oxide layer can result in weak or nonexistent solder joints. As a result, many fixed partial denture frameworks using base metal are cast in one piece. While the literature on one-piece castings is somewhat equivocal, many feel that the fit of the castings is definitely compromised. Also, it is often essential to section, index, and solder units because they simply do not fit. This can be difficult with base metal alloys.

Biocompatibility

While patients can be theoretically allergic to almost any element in a casting alloy, even gold, the major elements that are of interest in terms of biocompatibility are nickel and beryllium. It is estimated that approximately 22% of women are allergic to nickel. The incidence of nickel allergy in men is less than 10%. The major reason for the difference in incidence between the sexes is thought to be that many women have pierced ears and wear costume jewelry. Much of this jewelry is nickel based, and it is believed that this will induce the allergy.

The signs and symptoms of nickel allergy can be local or systemic. Often the presenting symptom is a rash or eczema on the arm or legs. Patients often do not associate such peripheral symptoms with an intraoral restoration and hence may suffer for prolonged periods before a diagnosis of nickel allergy is made. When use of a base metal alloy is contemplated, the patient should be specifically asked if he or she has any allergy to nickel or reaction to any metal.

Beryllium is primarily a potential problem for the laboratory technician where grindings containing beryllium can be the etiologic agent for a number of respiratory ailments. Proper ventilation and the routine wearing of a face mask can prevent such untoward events. Beryllium has also been shown to migrate toward the surface of restorations, and in that location can also dissolve in oral fluids. The clinical significance of these findings is unknown at this time but is a concern to some.

A similar situation may occur with the high palladium alloys. In a number of proprietary studies palladium has been shown to dissolve in oral fluids and be cytotoxic. This most frequently occurs when the combined concentration of gold and silver is less than 25% of the total alloy. Again the clinical significance of this is unknown.

Economic Considerations

Obviously the cost of a metal alloy needs to be considered. This can be even more important when the price of gold fluctuates extensively. Indeed the genesis of most of the research into alternative alloys, and many of the all-ceramic alternatives to metal-ceramics, was a gold price approaching $1000/ounce.

A pilot study conducted at the University of Southern California School of Dentistry in 1981 compared the price of a metal coping fabricated with different alloys. The price of gold at the time was close to $400/ounce. Fifty metal copings were collected at random, weighed, and an average weight calculated. The average price/coping/alloy could then be calculated. The results do not take into account the lower specific gravity of base metal alloys, which affords additional minor savings. Nor does it take into account the fact that copings made with one alloy could be thinner than those fabricated from another alloy. The data do indicate a significant differential in cost (Table 13.11).

Since 1981, the cost of noble metals has fluctuated considerably, but the price of gold has ranged around $1000 to $1600 an ounce.

That means the metal cost of laboratory work has at least doubled over that time, which has a huge effect on laboratory costs and subsequently raises the cost of restorative services to patients. Indeed, a major impetus for the development of all-ceramic alternatives to PFM is the laboratory costs.

Depending upon the philosophic orientation and sociologic makeup of a practice, the differences in cost of alloys may or may not be significant. Far more important would seem to be the predictability of an alloy in terms of castability, consistent fit, and lack of bond failure.

In summary, a host of metal alloys intended to be used with porcelain are currently available commercially. These have been classified according to both composition and the characteristics and physical properties of the major groups compared.

An analysis of the material presented reveals that one group of alloys, the high noble alloys, seems to have no deficiencies and scores high in all of the categories discussed. High noble alloys also happen to be cheaper than high gold alloys, although that is a secondary consideration. These alloys would seem to be the metals of choice. They are stronger and can be used in thinner section than the high gold alloys. They cast easily and accurately, and show fewer tendencies to distort on firing the porcelain. Porcelain bonding is very predictable with no discoloring of the porcelain. Biocompatibility is not a problem.

If cost was a major consideration, use of a palladium silver alloy with a porcelain low in sodium content would likely be a suitable choice. As is usually the case, proper manipulation of the alloy chosen is probably even more important than which alloy is chosen.

THE BOTTOM LINE

1. Porcelain-fused-to-metal crowns and fixed partial dentures continue to be important restorations and provide the best combination of reasonable esthetics with maximum longevity of available esthetic crown options.
2. Many different alloy systems with different properties and costs are available.
3. The dentist should choose which alloy is most appropriate for each restoration.
4. Some of the factors that must be considered when choosing an alloy include strength, ability to achieve excellent marginal integrity, ability to attain a predictable bond with porcelain, biocompatibility, and cost.
5. Base metal alloys are inexpensive but have significant problems with fit, porcelain bonding, and biocompatibility.
6. High gold alloys do not form dark oxides, and have the potential to provide improved esthetics for single crowns on anterior teeth.
7. High noble alloys are less expensive than high gold alloys and seem to be the alloy of choice for metal-ceramic restorations.

TABLE 13.11	Comparison of Costs for Different Alloys in 1981 and 2016	
Alloy	**Cost 1981**	**Cost 2016**
1. High gold	$50	$100
2. High noble	$26	$52
3. Palladium-silver	$17	$34
4. Base metal	$3	$6

Implant Materials

Dentists have tried for centuries to find a way to implant devices into the jaw bone to replace missing teeth. Many different approaches were tried but no material or technique proved successful until the 1970s. Up until that time, various forms of metal implants primarily fabricated from chrome-cobalt alloy had been used with some short-term success, but all failed in the long term. Blade implants, ramus-frame implants, and other configurations all failed eventually because of epithelial growth between the implant and surrounding bone and subsequent infection. The major problem with these implants was that the surgical site that was prepared was not sufficiently precise to provide initial intimate bone-implant proximity.

Vitreous carbon implants were introduced in the mid-1970s and showed great promise, but suffered the same fate as the implants described previously, as the shape of the implant was rectangular, which made it impossible to surgically prepare the site with sufficient precision.

The first successful implant system was the mandibular subperiosteal implant designed by Dr. Roy Bodine (Fig. 13.64). This chrome-cobalt implant was used with resorbed mandibles and demonstrated survival rates close to 20 years. With this system, an impression was made of the exposed mandible after raising a flap, and the implant framework was placed directly on the periosteum over the alveolar bone rather than in the mandible. These implant frameworks were restored with mandibular dentures that were secured to the metal framework with clips. While subperiosteal implants had acceptable survival rates, the frameworks eventually became infected and had to be removed. This removal often resulted in considerable morbidity, because bone had grown over the framework and had to be surgically removed before the framework could be removed. Maxillary superiosteal implants did not perform nearly as well as mandibular implants because of resorption of the maxillary alveolar process.

The major breakthrough with implants came as a result of Brånemark's research in Sweden. Brånemark was doing capillary research in animals using titanium cylinders to contain the specimens. When trying to remove the cylinders from the bony extremities of the animals in order to reuse them, the researchers discovered the cylinders were very difficult to remove and had in fact integrated into the bone. After several years of animal and human research, Brånemark introduced his system of root form titanium osseointegrated implants in the early 1980s. It is not hyperbole to state that this was one of the most important advances in the history of dentistry.

Brånemark's original clinical research was with "hybrid" prostheses, which consisted of five titanium implants placed in the anterior mandible between the mental foramina (Fig. 13.65). These implants were placed under a strict surgical protocol, then allowed to heal and integrate some time before restoration. The implants were splinted together and restored with a bar and arch-shortened mandibular denture. These restorations were opposed by a maxillary denture. Clinical results were outstanding with 95% implant survival and 100% prostheses survival at 5 years.

These original implants were composed of 99% commercially pure titanium and had machined surfaces. Many manufacturers developed and marketed a number of different implants with different designs, and data from current research cannot identify a "best" implant design. Several implant systems were introduced with "coatings" of hydroxyapatite and other formulations, but they performed poorly compared to titanium implants, primarily due to breakdown between the "coating" and the implant. Titanium-vanadium alloy implants have been used successfully and are stronger than commercially pure titanium implants, but appear to have no clinical advantage because fracture of implants is a very rare occurrence.

Manufacturers have experimented with different implant surfaces trying to create more rapid osseointegration. Most contemporary implants have microscopically "rough" surfaces, which seem to results in more rapid integration into the bone as indicated by "push-out tests." It is not known whether this is clinically significant.

Implants today are used to replace single teeth in all areas of the mouth, to restore multiple lost teeth with fixed partial dentures, and to support full-mouth reconstructions (Fig. 13.66). It is important to understand that Brånemark's original research with 95% survival at 5 years was done with five splinted implants in the anterior mandible. This is the best possible bone for implantation, so these results cannot be extrapolated to implants placed in other areas of the mouth. The least desirable bone for implantation is in the posterior maxilla.

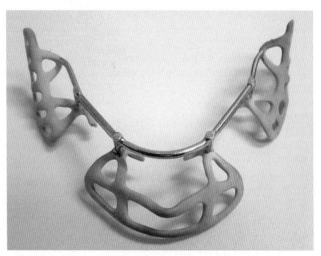

• **Fig. 13.64**　Mandibular subperiosteal implant framework.

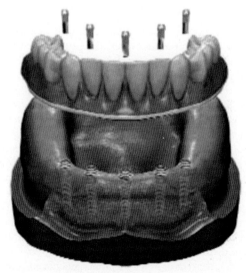

• **Fig. 13.65**　Illustration showing design of hybrid dental prosthesis.

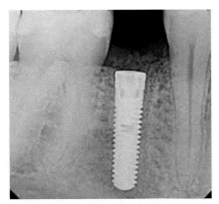

• **Fig. 13.66** Radiograph of single mandibular implant.

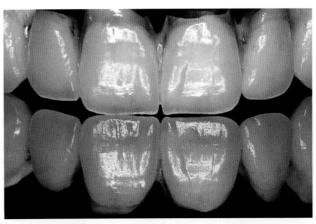

• **Fig. 13.67** Porcelain-fused-to-metal fixed prosthesis.

While data from Brånemark's original research cannot be used to predict survival of implants placed elsewhere in the mouth, it is clear that root form titanium implants have adequate survival rates to recommend routine use for the replacement of missing teeth. Restorations can be screw-retained to the implants or cement-retained. Many authorities prefer screw-retained restorations as this allows 100% retrieval, but this approach requires precise implant placement.

One issue that has come to light in recent years is the condition called periimplantitis, defined as periimplant bone loss accompanied by suppuration. The incidence of periimplantitis seems to be significantly higher than originally reported and seems to primarily occur in patients who originally lost their teeth to periodontitis and who smoke. In these patients, the decision to extract teeth and replace them with implants should be undertaken with an abundance of caution.

THE BOTTOM LINE

1. The advent of predictable osseointegration with titanium root-form implants is one of the most important advances in restorative dentistry.
2. Contemporary implants have acceptable survival rates and should be considered as the primary approach for the replacement of missing teeth.
3. No "best" implant design has been determined by clinical research.
4. Coated implants have not survived as well as noncoated implants.
5. Periimplantitis is a serious complication of implant therapy.
6. Smokers who lost their teeth due to periodontal disease are especially at risk for periimplantitis.

Evolution of All-Ceramic Crowns

New ceramic systems continue to be introduced to the profession at exponential rates. It is critical that clinicians understand how these systems have evolved since the mid-1980s and that they understand the deficiencies of many of these systems so they can more effectively evaluate the potential of new systems as they are introduced to the market. The three major concerns with new systems are as follows:

1. What is the real esthetic potential of the system compared to available tried and true systems?
2. What is a reasonable potential life span for the new system? This can be difficult to determine because improvements in

physical properties do not necessarily translate into improved longevity. Keep in mind that ceramics do not fail because they are not strong enough; they fail because it is not known how to manufacture flaw-free restorations. Those flaws, called Griffith flaws, tend to propagate over time and result in fatigue failure.

3. What clinical situations are recommended for the new system? Can fixed partial dentures made with this system reasonably be expected to survive? Should its use be limited to anterior teeth or can it be used in molars?

This section has been written to describe the main features of the different ceramic systems as they were introduced to the profession. It is not our intent to examine each system in great detail, but to highlight the important features that led to success or failure. It is also not intended to be all-inclusive but will focus on the major players.

The first esthetic crown was the porcelain jacket crown (PJC) introduced to the profession circa 1910 by Land. To fabricate this crown, a platinum foil was adapted to the die using a tinner's joint. This foil was used as a scaffold to carry the porcelain into the porcelain oven where it was fired and the foil later removed. The PJC had good esthetics, but poor marginal integrity and a short life span. They were cemented in place using different shades of silicophosphate cement. The major deficiency of the PJC was the fact they frequently fractured 1 or 2 years after placement.

In 1962, Weinstein-Katz and Weinstein filed the patent for the first metal-ceramic crown system.[99] At the time, a porcelain-fused-to-metal (PFM) was known as a "Ceramco." It became popular in the late 1960s, but dentists knew little about the important preparation details required to produce a truly esthetic restoration (Fig. 13.67). Dentists did not understand the space requirements needed for layers of metal, opaque porcelain, body, and incisal porcelains and thus most preparations were underprepared. They knew nothing about cervical margin design. Laboratory technicians were also unaware of many of the important details of fabrication. The dental profession and laboratory industry learned about PFMs by trial and error. This resulted in many restorations that lacked the expected esthetic potential and frequent fracturing of the feldspathic porcelain veneer from the metal coping.

In the mid-1970s, individuals such as John McLean, Jack Preston, Lloyd Miller, and Jack Nicholls began to do research that guided the profession in producing PFMs that had improved esthetics and great clinical longevity.

One excellent systematic review published in 1989 indicated the failure rate with PFMs is 5% at 11 years.[101] Several other studies have shown similar results.[102] Such data must be considered when assessing the utility of new ceramic systems. Numerous ceramic systems have been introduced to the profession (Fig. 13.68). Almost all of these systems have been brought to market with almost no clinical testing. It is also important to repeat the fact that laboratory testing of physical and mechanical properties and load-to-failure testing yields little useful information about expected clinical performance. Thus it is clear that clinical dentists are carrying out the essential clinical trials for the manufacturers.

In 1978 McLean introduced the aluminous core PJC.[103] This restoration used twin platinum foils for fabrication. One foil was used as a die spacer and the other was tin plated and used to form the core with aluminous core porcelain. This was veneered with compatible low-alkali porcelain. The laboratory technique was very demanding, which limited its commercial adaptation. In 1984 Donovan introduced a simplified single foil technique for fabricating aluminous core PJCs, but this simplified technique also failed to catch on.[104]

The twin-foil crown by McLean was the first in a series of foil-supported restorations that attempted to improve clinical longevity by reducing the number of microscopic defects on the internal portion of the crown. Shorer introduced the Renaissance foil system, which used a pleated noble metal foil and a gold colored bonding agent. Asami Tanaka had a similar system with his Sunrise crown. These foil-supported restorations had poor survival data, primarily because the foil took the form of the tooth preparation and frequently there were excesses of unsupported porcelain. The industry standard is that there should never be more than 2 mm of unsupported porcelain, regardless of the core material. With foil-supported crowns this is difficult to achieve in the majority of cases.

In 1993, Shorer and Whiteman introduced the Captek system. Captek is an interesting technology that forms a noble metal coping without casting or machining. A wax sheet containing a powdered metal alloy of 88% gold is adapted to a refractory die and heated in an oven until the wax melts and the metal coalesces into a porous coping. A second wax sheet containing platinum is adapted over the coping and heated. The wax melts and the platinum enters the gold coping by capillary action (hence "Captek"). The gold color of the coping results in excellent esthetics and the platinum provides strength to resist metal flexure. The major deficiency of Captek is the inability to provide adequate support for the veneering ceramic, again because the coping takes on the form of the tooth preparation and few preparations are ideal.

In 1983, Sozio and Riley introduced the Cerestore crown, also called the "shrink-free" ceramic crown.[105] This product used an extremely accurate epoxy-resin die system, on which was injected a high strength alumina-ceramic core. This core did not shrink on sintering and was quite opaque, which resulted in unesthetic cervical opacity. The core could be colored intrinsically and was overlayed with a relatively translucent veneering ceramic. The Cerestore crown

system had a relatively short time on the market, partially due to the inherent cervical opacity, which resulted in limiting the esthetic outcome to that attained with metal-ceramic restorations with porcelain labial margins, and partially, due to early clinical failures with fracture.

Experiences with Cerestore taught us one important principle: If an all-ceramic crown system uses an opaque core to improve fracture strength, the esthetic result achieved by that system will be no better than the esthetics achieved with metal-ceramics!

About the same time as Cerestore entered the marketplace, Adair and Grossman from the Dow Corning Company introduced Dicor, which was marketed as the "castable" ceramic crown.[106] Dicor crowns were waxed, invested, and cast using a glasslike material that was very translucent. The restoration was then given a specific heat treatment called "ceraming," which induced a change in crystalline structure and made it slightly less translucent. Then a thin film of extrinsic stain was painted on the crown to attain the desired shade.

Dicor was the first example of a "monolithic" crown system where the final esthetic result was attained by applying a thin layer of extrinsic coloration (Fig. 13.69). In general, such monolithic restorations lack depth and have a high level of surface or specular reflection. Such restorations often experience a high incidence of metamerism where the restoration appears one color with certain light sources and a very different color in different light sources. Thus the major deficiency of Dicor was the inability to achieve intrinsic coloration. Fracture rates for Dicor crowns were also relatively high.

Originally Dicor crowns were intended to be cemented with different shades of zinc-phosphate cement. However, Malament discovered that fracture rates could be improved if Dicor crowns were etched internally and bonded in place with resin cements. The combination of high fracture rates and poor esthetics led to the early demise of Dicor, however.

Experiences with Dicor taught us two important principles: First, monolithic crowns do not allow intrinsic coloration and provide depth of color in the same manner as layered crowns; second, the clinical performance of ceramic crowns can be improved by etching and bonding.

To overcome the esthetic disadvantages of Dicor, Willi Geller introduced the Willi Glass crown in 1987.[107] Willi Glass used an internal translucent core of Dicor, about 0.75 mm thick. This was veneered with Vitadur N ceramic. Willi Glass was undoubtedly the most esthetic restoration ever made available to the profession. However, it had a relatively short clinical life span and suffered

1. Feldspathic PJC
2. Aluminous Core PJC
3. Foil Reinforced
4. Captek
5. Cerestore
6. Dicor
7. High-Ceram
8. Willi's Glass
9. IPS Empress
10. Optec
11. Empress II
12. IPS Eris
13. IPS e.Max
14. Inceram (spinell, alumina, zirconia)
15. Procera All-Ceram
16. Zirconia cored materials

• **Fig. 13.68** Major ceramic systems used in restorative dentistry.

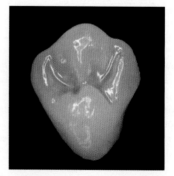

• **Fig. 13.69** Ceramic restoration by Dicor.

from catastrophic fracture. This was partially because the Dicor core was not strong enough at that thickness, and partially due to thermal incompatibilities of the Dicor core and the veneering porcelain.

In the late 1980s, Wholwend and Scharer introduced the original IPS Empress leucite reinforced ceramic system (Fig. 13.70).[108] This system introduced the concept of hot pressing the ceramic, which has the potential to reduce the number of microscopic defects in the ceramic crown.

IPS Empress crowns can be fabricated in two different ways. Monolithic IPS Empress crowns can be waxed, pressed, and stained. These monolithic restorations suffer from issues discussed previously and do not provide optimum esthetics on anterior teeth. Layered IPS Empress, with a leucite reinforced core and matched veneering porcelain, provides the most esthetic and durable ceramic option currently available for restoring anterior teeth. Clinical trials have indicated 95% survival of bonded, layered IPS Empress crowns on anterior teeth. Survival rates drop considerably with crowns on posterior teeth.

It is critical to understand that this high survival for IPS Empress crowns on anterior teeth is only achieved if they are internally etched and bonded in place. There are three approaches to accomplishing this. The first is the traditional approach of bonding the restoration in place using a fourth-generation or fifth-generation etch-and-rinse dentin bonding agent (DBA) and a dual cure resin cement. One problem with this approach is if the DBA is cured prior to cementation, the thickness of the cured DBA may prevent complete seating of the crown. Alternatively, if the DBA is cured after seating the crown at the same time as the dual cure cement, the hydraulic pressure generated during seating will likely collapse the collagen bundles and significantly compromise the hybrid layer and dentin bonding.

A second approach is to use Paul and Magne's immediate dentin sealing technique.[109] With this technique the dentin is sealed with a fourth-generation DBA immediately *after* tooth preparation, prior to making the impression. Thus the film thickness of the DBA is of no importance, and the tooth is sealed during the provisional phase. The sealed preparation must be isolated with Vaseline when making the provisional restoration to prevent bonding of the provisional to the dentin. The oxygen-inhibited layer of the DBA can also distort impressions, and the surface of the DBA must be carefully cleaned prior to cementation. This immediate dentin sealing technique results in much higher dentin bonds than are created when bonding at the cementation stage.

The third approach to bonding etched IPS Empress restorations in place is to use a self-adhesive resin cement. These cements do not produce a hybrid layer and strong bonds to dentin, but do provide an excellent seal. The long-term effect on crown survival with use of self-etching cements is not known.

Leucite-reinforced ceramic systems similar to IPS Empress (Optec HSP, Authentic) have appeared on the market. Optec HSP was a spectacularly unsuccessful product, which illustrates another important principle: *Every ceramic system, even if similar to another successful system, must generate its own clinical data to support use of the system.*

In the early 1990s, Vita introduced the In-Ceram system, utilizing slip-casting with infiltrated glass. Three different forms exist: In-Ceram Spinell, In-Ceram Alumina, and In-Ceram Zirconia. Spinell is the most translucent but has not performed well in clinical trials. Zirconia is the least translucent and has the same translucency as metal; it therefore has limited esthetic potential. In-Ceram Alumina has decent esthetic potential and has been used

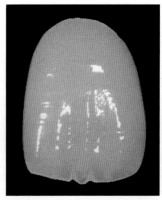

• **Fig. 13.70** Leucite-reinforced glass ceramic crowns (IPS Empress).

successfully for single crowns. These systems have not captured a major share of the market to date.

Nobel Biocare introduced Procera Allceram to the market in the 1990s. This system used a milled alumina or zirconia core veneered with low fusing ceramic. Crowns made with this system had inferior marginal integrity and a high incidence of chipping of the veneering ceramic because of lack of support of the ceramic by the core.

The next major system to appear on the market was IPS Empress II. It was introduced as a lithium disilicate reinforced material that was so strong it could be predictably used to fabricate three-unit fixed partial dentures. In this regard, IPS Empress II was a complete disaster. One local dental laboratory (Drake Dental Lab, Charlotte, NC) fabricated 360 IPS Empress II fixed partial dentures using Ivoclar's specification for connector height, and at 3 years, the failure rate due to fracture was 75% (personal communication; David Avery, Drake Dental Laboratory).

It should be noted that IPS Empress II was a lithium disilicate material and was not really related to the original IPS Empress, which was leucite reinforced. Part of the problem with IPS Empress II was that the veneering ceramic was not properly matched to the lithium disilicate core. This was corrected in a later version called IPS Eris. IPS Eris has shown promise for single crowns but should *not* be used for fabricating all-ceramic fixed partial dentures. IPS Eris has largely been made irrelevant with the introduction of IPS e.max, which is an optimized lithium disilicate material.

IPS e.max is a lithium disilicate material that was introduced in 2009 (Fig. 13.71). It can be pressed or machined and can be used as a monolithic material or layered. Monolithic IPS e.max has relatively high flexural strength of 360 to 400 MPa compared to IPS Empress, which has a flexural strength of approximately 160 MPa. Layered IPS e.max has approximately half the flexural strength as the monolithic form. No long-term clinical trials have been published at this point, but information gleaned from remake data from three commercial laboratories and over 21,000 IPS e.max monolithic and layered single crowns indicates the fracture rate at about 4 years is only 1%. As would be expected, layered IPS e.max crowns have better esthetic potential than monolithic crowns, but the monolithic crowns are stronger.

It should again be noted that higher strength does not automatically result in improved clinical performance, primarily because all-ceramic crowns do not fail because they are not strong enough. They fail because it is difficult to fabricate them without

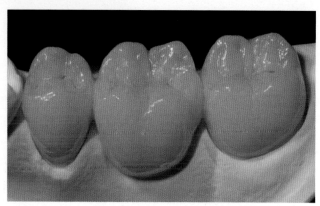

• **Fig. 13.71** Lithium disilicate (IPS e.max) ceramic fixed dental prosthesis.

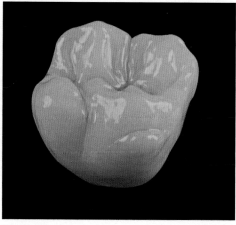

• **Fig. 13.72** Monolithic full contour zirconia restoration.

incorporating microscopic defects called Griffith flaws, and it is the propagation of these defects that results in catastrophic failure.

In the late 1990s, zirconia-based materials were introduced to the profession. The original restorations were cored with yttria-stabilized zirconia oxide and veneered with a compatible ceramic. Zirconia is a very strong material with flexural strengths as high as 1400 MPa. In clinical trials with these materials, core fracture was extremely rare even with posterior fixed partial dentures. However, the "Achilles heel" with these layered restorations was chip fracture of the veneer. The fractures did not occur at the interface between the core and the veneer, but rather were cohesive fractures in the body of the ceramic veneer. One clinical trial of over 900 crowns estimated that layered zirconia crowns fractured at a rate five times higher than that of metal-ceramic crowns.

There are two potential causes for this high incidence of veneer fracture. Because the core is computer designed and manufactured from a scan of the tooth preparation, it is highly likely that adequate support of the veneering porcelain is not provided by the core. This problem may have been solved by creating software that produces a virtual full-contour wax-up and then cuts that back to provide a core with optimal support. The second cause is the extremely poor thermal conductivity of the core material. Basically the core cools very slowly on removal from the porcelain oven and the veneering ceramic cools past its glass transition temperature while the core slowly continues to cool. This creates stress in the veneering ceramic, which causes it to fracture under occlusal loads. This problem may have been solved by using prolonged cooling times.

The reason core fracture is so rare with zirconia is that zirconia possesses a property called transformation toughening. When a defect begins to propagate, the material surrounding the defect undergoes a transformation from the tetragonal to the monoclinic phase, and this transformation is accompanied by a slight expansion, which effectively pinches off the defect and prevents it from propagating.

A relatively new zirconia restoration has been introduced in recent years. It is called monolithic zirconia or full contour zirconia (Fig. 13.72). This is basically a core of zirconia milled into a full crown and then either glazed or polished. Based on studies of layered zirconia, where core fracture is extremely rare, these restorations may reasonably be expected to have high survival rates. One major advantage of monolithic zirconia is that very conservative tooth preparations can be used because of the strength of the material. On molars, preparations similar to those used for cast gold crowns will suffice.

Full contour zirconia restorations are also relatively inexpensive. This is partially because they are designed and manufactured digitally. In an era where the price of gold is over or close to $1600/ounce, this low cost benefit is a real advantage.

There is no question that the esthetic results achieved with these restorations is compromised, but they are acceptable for molars and perhaps mandibular incisors. Research has shown that the best surface for full contour zirconia crowns is a polished surface. This polished surface is relatively kind to opposing enamel.

Recall that the preceding information is not meant to be either all-inclusive or a detailed description of available ceramic systems. Rather it is an overview of how these systems evolved with a brief description of the important features of the major players. More detailed descriptions will be given in subsequent chapters.

THE BOTTOM LINE

1. Many different ceramic systems have been introduced to the dental profession over the past 30 years.
2. All have been brought to market with little or no clinical testing.
3. Ceramic materials do not fracture because of a lack of strength. They fracture due to defect propagation and fatigue.
4. Because of #3, physical properties testing and load-to-failure studies yield little useful information on potential clinical survival rates.
5. Clinical trials or fatigue testing under water are the only appropriate means of predicting clinical survival of ceramic crowns.
6. Most of the ceramic systems introduced since 1980 have been clinical failures.
7. The current cost of gold is a major factor in the cost of restoring teeth with metal-ceramics.
8. Many all-ceramic systems, especially full contour zirconia, are cost-effective compared to PFM.
9. Monolithic crowns have good strength but relatively poor esthetics.
10. Layered restorations have good esthetic potential but reduced strength.
11. Current available systems that clinicians should consider are:
    a. Metal-ceramics: Reasonable esthetics, longest life span
    b. IPS Empress: Esthetics, anterior teeth only
    c. IPS e.max: Esthetic potential, potential longevity
    d. Layered and full contour zirconia: Potential longevity, cost

Contemporary Ceramic Materials

Since the early 1980s, many different ceramic systems have been brought to market. None of the systems had advanced clinical testing before coming to market and most systems failed primarily due to premature catastrophic fracture (Fig. 13.73). The driving force behind these new systems was twofold: Many clinicians were disappointed with the esthetic results they obtained with metal-ceramic restorations and hoped to obtain better esthetic results by using metal-free restorations. With some systems, improved esthetic results were obtained, but the price that was paid significantly reduced longevity. The second driving factor was the cost of noble metals. In 2016, the cost of gold ranged from $1200 to $1600 an ounce. This resulted in skyrocketing laboratory costs in a market that was not favorable to raising compensatory fees. Some of the newer systems offer significant savings in laboratory costs, partially due to nonuse of metal but also because many of these restorations can be fabricated digitally thus reducing labor costs.

There are a number of reasons why dentists fail to obtain predictable esthetics with metal-ceramic restorations and most of them are operator related. Most dentists tend to underprepare teeth that are to be restored with metal-ceramic crowns, and do not provide the laboratory technician sufficient room for the metal substructure, opaque layer and body, and incisal porcelain. Many use outdated cervical margin designs, and soft tissue management is generally poor, resulting in a high incidence of inadequate impressions.[110,111] Many dentists opt to send their laboratory work overseas and accept low-quality restorations in the name of cost reduction.

It is clear that with proper tooth preparation and soft tissue management, coupled with working with a decent ceramist, very esthetic restorations can be fabricated using metal-ceramics. Metal-ceramic restorations remain the gold standard for esthetic indirect crown systems because they provide a combination of reasonable esthetics with maximum longevity. Data from a number of clinical trials indicate that 95% of metal-ceramic restorations are in service 10 to 15 years after placement.[101]

As mentioned, early ceramic systems suffered from premature catastrophic fracture. This led Schärer and McLean to postulate that before a clinician uses a new ceramic system, he or she should be provided data from independent clinical trials that demonstrate a survival rate of no less than 95% at 5 years.[112] This demonstrates that they are not holding ceramic restorations to the same survival rate as metal-ceramic restorations, but they expect a reasonable survival rate for the economic survival of the restorative dentist.

It is reasonable for a clinician to adhere to Schärer's criteria, but the truth is that in order to publish a properly conducted 5-year clinical trial, it requires almost 10 years (Fig. 13.74)!

Thus even though manufacturers are diligently conducting such trials, information on investigated materials does not get into the hands of practicing dentists until many years after the materials are brought to market. An interesting approach to bring clinically relevant data to the market in a timelier manner will be described later in this section.

There are three major materials that have captured a significant portion of the ceramic market in 2017 that have not had properly conducted clinical trials published before they were widely used clinically. These three materials include leucite-reinforced IPS Empress (Ivoclar), lithium disilicate–reinforced IPS e.max (Ivoclar), and zirconia-based systems (many manufacturers). All of these materials can be used in the monolithic state or layered. Zirconia materials can be used layered in the partially stabilized state and monolithic in both the partially stabilized and fully stabilized state.

Monolithic ceramic restorations have relatively poor esthetic results but seem to provide longer clinical survival rates. With monolithic ceramic restorations, all of the color is on the surface, resulting in high surface reflectivity and specular reflection, a high incidence of metamerism, and no depth effect. Monolithic crowns are *not* suitable for maxillary anterior teeth. Layered restorations provide significantly improved esthetic results but lower survival rates.

The leucite-reinforced IPS Empress system was really the first successful ceramic system on the market appearing after an imposing list of failed systems. Layered IPS Empress should only be used on anterior teeth as clinical trials have demonstrated high failure rates on posterior teeth.[113] Monolithic Empress should not be used. IPS Empress can be pressed or milled, and the usual procedure is to press a leucite core and veneer it with the matched ceramic. Layered IPS Empress crowns must be etched with hydrofluoric acid and bonded in place with either dual-cure resin cements/bonding or self-adhesive resin cements. Fewer and fewer dental laboratories are fabricating these restorations today, and even though the esthetic results are excellent and survival on maxillary anterior teeth is satisfactory, their use in contemporary clinical dentistry is limited.

The material named IPS e.max is a lithium disilicate reinforced ceramic that can be used both in the monolithic state and layered.

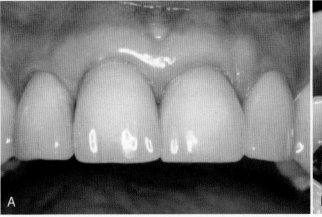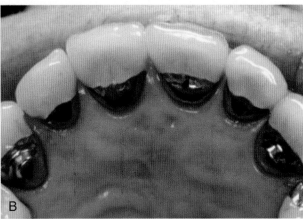

• **Fig. 13.73**   A and B, Metal-ceramic restorations after 21 years.

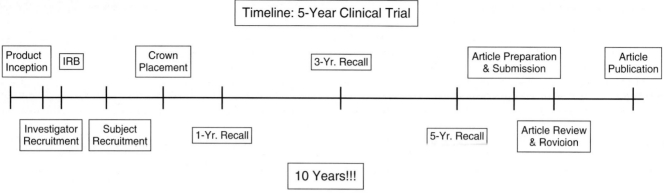

• **Fig. 13.74** Timeline outlining time required for publishing properly conducted 5-year clinical trial.

TABLE 13.12	Mechanical Properties of Leucite Reinforced, Lithium Disilicate, and Zirconia			
Material	Flexural Strength (MPa)	Elastic Modulus (GPa)	Hardness (VHN)	Reference
Leucite reinforced glass ceramic (Empress)	160	96	550	(Aboushelib et al., 2007a)
Lithium disilicate (IPS e.max)	400	95	5800	(Ivoclar, Vivadent)
Zirconia (Y-TZP)	800–1500	210	1200	(Piconi and Maccauro, 1999)

TABLE 13.13	Thermal Conductivity of Zirconia Compared to Other Material	
Material		**Thermal Conductivity W/(mK)**
Silver		429
Gold		318
Gold alloy		200
Base metal		40
Alumina		30
Zirconia		2

Most of what is known about the clinical performance with IPS e.max is with monolithic restorations. Monolithic e.max has a significantly higher flexural strength than IPS Empress at 400 MPa versus 160 MPa (Table 13.12). The flexural strength of layered e.max is about half of the monolithic form, which has been validated with both fatigue studies and clinical data.[114,115] It is important to remember that ceramic crowns fail by defect propagation, and it is likely that the clinical success of e.max restorations is a result of incorporating fewer inherent defects through pressing and milling the restorations. As impressive as the gain in flexural strength of monolithic e.max versus IPS Empress is, it pales in comparison to the flexural strength of monolithic zirconia, which has a flexural strength of 1500 MPa versus 400 MPa for e.max.

Zirconia restorations were first introduced to the profession as partially stabilized (yttria) zirconia oxide cores layered with a veneering ceramic. Initial clinical data established that the cores rarely fractured, but there was a high incidence of chip fractures of the veneering ceramic.[116] It was estimated that the incidence of veneer fracture with layered zirconia was five times that of metal-ceramic restorations. The low incidence of core fracture could be attributed to the property of transformation toughening (Fig. 13.75).

When a defect begins to propagate in a zirconia core, the materials immediately surrounding the defect change from the tetragonal to the monoclinic form of zirconia. This results in a slight expansion, which effectively "pinches off" the propagating defect.

Veneer chipping is likely caused by two issues. First, the high strength cores were originally fabricated by scanning the die of the tooth preparation and then a core of uniform thickness was milled. This core would follow the shape of the die and does not in any way account for the thickness of the veneering ceramic. The industry standard for support of the veneering ceramic is that the veneering ceramic should never exceed a thickness of 2 mm. New software that first produces a virtual full-contour image of the anticipated final restoration and then cuts back that restoration, to provide a core with optimum support of the veneering ceramic, should solve the support problem.

The second issue with veneer chipping is the thermal conductivity of zirconia. It is very low, perhaps 100 to 200 times lower than the conductivity of metals used to bond to porcelain (Table 13.13).

The net result of this is, as the layered ceramic unit exits the porcelain oven, the veneering ceramic cools first, below its glass transition temperature while the core very slowly continues to cool and shrink. This creates stress in the veneering ceramic, which is expressed clinically some time later by chip fracture. Slower cooling protocols have been introduced for firing layered zirconia restorations, and it is anticipated this will significantly reduce the incidence of chipping.[8]

One other solution to veneer chipping is being used by many dental laboratories. There is a substantial volume of anecdotal evidence that veneer chipping with Noritake veneering ceramic (Kuraray America, Inc.) is almost nonexistent. Clinicians would be wise to specify use of Noritake veneering ceramic when prescribing layered zirconia restorations.

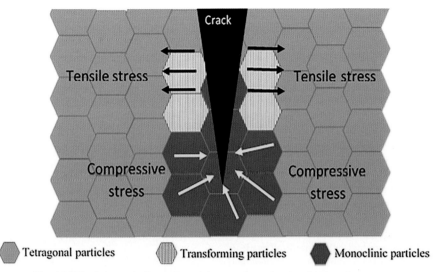

• **Fig. 13.75** Schematic illustration of the transformation toughening phenomenon.

A relatively new form of zirconia has become extremely popular in recent years despite a complete lack of clinical data on survival. Monolithic partially stabilized zirconia (also called full contour zirconia) has grabbed a huge share of the world market for indirect esthetic crowns. The rationale for this restoration is that in clinical trials of layered zirconia restorations core fracture is a relatively rare occurrence. A monolithic zirconia crown is essentially a core with a glazed or polished surface, and thus is expected to display good survival rates.

One major advantage of partially stabilized monolithic zirconia is that crowns can be fabricated with significantly more conservative tooth preparations compared to those needed for metal-ceramic and lithium disilicate crowns. The exact tooth reduction required is unknown at this time, but a 1-mm occlusal reduction with axial reduction of 0.75 mm and a well-defined chamfer margin seem appropriate. A second advantage is that numerous fatigue wear studies indicate that polished zirconia is extremely kind to opposing tooth structure. A third and apparently compelling advantage of these restorations is that they are very inexpensive.

One significant disadvantage related to partially stabilized monolithic zirconia is that it is relatively opaque. The color can be improved using glazes and external colorants, but the overall esthetic result is mediocre at best (Fig. 13.76).

The esthetic results are likely acceptable in the molar regions for all but the most demanding of patients, but they are likely contraindicated for routine use in the maxillary anterior area.

The relative opacity has resulted in the introduction of a new zirconia-based system: fully stabilized monolithic zirconia (Bruxzir Anterior, Glidewell Laboratory). These materials consist of zirconia oxide fully stabilized with yttria (8–12 wt%). They also contain cubic zirconia of up to 53% and are slightly less opaque than partially stabilized zirconia. This improvement in opacity is likely not within the realm of human perception and is accompanied by a 50% reduction in flexural strength. Clinicians are advised to adopt this new technology with extreme caution. There is no clinical track record, improvements in translucency are minimal, and the reduction in flexural strength is significant.

In the absence of properly conducted clinical trials on the previously discussed ceramic systems, another approach has been used to generate timely clinical data on the survival of these restorations. Dental laboratories often warranty their crowns for 5 years

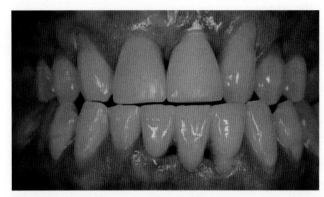

• **Fig. 13.76** Monolithic zirconia fixed dental prosthesis. (Case courtesy Dr. Vilhelm G. Ólafsson.)

and have meticulous data on remakes with these new ceramic systems. Assuming that most patients would return to their original dentists when experiencing premature failure with a ceramic crown to take advantage of the warranty, and assuming the dentists will return that restoration for remake to the same laboratory, examination of remake data provides insights of short-term to medium-term performance of large numbers of ceramic crowns.

This "laboratory survey" approach has provided 4-year data on over 21,000 lithium disilicate (e.max) restorations and 5-year data for over 71,000 monolithic and layered zirconia (partially stabilized) restorations.[117,118] The surveys found all three types of restoration had survival rates that would easily meet and exceed the Schärer criteria. Monolithic e.max single crowns fractured at a rate of 0.91% at 4 years, with layered e.max single crowns exhibiting double the fracture rate at 1.81%, which is still well below Schärer's criteria. Monolithic zirconia single crowns had an even lower rate of fracture (0.71%) at 5 years. Layered zirconia single crowns had a four to five times higher fracture rate at 3.24% at 5 years. These restorations were fabricated prior to initiation of the new protocols expected to reduce the chip fracture rate of layered zirconia restorations. One other result of note was the fracture rate of e.max inlays/onlays, which was 1.01% at 4 years.

A note on bonding zirconia. Zirconia cores cannot be effectively etched with any known acid. Zirconia restorations are best used with tooth preparations with adequate resistance and retention form, and should be cemented with resin-modified glass ionomer or self-adhesive resin cement. A number of different protocols have been developed for "bonding" zirconia restorations. All of these protocols involve air particle abrasion, use of a primer with MDP monomer and silane, and use of dual-cure resin cement. The bonds achieved with these protocols are initially weak and get weaker with artificial aging. There is a definite risk in use of air particle abrasion with zirconia restorations as some studies have demonstrated significant conversion of the core to the monoclinic form and substantial weakening after air particle abrasion.

Zirconia seems to have a strong affinity for proteins found in saliva and blood. It is likely the internal portion of most zirconia crowns will be contaminated during try-in. These proteins cannot be removed with phosphoric acid. A routine procedure for cementing zirconia crowns is the use of a sodium hydroxide solution (Ivoclean, Ivoclar) for 20 seconds after try-in before cementation to effectively remove these proteins.

Indications

Clearly metal-ceramic restorations can continue to be recommended for indirect esthetic crown restorations. However, the promising short-term results demonstrated with lithium disilicate and zirconia based systems permit their rational use in specific clinical situations.

It would seem reasonable to consider use of monolithic partially stabilized zirconia crowns for a molar tooth, in part due to their substantially reduced costs, and also because a more conservative tooth preparation can be used. These restorations can be recommended for mandibular anterior teeth because they are usually not highly visible and a more conservative tooth preparation can be used.

Monolithic lithium disilicate crowns can be recommended for routine use on premolar teeth due to their excellent survival rates, adequate esthetic results, and reduced costs. Layered lithium disilicate crowns can be recommended for maxillary anterior teeth. Fully stabilized zirconia crowns should not be used at this time until clinical information is available on clinical survival.

THE BOTTOM LINE

1. Metal-ceramic restorations continue to provide an impressive combination of reasonable esthetic results coupled with excellent clinical longevity.
2. Most ceramic systems introduced to the market prior to 1988 were clinical failures.
3. Ceramic systems should be documented with independent clinical trials that demonstrate 95% survival at 5 years.
4. It takes about 10 years from product inception to publication of a 5-year clinical trial.
5. The "laboratory survey" approach is a good one for obtaining clinical short-term survival rates.
6. Monolithic zirconia and lithium disilicate materials have adequate short-term survival rates.
7. Early results with layered zirconia showed unacceptable levels of chip fractures of the veneering ceramic. These problems may be solved with new approaches for support of the veneer and new firing cycles.
8. Fully stabilized zirconia crowns marketed for anterior applications have minor improvements in translucency and significantly reduced flexural strength.
9. It is not practical with current protocols to "bond" zirconia restorations. Zirconia restorations require traditional resistance and retention for and should be cemented with RMGI or self-adhesive resin cement.

References

1. Gordon SM, Dionne RA: The integration of clinical research into dental therapeutics: making treatment decisions. *J Am Dent Assoc* 136(12):1701–1708, 2005.
2. Kelly JR: Evidence based decision making: Guide to reading the dental materials literature. *J Prosthet Dent* 95(2):152–160, 2006.
3. Donovan TE: The selection of contemporary restorative materials: anecdote vs. evidence-based? *J Calif Dent Assoc* 34(2):129–134, 2006.
4. Donovan TE: Evidence-based Dentistry, dentists, and dental materials. *J Calif Dent Assoc* 34(2):118–120, 2006.
5. Lang LA, Teich ST: A critical appraisal of evidence-based dentistry: the best available evidence. *J Prosthet Dent* 111(6):485–492, 2014.
6. Greener EH: Amalgam—yesterday, today, and tomorrow. *Oper Dent* 4(1):24–35, 1979.
7. Eames WB, Sieweke JC, Wallace SW, et al: Elastomeric impression materials: effect of bulk on accuracy. *J Prosthet Dent* 41(3):304–307, 1979.
8. Tan JP, Sederstrom D, Polansky JR, et al: The use of slow heating and slow cooling regimens to strengthen porcelain fused to zirconia. *J Prosthet Dent* 107(3):163–169, 2012.
9. Wilson AD: Specification test for the solubility and disintegration of dental cements: a critical evaluation of its meaning. *J Dent Res* 55(5):721–729, 1976.
10. Heintze SD, Ruffieux C, Rousson V: Clinical performance of cervical restorations—a meta-analysis. *Dent Mater* 26(10):993–1000, 2010.
11. Kelly JR: Clinically relevant approach to failure testing of all-ceramic restorations. *J Prosthet Dent* 81(6):652–661, 1999.
12. Heintze SD: Clinical relevance of tests on bond strength, microleakage and marginal adaptation. *Dent Mater* 29(1):59–84, 2013.
13. Mahler DB, Terkla LG, Van Eysden J, et al: Marginal fracture vs mechanical properties of amalgam. *J Dent Res* 49(6 Suppl):1452–1457, 1970.
14. Summitt JB, Burgess JO, Berry TG, et al: The performance of bonded vs. pin-retained complex amalgam restorations: a five-year clinical evaluation. *J Am Dent Assoc* 132(7):923–931, 2001.
15. Leinfelder K: The enigma of dental amalgam. *J Esthet Restor Dent* 16(1):3–5, 2004.
16. Innes DBK, Youdelis WV: Dispersion strengthened amalgams. *J Can Dent Assoc* 29:587–592, 1963.
17. Donovan TE, Handlers JP: A rational policy on the use of dental amalgam. *CDA J* 12(2):10–12, 1984.
18. Bauer JG, First HA: The toxicity of mercury in dental amalgam. *CDA J* 10(6):47–61, 1982.
19. Souder W, Sweeney AB: Is mercury poisonous in dental amalgam restorations? *Dental Cosmos* 73(12):1145–1152, 1931.
20. Hoover AW, Goldwater LJ: Absorption and excretion of mercury in man. X. Dental amalgams as a source of urinary mercury. *Arch Environ Health* 12(4):506–508, 1966.
21. Frykholm KO: On mercury from dental amalgam: its toxic and allergic effects, and some comments on occupational hygiene. *Acta Odontol Scand* 15(7):56–83, 1957.
22. Svare CW, Peterson LC, Reinhardt JW, et al: The effect of dental amalgams on mercury levels in expired air. *J Dent Res* 60(9):1668–1671, 1981.
23. Vimy MJ, Lorscheider FL: Intra-oral air mercury released from dental amalgam. *J Dent Res* 64(8):1069–1071, 1985.
24. Abraham JE, Svare CW, Frank CW: The effect of dental amalgam restorations on blood mercury levels. *J Dent Res* 63(1):71–73, 1984.

25. Eggleston DW, Nylander M: Correlation of dental amalgam with mercury in brain tissue. *J Prosthet Dent* 58(6):704–707, 1987.

26. Nylander M, Friberg L, Lind B: Mercury concentrations in the human brain and kidneys in relation to exposure from dental amalgam fillings. *Swed Dent J* 11(5):179–187, 1987.

27. Mackert JR, Jr: Dental amalgam and mercury. *J Am Dent Assoc* 122(8):54–61, 1991.

28. Vimy MJ, Lorscheider FL: Serial measurements of intra-oral air mercury: estimation of daily dose from dental amalgam. *J Dent Res* 64(8):1072–1075, 1985.

29. Mackert JR, Jr: Factors affecting estimation of dental amalgam mercury exposure from measurements of mercury vapor levels in intra oral and expired air. *J Dent Res* 66(12):1775–1780, 1987.

30. Berglund A: Estimation by a 24-hour study of the daily dose of intra-oral mercury vapor inhaled after release from dental amalgam. *J Dent Res* 69(10):1646–1651, 1990.

31. Consumers Union: The mercury in your mouth. *Consum Rep* 56:316–317, 1991.

32. Mackert JR, Jr, Berglund A: Mercury exposure from dental amalgam fillings: absorbed dose and the potential for adverse health effects. *Crit Rev Oral Biol Med* 8(4):410–436, 1997.

33. Molin M, Bergman B, Marklund SL, et al: Mercury, selenium, and glutathione peroxidase before and after amalgam removal in man. *Acta Odontol Scand* 48(3):189–202, 1990.

34. Langan DC, Fan PL, Hoos AA: The use of mercury in dentistry: a critical review of the recent literature. *J Am Dent Assoc* 115(6):867–880, 1987.

35. Brodsky JB, Cohen EN, Whitcher C, et al: Occupational exposure to mercury in dentistry and pregnancy outcome. *J Am Dent Assoc* 111(5):779–780, 1985.

36. Eggleston DW: Effect of dental amalgam and nickel alloys on T-lymphocytes: preliminary report. *J Prosthet Dent* 51(5):617–623, 1984.

37. Mackert JR, Jr, Leffell MS, Wagner DA, et al: Lymphocyte levels in subjects with and without amalgam restorations. *J Am Dent Assoc* 122(3):49–53, 1991.

38. Saxe SR, Snowdon DA, Wekstein MW, et al: Dental amalgam and cognitive function in older women: findings from the Nun Study. *J Am Dent Assoc* 126(11):1495–1501, 1995.

39. Saxe SR, Wekstein MW, Kryscio RJ, et al: Alzheimer's disease, dental amalgam and mercury. *J Am Dent Assoc* 130(2):191–199, 1999.

40. Clarkson TW, Magos L, Myers GJ: The toxicology of mercury–current exposures and clinical manifestations. *N Engl J Med* 349(18):1731–1737, 2003.

41. Hujoel PP, Lydon-Rochelle M, Bollen AM, et al: Mercury exposure from dental filling placement during pregnancy and low birth weight risk. *Am J Epidemiol* 161(8):734–740, 2005.

42. Lygre GB, Haug K, Skjaerven R, et al: Prenatal exposure to dental amalgam and pregnancy outcome. *Community Dent Oral Epidemiol* 44(5):442–449, 2016.

43. National Center for Toxicological Research, U.S. Food and Drug Administration: White Paper: FDA Update/Review of Potential Adverse Health Risks Associated with Exposure to Mercury in Dental Amalgam, 2009. [WWW page]. http://www.fda.gov/MedicalDevices/ProductsandMedicalProcedures/DentalProducts/DentalAmalgam/ucm171117.htm.

44. U.S. Public Health Service: Dental Amalgam: A Scientific Review and Recommended Public Health Service Strategy for Research, Education and Regulation. Final Report of the Subcommittee on Risk Management of the Committee to Coordinate Environmental Health and Related Programs, 1993. [WWW page]. http://www.health.gov/environment/amalgam1/ct.htm.

45. National Council Against Health Fraud: Position paper on amalgam fillings, 2002. [WWW page]. http://www.ncahf.org/pp/amalgampp.pdf.

46. Life Sciences Research Organization, Inc.: Little evidence to link mercury fillings to human health problems, 2004. [WWW page]. http://www.lsro.org/presentation_files/amalgam/amalgam_pressrelease.pdf.

47. Bellinger DC, Trachtenberg F, Barregard L, et al: Neuropsychological and renal effects of dental amalgam in children: a randomized clinical trial. *JAMA* 295(15):1775–1783, 2006.

48. DeRouen TA, Martin MD, Leroux BG, et al: Neurobehavioral effects of dental amalgam in children: a randomized clinical trial. *JAMA* 295(15):1784–1792, 2006.

49. Soncini JA, Maserejian NN, Trachtenberg F, et al: The longevity of amalgam versus compomer/composite restorations in posterior primary and permanent teeth: findings From the New England Children's Amalgam Trial. *J Am Dent Assoc* 138(6):763–772, 2007.

50. Maserejian NN, Trachtenberg FL, Assmann SF, et al: Dental amalgam exposure and urinary mercury levels in children: the New England Children's Amalgam Trial. *Environ Health Perspect* 116(2):256–262, 2008.

51. Bellinger DC, Trachtenberg F, Zhang A, et al: Dental amalgam and psychosocial status: the New England Children's Amalgam Trial. *J Dent Res* 87(5):470–474, 2008.

52. Donovan T, Simonsen RJ, Guertin G, et al: Retrospective clinical evaluation of 1,314 cast gold restorations in service from 1 to 52 years. *J Esthet Restor Dent* 16(3):194–204, 2004.

53. Wilson AD, Kent BE: A new translucent cement for dentistry. The glass ionomer cement. *Br Dent J* 132(4):133–135, 1972.

54. Bowen RL: Use of epoxy resins in restorative materials. *J Dent Res* 35(3):360–369, 1956.

55. Buonocore MG: A simple method of increasing the adhesion of acrylic filling materials to enamel surfaces. *J Dent Res* 34(6):849–853, 1955.

56. Wieczkowski G, Jr, Joynt RB, Klockowski R, et al: Effects of incremental versus bulk fill technique on resistance to cuspal fracture of teeth restored with posterior composites. *J Prosthet Dent* 60(3):283–287, 1988.

57. Roggendorf MJ, Kramer N, Appelt A, et al: Marginal quality of flowable 4-mm base vs. conventionally layered resin composite. *J Dent* 39(10):643–647, 2011.

58. Flury S, Hayoz S, Peutzfeldt A, et al: Depth of cure of resin composites: is the ISO 4049 method suitable for bulk fill materials? *Dent Mater* 28(5):521–528, 2012.

59. Han SH, Park SH: Comparison of Internal Adaptation in Class II Bulk-fill Composite Restorations Using Micro-CT. *Oper Dent* 2016.

60. Czasch P, Ilie N: In vitro comparison of mechanical properties and degree of cure of bulk fill composites. *Clin Oral Investig* 17(1):227–235, 2013.

61. Alrahlah A, Silikas N, Watts DC: Post-cure depth of cure of bulk fill dental resin-composites. *Dent Mater* 30(2):149–154, 2014.

62. Ilie N, Bucuta S, Draenert M: Bulk-fill resin-based composites: an in vitro assessment of their mechanical performance. *Oper Dent* 38(6):618–625, 2013.

63. van Dijken JW, Pallesen U: A randomized controlled three year evaluation of "bulk-filled" posterior resin restorations based on stress decreasing resin technology. *Dent Mater* 30(9):e245–e251, 2014.

64. Moorthy A, Hogg CH, Dowling AH, et al: Cuspal deflection and microleakage in premolar teeth restored with bulk-fill flowable resin-based composite base materials. *J Dent* 40(6):500–505, 2012.

65. Unterbrink GL: Muessner R: Influence of light intensity on two restorative systems. *J Dent* 23(3):183–189, 1995.

66. Feilzer AJ, De Gee AJ, Davidson CL: Setting stress in composite resin in relation to configuration of the restoration. *J Dent Res* 66(11):1636–1639, 1987.

67. Johnson GH, Lepe X, Zhang H, et al: Retention of metal-ceramic crowns with contemporary dental cements. *J Am Dent Assoc* 140(9):1125–1136, 2009.

68. Burgess JO, Gallo JR: Treating root-surface caries. *Dent Clin North Am* 46(2):385–404, vii-viii, 2002.

69. Simonsen RJ, Calamia JR: Tensile bond strength of etched porcelain. *American Academy of Dental Research* (AADR); 1983 Mar 1. *Sage* 1983.

70. Horn HR: Porcelain laminate veneers bonded to etched enamel. *Dent Clin N Am* 27(4):671–684, 1983.

71. Friedman MJ: A 15-year review of porcelain veneer failure–a clinician's observations. *Compend Contin Educ Dent* 19(6):625–628, 630, 632 passim; quiz 638, 1998.

72. Weiner RS, Weiner LK, Kugel G: Teaching the use of bases and liners: a survey of North American dental schools. *J Am Dent Assoc* 127(11):1640–1645, 1996.

73. Hilton TJ: Cavity sealers, liners, and bases: current philosophies and indications for use. *Oper Dent* 21(4):134–146, 1996.

74. Samet N, Shohat M, Livny A, et al: A clinical evaluation of fixed partial denture impressions. *J Prosthet Dent* 94(2):112–117, 2005.

75. Cho GC, Chee WW: Distortion of disposable plastic stock trays when used with putty vinyl polysiloxane impression materials. *J Prosthet Dent* 92(4):354–358, 2004.

76. Chee WW, Donovan TE: Fine detail reproduction of very high viscosity poly(vinyl siloxane) impression materials. *Int J Prosthodont* 2(4):368–370, 1989.

77. Federick DR, Caputo A: Comparing the accuracy of reversible hydrocolloid and elastomeric impression materials. *J Am Dent Assoc* 128(2):183–188, 1997.

78. de Araujo PA, Jorgensen KD: Effect of material bulk and undercuts on the accuracy of impression materials. *J Prosthet Dent* 54(6):791–794, 1985.

79. Klooster J, Logan GI, Tjan AH: Effects of strain rate on the behavior of elastomeric impression. *J Prosthet Dent* 66(3):292–298, 1991.

80. Donovan TE, Chee WW: A review of contemporary impression materials and techniques. *Dent Clin North Am* 48(2):vi–vii, 445-470, 2004.

81. Kanehira M, Finger WJ, Endo T: Volatilization of components from and water absorption of polyether impressions. *J Dent* 34(2):134–138, 2006.

82. Chew CL, Chee WW, Donovan TE: The influence of temperature on the dimensional stability of poly (vinyl siloxane) impression materials. *Int J Prosthodont* 6(6):528–532, 1993.

83. Johnson GH, Lepe X, Aw TC: The effect of surface moisture on detail reproduction of elastomeric impressions. *J Prosthet Dent* 90(4):354–364, 2003.

84. Petrie CS, Walker MP, O'Mahony AM, et al: Dimensional accuracy and surface detail reproduction of two hydrophilic vinyl polysiloxane impression materials tested under dry, moist, and wet conditions. *J Prosthet Dent* 90(4):365 372, 2003.

85. Christensen GJ: Now is the time to change to custom impression trays. *J Am Dent Assoc* 125(5):619–620, 1994.

86. Bomberg TJ, Hatch RA, Hoffman W, Jr: Impression material thickness in stock and custom trays. *J Prosthet Dent* 54(2):170–172, 1985.

87. Cho GC, Donovan TE, Chee WW, et al: Tensile bond strength of polyvinyl siloxane impressions bonded to a custom tray as a function of drying time: Part I. *J Prosthet Dent* 73(5):419–423, 1995.

88. Williams PT, Jackson DG, Bergman W: An evaluation of the time-dependent dimensional stability of eleven elastomeric impression materials. *J Prosthet Dent* 52(1):120–125, 1984.

89. Chee WW, Donovan TE: Polyvinyl siloxane impression materials: a review of properties and techniques. *J Prosthet Dent* 68(5):728–732, 1992.

90. Kahn RL, Donovan TE: A pilot study of polymerization inhibition of poly (vinyl siloxane) materials by latex gloves. *Int J Prosthodont* 2(2):128–130, 1989.

91. Kahn RL, Donovan TE, Chee WW: Interaction of gloves and rubber dam with a poly(vinyl siloxane) impression material: a screening test. *Int J Prosthodont* 2(4):342–346, 1989.

92. Chee WW, Donovan TE, Kahn RL: Indirect inhibition of polymerization of a polyvinyl siloxane impression material: a case report. *Quintessence Int* 22(2):133–135, 1991.

93. Kimoto K, Tanaka K, Toyoda M, et al: Indirect latex glove contamination and its inhibitory effect on vinyl polysiloxane polymerization. *J Prosthet Dent* 93(5):433–438, 2005.

94. de Camargo LM, Chee WW, Donovan TE: Inhibition of polymerization of polyvinyl siloxanes by medicaments used on gingival retraction cords. *J Prosthet Dent* 70(2):114–117, 1993.

95. Amaya SP, Delgado AJ, Donovan TE: Inhibition of polymerization of contemporary polyvinyl siloxane impression materials by latex-free products. *Forum Fam Plan West Hemisph* 2:12–19, 2014.

96. Rudd KD, Morrow RM, Strunk RR: Accurate alginate impressions. *J Prosthet Dent* 22(3):294–300, 1969.

97. Rudd KD, Morrow RM, Range AA: Accurate casts. *J Prosthet Dent* 21(5):545–554, 1969.

98. Taggart WH: *A new and accurate method of making gold inlays*, Philadelphia, 1907, SS White Dental Manufacturing Company.

99. Weinstein M, Katz S, Weinstein AB: Porcelain covered metal-reinforced teeth. U.S. Patent No. 3,052,983, 1962.

100. Donovan TE, White LE: Evaluation of an improved centrifugal casting machine. *J Prosthet Dent* 53(5):609–612, 1985.

101. Leempoel PJ, Van't Hof MA, de Haan AF: Survival studies of dental restorations: criteria, methods and analyses. *J Oral Rehabil* 16(4):387–394, 1989.

102. Reitemeier B, Hansel K, Kastner C, et al: A prospective 10-year study of metal ceramic single crowns and fixed dental prosthesis retainers in private practice settings. *J Prosthet Dent* 109(3):149–155, 2013.

103. McLean JW, Jeansonne EE, Bruggers H, et al: A new metal-ceramic crown. *J Prosthet Dent* 40(3):273–287, 1978.

104. Donovan TE, Adishian S, Prince J: The platinum-bonded crown: a simplified technique. *J Prosthet Dent* 51(2):273–275, 1984.

105. Sozio RB, Riley EJ: The shrink-free ceramic crown. *J Prosthet Dent* 49(2):182–187, 1983.

106. Adair PJ, Grossman DG: The castable ceramic crown. *Int J Periodontics Restorative Dent* 4(2):32–46, 1984.

107. Geller W, Kwiatkowski SJ: The Willi's glas crown: a new solution in the dark and shadowed zones of esthetic porcelain restorations. *Quintessence Dent Technol* 11(4):233–242, 1987.

108. Wohlwend A, Scharer P: The Empress technique: A new technique for the fabrication of full ceramic crowns, inlays, and veneers. *Quintessence Int* 16:966–978, 1990.

109. Magne P, Kim TH, Cascione D, et al: Immediate dentin sealing improves bond strength of indirect restorations. *J Prosthet Dent* 94(6):511–519, 2005.

110. Donovan TE, Chee WW: Cervical margin design with contemporary esthetic restorations. *Dent Clin North Am* 48(2):vi, 417-431, 2004.

111. Donovan TE, Cho GC: Predictable aesthetics with metal-ceramic and all-ceramic crowns: the critical importance of soft-tissue management. *Periodontol 2000* 27:121–130, 2001.

112. Scharer P: All-ceramic crown systems: clinical research versus observation in supporting claims. *Signature* 1:1996.

113. Fradeani M, Aquilano A: Clinical experience with Empress crowns. *Int J Prosthodont* 10(3):241–247, 1997.

114. Zhao K, Pan Y, Guess PC, et al: Influence of veneer application on fracture behavior of lithium-disilicate-based ceramic crowns. *Dent Mater* 28(6):653–660, 2012.

115. Zhao K, Wei YR, Pan Y, et al: Influence of veneer and cyclic loading on failure behavior of lithium disilicate glass-ceramic molar crowns. *Dent Mater* 30(2):164–171, 2014.

116. Denry I, Kelly JR: State of the art of zirconia for dental applications. *Dent Mater* 24(3):299–307, 2008.

117. Sulaiman TA, Delgado AJ, Donovan TE: Survival rate of lithium disilicate restorations at 4 years: A retrospective study. *J Prosthet Dent* 114(3):364–366, 2015.

118. Sulaiman TA, Abdulmajeed AA, Donovan TE, et al: Fracture rate of monolithic zirconia restorations up to 5 years: A dental laboratory survey. *J Prosthet Dent* 116(3):436–439, 2016.

Index

Page numbers followed by b indicate boxes; f, figures; t, tables; and e, online only materials.

511